Edited by Jean Cornier,
Andrew Owen, Arno Kwade,
and Marcel Van de Voorde

Pharmaceutical Nanotechnology

Further Volumes of the Series "Nanotechnology Innovation & Applications"

Axelos, M. A. V. and Van de Voorde, M. (eds.)

Nanotechnology in Agriculture and Food Science

2017

Print ISBN: 9783527339891

Fermon, C. and Van de Voorde, M. (eds.)

Nanomagnetism

Applications and Perspectives

2017

Print ISBN: 9783527339853

Mansfield, E., Kaiser, D. L., Fujita, D., Van de Voorde, M. (eds.)

Metrology and Standardization for Nanotechnology

Protocols and Industrial Innovations

2017

Print ISBN: 9783527340392

Meyrueis, P., Sakoda, K., Van de Voorde, M. (eds.)

Micro- and Nanophotonic Technologies

2017

Print ISBN: 9783527340378

Müller, B. and Van de Voorde, M. (eds.)

Nanoscience and Nanotechnology for Human Health

2017

Print ISBN: 9783527338603

Puers, R., Baldi, L., van Nooten, S. E., Van de Voorde, M. (eds.)

Nanoelectronics

Materials, Devices, Applications

2017

Print ISBN: 9783527340538

Raj, B., Van de Voorde, M., Mahajan, Y. (eds.)

Nanotechnology for Energy Sustainability

2017

Print ISBN: 9783527340149

Sels, B. and Van de Voorde, M. (eds.)

Nanotechnology in Catalysis

Applications in the Chemical Industry, Energy Development, and Environment Protection

2017

Print ISBN: 9783527339143

Edited by Jean Cornier, Andrew Owen,
Arno Kwade, and Marcel Van de Voorde

Pharmaceutical Nanotechnology

Innovation and Production

WILEY-VCH
Verlag GmbH & Co. KGaA

Volume Editors

Dr. Jean Cornier
vdlconsult
Seumestr. 7
81379 München
Germany

Prof. Andrew Owen
University of Liverpool
Department of Molecular & Clinical Pharmacology
Ashton Street
Liverpool, L69 3GE
UK

Prof. Arno Kwade
TU Braunschweig
Partikeltechnik
Volkmaroder Str. 5
38104 Braunschweig
Germany

Prof. Dr. Dr. h.c. Marcel H. Van de Voorde
Member of the Science Council
of the French Senate and National Assembly, Paris
Rue du Rhodania, 5
BRISTOL A, Appartement 31
3963 Crans-Montana
Switzerland

Series Editor

Prof. Dr. Dr. h.c. Marcel H. Van de Voorde
Member of the Science Council
of the French Senate and National Assembly, Paris
Rue du Rhodania, 5
BRISTOL A, Appartement 31
3963 Crans-Montana
Switzerland

Cover credits: Pills bottom and background: fotolia_© Sven Bähren
3D pill top right with nanostructure inside: © mauritius-images

Library of Congress Card No.: applied for

British Library Cataloguing-in-Publication Data
A catalogue record for this book is available from the British Library.

Bibliographic information published by the Deutsche Nationalbibliothek
The Deutsche Nationalbibliothek lists this publication in the Deutsche Nationalbibliografie; detailed bibliographic data are available on the Internet at http://dnb.d-nb.de.

Print ISBN: 978-3-527-34054-5
ePDF ISBN: 978-3-527-80067-4
ePub ISBN: 978-3-527-80069-8
Mobi ISBN: 978-3-527-80070-4
oBook ISBN: 978-3-527-80068-1

Cover Design Adam Design
Typesetting Thomson Digital, Noida, India
Printing and Binding Markono Print Media Pte Ltd, Singapore
Printed on acid-free paper

*Thanks to my wife for her patience with me spending
many hours working on the book series through
the nights and over weekends.
The assistance of my son Marc Philip related to the complex
and large computer files with many sophisticated scientific
figures is also greatly appreciated.*

Marcel Van de Voorde

Series Editor Preface

Since years, nanoscience and nanotechnology have become particularly an important technology areas worldwide. As a result, there are many universities that offer courses as well as degrees in nanotechnology. Many governments including European institutions and research agencies have vast nanotechnology programmes and many companies file nanotechnology-related patents to protect their innovations. In short, nanoscience is a hot topic!

Nanoscience started in the physics field with electronics as a forerunner, quickly followed by the chemical and pharmacy industries. Today, nanotechnology finds interests in all branches of research and industry worldwide. In addition, governments and consumers are also keen to follow the developments, particularly from a safety and security point of view.

This books series fills the gap between books that are available on various specific topics and the encyclopedias on nanoscience. This well-selected series of books consists of volumes that are all edited by experts in the field from all over the world and assemble top-class contributions. The topical scope of the book is broad, ranging from nanoelectronics and nanocatalysis to nanometrology. Common to all the books in the series is that they represent top-notch research and are highly application-oriented, innovative, and relevant for industry. Finally they collect a valuable source of information on safety aspects for governments, consumer agencies and the society.

The titles of the volumes in the series are as follows:

Human-related nanoscience and nanotechnology

- *Nanoscience and Nanotechnology for Human Health*
- *Pharmaceutical Nanotechnology*
- *Nanotechnology in Agriculture and Food Science*

Nanoscience and nanotechnology in information and communication

- *Nanoelectronics*
- *Micro- and Nanophotonic Technologies*
- *Nanomagnetism: Perspectives and Applications*

Nanoscience and nanotechnology in industry

- Nanotechnology for Energy Sustainability
- Metrology and Standardization of Nanomaterials
- Nanotechnology in Catalysis: Applications in the Chemical Industry, Energy Development, and Environmental Protection

The book series appeals to a wide range of readers with backgrounds in physics, chemistry, biology, and medicine, from students at universities to scientists at institutes, in industrial companies and government agencies and ministries.

Ever since nanoscience was introduced many years ago, it has greatly changed our lives – and will continue to do so!

March 2016 *Marcel Van de Voorde*

About the Series Editor

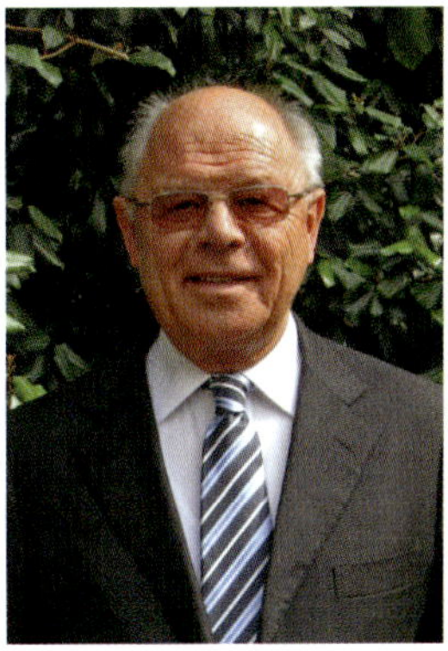

Marcel Van de Voorde, Prof. Dr. ir. Ing. Dr. h.c., has 40 years' experience in European Research Organisations, including CERN-Geneva and the European Commission, with 10 years at the Max Planck Institute for Metals Research, Stuttgart. For many years, he was involved in research and research strategies, policy, and management, especially in European research institutions.

He has been a member of many Research Councils and Governing Boards of research institutions across Europe, the United States, and Japan. In addition to his Professorship at the University of Technology in Delft, the Netherlands, he holds multiple visiting professorships in Europe and worldwide. He holds a doctor honoris causa and various honorary professorships.

He is a senator of the European Academy for Sciences and Arts, Salzburg, and Fellow of the World Academy for Sciences. He is a member of the Science Council of the French Senate/National Assembly in Paris. He has also provided executive advisory services to presidents, ministers of science policy, rectors of Universities, and CEOs of technology institutions, for example, to the president and CEO of IMEC, Technology Centre in Leuven, Belgium. He is also a Fellow of various scientific societies. He has been honored by the Belgian King and European authorities, for example, he received an award for European merits in Luxemburg given by the former President of the European Commission. He is author of multiple scientific and technical publications and has coedited multiple books, especially in the field of nanoscience and nanotechnology.

Contents

Foreword

Albert Einstein once remarked: "Look deep into nature, and then you will understand everything better." Beginning with the idea that most people would not believe in, nanotechnology has allowed us – literally – to look deep into the functioning of biological mechanisms at molecular level and thereby define new pathways for diagnosis and treatment of human disease. The nanotechnology-based production of pharmaceuticals therefore has the potential to revolutionize the treatment of human disease, facilitate changes in future healthcare systems by enabling more personalized, predictive, preventive, regenerative, and even remote (tele)medicine, and has a major impact on the survival of the human race.

The book gives a thorough overview of the science and technology in the nanopharmacy spectrum worldwide, and it also clearly highlights the research requirements that Europe needs to undertake during the next decade if it is to achieve invaluable breakthroughs in this fascinating field of nanopharmacy – breakthroughs that will enable Europe to place itself among the top-ranking competitive industrial regions in the world.

This is because nanotechnologies provide the tools for analysis and manipulation of biological processes at the nanoscale, which is where diseases take root and progress. The result is an increasingly better understanding of the molecular biology of disease leading to new targets for more specific and earlier diagnostic and therapeutic strategies.

This publication – which gives me genuine pleasure to introduce to you – is perhaps the first time that Europe and the wider world have a unique opportunity. This is both to assess the current state of the art and to provide the larger nanomedicine community with new resources and strategies. It will make the best of European and international innovation so as to generate a highly competitive industrial sector. At the forefront is the very latest thinking in fundamental research, characterization and safety issues of nanotechnology as applied to the development of new drugs and treatments for medicine. This will help to meet the enormous challenge of bringing new innovative, safe, and cost-effective products to the patient in as short a time frame as possible. There is strong emphasis on patient needs and concerns, including personalized approaches that will make for new, efficient, and effective solutions for healthcare.

Applications of nanotechnology for healthcare perhaps best exemplify how interdisciplinary research is vital for future success. This is because all disciplines and their stakeholders are represented in this work: beginning with the laboratory-based scientists and including regulators, representatives from industry, and most important of all representatives from society at large. All play an equal part in delivering the appropriate benefits at the right time at the right price to the right patient.

Only collaborations, such as those represented in this publication, will bring new discoveries from science into products that generate greater economic value through more rapid societal use. It is literally the attention to such small details that can make this happen, for Albert Einstein also remarked: "Whoever is careless with the truth in small matters cannot be trusted with important matters."[1)]

This publication is a great initiative and will give an impetus to the entire nanopharmacy community in Europe. For this reason, I believe that this book should find a large distribution facilitating a broad debate between all policy-making bodies and research institutes in Europe.

Director-General, Publications Office,
European Commission, Luxembourg

Rudolf Walter Strohmeier

1) 2010, The Ultimate Quotable Einstein, Edited by Alice Calaprice, Section: On Humankind, Quote Page 187 and 188, Princeton University Press, Princeton, New Jersey.

Industrial Requirement on Nanopharmacy Research

Information on "nanotechnology" is proliferating within the scientific literature and media. In the field of pharmacy and medicine alone, the number of publications on nanotechnology has increased substantially over the past two decades. Searching the chemical database on CAS controlled terms for entries on "nano" in combination with medicine, pharmaceuticals, therapeutics, or formulations resulted in only eight publications in 1995. Since then the number of publications has jumped to 173 in 2005 and over 1400 in 2015. Therefore, nanotechnology in pharmacy became a very important field for academic and industrial research and development.

Nano-relevant techniques and applications are very diverse; they range from nanosized crystals of pharmaceutical drug substances to lipid carriers of submicrometer range, to functionalized particles for targeting, to particles for nucleotide or peptide delivery, among others. The abundance of technological options and possible applications appears to be overwhelming, and sometimes confusing. In this "gold rush" for an emerging key technology of the twenty-first century, it seems to be the right time to pause, take stock of the scientific basis for nanotechnology-enabled progress, and take a systematic and holistic view of emerging applications.

For these reasons, *Pharmaceutical Nanotechnology* starts by providing the reader with an understanding of the fundamental basic and applied sciences of nanotechnology in the context of pharmaceutical applications. This includes challenges associated with GMP manufacturing, scale-up, methods for characterization, and potential occupational and environmental safety issues. It is recognized that current and future applications of nanotechnology are at very different stages of maturity. Consequently, the book also provides the course of pharmaceutical drug development in a systematic manner. Opportunities and challenges are also addressed from the perspective of early discovery, preclinical and clinical development, to regulation and commercialization.

Throughout this journey, the reader will realize that nanotechnology is not a vague vision of a miracle technology that might come up in some distant future, but is already a reality in a substantial number of commercial products, including oral, dermatological, and parenteral treatments. On the other hand, the potential utility of nanotechnology in pharmacy is by far not fully exploited.

New findings and concepts continue to emerge as is illustrated by over 320 new patent applications in the field of pharmaceutical and medical applications of nanotechnology in 2015 alone. Nanotechnology may play a crucial role in drug targeting and cellular delivery, oral and intravenous delivery of insoluble compounds, topical delivery to the lung, eye, and skin, diagnostic applications, and many other areas. The key to these new applications still lies in new research and sound science is still needed to elucidate mechanisms that underpin observed benefits. Despite the large number of publications, we still need a better and deeper understanding of the principles for preparation, characterization, and fate of nanoparticles in the body as well as in the environment.

Pharmaceutical nanotechnology still has the opportunity to avoid mistakes that have been made in the development and introduction of previous groundbreaking technologies. Researchers have previously been very enthusiastic about new opportunities, but the public were not brought on the journey, and sometimes unfounded worries about adverse effects are common. Therefore, *Pharmaceutical Nanotechnology* also addresses nanotoxicology and safety and ethical and societal aspects as integrated components of research and development of nanopharmaceutical products.

As demonstrated by the impressive list of contributors to this book, the challenges will hardly be met by a single inventor or institution. The topics are so diverse that they require multifunctional capabilities and collaborations in early laboratory research, pharmaceutical formulation, process engineering, material characterization, clinical evaluation and implementation, and regulatory and intellectual property considerations. *Pharmaceutical Nanotechnology* brings all these disciplines together to give a cross-cutting and in-depth review of this stimulating new field and is a very helpful basis for students and a base for academic research as well as provides industry with excellent innovation ideas. I wish the readers inspiring insights into the exciting field of the smallest particles.

Chief Scientist of Chemical & Pharmaceutical Development, *Peter Serno*
Bayer Pharma AG, Berlin

Head of Chemical & Pharmaceutical Development, *Olaf Queckenberg*
Bayer Pharma AG, Wuppertal

Introduction

Pharmaceutical Nanotechnology aims at applying nanotechnology to drug therapy of diseases and medical diagnostics. More exactly it involves the preparation and delivery of therapeutic substances in the molecular and nanometer size range to the expected site of action in the human body, reaching maximum efficacy while alleviating undesirable side effects at healthy organs and tissues. The importance of this emerging field of research and developments relies on the fact that nearly all present medicines exhibit poor pharmacokinetics and bioavailability characteristics, and instead of specifically concentrating and acting at their target sites they widely distribute within the body. Pharmaceutical Nanotechnology requires very specific knowledge on many topics such as drug formulation, drug delivery, route of administration, specific targeting, imaging, and diagnosis, and so on. Research in this field requires a multidisciplinary approach, involving pharmacists, material and chemical engineers, cellular biologists, and biophysicists as well as ICT specialists and medical specialists.

The goal of this unique book is to present an overall picture of the use of nanotechnology in pharmacy. It is designed to be a reference textbook on the application of nanotechnology in the development of nanostructures for therapeutic use. Focus is placed on the manufacturing and researching of candidate nanostructures as well as their translation into marketable medicines by industry. We also review the most interesting and promising developments in this emerging but fast developing field.

Following this brief introduction, Part One consists of Chapters 1–5 that give an *entry to the Nanopharmacy revolution* by addressing the history, potential, challenges, and most recent developments and applications of nanotechnology in pharmacy.

In Part Two, *a systematic review of the fundamentals of nanopharmacy* is performed with a description of the used nanostructures, their characterization methods, and a detailed overview of the preparation and manufacturing methods and issues. Established processes as well as new exploratory methods are separately reviewed and concrete actual examples of utilization given. All relevant aspects are being addressed including scale-up and occupational health.

Part Three reviews *the various steps in the development of a new nanodrug.* It includes the use of nanotools and models in drug discovery, drug targeting and design strategies, and nonclinical and clinical studies. Emphasis is laid on nanotoxicology and nanosafety aspects as well as regulatory issues for translation to the clinic of the most promising nanostructures. As the introduction of these new medicines may be controversial, ethical and societal aspects are also addressed in a specific chapter.

In Part Four, *key medical applications of nanodrugs* are reviewed. Diagnostics and imaging use and physical methods for treatment are first described. In the several following chapters and through the description of the various delivery routes in the body, main treatment areas such as cancer or infectious and neurodegenerative diseases are explained.

Finally, Part Five describes *market prospects and industrial commercialization aspects* with special focus on the commercial translation and its bottlenecks like the protection of intellectual property. Actual information about current commercialized products and market figures are also provided.

The chapters are written by leading researchers in pharmacy, biology, chemistry, physics, engineering, and medicine as well as law and social science from academia, industry, national/international laboratories, and government agencies in Europe, Israel, and the United States.

It is expected that this book will become a standard work for pharmacists and the pharmaceutical industry but also a database and a reference for scientists, researchers, and students, as well as for agencies, government, and regulatory authorities.

This book may bring inspiration for scientists, new ideas for drug developers, innovation in industry, and guidelines for toxicologists and finally will result in the establishment of guidelines for agencies and government authorities to establish safe rules in using this new promising technology. The book may result in breakthroughs in the pharmaceutical nanotechnology in such a way that medical doctors may cure life-threatening diseases such as cancer or infections with nanotechnology-based medicines, and thus in the welfare of the society.

Jean Cornier
Andrew Owen
Arno Kwade
Marcel Van de Voorde

Part One
Entry to the Nanopharmacy Revolution

1
History: Potential, Challenges, and Future Development in Nanopharmaceutical Research and Industry

Albertina Ariën[1] and Paul Stoffels[2]

[1]Pharmaceutical Development and Manufacturing Sciences, Drug Product Development, Janssen Pharmaceutical Research & Development, Turnhoutseweg 30, Beerse, Belgium
[2]Chief Scientific Officer, Johnson & Johnson

Since the advent in 1906 of Dr. P. Erlich's magic bullets that would lookfor specific disease-causing agents in the human body, many therapies have been developed to increase the delivery of drugs to the target site. Nanoparticle-based delivery systems provide new opportunities to overcome the limitations associated with traditional drug therapy and aim to achieve both therapeutic and diagnostic functions in the same platform. These nanocarriers allow targeting of the medication to the site of action and release the drug in a controllable manner. Other features linked to nanopharmaceuticals are increased drug loading, increased bioavailability, enhanced efficacy, and increased safety. The nanocarriers are designed to be biocompatible and biodegradable.

A wide range of therapies are nowadays on the market or in late-stage development for the treatment of serious conditions such as cancer and infectious diseases [1,2]. Therapies include carriers of nanopharmaceuticals such as liposomes, lipid-based formulations such as solid lipid nanoparticles, nanocrystals, polymer-based nanoformulations, protein–drug conjugate nanoparticles, surfactant-based nanoformulations, metal-based nanoparticles such as iron oxide or gold nanoparticles, dendrimers, virosomes, and modified viruses.

The first product on the market employing nanotechnology was Doxil® that received US-FDA approval in 1995 for the treatment of AIDS-related Kaposi's sarcoma [3]. Doxil® are stealth liposomes encapsulating about 10 000 doxorubicin molecules [3,4]. Encapsulation minimizes side effects, such as cardiotoxicity, neutropenia, vomiting, myelosuppression, and alopecia, which are associated with high doses of free doxorubicin [5]. The incorporation of lipid and specifically cholesterol increases the bilayer cohesiveness and reduces leakage. The liposomes are designed by their size of approximately 100 nm and their pegylated surface to target to solid tumors via EPR effect (enhanced permeability and retention effect) and reduce toxicity to healthy tissues.

Pharmaceutical Nanotechnology: Innovation and Production, First Edition. Edited by Jean Cornier, Arno Kwade, Andrew Owen, and Marcel Van de Voorde.

1.1 Nanopharmaceuticals in Cancer Therapy

Since, nanopharmaceuticals have become valuable arsenals in cancer therapy with enhancement of drug efficacy and decreased side effects. The efficiency of drug or gene delivery to a tumor site is dependent on the physicochemical properties of the delivery platform and a range of physiologically imposed design constraints, including clearance by the mononuclear phagocyte system and extravasation from circulation at the tumor site by the EPR effect.

The nanofeature of the pharmaceuticals contributes to enhanced solubility and chemical stability of the compounds along with potential protection from degradation by encapsulation into nanocarriers or coupling to synthetic polymers. Nanoparticle biodistribution and uptake by the reticuloendothelial system warranted the design of nanoparticles to evade rapid uptake such as lipid liposomes, albumin carriers, and PEGylation. PEGylation and conjugation to albumin respectively resulted in prolonged circulation and enhanced biodistribution of compounds, while the small size of nanopharmaceuticals led to improved tumor tissue accumulation [6].

Nanopharmaceuticals have improved biodistribution and targeting features as well as the potential of stimuli-sensitive microenvironments payload release. These collective features have led to the development of nanoparticle therapeutics of large antibody–drug conjugates (brentuximab vedotin and trastuzumab emtansine [6]) and small-molecule platforms such as liposomes (Doxil, DaunoXome, DepoCyt, Marqibo, Mepact, Myocet, Lipoplatin), polymeric nanoparticles (Eligard, Genexol, Opaxio, Zinostatin stimalamer), albumin nanoparticles (Abraxane), and metal-based nanoformulations (NanoTherm) [1,7].

Brentuximab vedotin and trastuzumab emtansine are antibody–drug conjugates (ADCs) with an anticancer drug conjugated to a targeting molecule. Brentuximab targets the protein CD30, a glycosylated phosphoprotein expressed by B cells, including B-cell lymphomas, some leukemias, and melanoma cancer stem cells [8–10]. Trastuzumab targets the human epidermal growth factor receptor 2 (HER2) overexpressed in HER2-positive breast cancer [11,12]. Monomethyl auristan E (MMAE) (brentuximab vedotin) and mertansine (trastuzumab emtansine) are too toxic to be used alone and hence coupling to a targeting antibody reduces toxic side effects. Several drug molecules are conjugated to each antibody via a valine–citrulline cleavable linker (brentuximab vedotin) or covalent linkage (trastuzumab emtansine) that is enzymatically degraded in endosomes following uptake. The relatively small number of approved ADCs highlights the difficulty in the development of nanotherapeutics to the clinic.

Since the introduction of Doxil on the market, many other liposomal formulations are developed [13]. More advanced liposomal carriers are designed to release their drug triggered by internal stimulus such as changes of pH or oxygen level or external stimulation such as local heating. Thermosensitive liposomes, such as ThermoDox, can release their payload in the tumor region with local heating owing to the gel-to-liquid crystalline phase change of the lipids at about 42 °C, a temperature that can be reached by local hyperthermia [13].

Another nanotherapeutic using temperature to induce tumor cell destruction or sensitization is NanoTherm, 15-nm-sized superparamagnetic iron oxide nanoparticles (SPION) coated with aminosilane. These nanoparticles are introduced directly in solid brain tumors and are exposed to a magnetic field that changes its polarity up to 100 000 times per second generating a local increase in temperature. Depending on the duration of exposure to the alternating magnetic field, the tumor cells may be destroyed or sensitized for further chemotherapy. Through the aminosilane coating, the nanoparticles remain localized, which allows repeated treatments [14].

Nanoparticle albumin-bound (nab™) technology is a nanotechnology-based drug delivery platform that exploits the natural properties of albumin to achieve a safe, solvent-free, efficient, and targeted drug delivery. Abraxane, or nab-paclitaxel, is a cremophor-free, albumin-bound 130-nm particle form of paclitaxel. The paclitaxel and albumin are not covalently linked but rather associated through hydrophobic interactions [15]. The particles of paclitaxel are in a noncrystalline, amorphous, readily bioavailable state, allowing for rapid drug release from the particles following intravenous administration. The albumin is thought to facilitate endothelial transcytosis and to play a role in preferential intratumoral accumulation of paclitaxel through its binding to SPARC (secreted protein acid and rich cysteine), a glycoprotein overexpressed in many tumors [15].

Nanopharmaceuticals have benefited from the concept of site-specific delivery. Active targeting of a nanoparticle is a way to minimize uptake in normal tissue and increase accumulation in a tumor. Active targeting can be achieved by linking, to the surface of the nanopharmaceuticals, molecules that bind specifically to surface membrane proteins that are upregulated in cancer cells [16]. These so-called targeting molecules are typically antibodies [17], antibody fragments [18], aptamers [19], or small molecules. Monoclonal IgG antibodies are widely used for protein recognition and targeting, since they have two epitope binding sites, high selectivity, and high binding affinity. Fab2 fragments of the antibodies retain both antigen-binding sites. Aptamers are folded single-strand oligonucleotides, usually 25–100 nucleotides in length (8–25 kDa) that bind to molecular targets [19]. Small molecules for targeting include peptides, growth factors, carbohydrates, ureas, and receptor ligands [20]. The interested reader is referred to Chapter 16 “Drug Targeting in Nanomedicine and Nanopharmacy: A Systems Approach” to read more on this topic.

1.2 Nanoparticles Actively Using the Host Machinery

Apart from cancer therapy, nanoparticles have become very valuable in vaccine therapy. Vaccine nanotechnology *avant la lettre* are the aluminum particles traditionally used as adjuvants, since most proteins are poorly immunogenic when administered alone. Strong adaptive immune responses to protein antigens typically require the antigen to be administered together with an adjuvant. Adsorption of the antigen on aluminum particles, either aluminum phosphate or aluminum hydroxide, transforms soluble antigens into particulate material. This form delays the release of the antigen and enhances the immune response by specifically activating macrophages and, additionally makes the antigen more prone to uptake by these antigen-presenting cells. Although used successfully since the 1930s, this approach does not work for every antigen, for example, tuberculosis and malaria. There is also some public concern regarding the ability of aluminum to translocate to the brain.

A more innovative approach to enhance the immune response is to integrate the antigen in liposomes. These virosomes consist of unilamellar phospholipid membrane nanovesicles incorporating virus-derived glycoproteins, 100–150 nm in diameter. The first commercial product based on this technology has been InflexalV®. The principle was to deliver influenza antigens within a nanostructure resembling a native influenza virus, but deprived of its genetic material and therefore of its *in vivo* replication capability. The preparation of virosomes [21,22] is based on virus dissolution, followed by a detergent removal procedure leading to the reconstitution of virus-like particles containing only the main virus antigens embedded in a lipid bilayer. Neither viral DNA nor core proteins are present in the final product. Properly formed virosomes retain the cell binding and membrane fusion properties of the native virus, mimicking the natural infection mechanism. This property, together with the particulate nature of virosomes, gives these structures the capability of triggering a broad immune response, involving both major histocompatibility complexes, MHC-I and MHC-II, while preventing the response against the structures themselves [23–25]. These nanoparticles are therefore considered an efficient delivery system, obsoleting the need for an extra adjuvant. Importantly, virosomes have a solid safety track record, as demonstrated during almost two decades of use. Due to versatility of this technology, flu vaccination was not the only application of this technology. The advantage of these reconstituted influenza virosomes is that the influenza glycoproteins embedded in the lipid bilayer activate macrophages and mediate membrane fusion and endocytosis. This leads to an accelerated cellular and humoral response [26,27]. The adjuvanting effect of influenza-derived virosomes was also exploited for the delivery of hepatitis A antigens (Epaxal®). Extensive clinical and postmarketing monitoring showed that Epaxal has an improved safety profile compared to an aluminum-adsorbed vaccine, while inducing a similar immune response. The difficulties with the stability of such virosomal structures have been recently overcome optimizing the formulation, allowing frozen as well as 4 °C long-term storage [28].

In contrast to these human-designed nanoparticles, Nature has provided us with surprisingly elegant nanopharmaceuticals, but only recently do we have the technology to unlock its potential. Millions of years of evolution have perfected viruses in their ability to infect host cells and express their viral genes. Although the viral replication materializes at the expense of the host cell, not all viruses are as pathogenic. For example, wild-type (wt) adenovirus typically causes only mild symptoms and is cleared by the immune system in healthy individuals. The relatively large icosahedral particles (about 80 nm) are proficient in transferring their linear double-stranded DNA to host cells. Scientists have taken advantage of this feature by deleting part of the viral genome (the E1 gene) and replacing it by a gene of choice. The resultant replication-deficient virus is a very efficient delivery device for any gene of interest, expressing high levels of the encoded protein. Originally explored for gene therapy purposes, it became soon apparent that E1-deleted adenoviruses coexpress low levels of viral proteins after cell transduction. This leads to an unexpectedly broad immune response, including local chemokine and cytokine responses. Transduced cells are rapidly cleared rendering the transgenic protein production transient. Although less suitable for gene therapy, this holds great promise for vaccination purposes. As opposed to one bolus injection of antigen in classical vaccines, recombinant adenoviruses use the cell machinery to produce the antigens *in vivo* over a period of a few weeks. This substantial but transient *in vivo* production supported by the immunogenic properties of adenoviruses lead to a robust and more balanced T- and B-cell immune response. Some infectious diseases that are unresponsive to traditional vaccines, such as Ebola or HIV, may finally be overcome using this technology [29–31]. In addition to prophylactic use, adenoviruses are currently also investigated for therapeutic use, for example in HPV infection, a major cause of cervical cancer. There are, however, two drawbacks that need to be addressed to use this next generation of vaccines to improve global health. First, one advantage of adenoviruses is also a potential problem. Its immunogenic character will lead to neutralizing antibodies against the vector requiring alternate vectors that show less preexisting immunity [32–34]. The second challenge is viral stability. Adenoviruses are sensitive to degradation during storage due to physical and chemical instability. Therefore, most adenoviruses are formulated as lyophilized products or as liquid formulations to be stored at −80 °C. However, recent advances have shown that with new and tailored formulations, it is possible to stabilize these complex biological structures to provide 2–3 year stability upon storage at 4 °C [35].

In recent years, significant progress has also been made in the field of viral gene therapy. After a few vector-related adverse events in the past, more suitable vectors have been further optimized for gene transfer applications. A wide range of target tissue is now in scope (e.g., muscle, liver, eye, salivary glands, and joint) and almost 1900 clinical trials [36] are ongoing in fields like cancer (e.g., gynecological and lung), neurological disorders (e.g., Alzheimer's), inflammatory diseases (e.g., rheumatoid arthritis), monogenic disorders (e.g., hemophilia A and B), ocular disorders (e.g., macular degeneration), and diabetes. A vector that appears to be particularly promising is adeno-associated virus (AAV). The first gene therapy product approved by the EMA in 2012 for lipoprotein lipase deficiency used this vector [37]. Originally discovered as a contaminant in adenovirus batches, AAV is now widely acknowledged for application in gene therapy. AAV is small compared to adenovirus, also nonenveloped but a single-stranded DNA virus from the family of parvoviruses. They are nontoxic and nonpathogenic in humans. The key advantage of recombinant AAV, replication incompetent, is that the absence of viral gene expression minimizes host immune responses. This allows stable gene transfer and long-term transgene expression. Using specific AAV serotypes allows tailoring of the tropism to the target organ. Further optimization can be done using tissue-specific promoters and codon-optimized transgenes. Difficulties with cumbersome AAV production and purification techniques have been overcome [38–40], but a point of concern remains the physically small transgene packaging capacity in AAVs limiting its use to relatively small genes. Recently, also RNA molecules and oligonucleotides based on RNA interference have proven their potential in gene therapy applications [41]. Liposomes incorporating nucleic acids or virus vector-mediated gene therapy can be used to downregulate specific cellular protein expression through RNA interference or microRNA production.

1.3 Nanopharmaceuticals for Oral Administration and Long-Acting Injectable Therapy

Although most research and commercial nanoparticles are administered parenterally, nanoparticles also have proven to enable oral drug delivery by increasing oral bioavailability. In recent years, advances in drug discovery and combinatorial chemistry have led to many potential drug candidates that can be characterized by poor aqueous solubility and hence low bioavailability [42]. Because of the large increase in surface area at smaller particle sizes, the dissolution rate and solubility of nanoparticulate drugs are significantly increased as described by respectively the Noyes–Whitney and Ostwald–Freundlich equations [42,43].

Particle size reduction techniques for small molecule APIs (active pharmaceutical ingredients) can be classified as “top-down” or “bottom-up” processes. Top-down processes are characterized by the milling of coarse particles into smaller particles, usually to a size range of 200–500 nm. Bottom-up nanoparticles are generated by controlled crystallization of a supersaturated solution. The most widely used top-down technique is wet media milling [44]. In this technique, drug crystals are reduced in particle size through the combination of high-energy shear and impact forces of the milling beads on the coarse drug particles. The nanoparticles that are generated are stabilized in the liquid phase by polymers or surfactants. The technology is proven to be scalable from discovery scale using as little as 10 mg API up to commercial manufacture [45]. Another technique that is frequently used to generate nanoparticles is high-pressure homogenization [46]. The nanoparticle suspensions that are formed can easily be further processed using techniques such as spray-drying, freeze-drying, or granulation to form solid oral tablets or fill into capsules [44]. The interested reader can learn more about particle size reduction techniques in Chapter 9 "Overview of Techniques and Description of Established Processes" and Chapter 12 "Scale-Up and cGMP Manufacturing of Nanodrug Delivery Systems for Clinical Investigations".

Multiple products, such as rapamycin, fenofibrate, aprepitant, and megasterol acetate, are on the market using the NanoCrystal® technology or the DissoCube® technology. The benefit of these nanoproducts over their conventional counterparts is that the dose can be significantly reduced and/or the food effect is much less pronounced [47]. The interested reader can learn more about oral applications of nanodrugs in Chapter 24 "Nanodrugs in Medicine and Healthcare: Oral Delivery."

Nanosuspension generated by particle-size reduction can also be used for parenteral applications to promote long-acting injectable therapies and enhance the amount of drug that can be administered. This approach is already frequently used in preclinical studies but commercial and clinical applications remain limited [42,48]. The only commercial application currently is paliperidone palmitate injectable formulation (Invega Sustenna) that is a slow-release intramuscular injectable formulation for the treatment of patients with schizophrenia [49]. This therapy offers the opportunity of improved adherence and simplified medication regimen over the oral therapy that needs to be dosed daily. Although no longer nanoparticles, Invega Trinza uses the same technology to obtain particles showing a 3 month sustained release profile, further improving patient's quality of life. A number of other nanoparticles are currently under clinical evaluation such as thymectacin (Theralux, Celmed) and a combination therapy of cabotegravir (GlaxoSmithKline) and Rilpivirine (Janssen). The combination therapy of the two long-acting HIV therapies that are dosed every 4 or 8 weeks has shown to be comparable in maintaining viral suppression rates to a three-drug oral therapy of cabotegravir and two nucleoside reverse transcriptase inhibitors (ViiV Healthcare) [50]. This therapy offers great opportunities in developing countries where distribution and procurement of drugs is precarious and where adherence to daily oral therapy remains strikingly low for many reasons such as stigma against HIV. Data from studies in nonhuman primates have also shown great potential of the long-acting therapy in the prevention of HIV and may present a useful alternative for HIV preexposure prophylaxis (PrEP) [51].

Long-acting injectable formulations do not only lead to improved patient comfort but also have the potential to increase therapeutic compliance and efficacy even when patients cannot autonomously or reliably take their medication (e.g., due to disability/morbidity) or have limited access to medication such as in developing countries. The controlled release rate translates into lower variability in plasma drug concentrations, often reducing adverse effects, which in turn contributes to better clinical outcome. This is especially relevant for the treatment of chronic viral or bacterial infections in developing countries such as HIV, tuberculosis, malaria, and dengue. The failure to maintain minimal inhibitory concentrations could rapidly lead to incomplete viral suppression and ultimately drug resistance [52].

1.4 Bridging Future Nanomedicines to Commercialization

A lot of nanotherapeutics have already gained market access worldwide. Although for nanopharmacy to show its full potential in healthcare industry, a number of challenges remain to be addressed:

- Stabilization of nanotherapeutics remains challenging. Further understanding on the principles governing physical stability of these colloidal drugs and prevention of specific degradation routes, for example, by formulation, remains to be elucidated.
- The scale-up and manufacturing of nanotherapeutics remains variable. Process control is challenging and concerns related to the unpredictable impact of small variations to chemistry, manufacturing, and control (CMC) on the *in vivo* faith of the nanodrugs require tight controls of physicochemical properties of individual drug batches. Well-defined analytical tools that allow the full characterization of the nanoparticles' safety, efficacy, and quality need further development. Existing *in vitro* techniques have limitations in a way that *in vitro in vivo* correlation (IVIVC) cannot be performed easily and extensive bioequivalence testing is still needed. It would be great if novel *in vitro* methods become available that are straightforward to use and are predictive of the *in vivo* behavior. The interested reader can learn more about developments in this field in Chapter 12 "Scale-Up and cGMP Manufacturing of Nanodrug Delivery Systems for Clinical Investigations," Chapter 17 "Nanoparticle Toxicity: General Overview and Insights Into Immunological Compatibility," and Chapter 15 "Computational Predictive Models for Nanomedicine."
- Toxicity related to nanotherapeutics remains to be further unraveled. Nanoparticles are developed in many cases to reduce toxicity of the drug by enhanced targeting or shielding from healthy tissue. New materials such as dendrimers may be employed as carriers. Although knowledge about the potential toxicity of these, more recent nanocarriers themselves remain to be elucidated as well as the potential new toxicities that may develop because of the small size of the dosage form. Existing toxicological assessment is developed for conventional dosage forms; appropriate tests to fully understand the toxicity of nanoparticles need further development [53]. Therefore, regulatory hurdles to establish long-term safety of nanotherapeutics remain high with the need for accountability for biodistribution, mass balance, long-term residence, and ultimate elimination. The interested reader can learn more about this topic in Chapter 17 "Nanoparticle Toxicity: General Overview and Insights Into Immunological Compatibility" and Chapter 18 "An Overview of Nanoparticle BioBiocompatibility for Their Use in Nanomedicine."
- Sophisticated methods for the detection and more exact quantitation and biocompatibility of the nanoparticles in tissues need further development and validation to assess short- and long-term potential toxicities.

In order to bridge these knowledge gaps, long-term collaborations between industry and universities are very important. Such collaborations allow the scientific experts at universities to unravel the knowledge gaps that restrain industry in their ability to develop robust nanopharmaceuticals with predictable physicochemical and biological properties that ensure its quality, safety, and efficacy that are required to gain regulatory approval. Governmental policies providing a predictable and stable environment of funding and regulations nourishing such long-term partnerships have shown to be crucial for the success of these interactions. Indeed, successful collaborations are built around a common vision, strong professional relationships and trust, and shared benefits that allow bridging the cultural differences between the academic and industrial world [54]. It will also contribute to the translation of great innovative ideas with a lot of promise for the society to robust products that can be commercialized. Indeed, currently a great culture of promise exists around nanopharmacy in academia and small start-ups but they face a lot of challenges to manufacture first batches of innovative nanotherapeutics according to good manufacturing practices that can be evaluated in clinical trials and translated into commercial products beneficial for the society.

A close interaction between different stakeholders, such as researchers, patient groups, healthcare providers, regulators, and society, will also help in advancing the impact of nanotherapeutics on global public health. Current studies suggest that there is skepticism about the safety of nanotechnology and its impact to the environment, while others see great potential for the treatment and prevention of diseases such as cancer [55]. More research driven by innovators across different disciplines is needed to continuously address knowledge gaps regarding potential health and safety implications of nanopharmaceuticals in a way more information becomes available regarding its impact on health outcomes and overall health care cost. The interested reader is referred to Chapter 21 "Social Studies of Nanopharmacy" to read more on this topic.

A better understanding of the physicochemical and biological parameters affecting the quality, safety, and efficacy of the nanopharmaceuticals will also enable "follow-on" nanotherapeutics to gain easier access to the market. Currently, nanotherapeutic product applications are assessed under conventional regulatory framework and it is extremely challenging to develop nanosimilars that could be approved after the innovator patents expiration. Therefore, the regulatory authorities have established an *ad hoc* expert group that gives guidance and drafted a number of reflection papers that give scientific and regulatory guidance for the development of follow-on nanotherapeutics and emerging next-generation nanotherapeutics [56]. In addition, innovators developing nanotherapeutics are encouraged to seek regulatory agency's advice on the appropriate tests and studies to be performed during the development of a novel nanotherapeutic. The interested reader can read more in Chapter 20 "Regulatory Issues in Nanomedicines."

1.5 Future Outlook

The use of nanotechnology in the pharmaceutical industry has already shown great potential in increasing bioavailability, reducing toxicity, and side effects of existing drugs and in improving overall health, adherence, and comfort of patients. The technology is set to spread rapidly. Many more new nanotherapeutics using GRAS (Generally Recognized as Safe) or new materials are currently in various stages of development going from early discovery to late-stage clinical trials. Although nanotherapeutics are usually administered intravenously, recent clinical studies have also shown great potential if dosed subcutaneously, dermally, or as aerosols [13,57]. While in the past nanotherapies were mainly used as vaccine or cancer therapy, current advancements encompass all major disease areas, such as Alzheimer's disease, rheumatoid arthritis, diabetes, gene therapy, infectious diseases, and many others. The future technologies exploit further cell-specific targeting enabled by advancements made in the understanding of how the molecular buildup of diseased organs differentiate from healthy tissue and how nanotherapeutics interact in the body. In addition, developments in manufacturing technologies will enable more efficient loading of drugs in the nanoparticles and even enable loading of two or more therapeutic agents into one nanocarrier as, for example, in nanoparticles prepared by the layer-by-layer technology [58]. Although the biggest leap forward in patient care that is trending more and more toward personalized medicine, and the detection, diagnosis, and prevention of diseases can be expected by the combination of nanotherapeutics with other nanotechnologies, including nanobots, cell therapy, nanodevices, sensory feedback, enhanced imaging, and others. Such combinations will undoubtedly revolutionize medical care and provide enormous benefit to the patient and society in the management of health, disease, and potentially aging. However, strong research efforts in an intensive cooperation of industry and universities are required to develop such revolutionizing combinations.

Acknowledgments

The authors wish to thank Abla Creasey and Janik Adriaansen for their contributions to this chapter. The authors also wish to acknowledge Peter Pruuost, Stef Heylen, and Dirk De Smaele for their valued input in reviewing this chapter.

References

1 Weissig, V., Pettinger, T.K., and Murdock, N. (2014) Nanopharmaceuticals (Part I): products on the market. *Int. J. Nanomedicine*, **9**, 4357–4373.

2 Sundar, S. and Prajapati, V.K. (2012) Drug targeting to infectious diseases by nanoparticles surface functionalized with special biomolecules. *Curr. Med. Chem.*, **19**, 3196–3202.

3 Barenholz, Y. (2012) Doxil® – the first FDA-approved nano-drug: lessons learned. *J. Control. Release*, **160**, 117–134.

4 Barenholz, Y. (2010) From nanotechnology to nano-drugs: our Doxil™ experience, Unither Nanomed, Feb. 25, 2010.

5 O'Brien, M.E.R., Wigler, N., Inbar, M., Rosso, R., Grischke, E., Santoro, A.,

Catane, R., Kieback, D.G., Tomczak, P., Ackland, S.P., Orlandi, F., Mellars, L., Alland, L., and Tendler, C. (2004) Reduced cardiotoxicity and comparable efficacy in a phase III trial of pegylated liposomal doxorubicin HCl (CAELYX™/Doxil®) versus conventional doxorubicin for first-line treatment of metastatic breast cancer. *Ann. Oncol.*, **15**, 440–449.

6 Dawidczyk, C.M., Kim, C., Park, J.H., Russell, L.M., Lee, K.H., Pomper, M.G., and Searson, P.C. (2014) State-of-the-art in design rules for drug delivery platforms: lessons learned from FDA-approved nanomedicines. *J. Control. Release*, **187**, 133–144.

7 Miele, E., Spinelli, G.P., Miele, E., Tomao, F., and Tomao, S. (2009) Albumin-bound formulation of paclitaxel (Abraxane ABI-007) in the treatment of breast cancer. *Int. J. Nanomedicine*, **4**, 99–105.

8 Mullard, A. (2013) Maturing antibody-drug conjugate pipeline hits 30. *Nat. Rev. Drug Discov.*, **12**, 329–332.

9 Sassoon, I. and Blanc, V. (2013) Antibody-drug conjugate (ADC) clinical pipeline: a review. *Methods Mol. Biol.*, **1045**, 1–27.

10 Sievers, E.L. and Senter, P.D. (2013) Antibody-drug conjugates in cancer therapy. *Annu. Rev. Med.*, **64**, 15–29.

11 Verma, S., Miles, D., Gianni, L., Krop, I.E., Welslau, M., Baselga, J., Pegram, M., Oh, D.-Y., Diéras, V., Guardino, E., Fang, L., Lu, M.W., Olsen, S., and Blackwell, K. (2012) Trastuzumab emtansine for HER2-positive advanced breast cancer. *N. Engl. J. Med.*, **367**, 1783–1791.

12 Lu, D., Burris, H.A., Wang, B., Dees, E.C., Cortes, J., Joshi, A., Gupta, M., Yi, J.-H., Chu, Y.-W., Shih, T., Fang, L., and Girish, S. (2012) Drug interaction potential of trastuzumab emtansine (T-DM1) combined with pertuzumab in patients with HER2-positive metastatic breast cancer. *Curr. Drug Metab.*, **13**, 911–922.

13 Fan, Y. and Zhang, Q. (2013) Development of liposomal formulations: from concept to clinical investigations. *Asian J. Pharm. Sci.*, **8**, 81–87.

14 Gobbo, O.L., Sjaastad, K., Radomski, M.W., Volkov, Y., and Prina-Mello, A. (2015) Magnetic nanoparticles in cancer theranostics. *Theranostics*, **5** (11), 1249–1263.

15 Hawkins, M.J., Soon-Shiong, P., and Desai, N. (2008) Protein nanoparticles as drug carriers in clinical medicine. *Adv. Drug Deliv. Rev.*, **60**, 876–885.

16 Hanahan, D. and Weinberg, R.A. (2011) Hallmarks of cancer: the next generation. *Cell*, **144**, 646–674.

17 Chames, P., Van Regenmortel, M., Weiss, E., and Baty, D. (2009) Therapeutic antibodies: successes, limitations and hopes for the future. *Br. J. Pharmacol.*, **157**, 220–233.

18 Holliger, P. and Hudson, P.J. (2005) Engineered antibody fragments and the rise of single domains. *Nat. Biotechnol.*, **23**, 1126.

19 Hu, M. and Zhang, K. (2013) The application of aptamers in cancer research: an up-to-date review. *Future Oncol.*, **9**, 369–376.

20 Weissleder, R., Kelly, K., Sun, E.Y., Shtatland, T., and Josephson, L. (2005) Cell-specific targeting of nanoparticles by multivalent attachment of small molecules. *Nat. Biotechnol.*, **23**, 1418–1423.

21 Metsikkö, K., vanMeer, G., and Simons, K. (1986) Reconstitution of the fusogenic activity of vesicular stomatitis virus. *EMBO J.*, **5** (13), 3429–3435.

22 Stegmann, T., Morselt, H.W., Booy, F.P., van Breemen, J.F., Scherphof, G., and Wilschut, J. (1987) Functional reconstitution of influenza virus envelopes. *EMBO J.*, **6** (9), 2651–2659.

23 Huckriede, A., Bungener, L., Stegmann, T., Daemen, T., Medema, J., Palache, A.M., and Wilschut, J. (2005) The virosome concept for influenza vaccines. *Vaccine*, **8** (23 Suppl. 1), S26–S38.

24 Cusi, M.G. (2006) Applications of influenza virosomes as a delivery system. *Hum. Vaccin.*, **2** (1), 1–7.

25 Moser, C., Amacker, M., Kammer, A.R., Rasi, S., Westerfeld, N., and Zurbriggen, R. (2007) Influenza virosomes as a combined vaccine carrier and adjuvant system for prophylactic and therapeutic immunizations. *Expert Rev. Vaccines*, **6** (5), 711–721.

26 Bungener, L., Serre, K., Bijl, L., Leserman, L., Wilschut, J., Daemen, T., and Machy, P. (2002) Virosome-mediated delivery of protein antigens to dendritic cells. *Vaccine*, **22, 20** (17–18), 2287–2295.

27 Bungener, L., Huckriede, A., de Mare, A., de Vries-Idema, J., Wilschut, J., and Daemen, T. (2005) Virosome-mediated delivery of protein antigens *in vivo*: efficient induction of class I MHC-restricted cytotoxic T lymphocyte activity. *Vaccine*, **23** (10), 1232–1241.

28 Adriaansen, J. and Doro, F. (2015) Improved formulations for virosomes. Patent WO2015091798 A3 filed Dec. 18, 2014 and issued Aug. 27, 2015.

29 Mennechet, F.J., Tran, T.T., Eichholz, K., van de Perre, P., and Kremer, E.J. (2015) Ebola virus vaccine: benefit and risks of adenovirus-based vectors. *Expert Rev. Vaccines*, **14** (11), 1471–1478.

30 Barouch, D.H., Alter, G., Broge, T., Linde, C., Ackerman, M.E., Brown, E.P., Borducchi, E.N., Smith, K.M., Nkolola, J.P., Liu, J., Shields, J., Parenteau, L., Whitney, J.B., Abbink, P., Ng'ang'a, D.M., Seaman, M.S., Lavine, C.L., Perry, J.R., Li, W., Colantonio, A.D., Lewis, M.G., Chen, B., Wenschuh, H., Reimer, U., Piatak, M., Lifson, J.D., Handley, S.A., Virgin, H.W., Koutsoukos, M., Lorin, C., Voss, G., Weijtens, M., Pau, M.G., and Schuitemaker, H. (2015) HIV-1 vaccines. Protective efficacy of adenovirus/protein vaccines against SIV challenges in rhesus monkeys. *Supramol. Sci.*, **349** (6245), 320–324.

31 Barouch, D.H., Stephenson, K.E., Borducchi, E.N., Smith, K., Stanley, K., McNally, A.G., Liu, J., Abbink, P., Maxfield, L.F., Seaman, M.S., Dugast, A.S., Alter, G., Ferguson, M., Li, W., Earl, P.L., Moss, B., Giorgi, E.E., Szinger, J.J., Eller, L.A., Billings, E.A., Rao, M., Tovanabutra, S., Sanders-Buell, E., Weijtens, M., Pau, M.G., Schuitemaker, H., Robb, M.L., Kim, J.H., Korber, B.T., and Michael, N.L. (2013) Protective efficacy of a global HIV-1 mosaic vaccine against heterologous SHIV challenges in rhesus monkeys. *Cell*, **155** (3), 531–539.

32 Geisbert, T.W., Bailey, M., Hensley, L., Asiedu, C., Geisbert, J., Stanley, D., Honko, A., Johnson, J., Mulangu, S., Pau, M.G., Custers, J., Vellinga, J., Hendriks, J., Jahrling, P., Roederer, M., Goudsmit, J., Koup, R., and Sullivan, N.J. (2011) Recombinant adenovirus serotype 26 (Ad26) and Ad35 vaccine vectors bypass immunity to Ad5 and protect non-human primates against ebola virus challenge. *J. Virol.*, **85** (9), 4222–4233.

33 Barouch, D.H., Liu, J., Li, H., Maxfield, L.F., Abbink, P., Lynch, D.M., Iampietro, M.J., SanMiguel, A., Seaman, M.S., Ferrari, G., Forthal, D.N., Ourmanov, I., Hirsch, V.N., Carville, A., Mansfield, K.G., Stablein, D., Pau, M.G., Schuitemaker, H., Sadoff, J.C., Billings, E.M., Rao, M., Robb, M.L., Kim, J.H., Marovich, M.A., Goudsmit, J., and Michael, N.L. (2012) Vaccine protection against acquisition of neutralization-resistant SIV challenges in rhesus monkeys. *Nature*, **482** (7383), 89–93.

34 Johnson, J.A., Barouch, D.H., and Baden, L.R. (2013) Nonreplicating vectors in HIV vaccines. *Curr. Opin. HIV AIDS*, **8** (5), 412–420.

35 Adriaansen, J. (2015) Improved adenovirus formulations. Patent WO2015040002 A1, filed Sept. 16, 2014 and issued March 26, 2015.

36 Ginn, S.L., Alexander, I.E., Edelstein, M.L., Abedi, M.R., and Wixon, J. (2013) Gene therapy clinical trials worldwide to 2012: an update. *J. Gene Med.*, **15** (2), 65–77.

37 Gaudet, D., Méthot, J., Déry, S., Brisson, D., Essiembre, C., Tremblay, G., Tremblay, K., de Wal, J., Twisk, J., van den Bulk, N., Sier-Ferreira, V., and van Deventer, S. (2013) Efficacy and long-term safety of alipogene tiparvovec (AAV1-LPLS447X) gene therapy for lipoprotein lipase deficiency: an open-label trial. *Gene Ther.*, **20** (4), 361–369.

38 Xie, Q., Hare, J., Turnigan, J., and Chapman, M.S. (2004) Large-scale production, purification and crystallization of wild-type adeno-associated virus-2. *J. Virol. Methods*, **122** (1), 17–27.

39 Smith, R.H., Ding, C., and Kotin, R.M. (2003) Serum-free production and column purification of adeno-associated virus type 5. *J. Virol. Methods*, **114** (2), 115–124.

40 Kaludov, N., Handelman, B., and Chiorini, J.A. (2002) Scalable purification of adeno-associated virus type 2, 4, or 5 using ion-exchange chromatography. *Hum. Gene Ther.*, **13** (10), 1235–1243.

41 Lundstrom, K. (2015) Special issue: Gene therapy with emphasis on RNA interference. *Viruses*, **7** (8), 4482–4487.
42 Williams, H.D., Trevaskis, N.L., Charman, S.A., Shanker, R.M., Charman, W.N., Pouton, C.W., and Porter, C.J.H. (2013) Strategies to address low drug solubility in discovery and development. *Pharmacol. Rev.*, **65**, 315–499.
43 Cavalli, R. and Leone, F. (2013) Nanosuspensions A versatile drug delivery platform. *Chim. Oggi.*, **31** (4), 46–49.
44 Merisko-Liversidge, E., Liversidge, G.G., and Cooper, E.R. (2003) Nanosizing: a formulation approach for poorly-water-soluble compounds. *Eur. J. Pharm. Sci.*, **18**, 113–120.
45 Van Eerdenbrugh, B. (2008) Top-down production of drug nanocrystals: nanosuspension stabilization, miniaturization and transformation into solid products. Thesis, Group Biomedical Sciences, Faculty of Pharmaceutical Sciences, Katholieke Universiteit Leuven, Leuven, Belgium.
46 Möschwitzer, J. and Müller, R.H. (2006) New method for the effective production of ultrafine drug nanocrystals. *J. Nanosci. Nanotechnol.*, **6** (9–10), 3145–3153.
47 Timpe, C. (2013) Oral nanocrystal products and nanotube drug delivery. *Chim. Oggi.*, **31** (4), 40–45.
48 Williams, P.E., Crauwels, H.M., and Basstanie, E.D. (2015) Formulation and pharmacology of long-acting rilpivirine. *Curr. Opin. HIV AIDS*, **10** (4), 233–238.
49 Kramer, M., Litman, R., Hough, D., Lane, R., Lim, P., Liu, Y., and Eerdekens, M. (2010) Paliperidone palmitate, a potential long-acting treatment for patients with schizophrenia. Results of a randomized, double-blind, placebo-controlled efficacy and safety study. *Int. J. Neuropsychopharmacol.*, **13**, 635–647.
50 ViiV Healthcare (2015) ViiV Healthcare announces positive headline results from a study of two drug injectable regimen for HIV maintenance therapy. London, 3 November 2015.
51 Radzio, J., Spreen, W., Yueh, Y.L., Mitchell, J., Jenkins, L., García-Lerma, J.G., and Heneine, W. (2015) The long-acting integrase inhibitor GSK744 protects macaques from repeated intravaginal SHIV challenge. *Sci. Transl. Med.*, **7** (270), 270ra5.
52 Descamps, D., Flandre, P., Calvez, V., Peytavin, G., Meiffredy, V., Collin, G., Delaugerre, C., Robert-Delmas, S., Bazin, B., Aboulker, J.P. *et al.* (2000) Mechanisms of virologic failure in previously untreated HIV-infected patients from a trial of induction-maintenance therapy. Trilège (Agence Nationale de Recherches sur le SIDA 072) Study Team. *JAMA*, **283**, 205–211.
53 De Jong, W.H. and Borm, P.J.A. (2008) Drug delivery and nanoparticles: applications and hazards. *Int. J. Nanomedicine*, **3** (2), 133–149.
54 Edmondson, G., Valigra, L., Kenward, M., Hudson, R.L., and Belfield, H. (2012) Making industry-university partnerships work: lessons from successful collaborations, Science|Business Innovation Board AISBL.
55 Pautler, M. and Brenner, S. (2010) Nanomedicine: promises and challenges for the future of public health. *Int. J. Nanomedicine*, **5**, 803–809.
56 Hafner, A., Lovric, J., Lakos, G.P., and Pepic, I. (2014) Nanotherapeutics in the EU: an overview on current state and future directions. *Int. J. Nanomedicine*, **9**, 1005–1023.
57 Uchechi, O., Ogbonna, J.D.N., and Attama, A.A. (2014) Nanoparticles for dermal and transdermal drug delivery, in *Nanotechnology and nanomaterials "Application of Nanotechnology in Drug Delivery"* (ed. A. Demir Sezer), Intech, pp. 193–235.
58 Denga, Z.J., Mortona, S.W., Ben-Akivaa, E., Dreadena, E.C., Shopsowitza, K.E., and Hammond, P.T. (2013) Layer-by-layer nanoparticles for systemic codelivery of an anticancer drug and siRNA for potential triple-negative breast cancer treatment. *ACS Nano*, **7** (11), 9571–9584.

2
Nanoscale Drugs: A Key to Revolutionary Progress in Pharmacy and Healthcare

Simon Sebastian Raesch,[1] Marina Poettler*,[2] Christoph Alexiou,[2] and Claus-Michael Lehr[1,3]*

[1]Helmholtz Institute for Pharmaceutical Research Saarland (HIPS), Helmholtz Centre for Infection Research (HZI), Department of Drug Delivery, Campus E8.1, 66123 Saarbrücken, Germany
[2]University Hospital Erlangen, Department of Otorhinolaryngology, Head and Neck Surgery, Section for Experimental Oncology and Nanomedicine (SEON), Else Kröner-Fresenius Professorship, Glueckstrasse 10a, 91054 Erlangen, Germany
[3]Saarland University, Department of Pharmacy, Campus A4.1, 66123 Saarbrücken, Germany

2.1
Introduction

2.1.1
Setting the Stage

Nanopharmaceuticals are defined as nanoscale assemblies, which can be relatively simple, resembling nanoparticles (NPs), nanoemulsions or polymer conjugates, or complex like multicomponent systems containing drugs, proteins or genes, and a selection of targeting ligands and signal systems to enable *in vitro* or *in vivo* detection [1].

Nanotechnology is thought to be the key technology of the twenty-first century. Thus, nanomedicine and its implementation in the health care system represent a vast potential for medical diagnosis and therapy. Nanomaterials used for medicine purposes are actually plausible, since the human body consists of nanostructures and processes within the body function on nanobasis including the development of diseases in cells. Here, nanomaterials can take advantage of cellular machineries to facilitate the delivery of drugs. Hence, nanopharmaceuticals offer a huge platform to directly combat targeted disease pattern. NPs comprising conjugated, encapsulated, absorbed, or dispersed drugs have exclusive characteristics that can improve the performance in different dosage forms. Nanopharmaceuticals can improve solubility and dissolution, modulate interactions with biological surfaces, and also control drug release. The implementation of

*Contributed equally.

Pharmaceutical Nanotechnology: Innovation and Production, First Edition. Edited by Jean Cornier, Arno Kwade, Andrew Owen, and Marcel Van de Voorde.

nanotechnology thus allows to enhance bioavailability and to alter pharmacokinetics and drug disposition in order to increase therapeutic efficacy and decrease side effects [2,3]. Additionally, size, shape, and surface characteristics of NPs can be varied, allowing achieving target or facilitating transport across biological barriers. By attaching ligands such as antibodies or aptamers bound to the surface of particles, site-specific ("active") targeting can be realized, or by using guidance in form of magnetic NPs. Nanomaterial-based drug delivery could in that way reduce the drug dose required to realize therapeutic advantage, which would consecutively bate the costs and/or lessen side effects linked to specific drugs.

The fact that our society grows older with the desire to stay healthy and mobile, together with amplified occurrence of diseases, such as cancer, diabetes, atherosclerosis, cardiovascular diseases, or Alzheimer's disease, is still a challenge for medicine today. Therefore, nanopharmacy opens new horizons for diagnosis, imaging, and therapy. Although several applications are developed or are even on market, nanopharmacy is still referred to as rather young and emerging technology.

2.1.2
Definition and Size Aspects

When it comes to defining what nanomaterials in general are, the response much depends on the community that is asked. Historically, nanomaterials itself have been first defined by physicists and material scientists, and subsequently most definitions of nanomaterials are based on the nano-specific physical peculiarities, such as optical and electronic properties, which are typically observed below 100 nm [4]. The European Commission defined nanomaterials as "A natural, incidental or manufactured material containing particles, in an unbound state or as an aggregate or as an agglomerate and where, for 50% or more of the particles in the number size distribution, one or more external dimensions is in the size range 1 nm–100 nm" [5]. Most other standards also require at least one (SCCP) [6] or two dimensions (ASTM, NIOSH) [7,8], or the diameter (ISO) [9] to be in the range between 1 and 100 nm and all of them have in common that they define NPs as such. In terms of intended use, the definition of the European Science Foundation, which expands the term of nanomedicine to particles of up to *hundreds of nanometers* [10], is more reasonable for the definition of NPs for the pharmaceutical delivery of drugs [11]. This is accounted for by the fact that the delivery of active pharmaceutical ingredients (APIs) requires the formulation of a certain dose within the particle, that is, the volume of the particle. By decreasing the size of a NP, its volume decreases to the third power. This means to deliver the same dose with a particle that is ten times smaller in diameter, the number of particles is increased by 1000. Reasonable amounts of drug can consequently only be delivered by NPs of a certain size and 100 nm therefore rather represents in practice a lower than an upper size limit. A diameter of 200–300 nm is thus often regarded as a suitable and common size for pharmaceutical nanocarriers. However, how the regulation of nanopharmaceuticals by drug agencies is realized differs among the latter [12] and will be discussed in another part of this book.

2.1.3
Nanopharmacy: Interdisciplinary Medicine

While a typical pharmaceutical product comes already in touch with a broad range of specialists during its evolution from a new molecular entity to an applicable formulation, developing nanopharmaceuticals requires *per se* even more disciplines to work together. In addition to the established biopharmaceutical parameters of the API, that is, solubility and permeability, the colloidal properties of the nanocarrier come into the play as well. The latter determine how biological barriers are being crossed, how they interact with biomolecules and cells, how they can be loaded with drugs, and how the drug is being released. Nanopharmaceuticals often require new approaches to determine these effects, necessitating adequate analytical approaches to reliably ensure safety and consistency of the product. Technically, these approaches are often very similar to those of so-called nanotoxicology, a discipline concerned with the safety and potential risks of nanomaterials for nonpharmaceutical applications.

The urge to formulate drugs in the nanoscale is based on two different reasons: First of all, newly developed drug molecules nowadays not only come with the gift of high activity toward a specific target but often as well with poor ADME profiles. Especially, since easily degradable biomacromolecules, such as polypeptides and polynucleotides, have emerged as a result from advancements in biotechnology, the need for formulations that can deliver these substances to the target site has increased. Due to their large and often fragile structure, biopharmaceuticals are subject to fast degradation/elimination, and lack the ability to permeate over biological barriers. Therefore, they are typically applied parenterally, which has never been the most favorable application route. Even direct intravenous injection, however, which for conventional drugs provides fastest and most complete bioavailability, cannot ensure the delivery of DNA/RNA for gene therapy. The success of any future gene therapy will highly depend on the vector reaching intracellular compartments, such as cytoplasm or nucleus, and therefore requires the controlled passage of several biological barriers. On the other hand, such macromolecular biopharmaceuticals offer the most promising perspectives when it comes to actually curing chronic diseases by genetically inhibition or reprogramming of cells.

Apart from that, nanotechnology also offers great possibilities to expand the lifetime of established drugs, by enhancing the pharmacokinetic profile by increasing solubility, bioavailability, and offering sustained release, or even the targeted delivery by complex NPs. Moreover, nanotechnology also offers advantages as a tool for diagnosis or for vaccination strategies and combinations thereof (see Figure 2.1).

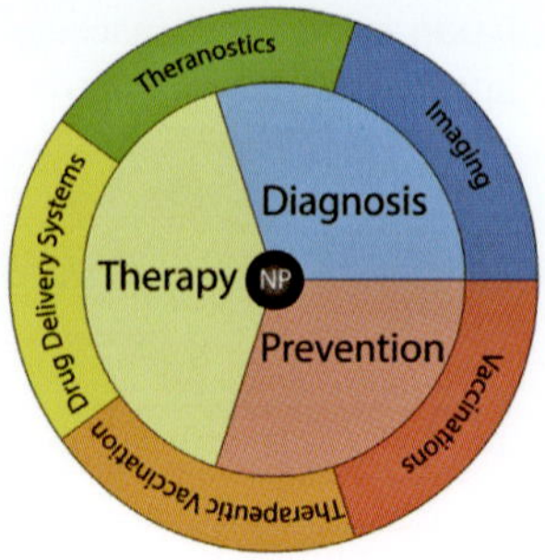

Figure 2.1 Fields of application for nanopharmaceuticals.

2.2 Nanopharmacy Concepts to Improve the Safety and Efficacy of Medicines

2.2.1 Overcoming the Solubility Barrier

As a consequence of contemporary drug discovery approaches and high-throughput screening, the lipophilicity of candidate drugs has steadily increased, leading to poor water solubility and thus limited bioavailability. The need for technologies that make the administration of nonwater-soluble drugs feasible has resulted in the development of methods that increase the surface of the API immensely, in order to accelerate dissolution and enhance therewith bioavailability. One approach is the general principle of "nanosizing": by decreasing the particle size, the relative surface area increases, which positively influences the dissolution rate as well as the solubility [13]. Nanosized drugs are therefore popular for improving oral drug delivery, and some of such products have already reached the market. Another way to improve solubility has been found in terms of adsorbing water insoluble APIs onto the large surface of mesoporous (2–50 nm pore size) particles [14]. Such particles may therefore be considered as nano-structured, even when the particle size is larger than 1 μm. Mesoporous silica particles such as MCM-41 have an immense inner surface area, on which APIs ban be bound and can additionally be modified to act as Trojan horses, that release their cargo at the desired site of action [15].

2.2.2 Controlling Drug Release

Talking about different ways of drug delivery also raises the question how drugs are being released from their carrier. The microenvironment of a tumor, for instance, is once more different from healthy tissue: due to a higher metabolic turnover, tumor cells use more oxygen and nutrients, whereby glycolysis is stimulated to produce more energy, which makes the environment acidic [16] and the tendency to lower pH values can also be found in inflamed tissue. Nowadays, drugs are mostly given systemically; this may lead to a high peak plasma concentration, followed by rapid elimination. Controlled drug release gives us the opportunity to overcome this burden and allows keeping drug concentrations within the therapeutic window over a prolonged period of time. In this context, at least two categories can be discriminated: sustained and stimuli-responsive release.

2.2.2.1 Sustained Release

The purpose of sustained release is to make a specific amount of drug available over a certain period of time. This makes particular sense for such molecules that, once released, will be quickly metabolized or otherwise eliminated from the body. One method to attain sustained release is to avoid the entering of the drug molecules to aqueous surrounding for a controlled period of time. This can be achieved either by diffusion control by an insoluble polymer cover or by degradation control of the nanocarrier [17].

Diffusion-Controlled Release

Here, the drug is encapsulated within the nanocarrier and restricted to go in the aqueous surrounding by a membrane or the particle structure itself. The drug release rate depends on this membrane and its composition.

Erosion-Controlled Release

The big advantage with degradable or erodible nanocarriers is that they can also be easily eliminated from the body after the drug has been released. The drug release kinetics can be managed by vigilant design of the encapsulation procedures and polymers to modify the erosion. The most prominent representatives are polyesters of lactic (PLA) and glycolic acid (PGA) as well as copolymers thereof (PLGA, i.e., poly(lactic-*co*-glycolic acid)) that are degraded via hydrolytic disruption. Hence, they can be easily metabolized and eliminated from the body as carbon dioxide and water [18].

2.2.2.2 Stimuli-Responsive Release

Stimuli-responsive release is a very important tool when it comes to diseases such as cancer. As tumorigenesis and cancer progression depend on daily treatment, it requires adequate control and management of drug release and profiles [19]. Two types of stimuli induction can be distinguished: internal and external stimuli. Whereby internal stimuli include pH value, enzymatic activity, and concentration of ions or small molecules, and external stimuli are magnetic field, heat, ultrasound, electric field, or light [20].

pH-Induced Release

Diseases such as cancer or inflammation are associated with a change of pH in their environment. This can be utilized to trigger the release of a drug in this pathological acidic surrounding. Three different mechanisms can be used to induce pH-sensitive drug release from a nanocarrier: pH-reactive PEG-detachment, unsteady acid bonds in polymers of carriers, and proton-accepting groups. Various nanocarriers have been designed in that way, based on, for example, lipids, polymers, polypeptides, and polysaccharides. When reaching their acidic target, these functionalized nanocarriers can accept protons and make conformational changes either via aggregation/precipitation, destabilization, or disruption depending on the pH. This can take place intra- and extracellularly [21].

Enzyme-Dependent Release

Among the vast selection of enzymatic activities, one is to break chemical bonds, triggering the destruction, or disassembly of a structure. As in certain diseases some enzymes are overexpressed, this can be exploited to trigger drug release from a nanocarrier. Several different nanocarrier systems have been designed with enzyme-sensitive polymers as cross-links, enabling targeted drug release at the inflammation or tumor site, including porous silica NPs, hydrogels micelles, or liposomes [22]. Interestingly, sequences, scissile by matrix metalloproteinases, have been used as ties between PEG molecules, iron oxide, or polymeric NPs [23].

Photosensitive Release

Here, functional groups bound to NPs can change their conformation when irradiated by light (UV or infrared), including nitrobenzene, pyrene, azobenzene, or cinnamoyl groups [24]. For example, the azobenzene group can be switched from *trans* to *cis* when irradiated by UV light and from *cis* to *trans* by visible light allowing a remote control by light [25]. Hydrogels with polypyrrole NPs are used as photothermal transducers and are activated by near-infrared-light irradiation to release neuro-active substances [26]. Furthermore, hypericin-bearing magnetic iron oxide NPs are under investigation for photodynamic therapy [27].

Thermoresponsive Release

Pathological conditions such as inflammation, cancer, or infections can also be used for controlled drug release. Thermosensitive nanocarriers for drug delivery are normally liposomes or NPs composed of thermosensitive polymers [28].

2.2.3
Overcoming Biological Barriers

Aside from the promise of controlled release and improved metabolic stability for pharmaceuticals, another main principle that speaks of the use of nanopharmaceuticals is the potential to overcome biological barriers. This is of particular importance for macromolecular biopharmaceuticals, such as peptides and nucleotides, eventually even allowing their noninvasive ("needle-free") administration.

2.2.3.1 Epithelial–Endothelial Barriers

Oral Drug Delivery: Gastrointestinal Mucosa

Oral administration is not only the most favorable route to make drugs systemically available, but also displays a possibility to topically deliver drugs to the intestine [29]. As the intestine is commonly affected by infections and other diseases such as Morbus Crohn, causing an accelerated gastrointestinal passage, the delivery of anti-infective or anti-inflammatory drugs in nanoparticulate formulations with extended residence time is a challenge, a classical pharmaceutical formulation cannot achieve. By using nanopharmaceuticals, which can penetrate the mucosa, such delivery is, however, feasible [30]. This is peculiarly true in case of inflammatory bowel diseases, in which, similar to the EPR effect, small particles can permeate through the defective epithelial layer caused by disrupted junctions (Figure 2.2) [31].

However, in case of systemic delivery across an intact mucosa, nanocarriers need not only to pass the mucus layer of the intestine, but also the tight epithelium. Additionally and regardless of the target, orally administered nanocarriers need to survive the passage through the rather "inconvenient" environment of the stomach. Although this can be solved with encapsulation of the nanocarrier within a secondary formulation, it could be shown that not only a variety of nanopharmaceuticals such as liposomes, SLN, and polymeric NPs can be designed to resists these conditions [32,33], but furthermore are also able to deliver instable (macro)molecules, for example, heparin [34], paclitaxel [33], or insulin [35] to the systemic circulation and can be used for vaccines delivery [36].

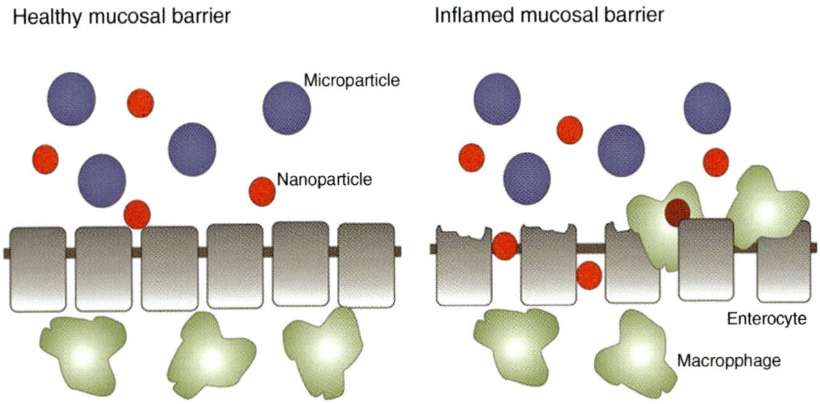

Figure 2.2 Proposed mechanism of the size dependent accumulation of particles in the inflamed intestinal mucosa. Small enough particles may accumulate in the gaps between epithelial cells or be taken up by invading immune cells. (Reprinted with permission from Ref. [29], © 2012 Elsevier B.V.)

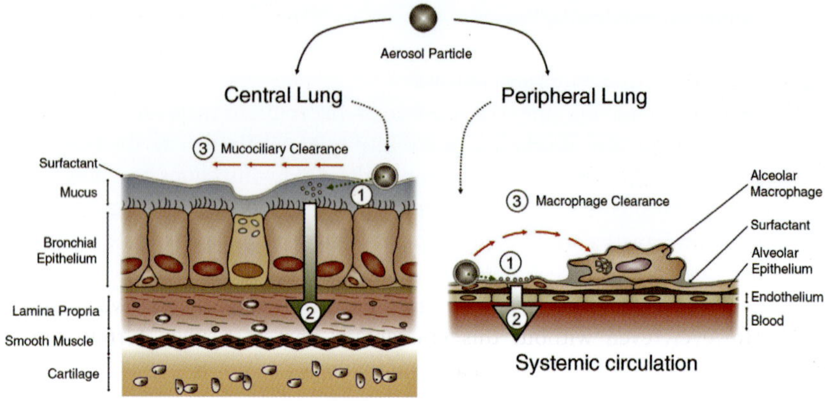

Figure 2.3 Cellular and non-cellular barriers of the lung: after landing on lung lining fluids (1) the drug (or eventually entire particles) must cross the pulmonary epithelium (2) in order to reach the underlying tissue or the systemic circulation, respectively. Besides, inhalation nanopharmaceuticals must also overcome effective clearance processes (3) provided by either mucus in the central lung (bronchi) or by macrophages in the peripheral lung (alveoli). (Reprinted with permission from Ref. [39], © 2014 Elsevier B.V).

Pulmonary Drug Delivery: Air–Blood Barrier

The lungs are one the most obvious target for nanopharmaceuticals, as airborne particles in the nanoscale are capable of following the thin conducting airways and deposit depending on their size in different parts of the lung [37]. This is not only beneficial for a variety of acute and chronic diseases that affect the lung, with its enormous inner surface of $\sim 100\,m^2$ [38], but the lung also gives the opportunity to deliver drugs systemically without first pass effect through the thin blood–air barrier. Due to the large amounts of air that are inhaled, the lung has thankfully very efficient clearance mechanisms to maintain its proper functioning, which, however, make the delivery by particles challenging (Figure 2.3).

In order to successfully deliver NPs to the lungs, the formulation needs to meet apparent size/shape criteria, depending on the desired site of deposition. NPs smaller than 100 nm have been shown to reach the deep lung easily; though can as easily be exhaled again [40]. The generation of such small aerosol particles, however, is not yet feasible, to gain the advantage of nanoparticulate delivery systems in the lung anyway, primary NPs need to be incorporated into microparticles that effectively reach the deep lung to be released after deposition. The high humidity along the conducting airways can interfere with the deposition, and influence the size and shape of the particles. Once the particle has deposited, it still faces a difficult environment and only a very low volume of liquid that is available to solve drugs and excipients [41]. Besides the mucus layer of the upper lung, which is discussed later, different mechanisms of disposition are observable in the lungs. In the respiratory zone, particles are typically taken up by alveolar macrophages, which then again migrate into the regions of mucociliary clearance. Macrophages themselves can be a target in the lungs, since there are several infections that manifest intracellularly, with the most known one being tuberculosis. The delivery of NPs releasing their cargo inside macrophages to reach the encapsulated pathogens is highly relevant due to the lack of efficient anti-infectives [42–44].

Single molecules, but also NPs have the ability to permeate through the epithelial layer into the systemic circulation [45], nevertheless, there is no such nanopharmaceutical on the market. This might be due to the fact, that the mechanisms that lead to uptake or permeation in the lung are not yet understood. However, even without this knowledge, nanoparticulate formulations have been shown to be effective. In a mouse model, a genome editing RNA was successfully delivered by aerolization in a chitosan-coated PLGA carrier to the deep lung where it corrected deficiency of surfactant protein B [46]. The use of *in vitro* test systems for the epithelial barrier of the lungs is nevertheless reasonable, confronted with the immense number of lung-targeted nanopharmaceuticals that are developed [47].

Transdermal Drug Delivery: Skin

The skin might be – not only for nanopharmaceuticals – the most difficult barrier to overcome due to its highly impermeable "brick and mortar" setup of the stratum corneum, which ensures a dense packing of corneocytes within intercellular lipids [48]. Topically administered drugs such as steroids, have been shown to be improvable by nanoparticulate formulations such as the micellar estradiol Estrasorb® [49,50]. Due to the high concentration of dendritic cells, the skin is also a popular target for vaccinations. Aiming at the relinquishment of needles, a few technologies were developed to increase transcutaneous permeability of larger molecules, such as ultrasound, electroporation, and PowderJect. Without the use of these additional technologies, the penetration of intact NPs is hardly possible [51], although permeation was reported *in vivo/vitro* depending on residence time and particle size [52]. A gate for vaccine delivery through the intact skin without the application of external forces was found in transfollicular transport [53,54]. Recent studies confirmed that the delivery of antigens incorporated in chitosan-PLGA NPs over the follicular provokes an immune response [55] without perturbating the normal skin barrier function, suggesting that it might be worthwhile looking further into nanoparticle-based needle-free transcutaneous vaccinations (Figure 2.4).

Drug Delivery to the Central Nervous System: Blood–Brain Barrier

In order to prevent pathogens and neurotoxic substances from entering the central nervous system, the body has developed a boundary that establishes two separated compartments, with the blood on the one side and the cerebrospinal fluid on the other side. The endothelium of the blood–brain barrier displays a highly efficient filter for molecules and particles (Figure 2.5). In principle, only very small or hydrophobic molecules are allowed to permeate the blood–brain

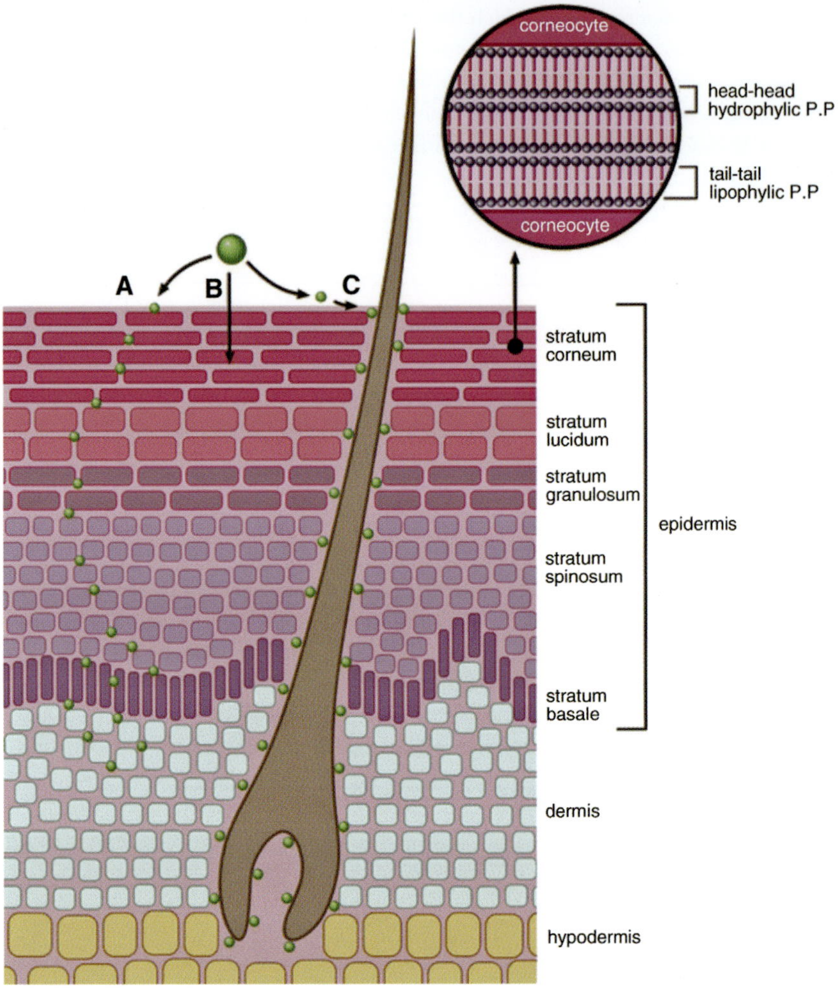

Figure 2.4 Schematic illustrations of the skin and main penetration routes, insert showing the lipid bilayers between corneocytes. Route A: across the lipid bilayers (intercellular route); Route B: across the corneocytes and lipid bilayers (intracellular route); Route C: along hair follicles and sweat glands. (Reprinted with permission from Ref. [56], © 2010 Elsevier B.V.)

barrier passively, while larger and hydrophilic molecules are restricted as well as particles, necessary exceptions are transported actively [57].

The desire to reach the cerebrospinal fluid is not only based on the need to deliver agents, which act on the central nervous system itself, such as antidepressants, analgesics, anticonvulsants, and so on, but also in order to reach brain tumors, which are not accessible without invasive high-risk methods. Which properties are required for nanocarriers in order to successfully cross this barrier and not to be quickly expelled from the cerebrospinal fluid is still being

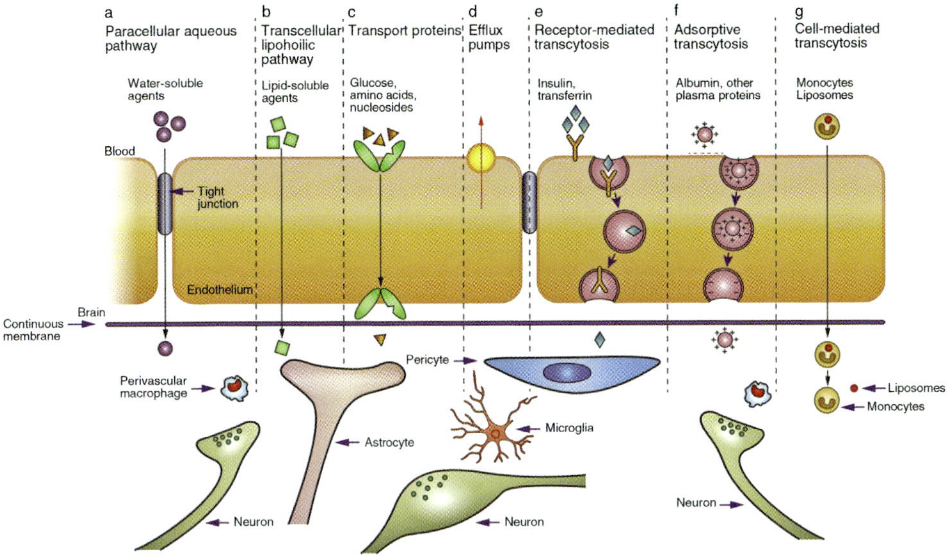

Figure 2.5 Transport routes across the blood–brain barrier. Pathways "a"–"f" are commonly for solute molecules; and the route "g" involves monocytes, macrophages, and other immune cells and can be used for any drugs or drugs-incorporated liposomes or NPs. (Reprinted with permission from Ref. [57], © 2012 Elsevier B.V.)

discussed [58,59]. However, liposomes, SLNs, and polymeric NPs have been applied successfully – some by rational surface modifications – for CNS delivery [60]. Kreuter *et al.* found a dexterous way to trick the blood–brain barrier by grafting certain polymers or proteins on the surface of nanocarriers [61].

Another possibility for giving nanopharmaceuticals access to the cerebrospinal fluid is making the endothelium of the blood–brain barrier more permeable. This can be achieved either by physical, chemical, or by biological stimuli. The most promising tools to achieve an increased permeability of the blood–brain barrier are the external application of ultrasound or by local heating. Although this has been applied successfully [62], as a disturbed barrier function also comes with an influx of unwanted neurotoxic substances and possibly an efflux of neoplastic cells, these techniques are used reluctantly.

2.2.3.2 **Noncellular Barriers**

Beside the epithelial/endothelial barriers that nanocarriers encounter and need to be crossed, the body is far from being clear of obstacles. The way to, or the residence time at the portal of entry can already be a challenge for the design of a suitable formulation. Ophthalmic drug delivery is a perfect example where drug formulations are physically removed from the site of application if not appropriately enhanced for mucoadhesion. Aside this physical clearance, however, other barriers need to be crossed or circumvented before a NP even comes into touch with a cell layer.

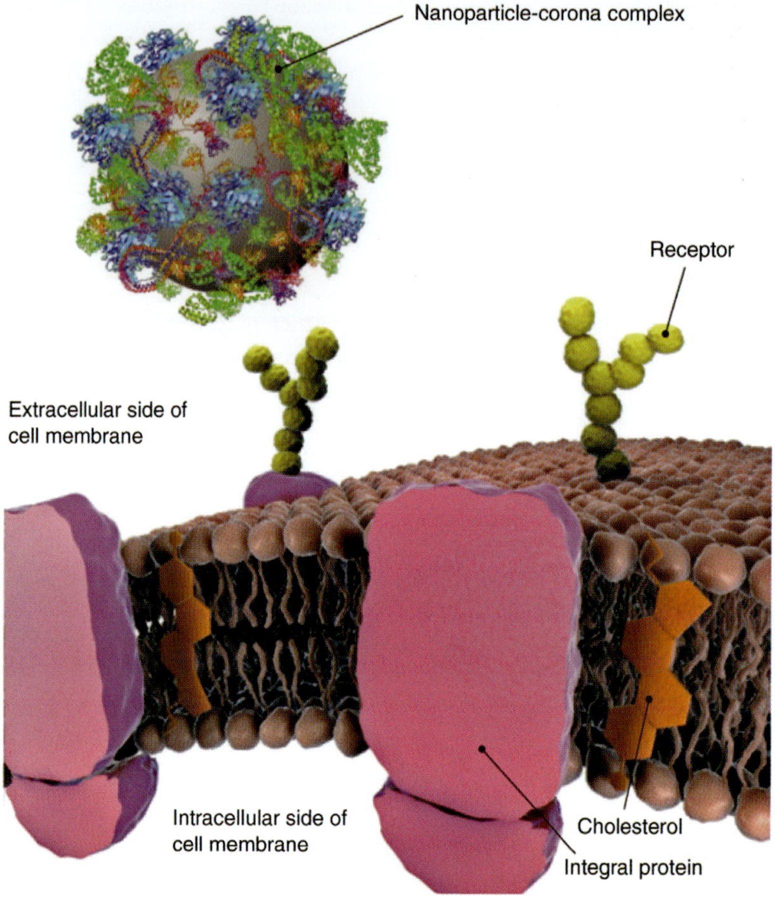

Figure 2.6 It is the NP–corona complex, rather than the bare NP, that interacts with biological machinery, here with a cell membrane receptor. (Reprinted with permission from Ref. [54], © 2012 Elsevier B.V.)

Immunological Barriers: The Nanoparticle Corona

The term "nanoparticle corona" was minted by K. A. Dawson in 2007 for the long-known process of pathogen opsonization that also occurs to NPs in a similar manner after contact with a biological fluid and influences the further fate of the NPs [63] (Figure 2.6). In plasma, as the most prominent extracellular fluid, it could be shown that active targeting ligands, which might be able to direct NPs toward a target *in vitro*, are influenced by the presence of the corona, leading to a different performance *in vivo* due to the masking of the ligands by blood proteins [64]. This adsorption is hindered in the presence of hydrophilic polymers (e.g., PEG) on the NP surface. They are consequently not as fast being recognized by the reticuloendothelial system, therewith remaining in circulation for an exceeded period [65,66]. Another possibility to make favorable use of the corona was nicely shown by Kreuter *et al.*, who found that by functionalizing NPs with polysorbate 80, apolipoprotein E and B enrich in the corona, which again leads to a an increased transport across the blood–brain barrier, possibly by using the transport pathway for lipoproteins [61].

Additionally, the adsorbed proteins can also change NP properties such as aggregation behavior [67], which subsequently alters the biological response. Most researchers are in the meantime aware of this NP corona and therefore test the targeting capabilities of their newly produced NPs under relevant conditions or even try to influence the corona in a beneficial manner [68,69].

The activation of the reticuloendothelial system occurs by opsonization of intruding NPs in the blood stream. Similarly, other portals of entry into the human body that are covered by a biological fluid also possess the ability to cover the surface of NPs with biomolecules. Thus, the modified surface makes the particle accessible to other clearance mechanisms. The corona that forms around NPs after contact with the pulmonary surfactant in the alveolar lining fluid of the deep lung has started to concern researchers, as here not only the solely biochemical composition of the adsorbed unique corona plays a role in the fate of NPs [70], but also the subsequent interaction with the membranous phospholipids [71], altering the interaction of NPs with cells *in vivo* [72]. Also, orally administered NPs will obviously interact with all present substances in the gastrointestinal act, though this complex is not yet elucidated at all.

Mucus and Biofilms

In order to at least remain at the desired site of action, NPs in the upper lung need to cope with the mucus layer that protects the epithelia. Together with entrapped particles, mucus is continuously transported toward the throat by ciliary movement. Mucosa-based entries to the body are the rule rather than the exception and the physical obstacle of mucus therefore needs to be considered in the design of nanopharmaceuticals that are intended to reach the cells underneath unimpaired. Mucus displays a barrier for intruding particles, pathogens, and nanopharmaceuticals, which filters by interaction and size [73]. In order to overcome this barrier, particles must either be very small and not interacting with the mucins or capable of disrupting the tight mucin network for example, by mucolytic activity [74,75]. Similar to mucus, bacterial biofilms exhibit an additional barrier for nanocarriers aiming at the delivery of antibacterial agents [76].

2.2.4 Targeting

Nanopharmaceuticals, different to the free drug, do not have to rely on either passive transport into a cell or across a barrier. Their way through the body can be influenced by a rational particle design, aiming for a targeted delivery to the site of action. There are multiple systems for targeted drug delivery, including biological substances as albumin, phospholipids for liposomes or gelatin, chemical substances as polymers, or solid metal NPs [77]. Nanocarriers can be designed to transport drugs *via* adsorption or attachment on the surface, dissolution within the matrix of the particle, or encapsulation in a polymer lipid [77,78]. In that way, drugs can be transported safely until they reach the area of interest, thereby reducing side effects on healthy tissue [78]. Generally, a distinction between two kinds of targeting is distinguished; active and passive targeting.

2.2.4.1 **Active Targeting**

While using active targeting, several advantages can be capitalized by attaching ligands to the nanocarriers surface by appropriate coupling chemistry. These ligands include small molecules, antibodies, peptides, and aptamers, which bind to specific receptors only [79]. Therefore, only specific cells will be recognized by ligand–receptor interactions. To yield the best outcome, receptors have to be chosen which are expressed mostly on targeted cells, for example, tumor cells, to spare healthy cells. NPs with their carried-on drug will then be internalized by the cell by receptor-mediated endocytosis and stored within endosomes or lysosomes. These endosomes are translocated to distinct organelles where the drug can be released for instance via enzymatic activity or pH. Nevertheless, specific active targeting or induced drug release is currently not used in clinics [80].

2.2.4.2 **Passive Targeting**

Passive targeting does not involve receptor-specific ligands, but takes advantage of the pathophysiological characteristics of diseased cells and tissues, for example, tumor vasculature. Tumor vessels tend to be more unorganized, gap junctions of endothelial cell are enlarged, and therefore the structure is more leaky than in normal vessels, making it easier to penetrate through. This enables the so-called EPR (enhanced permeability and retention) effect, which allows large molecules and particles up to 400 nm to accumulate in the tumor environment [81]. Although passive targeting approaches score in clinical therapy, this concept also has some limitations. First of all, the random approach makes it problematic to control this process precisely. Second, targeting all cells inside a tumor is also difficult, because the drug may not reach each cell. Furthermore, not all tumors are highly vascularized, so the EPR effect cannot be exploited [82].

2.3 Technical Realization of Nanopharmaceuticals

The possibilities of how an advanced nanopharmaceutical can be designed are sheer endless, as almost all technologies can be combined with each other and not all developed carrier systems unambiguously belong to one group only. The following distinction between different nanocarriers must therefore be arbitrary and should not be regarded as complete. An overview is given in Figure 2.7.

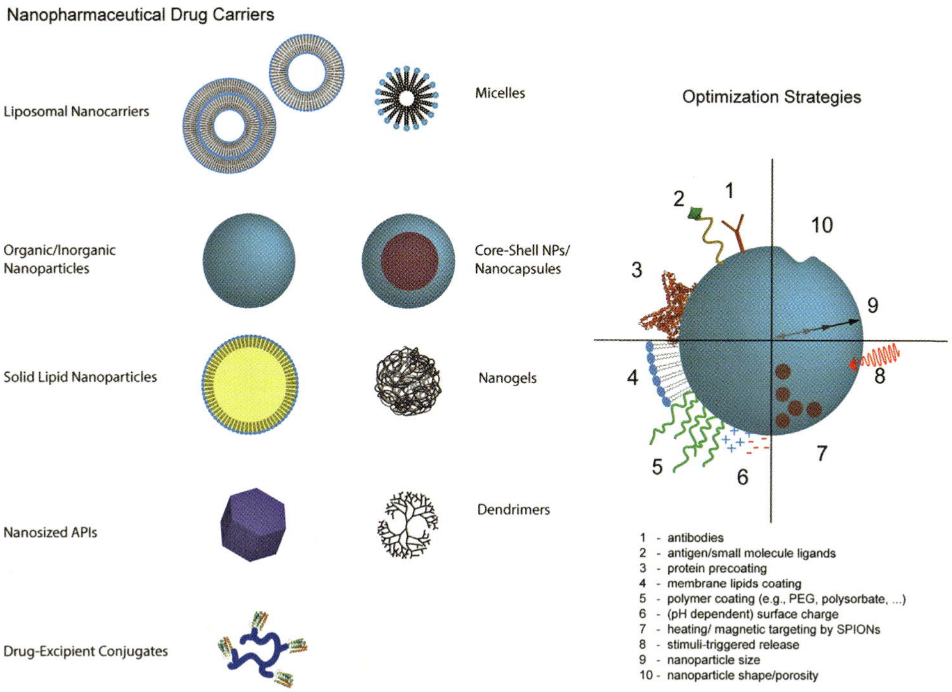

Figure 2.7 Most common nanopharmaceuticals and optional modifications.

2.3.1 Nanosized APIs

The simplest composition of a NP for drug delivery consists to 100% of the API alone and, as a pure drug NP, achieves maximal loading. Such nanocrystals, as they are often referred to, have been originally developed to overcome the poor solubility of an active compound and have proven to be successful. Although Rapamune® hit the market as one of the first nanopharmaceuticals in 1999, it perfectly shows how the classical nano properties, that is, surface/volume ratio can make a pharmaceutical feasible that otherwise would have been not. The road to this formulation started with the practical insoluble molecule and lead over an oral lipid-based solution, which still showed very poor and highly variable bioavailability [83], to the formulation of a tablet that consists of compressed nanocrystals. Some other nanocrystals have followed Rapamune® such as the antiemetic Emend®, the fenofibrate formulations Tricor® and Triglide®, and the progesterone derivative Megace ES®, all of which are produced in a top-down approach by nanomilling of bulk material, the NanoCrystal® technology, except for Triglide® that relies on high pressure homogenization [84]. Bottom-down techniques, that is, crystallization are not yet commonly used for the commercial production of nanocrystals. Nanocrystals surely can be combined with other nanotechnologies, such as surface-coating to improve the delivery or stability of the drug [85].

2.3.2 Organic Nanocarriers

2.3.2.1 Lipid-Based Nanocarriers

Doxil®, or Caelyx® as it is marketed outside the United States, was in 1997 not only the first FDA-approved nanopharmaceutical but has recently become the first, of which a generic form has been approved (Lipodox®) [86]. This formulation of the anthracycline doxorubicin is made up of unilamellar liposomes <100 nm, stabilized with PEG. It not only makes use of the EPR effect to passively target tumors, which is accompanied with a decreased cardiotoxicity and nephrotoxicity in comparison to the free drug, but also hides itself behind a "stealth" effect of PEGylation, marketed as STEALTH® liposomes, to increase residence time [66].

Liposomes consist of phospholipids, that organize themselves to one or more spherical bilayers. Due to the amphiphilic nature, liposomes can entrap both hydrophilic and hydrophobic compounds. Their properties such as permeability, charge, residence time, cell interactions, and so on are dramatically influenced by the deployed lipids and preparation method [87]. While most marketed formulations need to be injected, liposomes have also been successfully used for pulmonary, transdermal, and oral administration [88]. They have been shown to be functionalizable for active targeting, for stimuli-triggered and sustained release, and being able to deliver not only cytotoxic agents but also anti-infectives (e.g., AmBisome®), small molecules as well as macromolecules, and even vaccines [42,89,90]. Their downside, however, is a burst drug release together with low trigger control of drug release, low drug integration efficiency, and poor storage stability.

Beside liposomes, other lipid-based formulations are of interest for drug delivery: solid lipid nanoparticles (SLNs) consist of a surfactant-stabilized lipid core, solid at body temperature, in which the drug is incorporated. Typically, the used lipids are well-known pharmaceutical excipients such as single triglycerides, waxes, long-chain alcohols, or mixtures thereof. As an improved variation of SLNs, nanostructured lipid carriers (NLCs) have been developed from mixtures of lipids that possess different melting points. Advantages of SLNs/NLCs are for example the easy upscaling process, the absence of organic solvents in the production, and biodegradability [91]. Although initially used for transdermal application, SLNs/NLCs are successfully studied as mucus-penetrating vesicles for the delivery to the lungs [92,93] and the gastrointestinal tract [94], but also for permeation across the cornea [95] and the blood–brain barrier [96], suggesting their great potential for future controlled-release formulations of poorly soluble and instable APIs.

2.3.2.2 Polymer-Based Nanocarriers

The first polymeric nanopharmaceutical on the market was the polypeptide mixture Copaxone® (approved 1996 by the FDA). Its formulation, however, possesses no activity or advantages that can be attributed to its size and is therefore not discussed any further [97]. One of the most promising technologies in the pipeline might be ACCURINS® that relies on a stealth effect, targeting ligands, and sustained release from a polymer core [98]. On a lab scale, however, polymeric NPs are explored in innumerable variations and thus for the preparation likewise exist numerous methods, including nanoprecipitation, single/double emulsion solvent evaporation, nanospray drying, and so on [99]. Among others, the most commonly used polymers due to their biocompatibility are PEG, PLGA, PLA/poly-ε-caprolactone (PCL), starch, cellulose, alginate, gelatin, and chitosan [100]. Especially the latter is being explored intensively due to its anti-infective and mucoadhesive properties and its capability to bind DNA/RNA based on its positive charge [101–103]. Polymeric NPs, loaded with either hydrophilic or hydrophobic drugs can be made up of only one polymer or combinations, like oppositely charged polymers which form agglomerates or core-shell particles or layer-by-layer particles where one polymer is coated on top the other (or on an inorganic core) [99]. By using polymers with free reactive groups on the surface, particles can be functionalized with small molecules, drugs, proteins such as antibodies or antigens, the options are endless.

Block copolymers with hydrophilic and hydrophobic features allow the formation of polymeric micelles or polymerosomes. This is implemented for example, in Genexol-PM®, a paclitaxel formulation that avoids the use of cytotoxic Cremophor EL®, by deploying PEG–PLGA for the stabilization of the API within micelles. It has been approved in South Korea for treatment of nonsmall cell lung cancer and was demonstrated to be more effective as Taxol *in vitro* as well as *in vivo* [104].

By grafting polymers to drug molecules, the blood circulation time of drugs can be seriously improved. Conjugation with the water-soluble polymer PEG delays the digestion of especially peptide or protein drugs dramatically and has already resulted in a variety of peptides being marketed in their PEGylated form (e.g., Neulasta® = PEG-filgrastim, Oncaspar® = PEG-asparaginase, and Mircera® = PEG-Epoetin beta).

2.3.2.3 Protein-Based Nanoparticles

In order to reduce toxic effects of surfactants that are used to stabilize hydrophobic drugs, they can also be formulated with proteins. The most well-known one is Abraxane®, which uses the so-called nab® technology (nanoparticle albumin-bound). It is approved for metastatic breast cancer and advanced pancreatic cancer treatment and is furthermore considered for treatment of several other cancer entities including nonsmall cell lung cancer, gastric cancer, or malignant melanoma [105].

2.3.3 Inorganic Nanoparticles

Due to their exceptional properties, superparamagnetic iron oxide nanoparticles (SPIONs) are mainly explored for cancer treatment purposes. SPIONs have been in use as imaging agents for magnet resonance imaging. Moreover, they can be used as drug carriers for magnetic drug targeting (MDT) or they can be heated with an external alternating magnetic field, which is known as the hyperthermia effect. Just last year (2015) the use of superparamagnetic iron oxide particles for thermal ablation of brain tumors was initiated in Germany (NanoTherm®). The aminosilane-coated iron oxide NPs, however, require to be directly injected into the tumor. Used as drug carriers, SPIONs can be functionalized with distinct coatings, including phospholipids, polysaccharides, peptides, proteins, or fatty acids to establish biocompatibility [106,107]. Drugs can be loaded on functionalized SPIONs that can in turn be magnetically guided to the area of interest for example, a tumor [108]. The most feasible tumor models *in vivo* is the VX2 rabbit tumor model, where IA-MDT can be performed accordingly, whereby in a large preclinical animal study the efficiency could be demonstrated impressively [109]. The main advantages of SPIONs over classical cancer therapies would be the minimal intrusiveness and much less side effects, as well as the approachability of concealed tumors. Furthermore, MDT can be translated to a variety of diseases, including arteriosclerosis [110], diabetes [111], or infections [112]. Commercially available SPIONs are used as contrast agents, Lumirem® for lymph node or liver metastases, or Feraheme® and Rienso® for treatment of anemia [113].

NPs made from metals, such as gold, have emerged as promising drug carriers, because they can provide distinct features, such as low toxicity, inertness, simple synthesis, and large surface area. Furthermore, they can very easily be functionalized with surface coatings; thereby drug loading in abundance can be enabled to accumulate drugs for sustained or controlled release [114]. However, various questions about their biodistribution and pharmacokinetics still need to be addressed.

Other inorganic materials that are currently under investigation for nanopharmaceuticals include ceramics, such as alumina or silica, and carbon-based NPs. Beside these pharmaceutical applications, inorganic NPs are already established excipients in cosmetic preparations, such as sunscreen, and in dentistry.

2.4 Safety of Nanopharmaceuticals

While unlocking the full potential of nanotechnology in medicine and healthcare, the highest priority should still lay on safety and toxicity. A responsible development of nanopharmaceuticals should ensure no harm on environment, health, and safety (EHS). Nanosized objects are often man-made, either incidentally or on purpose, but also occur naturally, like in sea spray or volcanic ash. They are not *per se* dangerous and, NPs utilized for drug delivery are mostly less toxic compared to the drug they deliver. Nevertheless, potential risks of nanopharmaceuticals have to be evaluated [115].

Every pharmaceutical product needs a toxicological evaluation and the therapeutic index needs to be set to ensure that the dose used is efficient but not overly toxic. This certainly applies to nanopharmaceuticals to a special degree, as they can have additional effects in comparison to the pure drug. Most toxicological assays used for normal pharmaceuticals, however, are not suitable for nanopharmaceuticals and therefore new methods and assays are required and new regulations need to be set, strongly depending on different types of NPs. Also it must be emphasized, that effects of environmental NPs arise mostly in diseased people, while these are tested solitary in healthy individuals, eventual toxic effects may not become aware for a long time. Due to the specific physicochemical properties of NPs compared to the bulk material their behavior within the body may differ, including blood circulation time, organ or tissue distribution, or transfer of the blood–brain barrier. Basic knowledge on the interaction of NPs on tissue and cellular level need to be further examined as well as pharmacokinetics and distribution studies. By utilizing NPs as drug carriers the toxicity of some drugs can be reduced, the carrier itself needs to be characterized for its own toxicity [116]. Hence, nanotoxicity also depends on the administration route, in which extend organs, tissues, and cell can be reached. For instance, above 100 nm lipid, NPs are well tolerated when applied dermally, this could dramatically change when they are given intravenous. Thus, a better understanding of the interaction of NPs with biological systems will improve nanosafety immensely. A direct collaboration between nanotoxicologist and those designing nanocarriers would be the key to ensure safety of nanopharmaceuticals.

Based on these new needs for the assessment of nanosafety, Keck and Mueller proposed a Nanopharmaceutical Classification System (NCS [117]) to be able to judge the potential risks of novel nanocarriers based on their size (above/below 100 nm) and persistency (biodegradability) of the substance it is made up of, similar to the Biopharmaceutics Classification System. Clearly, their size influences the biological properties of NPs in various ways, which also may affect their safety or potential toxicity [118]. Alternatively, to classify the safety of a given nanomaterials, its intrinsic toxicity can be used as a first parameter, with the second parameter being its solubility/bioresistance (see Figure 2.8). According to those two parameters, any product or material can be classified into class I–IV, allowing to predict whether the nanosize is likely to change the safety/toxicity in comparison to larger particles of the same material or not. For class I materials, additional safety testing could possibly be waived. For class II and III, some additional testing might be advisable, because changes in the safety of the nanomaterial compared to the non-nano material cannot be excluded. For class IV materials, however, the safety of nanoproducts is very likely to be different to the bulk material [119,120].

2.5 Present and Future of Nanopharmacy

Forecasts predict a persistent growth of the global nanopharmaceuticals market and industry with a CAGR (current annual growth rate) of 11% until 2019 mainly

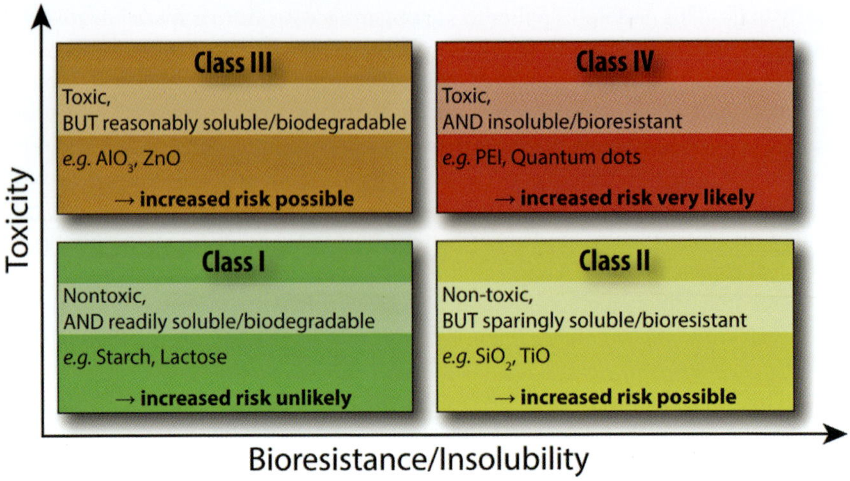

Figure 2.8 Safety classification system for nanoproducts and materials based on their "non-nano" forms. (Adapted from Ref. [120].)

focusing on submarkets of the CNS and cardiovascular treatment. In 2014, nanomedicine used for cancer-treating purposes had the highest amount with a market share of 33%. It will continue growing with 12% CARG until 2019 and 8% from 2019 to 2025, still cardiovascular and CNS will grow fastest until 2025 with a CARG of 11% [121]. Six different therapeutic submarkets can be considered as important within the overall world marked for nanopharmaceuticals:

- Malignant diseases
- Cardiovascular conditions
- Central nervous system (CNS) disorders
- Infectious diseases
- Inflammation
- Other applications of nanotechnology, for example, regenerative medicine

The aim of nanopharmacy is to formulate NPs that can be used in clinics for treatment of these diseases. As personalized medicine is on the cutting-edge, well-defined evaluation pathways for nanomedicine products need to be in clear view of regulatory systems. In nanopharmacy now we can divide two parts, one where nanocarriers are already used in clinics as liposomes or albumin NPs and the other where NPs are in preclinical development phase. To convert these NPs from basic research into pharmaceutical products, a better understanding of the interaction of NPs with biological environs is pivotal. Biodistribution, which is tightly linked to the ability of NPs to cross biological barriers, as well as toxicological aspects to support risk calculation and safety purposes must be evaluated critically. A database of NPs should include physicochemical characterization, for example, shape, size, material, and biological aspects as blood circulation time, immune response, toxicological assays, and so on. One should also take in consideration that the scaling up process might further influence NP properties. The translation from the laboratory to manufacturing process would benefit immensely from such a database.

With a combined liaison of experts from different fields, including science, medicine, pharmacy, material research, physics, engineering, and biotechnology, the translation of NPs from basic research to commercially available product would be boosted extremely. Detailed comprehension of threats and welfares in nanotechnology applications in medicine is crucial for regulators, drug creators, and the patients, who should be the beneficiaries in new drug delivery technologies.

References

1 Weissig, V. and Guzman-Villanueva, D. (2015) Nanopharmaceuticals (part 2): products in the pipeline. *Int. J. Nanomed.*, **10**, 1245–1257.

2 Etheridge, M.L. *et al.* (2013) The big picture on nanomedicine: the state of investigational and approved nanomedicine products. *Nanomedicine*, **9** (1), 1–14.

3 Wong, I.Y., Bhatia, S.N., and Toner, M. (2013) Nanotechnology: emerging tools for biology and medicine. *Genes Dev.*, **27** (22), 2397–2408.

4 Emerich, D.F. and Thanos, C.G. (2006) The pinpoint promise of nanoparticle-based drug delivery and molecular diagnosis. *Biomol. Eng.*, **23** (4), 171–184.

5 European Commission (2011) Commission recommendation of 18 October 2011 on the definition of nanomaterial. *Official J. Eur. Union*, **50**, 38–40.

6 Scientific Committee on Consumer Products (SCCP) (2007) Opinion on Safety of Nanomaterials in Cosmetic Products.

7 ASTM International (2012) Standard Terminology Relating to Nanotechnology.

8 National Institute for Occupational Safety and Health (NIOSH) (2009) Approaches to Safe Nanotechnology: Managing the Health and Safety Concerns Associated with Engineered Nanomaterials, in 2009-125.

9 International Organization for Standardization (ISO) (2015) Nanotechnologies—Vocabulary—Part 2: Nano-objects, in ISO/TS 80004-2:2015.

10 European Science Foundation, Scientific Forward Look on Nanomedicine (2005) in European Science Foundation Policy Briefing.

11 Duncan, R. and Gaspar, R. (2011) Nanomedicine(s) under the microscope. *Mol. Pharm.*, **8** (6), 2101–2141.

12 Sainz, V. *et al.* (2015) Regulatory aspects on nanomedicines. *Biochem. Biophys. Res. Commun.*, **468** (3), 504–510.

13 Merisko-Liversidge, E., Liversidge, G.G., and Cooper, E.R. (2003) Nanosizing: a formulation approach for poorly-water-soluble compounds. *Eur. J. Pharm. Sci.*, **18** (2), 113–120.

14 Bharti, C. *et al.* (2015) Mesoporous silica nanoparticles in target drug delivery system: a review. *Int. J. Pharm. Investig.*, **5** (3), 124–133.

15 Argyo, C. *et al.* (2014) Multifunctional mesoporous silica nanoparticles as a universal platform for drug delivery. *Chem. Mater.*, **26** (1), 435–451.

16 Pelicano, H. *et al.* (2006) Glycolysis inhibition for anticancer treatment. *Oncogene*, **25** (34), 4633–4646.

17 Robitzki, A.A. and Kurz, R. (2010) Biosensing and drug delivery at the microscale: novel devices for controlled and responsive drug delivery. *Handb. Exp. Pharmacol.*, (197), 87–112.

18 Yang, F. *et al.* (2015) Controlled drug release and hydrolysis mechanism of polymer-magnetic nanoparticle composite. *ACS Appl. Mater Interfaces*, **7** (18), 9410–9419.

19 Bandhavkar, S. (2016) Cancer stem cells: a metastasizing menace! *Cancer Med.*, **5** (4), 649–655.

20 Mo, R., Jiang, T., and Gu, Z. (2014) Recent progress in multidrug delivery to cancer cells by liposomes. *Nanomedicine (Lond)*, **9** (8), 1117–1120.

21 Kanamala, M. *et al.* (2016) Mechanisms and biomaterials in pH-responsive tumour targeted drug delivery: a review. *Biomaterials*, **85**, 152–167.

22 Ku, T.H. *et al.* (2011) Controlling and switching the morphology of micellar nanoparticles with enzymes. *J. Am. Chem. Soc.*, **133** (22), 8392–8395.

23 van Rijt, S.H. *et al.* (2015) Protease-mediated release of chemotherapeutics from mesoporous silica nanoparticles to *ex vivo* human and mouse lung tumors. *ACS Nano*, **9** (3), 2377–2389.

24 Xiao, H. *et al.* (2014) Photosensitive Pt(IV)-azide prodrug-loaded nanoparticles exhibit controlled drug release and enhanced efficacy *in vivo*. *J. Control. Release*, **173**, 11–17.

25 Liang, X. *et al.* (2008) Light driven open/close operation of an azobenzene-modified DNA nano-pincette. *Nucleic Acids Symp. Ser. (Oxf.)*, (52), 697–698.

26 Li, W. *et al.* (2015) Remote modulation of neural activities via near-infrared triggered release of biomolecules. *Biomaterials*, **65**, 76–85.

27 Unterweger, H. *et al.* (2015) Hypericin-bearing magnetic iron oxide nanoparticles for selective drug delivery in photodynamic therapy. *Int. J. Nanomedicine*, **10**, 6985–6996.

28 Matanovic, M.R., Kristl, J., and Grabnar, P.A. (2014) Thermoresponsive polymers: insights into decisive hydrogel characteristics, mechanisms of gelation, and promising biomedical applications. *Int. J. Pharm.*, **472** (1–2), 262–275.

29 Collnot, E.M., Ali, H., and Lehr, C.M. (2012) Nano- and microparticulate drug carriers for targeting of the inflamed intestinal mucosa. *J. Control. Release*, **161** (2), 235–246.

30 Schmidt, C. *et al.* (2013) Nano- and microscaled particles for drug targeting to inflamed intestinal mucosa: a first *in vivo* study in human patients. *J. Control. Release*, **165** (2), 139–145.

31 Vong, L.B. *et al.* (2012) An orally administered redox nanoparticle that accumulates in the colonic mucosa and reduces colitis in mice. *Gastroenterology*, **143** (4), 1027–1036. e3.

32 Zhang, X. *et al.* (2014) Biotinylated liposomes as potential carriers for the oral delivery of insulin. *Nanomedicine*, **10** (1), 167–176.

33 Jain, S. *et al.* (2012) Polyelectrolyte stabilized multilayered liposomes for oral delivery of paclitaxel. *Biomaterials*, **33** (28), 6758–6768.

34 Kim, S.K. *et al.* (2006) Oral delivery of chemical conjugates of heparin and deoxycholic acid in aqueous formulation. *Thromb. Res.*, **117** (4), 419–427.

35 Mukhopadhyay, P. *et al.* (2015) pH-sensitive chitosan/alginate core-shell nanoparticles for efficient and safe oral insulin delivery. *Int. J. Biol. Macromol.*, **72**, 640–648.

36 Sarti, F. *et al.* (2011) *In vivo* evidence of oral vaccination with PLGA nanoparticles containing the immunostimulant monophosphoryl lipid A. *Biomaterials*, **32** (16), 4052–4057.

37 Patton, J.S. and Byron, P.R. (2007) Inhaling medicines: delivering drugs to the body through the lungs. *Nat. Rev. Drug Discov.*, **6** (1), 67–74.

38 Patton, J.S. (1996) Mechanisms of macromolecule absorption by the lungs. *Adv. Drug. Deliv. Rev.*, **19** (1), 3–36.

39 de Souza Carvalho, C., Daum, N., and Lehr, C.M. (2014) Carrier interactions with the biological barriers of the lung: advanced *in vitro* models and challenges for pulmonary drug delivery. *Adv. Drug. Deliv. Rev.*, **75**, 129–140.

40 Yang, W., Peters, J.I., and Williams J 3rd, R.O. (2008) Inhaled nanoparticles: a current review. *Int. J. Pharm.*, **356** (1–2), 239–247.

41 Bastacky, J. *et al.* (1995) Alveolar lining layer is thin and continuous: low-temperature scanning electron-microscopy of rat lung. *J. Appl. Physiol.*, **79** (5), 1615–1628.

42 Labouta, H.I. *et al.* (2015) Bacteriomimetic invasin-functionalized

nanocarriers for intracellular delivery. *J. Control. Release*, **220** (Pt A), 414–424.
43 Armstead, A.L. and Li, B. (2011) Nanomedicine as an emerging approach against intracellular pathogens. *Int. J. Nanomedicine*, **6**, 3281–3293.
44 Dube, A. *et al.* (2014) Multimodal nanoparticles that provide immunomodulation and intracellular drug delivery for infectious diseases. *Nanomedicine*, **10** (4), 831–838.
45 Oberdoerster, G., Oberdoerster, E., and Oberdoerster, J. (2005) Nanotoxicology: an emerging discipline evolving from studies of ultrafine particles. *Environ. Health Perspect.*, **113** (7), 823–839.
46 Mahiny, A.J. *et al.* (2015) *In vivo* genome editing using nuclease-encoding mRNA corrects SP-B deficiency. *Nat. Biotechnol.*, **33** (6), 584–586.
47 Hittinger, M. *et al.* (2015) Preclinical safety and efficacy models for pulmonary drug delivery of antimicrobials with focus on *in vitro* models. *Adv. Drug. Deliv. Rev.*, **85**, 44–56.
48 Michaels, A.S., Chandrasekaran, S.K., and Shaw, J.E. (1975) Drug permeation through human skin: theory and *in vitro* experimental measurement. *AIChE J.*, **21** (5), 985–996.
49 Simon, J.A. and Group, E.S. (2006) Estradiol in micellar nanoparticles: the efficacy and safety of a novel transdermal drug-delivery technology in the management of moderate to severe vasomotor symptoms. *Menopause*, **13** (2), 222–231.
50 Uchechi, O., Ogbonna, J.D.N., and Attama, A.A. (2014) Nanoparticles for dermal and transdermal drug delivery, in *Application of Nanotechnology in Drug Delivery* (ed. A.D. Sezer), InTech, Rijeka, Croatia, pp. 193–235.
51 Watkinson, A.C. *et al.* (2013) Nanoparticles do not penetrate human skin: a theoretical perspective. *Pharm. Res.*, **30** (8), 1943–1946.
52 Labouta, H.I. and Schneider, M. (2013) Interaction of inorganic nanoparticles with the skin barrier: current status and critical review. *Nanomedicine*, **9** (1), 39–54.
53 Mathes, C. *et al.* (2016) Nanocarriers for optimizing the balance between interfollicular permeation and follicular uptake of topically applied clobetasol to minimize adverse effects. *J. Control. Release*, **223**, 207–214.
54 Lademann, J. *et al.* (2013) Drug delivery with topically applied nanoparticles: science fiction or reality. *Skin Pharmacol. Physiol.*, **26** (4–6), 227–233.
55 Mittal, A. *et al.* (2015) Inverse micellar sugar glass (IMSG) nanoparticles for transfollicular vaccination. *J. Control. Release*, **206**, 140–152.
56 Braakhuis, H.M. *et al.* (2015) Progress and future of *in vitro* models to study translocation of nanoparticles. *Arch. Toxicol.*, **89** (9), 1469–1495.
57 Chen, Y. and Liu, L. (2012) Modern methods for delivery of drugs across the blood-brain barrier. *Adv. Drug. Deliv. Rev.*, **64** (7), 640–665.
58 Voigt, N. *et al.* (2014) Surfactants, not size or zeta-potential influence blood-brain barrier passage of polymeric nanoparticles. *Eur. J. Pharm. Biopharm.*, **87** (1), 19–29.
59 Jo, D.H. *et al.* (2015) Size, surface charge, and shape determine therapeutic effects of nanoparticles on brain and retinal diseases. *Nanomedicine*, **11** (7), 1603–1611.
60 Alyautdin, R. *et al.* (2014) Nanoscale drug delivery systems and the blood-brain barrier. *Int. J. Nanomedicine*, **9**, 795–811.
61 Kreuter, J. *et al.* (2002) Apolipoprotein-mediated transport of nanoparticle-bound drugs across the blood-brain barrier. *J. Drug Target.*, **10** (4), 317–325.
62 Aryal, M. *et al.* (2015) Multiple sessions of liposomal doxorubicin delivery via focused ultrasound mediated blood-brain barrier disruption: a safety study. *J. Control. Release*, **204**, 60–69.
63 Cedervall, T. *et al.* (2007) Understanding the nanoparticle-protein corona using methods to quantify exchange rates and affinities of proteins for nanoparticles. *Proc. Natl. Acad. Sci. USA*, **104** (7), 2050–2055.
64 Salvati, A. *et al.* (2013) Transferrin-functionalized nanoparticles lose their targeting capabilities when a biomolecule corona adsorbs on the surface. *Nat. Nanotechnol.*, **8** (2), 137–143.

65 Gref, R. *et al.* (2000) 'Stealth' corona-core nanoparticles surface modified by polyethylene glycol (PEG): influences of the corona (PEG chain length and surface density) and of the core composition on phagocytic uptake and plasma protein adsorption. *Colloids Surf. B*, **18** (3–4), 301–313.

66 Lasic, D.D. and Needham, D. (1995) The "Stealth" liposome: a prototypical biomaterial. *Chem. Rev.*, **95** (8), 2601–2628.

67 Moerz, S.T. *et al.* (2015) Formation mechanism for stable hybrid clusters of proteins and nanoparticles. *ACS Nano*, **9** (7), 6696–6705.

68 Ritz, S. *et al.* (2015) Protein corona of nanoparticles: distinct proteins regulate the cellular uptake. *Biomacromolecules*, **16** (4), 1311–1321.

69 Polyak, B. and Cordovez, B. (2016) How can we predict behavior of nanoparticles *in vivo*? *Nanomedicine (Lond)*, **11** (3), 189–192.

70 Ruge, C.A. *et al.* (2012) The interplay of lung surfactant proteins and lipids assimilates the macrophage clearance of nanoparticles. *PLoS One*, **7** (7), e40775.

71 Raesch, S.S. *et al.* (2015) Proteomic and lipidomic analysis of nanoparticle corona upon contact with lung surfactant reveals differences in protein, but not lipid composition. *ACS Nano*, **9** (12), 11872–11885.

72 Schleh, C., Kreyling, W.G., and Lehr, C.M. (2013) Pulmonary surfactant is indispensable in order to simulate the *in vivo* situation. *Part. Fibre Toxicol.*, **10** (1), 6.

73 Kirch, J. *et al.* (2012) Optical tweezers reveal relationship between microstructure and nanoparticle penetration of pulmonary mucus. *Proc. Natl. Acad. Sci. USA*, **109** (45), 18355–18360.

74 Ensign, L.M., Cone, R., and Hanes, J. (2012) Oral drug delivery with polymeric nanoparticles: the gastrointestinal mucus barriers. *Adv. Drug Deliv. Rev.*, **64** (6), 557–570.

75 Dunnhaupt, S. *et al.* (2015) Nano-carrier systems: strategies to overcome the mucus gel barrier. *Eur. J. Pharm. Biopharm.*, **96**, 447–453.

76 Peulen, T.O. and Wilkinson, K.J. (2011) Diffusion of nanoparticles in a biofilm. *Environ. Sci. Technol.*, **45** (8), 3367–3373.

77 Natarajan, J.V. *et al.* (2014) Sustained-release from nanocarriers: a review. *J. Control. Release*, **193**, 122–138.

78 Mudshinge, S.R. *et al.* (2011) Nanoparticles: emerging carriers for drug delivery. *Saudi Pharm. J.*, **19** (3), 129–141.

79 Silva, A.C. *et al.* (2015) Delivery systems for biopharmaceuticals. Part I: nanoparticles and microparticles. *Curr. Pharm. Biotechnol.*, **16** (11), 940–954.

80 Bae, Y.H. and Park, K. (2011) Targeted drug delivery to tumors: myths, reality and possibility. *J. Control. Release*, **153** (3), 198–205.

81 Cerqueira, B.B. *et al.* (2015) Nanoparticle therapeutics: technologies and methods for overcoming cancer. *Eur. J. Pharm. Biopharm.*, **97** (Pt A), 140–151.

82 Jain, R.K. (1994) Barriers to drug delivery in solid tumors. *Sci. Am.*, **271** (1), 58–65.

83 Zimmerman, J.J. *et al.* (1999) The effect of a high-fat meal on the oral bioavailability of the immunosuppressant sirolimus (rapamycin). *J. Clin. Pharmacol.*, **39** (11), 1155–1161.

84 Müller, R. and Junghanns, J.U. (2008) Nanocrystal technology, drug delivery and clinical applications. *Int. J. Nanomed.*, **3** (3), 295–309.

85 Lu, Y., Li, Y., and Wu, W. (2016) Injected nanocrystals for targeted drug delivery. *Acta Pharm. Sin. B*, **6** (2), 106–113.

86 Barenholz, Y. (2012) Doxil® – the first FDA-approved nano-drug: lessons learned. *J. Control. Release*, **160** (2), 117–134.

87 Soema, P.C. *et al.* (2015) Predicting the influence of liposomal lipid composition on liposome size, zeta potential and liposome-induced dendritic cell maturation using a design of experiments approach. *Eur. J. Pharm. Biopharm.*, **94**, 427–435.

88 Pattni, B.S., Chupin, V.V., and Torchilin, V.P. (2015) New developments in liposomal drug delivery. *Chem. Rev*, **115** (19), 10938–10966.

89 Gordon, S. *et al.* (2012) Chitosan hydrogels containing liposomes and

cubosomes as particulate sustained release vaccine delivery systems. *J. Liposome Res.*, **22** (3), 193–204.

90 Schwendener, R.A. (2014) Liposomes as vaccine delivery systems: a review of the recent advances. *Ther. Adv. Vaccines*, **2** (6), 159–182.

91 Müller, R.H. *et al.* (2016) Nanostructured lipid carriers (NLC): the second generation of solid lipid nanoparticles. *Adv. Pharm. Bull.* **5** (3), 161–185.

92 Nafee, N. *et al.* (2014) Antibiotic-free nanotherapeutics: ultra-small, mucus-penetrating solid lipid nanoparticles enhance the pulmonary delivery and anti-virulence efficacy of novel quorum sensing inhibitors. *J. Control. Release*, **192**, 131–140.

93 Weber, S., Zimmer, A., and Pardeike, J. (2014) Solid lipid nanoparticles (SLN) and nanostructured lipid carriers (NLC) for pulmonary application: a review of the state of the art. *Eur. J. Pharm. Biopharm.*, **86** (1), 7–22.

94 Yuan, H. *et al.* (2013) Improved transport and absorption through gastrointestinal tract by PEGylated solid lipid nanoparticles. *Mol. Pharm.*, **10** (5), 1865–1873.

95 Hao, J. *et al.* (2014) Fabrication of a composite system combining solid lipid nanoparticles and thermosensitive hydrogel for challenging ophthalmic drug delivery. *Colloids Surf. B Biointerfaces*, **114**, 111–120.

96 Gastaldi, L. *et al.* (2014) Solid lipid nanoparticles as vehicles of drugs to the brain: current state of the art. *Eur. J. Pharm. Biopharm.*, **87** (3), 433–444.

97 Schrempf, W. and Ziemssen, T. (2007) Glatiramer acetate: mechanisms of action in multiple sclerosis. *Autoimmun. Rev.*, **6** (7), 469–475.

98 Ashton, S. *et al.* (2016) Aurora kinase inhibitor nanoparticles target tumors with favorable therapeutic index *in vivo*. *Sci. Transl. Med.*, **8** (325), 325ra17.

99 Rao, J.P. and Geckeler, K.E. (2011) Polymer nanoparticles: preparation techniques and size-control parameters. *Prog. Polym. Sci.*, **36** (7), 887–913.

100 Kamaly, N. *et al.* (2012) Targeted polymeric therapeutic nanoparticles: design, development and clinical translation. *Chem. Soc. Rev.*, **41** (7), 2971–3010.

101 Qi, L. *et al.* (2004) Preparation and antibacterial activity of chitosan nanoparticles. *Carbohydr. Res.*, **339** (16), 2693–2700.

102 Pan, Y. *et al.* (2002) Bioadhesive polysaccharide in protein delivery system: chitosan nanoparticles improve the intestinal absorption of insulin *in vivo*. *Int. J. Pharm.*, **249** (1–2), 139–147.

103 Nafee, N. *et al.* (2007) Chitosan-coated PLGA nanoparticles for DNA/RNA delivery: effect of the formulation parameters on complexation and transfection of antisense oligonucleotides. *Nanomedicine*, **3** (3), 173–183.

104 Ahn, H.K. *et al.* (2014) A phase II trial of Cremorphor EL-free paclitaxel (Genexol-PM) and gemcitabine in patients with advanced non-small cell lung cancer. *Cancer Chemother. Pharmacol.*, **74** (2), 277–282.

105 Kundranda, M.N. and Niu, J. (2015) Albumin-bound paclitaxel in solid tumors: clinical development and future directions. *Drug Des. Devel. Ther.*, **9**, 3767–3777.

106 Zaloga, J. *et al.* (2016) Pharmaceutical formulation of HSA hybrid coated iron oxide nanoparticles for magnetic drug targeting. *Eur. J. Pharm. Biopharm.*

107 Zaloga, J. *et al.* (2014) Development of a lauric acid/albumin hybrid iron oxide nanoparticle system with improved biocompatibility. *Int. J. Nanomedicine*, **9**, 4847–4866.

108 Lyer, S. *et al.* (2010) Visualisation of tumour regression after local chemotherapy with magnetic nanoparticles – a pilot study. *Anticancer Res.*, **30** (5), 1553–1557.

109 Tietze, R. *et al.* (2013) Efficient drug-delivery using magnetic nanoparticles: biodistribution and therapeutic effects in tumour bearing rabbits. *Nanomedicine*, **9** (7), 961–971.

110 Cicha, I. (2015) Thrombosis: novel nanomedical concepts of diagnosis and treatment. *World J. Cardiol.*, **7** (8), 434–441.

111 Wang, P. *et al.* (2014) GLP-1R-targeting magnetic nanoparticles for pancreatic islet imaging. *Diabetes*, **63** (5), 1465–1474.
112 Pera, N.P. *et al.* (2010) Detection of pathogenic *Streptococcus suis* bacteria using magnetic glycoparticles. *Org. Biomol. Chem.*, **8** (10), 2425–2429.
113 Schutz, C.A. *et al.* (2013) Therapeutic nanoparticles in clinics and under clinical evaluation. *Nanomedicine (Lond)*, **8** (3), 449–467.
114 Zhang, X. (2015) Gold nanoparticles: recent advances in the biomedical applications. *Cell Biochem. Biophys*, **72** (3), 771–775.
115 Wagner, S. *et al.* (2014) Spot the difference: engineered and natural nanoparticles in the environment – release, behavior, and fate. *Angew. Chem., Int. Ed.*, **53** (46), 12398–12419.
116 Shvedova, A., Pietroiusti, A., and Kagan, V. (2016) Nanotoxicology ten years later: lights and shadows. *Toxicol. Appl. Pharmacol.*, **299**, 1–2.
117 Keck, C.M. and Mueller, R.H. (2013) Nanotoxicological classification system (NCS) – a guide for the risk-benefit assessment of nanoparticulate drug delivery systems. *Eur. J. Pharm. Biopharm.*, **84** (3), 445–448.
118 Hillaireau, H. and Couvreur, P. (2009) Nanocarriers' entry into the cell: relevance to drug delivery. *Cell. Mol. Life Sci.*, **66** (17), 2873–2896.
119 Lehr, C.-M. and Groß, H. (2014) Wirksamere und sichere medikamente mit hilfe der nanotechnologie. *Nanotechnologie Aktuell*, **7**, 112–116.
120 Barthold, S. *et al.* (2015) Overview of inhaled nanopharmaceuticals, in *ISAM Textbook of Aerosol Medicine* (eds B. Rothen-Rutishauser and R. Dhand), International Society for Aerosols in Medicine, pp. 330–351.
121 Visiongain (2015) Nanopharmaceutical Industry and Market: Companies, Products, R&D and Revenue Forecasts 2015–2025. Pharma report 131.

3
The Emergence of Nanopharmacy: From Biology to Nanotechnology and Drug Molecules to Nanodrugs

Marilena Hadjidemetriou, Zahraa Al-Ahmady, Mariarosa Mazza, and Kostas Kostarelos

Nanomedicine Lab, Faculty of Medical and Human Sciences, University of Manchester, AV Hill Building, Manchester M13 9PT, United Kingdom.

3.1
Introduction

Nanopharmaceuticals consist of a pharmaceutically active molecule or substance ("pharmacon") adsorbed onto, conjugated to, or encapsulated within a nanoscale-based material, the size of which falls into a size range similar to intra- and extracellular biological structures [1]. The principal goal of *nanopharmacy* is to create novel agents with improved therapeutic efficacy utilizing nanoscience. This can be achieved either by using novel therapeutic molecules (small molecules, proteins, peptides, nucleic acids) or by reformulating existing ones (i.e., poorly soluble drugs and antibodies) [2,3]. In most cases, the broader aim is to increase the bioavailable drug concentration at the desired (e.g., target) site, while simultaneously minimizing toxic responses by reducing off-target effects [4,5]. Nanopharmaceuticals have been developed to address conditions for which traditional pharmaceutical treatments are ineffective (e.g., antibacterial resistance), diseases for which therapies are available but should be more adjusted to the patient's needs (cardiovascular diseases, cancer) and diseases for which therapeutic interventions are not available (e.g., stroke and Alzheimer's disease) [6].

Nanoparticles are of immense scientific interest because their properties differ from the bulk material or the isolated atoms and molecules used to fabricate or assemble them. For example, gold nanoparticles have different optical properties from atomic gold, as they are highly efficient in absorbing and scattering light. Gold nanoparticle size also commonly influences the light-induced collective oscillation of electrons on the metal surface, a phenomenon known as surface plasmon resonance. With increased gold nanoparticle size, the surface plasmon resonance wavelength shifts to longer wavelengths. This unique property is only one example that has been exploited in cancer research for the development of multiple imaging, diagnostic, and therapeutic purposes [7]. Nanopharmacy

Pharmaceutical Nanotechnology: Innovation and Production, First Edition. Edited by Jean Cornier, Arno Kwade, Andrew Owen, and Marcel Van de Voorde.

requires the interdisciplinary contribution from fields ranging from chemical sciences to biology and from physics to pharmacology. This is not entirely unexpected, since different and new scientific disciplines evolve constantly. Gene therapy is another example of a research field waiting to mature into a clinical discipline, where various disciplines need to converge toward the achievement of the same goal: effective delivery of biologically active nucleic acid sequences for the genetic treatment or alleviation of various pathological conditions.

The design of delivery systems is largely dependent on a variety of factors that are intricately related to each specific therapeutic or diagnostic application. The ability to fine-tune the pharmacological properties (biodistribution, tissue uptake, and pharmacokinetics) of biologically active molecules through their reformulation using nanomaterials is considered of utmost importance. There are various technologies and approaches that allow such fine-tuning and optimization. First, the route of administration affects nanoparticle biodistribution and provides an initial level of targeting. Second, surface functionalization of nanoparticles with specific moieties modifies their pharmacokinetic profile (e.g., PEGylation). Tissue uptake and cellular internalization of nanoparticles can also be controlled by decorating the outer surface of nanoparticles with targeting moieties. This can take place through molecular surface modifications, either in the form of chemically conjugated targeting ligands or proteins adsorbed from the local environment, that have the ability to dramatically alter the nature of the cellular interactions. Lastly, the engineering of nanoparticles designed to release their payload in response to various stimuli, can also provide an alternative method to target specific tissues [3,8]. The potential of nanopharmacy is challenged though from the high expectations linked to new discoveries, rapid nanotechnology advancements, and the need for short-term deliverables. Sensationalism is also another challenge. Components represented as *"nano"* commonly attain either the connotation of a "wonder" technology, full of promises of revolutionizing therapy, or in direct contrast, as an unparalleled threat to safety. Both connotations have very little basis in scientific reality, and do not take into consideration that some of the most stringent requirements for therapeutic efficacy and safety already govern the approval of new nanopharmaceuticals in a process that can lasts for decades. The clinical translation of multicomponent, sophisticated nanodrugs with chemical and biological functionalizations, such as targeting moieties, remains challenging and requires the use of already existing safety, efficacy, and quality assessments tools as well as the development of new testing strategies [6].

In short, nanopharmacy is an emergent, multidisciplinary field with great potential and expectations, however, will require time and persistent investment in order to allow maturation into clinical reality. A plethora of studies at the preclinical and clinical levels are currently carried out for new nanopharmaceuticals, some of which may have different and intriguing mode of action due to complex mechanisms involving the interplay among mechanical, chemical, pharmacological, and immunological components. This chapter aims to offer an overview of how nanotechnology advances can impact the design and development of novel pharmacological agents and contribute to the emerging field of nanopharmacy.

3.2 First Generation of Nanopharmaceuticals: From Drug Molecules to Nanodrugs

Early efforts in *nanopharmacy* were focused on improving the properties of already existing therapeutic agents, aiming to improve their pharmacokinetics, reduce the adverse effects arising from them, and specifically target them at the site of action. A multitude of materials has been investigated as drug delivery systems, including biological substances, such as proteins and phospholipids, as well as chemical substances, such as polymers, metals, carbon, and silica [9]. This section, based on the example of two clinically used anticancer agents, doxorubicin and paclitaxel, will highlight the major advantages associated with the formulation of therapeutic agents into nanoparticle-based moieties.

Nanoscale delivery systems have been explored for a diverse range of applications, with oncology being the most notable beneficiary to date. One of the major challenges to the treatment of solid tumors is the accumulation of the drug at the target tissue, while avoiding healthy tissue damage. The encapsulation of chemotherapeutic agents inside nanocarriers has been an established strategy to reduce the drug-associated toxicity to normal tissues and to simultaneously increase their accumulation into highly vascularized solid tumors [10,11]. Nanocarriers selectively accumulate into the tumor tissue as a result of the pathophysiological characteristics of the tumor, namely, leaky vasculature and poor lymphatic drainage. This phenomenon is known as enhanced permeability and retention (EPR) effect (Figure 3.1a) [12,13]. Key to the passive accumulation of nanocarriers at the tumor site is their long blood circulation time. Nanoparticles are recognized as foreign bodies and are opsonized by the cells of the reticuloendothelial system (mononuclear phagocyte system, MPS), and thus the availability of the drug at the required site is diminished [14,15]. A major breakthrough was the surface coating of nanoparticles with the hydrophilic polymer polyethylene glycol (PEG), which imparts steric stabilization and reduces the interaction of NPs with serum proteins, resulting in a substantial increase in the circulation time [16,17]. Because of the ability of these nanocarriers to avoid uptake by the MPS cells, they were termed "stealth" drug delivery systems.

Among the nanosized drug delivery systems, liposomes were the first and the most extensively used nanopharmaceuticals for cancer therapy [18]. Liposomes can be described as "spherical phospholipid vesicles consisting of one or more concentric lipid bilayers enclosing an aqueous core" [19]. Their ability to encapsulate hydrophilic molecules in their aqueous inner space [20] as well as hydrophobic molecules in their phospholipid bilayer membranes [21], makes them very attractive as drug delivery systems. They are now considered to be the most clinically established nanotechnology platform, with more than

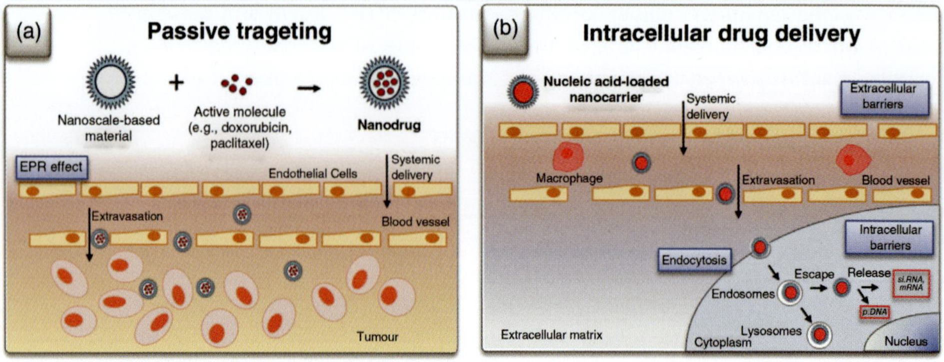

Figure 3.1 From drug molecules to nanodrugs. (a) Passive targeting of nanodrugs-EPR effect. Nanocarriers selectively accumulate into the tumor tissue as a result of the pathophysiological characteristics of the tumor, namely, leaky vasculature and poor lymphatic drainage, phenomenon known as enhanced permeability and retention effect (EPR). (b) Intracellular targeting. After intravenous injection, the vector: nucleic acid complex is distributed to organs via blood circulation and simultaneously undergoes elimination. In addition, cells of the reticuloendothelial system attempt to degrade and eliminate the vector, which is recognized as foreign. After extravasation, the vector is transported across the interstitial space to the target cells, where it has to cross the cell membrane barrier, translocate into the cytoplasm, and release its cargo to its intracellular therapeutic site. To exert its action, DNA has ultimately to reach the nucleus of the target cell, while the action of RNA molecules occurs in the cytoplasm.

12 liposome-based drugs approved for clinical use and many more in various stages of clinical trials [1,18]. Their success can be attributed to their ability to extensively accumulate into regions of enhanced vascular permeability and for their ability to reduce the side effects of encapsulated drugs [22]. The significant reduction in the cardiotoxicity of the anticancer agent doxorubicin (anthracycline antibiotic) after its encapsulation in PEGylated liposomes led to the development of the first nanodrug, Doxil®, approved by the FDA in 1995 for the treatment of AIDS-related Kaposi's sarcoma [23]. PEGylated liposomal doxorubicin shows superiority to free doxorubicin clinical performance owing to (a) prolonged circulation time due to the surface functionalization of liposomes with PEG, (b) stable retention of the drug inside the liposomes while in circulation, (c) increased tumor accumulation attributed to the EPR effect, and (d) decreased cardiac toxicity [23,24].

In addition to the adverse effects, the use of conventional drugs is often hindered by their insolubility in aqueous solutions [25]. The conversion of poor water-soluble drugs into nanodrugs, by their conjugation with macromolecular polymers or proteins, has been a successful strategy to avoid the use of organic solvent-based formulations, often associated with serious and dose-limiting toxicities. An example of a highly hydrophobic drug, successfully formulated into nanoscale delivery systems, is the anticancer agent paclitaxel. Abraxane®, albumin-based, 130-nm-sized nanoparticles conjugated with paclitaxel was licensed in 2005 for the treatment of metastatic breast cancer and in 2012 as a first-line treatment for advanced nonsmall-cell lung cancer. Albumin-based nanoparticles, similarly to other nanocarriers, passively accumulate at the side of solid tumors, via the EPR effect. In addition, dissociation of albumin nanoparticles into individual drug-bound albumin molecules has been found to facilitate specific albumin-receptor-mediated uptake by the endothelial cell walls of tumor microvessels that further increases the intratumor concentration of paclitaxel [26–28]. Another nanosystem developed for the delivery of paclitaxel is Opaxio®, approved in 2012 for the treatment of glioblastoma. Opaxio®, consists of paclitaxel covalently linked to solid polymer-based nanoparticles, composed of poly(L-glutamic acid). When bound to the polymer, then paclitaxel is inactive, thus, preventing paclitaxel-associated toxicity to healthy tissues. The success of this formulation is based on the enzymatic hydrolysis of the polymer after the accumulation of the nanoparticles inside the solid tumor, which results in the release of active paclitaxel from the polymeric backbone [29,30].

In addition to albumin- and polymer-based solid nanoparticles, micelles provide an alternative for parenteral administration of poorly water-soluble drugs. Micelles are self-assembled spherical nanoparticles with a hydrophobic core and a hydrophilic shell, made of amphiphilic copolymers [31]. An example of micellar formulation product available in the market is Genexol-PM, approved in South Korea for breast cancer and small-cell lung cancer. Genexol-PM consists of 20–50 nm micelles formed by the self-assembly of polyethylene glycol and polylactide polymers, the core of which contains paclitaxel. The co-polymer increases the water solubility of paclitaxel and allows delivery of higher doses than those achievable with paclitaxel alone [32].

In brief, the conversion of therapeutic molecules into nanodrugs requires a comprehensive understanding of both, the nanomaterial design and disease pathophysiology. Nanosized delivery systems offer the opportunity to reformulate conventional active molecules in order to improve their bioavailability, efficacy, and toxicity profile.

3.2.1 Making New Therapies Happen: The Example of Nucleic Acid Therapeutics

Besides improving the efficacy of already established therapeutic molecules, nanotechnology has enabled the development of new therapies. The example of gene therapy is a great case to illustrate the pivotal role of nanotechnology for the clinical translation of novel therapeutic strategies. Gene therapy can be described as the exogenous introduction of nucleic acids (DNA or RNA) into specific host cells, to intentionally modulate gene expression in order to treat or prevent pathological conditions. The treatment of inherited monogenic diseases caused by a single-gene defect by the introduction of a functional copy of the gene represents the prototype of gene therapy and has been referred to as "gene replacement." Other gene manipulation strategies are now at the preclinical stage of investigation, including gene knockdown by RNA interference (RNAi), gene addition, and gene editing with enormous therapeutic potential [33]. From the drug delivery point of view, nucleic acids have unfavorable physicochemical characteristics as therapeutic agents and the use of a delivery vector is a necessity for their clinical application [34].

One of the main challenges for the systemic delivery of nucleic acids is their short half-life due to the degradation by serum nucleases. In addition, the high molecular weight and negative charge of unmodified nucleic acids hamper their cellular uptake. The administration of nucleic acids requires the development of safe and efficient delivery vectors with the ability to target nucleic acids to the region of interest provide protection from nuclease degradation, shield recognition by the immune system, and limit excretion through the kidneys. The two main approaches for nucleic acid therapy are based on viral and nonviral delivery vectors, with ~70% of gene therapy clinical trials carried out so far using modified viruses, such as retroviruses, lentiviruses, adenoviruses, and adeno-associated viruses [35,36].

The ability of viruses to insert their genetic information into mammalian host cells has been successfully utilized for gene delivery. Viral nanoparticles used in gene therapy are engineered from viruses by replacing most of their pathogenic genes with a therapeutic gene cassette, while retaining their infectious nature [37]. The world's first gene therapeutics, Gendicine and Oncorine (adenoviral-vector based), were approved in China, for the treatment of neck and head cancer, in 2003 and 2006, respectively. In 2012, the European Medicines Agency recommended for the first time a gene therapy product, Glybera (adeno-associated viral vector based), for the treatment of lipoprotein lipase deficiency. Although, viral vectors have substantially advanced nucleic acid delivery, several limitations are associated their use, including their immunogenicity, mutagenesis after random integration into the host genome, limited nucleic acid capacity, and difficulty of vector production. Synthetic nonviral vector systems have the potential to address many of these limitations, particularly with respect to safety. Size-independent delivery of nucleic acids, simpler quality control, and ease of preparation are some of the advantages that nonviral vectors can offer. However, only few nonviral vectors have progressed into clinical trials, and none of these vectors has been approved by regulatory authorities. This is mainly due to the compromised therapeutic efficiency of nonviral vectors compared to viral vectors [35].

Liposomes were the first nonviral gene delivery systems to reach clinical trials. It was first described, in 1980, that liposomes could entrap and deliver DNA to monkey kidney cells [38]. Few years later, Felgner *et al.* demonstrated that synthetic cationic liposomes could complex DNA and facilitate efficient transfection of various mammalian cell lines [39]. Since then, the development of nonviral vectors is rapidly expanding, with a broad spectrum of nanoconstructs being under preclinical investigation, including polymeric nanoparticles, carbon-based materials [40], and peptides [41]. Among the various synthetic vectors, cationic lipids and polymers are the most studied nonviral delivery vesicles so far with few being currently under clinical investigation [42]. Liposomes, formed from the cationic lipid DOTAP and cholesterol, have been well characterized as gene delivery systems and have progressed in clinical trials. For example, DOTAP–cholesterol complexed with a plasmid encoding a tumor suppressor protein, FUS1, is currently in phase II for the treatment of nonsmall-cell lung cancer [43]. Polyethylenimine (PEI) is among the most studied polymeric materials for gene delivery. PEI–DNA complexes are currently in stages I and II of clinical trials for local gene therapy of ovarian, pancreatic, and bladder cancers [42,44,45]. To improve its stability and biocompatibility, PEI has been also modified with other polymers. A PEG–PEI–cholesterol lipopolymer, complexed with plasmid DNA encoding the human gene for interleukin 12 (IL-12), is currently under clinical investigation for ovarian and colorectal cancer treatment [46,47].

Despite the significant efforts, nonviral gene therapy is still clinically challenging and requires a better understanding of the fate of nanodrugs after administration. The barriers for effective delivery of nucleic acids by synthetic vectors depend on the target organ and on the route of administration. In general, local administration has fewer barriers compared with systemic delivery. After intravenous injection, the vector–nucleic acid complex is distributed to organs via blood circulation and simultaneously undergoes elimination. In addition, cells of the reticuloendothelial system attempt to degrade and eliminate the vector, which is recognized as foreign. After extravasation, the vector is transported across the interstitial space to the target cells, where it has to cross the cell membrane barrier, translocate into the cytoplasm, and release its cargo to its intracellular therapeutic site. To exert its action, DNA has ultimately to reach the nucleus of the target cell, while the action of RNA molecules occurs in the cytoplasm (Figure 3.1b) [34].

The need to develop vectors for nucleic acid-based therapeutics initiated the idea of organelle-specific drug delivery, as an attractive strategy to increase the therapeutic index of a drug. Intracellular targeting has been recently attempted for other novel therapeutic molecules, including the delivery of proapoptotic compounds to mitochondria, and the delivery of enzymes to defective lysosomes [48–50]. Although in its infancy stages, the intracellular spatial control of drug-containing nanoparticles is expected to sharply increase the therapeutic efficacy of nanodrugs and thus allow their clinical application.

3.2.1.1 Making Nanodrugs Smarter: Multifunctional Nanodrugs

The first generation of nanodrugs described earlier was mainly designed to overcome a single challenge, for example, increase drug stability, prolong plasma circulation half-life, or the need to passively target specific organs taken the advantage of the accompanied pathological changes [1]. Advances in the development of pharmaceutical nanotechnology has led to possibility of engineering multifunctional nanodrugs that can perform more than one task (concurrently or sequentially) [51,52] to efficiently deliver their payload (single or multiple) [53,54] to the target site. For the purpose of this chapter, multifunctional nanodrugs have been classified into three main categories: targeted, responsive, and diagnostic/theranostic nanodrugs.

Targeted Nanodrugs

Actively targeted nanodrugs represent the first group of multifunctional nanodrugs and can be accomplished by the attachment of targeting ligands on their outer surface, such as monoclonal antibodies, antibody fragments, peptides, and aptamers. It has been well established that the best way to prevent shielding of the targeting ligand by the polymeric coating layer (e.g., PEG) is to chemically attach the targeting moiety to the distal end of the polymer chain that is coating these nanodrugs (Figure 3.2a) [55]. An example of such actively targeted nanodrug is PEGylated doxorubicin-loaded liposomes that have human epidermal receptor 2 (HER2) monoclonal antibody attached to their surface [56]. These liposomes were successfully used to target HER2-overexpressing tumor cells in mice [56] and are currently under phase I/II clinical testing for HER2-positive breast cancer patient [57,58].

It is important to clarify that active targeting of long circulating nanodrugs is not necessarily independent from passive targeting and in most of the cases

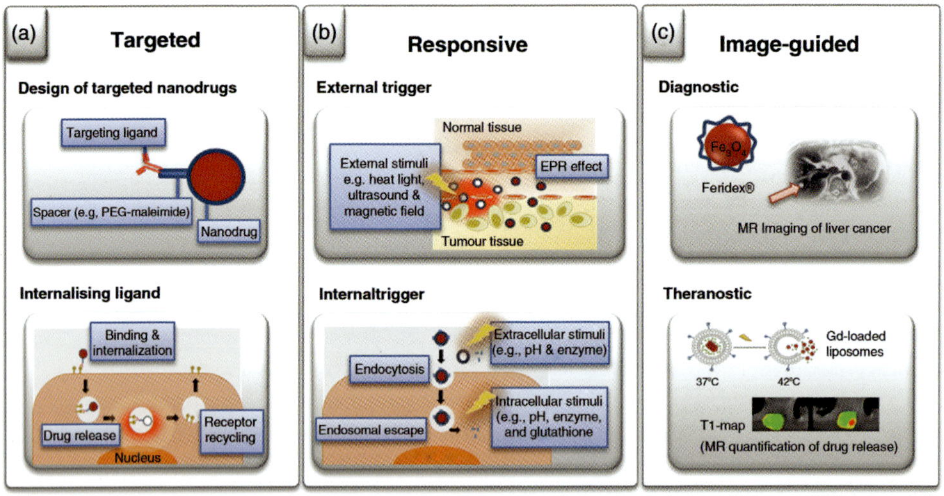

Figure 3.2 Making nanodrugs smarter (a) targeted nanodrugs. The ideal design of targeted nanodrugs is to attach the targeting ligand to the distal end of the polymeric coating layer in order to reserve its binding capacity. After binding with target cells, activation of receptor-mediated uptake process of nanodrug occurs, carrying therapeutic payload into the target cell. (b) Responsive nanodrugs are designed to release their cargo in the vicinity of the target tissue (such as a tumor) in response to external stimuli (such as heat) or internal stimuli (such as a change in pH). (c) Image-guided nanodrugs. The selective uptake of Feridex® nanoparticles by normal hepatic cells compared to tumor cells, allows malignant tissue to be easily distinguished by appearing as a bright spot compared to the surrounding normal tissue. Encapsulation of MR contrast agents that can change signal intensity based on the interaction with surrounding water molecules allows real-time monitoring of drug release. The increase in MR signal after release of encapsulated MR contrast agent and drug from liposomes provides information about spatial and temporal drug release.

these two phenomena are closely connected. This is because the accumulation of targeted nanodrugs to the pathological tissue is mainly dependent of the EPR effect (passive targeting), while the interaction with the target cell will be driven by ligand-mediated interaction (active targeting) [52]. Therefore, any improvement in therapeutic activity is not due to higher accumulation of actively targeted nanodrugs in the diseased site *per se*, but due to the activation of receptor-mediated uptake process (cellular internalization) of nanodrugs carrying therapeutic payload into the target cells [59]. As a result, the premature loss of the therapeutic payload prior to binding and uptake by target cells (drug retention/stability) [60] and the rate of drug release (bioavailability) [61] are very crucial to increase the therapeutic activity compared to nontargeted nanodrugs. In the case of HER2-targeted liposomes, for example, previous studies in mice have shown that their overall tumor accumulation did not increase compared to nontargeted liposome. However, the intratumoral microdistribution and cellular localization of targeted anti-HER2 liposomes were different due to their cellular internalization capacity. Significant fraction of HER2-targeted liposomes was observed within cancer cells, compared to nontargeted liposomes mainly found in stromal cells [56]. There are many factors that affect the efficiency of targeted nanodrugs such as vascular permeability, tissue penetrability, binding site barrier, receptor density, targeting ligands affinity to their target, and interaction with plasma proteins [62]. Therefore, targeted nanodrugs have shown to have the best therapeutic effect when directed toward easily reached target, such as tumor vasculature, micrometastasis, blood cancer [63], and when combined with permeability enhancers [51,63]. The clinical progress of targeted nanodrugs has been much slower compared to nontargeted ones and only few examples have progressed into the clinic such as HER2-targeted liposomal doxorubicin (MM-302) for HER2-positive breast cancer (Phase I/II) [57,58] and Docetaxel-loaded polymeric nanodrugs targeted against prostate-specific membrane antigen (Phase I/II) [64]. The main reason behind that is the substantial increase in the manufacturing cost, such as the production of high-quality antibodies. The therapeutic benefits achieved from targeted nanodrugs have to be considerably higher than what can be achieved from nontargeted counterparts to justify their approval [18].

Responsive Nanodrugs

The second group of multifunctional nanodrugs combine responsive functionality to several stimuli. This can be achieved by the inclusion of specific components that respond (in a "smart," responsive manner) to different types of stimuli that can change their properties or behavior (Figure 3.2b). Smart nanodrugs can be designed to respond to triggers at the cellular levels, such as pH-sensitive nanodrugs to trigger the release of their payload in the late endosome or lysosomes or to facilitate the escape from the lysosome to the cytoplasm. Alternatively, many other formulations were designed to take advantage of the specific microenvironmental changes at the tissue level of certain pathological conditions such as low interstitial pH [65], changes in the level of certain enzymes (phospholipase A2 [66] and matrix metalloproteinases [67]), or alteration in the level of glutathione (redox-responsive nanodrugs) [68]. Among these pathological changes, neoplastic conditions remained the main focus in addition to other diseases such as inflammation, infection, and ischemia [52]. Stimuli-responsive nanodrugs can also respond to external triggers from outside the body (external stimuli), for example, changes in temperature, light, magnetic field, or ultrasound [69]. Interest in designing stimuli-responsive nanodrugs increased with the realization that more efficient delivery strategies are needed. One example on that is the need to provide a tailored release profile (triggered release) with excellent control on the time, duration, and site of drug release. This is mainly because the early generation of nanodrugs, such as Doxil, has been clinically approved to reduce drug-associated toxicity rather than improving efficacy [70].

The concept of stimuli-responsive nanodrugs was first suggested in late 1970s, and was based on hyperthermia (external trigger) induced-release of methotrexate from thermosensitive liposomes. That early example was demonstrated to be four times more efficient to deliver drug to heated tumor compared to nonheated control tumors [71]. Shortly after, many other examples of smart responsive nanodrugs followed [69,72–74]. In another widely explored type of responsive nanoparticle-based approach, the acidic environment of some tumor interstitial spaces [65] or endosomes has been utilized to design pH-sensitive systems. The inclusion of pH-sensitive components is essential in the design of this type. PEGylated poly(L-histidine) copolymer self-assembles into a stable form of polymeric micelles at neutral pH, but as the pH drops to 6.5 or less, protonation of histidine residues in the poly(L-histidine) block occurs resulting in destablization of the micelle structure and release of the incorporated drug. The generation of high local drug concentration in the tumor interstitium or at the cellular level has proved to be effective when resistance to certain drugs is likely to happen, for example, due to drug efflux [75,76]. Redox-responsive nanodrugs is another type of smart systems that respond to the differences in the redox potential such as the changes in glutathione level. Glutathione level increases significantly by more than 100-fold intracellularly compared to extracellular environment and in tumor tissue compared to healthy ones [68,77]. Disulfide bonding is one of the most widely used chemical strategy in the design of redox-responsive nanodrugs, since it is prone to rapid cleavage by glutathione to attain redox sensitivity [77]. Many examples have been described in this regard by the inclusion of disulfide bonds either in the core [78] or in the shell [79] of micelles and the lipid component of liposomes [74] that lead to rapid structural disassembly and release of encapsulated drugs. Although conceptually promising, in practice only a few examples of responsive nanodrugs have progressed to clinical evaluation. In particular, internal triggers are often seen harder to control because of the variability from one patient to another or even within the same tissue, such as the variability in the degree of pH changes at the tumor site. On the other hand, external triggers could be better controlled and indeed most of the progress that has been made in responsive systems has been in that area [69]. To that end, we would like to mention two examples of externally triggered nanodrugs, currently in clinical trials. These two examples are similar in concept, but very different in design. The first example is ThermoDox®, a liposomal doxorubicin formulation that releases drug in response to external mild hyperthermia (41–45 °C) [80]. The responsive nature of ThermoDox® is based on the presence of lipids, such as dipalmitoylphosphatidylcholine and lysolipids, with a suitable phase transition temperature that undergo changes from gel-to-liquid phase and stabilize long-lasting pores in the liposomal membrane for the drug to be released, in response to mild increase in temperature [81]. These changes in the liposomal structure lead to ultrafast release of encapsulated drug in the tumor vasculature [82] and showed efficient tumor growth control in several tumor models in mice [83,84] and currently been tested in human patients [85]. Initial data from phase III clinical trial for hepatocellular carcinoma (HCC) with optimum radiofrequency ablative heating have shown 58% improvement in overall survival [86,87]. ThermoDox® is also currently clinically tested with other external heating techniques such as high-intensity focused ultrasound (HIFU) for HCC [88] or with external microwave hyperthermia for recurrent chest wall breast cancer. NanoTherm® is another example of an externally responsive nanodrug that has advanced to clinical testing for magnetic thermal ablation. NanoTherm® consists of aminosilane-coated superparamagnetic iron oxide nanoparticles with 15 nm core diameter. It is important to stress here that the nanomaterial (iron oxide nanopartciles) is playing the key therapeutic role in this example. In this particular case, the nanodrugs is directly introduced into the solid tumor mass and externally activated by external exposure to alternating magnetic field. The changes in the polarity of the applied magnetics force up to hundred thousand times per second caused the iron-oxide nanoparticles to significantly increase their core temperature. The temperature in the tumor can be controlled by changing the duration of exposure to the oscillating magnetic field to achieve intratumoral temperature in the ablative region (>50 °C) that can directly destroy cancer cells. NanoTherm® is currently clinically tested for glioblastoma multiforme [89] and prostate cancer [90].

Diagnostic/Theranostic Nanodrugs

The third group of multifunctional nanodrugs comprises those having additional imaging functionality either for diagnostic purposes only or in combination with therapy (theranostics) (Figure 3.2c). The inclusion of imaging component in the design of nanodrugs enables not only the track of their pharmacokinetics, accumulation in the target organ and off-target (healthy tissues), but also allows the efficacy of the therapy to be monitored noninvasively and in real time [54]. Due to the significant potential this group of nanodrugs holds, many examples of nanodrugs for image-guidance and theranostic purposes have been reported and the progress is still exponential. Although widely different in functionality, the design of these nanodrugs can be divided into two main categories: (a) those based on traditional nanodrugs (such as liposomes and micelles) that can be functionalized with contrast imaging modalities [53]; and (b) those that are built on a template nanoparticle, such as gold and iron oxide, that have intrinsic imaging properties but can be further modified with a second imaging modality or therapeutic molecule [52,91].

Diagnostic These types of nanodrugs include those designed for purely diagnostic purposes, utilizing the potential diagnostic advantages offered compared to low-molecular-weight contrast agents. These possible benefits can be summarized as (a) flexibility in the chemical composition and size to improve biocompatibility; (b) improved biological stability and reduced clearance rate to prolong the time window for imaging; (c) capability of active targeting via surface modification with specific ligands; and (d) ability to design multifunctional contrast agents by using a combination of more than one contrast agent, for example, for magnetic and optical imaging [92]. Feridex®, a colloidal aqueous dispersion of iron oxide nanoparticles associated with dextran that was approved by the FDA for magnetic resonance (MR) imaging. The size and paramagnetic properties of iron oxide nanoparticles offer unique advantages compared to other MR contrast agents such as gadolinium chelates. Feridex® nanoparticles are between 80 and 150 nm, therefore, their renal clearance is reduced and their uptake is diverted toward the reticuloendothelial system resulting in rapid accumulation in the liver and spleen. Consequently, hepatic imaging was the first application of these nanoparticles for detection of hepatic cancer [93]. In addition, the uptake of iron oxide nanoparticles by activated inflammatory cells such as macrophages and activated microglia makes them excellent contrast agent for imaging inflammatory processes associated with some pathologies such as multiple sclerosis, stroke, and brain tumors [91].

Theranostic One of the key advantages that nanodrugs offer is improved localization of the therapeutic molecules to the target site, particularly after systemic administration. Determination of their pharmacokinetic profile and accumulation into target sites is of significant usefulness [54]. An example of this is the use of radioactive isotope indium-111 to label PEGylated liposomes to monitor their accumulation in the tumor tissue in patients with different cancer types such as breast, head and neck, and Kaposi's sarcoma [94]. This technology has been able to demonstrate in real time that 50% of the PEGylated liposomes were still in systemic circulation 48 h after administration. It also proved that radiolabeled liposomes localized efficiently into the tumor, but the level of accumulation varied considerably from one tumor type to another [94]. In the case of doxorubicin-loaded PEGylated liposomes, a significant percentage of liposomes can be taken up by circulating and tumor-associated macrophages. Since these macrophages are known to play an important role in the clearance mechanism of liposomes, the direct cytotoxic effect of drug-loaded liposomes on the macrophages (following drug release inside the macrophages) can extensively change the pharmacokinetics and distribution of liposomes [95]. The use of theranostic nanodrugs can also guide the patient selection process in clinical practice (personalized medicine). This will help to justify only those patients that show evidence of high drug accumulation in the desired target site, and good therapeutic response to the initial treatment cycles, should be considered for continuation. Otherwise, replacement or adding alternative therapeutic options should be taken into account [54].

Another important advantage that theranostic nanodrugs offer is the ability to monitor drug release. In order for a nanodrug to be therapeutically effective, the encapsulated drug should be released once accumulated at the pathological site. MR contrast agents such as gadolinium and manganese have been highly useful for this purpose as their signal depends on the interaction with the surrounding water molecules. The MR signal generated can vary significantly when these agents are encapsulated within a nanoparticle (limited interaction with water molecules), compared to that obtained after the release of the contrast agent (free interaction with water molecules). One such example are paramagnetic temperature-responsive liposomes, consisting of Gd(HPDO3A) – a clinically approved MR contrast agent (ProHance®) – coencapsulated with doxorubicin inside the aqueous space of liposomes [96,97]. The expectation is that even more efforts will be invested in developing theranostic nanodrugs, and that these systems and strategies will contribute substantially to realizing the potential of personalized medicine.

3.3 Conclusion

Nanopharmacy as new discipline brings together the chemical, physical, and engineering sciences with pharmaceutical sciences aiming to generate nanoscale systems of diagnostic and therapeutic value. Initial efforts intended to improve the performance of already existing therapeutics. The conversion of therapeutic agents to nanodrugs requires a comprehensive understanding of both nanomaterial design and disease pathophysiology. The encapsulation of chemotherapeutics into nanosized delivery systems has been a successful strategy to obtain high drug accumulation in target disease sites and decreased off-target drug-associated toxicities. In addition, reformulation of poorly soluble drugs into nanosized particles (e.g., Abraxane) has enabled the development of therapies for cancer by improving drug bioavailability.

Besides improving the efficacy of already established therapeutic molecules, the application of nanotechnology in pharmaceutical science has enabled the development of new therapies. Nanomedicine-based gene therapy has opened the avenue to treat disorders by delivering nucleic acids intracellularly. Smart nanodrugs of different chemistry are being developed to enable targeting and design of responsive nanoparticles to microenvironment changes (pH, enzymes) or external stimuli (temperature, light, magnetic fields). Incorporation of the imaging component in the development of nanomedicines is increasing the potential to couple therapy with diagnostic capabilities. Imaging modalities have opened up an entirely new avenue to design sophisticated nanopharmaceuticals that can simultaneously achieve diagnosis and therapy.

Due to the complexity of their mode of action, the assessment of safety and risk/benefit of new nanopharmaceuticals remains challenging at the present: new tools for nanocharacterization and testing strategies for quality and safety assessments remain to be defined. Undoubtedly, the emergence of nanopharmacy will contribute to solution of unmet needs in the development of new nanoscale technologies, aiming to improve clinical outcomes in a variety of clinical settings. At present, the major field of application is in oncology; however, nanomedicines will most likely have many more possibilities in the treatment of neurology [98] and immune disorders [99].

References

1 Weissig, V., Pettinger, T.K., and Murdock, N. (2014) Nanopharmaceuticals (part 1): products on the market. *Int. J. Nanomedicine*, **9**, 4357–4373.

2 Langer, R. and Weissleder, R. (2015) Nanotechnology. *JAMA*, **313**, 135–136.

3 Cheng, C.J., Tietjen, G.T., Saucier-Sawyer, J.K., and Saltzman, W.M. (2015) A holistic approach to targeting disease with polymeric nanoparticles. *Nat. Rev. Drug Discov.*, **14**, 239–247.

4 Wong, I.Y., Bhatia, S.N., and Toner, M. (2013) Nanotechnology: emerging tools for biology and medicine. *Gene Dev.*, **27**, 2397–2408.

5 Xu, X., Ho, W., Zhang, X., Bertrand, N., and Farokhzad, O. (2015) Cancer nanomedicine: from targeted delivery to combination therapy. *Trends Mol. Med.*, **21**, 223–232.

6 Bremer-Hoffmann, S., Amenta, V., and Rossi, F. (2015) Nanomedicines in the European translational process. *Eur. J. Nanomedicine*, **7**, 135–268.

7 Huang, X. and El-Sayed, M.A. (2010) Gold nanoparticles: optical properties and implementations in cancer diagnosis and photothermal therapy. *J. Adv. Res.*, **1**, 13–28.

8 Kostarelos, K. (2003) Rational design and engineering of delivery systems for therapeutics: biomedical exercises in colloid and surface science. *Adv. Colloid Interface Sci.*, **106**, 147–168.

9 Onoue, S., Yamada, S., and Chan, H.K. (2014) Nanodrugs: pharmacokinetics and safety. *Int. J. Nanomedicine*, **9**, 1025–1037.

10 Peer, D., Karp, J.M., Hong, S., FaroKHzad, O.C., Margalit, R., and Langer, R. (2007) Nanocarriers as an emerging platform for cancer therapy. *Nat. Nanotechnol.*, **2**, 751–760.

11 Davis, M.E., Chen, Z.G., and Shin, D.M. (2008) Nanoparticle therapeutics: an emerging treatment modality for cancer. *Nat. Rev. Drug Discov.*, **7**, 771–782.

12 Matsumura, Y. and Maeda, H. (1986) A new concept for macromolecular therapeutics in cancer chemotherapy: mechanism of tumoritropic accumulation of proteins and the antitumor agent smancs. *Cancer Res.*, **46**, 6387–6392.

13 Maeda, H. (2001) The enhanced permeability and retention (EPR) effect in tumor vasculature: the key role of tumor-selective macromolecular drug targeting. *Adv. Enzyme Regul.*, **41**, 189–207.

14 Gregoriadis, G. and Neerunjun, D.E. (1974) Control of the rate of hepatic uptake and catabolism of liposome-entrapped proteins injected into rats. Possible therapeutic applications. *Eur. J. Biochem.*, **47**, 179–185.

15 Iyer, A.K., Khaled, G., Fang, J., and Maeda, H. (2006) Exploiting the enhanced permeability and retention effect for tumor targeting. *Drug Discov. Today*, **11**, 812–818.

16 Allen, T.M. and Hansen, C. (1991) Pharmacokinetics of stealth versus

conventional liposomes: effect of dose. *Biochim. Biophys. Acta*, **1068**, 133–141.
17 Allen, T.M., Hansen, C., Martin, F., Redemann, C., and Yau-Young, A. (1991) Liposomes containing synthetic lipid derivatives of poly(ethylene glycol) show prolonged circulation half-lives *in vivo*. *Biochim. Biophys. Acta*, **1066**, 29–36.
18 Allen, T.M. and Cullis, P.R. (2013) Liposomal drug delivery systems: from concept to clinical applications. *Adv. Drug Deliv. Rev.*, **65**, 36–48.
19 Bangham, A.D. and Horne, R.W. (1964) Negative staining of phospholipids and their structural modification by surface-active agents as observed in electron microscope. *J. Mol. Biol.*, **8** (5), 660–668.
20 Li, X., Hirsh, D.J., Cabral-Lilly, D., Zirkel, A., Gruner, S.M., Janoff, A.S., and Perkins, W.R. (1998) Doxorubicin physical state in solution and inside liposomes loaded via a pH gradient. *Biochim. Biophys. Acta*, **1415**, 23–40.
21 Koudelka, S. and Turanek, J. (2012) Liposomal paclitaxel formulations. *J. Control Release*, **163**, 322–334.
22 Gabizon, A., Catane, R., Uziely, B., Kaufman, B., Safra, T., Cohen, R., Martin, F., Huang, A., and Barenholz, Y. (1994) Prolonged circulation time and enhanced accumulation in malignant exudates of doxorubicin encapsulated in polyethylene-glycol coated liposomes. *Cancer Res.*, **54**, 987–992.
23 Barenholz, Y. (2012) Doxil® – the first FDA-approved nano-drug: lessons learned. *J. Control Release.*, **160**, 117–134.
24 Gabizon, A., Shmeeda, H., and Barenholz, Y. (2003) Pharmacokinetics of pegylated liposomal doxorubicin: review of animal and human studies. *Clin. Pharmacokinet.*, **42**, 419–436.
25 De Jong, W.H. and Borm, P.J. (2008) Drug delivery and nanoparticles: applications and hazards. *Int. J. Nanomedicine*, **3**, 133–149.
26 Desai, N., Trieu, V., Yao, Z., Louie, L., Ci, S., Yang, A., Tao, C., De, T., Beals, B., Dykes, D., Noker, P., Yao, R., Labao, E., Hawkins, M., and Soon-Shiong, P. (2006) Increased antitumor activity, intratumor paclitaxel concentrations, and endothelial cell transport of cremophor-free, albumin-bound paclitaxel, ABI-007, compared with cremophor-based paclitaxel. *Clin. Cancer Res.*, **12** (4), 1317–1324.
27 Gradishar, W.J. (2006) Albumin-bound paclitaxel: a next-generation taxane. *Expert Opin. Pharmacother.*, **7**, 1041–1053.
28 Green, M.R., Manikhas, G.M., Orlov, S., Afanasyev, B., Makhson, A.M., Bhar, P., and Hawkins, M.J. (2006) Abraxane, a novel Cremophor-free, albumin-bound particle form of paclitaxel for the treatment of advanced non-small-cell lung cancer. *Ann. Oncol.*, **17**, 1263–1268.
29 Li, C., Yu, D.F., Newman, R.A., Cabral, F., Stephens, L.C., Hunter, N., Milas, L., and Wallace, S. (1998) Complete regression of well-established tumors using a novel water-soluble poly(L-glutamic acid) paclitaxel conjugate. *Cancer Res.*, **58**, 2404–2409.
30 Jeyapalan, S., Boxerman, J., Donahue, J., Goldman, M., Kinsella, T., Dipetrillo, T., Evans, D., Elinzano, H., Constantinou, M., Stopa, E., Puthawala, Y., Cielo, D., Santaniello, A., Oyelese, A., Mantripragada, K., Rosati, K., Isdale, D., and Safran, H. (2014) Paclitaxel poliglumex, temozolomide, and radiation for newly diagnosed high-grade glioma: a Brown University Oncology Group Study. *Am. J. Clin. Oncol.*, **37** 444–449.
31 Cho, H., Lai, T.C., Tomoda, K., and Kwon, G.S. (2015) Polymeric micelles for multi-drug delivery in cancer. *AAPS Pharm. Sci. Tech.*, **16**, 10–20.
32 Kim, T.Y., Kim, D.W., Chung, J.Y., Shin, S.G., Kim, S.C., Heo, D.S., Kim, N.K., and Bang, Y.J. (2004) Phase I and pharmacokinetic study of Genexol-PM, a cremophor-free, polymeric micelle-formulated paclitaxel, in patients with advanced malignancies. *Clin. Cancer Res.*, **10**, 3708–3716.
33 Wang, D. and Gao, G. (2014) State-of-the-art human gene therapy: part II. Gene therapy strategies and clinical applications. *Discovery Medicine*, **18**, 151–161.
34 Kostarelos, K. and Miller, A.D. (2005) Synthetic, self-assembly ABCD nanoparticles, a structural paradigm for viable synthetic non-viral vectors. *Chem. Soc. Rev.*, **34**, 970–994.

35 Nguyen, J. and Szoka, F.C. (2012) Nucleic acid delivery: the missing pieces of the puzzle? *Acc. Chem. Res.*, **45**, 1153–1162.
36 Ginn, S.L., Alexander, I.E., Edelstein, M.L., Abedi, M.R., and Wixon, J. (2013) Gene therapy clinical trials worldwide to 2012 – an update. *J. Gene Med.*, **15**, 65–77.
37 Wang, D. and Gao, G. (2014) State-of-the-art human gene therapy: part I. Gene delivery technologies. *Discov. Med.*, **18**, 67–77.
38 Fraley, R., Subramani, S., Berg, P., and Papahadjopoulos, D. (1980) Introduction of liposome-encapsulated SV40 DNA into cells. *J. Biol. Chem.*, **255**, 10431–10435.
39 Felgner, P.L., Gadek, T.R., Holm, M., Roman, R., Chan, H.W., Wenz, M., Northrop, J.P., Ringold, G.M., and Danielsen, M. (1987) Lipofection: a highly efficient, lipid-mediated DNA-transfection procedure. *Proc. Natl. Acad. Sci. USA*, **84**, 7413–7417.
40 Podesta, J.E., Al-Jamal, K.T., Herrero, M.A., Tian, B., Ali-Boucetta, H., Hegde, V., Bianco, A., Prato, M., and Kostarelos, K. (2009) Antitumor activity and prolonged survival by carbon-nanotube-mediated therapeutic siRNA silencing in a human lung xenograft model. *Small*, **5**, 1176–1185.
41 Mazza, M., Hadjidemetriou, M., de Lazaro, I., Bussy, C., and Kostarelos, K. (2015) Peptide nanofiber complexes with siRNA for deep brain gene silencing by stereotactic neurosurgery. *ACS Nano*, **9**, 1137–1149.
42 Yin, H., Kanasty, R.L., Eltoukhy, A.A., Vegas, A.J., Dorkin, J.R., and Anderson, D.G. (2014) Non-viral vectors for gene-based therapy. *Nat. Rev. Genet.*, **15**, 541–555.
43 Lu, C., Stewart, D.J., Lee, J.J., Ji, L., Ramesh, R., Jayachandran, G., Nunez, M.I., Wistuba, I.I., Erasmus, J.J., Hicks, M.E., Grimm, E.A., Reuben, J.M., Baladandayuthapani, V., Templeton, N.S., McMannis, J.D., and Roth, J.A. (2012) Phase I clinical trial of systemically administered TUSC2(FUS1)-nanoparticles mediating functional gene transfer in humans. *PLoS One*, **7**, e34833.
44 Gofrit, O.N., Benjamin, S., Halachmi, S., Leibovitch, I., Dotan, Z., Lamm, D.L., Ehrlich, N., Yutkin, V., Ben-Am, M., and Hochberg, A. (2014) DNA based therapy with diphtheria toxin-A BC-819: a phase 2b marker lesion trial in patients with intermediate risk nonmuscle invasive bladder cancer. *J. Urol.*, **191**, 1697–1702.
45 Buscail, L., Bournet, B., Vernejoul, F., Cambois, G., Lulka, H., Hanoun, N., Dufresne, M., Meulle, A., Vignolle-Vidoni, A., Ligat, L., Saint-Laurent, N., Pont, F., Dejean, S., Gayral, M., Martins, F., Torrisani, J., Barbey, O., Gross, F., Guimbaud, R., Otal, P., Lopez, F., Tiraby, G., and Cordelier, P. (2015.) First-in-man phase 1 clinical trial of gene therapy for advanced pancreatic cancer: safety, biodistribution, and preliminary clinical findings. *Mol. Ther.*, **23**, 779–789.
46 Anwer, K., Kelly, F.J., Chu, C., Fewell, J.G., Lewis, D., and Alvarez, R.D. (2013) Phase I trial of a formulated IL-12 plasmid in combination with carboplatin and docetaxel chemotherapy in the treatment of platinum-sensitive recurrent ovarian cancer. *Gynecol. Oncol.*, **131**, 169–173.
47 Alvarez, R.D., Sill, M.W., Davidson, S.A., Muller, C.Y., Bender, D.P., DeBernardo, R.L., Behbakht, K., and Huh, W.K. (2014) A phase II trial of intraperitoneal EGEN-001, an IL-12 plasmid formulated with PEG-PEI-cholesterol lipopolymer in the treatment of persistent or recurrent epithelial ovarian, fallopian tube or primary peritoneal cancer: a gynecologic oncology group study. *Gynecol. Oncol.*, **133**, 433–438.
48 Sakhrani, N.M. and Padh, H. (2013) Organelle targeting: third level of drug targeting. *Drug Des. Devel. Ther.*, **7**, 585–599.
49 Biswas, S. and Torchilin, V.P. (2014) Nanopreparations for organelle-specific delivery in cancer. *Adv. Drug Deliv. Rev.*, **66**, 26–41.
50 Paulo, C.S., Pires das Neves, R., and Ferreira, L.S. (2011) Nanoparticles for intracellular-targeted drug delivery. *Nanotechnology*, **22**, 494002.
51 Al-Ahmady, Z.S., Chaloin, O., and Kostarelos, K. (2014) Monoclonal antibody-targeted, temperature-sensitive liposomes: *in vivo* tumor chemotherapeutics in combination with

mild hyperthermia. *J. Control. Release*, **196**, 332–343.

52 Torchilin, V.P. (2014) Multifunctional, stimuli-sensitive nanoparticulate systems for drug delivery. *Nat. Rev. Drug Discov.*, **13**, 813–827.

53 Lozano, N., Al-Ahmady, Z.S., Beziere, N.S., Ntziachristos, V., and Kostarelos, K. (2015) Monoclonal antibody-targeted PEGylated liposome-ICG encapsulating doxorubicin as a potential theranostic agent. *Int. J. Pharm.*, **482**, 2–10.

54 Lammers, T., Aime, S., Hennink, W.E., Storm, G., and Kiessling, F. (2011) Theranostic nanomedicine. *Acc. Chem. Res.*, **44**, 1029–1038.

55 Moreira, J.N., Ishida, T., Gaspar, R., and Allen, T.M. (2002) Use of the post-insertion technique to insert peptide ligands into pre-formed stealth liposomes with retention of binding activity and cytotoxicity. *Pharm. Res.*, **19**, 265–269.

56 Kirpotin, D.B., Drummond, D.C., Shao, Y., Shalaby, M.R., Hong, K., Nielsen, U.B., Marks, J.D., Benz, C.C., and Park, J.W. (2006) Antibody targeting of long-circulating lipidic nanoparticles does not increase tumor localization but does increase internalization in animal models. *Cancer Res.*, **66**, 6732–6740.

57 ClinicalTrials.gov (2015) Safety and Pharmacokinetic Study of MM-302 in Patients With Advanced Breast Cancer (NCT01304797). Available at https://clinicaltrials.gov/ct2/show/NCT01304797?term=mm302&rank=1.

58 ClinicalTrials.gov (2016) MM-302 Plus Trastuzumab vs. Chemotherapy of Physician's Choice Plus Trastuzumab in HER2-Positive Locally Advanced/Metastatic Breast Cancer Patients (HERMIONE) (NCT02213744). Available at https://clinicaltrials.gov/ct2/show/NCT02213744?term=mm302&rank=2.

59 Sapra, P. and Allen, T.M. (2002) Internalizing antibodies are necessary for improved therapeutic efficacy of antibody-targeted liposomal drugs. *Cancer Res.*, **62**, 7190–7194.

60 Vingerhoeds, M.H., Steerenberg, P.A., Hendriks, J.J., Dekker, L.C., Van Hoesel, Q.G., Crommelin, D.J., and Storm, G. (1996) Immunoliposome-mediated targeting of doxorubicin to human ovarian carcinoma *in vitro* and *in vivo*. *Br. J. Cancer*, **74**, 1023–1029.

61 Sapra, P. and Allen, T.M. (2004) Improved outcome when B-cell lymphoma is treated with combinations of immunoliposomal anticancer drugs targeted to both the CD19 and CD20 epitopes. *Clin. Cancer Res.*, **10**, 2530–2537.

62 Hadjidemetriou, M., Al-Ahmady, Z., Mazza, M., Collins, R.F., Dawson, K., and Kostarelos, K. (2015) *In vivo* biomolecule corona around blood-circulating, clinically used and antibody-targeted lipid bilayer nanoscale vesicles. *ACS Nano*, **9**, 8142–8156.

63 Lammers, T., Kiessling, F., Hennink, W.E., and Storm, G. (2012) Drug targeting to tumors: principles, pitfalls and (pre-) clinical progress. *J. Control. Release*, **161**, 175–187.

64 ClinicalTrials.gov (2016) A Phase 2 Study to Determine the Safety and Efficacy of BIND-014 (Docetaxel Nanoparticles for Injectable Suspension), Administered to Patients With Metastatic Castration-Resistant Prostate Cancer (NCT01812746). Available at https://clinicaltrials.gov/ct2/show/NCT01812746?term=bind-014&rank=1.

65 Wojtkowiak, J.W., Verduzco, D., Schramm, K.J., and Gillies, R.J. (2011) Drug resistance and cellular adaptation to tumor acidic pH microenvironment. *Mol. Pharmaceutics*, **8**, 2032–2038.

66 Andresen, T.L., Jensen, S.S., Kaasgaard, T., and Jorgensen, K. (2005) Triggered activation and release of liposomal prodrugs and drugs in cancer tissue by secretory phospholipase A2. *Curr. Drug Deliv.*, **2**, 353–362.

67 Sarkar, N., Banerjee, J., Hanson, A.J., Elegbede, A.I., Rosendahl, T., Krueger, A.B., Banerjee, A.L., Tobwala, S., Wang, R., Lu, X., Mallik, S., and Srivastava, D.K. (2008) Matrix metalloproteinase-assisted triggered release of liposomal contents. *Bioconjug. Chem.*, **19**, 57–64.

68 Torchilin, V. (2009) Multifunctional and stimuli-sensitive pharmaceutical nanocarriers. *Eur. J. Pharm. Biopharm.*, **71**, 431–444.

69 Mura, S., Nicolas, J., and Couvreur, P. (2013) Stimuli-responsive nanocarriers for drug delivery. *Nat. Mater.*, **12**, 991–1003.
70 O'Brien, M.E., Wigler, N., Inbar, M., Rosso, R., Grischke, E., Santoro, A., Catane, R., Kieback, D.G., Tomczak, P., Ackland, S.P., Orlandi, F., Mellars, L., Alland, L., and Tendler, C. (2004) Reduced cardiotoxicity and comparable efficacy in a phase III trial of pegylated liposomal doxorubicin HCl (CAELYX/Doxil) versus conventional doxorubicin for first-line treatment of metastatic breast cancer. *Ann. Oncol.*, **15**, 440–449.
71 Weinstein, J.N., Magin, R.L., Yatvin, M.B., and Zaharko, D.S. (1979) Liposomes and local hyperthermia: selective delivery of methotrexate to heated tumors. *Supramol. Sci.*, **204**, 188–191.
72 Al-Ahmady, Z.S., Scudamore, C.L., and Kostarelos, K. (2015) Triggered doxorubicin release in solid tumors from thermosensitive liposome-peptide hybrids: critical parameters and therapeutic efficacy. *Int. J. Cancer*, **137**, 731–743.
73 Al-Ahmady, Z.S., Al-Jamal, W.T., Bossche, J.V., Bui, T.T., Drake, A.F., Mason, A.J., and Kostarelos, K. (2012) Lipid-peptide vesicle nanoscale hybrids for triggered drug release by mild hyperthermia *in vitro* and *in vivo*. *ACS Nano*, **6**, 9335–9346.
74 Goldenbogen, B., Brodersen, N., Gramatica, A., Loew, M., Liebscher, J., Herrmann, A., Egger, H., Budde, B., and Arbuzova, A. (2011) Reduction-sensitive liposomes from a multifunctional lipid conjugate and natural phospholipids: reduction and release kinetics and cellular uptake. *Langmuir*, **27**, 10820–10829.
75 Kim, D., Gao, Z.G., Lee, E.S., and Bae, Y.H. (2009) *In vivo* evaluation of doxorubicin-loaded polymeric micelles targeting folate receptors and early endosomal pH in drug-resistant ovarian cancer. *Mol. Pharmaceutics*, **6**, 1353–1362.
76 Kim, D., Lee, E.S., Oh, K.T., Gao, Z.G., and Bae, Y.H. (2008) Doxorubicin-loaded polymeric micelle overcomes multidrug resistance of cancer by double-targeting folate receptor and early endosomal pH. *Small*, **4**, 2043–2050.
77 Saito, G., Swanson, J.A., and Lee, K.D. (2003) Drug delivery strategy utilizing conjugation via reversible disulfide linkages: role and site of cellular reducing activities. *Adv. Drug Deliv. Rev.*, **55**, 199–215.
78 Li, Y., Xiao, K., Luo, J., Xiao, W., Lee, J.S., Gonik, A.M., Kato, J., Dong, T.A., and Lam, K.S. (2011) Well-defined, reversible disulfide cross-linked micelles for on-demand paclitaxel delivery. *Biomaterials*, **32**, 6633–6645.
79 Wen, H.Y., Dong, H.Q., Xie, W.J., Li, Y.Y., Wang, K., Pauletti, G.M., and Shi, D.L. (2011) Rapidly disassembling nanomicelles with disulfide-linked PEG shells for glutathione-mediated intracellular drug delivery. *Chem. Commun.*, **47**, 3550–3552.
80 Landon, C.D., Park, J.Y., Needham, D., and Dewhirst, M.W. (2011) Nanoscale drug delivery and hyperthermia: the materials design and preclinical and clinical testing of low temperature-sensitive liposomes used in combination with mild hyperthermia in the treatment of local cancer. *Open Nanomed. J.*, **3**, 38–64.
81 Needham, D., Park, J.Y., Wright, A.M., and Tong, J. (2013) Materials characterization of the low temperature sensitive liposome (LTSL): effects of the lipid composition (lysolipid and DSPE-PEG2000) on the thermal transition and release of doxorubicin. *Faraday Discuss.*, **161**, 515–534.
82 Manzoor, A.A., Lindner, L.H., Landon, C.D., Park, J.Y., Simnick, A.J., Dreher, M.R., Das, S., Hanna, G., Park, W., Chilkoti, A., Koning, G.A., ten Hagen, T.L., Needham, D., and Dewhirst, M.W. (2012) Overcoming limitations in nanoparticle drug delivery: triggered, intravascular release to improve drug penetration into tumors. *Cancer Res.*, **72**, 5566–5575.
83 Kong, G., Anyarambhatla, G., Petros, W.P., Braun, R.D., Colvin, O.M., Needham, D., and Dewhirst, M.W. (2000) Efficacy of liposomes and hyperthermia in a human tumor xenograft model: importance of triggered drug release. *Cancer Res.*, **60**, 6950–6957.
84 Yarmolenko, P.S., Zhao, Y., Landon, C., Spasojevic, I., Yuan, F., Needham, D., Viglianti, B.L., and Dewhirst, M.W. (2010) Comparative effects of thermosensitive doxorubicin-containing liposomes and

hyperthermia in human and murine tumours. *Int. J. Hyperthermia*, **26**, 485–498.

85 Celsion.com (2015) Optima Study Highlighted at ILCA Symposium. Available at http://celsion.com/docs/OPTIMA_Study_ ILCA_Symposium.

86 Celsion.com (2015) THERMODOX®. Available at http://celsion.com/docs/technology_thermodox.

87 ClinicalTrials.gov (2016) A Study of ThermoDox™ in Combination With Radiofrequency Ablation (RFA) in Primary and Metastatic Tumors of the Liver (NCT00441376). Availabel at https://clinicaltrials.gov/ct2/show/NCT00441376?term=thermodox&rank=3.

88 ClinicalTrials.gov (2016) Targeted Chemotherapy Using Focused Ultrasound for Liver Tumours (TARDOX) (NCT02181075). Available at https://clinicaltrials.gov/ct2/show/NCT02181075?term=thermodox&rank=4.

89 Maier-Hauff, K., Rothe, R., Scholz, R., Gneveckow, U., Wust, P., Thiesen, B., Feussner, A.von, Deimling, A., Waldoefner, N., Felix, R., and Jordan, A. (2007) Intracranial thermotherapy using magnetic nanoparticles combined with external beam radiotherapy: results of a feasibility study on patients with glioblastoma multiforme. *J. Neurooncol.*, **81**, 53–60.

90 Johannsen, M., Thiesen, B., Wust, P., and Jordan, A. (2010) Magnetic nanoparticle hyperthermia for prostate cancer. *Int. J. Hyperthermia*, **26**, 790–795.

91 Wang, Y.X. (2011) Superparamagnetic iron oxide based MRI contrast agents: current status of clinical application. *Quant. Imaging Med. Surg.*, **1**, 35–40.

92 Weissig, V. and Guzman-Villanueva, D. (2015) Nanopharmaceuticals (part 2): products in the pipeline. *Int. J. Nanomedicine*, **10**, 1245–1257.

93 Clement, O., Siauve, N., Cuenod, C.A., and Frija, G. (1998) Liver imaging with ferumoxides (Feridex): fundamentals, controversies, and practical aspects. *Top. Magn. Reson. Imaging*, **9**, 167–182.

94 Harrington, K.J., Mohammadtaghi, S., Uster, P.S., Glass, D., Peters, A.M., Vile, R.G., and Stewart, J.S. (2001) Effective targeting of solid tumors in patients with locally advanced cancers by radiolabeled pegylated liposomes. *Clin. Cancer Res.*, **7**, 243–254.

95 Dams, E.T., Laverman, P., Oyen, W.J., Storm, G., Scherphof, G.L., van Der Meer, J.W., Corstens, F.H., and Boerman, O.C. (2000) Accelerated blood clearance and altered biodistribution of repeated injections of sterically stabilized liposomes. *J. Pharmacol. Exp. Ther.*, **292**, 1071–1079.

96 de Smet, M., Heijman, E., Langereis, S., Hijnen, N.M., and Grull, H. (2011) Magnetic resonance imaging of high intensity focused ultrasound mediated drug delivery from temperature-sensitive liposomes: an *in vivo* proof-of-concept study. *J. Control. Release*, **150**, 102–110.

97 de Smet, M., Langereis, S., van den Bosch, S., and Grull, H. (2010) Temperature-sensitive liposomes for doxorubicin delivery under MRI guidance. *J. Control. Release*, **143**, 120–127.

98 Gendelman, H.E., Anantharam, V., Bronich, T., Ghaisas, S., Jin, H.J., Kanthasamy, A.G., Liu, X.M., McMillan, J., Mosley, R.L., Narasimhan, B., and Mallapragada, S.K. (2015) Nanoneuromedicines for degenerative, inflammatory, and infectious nervous system diseases. *Nanomed. Nanotechnol.*, **11**, 751–767.

99 Gharagozloo, M., Majewski, S., and Foldvari, M. (2015) Therapeutic applications of nanomedicine in autoimmune diseases: from immunosuppression to tolerance induction. *Nanomedicine*, **11**, 1003–1018.

4 Understanding and Characterizing Functional Properties of Nanoparticles

Ester Polo, Valentina Castagnola, and Kenneth A. Dawson

University College Dublin, School of Chemistry and Chemical Biology, Centre for BioNano Interactions, Belfield, Dublin 4, Ireland

4.1 Introduction

While characterization of particles in general, and nanoparticles in particular, is a well-developed arena, and in some aspects mature field of science, typically measurements of properties have been developed with a purely physiochemical perspective in mind. Particle size, to some degree surface zeta potential, chemical composition, and shapes, and other obvious properties are captured with increasing ease, and many commercial instruments are available, or being developed for broad use [1–3].

We believe that a major limiting feature in translating nanotechnology into concrete achievements in such fields as nanomedicine targeting has been, and is increasingly, our lack of understanding, and control, of the detailed relationship between (mainly) surface and shape information, and biological outcomes [4–7].

Thus, in strong contrast to successful efforts to characterize the materials properly, the understanding and means to characterize those specific features that affect the biological function of nanoparticles have been much less well understood and little developed. Above all, there has been a lack of understanding and conceptual framework. This is a profound matter for, while characterization is at first sight, a simple matter of "measurement of properties," this is a mistaken conception for this arena. Deeper reflection on the lessons of the history of science suggests that progress here is a central driver for the advancement of the science and technology that underlies bionanoscience, nanomedicine, and many other aspects of the safety of all products and medicines involving the nanoscale [8]. Succinctly put, some fields are lucky enough to lead to rapid "discoveries" that revolutionize our world. A good example is the discovery of the drug penicillin [9]. Others however begin with an observation of "interesting effects," which are progressively mastered over a generation,

Pharmaceutical Nanotechnology: Innovation and Production, First Edition. Edited by Jean Cornier, Arno Kwade, Andrew Owen, and Marcel Van de Voorde.

leading to broad and deep innovations. The introduction of semiconductors and (possibly) superconductors is an example of the latter [10–14].

While it is not yet late for radical discovery to take place in the applications of nanotechnology (indeed, there are some promising signs of specific events there), the broad experience is likely to be closer to that of semiconductors, and other technology examples where the effects are progressively understood, and systematically connected back to detailed material properties [15,16]. We believe that such measurement and interpretation of effects and the properties that lead to them will progressively become the core of the scientific and technological advance.

A much later development, while hardly disconnected and certainly just as important to a maturing technology, is the "standardization" of such measurements [17,18]. The two issues are sometimes conflated, or confused. They are quite different. The former is now critically urgent if we are to identify and develop practically useful medical technologies. The latter, equally important, has been quite successful in terms of physical measurement, and can be developed with further prudent and measured reflection.

In truth, in this arena, we are still struggling with the challenge of mastering the connection between material cause and biological effects [19,20]. We consider that the understanding of those is (in the absence of widespread and facile discovery) becoming the major driver for development. Perhaps this was always likely to be so here, where biology is brought into contact a new universe of objects on the biologically active size scale. Possibly full acceptance of it awaited a cool and measured assessment of the events: that is occurring now. But one should not misread the situation. We have in our hands biological effects we do not know how to control, but which have at least the broad and enduring significance seen in semiconductors.

To understand why different opinions on these topics may persist for several more years, it is necessary to understand that for some, nanotechnology is now a maturing arena, while for others the story has just begun, and the best, by far, has yet to come. Both are correct, but are driven from completely different understandings. From the perspective of aspirations for facile and fortuitous "discovery" based on trial and error, it may be true that the coming few years could be considered a maturation of that process. From a broader and deeper perspective, with a full awareness of the biological mechanisms we now find ourselves able to prompt, if not yet fully control, the analogy with semiconductors is helpful. Those close to the science will be clear that the best science and the most enduring practical impacts from a growing capacity and strength are all yet to come. The challenge will now be to effectively communicate that, and sustain the means to deliver it.

With a view to clarifying some of this discussion for a broader audience, reflect for a moment on how proteins and the other key naturally occurring nanoparticles within living systems are all carefully recognized mainly at their surface, and have directed biological tasks [21,22]. However, the fidelity with which biological systems manage this recognition is extraordinarily effective, and must be, for that is how organisms defend against infection, and other foreign body threats [23,24]. There was, and is, every reason to expect this is a subtle issue, where details and exquisite control matter. We require a high level of commitment to understand how to engage with those systems, and how to engineer correctly the interface of materials, to allow us to do this in a controlled manner. That is now happening.

While this cannot be discussed here, we consider there are very solid grounds to hope that within a generation there could emerge a deep, durable understanding of the science, feeding a world-changing space of applications. However, this will have to be wrought by persistent, disciplined efforts, where depth of understanding, rather than simply more new ideas will be required. There will be few shortcuts, and executional excellence will be central. Here, we will lay out the background, and overview of the situation, and point out where we believe the major future developments are required.

4.1.1
Key Concepts: Size Matters, Biological Interactions

We do not know yet all of the material properties that affect the biology. The timing of the discussion is useful however, for we do know some, and the general shape of things to come is clarifying. Only now have we an emerging conceptual framework, against which progress can be measured, and hypotheses tested. Here, we will focus on the most clear properties (which increasingly we consider to be size, shape, and surface character) that determine the biology [25–29]. Many other specific factors for specific materials could also be relevant, but those are central.

The reasons that, two decades in, we are still discussing this question is partly technical, partly a consequence of the challenge in bridging such varied communities, partly driven by initial excitement that in itself (isolated from more fundamental understanding) nanotechnology would easily lead to new biomedical outcomes [8,30,31]. In part, it is just because this is a very new and interdisciplinary field, and in scientific terms we are still at an early stage. Thus, it has been easier to make progress in characterizing nanomaterials in general terms, than in identifying the key parameters defining the outcomes.

Now we need to both clarify, and fundamentally enlarge our vision, to accommodate the mission of understanding what must be characterized and linked to biological outcomes. It is therefore worth briefly returning to the foundations of our enduring commitment to this arena, and recapitulating the central issues.

The nanoscale is the "natural" scale of many key elements of biology and biological function. Cells barriers and organs function, signal, communicate, and transfer materials using active nanoscale processes fueled by the cellular energy and rarely involve diffusive motion [5,32–34]. Those processes are all highly regulated, and subjected to detailed monitoring within cells, and other organizational levels [35–37]. Proteins are nanoparticles (low-density lipoprotein is about 30 nm, transferrin about 5 nm, and fibrinogen about 8 nm [38]), and a living organism is to a very large degree a very complex and sophisticated nanoparticle processor.

Beneath some size (the specifics depend on the material) typically around 1 nm, nanoparticles begin to interact at cell level by processes more typical of molecules, for example, partition and equilibration by diffusive motion [27,39]. For sizes much larger (again dependent on the details) than some hundreds of nanometers, recognition-regulated entry into cells by active processes diminishes and more generic sweeping by first-line immune cells become important [28,40].

For sizes involving some tens of nanometers, all of the endogenous trafficking, and other active processes, the nanoparticles may be essentially recognized as biological entities, and become part of the whole biological process, in many complex ways [22,41,42]. This is the only size range where this can occur.

It is difficult to overstress the importance of this point. Every beginning student of the field should reflect deeply and often on this point. It removes the importance of this field as only being relevant for a specific time and place in development. Many other scientific fashions, and "hot" spots of development, are best understood as specific to given communities for specific times. Here the issues are different, broader, and more durable. In the many decades to come, as our capacity to engineer objects on this size-scale develops, and most important, as our understanding and purpose refine, none can doubt that the capacity for mankind to predictively operate and design functional entities at the same scale as biological processing machinery will have enduring value. As with semiconductors, intended one day to change the world, we may be absolutely secure in the knowledge this field will benefit all around us enormously. This means the field of bionanoscale interactions belongs not to us, and our communities as they are today, but to the course of historical development of science. This is important. It needs to be restated. It will distill, purify, and inspire the right kind of effort for the decades to come.

These factors also mean that ultimate achievement in the field is also, reassuringly, unavoidable, whatever we in our generation achieve. Biological law defines that we are working in the right size regime. There will never be another, for those kinds of processes.

There remains the simple point that one key property controlling the impact on biological process is simply size [7,21,26,27]. However, this is merely an enabling property. Within reasonable ranges of size (as outlined above) we are in a regime where objects are recognized and processed using the endogenous mechanisms of the cell. At every level of biological activity, there are systems to interrogate, analyze, and decide on the fate of nanoscale objects. The real questions now involve how key material properties of size, shape, and surface may be exquisitely controlled to face this complex cellular interrogation process with the respects it expects and deserves.

4.1.2 Link Between Material Properties and Characterization for Differing Timescales of Biological Interaction

To understand which properties (besides size) are important in determining biological interactions, it is necessary to decide on the timescale under consideration. The understanding of these multiple timescales, and their role, is central to the framing of meaningful scientific investigations. Above all, it is necessary to resolve this question in order to meaningfully "characterize" a nanomaterial. The relevant characteristics are different, depending on the timescale of interest. Our aim here will be to point toward what really needs to be advanced in terms of understanding and the nature of the characterization required in each of these elements.

4.1.2.1 Early Times

By early times, we mean those that determine key outcomes in tissue culture experiments, as well as early *in vivo* phenomena such as liver accumulation, and early immunological responses [43]. Key elements of these outcomes are decided within some hours. Here the key concept is biological recognition of the nanoparticle surface presentation, driven by receptors, whether expressed on the cell or barrier surface, or intracellular. Still, there are likely other aspects of the nanoparticle, in particular we believe its "shape" can also be recognized at early stages, biologically [44]. Less about this aspect is known, at the moment.

To give explicit examples, we believe that when nanoparticles come into contact with a biological milieu they adsorb to some biomolecules from the environment [22,45]. For highly adsorbing surfaces, this leads to a long-lived surface adsorption of biomolecules (See Figure 4.1). Often the inner layer is tightly bound the hard corona with biomolecular timescales of hours, and subsequent ones less so (the soft corona) with exchange times of seconds. These numbers are only guidelines for typical classes of materials [46].

We believe that biological recognition of those adsorbed biomolecules can take place when the residence time exceeds the timescales required for the early stage of receptor-initiated action such as recruitment of membrane machinery (adapter proteins and others), potentially requiring several minutes. This means that often, but perhaps not always, it will be the innermost strongly adsorbed biomolecular layer that will provide the biological identity at early stages of evolution of the nanoparticle that has been internalized by humans or animals [47].

For nanoparticles that have been modified by a low adsorbing polymer (for example PEGylation), to which, potentially an additional ligand has been added for targeting, the situation is potentially more complex [28,48]. The "hard" corona, in this sense of long-lived molecular layer, is then clearly partly composed of the polyethylene glycol, linker and grafting moieties, the grafted ligand, and any residual bare nanoparticle surface accessible. However, it is believed that for many specific designs there is also significant residual biomolecular adsorption and other nonspecific involvement of biomolecules over timescales that

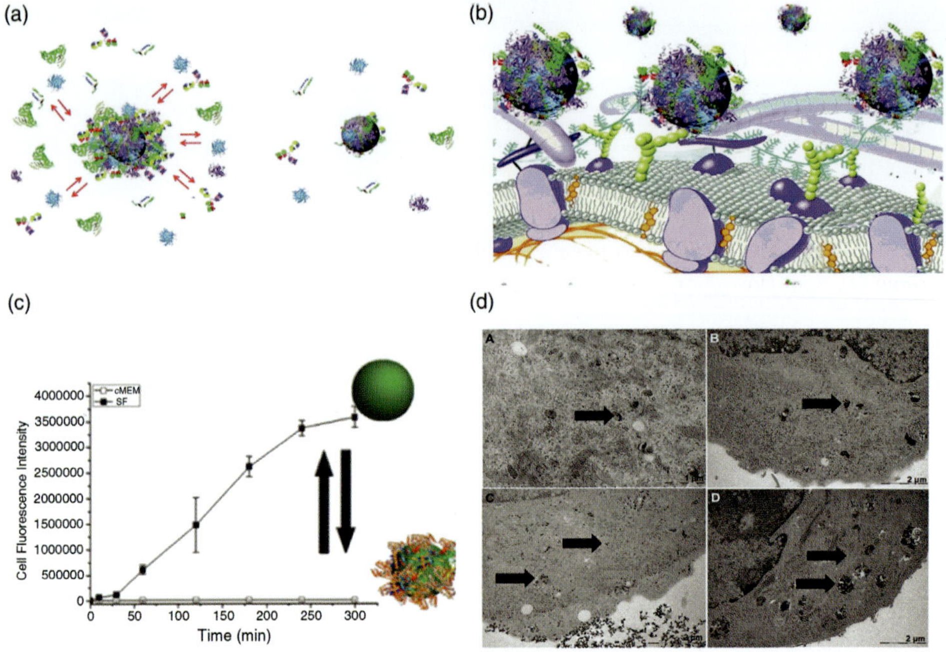

Figure 4.1 (a) Dynamic (soft) and hard corona. (b) It is the nanoparticle–corona complex, rather than the bare nanoparticle, that interacts with biological machinery, here with a cell membrane receptor [45]. (c) Silica nanoparticles exposed to cells in the absence of serum have a stronger adhesion to the cell membrane and higher internalization efficiency, in comparison when a preformed corona is present on their surface. (d) Transmission electron microscopy images of A549 cells exposed to 100 µg/mL 50 nm silica nanoparticles in complete and serum-free medium for 4 h (a and c, respectively) and 24 h (b and d, respectively). The arrows indicate some of the NPs in the cells [37].

could be biologically recognized [49]. This would suggest that the polyethylene glycol, linker, and ligand could all take part in early recognition events, leading to a potentially complex outcome [48,50]. Still, while the situation may be complex, at least we have a well-defined concept of relevant characterization required to understand, and ultimately link to biological outcomes [29]. If we achieve this, we will be able to understand and increasingly control such deeply important topics as nanoscale immunology and nanoparticle biodistributions.

4.1.2.2 **Degradation of Surface**

At intermediate times, the key issues to think about and characterize may be degradation kinetics of the surface layers within lysosomes and phagosomes inside the cell [51,52]. This is the usual role of those organelles and although there is some small possibility for particles to be released from the lysosomes (by processes not yet fully understood) the experience we are building suggests that this intracellular degradation of the surface layer of say biomolecules occurs possibly over many hours and days [53]. Thus, while aspects such as size and shape can continue to exercise a major effect on the biological interactions, a significant element of the biological processing now involves the chemical degradation, or intracellular attempts to do so [54]. It is perhaps sufficient to stress that the degradation pathway leads to both degradative products (needing attention and clarification), and secondary metabolites, but that in addition the actual process of degradation may also have a cellular regulatory effect. In the most extreme cases, of slowed or inappropriate degradative processes, possibly driven by specific anomalous surface chemistries, difficulties in fully degrading the particle could lead to longer term damage, manifested for example in chronic or long-term exposures [55]. Clearly, the key things to characterize here are completely different from the short-term effects. They include the nature of the nanoparticle surface in the degradative environment, the surface degradation chemistry occurring, and the degradative products and rate of production of these. Some very limited progress has been made here, but for those concerned about safety of nanoparticles this is clearly an important issue [56].

4.1.2.3 Long Timescales

Nanoparticles, initially recognized will often be accumulated in the degradative organelles of cells, within which the long-lived coating will be degraded off within some hours. For very slowly degrading (rather than rapidly dissolving) nanoparticles, this then leaves the nanoparticle surface in contact with the multitude of enzymes and other biomolecules in the lysosome or phagosome. The understanding of nanomaterial recognition over much longer times, involving weeks or months (or longer) is very poorly developed, but it will be important for a substantive and durable understanding of nanomaterial safety for non or solely degrading materials. It will require some new ways of thinking, because the organelles involved (e.g., phagosomes and lysosomes) were not designed to, and are only rarely required to, process such resistant nanoscale foreign materials. Tissue culture approaches are not well evolved to accommodate such challenges, and *in vivo* studies rarely share much light on the nature of the mechanisms involved. In general however we now have some perspective in our thinking here. Biological processes are framed to restore themselves to their resting levels, or homeostasis. Thus, if nanoparticles are not successfully degraded, there is the possibility that ongoing biodegradative processes will be closed down, and possibly limited long-term impacts will result. On the contrary, however, should there be residual degradative activity, and processes fail to close down, then there is a significant possibility that they will lead to some form of cellular damage. That may have safety implications. The means to characterize and investigate this require development. Those that will reflect deeply on the future will see this as one of the most challenging, and most necessary activity, because relatively unattended element. We believe that we see how this may be approached, but as we write at this date, little depth has been achieved.

4.1.2.4 Priorities

However, medium- and long-term issues are unlikely to set the immediate and major course of development for nanomedicine achievement. For that we will need to show that we can drive qualitatively new therapeutic outcomes. For that to occur, of most interest are a few arenas where most other technologies have been slow to succeed, but where nanotechnology will. Among the most important of those areas of focus is the concept of therapeutic targeting to specific sites (in organs, tissues, cells), or specific actions within, for example, the immune and other systems. Nanoparticle capacity to target these in a controlled manner will be a defining achievement for our generation, or a later one. For that to occur we will need to more fully master the issue of nanoscale recognition. There is no choice. It will not happen accidently. However, it can be done.

4.2 The Approach to Characterization

By organizing our presentation in this manner, we hope that having clarified the nature of the challenge involved in different contexts and different timescales, we will be able to more clearly focus on the nature of the characterization required. Here, we are seeking to reverse the usual approach. That is, instead of assessing and using the methodologies and instrumental capacities, we currently have, we wish to more strongly highlight what is missing as a means to light the way to the methods and instruments that need to be advanced.

4.2.1 The Nature of Early-Stage Biological Recognition

After a slow start, we are making progress here, and are now at the point that we can begin to understand the overall challenges, as well as specific approaches to address them. We would like to restate the fact that such biological recognition is often driven by receptors located on cells, endothelia, biological barriers, and other locations. It underlies many key aspects from biodistribution, immunological responses, targeting, and other aspects. While there may be exceptional and specific technologies, and treatments that enable us to overcome the biological processes thereby giving access to all compartments, these will be narrowly defined and likely narrowly applied. It is no longer credible to imagine that we can master targeted medicines without mastering recognition [57].

If one accepts those broad conclusions, then the implications are clear. It is difficult to imagine we can either master the principle of targeting or regulate and ultimately market it in products, unless we can characterize it. Thus, as a leading priority, we need methods both to construct (and characterize) more precise organization of biomolecules and for example, the protein epitopes or other functional motifs, on the surfaces of particles [58]. Very simply put, it matters little what is grafted or adsorbed on a nanoparticle surface if it is not presented in a manner useful to be seen by relevant receptors [49].

Some new methods are already emerging that enable us to study those questions. They must go much further, and be applied widely.

4.2.1.1 Epitope and Recognition Motif Mapping

These methods currently rely on the mapping out of recognition motifs based on antibodies, in a manner rather similar to immune gold or immunofluorescence mapping of proteins. They can be considerably advanced by paring down the recognition motif to make it more compact, and use of more advanced labeling strategies.

Crucially however, they all now seem to point to the same fundamental point. Unlike protein molecules, which are essentially identical to each other, different nanoparticles made by current approaches have very different organizations, even within the same sample. The biological recognition of those differences we believe underlies many subtle and complex differences in the biology observed. While some degree of variation between particles may even be of some value in medicines, at the moment it is entirely uncontrolled and uncharacterized. This cannot lead to long-term success. Indeed, early results that are emerging from them suggest that many current ligation strategies may simply be wholly inadequate. Our informal explorations, while far from general, suggest that current fabrications can lead the great majority of nominally functional targeting agents to be so poorly disposed and oriented as to be unavailable for purpose. Indeed, while it is still not established, and certainly not yet a universally held view, we are beginning to form an opinion that even relatively conventional formulations of targeted nanomedicines (which have nearly universally failed to reach the market) have not been given a fair chance to succeed. Succinctly put, they have been undermined by the execution, rather than the concept. The outcome of this discussion as it evolves could have profound implications for our perceptions of how successful nanotechnology is, or can be, in delivering therapeutics (Figure 4.2).

4.2.1.2 Forces, Dynamics, and Other Processes at Bio-Nano interface

While we have sought to lay out concepts and not focus on details, it is worth commenting on directions of implementation of these ideas using different technologies. This is much to be encouraged, and it should be done so in the context of what is actually required, rather than what is incrementally possible. The examples we give here are not yet fully evolved, and by no means are they sufficient. They merely illustrate arenas where we seek (and are now beginning to get) precise and detailed (e.g., interaction) data, rather than generic average properties. They make contact with the concepts of biology, rather than only broad characterization.

For instance, promising directions suggest that it will be possible to apply ultrasensitive oscillators (advanced from conventional quartz crystal microbalance, QCM) to measure the biophysicochemical interactions of nanoparticles

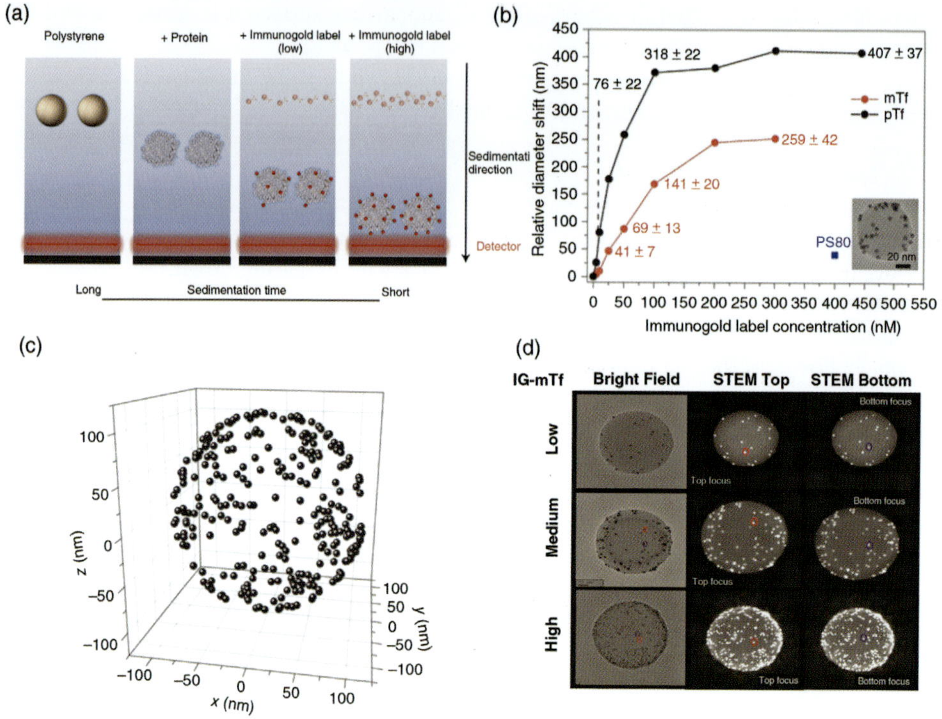

Figure 4.2 (a) Schematic representation of the use of DCS to measure immunogold labeling. The addition of proteins or immunogold labels increases the net density and hydrodynamic radius of the particles. The net effect for the polystyrene nanoparticles is a reduction in the sedimentation time in a disc centrifuge, causing them to reach the detector faster. (b) Transferrin protein (Tf) was adsorbed onto 200 nm polystyrene particles, appropriate monoclonal antibodies (for an epitope proximate to the transferrin receptor-binding region) and polyclonal antibodies were adsorbed onto 5 nm gold nanoparticles. The immunogold labels has been titrated against the transferrin-coated polystyrene particles and observed the change in size of the complex using differential centrifugal sedimentation (DCS). (c) Three-dimensional reconstruction of immunogold label positions on a 200 nm transferring-coated nanoparticle. (d) Bright field images and STEM images of 200 nm transferring-coated nanoparticles with different amounts of immunogold labels (low, medium, and high) [58].

and biomolecules, and nanoparticles with cell receptors, and determine the amount of various substances in individual nanoparticles. Furthermore, light trapping enable to measure forces within narrow channels for even small nanoparticles. Crucially, these all give detailed microscopic information, relevant to biological interactions, not just a general form of characterization.

QCM is a very sensitive technology for measuring surface properties, capable to detect changes in mass at a molecular level. It has long been one of the most effective instruments for determining binding affinity of molecules. As a molecule flows over the quartz crystal and is recognized by compounds functionalized on the surface, the crystal vibration energy changes. This change can be used to characterize real time, label free interactions between molecules. Now not only various biomolecules, but also intact cells have been immobilized on QCM sensor surface, which allows a direct and quantitative measurement of nanoparticle–cell interactions in a biologically relevant milieu. In particular, the possibility to flow particles through a microfluidic system in contact with the sensor surface make this system closer to the *in vivo* scenario, in a physiologically relevant environment (Figure 4.3) [59,60].

Other very sensitive systems of detection such as MEMS (micro electromechanical systems) sensor can be used to characterize nanoparticles and their interactions. In this case, a minute cantilever that resonates with a particular frequency is used. Once again a microfluidic system is used to push the sample through a channel embedded in the cantilever. The measure of a shift in the frequency of resonance, via a laser focused on the tip of the cantilever, gives an accurate and precise measurement of the particle's buoyant mass in the sample

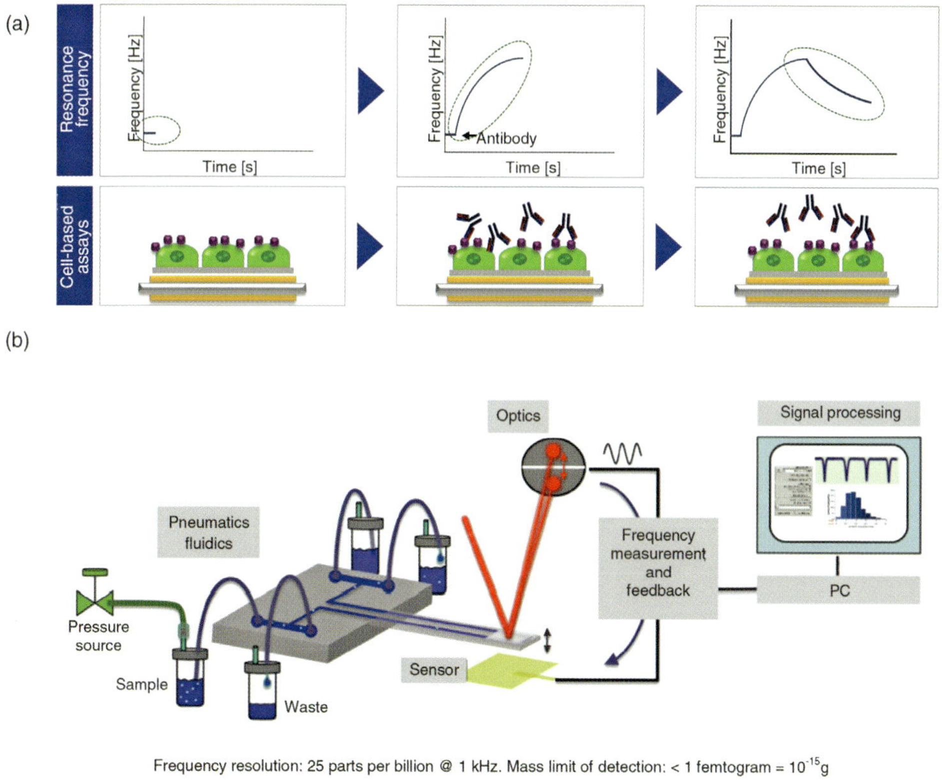

Figure 4.3 (a) Scheme of the binding curves related to recognition of receptors on the cell surface in flow by quartz crystal microbalance. (b) Scheme of resonant mass measurement instrument setup.

– whether positive or negative [61]. Such approaches will allow us to really measure how much of a substance is on a particle surface, rather than the averaged measurements made today.

Also light trapping opens the way to novel particle characterization possibilities including even the ability to obtain relevant interactions of single NPs. Near-field light scattering (NLS) is an emerging technique used to measure nanoparticle surface properties that came about because of a limitation in zeta potential instruments that can only measure in the electrostatic regime. NLS, on the other hand directly measures all interfacial forces combining two established techniques, optical tweezing and total internal reflection microscopy (TIRM) [62,63]. In optical tweezing, a waveguide (WG) transports the light from a laser source through the experimental chamber and the propagated light generates an exponentially decaying field (evanescent field) that extends above the WG. When a NP passes close to the WG, it is trapped by an optical force that is a result of the sharp gradient in the light intensity. This trapping force pulls the NPs toward the surface of the WG and together with the repulsive interaction of the NPs with the surface of the WG creates a potential well in the z direction (Figure 4.4a). The closer is the NPs to the WG the more light it will scatter (as the light intensity decays from the WG to the medium) and this effect is used to measure the fluctuations (generated by the Brownian motion) around the minimum of the potential well. Using TIRM physics, the images of the particle over the course of a few seconds can be transformed to quantitatively reveal a particle's repulsive interaction with the surface [64]. From this, a histogram of the distances allows to measure the total force of the NP as a function of its separation to the WG. Strongly stabilized particles with good steric coatings will have stronger surface repulsion (Figure 4.4b). Though this technique is still very new, it has promise for carrying out accurate measurements in the relevant biological media adding real insight into the interactions there [65,66].

No such individual tools will alone satisfy the need. Many are required to evolve a deeper understanding of the microscopic details. But such example illustrates that evolution in the thinking is occurring, and that real progress toward delivery of the tools is occurring albeit later in the evolution of the field than desirable, and on a narrower bandwidth than is required for such a strategic arena. Still, innovative and dynamic thinking is emerging, and allowing us to highlight what is needed, and what is feasible.

4.2.2
The Nature of the Intracellular Bio-Nano Interface

We have stressed a lot the need to understand and characterize the biointerface outside cells. The reason is clear, and will remain the urgent priority in gaining the most basic control of biological interactions for targeting. While less clear, and much less discussed and advanced, the future will bring increasing focus on the nature of the intracellular bio-nano interface. The simplest considerations already suggest how some, but not necessarily all of the adsorbed interfacial

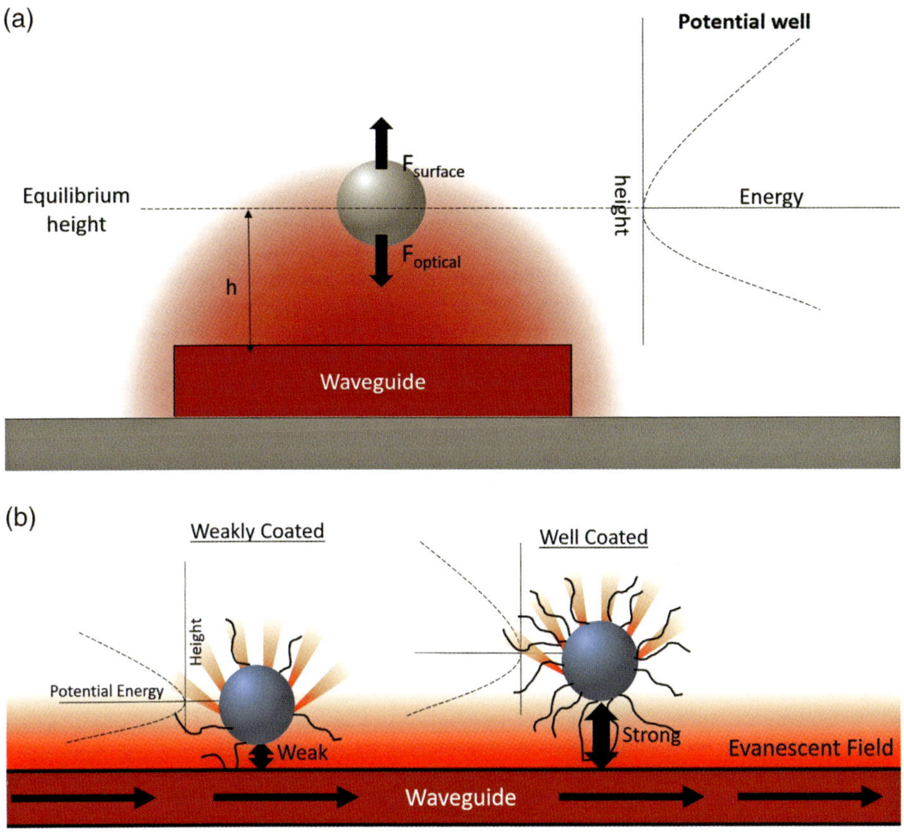

Figure 4.4 (a) Particles flowing in solution are captured by the optical field in the vicinity of the waveguide and the repulsive interaction of the NPs with the surface of the WG creates a potential well in the *z* direction. (b) The particles interact with the surface with different strength depending on their coating and surface properties.

components are carried far into the cell, continuing to define the intracellular interactions. Indeed there are also key interactions relevant in the degradative organelle, involving understanding both the physical interface as well as the chemistry at the interface as the degradative processes progress [51].

These are wholly new arenas of science, of deep value and significance to the creation of a real and durable field of bionanoscience. Fortunately, our job as teachers and motivators of those that follow will unfold naturally. The beauty and importance of the questions will inspire future generations of outstanding scientists to master them. They will build new conceptions of the intracellular nanomaterial–biological interface in much the same way as the twentieth century brought materials surface science from a primitive arena to one that today allows billions of tiny engineered surface features to drive our computers and mobile phones.

4.2.3
The Future of the Bio-Nano Interface, Bionanoscience, and Nanomedicine

The conclusion that fundamental bio-nano interface science is the key to bionanoscience, and that those are key to nanomedicine could perhaps even now be seen as an overstatement. However, if the past decade has taught us anything, it suggests at least that this is the direction our understanding is taking. Perhaps the most complex issue here is not science. While the science that needs to be done is deeply challenging, it is feasible, truly innovative, and will excite and inspire a new generation of scientists, who will be realistic and focused.

If one seeks a broader assessment, the challenges we face in developing this field are complex mixtures of science, technology, policy, and community. We have hitherto been at too early a stage of development for an easy and simple unity of opinion to drive the research agenda, though perhaps now one can see that begin to emerge. Until more recently, there has been an opinion that nanosciences and nanotechnology would lead rapidly, naturally almost effortlessly to many discoveries, cures, and advances. In fact, this was never highly likely if one considers that we are bringing together two formerly disjoint universes, biological processing of living organisms, and the engineered nanoscale together, the former having highly regulated and highly monitored active processes. It is perhaps more clear now, as we recognize that we are not engaged in fortuitous discovery of many new analogous of wonder drugs such as penicillin, but in the deeply disciplined and focused carving out of knowledge that allows us to control biological processes in radically new ways. Only now, perhaps is it possible to appreciate just how strategic is the knowledge, depth, and capacity to control these phenomena.

These conclusions are deeply important for communities, young researchers, and planners, for they suggest the shape of opportunity to come. For those less deeply involved in the science, the analogy with the valve semiconductor and the road to the computer chip is likely the key to understanding the future in this arena. There will be (very important) exceptions, but that is the central message.

Teachers and experienced researchers, though they will need to have the courage to remain firm and constant in vision, will have little trouble in explaining these issues to a new generation of scientists, for the science will speak for itself and they will judge for themselves. The best will conclude correctly, and this independent assessment will strengthen them as they face the real scientific challenges of the future. Still, young researchers may have to try harder to overcome the consequences of early promises, and the sense of a maturing era of "bonanza." They will need confidence to convince sponsors and funders that the best has yet to come, and that they now have the measure of the challenge, and the fidelity and drive to succeed. Policy makers and sponsors, having heard confusing signals, will face the most difficult challenges for being removed from direct experience of the phenomena; they will still have to interpret the messages. They will require courage and deeply balanced judgment to understand the complexity of the environment, both scientific and cultural, and remain confident. Some may be the unsung heroes of future success, for in their absence focused effort will be dramatically slowed, and confusion intervenes.

In science, though, we now begin to see the growth of interest in real depth of our understanding, substantive science, and the recognition of the power this confers. It is true that we see that it is hard work to mine such understanding. Such achievement is torn out of the unyielding rock of inviolable and immensely discerning biological law governing living processes, and requires that we bend our capacity to engineer the nanoscale to that need, for that law will not bend its will to casual exploration.

But now with the experience to be able to measure these events, we also know, with a confidence born of real insight, and achievement that nanoscience and nanotechnology will deliver on its promise. Of that, we have no doubt.

References

1 Jiang, J., Oberdörster, G., and Biswas, P. (2009) Characterization of size, surface charge, and agglomeration state of nanoparticle dispersions for toxicological studies. *J. Nanopart. Res.*, **11** (1), 77–89.

2 Domingos, R.F. *et al.* (2009) Characterizing manufactured nanoparticles in the environment: multimethod determination of particle sizes. *Environ. Sci. Technol.*, **43** (19), 7277–7284.

3 Murdock, R.C. *et al.* (2008) Characterization of nanomaterial dispersion in solution prior to *in vitro* exposure using dynamic light scattering technique. *Toxicol. Sci.*, **101** (2), 239–253.

4 Blanco, E., Shen, H., and Ferrari, M. (2015) Principles of nanoparticle design for overcoming biological barriers to drug delivery. *Nat. Biotechnol.*, **33** (9), 941–951.

5 Chou, L.Y., Ming, K., and Chan, W.C. (2011) Strategies for the intracellular delivery of nanoparticles. *Chem. Soc. Rev.*, **40** (1), 233–245.

6 Mitragotri, S., Burke, P.A., and Langer, R. (2014) Overcoming the challenges in administering biopharmaceuticals: formulation and delivery strategies. *Nat. Rev. Drug Discov.*, **13** (9), 655–672.

7 Albanese, A., Tang, P.S., and Chan, W.C. (2012) The effect of nanoparticle size, shape, and surface chemistry on biological systems. *Annu. Rev. Biomed. Eng.*, **14**, 1–16.

8 Mitragotri, S. *et al.* (2015) Accelerating the Translation of Nanomaterials in Biomedicine. *ACS Nano*, **9** (7), 6644–6654.

9 Chain, E. (1979) The early years of the penicillin discovery. *Trends Pharmacol. Sci.*, **1** (1), 6–11.

10 Lundskog, A. *et al.* (2014) Direct generation of linearly polarized photon emission with designated orientations from site-controlled InGaN quantum dots. *Light Sci. Appl.*, **3**, e139.

11 Roh, D.K. *et al.* (2014) High efficiency solid-state dye-sensitized solar cells assembled with hierarchical anatase pine tree-like TiO_2 nanotubes. *Adv. Funct. Mater.*, **24** (3), 379–386.

12 Duan, X. *et al.* (2003) High-performance thin-film transistors using semiconductor nanowires and nanoribbons. *Nature*, **425** (6955), 274–278.

13 Ponce, F. and Bour, D. (1997) Nitride-based semiconductors for blue and green light-emitting devices. *Nature*, **386**, 351–359.

14 Grätzel, M. (2001) Photoelectrochemical cells. *Nature*, **414** (6861), 338–344.

15 Brongersma, M.L., Cui, Y., and Fan, S. (2014) Light management for photovoltaics using high-index nanostructures. *Nat. Mater.*, **13** (5), 451–460.

16 Malinkiewicz, O. *et al.* (2014) Perovskite solar cells employing organic charge-transport layers. *Nat. Photon.*, **8** (2), 128–132.

17 Hassellöv, M. *et al.* (2008) Nanoparticle analysis and characterization methodologies in environmental risk assessment of engineered nanoparticles. *Ecotoxicology*, **17** (5), 344–361.

18 Powers, K.W. *et al.* (2007) Characterization of the size, shape, and state of dispersion of nanoparticles for toxicological studies. *Nanotoxicology*, **1** (1), 42–51.

19 Lynch, I., Weiss, C., and Valsami-Jones, E. (2014) A strategy for grouping of nanomaterials based on key physico-chemical descriptors as a basis for safer-by-design NMs. *Nano Today*, **9** (3), 266–270.

20 Fadeel, B. *et al.* (2013) Bridge over troubled waters: understanding the synthetic and biological identities of engineered nanomaterials. *Wiley Interdiscip. Rev. Nanomed. Nanobiotechnol.*, **5** (2), 111–129.

21 Lundqvist, M. *et al.* (2008) Nanoparticle size and surface properties determine the protein corona with possible implications for biological impacts. *Proc. Natl. Acad. Sci.*, **105** (38), 14265–14270.

22 Monopoli, M.P. *et al.* (2012) Biomolecular coronas provide the biological identity of nanosized materials. *Nat. Nanotech.*, **7** (12), 779–786.

23 Dobrovolskaia, M.A. and McNeil, S.E. (2007) Immunological properties of engineered nanomaterials. *Nat. Nanotech.*, **2** (8), 469–478.

24 Dobrovolskaia, M.A., Germolec, D.R., and Weaver, J.L. (2009) Evaluation of nanoparticle immunotoxicity. *Nat. Nanotech.*, **4** (7), 411–414.

25 Black, K.C.L. *et al.* (2014) Radioactive 198Au-doped nanostructures with different shapes for *in vivo* analyses of their biodistribution, tumor uptake, and intratumoral distribution. *ACS Nano*, **8** (5), 4385–4394.

26 Dreaden, E.C. *et al.* (2012) Size matters: gold nanoparticles in targeted cancer drug delivery. *Ther. Deliv.*, **3** (4), 457–478.

27 Jiang, Y. *et al.* (2015) The Interplay of size and surface functionality on the cellular uptake of sub-10 nm gold nanoparticles. *ACS Nano*, **9** (10), 9986–9993.

28 Walkey, C.D. *et al.* (2012) Nanoparticle size and surface chemistry determine serum protein adsorption and macrophage uptake. *J. Am. Chem. Soc.*, **134** (4), 2139–2147.

29 Hristov, D.R. *et al.* (2015) Tuning of nanoparticle biological functionality through controlled surface chemistry and characterisation at the bioconjugated nanoparticle surface. *Scientific Rep.*, **5**, 17040.

30 Ferrari, M. (2005) Cancer nanotechnology: opportunities and challenges. *Nat. Rev. Cancer*, **5** (3), 161–171.

31 Shao, K. *et al.* (2015) Nanoparticle-based immunotherapy for cancer. *ACS Nano*, **9** (1), 16–30.

32 Ghosh, P. *et al.* (2010) Intracellular delivery of a membrane-impermeable enzyme in active form using functionalized gold nanoparticles. *J. Am. Chem. Soc.*, **132** (8), 2642–2645.

33 Jiang, W. *et al.* (2008) Nanoparticle-mediated cellular response is size-dependent. *Nat. Nanotech.*, **3** (3), 145–150.

34 Sandin, P. *et al.* (2012) High-speed imaging of Rab family small GTPases reveals rare events in nanoparticle trafficking in living cells. *ACS Nano*, **6** (2), 1513–1521.

35 dos Santos, T. *et al.* (2011) Quantitative assessment of the comparative nanoparticle-uptake efficiency of a range of cell lines. *Small*, **7** (23), 3341–3349.

36 Kim, J.A. *et al.* (2012) Role of cell cycle on the cellular uptake and dilution of nanoparticles in a cell population. *Nat. Nanotech.*, **7** (1), 62–68.

37 Lesniak, A. *et al.* (2012) Effects of the presence or absence of a protein corona on silica nanoparticle uptake and impact on cells. *ACS Nano*, **6** (7), 5845–5857.

38 Erickson, H.P. (2009) Size and shape of protein molecules at the nanometer level determined by sedimentation, gel filtration, and electron microscopy. *Biol. Proced. Online*, **11** (1), 32.

39 Huang, K. *et al.* (2012) Size-dependent localization and penetration of ultrasmall gold nanoparticles in cancer cells, multicellular spheroids, and tumors *in vivo*. *ACS Nano*, **6** (5), 4483–4493.

40 Zhang, S., Gao, H., and Bao, G. (2015) Physical principles of nanoparticle cellular endocytosis. *ACS Nano*, **9** (9), 8655–8671.
41 Mahmoudi, M. *et al.* (2011) Protein–nanoparticle interactions: opportunities and challenges. *Chem. Rev.*, **111** (9), 5610–5637.
42 Nel, A.E. *et al.* (2009) Understanding biophysicochemical interactions at the nano–bio interface. *Nat. Mater.*, **8** (7), 543–557.
43 Tenzer, S. *et al.* (2013) Rapid formation of plasma protein corona critically affects nanoparticle pathophysiology. *Nat. Nanotech.*, **8** (10), 772–781.
44 Hamad-Schifferli, K. (2015) Exploiting the novel properties of protein coronas: emerging applications in nanomedicine. *Nanomedicine*, **10** (10), 1663–1674.
45 Walczyk, D. *et al.* (2010) What the cell "sees" in bionanoscience. *J. Am. Chem. Soc.*, **132** (16), 5761–5768.
46 Monopoli, M.P. *et al.* (2011) Physical–chemical aspects of protein corona: relevance to *in vitro* and *in vivo* biological impacts of nanoparticles. *J. Am. Chem. Soc.*, **133** (8), 2525–2534.
47 Walkey, C.D. *et al.* (2014) Protein corona fingerprinting predicts the cellular interaction of gold and silver nanoparticles. *ACS Nano*, **8** (3), 2439–2455.
48 Schottler, S. *et al.* (2016) Protein adsorption is required for stealth effect of poly(ethylene glycol)- and poly (phosphoester)-coated nanocarriers. *Nat. Nanotech.*, **11** (4), 372–377.
49 Salvati, A. *et al.* (2013) Transferrin-functionalized nanoparticles lose their targeting capabilities when a biomolecule corona adsorbs on the surface. *Nat. Nanotech.*, **8** (2), 137–143.
50 Verhoef, J.J. *et al.* (2014) Potential induction of anti-PEG antibodies and complement activation toward PEGylated therapeutics. *Drug Discov. Today*, **19** (12), 1945–1952.
51 Bertoli, F. *et al.* (2014) Magnetic nanoparticles to recover cellular organelles and study the time resolved nanoparticle-cell interactome throughout uptake. *Small*, **10** (16), 3307–3315.
52 Hofmann, D. *et al.* (2014) Mass spectrometry and imaging analysis of nanoparticle-containing vesicles provide a mechanistic insight into cellular trafficking. *ACS Nano*, **8** (10), 10077–10088.
53 Stern, S.T., Adiseshaiah, P.P., and Crist, R.M. (2012) Autophagy and lysosomal dysfunction as emerging mechanisms of nanomaterial toxicity. *Part. Fibre Toxicol.*, **9** (1), 1–17.
54 Sabella, S. *et al.* (2014) A general mechanism for intracellular toxicity of metal-containing nanoparticles. *Nanoscale*, **6** (12), 7052–7061.
55 Donaldson, K. *et al.* (2010) Asbestos, carbon nanotubes and the pleural mesothelium: a review of the hypothesis regarding the role of long fibre retention in the parietal pleura, inflammation and mesothelioma. *Part. Fibre Toxicol.*, **7** (1), 1–17.
56 Soenen, S.J. *et al.* (2011) Cellular toxicity of inorganic nanoparticles: common aspects and guidelines for improved nanotoxicity evaluation. *Nano Today*, **6** (5), 446–465.
57 Mahon, E. *et al.* (2012) Designing the nanoparticle–biomolecule interface for "targeting and therapeutic delivery". *J. Control. Release*, **161** (2), 164–174.
58 Kelly, P.M. *et al.* (2015) Mapping protein binding sites on the biomolecular corona of nanoparticles. *Nat. Nanotech.*, **10** (5), 472–479.
59 Elmlund, L. *et al.* (2015) Study of the interaction of trastuzumab and SKOV3 epithelial cancer cells using a quartz crystal microbalance sensor. *Sensors*, **15** (3), 5884–5894.
60 Li, X. *et al.* (2015) Real-time and label-free analysis of binding thermodynamics of carbohydrate-protein interactions on unfixed cancer cell surfaces using a QCM biosensor. *Scientific Rep.*, **5**, 14066.
61 Weinbuch, D. *et al.* (2013) Micro-flow imaging and resonant mass measurement (archimedes) – complementary methods to quantitatively differentiate protein particles and silicone oil droplets. *J. Pharm. Sci.*, **102** (7), 2152–2165.
62 Mandal, S., Serey, X., and Erickson, D. (2009) Nanomanipulation using silicon photonic crystal resonators. *Nano Lett.*, **10** (1), 99–104.

63 Prieve, D.C. (1999) Measurement of colloidal forces with TIRM. *Adv. Colloid Interface Sci.*, **82** (1), 93–125.
64 Schein, P. *et al.* (2015) Nanophotonic force microscopy: characterizing particle–surface interactions using near-field photonics. *Nano Lett.*, **15** (2), 1414–1420.
65 Chen, Y.-F. *et al.* (2012) Controlled photonic manipulation of proteins and other nanomaterials. *Nano Lett.*, **12** (3), 1633–1637.
66 Yang, A.H. *et al.* (2009) Optical manipulation of nanoparticles and biomolecules in sub-wavelength slot waveguides. *Nature*, **457** (7225), 71–75.

5
Omics-Based Nanopharmacy: Powerful Tools Toward Precision Medicine

Daniel Rosenblum[1,2,3] *and Dan Peer*[1,2,3]

[1]*Tel Aviv University, George S. Wise Faculty of Life Sciences, Department of Cell Research and Immunology, Laboratory of NanoMedicine, Tel Aviv 69978, Israel*
[2]*Department of Materials Science and Engineering, The Iby and Aladar Fleischman Faculty of Engineering*
[3]*Tel Aviv University, Center for Nanoscience and Nanotechnology, Tel Aviv 69978, Israel*

5.1
Introduction

Cancer is still the second major cause of mortality in the United States [1] with around 1.6 million new cases in average per year [2]. The traditional cancer therapy, which involves surgery, radiation with or without chemotherapy, has some success in certain types of cancers; however, the heterogeneity between patients, and within a particular tumor, limits the success of common therapeutic approaches. Most of these therapeutic interventions lack specificity and thus majority of the anticancer drugs, as an example, can induce substantial side effects. In addition, when treatment fails or when relapse occurs, the absence of sustaining therapeutic modalities feedback slows down the decision making to change the strategy [3]. In the post genomic era, the growing knowledge and understanding of the human genome, epigenome, transcriptome, proteome, metabolome, and more recently the microbiome has led to the discovery of numerous biomarkers that can be used to detect early-stage cancers and to predict the disease progression, response, and clinical outcome [4].

Clinical bioinformatics and genome/xeome/transcriptome analysis are applied to guide the modern physicians to personalized the treatment and prescribe the appropriate drug(s) available from the arsenal of drugs to an individual at the appropriate timing. For instance, the dose of chemotherapeutic drugs given to patients is calculated based on the patient's body weight and surface area and often causing small to severe adverse effects. Novel understanding of metabolites (via metabolomics) on the position of drug-metabolizing enzymes could substantially improve the therapeutic outcome by manipulating the drug-dosing regime. Recent clinical data demonstrates that small changes in

Pharmaceutical Nanotechnology: Innovation and Production, First Edition. Edited by Jean Cornier, Arno Kwade, Andrew Owen, and Marcel Van de Voorde.

chemotherapeutic concentrations can make the difference between substantial tumor regression and intolerable adverse effects [5].

Novel therapeutics applying nanotechnology (defined here as nanoparticles of various shape, size, and made from various materials) encapsulating therapeutic payloads investigated for the last 20 years with more than 30 "nanodrugs" approved for clinical use and more than 300 under clinical investigation [6] are collectively termed in this chapter as nanopharmacy (NP).

Nanopharamcy, holds great promise for revolutionizing disease management with improve therapeutic outcome by maximizing the therapeutic effect and minimizing adverse effects [7,8].

Several lipid-based- and protein-based nanopharmacy are already clinically approved for clinical use in oncology (e.g., DOXIL™, Abraxne™, and Marqibo™, to name a few) and numerous products are under clinical evaluation [9,10]. Two of the more promising startegies currently in clinical trials are ALN-VSP and NK105. ALN-VSP is a SNALP (stable lipid–nucleic acid particle) [7] formulated with siRNAs targeting VEGF and kinesin spindle protein (KSP). ALN-VSP was recently reported to accomplish phase I clinical trial in patients with VEGF-overexpressing tumors (i.e., renal cell carcinoma (RCC), endometrial cancer, and angiosarcoma) [11]. The second nanocarrier NK105 is a paclitaxel-incorporating "core–shell-type" polymeric micellar formulation. NK105 was recently entered phase III clinical trials for the treatment of previously treated, advanced, or recurrent gastric cancer after successful phase II with overall response rates of 25% and mild toxicity [12].

Personalized medicine has the power of using NP in combination with molecular biomarkers ("OMICS" data) achieving improve prognosis and disease management as well as individualized drug selection and dosage profiling (pharmacotyping) to ensure maximal efficacy and safety [7]. Moreover, using NP with tumor biomarkers and pharmacotyping enables to generate multifunctional drug carriers containing targeting, therapeutic, and diagnostic moieties, which are tailor-made to specific individual [6,7]. These multifunctional NP can be guided and accumulated to disease-specific tissues or subpopulation of cells, for example, through conjugation with an appropriate antibody or natural ligand, thus increasing the effective dose of the drug at tumor site as well as accumulating an imaging agent for theranostic purposes.

5.2 Precision Medicine

Precision (also known as "personalized") medicine aims to individualize therapeutic interventions, based on *ex vivo*-obtained OMICS information (such as genomics, proteomics, lipidomics, and metabolomics) profiling together with *in vivo* imaging insights on the type, the stage, and the grade of the disease, as well as on the potential response of a particular patient to a specific treatment [13]. With next-generation sequencing (NGS) technologies, it is now possible to identify almost the majority of germline variants of an individual in an affordable cost and thus paving the path to clinicians to provide healthcare from an individual perspective [14].

5.2.1 Precision Oncology

The fast-growing knowledge of molecular understanding of the leading mutations that may result in transformation from a normal cell into cancerous cell and identification of tumor- specific biomarkers has been mostly contributed by large-scale "OMICS" strategies, paving the way for the development of pathway-specific drugs and novel molecular diagnostics [15–17]. More than twenty pathway-specific drugs are already clinically approved for use in breast cancer, some hematological malignancies, ovarian and colon cancers, few prominent examples of such drugs and their current use in precision cancer care will be discussed in this chapter. These pathway-specific drugs could generally be categorized into two major groups: The first group consists mainly on therapeutic monoclonal antibodies (mAbs), which could target an overexpressed or specific receptors on tumor cells and subsequently mediate cytotoxicity via antibody-dependent cell cytotoxicity (ADCC), complement-dependent cytotoxicity (CDC) mechanisms or by carrying a toxic factor (e.g., radioisotope, toxin, or small-molecule chemotherapeutic agent). The second group is small-molecules inhibitors, which specifically inhibit receptor signaling pathways or intracellular enzymatic activity and thus promoting apoptosis in the target tumor cells.

5.2.2 Therapeutic mAbs

From the generation of the first hybridoma by Milstein and co-workers and the first publication in 1975 till the approval of the first mAb in 1997 for B cell malignancies (anti-CD20 mAb, Rituxan®), vast activity has been documented both in pharmaceutical companies and in the academic world. Below we are reviewing several examples that have been well documented.

Human epidermal growth factor receptor 2 (HER2) is a tyrosine kinase receptor that is overexpressed in approximately 15–25% of primary human breast cancers, and is associated with poor clinical outcomes and aggressive tumor progression. The first commercially available HER 2 targeting agent was the monoclonal antibody trastuzumab (Herceptin®). The use of Herceptin® in combination with chemotherapy or as monotherapy for patients with metastatic disease or early-stage disease has proven to improve survival for patients with breast cancer overexpressing HER2. Several new targeting agents for $HER2^+$ breast tumors are under clinical evaluation, for example, MM-302 is a liposomal nanoscale carrier encapsulating doxorubicin (DOX) and conjugated to single-chain variable fragments (*scFv*) that target HER2-overexpressing cancer cells. The use of this nanocarrier attempting to limit off target toxicity to nonmalignant cells and reduce adverse effects. MM-302 is currently under phase II study evaluation in patients with HER-2 positive metastatic breast cancer after finishing a promising phase I clinical trial [18].

Colorectal cancer (CRC) is the third most common malignancy in both men and women and the fourth leading cause of cancer deaths, with over 1.2 million new cases and approximately 600 000 deaths annually worldwide [19]. Although CRC is highly manageable if diagnosed and surgically removed at early stages, the 5-year survival rate is under 10% in patients with metastatic disease [20]. Epidermal growth factor receptor (EGFR) has been found to be overexpressed in many solid tumors including CRC, therefore making it a substantial target for cancer therapy [21]. Two anti-EGFR antibodies have been approved for clinical use in metastatic CRC cetuximab (Erbitux®) and panitumumab (Vectibix®). Initially, when anti-EGFR antibodies were introduced to clinical practice, there was scarce knowledge on the molecular mechanism of action and of tumor resistance to these targeted compounds. Thus, when only 10–20% of randomly selected CRC patients responded to these anti-EGFR antibodies there was an urgent need to further understand the molecular basis of tumor resistance [22]. Later on, it has been demonstrated that mutations in Kirsten RAS (KRAS) and V-raf murine sarcoma viral oncogene homolog B1 (BRAF) in the EGFR pathway may confer resistance in CRC patients [22,23]. Colorectal tumors that absence the mutations in KRAS or BRAF display high sensitivity to cetuximab and panitumumab. Therefore, these selected patients are the most favorable for anti-EGFR therapy. However, although KRAS and BRAF seem as good negative predictive factors, these markers still remain unable to completely identify patients who will response to this therapy and the use of whole genome expression signatures might be beneficial for further characterization of more predictive biomarkers.

5.2.3
Therapeutic Small-Molecules Inhibitors

BRCA1 and BRCA2 are tumor suppressor proteins playing a key role in DNA repair through the homologous recombination (HR) mechanism. Germ-line mutations of BRCA1 and BRCA2 are fundamental defects in hereditary breast and ovarian cancers [24,25]. While HR mechanism can restore double-strand breaks precisely, other DNA repair mechanisms such as Base Excision Repair (BER) are insufficient for complete DNA repair, resulting in multiple genetic aberrations. Poly-ADP-ribose polymerase (PARP) is a family of enzymes essential for BER. When HR-defective cells (i.e., BRCA1/2-mutated breast or ovarian cancer cells) are treated with PARP inhibitors, the dual inhibition of these two DNA repairing mechanisms leads to "synthetic lethality" [24], resulting in the generation of unfixed DNA single- and double-strand breaks, collapsed replication forks and eventually to apoptosis [26]. Several PARP inhibitors are currently under different stages of clinical evaluation for patients with BRCA1/2 aberrations. Iniparib is a PARP 1 inhibitor currently under phase III clinical evaluations after concluding an open-label, phase II study on triple negative breast cancer patients. The addition of Iniparib to gemcitabine and carboplatin chemotherapy prolonged the median progression-free survival from 3.6 months to 5.9 months and the median overall survival from 7.7 months to 12.3 months [27].

5.2.4 Chimeric Antigen Receptors (CARs)

An emerging technology addressing personalized therapy is the chimeric antigen receptors (CARs) startegy. CAR is a technology for reprogramming autologous T-cell specificity and function toward tumor-associated antigens [28]. CARs are hybrid receptors comprising of a targeting ligand for a cell-surface molecule, the targeting moiety mostly consisting of a specific humanized scFv or a fragment antigen-binding (Fab) fused to one (first-generation CARs) or multiple (second or third generations) costimulatory or activating signaling endodomains (i.e., CD28, OX40, and 41BB) assembled to reprogram T-cell function [29,30]. The introduction of CARs to T cells provides them with a new specificity that is independent of the major histocompatibility complex (MHC) antigen – presenting context and do so without interrupting with the endogenous activity. Furthermore, due to its intrinsic costimulation activity, CARs do not compete with endogenous TCR–CD3 complex interaction, which is usually the rate-limiting step during TCR activation [31]. CARs have successfully been generated against a large number of cell surface determinants, including CD19 (which is the most advanced in the clinic), HER2, Disialoganglioside GD2, and Prostate-specific membrane antigen (PSMA) [28]. CARs are currently evaluated in approximately 25 phases 1/2 clinical studies for various malignancies, for example, CD19-specific and CD20-specific CARs for treating B-cell malignancies (i.e., follicular lymphoma, chronic lymphocytic leukemia (CLL), B-acute lymphoblastic leukemia, and many more) [www.clinicaltrials.gov]. One example of such a trial was recently conducted in the National Cancer Institute (NCI) evaluated the efficacy of CD19 CARs on seven patients, four with CLL, three with follicular lymphoma, and one with marginal zone lymphoma [32]. This study reported on one patient with a complete response, one with stable disease, and the remaining evaluable patients achieved partial responses. In addition, four of the seven patients treated with the CAR-modified T cells exhibited B-cell aplasia. However, several safety issues should be taken under consideration. The potential of the introduced promoter and the transgene cDNA that might cause genotoxicity and therefore the risk of cell transformation. Furthermore, CARs can potentially exhibits toxic effects by damaging normal tissues, mainly due to the fact that most CARs targets may also be expressed on the cell surface of normal cells or after tumor evolution might not be expressed on tumor cells after a certain time.

A sudden death of a patient at the NCI who received autologous HER2-specific T cells expressing a third-generation CAR along with IL2 is attributed to diminishing of normal lung cells expressing a low level of HER2. To address this issue, several methods of coexpression of CARs together with conditional viral or human suicide genes have been proposed (i.e., Herpes simplex virus type 1 thymidine kinase (HSV-1 TK), human TK, Fas, and inducible caspase 9) [33,34].

Current personalized therapies target a specific molecular marker in the tumor cells and thus neglecting the vast heterogeneity present within the primary tumor, between different metastases, between the various cell types within each metastasis, and between tumors of different patients [5,35,36]. Consequently, current treatment usually results in apparent partial or complete responses, which in most cases followed by a resistant tumor relapse and mortality of the patients.

In addition, the consequence of a specific therapy is not determined solely by the molecular variation within a certain tumor, pharmacokinetics, and drug metabolism – differences between patients results in changes of drug levels throughout the treatment and could also contribute to drug resistance. Thus, personalized treatment requires multilayers characterization of the molecular signatures of tumor cell subpopulations together with individualized pharmacotyping (Identify sequence variations in drug target proteins, drug-metabolizing enzymes, and drug transporters that could alter drug efficacy and drug adverse effects) to achieve maximal efficacy [7].

5.3 "OMICS" – New Era in Understanding Pathology

"OMICS" have driven the resolution of biology to an extraordinary high definition, passing from reductionism approach to a system-oriented approach. The rapid advancement of high-throughput technologies at the last decade (i.e., next-generation sequencing (NGS), mass spectrometry, and high-content analysis) makes it possible to examine biological systems at different levels from whole genome sequencing (WGS) or whole exome sequencing (WES) to whole metabolome and proteome with very high resolution and at affordable cost. The ability to carefully examine pathologies at different "omics" levels allows to stratify complex biological phenomena toward understanding of complex pathologies. Therefore, patients could be monitored regularly and personal profiles of multiple "omics," such as the genome, the epigenome, the transcriptome, the proteome, and the metabolome, be collected and integrated to molecular signatures representing the patient's physiological or pathological state at the specific time point when the sample is taken from the patient. These molecular signatures could enable physicians to individualize risk assessment, disease prevention, diagnosis, and therapy.

5.3.1 Next-Generation Sequencing (NGS)

NGS is a highly parallelized process that enables the sequencing of millions of molecules concomitantly. Several NGS technologies have been developed:

1) Pyrosequencing technology developed by 454 Life Sciences (now part of Roche), which use luciferase to read out signals as individual nucleotides are added to DNA templates.
2) Several types of technologies developed by Illumina sequencing use reversible dye-terminator techniques that add a single nucleotide to the DNA template in each cycle.
3) SOLiD sequencing by Life Technologies (ThermoScientific), which uses preferential ligation of fixed length oligonucleotides [37].

The application of NGS in cancer research, mainly through whole-genome sequencing, whole-exome technologies (WES), and RNA-seq, has produced a vast amount of data on the context and complexity of cancer genomic alterations, including point mutations, small insertions or deletions, copy number alternations, and structural differences. In recent years, dozens of NGS-based studies have been carried out providing a broad molecular characterization of different tumors. These studies succeeded to identify multiple genetic alterations contributing to oncogenesis, tumor progression and metastasis, and to expand our understanding of tumor heterogeneity and evolution [38]. One such study involved 510 breast cancer tumors using WES together with analyses of expression patterns, DNA methylation profiles, microRNA sequencing, and reverse-phase protein arrays found two novel protein-expression-defined subclasses and novel subtype-associated mutations. Deciphering new molecular patterns enable the identification of new therapeutic targets, better diagnostics, and treatment for these patients [39]. Similar efforts have yielded substantial achievements for ovarian carcinoma [40–42], colorectal cancer [43], squamous cell lung cancer [44], hepatocellular carcinoma [45], and so on.

An additional use of WGS is pharmacogenomics analysis. It is known and well documented in the literature that a particular drug may behave differently in terms of its efficacy when administered to different individuals. This is most likely due to differences in genomic and epigenetic profiles and different life styles [46]. Therefore, genetic data can be used to assign an appropriate drug at appropriate doses and thus reduce treatment's adverse effects.

5.3.2
The Identification of "Clear-Cut" Biomarkers Using State-of-the-Art Proteomics

A global human proteome project to map the human proteins was launched by The Human Proteome Organization. Improvements in mass spectrometry technologies have developed to a level such that it can be used to assess the complexity of the entire human proteome [47]. Mass Spectroscopy (MS)-based proteomic analysis was developed to become a robust strategy to discover new, protein-based biomarkers. The use of MS-derived protein patterns together with bioinformatics has enabled physicians and scientists to differentiate between pathologic states or even to carefully identify cancer patients from healthy subjects [48]. To this end, several MS strategies have been developed.

The first is surface-enhanced laser-desorption ionization time-of-flight MS (SELDI-TOF-MS). SELDI-TOF-MS can be used to analyze the masses of protein directly without enzymatic digestion [49]. A different approach uses a combination of MS and liquid chromatography (LC/MS), in a LC/MS analysis, the whole proteins repertoire in a biological sample are partially digested by proteases. Another strategy that is more extensively used is a matrix-assisted laser desorption ionization/time-of-flight (MALDI-TOF) mass spectrometry. MALDI-TOF is an extremely sensitive method that permits the detection of chemical and biological compounds (such as peptides or proteins) at a subfemtomole resolution [50]. MALDI-TOF can be used directly on biological samples in a rapid and automated procedure. These MS strategies have been successfully used to analyze various biological samples of different complexities, such as tissues, serum, plasma, and urine. SELDI-TOF-MS was used for identification of a new biomarker for the early detection of pancreatic and colon cancers by analyzing plasma samples [47,51].

Aberrant post-translational modifications of proteins play a pivotal role in oncogenesis of various malignancies due to the interference with different signaling cascades. One dominant example is aberrant phosphorylation predominantly of receptor tyrosine kinases (i.e., HER2 and EGFR); therefore, many efforts have been made on profiling, targeting, and inhibiting these phosphorylated proteins. Although the vast amount of data collected by high-throughput transcriptome technologies of the downstream transcriptional changes that follow respective stimuli or pathologic status, many critical events involved in cellular responses occurs at the post-translational protein modification level rather than in the changes in the transcription pattern. Lately, new MS-based technologies for the analysis of phosphoprotein expression profiles have been developed and became a powerful technology for quantitative phosphoproteomic analysis, which is essential for the understanding of cancer biology. However, currently, most of the studies analyzing large-scale phosphoproteom have been conducted on cell lines *in vitro* or in mouse models, further developments are needed in order to be able to deal with nonhomogeneous cell populations such as the one present in tumor biopsies.

Recently, two different strategies have been proposed to bring the knowledge gained from basic science closer to personalized medicine are the personal “OMICS” profiling and the “OMICS” profiling at single-cell resolution.

5.3.3
Personal OMICS Profiling

A recent study examined the ability of WGS of a healthy individual to estimate for disease risk by using integrated multiple “omics” data sets of this individual over time. The integrated personal omics profiling (iPOP) is a combined data sets of high-resolution WGS, transcriptomic, metabolomic, and proteomic profiles all from multiple samples taken over a 14-month period from a single 54 year individual. During that time the integrated analysis enabled to predispose individual's genetic disease risks, and to track the emergence of type 2 diabetes. Moreover, the patient was subjected to two viral infections during the experiment, which revealed extensive and dynamic changes mainly in the transcriptomes, between healthy states, in response to viral infections and recovery [52]. iPOP represents novel approach to personalized monitoring in real time of multidimensional "omics" of an individual and illustrates how traits associated with disease can be monitored in real time enable to identify varying physiological or pathological stages. In addition, this research illustrates the dynamic and complex nature of the human biological system, suggests that such longitudinal monitoring of patient's "omics" profile may be the future of disease monitoring and diagnosis.

5.3.4 Single-Cell Sequencing

Until the recent development of NGS technologies, the ability to study dissimilarities within a single tumor (intratumor heterogeneity) in high resolution was extremely limited [53]. Most NGS techniques that have been developed to date require DNA or RNA from a minimum of 10^5 cells [54]. This limitation becomes a major problem particularly when analyzing solid tumors, due to the vast heterogeneity rely within those tumors in addition to present of embedded noncancerous cells, such as leukocytes and fibroblasts [55]. When analyzing such complex mixture of different cells, the gene expression data obtained from tumor sequencing is often masked by the microenvironment cells, thus the "average" data obtained might be completely different from that of the individual tumor cell [56]. Therefore, the ability to analyze separately these distinct cell populations is critical for better understanding of tumor heterogeneity. The first study succeeded to analyze single tumor cells used breast cancer as a model [57]. In this study, the researchers have sequenced 100 single cells from distinct sections of human polygenic metastatic breast tumor revealing three distinct clonal subpopulations that probably represent sequential clonal expansions. In addition they sequenced an additional 100 single cells from a monogenomic primary breast tumor and from its' matched liver metastasis, demonstrating that a single clonal expansion formed the primary tumor and seeded the liver metastasis [58].

The results from several single-cell WGS/WES analyses of heterogeneous tumors provide scientists with a better observation of intratumor genetic landscape, the tumor's progression pathway(s), and on the metastatic process than previously used bulk tissue for sequencing. Additional in deep understanding and clinical evaluation of such platforms could improve the interpretation of tumor development and the identification of rare tumor cell subpopulations, which might counts for treatment failure and disease relapse [59]. Furthermore, better characterization of tumor subpopulations provides physicians with more tools to personalize the treatment and to target multiple tumor cells concomitantly and, thus minimize the risk of disease recurrence and treatment failure.

5.4 Nanomedicine

Nanomedicine has an immense potential to revolutionize personalized cancer diagnosis and therapy. Nanomedicines are being implemented to overcome several limitations of conventional chemotherapy such as nonspecific biodistribution, poor water solubility of most common chemotherapeutic drugs (i.e., Paclitaxel, cisplatin, and Doxetaxel), low therapeutic indices, and tumor multidrug resistance. The ability to create a wide range of nanocarriers that could encompass both hydrophilic and hydrophobic drugs concomitantly with different targeting moieties [6] (i.e., monoclonal antibodies, natural ligands, and aptamers), which in turn could direct and release the drugs in a specific location or target a specific cell subpopulation and contrast substances for precise molecular imaging makes nanocarriers the most suitable delivery platforms for personalized cancer care.

5.4.1 Personalized Oncology Using Nanomedicine

5.4.1.1 Passive Tissue Targeting vs. Active Cellular Targeting

Nanocarriers can carry their therapeutic payloads either passively or actively to target solid or hematological malignancies. Passive targeting occurs due to the unique characteristics of solid tumors blood vessels that allow nanocarriers (≈200 nm) to preferentially accumulate in the tumor due to the leaky tumor endothelial vessels at tumor site (compared to healthy vasculature) and defect in tumor lymphatic drainage, this phenomenon is known as the enhanced permeability and retention (EPR) effect. This approach first reached the clinic in the mid-1990s with the approval of DOXIL®, liposomal formulation of doxorubicin for refractory Kaposi's sarcoma, recurrent breast and ovarian cancers, and multiple myeloma [60–62]. Since the approval of DOXIL®, several therapeutic nanocarriers based on this strategy were approved for different malignancies, for example, Abraxane® – albumin-bound paclitaxel nanoparticles approved by the FDA in 2005 as a second-line chemotherapy for metastatic breast cancer. DaunoXome® – liposomal formulation of daunorubicin for the treatment of kaposi's sarcoma [3,63] and recently Marqibo® – liposomal formulation based on sphingomyelin and cholesterol entrapping vincristine sulfate that was designed to overcome the dosing and pharmacokinetic limitations of standard vincristine. Marqibo® has been demonstrated to have an increased circulation time, improved delivery to target tissues, and to facilitate dose escalation without increasing toxicity [64]. Although various novel nanocarriers based on passive targeting approaches are under clinical evaluation (i.e., NK105 [12] and CRLX101 [65]), they generally suffer from several limitations. Relying only on the EPR effect for tumor targeting disregards the variability in tumor vasculature within a single tumor or between different tumors, which in some cases, does not allow a sufficient amount of drug to reach the target site and thus decrease treatment efficacy and increase the risk for multiple drug resistance, where chemotherapy treatments fails due to intrinsic resistance of cancer cells toward one or more drugs or acquired resistance during the course of chemotherapy [6]. One suggested solution overcoming these limitations is to modify the nanocarriers to have a homing capability, so they could actively bind to specific targets on tumor cells. This binding is achieved by decorating the surface of the nanocarriers with targeting agents such as natural ligands (i.e., Folate and transferrin), monoclonal antibodies, aptamers, or tumor-specific targeting peptides [66]. Nanocarriers will recognize and specifically interact with the selected receptor on tumor cells, subsequently the bound carriers are internalized, escape from the endosome through different mechanisms [7] and the encapsulated drug is released within the cell cytoplasm. Alternatively, the particles can bind to the cells' membrane and release their payload into the cells by a simple diffusion acting as a slow-release drug depot.

The ability to conjugate a large variety of targeting entities, which are highly selective to target molecules that are exclusively expressed on tumor cells enable to specifically match the targeting entity to a specific biomarker on tumor cells according to personally analyzed "omics" profiling. In addition, active cellular targeting offers the advantages to improve drug therapeutic efficiency and to dramatically reduce toxicity and adverse effects, thus leading to possible novel therapeutic modalities in cancer management. Despite the extensive research done in the past two decades, to date no targeted particulate nanocarrier has been approved for clinical use. Nevertheless, several targeted particulate nanocarriers are currently under clinical evaluation and countless more are being developed. For example, Senzer *et al.* recently announced a successful phase I clinical study of SGT-53 a liposomal nanocarrier formulation targeted by a single-chain antibody fragment to the transferrin receptor delivering plasmid encoding a wild-type human p53 tumor suppressor protein [67]. The administration of SGT-53 to patients with advanced solid tumors resulted with disease stabilization in the majority of patients with minor adverse effects. Furthermore, they observed an accumulation of the transgene in metastatic tumors, but not in normal skin tissue, in a dose-related manner. In another study, PK-2 a polymeric HPMA linear nanocarrier containing doxorubicin (DOX) and targeted by N-linked galactosamine, which binds to the hepatic asialoglycoprotein receptor (ASGPR) was tested [68]. The DOX was linked to the nanocarrier via a tetrapeptide spacer (Gly–Phe–Leu–Gly), this spacer designed for specific cleavage by lysosomal cathepsins and was shown to release free DOX in the liver. Due to this controlled release mechanism, the drug could accumulate in its target site, the nucleus.

Targeting leukocytes possess a greater challenge, due to their dispersion in the body [69]. By coupling an anti-CD22 antibody fragment that target CD22 express on B cells to PEGylated DOX-loaded liposomes Tuscano *et al.* demonstrated an increase DOX accumulation in Non-Hodgkin's Lymphoma xenografts and increased survival over untargeted doxorubicin-loaded liposomes [70]. After administration, most nanosized liposomes were captured by the mononuclear phagocyte system (MPS) in the liver and spleen [69]. This elimination is due to the recognition by serum proteins (opsonins) and complement components, which prime liposomes for macrophage removal from the circulation. The advantages of targeted drug delivery for the preferential antitumor efficacy are not limited to liposomes. Saad *et al.* compared the therapeutic antitumor efficacy of three targeted or untargeted paclitaxel-loaded nanocarriers: linear polymer, dendrimer, or PEGylated liposomes. They demonstrated superior tumor accumulation and tumor suppression for all targeted delivery systems over untargeted ones and of free paclitaxel [71]. In another study conjugation of FDA approved humanized anti-HER2 antibody Herceptin (Genentech, San Francisco, CA) to paclitaxel PEGylated liposomes increased significantly the nanocarriers' accumulation in Xenograft human breast tumors and showed better therapeutic efficacy over untargeted paclitaxel liposomes [72].

5.4.2
RNAi: A powerful Approach for Cancer Personalized Therapy

RNA interference (RNAi) is a natural cellular mechanism of RNA-guided gene regulation [63]. RNAi is mediated by double-stranded RNA (dsRNA) that down-regulates the expression of specific set of genes through complementary sequences either by degrading specific messenger RNA (mRNA) or by blocking its translation [9]. RNAi has become a powerful tool in molecular biology as well as a therapeutic tool by introducing short hairpin RNA (shRNA) or synthetic small interfering RNAs (siRNAs) directly into the cell cytoplasm [73]. siRNAs are chemically synthesized dsRNAs of 19–23 base pairs with 2-nucleotides unpaired in the 5′- and 3′-ends [73,74]. Inside the cell cytoplasm, siRNAs are incorporated into RNA-induced silencing complex (RISC), a complex that unwinds the RNA duplex and discards the sense strand. The antisense RNA–RISC complex anneal to complementary target mRNA and cleave or block its translation [7,63]. The RISC–RNA complex is catalytic and the antisense strand is protected from degradation, thus the same RNA template can be used repetitively to eradicate many transcripts. In fact, gene knockdown occurs with picomolar concentrations of siRNA at the cytoplasm and show a therapeutic effect for up to 7 days in dividing cells and for several weeks in nondividing cells [75,76]. The power of RNAi in personalized medicine is achieved by designing sequence specific RNAi molecules such siRNAs to potentially silence any cellular target. RNAi-induced gene silencing possesses similar inhibitory effects of conventional pharmaceuticals, such as protein-based drugs (i.e., antibodies) and small molecules inhibitors. However, the inhibitory effects of these drugs are dependent on blocking their targets function, some disease-related molecules, primarily proteins, do not have enzymatic function or have a conformation that is not accessible to conventional drugs or small-molecule compounds, hence these targets are considered as "nondruggable." Several such "nondruggable" molecules have been successfully targeted by RNAi approach *in vivo* [77–80] demonstrating an exclusively allele-specific gene silencing [80,81].

Furthermore, by downregulation of target's gene at the transcript level amplified effect is achieved due to the fact that a single mRNA molecule translates to multiple copies of protein. The progress of "omics" technologies (reviewed above) contribute to further understanding of the basis of cancer oncogenesis and progression as well as the interaction of the transcriptomes with their environment, leading to identify disease-related genes and biomarkers, which in turn facilitating the design of novel individualized RNAi constructs accordingly [82]. Such strategies could be utilized for stemline the drug development process in personalized cancer care (see Figure 5.1 for more details).

The occurrence of drug resistance in cancer patients has driven the administration of drug combinations to treat cancer as an alternative to increased doses of chemotherapeutics associated with severe adverse effects [83]. Following the above paradigm, Chen *et al.* developed a liposome–polycation–hyaluronic acid nanocarrier targeted by GC4 (scFv selected by phage display against ovarian tumors), encapsulating three different siRNA and one miRNA against different proliferation, angiogenesis, and survival signaling pathways (i.e., Cmyc, MDM2, VEGF, and miR34a) achieving a 80% reduction in lung metastasis Xenograft mice [84].

These results emphasize the power of the modified mRNA technology and its potential to overcome the limitation of classical gene therapy in personalized cancer care.

5.5
Future Outlook

Although the substantial progress achieved already toward personalizing cancer treatment, the current personalized therapies targets a single specific molecular marker on tumor cells and thus neglecting the vast heterogeneity presents within the primary tumor, between different metastases, within each metastasis, and between tumors of different patients [5]. Consequently, current treatment usually results in apparent partial or complete responses, which in most cases follow by a resistant tumor relapse and mortality of the patients. In addition, the consequences of a specific therapy are not determined solely by the molecular variation within a certain tumor, pharmacokinetics and drug metabolism differences between patients result in changes of drug levels throughout the treatment could also contribute to therapy resistance. Therefore, personalized treatment requires multilayer characterization of the molecular signatures of tumor cell subpopulations together with individualized pharmacotyping (Identify sequence variations in drug target proteins, drug-metabolizing enzymes, and drug transporters that could alter drug efficacy and drug adverse effects) to achieve maximal efficacy [7].

The development and safety assessments of personalized drugs may lead to overwhelming costs compared with drugs that target a population of patients. One reasonable solution is to develop clinically approved, target-specific compounds for each of the known molecular targets attributed to cancer using

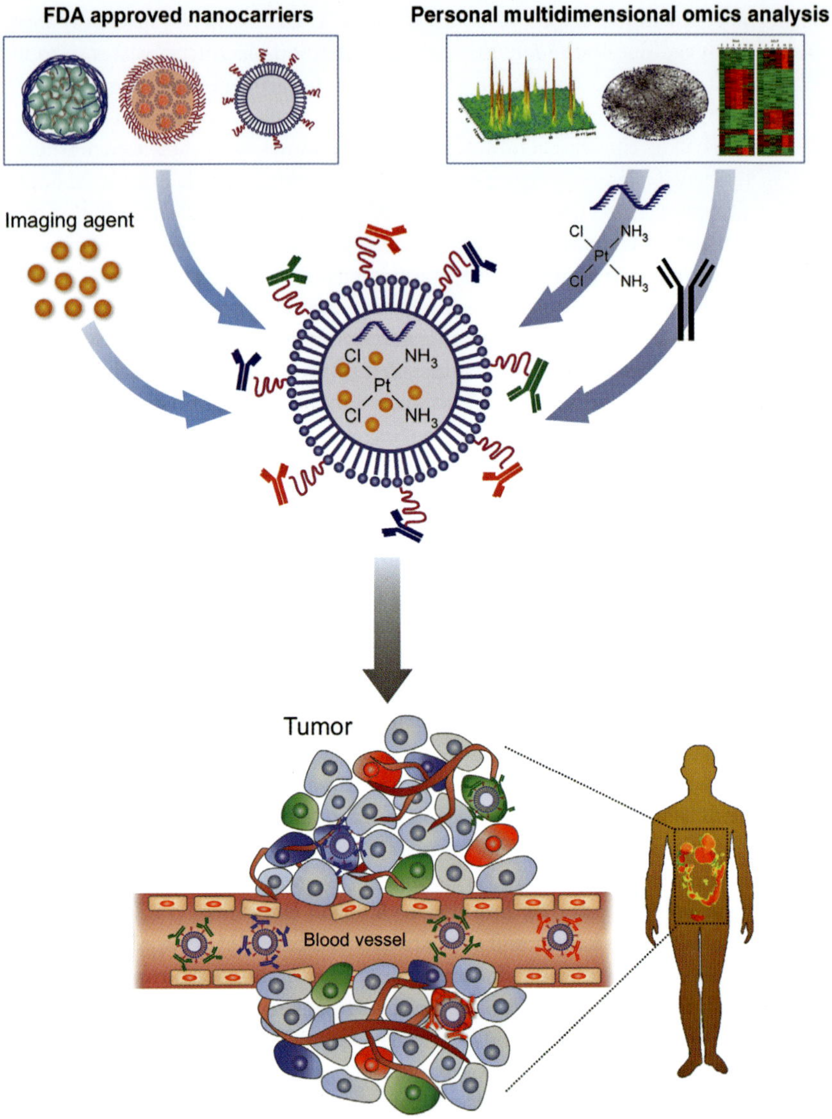

Figure 5.1 Schematic illustration of a personalized approach for future therapeutics. According to patient's personal multidimentional "omics" data (i.e., genomics, proteomics, and metabolomics), a tailor-made nanocarrier will be designed carrying appropriate therapeutic payloads together with an imaging agent optimized with triggered-release mechanisms. The theranostic nanocarrier will be decorated with multiple-targeting moieties against different tumor subpopulation to ensure maximal therapeutic effect. The therapeutic efficacy could be noninvasively monitored in real time, thus enable the clinician to assess the treatment tailored to each patient. (Reproduced from Ref. [35] with permission from Elsevier.)

consortium efforts such as made by the NCI's Cancer Target Discovery and Development Network, combination of these compounds could be tailor made for each individual at an acceptable cost.

Nanomedicine provides a unique opportunity to hinder devastating effects of cancer, which affects millions of people yearly. Nanomedicine technologies have already started revolutionizing cancer therapy since the introduction of first-generation nanocarriers in the mid-1990s, various novel and highly sophisticated nanocarriers demonstrating higher specificity, improved circulation time, decreased adverse effects, and higher efficacy both *in vitro* and *in vivo* have been developed and currently several actively targeted nanocarriers are under clinical evaluation. Moreover, the notion of simultaneous delivery of imaging and therapeutic agents using theranostics nanocarriers paves the way for early cancer diagnostic and precocious feedbacks on treatment effectiveness, without the need of detecting traditional end points (i.e., reduction in tumor size). Furthermore, the use of multiparameter "omics" data for precise molecular biomarkers recognition together with versatile drug-delivery nanocarriers, which could target concomitantly and specifically tumor cells subpopulations might overcome the tumor heterogeneity problem and thus minimize the risk for disease relapse. Ultimately, the combination of different targeting moieties, imaging agents, chemotherapeutic drugs, specific inhibitors, and RNAi may enable effective and controlled delivery of therapeutic agents in cancer patients together with non-invasive monitoring of the treatment in real time, thus empower clinicians to make decisions based on the therapeutic outcomes of individual patients, which will lead to a real personalized therapy. Notwithstanding this immense potential, the development and clinical use of nanomedicines for personalized therapy hold some major challenges and hurdles. Unforeseen toxicity toward synthetic nanomedicine still remains a major concern. Adequate and comprehensive understanding of the specific interactions between lipid and polymeric-based nanocarriers with the immune system both at the cellular and molecular levels might enable to assess the likelihood, mechanisms and severity of nanotoxicity that currently are not fully predictable using classic toxicological methods [82,85]. Another major challenge will be the scientific challenges of transferring nanomedicines from the lab scale into an initial proof-of-principle phases to validated, reliable and commercially approved products with proven efficacy and safety. To do so, collaborative efforts between academia and the pharmaceutical companies have to be further developed [86]. While these collaborations are still very limited and issues related to intellectual property will continue to be addressed, the collaborations already initialed will have long-term impacts on the field of nanomedicine. Further issue need to be considered is the regulatory requirements, which may also present a daunting hurdle for many nanomedicines. It will be crucial that regulatory authorities provide foreseeable and well-defined evaluation pathways for nanomedicines, in order to keep pace with rapidly developing personalized nanomedicines.

We envision that in a few years' time, clinicians would have the ability to choose from a large arsenal of clinically approved nanocarriers building blocks, which could be easily assembled in a combinatorial manner with the appropriate therapeutic agent, and targeting molecules all according to the patient's molecular characteristics attributed to multilevels "omics" information (Figure 5.1). Thus, enable clinicians to fulfill the full potential of personalized cancer therapy and achieve improved therapeutic outcomes all in a realistic cost.

Acknowledgments

This work was supported in part by the grants from the Lewis Family Trust, the Israeli Center of Research Excellence (I-CORE), Gene Regulation in Complex Human Disease, Center No 41/11; The DOTAN Center for hematological malignancies at Tel Aviv University; FTA: Nanomedicine for Personalized Theranostics, and by The Leona M. and Harry B. Helmsley Nanotechnology Research Fund awarded to D.P.

References

1 Donna, L. and Hoyert, J.X. (2012) Deaths: preliminary data for 2011. *Natl. Vital Stat. Rep.*, **61** (6), 1–64.
2 Siegel, R., Naishadham, D., and Jemal, A. (2013) Cancer statistics, 2013. *CA. Cancer J. Clin.*, **63** (1), 11–30.
3 Diou, O., Tsapis, N., and Fattal, E. (2012) Targeted nanotheranostics for personalized cancer therapy. *Expert Opin. Drug Del.*, **9** (12), 1475–1487.
4 Ludwig, J.A. and Weinstein, J.N. (2005) Biomarkers in cancer staging, prognosis and treatment selection. *Nat. Rev. Cancer*, **5** (11), 845–856.
5 Vogelstein, B. *et al.* (2013) Cancer genome landscapes. *Supramol. Sci.*, **339** (6127), 1546–1558.
6 Peer, D. *et al.* (2007) Nanocarriers as an emerging platform for cancer therapy. *Nat. Nanotechnol.*, **2** (12), 751–760.
7 Daka, A. and Peer, D. (2012) RNAi-based nanomedicines for targeted personalized therapy. *Adv. Drug Deliv. Rev.*, **64** (13), 1508–1521.
8 Elinav, E. and Peer, D. (2013) Harnessing nanomedicine for mucosal theranostics – a silver bullet at last? *ACS Nano*, **7** (4), 2883–2890.
9 Venditto, V.J. and Szoka, F.C. Jr. (2013) Cancer nanomedicines: so many papers and so few drugs! *Adv. Drug Deliv. Rev.*, **65** (1), 80–88.
10 Goldenberg, M.M. (2012) Pharmaceutical approval update. *P T*, **37** (12), 668–708.
11 Tabernero, J. *et al.* (2013) First-in-humans trial of an RNA interference therapeutic targeting VEGF and KSP in cancer patients with liver involvement. *Cancer Discov.*, **3** (4), 406–417.
12 Kato, K. *et al.* (2012) Phase II study of NK105, a paclitaxel-incorporating micellar nanoparticle, for previously treated advanced or recurrent gastric cancer. *Invest. New Drugs*, **30** (4), 1621–1627.
13 Hamburg, M.A. and Collins, F.S. (2010) The path to personalized medicine. *N. Engl. J. Med.*, **363** (4), 301–304.
14 Roberts, N.J. *et al.* (2012) The predictive capacity of personal genome sequencing. *Sci. Transl. Med.*, **4** (133), 133–158.
15 Gonzalez de Castro, D., Clarke, P.A., Al-Lazikani, B., and Workman, P. (2013) Personalized cancer medicine: molecular diagnostics, predictive biomarkers, and drug resistance. *Clin. Pharmacol. Ther.*, **93** (3), 252–259.
16 Landesman-Milo, D., Ramishetti, S., and Peer, D. (2015) Nanomedicine as an emerging platform for metastatic lung cancer therapy. *Cancer Metastasis Rev.*, **34** (2), 291–301.

17 Perevedentseva, E., Peer, D., Uvarov, V., Zousman, B., and Levinson, O. (2015) Nanodiamonds of laser synthesis for biomedical applications. *J. Nanosci. Nanotechnol.*, **15** (2), 1045–1052.

18 Reynolds, J.G. *et al.* (2012) HER2-targeted liposomal doxorubicin displays enhanced anti-tumorigenic effects without associated cardiotoxicity. *Toxicol. Appl. Pharmacol.*, **262** (1), 1–10.

19 Silvestri, A. *et al.* (2013) Individualized therapy for metastatic colorectal cancer. *J. Intern. Med.*, **274** (1), 1–24.

20 National Cancer Institute (2008) SEER Cancer Statistics Review, 1975–2005. National Cancer Institute, Bethesda, MD. Available at http://seer.cancer.gov/csr/1975_2005/.

21 Vecchione, L., Jacob, B., Normanno, N., Ciardiello, F., and Tejpar, S. (2011) EGFR-targeted therapy. *Exp. Cell Res.*, **317** (19), 2765–2771.

22 Di Nicolantonio, F. *et al.* (2008) Wild-type BRAF is required for response to panitumumab or cetuximab in metastatic colorectal cancer. *J. Clin. Oncol.*, **26** (35), 5705–5712.

23 Karapetis, C.S. *et al.* (2008) K-ras mutations and benefit from cetuximab in advanced colorectal cancer. *N. Engl. J. Med.*, **359** (17), 1757–1765.

24 Carey, L.A. and Sharpless, N.E. (2011) PARP and cancer – if it's broke, don't fix it. *N. Engl. J. Med.*, **364** (3), 277–279.

25 Sudo, T. (2012) Molecular-targeted therapies for ovarian cancer: prospects for the future. *Int. J. Clin. Oncol.*, **17** (5), 424–429.

26 Martin, S.A., Lord, C.J., and Ashworth, A. (2008) DNA repair deficiency as a therapeutic target in cancer. *Curr. Opin. Genet. Dev.*, **18** (1), 80–86.

27 O'Shaughnessy, J. *et al.* (2011) Iniparib plus chemotherapy in metastatic triple-negative breast cancer. *N. Engl. J. Med.*, **364** (3), 205–214.

28 Sadelain, M., Brentjens, R., and Riviere, I. (2009) The promise and potential pitfalls of chimeric antigen receptors. *Curr. Opin. Immunol.*, **21** (2), 215–223.

29 Louis, C.U. *et al.* (2011) Antitumor activity and long-term fate of chimeric antigen receptor-positive T cells in patients with neuroblastoma. *Blood*, **118** (23), 6050–6056.

30 Cartellieri, M. *et al.* (2010) Chimeric antigen receptor-engineered T cells for immunotherapy of cancer. *J. Biomed. Biotechnol.*, **2010**, 956304.

31 Davila, M.L., Brentjens, R., Wang, X.Y., Riviere, I., and Sadelain, M. (2012) How do CARs work? Early insights from recent clinical studies targeting CD19. *Oncoimmunology*, **1** (9), 1577–1583.

32 Kochenderfer, J.N. *et al.* (2012) B-cell depletion and remissions of malignancy along with cytokine-associated toxicity in a clinical trial of anti-CD19 chimeric-antigen-receptor-transduced T cells. *Blood*, **119** (12), 2709–2720.

33 Jena, B., Dotti, G., and Cooper, L.J. (2010) Redirecting T-cell specificity by introducing a tumor-specific chimeric antigen receptor. *Blood*, **116** (7), 1035–1044.

34 Ciceri, F. *et al.* (2009) Infusion of suicide-gene-engineered donor lymphocytes after family haploidentical haemopoietic stem-cell transplantation for leukaemia (the TK007 trial): a non-randomised phase I-II study. *Lancet Oncol.*, **10** (5), 489–500.

35 Rosenblum, D. and Peer, D. (2014) Omics-based nanomedicine: the future of personalized oncology. *Cancer Lett.*, **352** (1), 126–136.

36 Bogart, L.K. *et al.* (2014) Nanoparticles for imaging, sensing, and therapeutic intervention. *ACS Nano*, **8** (4), 3107–3122.

37 Pareek, C.S., Smoczynski, R., and Tretyn, A. (2011) Sequencing technologies and genome sequencing. *J. Appl. Genet.*, **52** (4), 413–435.

38 Shyr, D. and Liu, Q. (2013) Next generation sequencing in cancer research and clinical application. *Biol. Proced. Online*, **15** (1), 4.

39 Cancer Genome Atlas Network (2012) Comprehensive molecular portraits of human breast tumours. *Nature*, **490** (7418), 61–70.

40 Cancer Genome Atlas Research Network (2011) Integrated genomic analyses of ovarian carcinoma. *Nature*, **474** (7353), 609–615.

41 Patch, A.M. *et al.* (2015) Whole-genome characterization of chemoresistant ovarian cancer. *Nature*, **521** (7553), 489–494.

42 Holmes, D. (2015) Ovarian cancer: beyond resistance. *Nature*, **527** (7579), S217.

43 Cancer Genome Atlas Network (2012) Comprehensive molecular characterization of human colon and rectal cancer. *Nature*, **487** (7407), 330–337.

44 Cancer Genome Atlas Research Network (2012) Comprehensive genomic characterization of squamous cell lung cancers. *Nature*, **489** (7417), 519–525.

45 Totoki, Y. *et al.* (2011) High-resolution characterization of a hepatocellular carcinoma genome. *Nat. Genet.*, **43** (5), 464–469.

46 Ma, Q. and Lu, A.Y. (2011) Pharmacogenetics, pharmacogenomics, and individualized medicine. *Pharmacol. Rev.*, **63** (2), 437–459.

47 Ehmann, M. *et al.* (2007) Identification of potential markers for the detection of pancreatic cancer through comparative serum protein expression profiling. *Pancreas*, **34** (2), 205–214.

48 Petricoin, E.F., Zoon, K.C., Kohn, E.C., Barrett, J.C., and Liotta, L.A. (2002) Clinical proteomics: translating benchside promise into bedside reality. *Nat. Rev. Drug Discov.*, **1** (9), 683–695.

49 Honda, K. *et al.* (2013) Proteomic approaches to the discovery of cancer biomarkers for early detection and personalized medicine. *Jpn. J. Clin. Oncol.*, **43** (2), 103–109.

50 Cho, Y.T. *et al.* (2013) Matrix-assisted laser desorption ionization/time-of-flight mass spectrometry for clinical diagnosis. *Clin. Chim. Acta*, **415**, 266–275.

51 Murakoshi, Y. *et al.* (2011) Plasma biomarker discovery and validation for colorectal cancer by quantitative shotgun mass spectrometry and protein microarray. *Cancer Sci.*, **102** (3), 630–638.

52 Chen, R. *et al.* (2012) Personal omics profiling reveals dynamic molecular and medical phenotypes. *Cell*, **148** (6), 1293–1307.

53 Schubert, C. (2011) Single-cell analysis: The deepest differences. *Nature*, **480** (7375), 133–137.

54 Metzker, M.L. (2010) Applications of next-generation sequencing sequencing technologies – the next generation. *Nat. Rev. Genet.*, **11** (1), 31–46.

55 Marusyk, A. and Polyak, K. (2010) Tumor heterogeneity: causes and consequences. *BBA Rev. Cancer*, **1805** (1), 105–117.

56 Wang, D. and Bodovitz, S. (2010) Single cell analysis: the new frontier in 'omics'. *Trends Biotechnol.*, **28** (6), 281–290.

57 Navin, N. *et al.* (2011) Tumour evolution inferred by single-cell sequencing. *Nature*, **472** (7341), 90–94.

58 Hou, Y. *et al.* (2012) Single-cell exome sequencing and monoclonal evolution of a JAK2-negative myeloproliferative neoplasm. *Cell*, **148** (5), 873–885.

59 Lien, K.Y. *et al.* (2010) Rapid isolation and detection of cancer cells by utilizing integrated microfluidic systems. *Lab Chip*, **10** (21), 2875–2886.

60 Barenholz, Y. (2012) Doxil® – the first FDA-approved nano-drug: lessons learned. *J. Control. Release*, **160** (2), 117–134.

61 Barenholz, Y.C. and Peer, D. (2012) Liposomes, lipid biophysics, and sphingolipid research: from basic to translation research. *Chem. Phys. Lipids*, **165** (4), 363–364.

62 Barenholz, Y. and Peer, D. (2012) Liposomes and other assemblies as drugs and nano-drugs: from basic and translational research to the clinics. *J. Control. Release*, **160** (2), 115–116.

63 Peer, D. (2013) A daunting task: manipulating leukocyte function with RNAi. *Immunol. Rev.*, **253** (1), 185–197.

64 Silverman, J.A. and Deitcher, S.R. (2013) Marqibo® (vincristine sulfate liposome injection) improves the pharmacokinetics and pharmacodynamics of vincristine. *Cancer Chemother. Pharmacol.*, **71** (3), 555–564.

65 Weiss, G.J. *et al.* (2013) First-in-human phase 1/2a trial of CRLX101, a cyclodextrin-containing polymer-camptothecin nanopharmaceutical in patients with advanced solid tumor malignancies. *Invest. New Drugs*, **31** (4), 986–1000.

66 Perche, F. and Torchilin, V.P. (2013) Recent trends in multifunctional liposomal nanocarriers for enhanced tumor targeting. *J. Drug Deliv.*, **2013**, 705265.

67 Senzer, N. *et al.* (2013) Phase I study of a systemically delivered p53 nanoparticle in advanced solid tumors. *Mol. Ther.*, **21** (5), 1096–1103.

68 Seymour, L.W. *et al.* (2002) Hepatic drug targeting: phase I evaluation of polymer-bound doxorubicin. *J. Clin. Oncol.*, **20** (6), 1668–1676.

69 Peer, D. (2010) Induction of therapeutic gene silencing in leukocyte-implicated diseases by targeted and stabilized nanoparticles: a mini-review. *J. Control. Release*, **148** (1), 63–68.

70 Tuscano, J.M., Martin, S.M., Ma, Y., Zamboni, W., and O'Donnell, R.T. (2010) Efficacy, biodistribution, and pharmacokinetics of CD22-targeted pegylated liposomal doxorubicin in a B-cell non-Hodgkin's lymphoma xenograft mouse model. *Clin. Cancer Res.*, **16** (10), 2760–2768.

71 Saad, M. *et al.* (2008) Receptor targeted polymers, dendrimers, liposomes: which nanocarrier is the most efficient for tumor-specific treatment and imaging? *J. Control. Release*, **130** (2), 107–114.

72 Yang, T. *et al.* (2007) Antitumor effect of paclitaxel-loaded PEGylated immunoliposomes against human breast cancer cells. *Pharm. Res.*, **24** (12), 2402–2411.

73 Peer, D. and Lieberman, J. (2011) Special delivery: targeted therapy with small RNAs. *Gene Ther.*, **18** (12), 1127–1133.

74 Amarzguioui, M., Rossi, J.J., and Kim, D. (2005) Approaches for chemically synthesized siRNA and vector-mediated RNAi. *FEBS Lett.*, **579** (26), 5974–5981.

75 Peer, D., Park, E.J., Morishita, Y., Carman, C.V., and Shimaoka, M. (2008) Systemic leukocyte-directed siRNA delivery revealing cyclin D1 as an anti-inflammatory target. *Supramol. Sci.*, **319** (5863), 627–630.

76 Bartlett, D.W. and Davis, M.E. (2006) Insights into the kinetics of siRNA-mediated gene silencing from live-cell and live-animal bioluminescent imaging. *Nucleic Acids Res.*, **34** (1), 322–333.

77 Bertrand, J.R. *et al.* (2002) Comparison of antisense oligonucleotides and siRNAs in cell culture and *in vivo*. *Biochem. Biophys. Res. Commun.*, **296** (4), 1000–1004.

78 Zimmermann, T.S. *et al.* (2006) RNAi-mediated gene silencing in non-human primates. *Nature*, **441** (7089), 111–114.

79 Dorn, G. *et al.* (2004) siRNA relieves chronic neuropathic pain. *Nucleic Acids Res.*, **32** (5).

80 Shen, J. *et al.* (2006) Suppression of ocular neovascularization with siRNA targeting VEGF receptor 1. *Gene Ther.*, **13** (3), 225–234.

81 Miller, V.M. *et al.* (2003) Allele-specific silencing of dominant disease genes. *Proc. Natl. Acad. Sci. USA*, **100** (12), 7195–7200.

82 Moghimi, S.M., Peer, D., and Langer, R. (2011) Reshaping the future of nanopharmaceuticals: ad iudicium. *ACS Nano*, **5** (11), 8454–8458.

83 Wu, S. and Singh, R.K. (2011) Resistance to chemotherapy and molecularly targeted therapies: rationale for combination therapy in malignant melanoma. *Curr. Mol. Med.*, **11** (7), 553–563.

84 Chen, Y.C., Zhu, X.D., Zhang, X.J., Liu, B., and Huang, L. (2010) Nanoparticles modified with tumor-targeting scFv deliver siRNA and miRNA for cancer therapy. *Mol. Ther.*, **18** (9), 1650–1656.

85 Peer, D. (2012) Immunotoxicity derived from manipulating leukocytes with lipid-based nanoparticles. *Adv. Drug Deliv. Rev.*, **64** (15), 1738–1748.

86 Ratner, M. (2011) Pfizer reaches out to academia – again. *Nat. Biotechnol.*, **29** (1), 3–4.

Part Two
Fundamentals of Nanotechnology in Pharmacy

6
Nanostructures in Drug Delivery

Salma Nabil Tammam and Alf Lamprecht

Laboratory of Pharmaceutical Technology and Biopharmaceutics, University of Bonn, 53121, Germany

6.1
Introduction

Nanomedicine is an emerging specialty born from nanotechnology and is defined as the repair, monitoring, construction, and control of biological systems at the molecular level using nanostructures and has an enormous potential to improve healthcare. For drug delivery in particular, nanomedicine offers numerous advantages: improved delivery of poorly water-soluble drugs [1]; targeted delivery of drugs to particular tissue, cell [2,3], or even organelle [4,5]; improving drug absorption and bioavailability [6]; delivery of protein and macromolecule drugs to intracellular targets [7]; codelivery of two or more drugs (combination therapy) [8]; or a drug and an imaging modality (theranostics) [9]. Optimally nanostructures for drug delivery should include imaging molecules, a payload of drugs, ligands for site-specific targeting, a destabilizing mechanism allowing for tailored drug release at the desired site, and sensors that probe the efficacy of the drug in real time [10]. While such optimal formulation is yet to exist, on the way to achieving such complete formulation several rather promising classes of nanostructures have been developed.

6.2
Nanocarrier Classification

A wide range of nanostructures have been designed for drug delivery. Nanostructures or nanocarriers for drug delivery include liposomes, polymer or lipid particles, micelles, quantum dots, gold nanoparticles (AuNPs), silver NPs (AgNPs), silica NPs, and although not technically a nanocarrier, drug nanocrystals. As implied from their names, such nanostructures are based on rather unique assemblies of synthetic, natural, and biological components such as natural and

Pharmaceutical Nanotechnology: Innovation and Production, First Edition. Edited by Jean Cornier, Arno Kwade, Andrew Owen, and Marcel Van de Voorde.

synthetic polymers, metal ions, oils, and lipids [10]. Based on the material of synthesis, in a broad sense, nanostructures can be classified into inorganic and organic nanocarriers. Inorganic delivery systems comprise a wide variety of nanostructures, including metallic nanostructures and nonmetallic structures such as silica and carbon-based structures. Organic nanocarriers could be further classified into drug nanocrystals and matrix and vesicle nanocarriers (Figure 6.1).

6.2.1 Inorganic Nanostructures

A variety of different nanostructures composed of different metals have found use in nanomedicine. Gold, palladium, copper, iron, silver, platinum, selenium, and lanthanides [11,12] are examples of metals used in nanomedicine. Unlike other classes of nanostructures, apart from the more common nanospheres, metals have been used to synthesis a huge range of peculiar structures, such as hollow nanospheres, nanorods, nanocubes, nanoprisms, nanocrescents, nanopyramids, and many more [13,14]. It is therefore no wonder that a plethora of

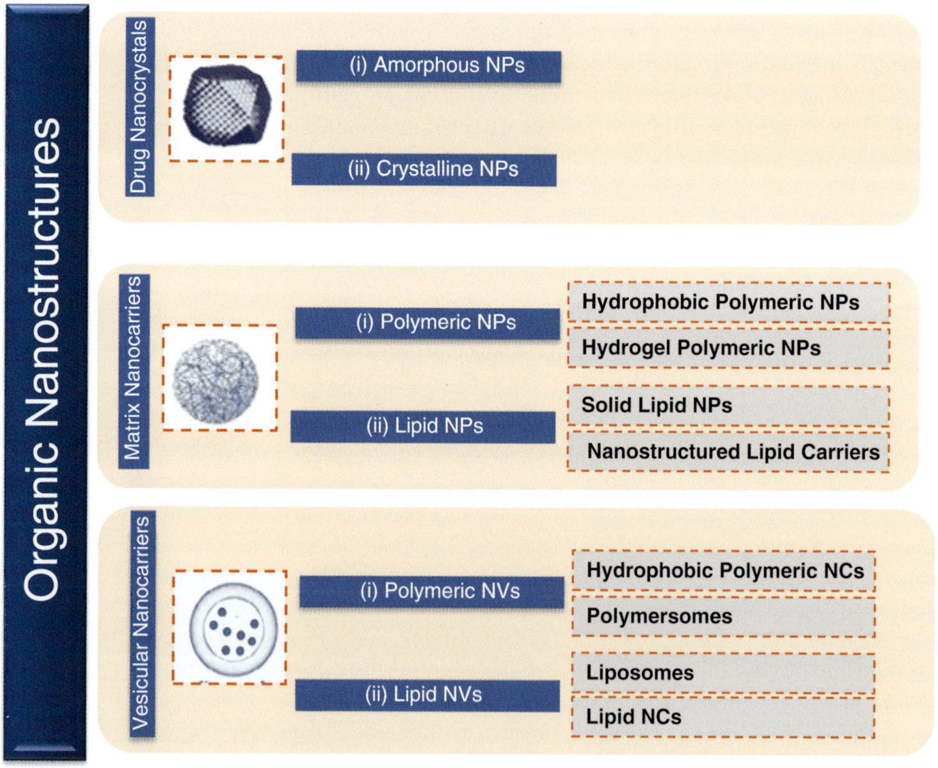

Figure 6.1 Organic nanostructure for drug delivery classification. NPs: nanoparticles; NCs: nanocapsules; NVs: nanovesicles.

various methods have been developed for metallic nanostructure synthesis. Metallic nanostructures could be generally synthesized by top-down and bottom-up approaches. As implied for its name, the bottom-up approach refers to the construction of the nanostructure atom-by-atom or molecule-by-molecule. In the top-down approach on the other hand bulk starting material is reduced in size using physical or chemical means [15,16]. Top-down synthetic approaches produce structures with surface imperfections. Such imperfections can have crucial impact on physical properties and surface chemistry of metallic nanostructures due to high aspect ratio [15]. Examples of top-down approaches include milling and attrition [17], laser ablation [18], and the exploding wire method [19]. Bottom-up approaches for metallic nanostructure synthesis could be broadly classified into physical, chemical, and biological methods and have been elegantly reviewed [14,15,20].

Apart from metals, carbon and silica are among the most popular nonmetals exploited in nanostructure synthesis for drug delivery. Fullerenes are hollow cage-like structures composed exclusively of carbon atoms. Although several fullerenes exist, by far the most popular is the buckyball or the C60 molecule. Composed of 60 carbon atoms arranged in the shape of a truncated icosahedron or a soccer ball, this cage-like molecule, emits photoluminescence that could be exploited in imaging technologies [21], is highly reactive enabling facile modification with therapeutic and targeting ligands [22] and could form complexes with other atoms and molecules such as nucleic acids and proteins making them interesting drug delivery vehicles [23,24] and possibly allowing co-therapy [22] and theranostic advantages [25]. Similarly, mesoporous silica nanostructures have the capability of hosting different guest molecules [26], such as drugs, macromolecular therapeutics, and imaging and contrast agents. Mesoporous silica nanostructures also offer the possibility of tailored drug release. For example, gate-like structures could be covalently anchored to the nanostructure's pore outlets, obstructing drug release via the mesopore entrances. Such nanogates allow drug release only when needed and in most cases in response to internal or external stimuli. For instance, the synthesis of a pH-responsive nanogated MSN using acetal group linked AuNPs as gates was recently reported. The hydrolysis of acetal linker at acidic pH liberates the AuNPs releasing the loaded drug. The latter is quiet desirable in the treatment of acidic targets, such as tumors and inflammatory tissues [27].

From a drug delivery perspective, inorganic structures are capable of drug targeting [28], assisting in simultaneous treatment and diagnosis [29], drug encapsulation (as opposed to surface attachment), and providing tunable drug release [30]. Also, due to their intrinsic surface plasmon resonance, AuNPs (and other metallic NPs) exhibit strongly enhanced visible and near-infrared light absorption, that is several orders of magnitude stronger than that of conventional laser phototherapy agents [31] and hence have been efficiently exploited in photothermal therapy [14]. However, for drug delivery, the nature of material is quite important and despite the increased potential of such NPs their long-term use is limited by their toxicity and nonbiodegradability [32].

Nonbiodegradability in particular would lead to long-term toxicity, as opposed to drugs/or carriers that cause transient toxicity and are then cleared by the body, ending the cascade of toxic events. For instance, after 28 days of oral exposure to AgNPs, silver was cleared from most organs after 8 weeks postdosing, but remarkable accumulation was found in the brain and testis of rats [33]. Similarly, 40 nm I.V. AuNPs were removed from the circulation primarily by Kupffer cells of the liver. Although the percentage of Au-containing Kupffer cells decreased with time, AuNP clusters within the cells markedly increased in size. The latter was a result of phagocytosis of damaged AuNP-containing Kupffer cells by nearby Kupffer cells, leading to further accumulation of AuNPs. Over a period of 6 months, only a 9% fall in the gold content was observed and it was concluded that even after the normal life span of the mouse, most of the gold nanoparticles will remain in the liver [34]. From a toxicity aspect, on several occasions, the administration of inorganic NPs has been reported to cause oxidative stress, DNA damage [35,36], and major damage in the liver, spleen, and lungs [37]. Also, blood clotting and hemolysis have been reported following intravenous administration [38]. In addition to the nature of the material, the nanostructure shape is a major determinant of its toxicity profile [32]. For example, chronic exposure to carbon nanotubes have been reported to cause epithelioid granulomatous lesions in the lung, persistent interstitial inflammation, aggregation of platelets *in vitro*, possibly enhancing vascular thrombosis, as well inducing apoptosis in models of human kidney and bronchi [39–43]. Similarly, gold nanorods show higher toxicity than gold nanospheres [44]. For such reason and despite their potential, the use of inorganic nanostructures in drug delivery has been quite limited in comparison to organic, spherical nanostructures. Nanostructures for drug delivery are essentially dosage forms and their formulation materials should principally be of approved pharmaceutical excipients, such as biodegradable and biocompatible polymers and lipids and organic materials.

6.2.2 Organic Nanostructures

6.2.2.1 Drug Nanocrystals

The term nanocrystal is generally applied to nanometric drug particles, despite the fact that based on the production technology, amorphous nanostructures could also be obtained [45]. Drug nanocrystals are composed of 100% drug and are accordingly free of carrier material [16]. Due to the increased surface area, drug nanocrystals are characterized by increased dissolution velocity compared to bulk drug. They also exhibit increased saturation solubility [46,47], as well as increased adhesive properties. Amorphous drug nanoparticles show enhanced solubility when compared to crystalline nanoparticles; however, preservation of amorphous state upon storage is complicated [45]. Apart from enhancing solubility, drug nanocrystals offer other advantages such as enhanced bioavailability and absorption rates, improved dose proportionally, and reduced intersubject variability [46,48,49]. In addition, owing to their small-size drug nanocrystal suspensions could be intravenously administered. "Per definition" their intravenous injection would lead to a 100% bioavailability [16]. Nanocrystals could also be successfully administered via several alternate routes that were not possible with bulk drug, such as dermal [50], pulmonary [51], and buccal [52] administration.

Several methods of drug nanocrystal synthesis have been developed. While the most popular methods are the bottom-up and top-down methods [16,45], recently methods combining both modalities have come into focus [47] (Figure 6.2). On the commercial front, top-down approaches are the most dominant [16,45]. Top-down production methods are basically high-energy processes in which drug particles are broken down to particles of smaller size by mills and homogenizers such as pearl milling and high-pressure homogenization using piston gap and jet stream homogenizers [16,45,47,53]. Rapamune®, Emend®, Tricor®, and Megace ES® are all examples of commercial drug nanocrystal-containing formulations prepared by the top-down approach, pearl milling [45]. Despite success on the commercial front, milling and homogenization-based techniques are time consuming, cannot reduce particle size below a certain limit (which in most of the cases is about 150–300 nm) and of concern are issues related to the solid-state changes of the milled product and chemical

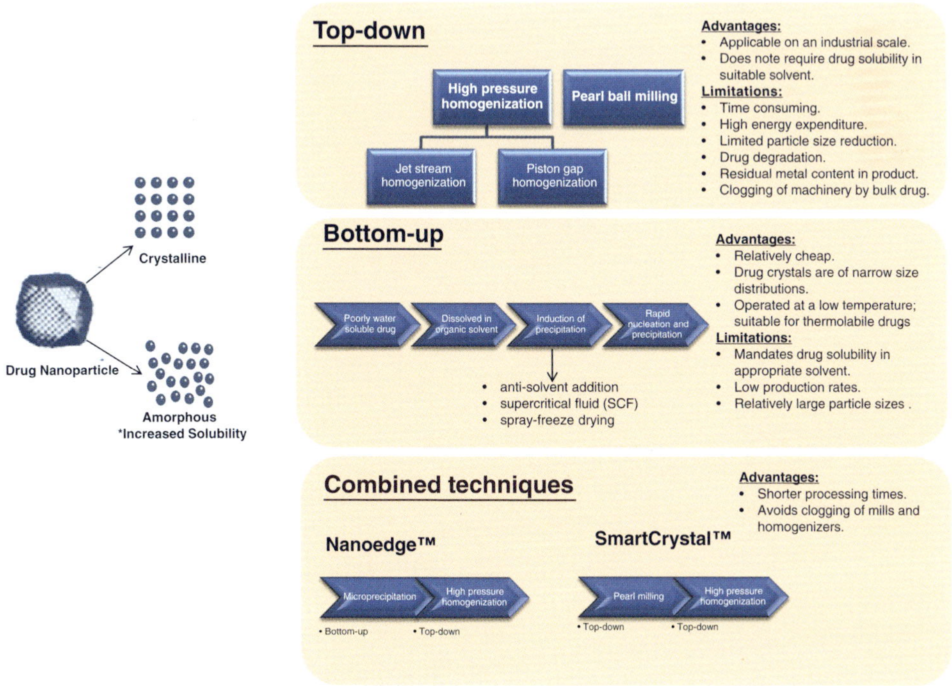

Figure 6.2 Drug nanocrystal classification and synthesis methods by top-down, bottom-up, and combinative techniques.

degradation [47]. Also, residual metal content is a potential issue with top-down processes [16].

Precipitation-based processes are examples of bottom-up techniques [47]. Precipitation-based methods are low-energy processes that do not require complicated machinery. They are less expensive, provide drug crystals with narrow size distributions, and could be operated at a low temperature, making them suitable for thermolabile drugs [47]. These methods mandate dissolving the drug in an appropriate solvent, after which nanocrystal formation occurs by precipitation of the drug by several methods such as by antisolvent addition [54], by using supercritical fluids (SCFs) [55], or by the removal of solvent for instance by spray-freeze drying [56]. Alternatively, precipitation could also be performed in conjunction with centrifugation (high-gravity precipitation) [57]. For precipitation methods in general, it is important to note that the formed nanocrystals still need to be stabilized to circumvent further growth in to the micrometer range. One method of doing so is performing precipitation in the presence of special polymers. This approach was successfully applied in the nanocrystallization of ibuprofen, itraconazole, and ketoconazole [58,59]. Moreover, the drug needs to be soluble in at least one solvent, which may be problematic for new drugs that are insoluble in both aqueous and organic media [45]. In addition, advanced techniques such as processing with supercritical fluid are relatively expensive [47]. Also, of the critical challenges the precipitation methods face are the low production rates, relatively large particle sizes (typically ~100–500 nm), and batch-to-batch variation [60]. Recent variations of the precipitation technique focused at reducing the nanocrystal size, show quite promising results in the lab [60,61]. On a more industrial level, in attempt to reduce limitations and complications seen with both the top-down and bottom-up approaches, combinative techniques were developed. For instance, to avoid long processing times and clogging of mills and homogenizers Baxter developed the first combinative method known as Nanoedge™ technology. NanoEdge™ starts with bottom-up microprecipitation, followed by top-down high-pressure homogenization [62]. Recently, several other combinative approaches have been developed, which combine precipitation by freeze drying or spray drying with high-pressure homogenization [63] or two top-down approaches such as low-energy pearl milling, followed by high-pressure homogenization (SmartCrystal™ technology) [64].

6.2.2.2 Matrix Systems

Matrix systems are very popular for drug delivery, particularly for sustained release formulations [65]. Such systems are solid monolithic structures in which drug molecules are dissolved, encapsulated, chemically bound, or adsorbed to a polymeric or lipid matrix. Matrix nanostructures in most cases lack a distinctive external wall [66,67].

Polymeric Matrix Nanocarriers

For pharmaceutical applications, biodegradability and biocompatibility of a polymer are of utmost importance. Biodegradation occurs when water penetrates the polymeric matrix, hydrolyzing and shortening the polymer chains, reducing their molecular weight (MW), and inducing metabolism of the fragments and NP erosion [68]. Biocompatibility is different than biodegradability and implies that a material is not toxic nor has deleterious effects on biological systems. However, it should be noted that biocompatibility does not entail biodegradability. For instance, poly(*N*-isopropyl acrylamide) is nontoxic, biocompatible but not biodegradable [68]. In this case, how such biocompatible nanocarriers are to be eliminated from the body should be considered to avoid tissue overloading with nondegradable polymers.

Hydrophobic Polymers Most of the polymers used in matrix NP formulation for drug delivery are hydrophobic. Examples of hydrophobic biodegradable polymers include poly(lactic acid) (PLA), poly(lactide-*co*-glycolic acid) (PLGA), poly (ε-caprolactone) (PCL), and poly(alkyl cyanoacrylates) (PACA), whereas other acrylate polymers such as eudragit and ethyl cellulose are examples of nonbiodegradable polymers [69]. NP synthesis from some acrylate polymers could be synthesized by polymerization. For instance, poly(methylmethacrylate) and poly (ethylcyanoacrylate) NPs could be synthesized via emulsion polymerization, whereas poly(alkylcyanoacrylate) NPs are formulated by interfacial polymerization [67]. However, in such case, the interactions between the drugs and the polymers being formed should be considered as well as their subsequent change in reactivity [70].

Owing to their hydrophobicity, emulsion based techniques are the most popular means of NP formulation from preformed hydrophobic polymers [71]. For the emulsion formation, the polymer and in most cases a hydrophobic drug are dissolved in an organic, halogenated solvent and emulsified in an aqueous medium containing a surfactant (o/w emulsion). The subsequent evaporation of the organic phase allows for nucleation of the polymer on the water–solvent interphase, and hardening of the nanoemulsion droplets to from nanoparticles [69,72]. Several other modalities of the emulsion–solvent evaporation technique have been used to allow for NP formation. These methods avoid the use of toxic halogenated solvents [71]. In the emulsion–solvent diffusion technique, the organic solvent used is partially water miscible and therefore the subsequent addition of water to the emulsion leads to solvent diffusion into the external phase, resulting in the formation of NPs. The organic solvent can then be eliminated under reduced pressure [73]. A variation of the emulsion–diffusion technique is the salting-out method. In this method, the drug and polymer are initially dissolved in a solvent such as acetone, and emulsified in an aqueous phase containing a surfactant and a salting out agent (such as magnesium chloride or calcium chloride). Upon dilution of the emulsion, the diffusion of acetone into the aqueous phase occurs thus inducing the formation of NPs [74]. Unfortunately, all of the aforementioned methods are not suitable for fragile molecule encapsulation, particularly protein and nucleic acid drugs. Due to the use of organic solvent, fragile drugs are exposed to hydrophobic interfaces (i.e., organic solvent and air) and subsequently suffer denaturation [75,76]. In addition to the denaturing conditions, emulsion-based methods also have other drawbacks. Despite high encapsulation efficiencies of hydrophobic drugs, emulsion-based techniques are traditionally recognized as unsuitable for water-soluble drugs [77]. In attempt to encapsulate hydrophilic drugs, w/o/w double emulsions are used in which the hydrophilic drug is initially dissolved in water, while the polymer is dissolved in a water-immiscible solvent. The drug-containing aqueous phase is emulsified in the polymeric organic solution. This primary w/o emulsion is emulsified again in a surfactant-containing aqueous phase, resulting in the formation of a w/o/w double emulsion. However, this method yields poor encapsulation efficiencies (EE) of small, low-molecular-weight (MW) drugs, because of their escaping tendency into the external aqueous phase [71,78]. The latter also holds for larger drugs such as proteins. Francis *et al.* [79] used the double emulsion–solvent evaporation technique for protein encapsulation in PLGA and eudragit NPs and observed that for NPs smaller than 470 nm protein encapsulation did not occur. Even for larger NPs, protein encapsulation was quite low and inhomogeneous [79].

Another major drawback of the emulsion-based technique is the associated toxicity imparted by the surfactants and residual organic solvents. Recent studies have shown the relatively high impact of the surfactant on a NPs surface properties and toxicity [80,81]. However, in some cases, the impactful effect of surfactants has been exploited in therapy. For instance, Singh *et al.* demonstrated that PLGA NPs prepared with Cremophor EL and cetyltrimethylammonium bromide as surfactants, demonstrated high P-glycoprotein modulatory activity, enhancing the cytotoxicity of doxorubicin in multidrug-resistant cancer [80]. The nanoprecipitation technique, also known as the solvent displacement method, is a non-emulsion-based method for NP formulation. In this method, two miscible liquids are used: the solvent, in which the drug and polymer are dissolved, and the nonsolvent. Nanoprecipitation occurs by rapid desolvation of the polymer when the polymer solution is added to the nonsolvent. Upon diffusion of the polymer-containing solvent into the dispersing medium, the polymer precipitates, entrapping the drug and leading to rapid NP formation. Nanoprecipitation is a single-step process that does not require the use of surfactants and yields NPs with narrow size distributions [69,71]. Similar to the emulsion–diffusion approach, the nanoprecipitation technique avoids the use to toxic halogenated solvents; however, still requires the use of volatile, organic solvents such as acetone and ethyl acetate. These solvents also limit the application of these methods to encapsulation of sensitive macromolecule and protein drugs [82]. In an attempt to synthesize organic solvent/surfactant-free NPs, Ali *et al.* synthesized Eudragit, PLGA, and poly(ethylene glycol) (PEG) modified PLGA NPs via a modified nanoprecipitation approach using PEG as a the solvent. The authors proved that NPs of different sizes could be obtained using the nontoxic PEG, and that the NPs were capable of preserving encapsulated protein activity [82].

Owing to their hydrophobicity and surface charge, polymeric NPs are rapidly opsonized following I.V. administration and cleared by the reticuloendothelial system (RES). Unless the purpose is to target the RES such as in the case of inflammation or some autoimmune diseases [69], these NPs have to be modified in a way allowing them to evade sequestration by the RES. Because hydrophilic, neutral particles show slower opsonization than hydrophobic charged ones [83], one widely used approach to slow opsonization and RES uptake is surface modification with long hydrophilic polymer chains and nonionic surfactants, which can block electrostatic and hydrophobic interactions. PEGs are the most effective and most commonly used of all the polymers tested [84].

Hydrophilic Polymers Chitosans, alginates, and gelatin are examples of hydrophilic polymers and produce hydrogel NPs. Hydrogel NPs contain more than 50% water of their total weight. Macroscopically they appear as solids, they do however behave as liquids on the molecular scale [85]. Chitosan NPs are formulated by covalent or ionic cross-linking. Ionic cross-linking involves the use of low MW polyanions such as tripolyphosphate (TPP) and is referred to as ionotropic gelation. NPs are formed in the ionotropic gelation method upon the addition of an alkaline TPP solution ($pH = 7–9$) into an acidic chitosan solution ($pH = 4–6$) through inter- and intramolecular linkages between TPP phosphates and chitosan amino groups. With different concentrations and added volumes of chitosan and TPP, NPs with varying characteristics can be obtained. Unlike chitosan, alginates are anionic and therefore any cationic species can initiate NP formation. Calcium chloride is received much attention in alginate NP formation. Emulsion-cross-linking, coacervation/precipitation, spray-freeze drying, the emulsion-droplet coalescence method, and sieving of chitosan–drug gels have also been used in chitosan NP synthesis [86].

Gelatin is a biodegradable, biocompatible protein polymer. Type A gelatin is derived from acid-cured tissue, whereas type B is obtained from alkali-cured tissue. The different production processes lead to a difference in the isoelectric point (pI), pH, and other properties of gelatin types A and B. While type A has an isoelectric point (pI) between 8 and 9 and is hence cationic at neutral pH, type B has a pI between 4.8 and 5.4 and is therefore anionic. Gelatin subtypes could therefore be exploited in loading of cationic and anionic drugs [87]. Similar to chitosan, gelatin NPs could be synthesized by several methods including w/o emulsions and coacervation-phase separation. Emulsion-based methods (as with hydrophobic polymers) are limited by the excessive use of surfactant and the large volume of oil phase. They also involve the use of covalent cross-linkers such as glutraldehyde making their synthesis quite harsh and increasing their toxicity [87,19]. In the layer-by-layer method, a gelatin core is synthesized initially by a two-step desolvation and cross-linking procedure. Briefly, gelatin is initially dissolved in water by gentle heating, and then precipitated by a nonsolvent such as acetone. The gel-like precipitate is redissolved in water acidified with HCl, precipitated once more by acetone and finally cross-linked by a very small amount of glutraldehyde. The sequential coating of polycations and polyanions is then conducted by layer-by-layer assembly where the formation of each layer may be monitored by changes in NP zeta potential [88].

Lipid Matrix Nanocarriers

Lipid-based nanocarriers are synthesized from physiological lipids or lipid molecules used as common pharmaceutical excipients [89]. Lipid NPs could be synthesized by high-pressure homogenization and similar to polymeric NPs by a variety of emulsion-based techniques [89,90]. Lipid nanoparticles with solid matrices are further divided into solid lipid nanoparticles (SLN) and nanostructured lipid carriers (NLC). In SLNs, the matrix is composed of lipids (or a blend of lipids) that are solid at room temperature and stabilized by a surfactant layer. While SLNs show improved physical stability (in comparison to lipid nanocapsules) are easily produced and up scaled and are of low cytotoxicity, they unfortunately exhibit low-drug loading and undesired agglomeration resulting in rapid drug release [10,91]. Such undesirable drug release generally occurs due to the SLNs highly crystalline lipid matrix. In SLNs, drugs are loaded in the lipid matrix in its molecular form between fatty acid chains. During production and storage, the formation and enhancement of the crystal structure often leads to drug expulsion [92]. NLCs (also known as the second generation of lipid nanoparticles) are comprised of a lipid core composed of a mixture of solid and liquid lipids [10,91]. As opposed to the highly organized lipid crystal matrix of SLNs, the lipid matrix of NLCs has a less organized crystalline lipid core or more of an amorphous structure, allowing for drug loading in both; molecular form and in clustered aggregates at lattice imperfections. Consequently, NLCs exhibit improved drug loading and reduced drug leakage [92]. Owing to their lipid interiors lipid NPs are generally considered more efficient for hydrophobic drug loading. Encapsulation of hydrophilic drugs is rather a challenging, due to partitioning of the drugs toward the aqueous phase [93]. Several researchers have however demonstrated that hydrophilic drug encapsulation is possible via careful selection of lipid type, particularly with regards to crystallization, hydrophilicity, and self-emulsifying properties of the lipid [93,94]. Similar to hydrophobic polymeric NPs, lipid NPs are also rapidly cleared by the RES and hence their PEGylation or modifications with hydrophilic polymers and surfactants is also required for a prolonged plasma half-life [95].

6.2.2.3 Vesicular Systems

AS opposed to matrix systems, vesicle-based nanocarriers are composed of a core-shell structure. They could be mononuclear or multi nuclear [66,96] and depending on the material of the shell could be either lipid vesicles such liposomes and lipid nanocapsules or polymeric capsules.

Polymeric Nanovesicles

Polymeric nanovesicles or nanocapsules fall in Limbo between nanoemulsion and nanospheres. NCs are emulsions with a solid shell, or nanospheres with liquid interiors [97]. Though in most cases the liquid core is of oily nature and hence used to incorporate hydrophobic drugs [98–100], NCs with aqueous cores have been reported and are known as polymersomes [101], due to their similarity to liposomes. Hydrophilic drugs could be encapsulated in the polymersome aqueous core. In contrast to liposomes (as will be discussed later), owing to the solid nature of the polymer shell, polymeric nanocapsules show an increased stability of the particles upon storage and reduced drug leakage [101]. Membrane viscosity and lateral diffusivity measurements [102,103] have led to the conclusion that membrane fluidity decreases with the increase in MW and polymer chain length [103]. Electromechanical stability also increases with membrane thickness [104] that is directly proportional to MW of the shell-forming material (polymers or lipids). Owing to their lower MW, phospholipid membranes rupture well before polymeric membranes. Prior to complete rupture, even when intact, permeation of water through the thick polymer membranes in polymersomes and nanocapsules is considerably reduced in comparison to lipid membranes and hence NCs show increased stability, reduced drug leakage and possibly decreased burst release than liposomes [76].

Compared to nanospheres, NCs have higher drug loading [99] and a lower polymeric content. The latter is particularly useful in the case of nonbiodegradable polymers. While release from NCs has been comparable to that of emulsions; mainly governed by its partition between the oil core and the external aqueous phase [99,105]. NCs have on different occasions demonstrated the ability to retard drug release. For instance, sustained pH responsive release of doxorubicin from poly (acrylic acid) (PAA)/*N*-isopropylacrylamide (NIPAm) nanocapsules was reported [106]. In general, release from NCs is a function of several parameters, of major importance is the shell thickness. Based on the polymer used, its concentration and the methods of synthesis, NCs with polymeric shells ranging from 1.5–20 nm have been reported [96]. Of the various methods available for NC synthesis, the double emulsification methods seem the most capable of providing sustained release NCs [96].

Interfacial deposition of preformed polymers is one of the most common methods for NC synthesis. In this method, the drug is initially dissolved in an organic water miscible solvent. Oil that is miscible with the solvent but immiscible with the mixture is then added to the drug solution. This mixture is then dispersed in an aqueous phase containing a surfactant. Upon mixing, the solvent diffuses into the aqueous phase inducing polymer aggregation around the oil droplet and NC formation [67]. Most of the emulsion-based techniques used to synthesis nanospheres could be optimized for NCs synthesis with addition of oil to the organic phase. The emulsion solvent diffusion technique is however an exception. Although Pisani *et al.* [107] were able to prepare NCs using the emulsion solvent evaporation technique, it is generally not recommended for nanoencapsulation. NCs do not resist direct evaporation of the solvent, possibly due to the mechanical stress induced by gas bubble formation inside the aqueous suspension [96].

Synthesis of polymersomes on the other hand is more closely related to liposome synthesis. Phase inversion (solvent switching) and polymer rehydration are two of the most popular techniques for polymersome synthesis. In the polymer rehydration technique, amphiphilic block copolymers are initially dissolved in an organic solvent, and a thin film is formed by evaporation of the solvent.

Subsequent film hydration leads to polymersome formation where water permeates through defects in the polymer layers causing polymer layer inflation and formation of bulges, which finally produce vesicles upon separation from the surface [101]. In the absence of organic solvent, due to their amphiphilic nature, block copolymers display a plethora of ordered morphologies, including lamellar phases. Hydration of the dry lamellae by aqueous solution leads to the formation of a stable dispersion of amphiphilic block copolymer aggregates. For amphiphiles in solution, a time-average molecular shape in the form of a cylinder, wedge, or cone entails whether membrane, cylindrical, or spherical morphologies will respectively form. This average molecular shape is dependent on of the hydrophilic fraction (f). For generating polymersomes in water, a phospholipid-like ratio of hydrophilic fraction to total mass: $f \approx 35 \pm 10\%$ is favored [108]. By changing the hydrophilic block fraction of an amphiphilic block copolymer, the morphology of the resultant structure in aqueous solution can be directed toward spherical micelles ($f > 50\%$), worm-like micelles ($40\% < f < 50\%$), or unilamellar polymer vesicles such as polymersomes ($25\% < f < 40\%$) [109]; enabling organic solvent-free synthesis of polymersomes. The latter would be quite useful in encapsulation of macromolecule drugs that normally suffer degradation upon exposure to hydrophobic interfaces.

In polymersome synthesis, the copolymers used are amphiphilic contain PEG or similar molecules, for such reason polymersomes are naturally stealthed [101]. Hydrophobic lipid capsules on the other hand require PEGylation to avoid rapid RES sequestration and elimination [97].

Lipid Nanovesicles

Liposomes Composed of a hydrophilic head group and two long hydrophobic tails, phospholipids are poorly soluble in water and therefore tend to self-assemble into bilayers. At the edge of a phospholipid bilayer increased energy exits due to the exposure of hydrophobic tails to water. To minimize this energy, the bilayer closes to form spherical vesicles eliminating the edges [110]. For such reason, phospholipids tend to form spherical vesicles in aqueous solutions known as liposomes. Liposomes consist of an aqueous core entrapped by one (unilamellar; ULVs) or more bilayers (multilamellar; MLVs) composed of natural or synthetic lipids. Liposomes could entrap a wide range of drugs; lipophilic drugs are entrapped in the lipid bilayer, whereas strongly hydrophilic drugs are located exclusively in the aqueous compartment. Drugs with intermediate hydro/lipophilicity partition between the lipid and aqueous phases, both in the bilayer and in the aqueous core [111].

Similar to polymersomes, liposomes are synthesized via the hydration of lipid films. Conventional methods of liposome synthesis include the Bangham method, the detergent depletion method, the ethanol/ether injection method, and the reverse-phase evaporation and emulsion-based methods [110,112]. Unfortunately, all of the aforementioned methods involve the organic solvents. Organic solvent-free synthesis includes agitating lipids in water to produce

MLVs. MLVs could then be subjected to several cycles of freeze-thawing in order to increase entrapment efficiencies for water-soluble drugs. ULVs could subsequently be obtained from the MLVs by sonication, French press or high-pressure homogenization techniques. Methods relying on supercritical fluids (SCFs) have also been developed. SCFs are gradually replacing organic solvents since they enable more efficient separation and purification. SCF-based methods such as supercritical fluid injection and decompression enables large-scale, organic solvent-free synthesis and more interestingly *in-situ* sterilization [112].

Liposomes allow drug encapsulation [111] rather than surface adsorption, protecting the loaded cargo from degradation. Liposomes could also coencapsulate several therapeutic and imaging agents making liposomal cotherapy [113] and theranostics [114] possible. Liposomes are rapidly eliminated *in-vivo* by the RES; however, their surface modification is quite simple, where PEGylated (stealthed) liposomes and immunoliposomes show tremendous success in targeted drug delivery, particularly in cancer [10]. Moreover, they are of low toxicity, immunogenicity, and are in most cases biodegradable and biocompatible [10]. Their main weak points lie in their stability and premature drug leakage *in vivo*. The latter is quite emphasized in liposomes composed of natural phospholipids such as egg or soybean phosphatidylcholine that form more permeable and less stable bilayers (first-generation liposomes). Liposomes formed from saturated phospholipids with long acyl chains (e.g., dipalmitoylphosphatidylcholine) [115] or those containing cholesterol [115] and sphingomyelin [116] form more rigid, impermeable bilayer structures and hence are more stable [117–119]. Such changes have led to a reduction in premature drug release. Further modifications have led to the synthesis of liposomes capable of drug release in response to internal stimuli; such as pH [120] or specific enzymes [121] or external stimuli such as heat [122] and/or low-frequency ultrasound [123].

Bolaamphiphiles (BA) are a novel class of lipids containing two hydrophilic domains located at both ends of the hydrophobic domain. Unlike conventional liposomes, BA vesicles contain monolayer membranes as opposed to bilayers. This aspect in particular makes BA vesicles more stable and less prone to drug leakage. However, as with phospholipids several different BAs exist and consequently could form different structures, some of them more stable than others. For instance, short-chain BAs form micelles, longer chain BAs form vesicles. However, if a diamide midsection is incorporated into the hydrophobic chain of BAs, shorter chains form vesicles whereas longer ones form fibers. Interestingly, replacing the diamide with a diester midsection leads to vesicle formation with both short- and long-chained BAs, both of which are more stable than vesicles made from BAs with diamide midsections and hence are more suitable for drug delivery [10,124].

Lipid Nanocapsules Lipid NCs composed of an oily core and a surfactant shell have also been developed for the delivery of lipophilic drugs [70,125]. These NCs are formulated from biocompatible excipients via an organic solvent free-phase inversion technique [100]. Generally, NC synthesis would involve; an oily phase (mainly medium chain triglycerides), a mixture of hydrophilic and lipophilic surfactants and a NaCl solution as the external phase [70]. In the phase inversion technique, the oil, surfactants, and salt water are initially mixed with a gradual rise in temperature leading to the formation of a w/o emulsion as determined by its low conductivity. The system is then cooled down leading to phase inversion and the formation of an o/w emulsion (high conductivity). An aqueous LNC suspension is obtained following dilution with water [126]. Due to the low solubility of hydrophobic drugs in the external aqueous phase during LNC preparation, EE is quite high [127]. Similar to other NCs, LNC also contain a low amount of excipients (relative to drug) compared to NP formulations [127]. It should however be noted that care has to be taken when considering the surfactant mixture for LNC preparations and that not all surfactant lead to LNC formation. For instance, it was shown that LNC preparation was not possible using Cremophor A6 as the sole surfactant as opposed to Cremophor A25. The underlying reason might be the higher hydrophobicity of the Cremophor A6 in comparison to Cremophor A25 and accordingly the polar head group was too short to undergo successful phase inversion upon temperature change. Accordingly, the affinities of the surfactant for the oily and aqueous phases have to be balanced for successful LNC formulation [125,128]. Similarly, LNC formulation is only possible for a range of excipient ratios where the optimal formulation would correspond to 20% oil phase, 20% surfactant, and 60% water phase [126].

Release from LNC also seems to follow zero-order kinetics where the release rate is mainly affected by drug lipid interactions and partitioning between the liquid oily core of the capsule and the external aqueous phase [125]. In that sense, release from LNC could be comparable to that of nanoemulsion or polymeric NCs with quite thin membranes since the LNC shell is presumably a "molecular monolayer" [125]. It is however notable that drug release rates from LNC could be somewhat controlled by the adjustment by favorable drug-lipid interactions.

Similar to polymersomes, LNCs are intrinsically stealthy, since most of the surfactants used contain PEG or similar hydrophilic parts [126,129]. Their stealthiness is further amplified by their rather small size sine LNCs are generally ≤100 nm making them even more invisible to RES sequestration [126,129]. Their small size also makes them optimum vehicles [100].

6.3 Drug Loading and Release

With the diversity in the available types and classes of nanostructures developed for drug delivery, comes the diversity in strategies for drug loading. In a broad sense, drugs could be either encapsulated within the nanostructure or bound to the surface either chemically or simply by adsorption. It is generally agreed upon that drug encapsulation, as opposed to surface binging offers protection of the loaded cargo from degradation by enzymatic attack, pH, or temperature variation [130]. Surface-bound drug could be attached to a nanostructure surface either via covalent linking or simply by adsorption through hydrophobic or electrostatic interactions for instance [131]. Covalent attachment mostly requires chemical modification possibly causing reduced drug release or incomplete intracellular processing of a drug or prodrug [131]. On the other hand, despite being rapid, simple and (in most cases) not needing preliminary modification, the possible displacement of the adsorbed drugs *in vivo* is a major problem with surface-adsorbed drugs [132]. Serum proteins in many cases have a higher affinity for the nanostructure surface than the drug and hence induce the premature release of drug. A number of studies conducted [133,134] using NPs with adsorbed antibodies have reported displacement of the antibodies by serum proteins. In the following sections, drug encapsulation rather than surface binding will be further discussed. For simplicity, drugs will be classified into three classes: hydrophobic drugs, hydrophilic drugs, and macromolecular dugs, including proteins, DNA, and RNA therapeutics.

6.3.1 Hydrophobic Drugs

Encapsulation of hydrophobic drug in hydrophobic polymeric NPs is quite efficient. Due to the similar hydrophobicity, drug polymer interaction is increased. Moreover, there is a reduced diffusion of the drug into the aqueous continuous phase, increasing EE. This is why emulsion-based methods generally lead to high EE of hydrophobic drugs [94]. Drug release from polymeric NPs occurs by a variety of mechanisms, including desorption of the surface-bound/adsorbed drug, diffusion through the NP matrix, NP matrix erosion, or a combination of both erosion and diffusion [135]. Even though the EE is quite high, release from matrix NPs is somehow uncontrollable, with most drugs exhibiting an initial burst release [100]. The diffusion of the drug molecules through the NP polymer matrix depends on the interaction of the drug with the polymeric matrix and surrounding medium, the MW and diffusion coefficient of the drug, its concentration throughout the polymer matrix and the distance the drug has to traverse from its location within the NP matrix to the external phase (NP size) [136]. Due to their larger surface-area-to-volume ratio, in smaller NPs most of the drug is located near the particle surface, leading to faster drug release [136]. Larger particles on the other hand, have large cores, allowing more drug to be encapsulated per particle [4] and giving slower release, since the drug would have to diffuse through a larger polymeric matrix to reach the external phase [136]. So increasing NP size will increase EE and reduce burst release, but all on the expense of NP cell uptake since smaller NPs exhibit several order of magnitude higher uptake than larger NPs [4]. Since polymer matrix degradation is a major player in a NPs release profile, increasing the polymer's MW would also retard release. For instance, the *in-vitro* release of estradiol from PLGA NPs decreased with increase in PLGA MW [137]. In order to tackle the burst release problem (independent of formulation), gel filtration to remove surface-bound drug and reduce burst release is also a possible approach [138].

Lipophilic drugs are generally unsuitable for injection [127], and hence their encapsulation into hydrophilic nanocarriers would be advantageous. Though more complicated than in hydrophobic polymers, the encapsulation of hydrophobic drugs is also possible in hydrophilic polymers. For instance, an EE of 73% was achieved for the hydrophobic cyclosporine A by dissolving it in an acetonitrile/water mixture (1:1) prior to its incorporation into chitosan solution and addition of the TPP in the ionotropic gelation method [139]. However, cyclosporine A is a polypeptide with a MW surpassing 1 kDa, whether the latter is applicable to smaller hydrophobic drugs is questionable. Via a modified version of the ionic gelation method, rifampicin was loaded into chitosan NPs with a high EE. To do so, an organic rifampicin solution was emulsified in a polymer surfactant solution forming an o/w emulsion. Cross-linking of the particles was then induced by addition of TPP. Interestingly, these NPs resulted in a mild initial burst release followed by a sustained release of rifampicin [140].

Lipid matrix NPs are also good alternatives for hydrophobic drug loading. It is well established that NLCs are quite efficient drug delivery vehicles, where they encapsulate lipophilic drugs with high EEs, provide sustained release, retain drug activity, and avoid drug leakage upon storage for long durations [92,141,142]. Although SLNs do suffer from relatively low EE and burst release, favorable interactions between drug and lipid could be exploited to increase EE and delay drug release. For instance, prednisolone-loaded SLNs were able to provide a sustained release of drug over period of five weeks. More interestingly, when an inner lipid matrix composed of cholesterol was used ≈84% drug was released as opposed to ≈37% only when compritol was used [143]. The latter is a sensible explanation behind the improved performance of SLNs since favorable drug lipid interaction is the reason as to why some LNC also exhibit a retardation in release of drugs [125].

Similar to biological membranes, liposomes have low permeability to hydrophilic drugs and high permeability to hydrophobic ones. For such reason, retention of highly hydrophobic drugs is problematic [144]. An example of such drugs is docetaxel. Zhigaltsev *et al.* have however modified docetaxel and demonstrated that a weak-base derivative can be actively loaded into liposomes using pH gradient loading techniques to achieve stable drug encapsulation and controlled drug release [145]. Polymeric nanocapsules provide a good alternative for hydrophobic drug encapsulation owing to their thicker, more rigid membranes [96,101]. Penicillin G was loaded into poly(butyl adipate) NCs reaching an EE of 77% by the double emulsion based method. The authors used two surfactants, Span and Tween, and reported that increasing Span concentration as an inner surfactant results in an increased entrapment of penicillin G mostly, since Span sealed the inner aqueous phase. Increasing Tween concentration as the outer surfactant enhanced the viscosity of external water phase, decreasing the rate of penicillin G diffusion from the inner water phase to the outer water phase synergistically increasing EE [146]. Liposomes and polymersomes both offer the advantage of coloading hydrophilic and lipophilic drugs at the same time.

However, as opposed to liposomes, encapsulation of hydrophobic drugs in polymersome membranes is more stable [76]. For instance, polymersomes coloaded with doxorubicin and taxol simultaneously allowed a higher maximum tolerated dose than the free drug cocktail, shrank tumors more effectively and more sustainably than free drug [147].

LNCs afford a relatively hydrophilic surface and an oily core allowing for encapsulation of hydrophobic drugs, while imparting an overall hydrophilicity to the drug/nanocarrier complex enabling I.V. administration of lipophilic drugs. The encapsulation of hydrophobic ibuprofen into 50 nm LNCs synthesized from biocompatible pharmaceutical excipients allowed for an EE of 94–98%, an increased AUC and half-life following I.V. administration and led to a prolongation of the pain relief for at least 2 h in comparison to drug solution [127]. High EE and a sustained release from LNCs were also obtained for amiodarone [100].

6.3.2 Hydrophilic Drugs

Encapsulation of low MW hydrophilic drugs in hydrophobic polymeric matrix NPs is quite low, due to escape of the drug molecules into the aqueous continuous phase [148]. Even with methods developed especially for hydrophilic molecules such as the w/o/w emulsion-based method, EE is still low [78]. Even if encapsulated, drug particles tend to form small clusters on the surface or within the polymer matrix just below the surface of the NPs, or merely adsorb onto the NP surface resulting in a high initial burst release [148,149]. Several approaches however were used to enhance encapsulation of water-soluble drugs in polymeric matrix NPs. These approaches include modifications to (1) the polymer, (2) the continuous aqueous phase, and (3) the drug. For example, modification of PLGA with mannose and PEG increased EE of amphotericin B where mannose-PLGA and mannose-PEG-PLGA NPs showed $\approx$1.3- and 1.5-fold increased encapsulation, respectively. Such increase in EE was attributed to the increased miscibility between the drug and modified polymer [150]. Making the aqueous phase less amenable to drug diffusion by addition of electrolytes or nonelectrolytes to the external water phase is also a possible approach. The electrolytes decrease the difference in osmotic pressure between the external and internal water phases, thereby retarding the leaching of hydrophilic drugs into the external phase [71]. Reducing drug solubility in the aqueous phase for instance by pH change also reduced drug diffusion into the external phase and increased EE of rhodamine 123 in PLGA NPs [151]. Changes to the drug itself include complexation with hydrophobic moieties that will increase the drug's overall hydrophobicity increasing interaction with the polymer. Such technique is known as hydrophobic ion-pairing (HIP) complexation. Almost 100% EE of gentamicin sulfate in PLGA NPs was achieved following complexation of anionic bis(2-ethylhexyl) sulfosuccinate sodium salt with cationic drug [152]. The water-in-oil (w/o) emulsion phase separation/coacervation provides high encapsulation efficiency of hydrophilic drugs [153]. Controlling the coacervation step is however, quiet challenging, and the method requires the costly handling of large quantities of oils [71]. Interestingly, over 90% EE for clodronate in Eudragit has been achieved by a modified solvent displacement method. Eudragit RL was initially dissolved in ethyl acetate whereas clodronate in water. Due to the partial miscibility of ethyl acetate with water, molecular dispersion of drug in the ethyl acetate/Eudragit phase was possible upon addition of the inner aqueous phase at a volume lower than the water saturation capacity of ethyl acetate. Due to electrostatic interaction between drug and polymer, the drug did not precipitate upon mixing with organic solvent and NP formation was possible [78].

One would generally assume that encapsulation of hydrophilic molecules would be more successful in hydrophilic polymers since the solubility of both the drug and the polymer in the same solvent would entail their facile interaction especially if they are of opposite charge. While the latter might be true for encapsulation of macromolecule drugs [4,154–156] (as detailed later), low MW drugs show much lower encapsulation efficiencies. For chitosan, NPs formulated by the ionotropic gelation method for instance; EE was ≈9% and 2–25% for doxorubicin hydrochloride [157,158] and 24% for sodium valproate [135]. The reason for such low efficiency is the rapid diffusion of the drug molecules from the aqueous solution filled pores into the aqueous continues phase [159]. Encapsulated drugs also seem to suffer significant burst release from hydrogel NPs [157]. It is also worth mentioning that owing to its cationic nature, encapsulation of cationic drugs such as doxorubicin is limited by repulsive interactions occurring between drug and polymer. Decreasing such interactions for instance by associating doxorubicin hydrochloride with anionic dextran sulfate, resulted in a twofold increase in EE [157]. However, whether such increase was simply attributed to the neutralization of cationic charge, or to the larger MW of the final drug–polyanion complex is questionable, since dextran sulfate is a very large molecule and hence would lead to entanglement of drug/polyanioin complex into the hydrogel net. The latter is underpinned by the fact that complexation with anionic phosphoric acid lead to an insignificant change in EE of doxorubicin, moreover while doxorubicin NPs exhibited burst release, doxorubicin–dextran sulfate NPs showed a much more sustained pattern [157]. Hydrophilic chitosan NPs could also be synthesized by the emulsion cross-linking method, in which a w/o emulsion is prepared by emulsifying of the chitosan/drug solution in an external oil phase. The emulsion is stabilized by a surfactant and is cross-linked by a cross-linking agent such as glutraldehyde to harden the droplets [86]. It is possible that the use of an external hydrophobic phase in which the drug is insoluble allows for improvement of low MW hydrophilic drug EE, since chitosan NPs prepared with such method show much higher EE; over 80% for theophylline, aspirin or griseofulvin [160]. Such results are not 100% conclusive though, since microparticles as opposed to NPs were formed and the increased EE may be attributed to the larger particle size as opposed to the use of an external oil phase.

Hydrophilic drugs could be tightly encapsulated within the aqueous cores of liposomes, albeit with low efficiencies [144]. Many of the current drugs are weak bases and can be loaded in response to pH gradients [161]. Antineoplastics, local anesthetics, and antihistamines have all been successfully loaded into preformed liposomes in response to an imposed proton gradient [161]. While ML liposomes provide better retardation of hydrophilic drug release, burst release of hydrophilic drugs is observed in UL liposomes [162]. Burst release is also seen in stimuli-responsive liposomes, where a large bolus of drug is released once the membrane is disrupted in response to the stimulus [163]. While the latter might be quiet useful when the trigger is only activated at the drug's target, for instance with-in a tumor [164]. Premature release will result in drug dumping at wrong location resulting in similar toxicities to large blouses of free drug. In comparison to lipids, polymers have higher MWs, the membrane of polymersomes is therefore thicker, stronger, and tougher making them more stable than liposomes [165]. While drug release retardation is relatively limited from polymersomes (in comparison to matrix NPs), thicker membranes generated via increasing polymer concentration during synthesis significantly slows down drug release [96].

For small drugs, with disregard to their hydro/lipophilicity, burst, uncontrolled release is a common dilemma. Covalent modification forms more stable conjugates and therefore uncontrolled release does not pose a problem, on the contrary the question as to how the drug will be released presents itself. Covalent modification could either be labile or nonlabile. For drug delivery, labile conjugates are a must to ensure drug release from the nanostructure at its site of action. Drug conjugation to nanostructures could be conducted directly or indirectly using linker molecules [69]. Examples of cross-linkers include the NHS ester-based amine-sulfhydryl cross-linkers; NS-succinimidyl iodoacetate (SIA), succinimidyl-4-(*N*-maleimidomethyl)cyclohexane-1-carboxylate (SMCC), and *N*-succinimidyl-3-(2-pyridyldithio)-propionate (SPDP). While SIA and SMCC form noncleavable bonds, SPDP conjugates contain reducible disulfide bonds that could be cleaved with cysteine sulfhydryls for example [4,166] and is hence better for drug conjugation [167]. Other cleavable cross-linkers include the amine–amine cross-linkers (3,3′-dithiobis(sulfosuccinimidyl propionate)) (DTSSP) that similar to SPDP are cleaved in the presence of thiols and (bis(2-(succinimidooxycarbonyloxy) ethyl)sulfone) (BSOCOES), which is cleaved in basic pH [168]. Apart from cross-linker molecules, direct conjugation is also possible. For instance, cisplatin was covalently conjugated to the hydrophobic segments of two block copolymer chains Bi(PEG-PLA) through an acid-sensitive hydrazone bond. The polymer cisplatin conjugates readily precipitated in aqueous solutions forming 100 nm NPs due to their very low critical micelle concentrations. The NPs exhibited high cisplatin loading, excellent acid-responsive drug release, and enhanced *in vitro* cytotoxicity against ovarian cancer cells [169].

6.3.3 Macromolecular Drugs

Similar to low MW hydrophilic drugs, EE of proteins and nucleic acid drugs in hydrophobic matrix NPs is quite low [79]. Also, since most of the cargo seems to either be adsorbed on the surface or loaded directly beneath the surface of

NP [79], such systems suffer from an undesirable burst release [170]. Modifications to the polymer, external aqueous phase (in emulsion based methods), and to the drug itself are also used in attempt to increase EE. For instance, PEGylation of PLGA was found to enhance EE of hydrophilic protein drugs prepared by the w/o/w emulsion-based method. During formulation of the primary emulsion, the PEG chains are directed toward the water phase containing the protein. This orientation avoids increased protein content with the water–organic solvent interface, and hence minimizes the interface-induced protein denaturation and aggregation [75]. Similarly, PEGylation of the protein itself also led to increased protein stabilization in PLGA NPs prepared by the double emulsion method [171]. However, nonspecific covalent attachment of a large PEG molecule can lead to changes in the protein structure and consequently its activity [172]. To enhance protein encapsulation, HIP complexation could also be applied. As a result of the increased hydrophobicity, the protein-containing HIP complex, partitioning into the polymeric matrix can be significantly enhanced during encapsulation, increasing EE, and reducing burst release [173–175]. Changes in the composition of the outer an inner water phase also have their impact on EE of macromolecule drugs in the w/o/w emulsion-based approach. Adding 5% NaCl or 15% glucose to the external water phase induced a significant increase in EE of protein drugs [176], similarly $CaCl_2$ was used to increase EE of plasmid DNA [177]. Adding bovine serum albumin (BSA) to the inner water phase increased the EE and preserved the activity of a siRNA [178] and the monoclonal antibody bevacizumab [179]. The increased EE was attributed to the reduced drug leakage and formation of more stable emulsions, due to the surfactant-like characteristics of BSA. Also, the ester backbone in polyester hydrophobic polymers is prone to autocatalytic degradation due to free carboxylic end groups [180]. Such degradation leads to acidification within the NP milieu that leads to degradation of fragile drugs and macromolecules [181]. Coencapsulation with bases such as magnesium hydroxide has been reported to help neutralize acidic pH in the NPs [180].

As opposed to low MW drugs are of larger size and are therefore entangled within the matrix of polymeric NPs exhibiting stronger encapsulation and a more retarded release [182]. Chitosan is an example of biodegradable polymer that has been extensively exploited in the encapsulation of macromolecules. Chitosan NP formulation by the ionotropic gelation method is devoid of organic solvents, where the incorporation of therapeutic molecules occurs via mild electrostatic interactions in aqueous, physiological conditions, preserving their activity [4]. The latter is obvious by the high EE, reduced burst, and improved sustained release of active macromolecular drugs from chitosan hydrogel NPs [4,154,183,184].

Polymersomes formed by film rehydration have been shown to incorporate transmembrane proteins in the bilayer as well as encapsulate proteins in the aqueous lumen, and in most cases retain their functional conformation [76]. Biodegradable polymersomes based on asymmetric PEG–PCL–PDEA triblock successfully encapsulated BSA, cytochrome C, lysozyme, ovalbumin, and immunoglobulin G with very high EE, drug:polymer ratio, were able to provide sustained release of protein and more importantly preserved activity of the released protein [185]. To synthesize these polymersomes, a copolymer solution in chloroform was evaporated to from a thin film, that was further dried under vacuum. The dry film was then rehydrated with the protein solution to form the polymersomes. It is possible that reduced interaction of the proteins with hydrophobic solvent circumvented protein denaturation [185]. Hydrophobic polymers tend to adsorb proteins strongly with an increased tendency to denature proteins at the initial protein-surface interphase. Due to the increased polarity of copolymers, they bind proteins less avidly resulting in better retention of activity [186]. This is a possible reason for the retention of protein activity in polymersomes as opposed to matrix NPs. This is most probably also the reason as to why PEGylation of PLGA or the protein leads to an increased retention of the proteins' activity [75,171].

6.4 General Discussion and Conclusions

While drug nanocrystals offer numerous advantages, they are unfortunately, incapable of *in-vivo* protection of the drug molecule from degradation, drug targeting to specific tissue or cell, providing tunable/tailored plasma or target tissue drug concentrations and they are also not capable of providing any prognostic/diagnostic edge. To impart all of those favorable aspects, drug loading (mainly by encapsulation) is quite important. While several nanostructures for drug delivery have been developed and optimized, an optimal delivery vehicle is yet to exist. Having said that, some nanostructures better fit certain tasks than others. For instance, for protein and macromolecular delivery, the use of polymeric hydrogel NPs seem like a more obvious solution than hydrophobic polymeric NPs or any other capsule carrier with an oily core. While the latter is an obvious example, it might be a harder decision in other cases. For instance, for hydrophobic drug delivery, both hydrophobic polymeric matrix NPs and NCs provide a high EE, however burst release is problematic for NPs but at the same time they do have increased stability relative to NCs. With the control of the polymer thickness layer, NCs could provide controlled drug release and avoid drug leakage, they are however less stable than matrix NPs. Similarly, if a sustained drug concentration in plasma is required or targeting of tumors using the enhanced permeation retention effect it is of utmost importance to use stealth NPs to avoid RES sequestration. Most of LNCs and polymersomes are intrinsically stealthy, LNCs are very efficient lipophilic drug carriers, whereas polymersomes have large aqueous cores making the first a better option for lipophilic drugs, whereas the second a preferable option for hydrophilic drugs. Figure 6.3 attempts to clarify the strengths weaknesses for each of the aforementioned discussed organic nanostructures for drug delivery. The choice of optimal formation would therefore depend on the nature of the drug, required release pattern, mode of administration, and final drug target. However, other parameters to consider would be the

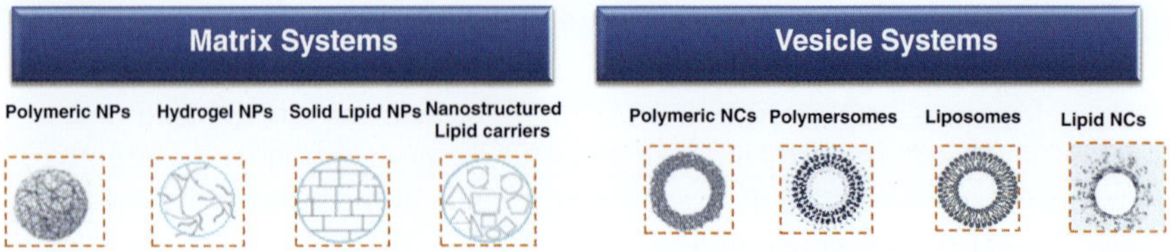

	Polymeric NPs	Hydrogel NPs	Solid Lipid NPs	Nanostructured Lipid carriers	Polymeric NCs	Polymersomes	Liposomes	Lipid NCs
Description	**Hydrophobic polymeric matrix**	**Hydrophilic polymeric matrix**	**Highly crystalline lipid matrix surrounded by surfactant layer**	**Less crystalline lipid matrix surrounded by surfactant layer**	**Polymer shell and an oily core**	**Copolymer shell and an aqueous core**	**Phospholipid bilayer shell and an aqueous core**	**Surfactant shell and an oily core**
Hydrophobic drug EE	High	Low	Low	High	High	Low	Low	High
Hydrophilic drug EE	Low	Low-moderate	Low	Low	Low	High	Low	Low
Macromolecule EE	Low	High	Low	Low	Low	Moderate-high	Low-moderate	Low
Excipient: drug ratio	High	High	High	High	Low	Low	Low	Low
Stealth	Low	Low-moderate	Low	Low	Low	High	Low	High
Stability	High	Moderate-high	High	High	Low	Low	Low	Low

Figure 6.3 Description and characteristics of organic nanostructures for drug delivery.

associated toxicity. While organic nanocarriers are far less toxic than their inorganic counterparts, toxicity of surfactants, residual organic solvents, and chemical cross-linkers all have to be considered. Also how the biocompatible, nonbiodegradable polymers are to be eliminated from the body. For some formulations and in some cases, case-to-case nanocarrier synthesis and design might also serve quite beneficial. Apart from the nanocarriers physicochemical properties, the fate of the nanocarrier in the body is dependent upon the patient health state and therefore a “one size fits all solution” may not work. In this case simple, rapid synthetic procedures that be tailored and conducted on spot in hospitals and clinics for critical cases would be rather interesting. On the other hand form an industrial point of view, focus would be on synthetic procedures that are cost efficient and could be easily scaled up allowing industrial application.

References

1 Merisko-Liversidge, E.M. and Liversidge, G.G. (2008) Drug nanoparticles: formulating poorly water-soluble compounds. *Toxicol. Pathol.*, **36** (1), 43–48.

2 Tian, Q., Zhang, C.-N., Wang, X.-H., Wang, W., Huang, W., Cha, R.-T., Wang, C.-H., Yuan, Z., Liu, M., Wan, H.-Y., and Tang, H. (2010) Glycyrrhetinic acid-modified chitosan/poly(ethylene glycol) nanoparticles for liver-targeted delivery. *Biomaterials*, **31** (17), 4748–4756.

3 Choi, C.H.J., Zuckerman, J.E., Webster, P., and Davis, M.E. (2011) Targeting kidney mesangium by nanoparticles of defined size. *Proc. Natl. Acad. Sci. USA*, **108** (16), 6656–6661.

4 Tammam, S., Azzazy, H.M., Breitinger, H.G., and Lamprecht, A. (2015) Chitosan

nanoparticles for nuclear targeting: the effect of nanoparticle size and nuclear localization sequence density. *Mol. Pharm.*, **12** (12), 4277–4289.
5 Marrache, S. and Dhar, S. (2012) Engineering of blended nanoparticle platform for delivery of mitochondria-acting therapeutics. *Proc. Natl. Acad. Sci. USA*, **109** (40), 16288–16293.
6 Shahbazi, M. and Santos, H. (2013) Improving oral absorption via drug-loaded nanocarriers: absorption mechanisms, intestinal models and rational fabrication. *Curr. Drug Metab.*, **14** (1), 28–56.
7 Tang, R., Kim, C.S., Solfiell, D.J., Rana, S., Mout, R., Velázquez-Delgado, E.M., Chompoosor, A., Jeong, Y., Yan, B., Zhu, Z.-J., Kim, C., Hardy, J.A., and Rotello, V.M. (2013) Direct delivery of functional proteins and enzymes to the cytosol using nanoparticle-stabilized nanocapsules. *ACS Nano*, **7** (8), 6667–6673.
8 Hu, C.-M.J. and Zhang, L. (2012) Nanoparticle-based combination therapy toward overcoming drug resistance in cancer. *Biochem. Pharmacol.*, **83** (8), 1104–1111.
9 Jokerst, J.V. and Gambhir, S.S. (2011) Molecular Imaging with theranostic nanoparticles. *Acc. Chem. Res.*, **44** (10), 1050–1060.
10 Puri, A., Loomis, K., Smith, B., Lee, J., Yavlovich, A., Heldman, E., and Blumentha, R. (2009) Lipid-based nanoparticles as pharmaceutical drug carriers: from concepts to clinic. *Crit. Rev. Ther. Drug Carrier Syst.*, **26** (6), 523–580.
11 Wang, C., Cheng, L., and Liu, Z. (2011) Drug delivery with upconversion nanoparticles for multi-functional targeted cancer cell imaging and therapy. *Biomaterials*, **32** (4), 1110–1120.
12 Mittal, A.K., Chisti, Y., and Banerjee, U.C. (2013) Synthesis of metallic nanoparticles using plant extracts. *Biotechnol. Adv.*, **31** (2), 346–356.
13 Xia, Y. and Halas, N.J. (2005) Shape-controlled synthesis and surface plasmonic properties of metallic nanostructures. *MRS bulletin.*, **30** (05), 338–348.
14 Dreaden, E.C., Alkilany, A.M., Huang, X., Murphy, C.J., and El-Sayed, M.A. (2012) The golden age: gold nanoparticles for biomedicine. *Chem. Soc. Rev.*, **41** (7), 2740–2779.
15 Thakkar, K.N., Mhatre, S.S., and Parikh, R.Y. (2010) Biological synthesis of metallic nanoparticles. *Nanomedicine*, **6** (2), 257–262.
16 Keck, C.M. and Müller, R.H. (2006) Drug nanocrystals of poorly soluble drugs produced by high pressure homogenisation. *Eur. J. Pharm. Biopharm.*, **62** (1), 3–16.
17 Yadav, T., Yadav, R., and Singh, D. (2012) Mechanical milling: a top down approach for the synthesis of nanomaterials and nanocomposites. *J. Nanosci. Nanotechnol.*, **2** (3), 22–48.
18 Mafuné, F., Kohno, J., Takeda, Y., and Kondow, T. (2001) Formation of gold nanoparticles by laser ablation in aqueous solution of surfactant. *J. Phys. Chem. B.*, **105** (22), 5114–5120.
19 Ju Park, E., Won Lee, S., Bang, I.C., and Park, H.W. (2011) Optimal synthesis and characterization of Ag nanofluids by electrical explosion of wires in liquids. *Nanoscale Res. Lett.*, **6** (1), 223.
20 Richards, R. and Bönnemann, H. (2005) Synthetic approaches to metallic nanomaterials, in *Nanofabrication Towards Biomedical Applications*, Wiley-VCH Verlag GmbH & Co. KGaA.
21 Kwag, D.S., Park, K., Oh, K.T., and Lee, E.S. (2013) Hyaluronated fullerenes with photoluminescent and antitumoral activity. *Chem. Commun.*, **49** (3), 282–284.
22 Fan, J., Fang, G., Zeng, F., Wang, X., and Wu, S. (2013) Water-dispersible fullerene aggregates as a targeted anticancer prodrug with both chemo- and photodynamic therapeutic actions. *Small*, **9** (4), 613–621.
23 Evstigneev, M.P., Buchelnikov, A.S., Voronin, D.P., Rubin, Y.V., Belous, L.F., Prylutskyy, Y.I., and Ritter, U. (2013) Complexation of C60 fullerene with aromatic drugs. *ChemPhysChem*, **14** (3), 568–578.
24 Montellano, A., Da Ros, T., Bianco, A., and Prato, M. (2011) Fullerene C_{60} as a

multifunctional system for drug and gene delivery. *Nanoscale*, **3** (10), 4035–4041.
25 Chen, Z., Ma, L., Liu, Y., and Chen, C. (2012) Applications of functionalized fullerenes in tumor theranostics. *Theranostics*, **2** (3), 238.
26 Vallet-Reg, M. (2012) Mesoporous silica nanoparticles: their projection in nanomedicine. *ISRN Mater. Sci.*, **2012**, 1–20.
27 Liu, R., Zhang, Y., Zhao, X., Agarwal, A., Mueller, L.J., and Feng, P. (2010) pH-responsive nanogated ensemble based on gold-capped mesoporous silica through an acid-labile acetal linker. *J. Am. Chem. Soc.*, **132** (5), 1500–1501.
28 Liu, H., Liu, T., Wu, X., Li, L., Tan, L., Chen, D., and Tang, F. (2012) Targeting gold nanoshells on silica nanorattles: a drug cocktail to fight breast tumors via a single irradiation with near infrared laser light. *Adv. Mater.*, **24** (6), 755–761.
29 Hayashi, K., Nakamura, M., Sakamoto, W., Yogo, T., Miki, H., Ozaki, S., Abe, M., Matsumoto, T., and Ishimura, K. (2013) Superparamagnetic nanoparticle clusters for cancer theranostics combining magnetic resonance imaging and hyperthermia treatment. *Theranostics*, **3** (6), 366–376.
30 Moon, G.D., Choi, S.-W., Cai, X., Li, W., Cho, E.C., Jeong, U., Wang, L.V., and Xia, Y. (2011) A New theranostic system based on gold nanocages and phase-change materials with unique features for photoacoustic imaging and controlled release. *J. Am. Chem. Soc.*, **133** (13), 4762–4765.
31 Huang, X., Jain, P., El-Sayed, I., and El-Sayed, M. (2008) Plasmonic photothermal therapy (PPTT) using gold nanoparticles. *Lasers Med. Sci.*, **23** (3), 217–228.
32 Khanna, P., Ong, C., Huat Bay, B., and Baeg, G. (2015) Nanotoxicity: an interplay of oxidative stress, inflammation and cell death. *Nanomaterials*, **5** (3), 1163–1180.
33 van der Zande, M., Vandebriel, R.J., Van Doren, E., Kramer, E., Herrera Rivera, Z., Serrano-Rojero, C.S., Gremmer, E.R., Mast, J., Peters, R.J.B., Hollman, P.C.H., Hendriksen, P.J.M., Marvin, H.J.P., Peijnenburg, A.A.C.M., and Bouwmeester, H. (2012) Distribution, elimination, and toxicity of silver nanoparticles and silver ions in rats after 28-day oral exposure. *ACS Nano*, **6** (8), 7427–7442.
34 Sadauskas, E., Danscher, G., Stoltenberg, M., Vogel, U., Larsen, A., and Wallin, H. (2009) Protracted elimination of gold nanoparticles from mouse liver. *Nanomedicine*, **5** (2), 162–169.
35 Misawa, M. and Takahashi, J. (2011) Generation of reactive oxygen species induced by gold nanoparticles under X-ray and UV irradiations. *Nanomedicine*, **7** (5), 604–614.
36 Eom, H.-J. and Choi, J. (2009) Oxidative stress of CeO_2 nanoparticles via p38-Nrf-2 signaling pathway in human bronchial epithelial cell, Beas-2B. *Toxicol. Lett.*, **187** (2), 77–83.
37 Chen, Y.-S., Hung, Y.-C., Liau, I., and Huang, G.S. (2009) Assessment of the *in vivo* toxicity of gold nanoparticles. *Nanoscale Res. Lett.*, **4** (8), 858–864.
38 Dobrovolskaia, M.A., Aggarwal, P., Hall, J.B., and McNeil, S.E. (2008) Preclinical studies to understand nanoparticle interaction with the immune system and its potential effects on nanoparticle biodistribution. *Mol. Pharm.*, **5** (4), 487–495.
39 Lam, C.-W., James, J.T., McCluskey, R., and Hunter, R.L. (2004) Pulmonary toxicity of single-wall carbon nanotubes in mice 7 and 90 days after intratracheal instillation. *Toxicol. Sci.*, **77** (1), 126–134.
40 Morimoto, Y., Horie, M., Kobayashi, N., Shinohara, N., and Shimada, M. (2012) Inhalation toxicity assessment of carbon-based nanoparticles. *Acc. Chem. Res.*, **46** (3), 770–781.
41 Radomski, A., Jurasz, P., Alonso-Escolano, D., Drews, M., Morandi, M., Malinski, T., and Radomski, M.W. (2005) Nanoparticle induced platelet aggregation and vascular thrombosis. *Br. J. Pharmacol.*, **146** (6), 882–893.
42 Cui, D., Tian, F., Ozkan, C.S., Wang, M., and Gao, H. (2005) Effect of single wall carbon nanotubes on human HEK293 cells. *Toxicol. Lett.*, **155** (1), 73–85.

43 Alazzam, A., Mfoumou, E., Stiharu, I., Kassab, A., Darnel, A., Yasmeen, A., Sivakumar, N., Bhat, R., and Al Moustafa, A.-E. (2010) Identification of deregulated genes by single wall carbon-nanotubes in human normal bronchial epithelial cells. *Nanomedicine*, **6** (4), 563–569.

44 Wang, S., Lu, W., Tovmachenko, O., Rai, U.S., Yu, H., and Ray, P.C. (2008) Challenge in understanding size and shape dependent toxicity of gold nanomaterials in human skin keratinocytes. *Chem. Commun.*, **463** (1–3), 145–149.

45 Junghanns, J.-U.A.H. and Müller, R.H. (2008) Nanocrystal technology, drug delivery and clinical applications. *Int. J. Nanomedicine*, **3** (3), 295–310.

46 Hanafy, A., Spahn-Langguth, H., Vergnault, G., Grenier, P., Tubic Grozdanis, M., Lenhardt, T., and Langguth, P. (2007) Pharmacokinetic evaluation of oral fenofibrate nanosuspensions and SLN in comparison to conventional suspensions of micronized drug. *Adv. Drug Deliv. Rev.*, **59** (6), 419–426.

47 Sinha, B., Müller, R.H., and Möschwitzer, J.P. (2013) Bottom-up approaches for preparing drug nanocrystals: formulations and factors affecting particle size. *Int. J. Pharm.*, **453** (1), 126–141.

48 Liversidge, G.G. and Cundy, K.C. (1995) Particle size reduction for improvement of oral bioavailability of hydrophobic drugs: I. absolute oral bioavailability of nanocrystalline danazol in beagle dogs. *Int. J. Pharm.*, **125** (1), 91–97.

49 Jinno, J.-i., Kamada, N., Miyake, M., Yamada, K., Mukai, T., Odomi, M., Toguchi, H., Liversidge, G.G., Higaki, K., and Kimura, T. (2006) Effect of particle size reduction on dissolution and oral absorption of a poorly water-soluble drug, cilostazol, in beagle dogs. *J. Control. Release*, **111** (1–2), 56–64.

50 Al Shaal, L., Muller, R., and Keck, C. (2010) Preserving hesperetin nanosuspensions for dermal application. *Pharmazie*, **65** (2), 86–92.

51 Sultana, S., Talegaonkar, S., Ali, R., Mittal, G., Ahmad, F.J., and Bhatnagar, A. (2012) Inhalation of alendronate nanoparticles as dry powder inhaler for the treatment of osteoporosis. *J. Microencapsul.*, **29** (5), 445–454.

52 Branham, M.L., Moyo, T., and Govender, T. (2012) Preparation and solid-state characterization of ball milled saquinavir mesylate for solubility enhancement. *Eur. J. Pharm. Biopharm.*, **80** (1), 194–202.

53 Salazar, J., Müller, R.H., and Möschwitzer, J.P. (2013) Performance comparison of two novel combinative particle-size-reduction technologies. *J. Pharm. Sci.*, **102** (5), 1636–1649.

54 Thorat, A.A. and Dalvi, S.V. (2012) Liquid antisolvent precipitation and stabilization of nanoparticles of poorly water soluble drugs in aqueous suspensions: recent developments and future perspective. *Chem. Eng. J.*, **181–182** (1), 1–34.

55 Zhang, J., Huang, Y., Liu, D., Gao, Y., and Qian, S. (2013) Preparation of apigenin nanocrystals using supercritical antisolvent process for dissolution and bioavailability enhancement. *Eur. J. Pharm. Sci.*, **48** (4–5), 740–747.

56 Hu, J., Johnston, K.P., and Williams, R.O. III (2003) Spray freezing into liquid (SFL) particle engineering technology to enhance dissolution of poorly water soluble drugs: organic solvent versus organic/aqueous co-solvent systems. *Eur. J. Pharm. Sci.*, **20** (3), 295–303.

57 Chiou, H., Li, L., Hu, T., Chan, H.K., Chen, J.C., and Yun, J. (2007) Production of salbutamol sulfate for inhalation by high-gravity controlled antisolvent precipitation. *Int. J. Pharm.*, **331** (1), 93–98.

58 Rasenack, N. and Müller, B. (2002) Dissolution rate enhancement by in situ micronization of poorly water-soluble drugs. *Pharm. Res.*, **19** (12), 1894–1900.

59 Rasenack, N. and Müller, B. (2002) Ibuprofen crystals with optimized properties. *Int. J. Pharm.*, **245** (1–2), 9–24.

60 Zhang, J., Li, Y., An, F., Zhang, X., Chen, X., and Lee, C. (2015) Preparation and size control of sub-100 nm pure nanodrugs. *Nano Lett.*, **15** (1), 313–318.

61 Kasai, H., Murakami, T., Ikuta, Y., Koseki, Y., Baba, K., Oikawa, H., Nakanishi, H., Okada, M., Shoji, M., Ueda, M., Imahori, H., and Hashida, M. (2012) Creation of pure nanodrugs and their anticancer properties. *Angew. Chem., Int. Ed.*, **51** (41), 10315–10318.

62 Kipp, J., Wong, J., and Doty, M. (2003) Microprecipitation method for preparing submicron nanosuspensions. US Patent 6,607,784 B2, 2003.

63 Salazar, J., Müller, R.H., and Möschwitzer, J.P. (2013) Performance comparison of two novel combinative particle size reduction technologies. *J. Pharm. Sci.*, **102** (5), 1636–1649.

64 Petersen, R. (2007) Nanocrystals for use in topical cosmetic formulations and method of production thereof. EP 2099420, filed Nov. 19, 2007 and issued Sept. 16, 2009.

65 Nokhodchi, A., Raja, S., Patel, P., and Asare-Addo, K. (2012) The role of oral controlled release matrix tablets in drug delivery systems. *Bioimpacts*, **2** (4), 175–187.

66 Singh, M.N., Hemant, K.S.Y., Ram, M., and Shivakumar, H.G. (2010) Microencapsulation: a promising technique for controlled drug delivery. *Res. Pharm. Sci.*, **5** (2), 65–77.

67 Letchford, K. and Burt, H. (2007) A review of the formation and classification of amphiphilic block copolymer nanoparticulate structures: micelles, nanospheres, nanocapsules and polymersomes. *Eur. J. Pharm. Biopharm.*, **65** (3), 259–269.

68 Mansour, H.M., Sohn, M., Al-Ghananeem, A., and DeLuca, P.P. (2010) Materials for pharmaceutical dosage forms: molecular pharmaceutics and controlled release drug delivery aspects. *Int. J. Mol. Sci.*, **11** (9), 3298.

69 Tammam, S.N., Azzazy, H.M.E., and Lamprecht, A. (2015) Biodegradable particulate carrier formulation and tuning for targeted drug delivery. *J. Biomed. Nanotechnol.*, **11** (4), 555–577.

70 Anton, N., Benoit, J.-P., and Saulnier, P. (2008) Design and production of nanoparticles formulated from nano-emulsion templates—a review. *J. Control. Release*, **128** (3), 185–199.

71 Sah, E. and Sah, H. (2015) Recent trends in preparation of poly(lactide-*co*-glycolide) nanoparticles by mixing polymeric organic solution with antisolvent. *J. Nanomaterials*, **2015**, 22.

72 Staff, R., Landfester, K., and Crespy, D. (2013) Recent advances in the emulsion solvent evaporation technique for the preparation of nanoparticles and nanocapsules, in *Hierarchical Macromolecular Structures: 60 Years after the Staudinger Nobel Prize II* (ed. V. Percec), Springer-Verlag Berlin Heidelberg, 329–344.

73 Moinard-Chécot, D., Chevalier, Y., Briançon, S., Beney, L., and Fessi, H. (2008) Mechanism of nanocapsules formation by the emulsion–diffusion process. *J. Colloid Interface Sci.*, **317** (2), 458–468.

74 Ibrahim, H., Bindschaedler, C., Doelker, E., Buri, P., and Gurny, R. (1992) Aqueous nanodispersions prepared by a salting-out process. *Int. J. Pharm.*, **87** (1), 239–246.

75 Li, Y.-P., Pei, Y.-Y., Zhang, X.-Y., Gu, Z.-H., Zhou, Z.-H., Yuan, W.-F., Zhou, J.-J., Zhu, J.-H., and Gao, X.-J. (2001) PEGylated PLGA nanoparticles as protein carriers: synthesis, preparation and biodistribution in rats. *J. Control. Release*, **71** (2), 203–211.

76 Christian, D.A., Cai, S., Bowen, D.M., Kim, Y., Pajerowski, J.D., and Discher, D.E. (2009) Polymersome carriers: from self-assembly to siRNA and protein therapeutics. *Eur. J. Pharm. Biopharm.*, **71** (3), 463–474.

77 Jelvehgari, M. and Montazam, S.H. (2012) Comparison of microencapsulation by emulsion-solvent extraction/evaporation technique using derivatives cellulose and acrylate-methacrylate copolymer as carriers. *Jundishapur. J. Nat. Pharm. Prod.*, **7** (4), 144–152.

78 Niebel, W., Walkenbach, K., Béduneau, A., Pellequer, Y., and Lamprecht, A. (2012) Nanoparticle-based clodronate delivery mitigates murine experimental colitis. *J. Control. Release*, **160** (3), 659–665.

79 Francis, D., Mouftah, S., Steffen, R., Beduneau, A., Pellequer, Y., and Lamprecht, A. (2015) Ion milling coupled field emission scanning electron microscopy reveals current misunderstanding of morphology of polymeric nanoparticles. *Eur. J. Pharm. Biopharm.*, **89**, 56–61.

80 Singh, M.S. and Lamprecht, A. (2016) P-glycoprotein inhibition of drug resistant cell lines by nanoparticles. *Drug Dev. Ind. Pharm.*, **42** (2), 325–331.

81 Wachsmann, P., Moulari, B., Béduneau, A., Pellequer, Y., and Lamprecht, A. (2013) Surfactant-dependence of nanoparticle treatment in murine experimental colitis. *J. Control. Release*, **172** (1), 62–68.

82 Ali, M.E. and Lamprecht, A. (2013) Polyethylene glycol as an alternative polymer solvent for nanoparticle preparation. *Int. J. Pharm.*, **456** (1), 135–142.

83 Aggarwal, P., Hall, J.B., McLeland, C.B., Dobrovolskaia, M.A., and McNeil, S.E. (2009) Nanoparticle interaction with plasma proteins as it relates to particle biodistribution, biocompatibility and therapeutic efficacy. *Adv. Drug Deliv. Rev.*, **61** (6), 428–437.

84 Owens, D.E. and Peppas, N.A. (2006) Opsonization, biodistribution, and pharmacokinetics of polymeric nanoparticles. *Int. J. Pharm.*, **307** (1), 93–102.

85 Lee, K.Y. and Yuk, S.H. (2007) Polymeric protein delivery systems. *Prog. Polym. Sci.*, **32** (7), 669–697.

86 Agnihotri, S.A., Mallikarjuna, N.N., and Aminabhavi, T.M. (2004) Recent advances on chitosan-based micro- and nanoparticles in drug delivery. *J. Control. Release*, **100** (1), 5–28.

87 Aramwit, P., Jaichawa, N., Ratanavaraporn, J., and Srichana, T. (2015) A comparative study of type A and type B gelatin nanoparticles as the controlled release carriers for different model compounds. *Materials Express*, **5** (3), 241–248.

88 Shutava, T.G., Balkundi, S.S., Vangala, P., Steffan, J.J., Bigelow, R.L., Cardelli, J.A., O'Neal, D.P., and Lvov, Y.M. (2009) Layer-by-layer-coated gelatin nanoparticles as a vehicle for delivery of natural polyphenols. *ACS Nano*, **3** (7), 1877–1885.

89 Almeida, A.J. and Souto, E. (2007) Solid lipid nanoparticles as a drug delivery system for peptides and proteins. *Adv. Drug Deliv. Rev.*, **59** (6), 478–490.

90 Das, S. and Chaudhury, A. (2011) Recent advances in lipid nanoparticle formulations with solid matrix for oral drug delivery. *AAPS PharmSciTech.*, **12** (1), 62–76.

91 Ali, M.E., McConville, J.T., and Lamprecht, A. (2015) Pulmonary delivery of anti-inflammatory agents. *Expert Opin. Drug Deliv.*, **12** (6), 1–17.

92 Wissing, S.A., Kayser, O., and Müller, R.H. (2004) Solid lipid nanoparticles for parenteral drug delivery. *Adv. Drug Deliv. Rev.*, **56** (9), 1257–1272.

93 Rohit, B. and Pal, K.I. (2013) A method to prepare solid lipid nanoparticles with improved entrapment efficiency of hydrophilic drugs. *Curr. Nanosci.*, **9** (2), 211–220.

94 Shah, M., Agrawal, Y.K., Garala, K., and Ramkishan, A. (2012) Solid lipid nanoparticles of a water soluble drug, ciprofloxacin hydrochloride. *Indian J. Pharm. Sci.*, **74** (5), 434–442.

95 Müller, R., Maaben, S., Weyhers, H., and Mehnert, W. (1996) Phagocytic uptake and cytotoxicity of solid lipid nanoparticles (SLN) sterically stabilized with poloxamine 908 and poloxamer 407. *J. Drug Target.*, **4** (3), 161–170.

96 Mora-Huertas, C.E., Fessi, H., and Elaissari, A. (2010) Polymer-based nanocapsules for drug delivery. *Int. J. Pharm.*, **385** (1–2), 113–142.

97 Kothamasu, P., Kanumur, H., Ravur, N., Maddu, C., Parasuramrajam, R., and Thangavel, S. (2012) Nanocapsules: the weapons for novel drug delivery systems. *Bioimpacts*, **2** (2), 71–81.

98 de Faria, T.J., Machado de Campos, A., and Lemos Senna, E. (2005) Preparation and characterization of poly(D,L-lactide) (PLA) and poly(D,L-lactide)-poly(ethylene glycol) (PLA-PEG) nanocapsules containing antitumoral agent methotrexate. *Macromol. Symp.*, **229** (1), 228–233.

99 Teixeira, M., Alonso, M.J., Pinto, M.M.M., and Barbosa, C.M. (2005) Development and characterization of PLGA nanospheres and nanocapsules containing xanthone and 3-methoxyxanthone. *Eur. J. Pharm. Biopharm.*, **59** (3), 491–500.

100 Lamprecht, A., Bouligand, Y., and Benoit, J.-P. (2002) New lipid nanocapsules exhibit sustained release properties for amiodarone. *J. Control. Release.*, **84** (1–2), 59–68.

101 Lee, J.S. and Feijen, J. (2012) Polymersomes for drug delivery: design, formation and characterization. *J. Control. Release*, **161** (2), 473–483.

102 Lee, J.C.-M., Santore, M., Bates, F.S., and Discher, D.E. (2002) From membranes to melts, rouse to reptation: diffusion in polymersome versus lipid bilayers. *Macromolecules*, **35** (2), 323–326.

103 Dimova, R., Seifert, U., Pouligny, B., Förster, S., and Döbereiner, H.-G. (2002) Hyperviscous diblock copolymer vesicles. *Eur. Phys. J. E.*, **7** (3), 241–250.

104 Aranda-Espinoza, H., Bermudez, H., Bates, F.S., and Discher, D.E. (2001) Electromechanical limits of polymersomes. *Phys. Rev. Lett.*, **87** (20), 208301.

105 Cruz, L., Soares, L.U., Costa, T.D., Mezzalira, G., da Silveira, N.P., Guterres, S.S., and Pohlmann, A.R. (2006) Diffusion and mathematical modeling of release profiles from nanocarriers. *Int. J. Pharm.*, **313** (1–2), 198–205.

106 Nan, J., Chen, Y., Li, R., Wang, J., Liu, M., Wang, C., and Chu, F. (2014) Polymeric hydrogel nanocapsules: a thermo and pH dual-responsive carrier for sustained drug release. *Micro. Nano. Lett.*, **6** (3), 200–208.

107 Pisani, E., Fattal, E., Paris, J., Ringard, C., Rosilio, V., and Tsapis, N. (2008) Surfactant dependent morphology of polymeric capsules of perfluorooctyl bromide: influence of polymer adsorption at the dichloromethane–water interface. *J. Colloid Interface Sci.*, **326** (1), 66–71.

108 Discher, D.E. and Ahmed, F. (2006) Polymersomes. *Annu. Rev. Biomed. Eng.*, **8**, 323–341.

109 Discher, D.E., Ortiz, V., Srinivas, G., Klein, M.L., Kim, Y., Christian, D., Cai, S., Photos, P., and Ahmed, F. (2007) Emerging applications of polymersomes in delivery: from molecular dynamics to shrinkage of tumors. *Prog. Polym. Sci.*, **32** (8–9), 838–857.

110 Patil, Y.P. and Jadhav, S. (2014) Novel methods for liposome preparation. *Chem. Phys. Lipids.*, **177**, 8–18.

111 Gulati, M., Grover, M., Singh, S., and Singh, M. (1998) Lipophilic drug derivatives in liposomes. *Int. J. Pharm.*, **165** (2), 129–168.

112 Meure, L.A., Foster, N.R., and Dehghani, F. (2008) conventional and dense gas techniques for the production of liposomes: a review. *AAPS PharmSciTech.*, **9** (3), 798–809.

113 Peng, Z., Wang, C., Fang, E., Lu, X., Wang, G., and Tong, Q. (2014) Co-delivery of doxorubicin and SATB1 shRNA by thermosensitive magnetic cationic liposomes for gastric cancer therapy. *PLoS ONE*, **9** (3), e92924.

114 Li, S., Goins, B., Zhang, L., and Bao, A. (2012) Novel multifunctional theranostic liposome drug delivery system: construction, characterization, and multimodality MR, near-infrared fluorescent, and nuclear imaging. *Bioconjugate Chem.*, **23** (6), 1322–1332.

115 Cullis, P.R. (1976) Lateral diffusion rates of phosphatidylcholine in vesicle membranes: eeffects of cholesterol and hydrocarbon phase transitions. *FEBS Lett.*, **70** (1–2), 223–228.

116 Webb, M.S., Harasym, T.O., Masin, D., Bally, M.B., and Mayer, L.D. (1995) Sphingomyelin-cholesterol liposomes significantly enhance the pharmacokinetic and therapeutic properties of vincristine in murine and human tumour models. *Br. J. Cancer.*, **72** (4), 896–904.

117 Immordino, M.L., Dosio, F., and Cattel, L. (2006) Stealth liposomes: review of the basic science, rationale, and clinical applications, existing and potential. *Int. J. Nanomedicine*, **1** (3), 297–315.

118 Akbarzadeh, A., Rezaei-Sadabady, R., Davaran, S., Joo, S., Zarghami, N., Hanifehpour, Y., Samiei, M., Kouhi, M., and Nejati-Koshki, K. (2013) Liposome: classification, preparation, and

applications. *Nanoscale Res. Lett.*, **8** (1), 1–9.
119 Allen, T.M. and Cullis, P.R. (2013) Liposomal drug delivery systems: from concept to clinical applications. *Adv. Drug Deliv. Rev.*, **65** (1), 36–48.
120 Samoshina, N.M., Liu, X., Brazdova, B., Franz, A.H., Samoshin, V.V., and Guo, X. (2011) Fliposomes: pH-sensitive liposomes containing a trans-2-morpholinocyclohexanol-based lipid that performs a conformational flip and triggers an instant cargo release in acidic medium. *Pharmaceutics*, **3** (3), 379–405.
121 Davidsen, J., Jørgensen, K., Andresen, T.L., and Mouritsen, O.G. (2003) Secreted phospholipase A2 as a new enzymatic trigger mechanism for localised liposomal drug release and absorption in diseased tissue. *Biochim. Biophys. Acta*, **1609** (1), 95–101.
122 Kneidl, B., Peller, M., Winter, G., Lindner, L.H., and Hossann, M. (2014) Thermosensitive liposomal drug delivery systems: state of the art review. *Int. J. Nanomedicine*, **9**, 4387–4398.
123 Schroeder, A., Avnir, Y., Weisman, S., Najajreh, Y., Gabizon, A., Talmon, Y., Kost, J., and Barenholz, Y. (2007) Controlling liposomal drug release with low frequency ultrasound: mechanism and feasibility. *Langmuir*, **23** (7), 4019–4025.
124 Popov, M., Linder, C., Deckelbaum, R.J., Grinberg, S., Hansen, I.H., Shaubi, E., Waner, T., and Heldman, E. (2010) Cationic vesicles from novel bolaamphiphilic compounds. *J. Liposome Res.*, **20** (2), 147–159.
125 Abdel-Mottaleb, M.M.A., Neumann, D., and Lamprecht, A. (2010) In vitro drug release mechanism from lipid nanocapsules (LNC). *Int. J. Pharm.*, **390** (2), 208–213.
126 Saulnier, P. and Benoit, J.P. (2006) Lipidic core nanocapsules as new drug delivery systems, in *Nanoparticulates as Drug Carriers* (ed. V.P. Torchilin), Imperial Collage Press, 213–224.
127 Lamprecht, A., Saumet, J.-L., Roux, J., and Benoit, J.-P. (2004) Lipid nanocarriers as drug delivery system for ibuprofen in pain treatment. *Int. J. Pharm.*, **278** (2), 407–414.
128 Anton, N., Gayet, P., Benoit, J.-P., and Saulnier, P. (2007) Nano-emulsions and nanocapsules by the PIT method: an investigation on the role of the temperature cycling on the emulsion phase inversion. *Int. J. Pharm.*, **344** (1–2), 44–52.
129 Lamprecht, A. and Benoit, J.-P. (2006) Etoposide nanocarriers suppress glioma cell growth by intracellular drug delivery and simultaneous P-glycoprotein inhibition. *J. Control. Release*, **112** (2), 208–213.
130 Gamboa, J.M. and Leong, K.W. (2013) *In vitro* and *in vivo* models for the study of oral delivery of nanoparticles. *Adv. Drug Deliv. Rev.*, **65** (6), 800–810.
131 Kim, C.K., Ghosh, P., Pagliuca, C., Zhu, Z.-J., Menichetti, S., and Rotello, V.M. (2009) Entrapment of hydrophobic drugs in nanoparticle monolayers with efficient release into cancer cells. *J. Am. Chem. Soc.*, **131** (4), 1360–1361.
132 Yu, M., Park, J., and Jon, S. (2012) Targeting strategies for multifunctional nanoparticles in cancer imaging and therapy. *Theranostics*, **2** (1), 3–44.
133 Illum, L., Jones, P.D.E., Kreuter, J., Baldwin, R.W., and Davis, S.S. (1983) Adsorption of monoclonal antibodies to polyhexylcyanoacrylate nanoparticles and subsequent immunospecific binding to tumour cells *in vitro*. *Int. J. Pharm.*, **17** (1), 65–76.
134 Kubiak, C., Manil, L., and Couvreur, P. (1988) Sorptive properties of antibodies onto cyanoacrylic nanoparticles. *Int. J. Pharm.*, **41** (3), 181–187.
135 Hamidi, M., Azadi, A., Mohamadi-Samani, S., Rafiei, P., and Ashrafi, H. (2012) Valproate-loaded hydrogel nanoparticles: preparation and characterization. *J. Appl. Polym. Sci.*, **124** (6), 4686–4693.
136 Lowman, A.M. and Hans, M.L. (2007) Chapter 30. Nanoparticles for drug delivery, in *Handbook of Nanoscience, Engineering, and Technology*, 2nd edn (eds A. William, I. Goddard, D.W. Brenner, S.E. Lyshevski, and G.E. Lafrate), CRC Press, 30-1–30-28.

137 Mittal, G., Sahana, D.K., Bhardwaj, V., and Ravi Kumar, M.N.V. (2007) Estradiol loaded PLGA nanoparticles for oral administration: effect of polymer molecular weight and copolymer composition on release behavior *in vitro* and *in vivo*. *J. Control. Release*, **119** (1), 77–85.

138 Dalpiaz, A., Leo, E., Vitali, F., Pavan, B., Scatturin, A., Bortolotti, F., Manfredini, S., Durini, E., Forni, F., Brina, B., and Vandelli, M.A. (2005) Development and characterization of biodegradable nanospheres as delivery systems of anti-ischemic adenosine derivatives. *Biomaterials*, **26** (11), 1299–1306.

139 De Campos, A.M., Sánchez, A., and Alonso, M.J. (2001) Chitosan nanoparticles: a new vehicle for the improvement of the delivery of drugs to the ocular surface. Application to cyclosporin A. *Int. J. Pharm.*, **224** (1–2), 159–168.

140 Patel, B.K., Parikh, R.H., and Aboti, P.S. (2013) Development of oral sustained release rifampicin loaded chitosan nanoparticles by design of experiment. *J. Drug Deliv.*, **2013**, 1–10.

141 Teeranachaideekul, V., Müller, R.H., and Junyaprasert, V.B. (2007) Encapsulation of ascorbyl palmitate in nanostructured lipid carriers (NLC) – effects of formulation parameters on physicochemical stability. *Int. J. Pharm.*, **340** (1–2), 198–206.

142 Tamjidi, F., Shahedi, M., Varshosaz, J., and Nasirpour, A. (2013) Nanostructured lipid carriers (NLC): a potential delivery system for bioactive food molecules. *Innov. Food Sci. Emerg. Technol.*, **19**, 29–43.

143 zur Mühlen, A., Schwarz, C., and Mehnert, W. (1998) Solid lipid nanoparticles (SLN) for controlled drug delivery – drug release and release mechanism. *Eur. J. Pharm. Biopharm.*, **45** (2), 149–155.

144 Bozzuto, G. and Molinari, A. (2015) Liposomes as nanomedical devices. *Int. J. Nanomedicine*, **10**, 975–999.

145 Zhigaltsev, I.V., Winters, G., Srinivasulu, M., Crawford, J., Wong, M., Amankwa, L., Waterhouse, D., Masin, D., Webb, M., Harasym, N., Heller, L., Bally, M.B., Ciufolini, M.A., Cullis, P.R., and Maurer, N. (2010) Development of a weak-base docetaxel derivative that can be loaded into lipid nanoparticles. *J. Control. Release*, **144** (3), 332–340.

146 Khoee, S. and Yaghoobian, M. (2009) An investigation into the role of surfactants in controlling particle size of polymeric nanocapsules containing penicillin-G in double emulsion. *Eur. J. Med. Chem.*, **44** (6), 2392–2399.

147 Ahmed, F., Pakunlu, R.I., Brannan, A., Bates, F., Minko, T., and Discher, D.E. (2006) Biodegradable polymersomes loaded with both paclitaxel and doxorubicin permeate and shrink tumors, inducing apoptosis in proportion to accumulated drug. *J. Control. Release*, **116** (2), 150–158.

148 Hoffart, V., Lamprecht, A., Maincent, P., Lecompte, T., Vigneron, C., and Ubrich, N. (2006) Oral bioavailability of a low molecular weight heparin using a polymeric delivery system. *J. Control. Rel.*, **113** (1), 38–42.

149 Thote, A.J. and Gupta, R.B. (2005) Formation of nanoparticles of a hydrophilic drug using supercritical carbon dioxide and microencapsulation for sustained release. *Nanomedicine*, **1** (1), 85–90.

150 Nahar, M. and Jain, N. (2009) Preparation, characterization and evaluation of targeting potential of amphotericin B-loaded engineered PLGA nanoparticles. *Pharm. Res.*, **26** (12), 2588–2598.

151 Kirthivasan, B., Singh, D., Bommana, M., Raut, S., Squillante, E., and Sadoqi, M. (2012) Active brain targeting of a fluorescent P-gp substrate using polymeric magnetic nanocarrier system. *Nanotechnology*, **23** (25), 255102.

152 Imbuluzqueta, E., Gamazo, H., and Lana, H. (2013) Hydrophobic gentamicin-loaded nanoparticles are effective against Brucella melitensis infection in mice. *Antimicrob. Agents Chemother*, **57** (7), 3326–3333.

153 Kumar, R.GT., Ramstack, J.M., Herbert, P., and Figa, M. (2012) Coacervation process. US Patent, EP2131815 A4, filed Mar. 19, 2008 and issued - - -.

154 Pan, Y., Li, Y.-j., Zhao, H.-Y., Zheng, J.-m., Xu, H., Wei, G., and Hao, J.-s. (2002) Bioadhesive polysaccharide in protein delivery system: chitosan nanoparticles improve the intestinal absorption of insulin *in vivo*. *Int. J. Pharm.*, **249** (1), 139–147.

155 Csaba, N., Köping-Höggård, M., and Alonso, M.J. (2009) Ionically crosslinked chitosan/tripolyphosphate nanoparticles for oligonucleotide and plasmid DNA delivery. *Int. J. Pharm.*, **382** (1), 205–214.

156 Mohammadpour Dounighi, N., Eskandari, R., Avadi, M., Zolfagharian, H., Mir Mohammad Sadeghi, A., and Rezayat, M. (2012) Preparation and *in vitro* characterization of chitosan nanoparticles containing Mesobuthus eupeus scorpion venom as an antigen delivery system. *J. Venom. Anim. Toxins*, **18** (1), 44–52.

157 Janes, K.A., Fresneau, M.P., Marazuela, A., Fabra, A., and Alonso, M.J. (2001) Chitosan nanoparticles as delivery systems for doxorubicin. *J. Control. Release*, **73** (2), 255–267.

158 Jain, N.K. and Jain, S.K. (2010) Development and *in vitro* characterization of galactosylated low molecular weight chitosan nanoparticles bearing doxorubicin. *AAPS PharmSciTech.*, **11** (2), 686–697.

159 Tahara, K., Yamamoto, K., and Nishihata, T. (1995) Overall mechanism behind matrix sustained release (SR) tablets prepared with hydroxypropyl methylcellulose 2910. *J. Control. Release*, **35** (1), 59–66.

160 Sankar, C., Rani, M., Srivastava, A., and Mishra, B. (2001) Chitosan based pentazocine microspheres for intranasal systemic delivery: development and biopharmaceutical evaluation. *Die Pharmazie*, **56** (3), 223–226.

161 Madden, T.D., Harrigan, P.R., Tai, L.C.L., Bally, M.B., Mayer, L.D., Redelmeier, T.E., Loughrey, H.C., Tilcock, C.P.S., Reinish, L.W., and Cullis, P.R. (1990) The accumulation of drugs within large unilamellar vesicles exhibiting a proton gradient: a survey. *Chem. Phys. Lipids.*, **53** (1), 37–46.

162 Nounou, M.M., El-Khordagui, L.K., Khalafallah, N.A., and Khalil, S.A. (2006) In vitro release of hydrophilic and hydrophobic drugs from liposomal dispersions and gels. *Acta Pharm.*, **56** (3), 311.

163 Blenke, E.O. (2012) Strategies for triggered drug release from liposomes: In search of “smart” lipids and “smart” triggers. Master of Science in Drug Innovation University of Utrecht.

164 Chen, Q., Tong, S., Dewhirst, M.W., and Yuan, F. (2004) Targeting tumor microvessels using doxorubicin encapsulated in a novel thermosensitive liposome. *Mol. Cancer Ther.*, **3** (10), 1311–1317.

165 Meng, F., Zhong, Z., and Feijen, J. (2009) Stimuli-responsive polymersomes for programmed drug delivery. *Biomacromolecules*, **10** (2), 197–209.

166 Yu, M.K., Park, J., Jeong, Y.Y., Moon, W.K., and Jon, S. (2010) Integrin-targeting thermally cross-linked superparamagnetic iron oxide nanoparticles for combined cancer imaging and drug delivery. *Nanotechnology*, **21** (41), 415102.

167 Derfus, A.M., Chen, A.A., Min, D.-H., Ruoslahti, E., and Bhatia, S.N. (2007) Targeted quantum dot conjugates for siRNA delivery. *Bioconjug. Chem.*, **18** (5), 1391–1396.

168 Thermo Scientific (2012) Thermo scientific pierce crosslinking technical handbook.

169 Aryal, S., Hu, C.-M.J., and Zhang, L. (2010) Polymer – cisplatin conjugate nanoparticles for acid-responsive drug delivery. *ACS Nano*, **4** (1), 251–258.

170 Luan, X., Skupin, M., Siepmann, J., and Bodmeier, R. (2006) Key parameters affecting the intial release (burst) and encapsulation effeciency of peptide-containing poly(lactide-*co*-glycolide) microparticles. *Pharm. Nanotechnol.*, **324** (2), 168–175.

171 Vasudev, S., Ahmad, S., Parveen, R., Ahmad, F., Anish, C., Ali, M., and Panda, A. (2011) Formulation of PEG-ylated L-asparaginase loaded poly (lactide-*co*-glycolide) nanoparticles: influence of pegylation on enzyme loading, activity and *in vitro* release. *Pharmazie*, **66** (12), 956–960.

172 Harris, J.M. and Chess, R.B. (2003) Effect of pegylation on pharmaceuticals. *Nat. Rev. Drug Discov.*, **2** (3), 214–221.
173 Gaudana, R., Gokulgandhi, M., Khurana, V., Kwatra, D., and Mitra, A.K. (2012) Design and evaluation of a novel nanoparticulate-based formulation encapsulating a HIP complex of lysozyme. *Pharm. Dev. Technol.*, **18** (3), 752–759.
174 Yang, L., Cui, F., Shi, K., Cun, D., and Wang, R. (2009) Design of high payload PLGA nanoparticles containing melittin/sodium dodecyl sulfate complex by the hydrophobic ion-pairing technique. *Drug Dev. Ind. Pharm.*, **35** (8), 959–968.
175 Sun, S., Liang, N., Yamamoto, H., Kawashima, Y., Cui, F., and Yan, P. (2015) pH-sensitive poly(lactide-*co*-glycolide) nanoparticle composite microcapsules for oral delivery of insulin. *Int. J. Nanomedicine*, **10**, 3489–3498.
176 Zhang, Z., Tongchusak, S., Mizukami, Y., Kang, Y.J., Ioji, T., Touma, M., Reinhold, B., Keskin, D.B., Reinherz, E.L., and Sasada, T. (2011) Induction of anti-tumor cytotoxic T cell responses through PLGA-nanoparticle mediated antigen delivery. *Biomaterials*, **32** (14), 3666–3678.
177 Cohen, H., Levy, R., Gao, J., Fishbein, I., Kousaev, V., Sosnowski, S., Slomkowski, S., and Golomb, G. (2000) Sustained delivery and expression of DNA encapsulated in polymeric nanoparticles. *Gene Ther.*, **7** (22), 1896–1905.
178 Cun, D., Foged, C., Yang, M., Frokjaer, S., and Nielson, H.M. (2010) Preparation and characterisation of poly(DL-lactide-*co*-glycolide) nanoparticles for siRNA delivery. *Int. J. Pharm.*, **390** (1), 70–75.
179 Varshochian, R., Jeddi-Tehrani, M., Mahmoudi, A.R. *et al.* (2013) The protective effect of albumin on bevacizumab activity and stability in PLGA nanoparticles intended for retinal and choroidal neovascularization treatments. *Eur. J. Pharm. Sci.*, **50** (3–4), 341–352.
180 Zhu, G., Mallery, S.R., and Schwendeman, S.P. (2000) Stabilization of proteins encapsulated in injectable poly (lactide-*co*-glycolide). *Nat. Biotech.*, **18** (1), 52–57.
181 Ibrahim, M.A., Ismail, A., Fetouh, M.I., and Göpferich, A. (2005) Stability of insulin during the erosion of poly(lactic acid) and poly(lactic-*co*-glycolic acid) microspheres. *J. Control. Release*, **106** (3), 241–252.
182 Elgadir, M.A., Uddin, M.S., Ferdosh, S., Adam, A., Chowdhury, A.J.K., and Sarker, M.Z.I. (2015) Impact of chitosan composites and chitosan nanoparticle composites on various drug delivery systems: a review. *J. Food Drug Anal.*, **23** (4), 619–629.
183 Huang, Z., Dong, L., Chen, J., Gao, F., Zhang, Z., Chen, J., and Zhang, J. (2012) Low-molecular weight chitosan/vascular endothelial growth factor short hairpin RNA for the treatment of hepatocellular carcinoma. *Life Sci.*, **91** (23–24), 1207–1215.
184 Bhattarai, N., Ramay, H.R., Gunn, J., Matsen, F.A., and Zhang, M. (2005) PEG-grafted chitosan as an injectable thermosensitive hydrogel for sustained protein release. *J. Control. Release*, **103** (3), 609–624.
185 Liu, G., Ma, S., Li, S., Cheng, R., Meng, F., Liu, H., and Zhong, Z. (2010) The highly efficient delivery of exogenous proteins into cells mediated by biodegradable chimaeric polymersomes. *Biomaterials*, **31** (29), 7575–7585.
186 Hermanson, G.T. (2013) Chapter 14 – Microparticles and nanoparticles, in *Bioconjugate Techniques (Third edition)* (ed. G.T. Hermanson), Academic Press, 549–588.

7
Characterization Methods: Physical and Chemical Characterization Techniques

Sven Even F. Borgos

SINTEF Materials and Chemistry, Dept. of Biotechnology and Nanomedicine, Sem Sælands v. 2A, N-7034 Trondheim, Norway

7.1
The Need for Nanomedicine-Specific Characterization

Nanomedicines owe much of their tremendous potential to their nanometer size range and surface structure. This implies that for any nanoparticles, a key characteristic is that their composition has a very high proportion of surface atoms, which can interact directly with the biological environment where they are intended to exert their effect. Also, their size range introduces some highly specific physicochemical constraints, for example, the high confinement of electrons in inorganic materials, which causes effects such as specific optical absorption through surface plasmons and high semiconductor bandgap. For organic nanoparticles, spontaneous self-ordered assembly can occur directly based on molecular size and other properties of the constituent molecules, for example, in the formation of crystalline domains in lipid nanoparticles, or the assembly of liposomes with a hydrophilic interior.

Nevertheless, the unique properties of nanomedicines also cause some unique challenges in their characterization. Their existence intermediate to small molecules on one hand and (nanostructured) solid phase on the other, means that classical analytical techniques developed and optimized for either of those compositional domains might not apply or might give erroneous answers. Some features with proven biological importance are inherently nanomedicine-specific as compared to traditional medicines, for example, size and surface charge, whereas other (e.g., drug release) can to some extent have parallels in other advanced drug formulations like prodrugs. The nanomedicine-specific analytical challenges are not just of academic interest, but rather have a very significant impact on the applicability of these medicines in the clinical setting. Regulatory frameworks are mostly developed for small molecule or protein drugs. This becomes critical when taking into account that before any new drug candidate can enter clinical trials, regulatory authorities demand data on drug safety. The European

Pharmaceutical Nanotechnology: Innovation and Production, First Edition. Edited by Jean Cornier, Arno Kwade, Andrew Owen, and Marcel Van de Voorde.

Commission recently acknowledged that the lack of established methods and structures to provide such preclinical data was one main bottleneck in the process of bringing promising nanomedical drugs to the market. This led to the establishment in 2015 of the European Nanomedicine Characterisation Laboratory (EU-NCL) under the H2020 funding program. The EU-NCL is a distributed platform consisting of a small number of core laboratories highly specialized in different aspects of nanomedicines characterization. It is based closely on concepts and experiences from the Nanotechnology Characterization Laboratory (NCL) established in 2004, by the U.S. National Cancer Institute (NCI). Whereas NCL, by mandate from its funding organization, is intended to address nanomedicines against cancer, the EU-NCL has a scope that encompasses all diseases, although cancer is at present by far the most frequent target for new nanomedicine candidates.

7.2
The Assay Cascade: From Basic Properties to Complex Interactions

The characterization of nanomedicines can pursue different endpoints and different levels of complexity. As coined by NCL, these complementary yet interconnected approaches have been loosely termed the *assay cascade*. It defines the three major areas that should be addressed in the assessment of nanomedicines before introduction into clinical trials; these are physicochemical (PCC), *in vitro* and *in vivo* characterization. The first level – physicochemical – is the fundamental description of the pristine nanoparticles, that is, before any interaction with the biological systems takes place. The methods used for this are also generally applicable to nonmedicinal nanomaterials and are widely applied in the physical and chemical sciences. The second level – *in vitro* – addresses the interactions with simple biological systems, mostly mammalian cell culture. This allows highly controlled and reproducible studies of the influence that is exerted by the nanoparticles on single cells, and notably the cellular toxicity effects. The third level – *in vivo* characterization – looks at pharmacokinetic, immunological, and toxicological profiling in animal models. This is the crucial measure for demonstrating the safety that regulators demand before clinical trials can be initiated, and this assay level gives information on the nanomedicines' complex interaction with the whole organ systems.

As described in the simplified schedule above, nanomedicines characterization could in theory progress in a sequential fashion, starting with PCC, going on to *in vitro* and finally *in vivo*, obtaining all relevant information at every stage. This, however, could be highly and unnecessarily resource intensive, as not all parameters are of equal relevance for all nanomaterials and formulations. The use of selected *in vitro* assays would, for instance, be justified based either on PCC characteristics or on specific *in vivo* effects. The *in vitro* assays can then help to elucidate which fundamental biological processes and signaling pathways are affected by a specific nanoparticle, and this should then be seen in light of the physicochemical properties measured on the pristine material. Such an approach

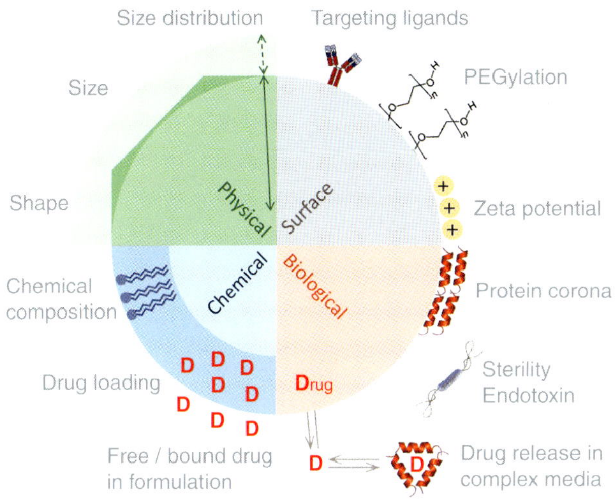

Figure 7.1 Overview of important physicochemical characteristics in nanomedicines.

would be particularly applicable where experience has been accumulated with a range of different nanomedicines, like in the case of the NCL. Indeed, the NCL has published a paper on "lessons learned" over its first decade of operation [1]. One prominent example of rational assay selection from the NCL is the introduction of a prescreening step for sterility and endotoxins before any other assays are run. This was based on the observation that a significant proportion of submitted materials contained endotoxins. These are compounds that induce a strong inflammatory response *in vivo* and their presence is unacceptable in the clinical setting. Thus, even the first PCC characterization of endotoxin-containing nanomedicines should not be initiated, as these will inevitably fail *in vivo*.

The current chapter will look at some major and promising nanomedicine physicochemical characterization techniques for pristine nanoparticles as well as their transformation upon initial contact with biological media. Although volume limits does not allow an exhaustive review of all relevant techniques, several recent reviews have looked at aspects of nanoparticle characterization [2–7] and the reader is referred to these for further in-depth information. A graphical summary of relevant characterization targets and parameters described in this chapter is shown in Figure 7.1.

7.3 Physicochemical Characterization of Pristine Nanoparticles

7.3.1 Size, Size Distribution, and Topology

Size might be seen as the defining feature of nanomedicines as a group, and has a significant effect on their interaction with cells [8]. As virtually all nanoparticles has some degree of polydispersity in their size, the ensemble size distribution of the sample population is of additional interest. Varenne *et al.* [9] recently performed a detailed comparative study of size determination for poly(isobutyl cyanoacrylate) nanoparticles decorated with dextran; this is a highly relevant model system for a range of nanomedicines, and the study compared the major techniques available at present. NP sizing techniques can essentially be classified in (i) batch particle size measurements, (ii) single particle size measurements, and (iii) separation-based size measurements.

7.3.1.1 **Batch Particle Sizing Techniques**

Dynamic light scattering (DLS) [10,11] has become probably the most commonly used technique for size determination due to its relative ease of application. DLS, also known as photon correlation spectroscopy (PCS), measures Brownian motion of nanoparticles in suspension. Size is calculated based on time-resolved analysis of scattered light from the nanoparticles. The autocorrelation function is used to calculate the particle diffusion coefficient, which is then related to the nanoparticle hydrodynamic diameter by the Stokes–Einstein relationship. Although less sensitive than, for example, static light scattering (see below), DLS works over a relatively broad concentration range and sizes of 1–1000 nm. DLS is mostly used in the bulk mode, that is, without sample prefractionation. This limits its applicability on samples with large degree of size heterogeneity, as scattered light intensity is proportional to particle radius to the sixth power, meaning the signal from small particles might not be discernible from noise in the presence of large particles. Some work has been done on the online coupling of DLS to, for example, field flow fractionation (see below) [12] or other separation techniques to overcome the above problem, although this generally comes at the cost of sensitivity. Also, as with all techniques that measure hydrodynamic radius, the result will be dependent on the solvent used, and in particular the presence of electrolytes.

Static light scattering (SLS), mostly in the form of multiangle light scattering (MALS), is a powerful sizing technique [11]. Although a batch technique *per se,* it is usually applied in conjunction with a separation step (size exclusion chromatography, field flow fractionation) and can provide direct measurements on both nanoparticle size and to some extent also shape. Notably, SLS measures the physical diameter of the nanoparticle, more specifically the radius of gyration, as opposed to DLS. The interaction of the particle surface with monochromatic light, generally from a laser source, will yield a characteristic scatter intensity distribution as a function of size and surface morphology [13]. For electrically conductive nanoparticles (e.g., Au, Ag), the induction of surface plasmons will lead to isotropic scattering and hence limit the applicability of MALS for sizing. The same surface plasmon phenomena will, however, enable the use of wavelength-specific light absorption for size estimation in conductive nanoparticles. This is commonly used, for example, for sizing of gold nanoparticles [14].

7.3.1.2 Single Particle Sizing Techniques

Nanoparticle tracking analysis (NTA) [15–17] is a relatively new technique, which is somewhat related to DLS in its operating principle. Whereas DLS measures a time development of the overall scattered light distribution from a sample volume, NTA tracks the Brownian motion of single particles in a two-dimensional liquid focal plane, thereby obtaining a translational diffusion coefficient. This can then be used to calculate particle size from the Stokes–Einstein equation when temperature and viscosity of the medium is known. Compared to DLS, the size resolution is significantly improved. Importantly, NTA has the added advantage of giving a direct measure of particle concentration in the bulk sample; this is nontrivial to obtain by most other methods.

Tunable resistive pulse sensing (TRPS) [18–20] is a nanopore-based technique that can be used to measure size (above approx. 50 nm), charge, and concentration. An elastomeric membrane is penetrated with a cone-shaped probe creating a size-tunable pore. When the pore is placed in a conductive liquid, passage of a nanoparticle through the pore can be detected as increased electrical resistance across the membrane. Larger particles will induce higher resistance, making the size measurement possible. The rate of nanoparticle translocation is dependent on particle concentration and electrophoretic mobility, and with appropriate tuning and calibration this will then give measurements on concentration and surface charge.

Transmission electron microscopy (TEM) is a very mature technology within the physical sciences, and the most frequently used electron microscopy technique for characterizing nanomaterials. It can provide spatial resolution down to <1 nm, thus giving a direct measure on both size and topology of the sample. An incident electron beam interacts with the sample to generate elastically and inelastically scattered electron that can be used to recreate the structure of the scattering sample. For inorganic nanoparticles, this is generally a robust imaging technology. For organic nanoparticles, however, or for inorganic nanoparticles that have interacted with biological systems, challenges exist with regards to the ultrahigh vacuum required, such as drying artifacts, and with electron contrast between the nanoparticle and adsorbed proteins. Cryogenic electron microscopy is among the developments that have improved the applicability to nanomedicines [21], as is cryo-electron tomography [22]. Recently, the field of liquid TEM is showing exciting potential for imaging of organic nanomaterials in their native state [23,24], as shown for liposomes [25] and polymeric nanoparticles [26] in aqueous environment. It should be noted that as TEM is an image-based technique, great caution has to be taken to avoid bias in the interpretation upon manual image analysis. Recent developments point toward automated, computational methods to improve the quantitative analysis of heterogeneous samples [27].

Atomic force microscopy (AFM) belongs to a set of techniques known as scanning probe microscopy, is capable of providing nondestructive topographical mapping of single nanoparticles with sub-Angstrom resolution in the *Z*-direction, and has a range of applications within nanomedicines characterization [28], among them size measurements [29]. AFM operates by scanning a flexible cantilever over the sample, making contact or near-contact with the sample surface through a sharp tip extending from the cantilever. Deflection of the cantilever, either static or by changes in resonance frequency, reflects interactions with the sample surface. It should be noted that lateral resolution is limited by the radius and shape of the cantilever tip, and mathematical deconvolution becomes a necessity. Nevertheless, AFM can provide very valuable size information alone or in complement with other sizing techniques [30]. Besides high-resolution imaging, this enables measurement of parameters such as adhesion, local elasticity, and stiffness as well as binding forces between individual biomolecules or individual nanoparticles [31–33].

Single particle inductively coupled plasma mass spectrometry (sp-ICP-MS) is a relatively new sizing technique made possible by improvements in mass spectrometer instrumentation, notably the sufficiently fast sampling rate. Lee *et al.* have demonstrated its applicability for sizing of nanoparticles from a wide range of elements [34]. The method relies on infusion of a nanoparticle suspension sufficiently dilute that only a single nanoparticle will be analyzed within the chosen sampling interval as a transient signal. The signal intensity is then directly proportional to the amount of the element under investigation in the analyzed nanoparticle. Whereas sp-ICP-MS does address the simultaneous detection of nanoparticle size and chemical identity, there are some limitation on the upper and lower size that can be analyzed by this method; for gold nanoparticles, the range 10–200 nm has been shown. Importantly, ICP-MS is not suited for quantification of the organic elements, such as C, H, N, and O, although the latest generation of instruments has brought S and P quantification into the interesting concentration range [35]. Nevertheless, very high sensitivity (commonly in the low- or sub-pg/ml range) can be obtained for most other elements, also in complex and environmental matrices [36]. Some work has been done on the online coupling to electrospray differential mobility analysis [37] to obtain real-time size separation before ICP-MS detection and thus improve on the size resolution achievable.

7.3.1.3 Separation- and Fractionation-Based Sizing Techniques

Field flow fractionation (FFF) is emerging as a very versatile and widely applicable set of techniques [38] for separation of nanoparticles and very large polymers, and has rapidly gained popularity. It has been used extensively in the characterization of nanomedicines [39,40], and the modality of asymmetric flow FFF (AF4) is of particular importance; for inorganic or composite nanoparticles with a density significantly different from the surrounding medium, centrifugal FFF (CF3) and sedimentation FFF (SdFFF) can give even better size resolution. FFF is based on the separation of analytes in a laminar liquid flow, where particle diffusion is counterbalanced by an externally applied separation field perpendicular to the direction of flow. The notable benefits of FFF for nanomedicines analysis include the very wide acceptable particle size range, low nm to about 1 μm in normal mode and further toward 100 μm in steric (inverse) mode. FFF being a purely liquid-based separation, absence of a stationary separation phase ensures that secondary separation effects are minimal, and it also means that shear forces on the analytes are negligible. Finally, the FFF separation principle allows for a very wide selection of mobile phases. Although elution time from the FFF channel will be directly related to size (AF4), or to a combination of size and other analyte parameters (CF3/SdFFF), the size resolution is generally low, necessitating the use of online detectors for measurement of size, as well as other parameters such as morphology or chemical composition. Detectors that are often coupled to FFF include MALS, UV/VIS absorbance, fluorescence and refractive index, and DLS and ICP-MS.

The perpendicular separation field applied in FFF has mostly been confined to a liquid flow field (AF4) or a centrifugal/gravitational field (CF3/SdFFF); for polymer analysis, thermal diffusion coefficient-based separation (thermal FFF, TF3/ThFFF) has been applicable [41]. Very recently, it was demonstrated that TF3 is able to separate polymeric micelles based on their chemical corona composition [42]; this is of relevance, since numerous nanomedicines are micellar formulations. The FFF separation based on either magnetic or electrical fields have been technically challenging; very recently, however, a report was published on combined electrical and asymmetric flow FFF (EAF4) [43], giving a promising outlook for FFF separation of nanomedicines and other large analytes based on their electrophoretic mobility. This is of significant interest, as net surface charge is an important parameter for the interaction of nanoparticles with biological systems.

Liquid chromatography (LC) has seen some use in separation of nanoparticles based on size, primarily as size exclusion chromatography (SEC), for example, [44], but also by high-performance LC and hydrodynamic chromatography (HDC) [45]. SEC is a very mature separation technique and has traditionally been used for separation of analytes based on size, although specific challenges arise with nanomaterials, such as degradation on-column, and unwanted secondary interactions with or irreversible adsorption to the stationary phase [46].

Analytical ultracentrifugation (AUC) measures real-time sedimentation of nanoparticles and other analytes by online optical detection of the centrifugal compartment, giving data on sedimentation equilibrium and sedimentation velocity. This is a versatile and powerful technique with high resolution [47] that has been applied for a range of medically relevant nanoparticles both inorganic and organic, providing information on numerous parameters, including size, density, shape, porosity, and molecular weight [48–50] as well as grafting density on the surface [51]. From a quality point of view, both repeatability and reproducibility between labs is generally good; however, some concerns have existed on the level of accuracy, recently prompting a large multilaboratory comparison of calibration accuracy and external references in AUC [52] that highlighted the need for careful calibration.

7.3.2 Surface Characteristics and Functionalization

7.3.2.1 Zeta (ζ) Potential

Surface charge of a nanoparticle is commonly expressed as zeta potential, which is the electrical potential between the stationary layer of solvent molecules adjacent to dispersed nanoparticles and the bulk solvent. This is an important parameter for several reasons: in the biological context, the effect on formation of the protein corona (Section 7.4.2) might be the most immediate concern. Also, nanoparticles with net surface charge close to zero are prone to agglomeration, which might affect dosing of the pristine nanoparticles to the biological system. Environmental factors such as pH, ionic strength, and adsorbed biomolecules all affect the zeta potential. Surface charge is generally an important parameter in the interaction between nanoparticles and cells, for example, on platelet aggregation [53].

Zeta potential is mostly measured by two methods: either electrophoretic light scattering (ELS)[54] or tunable resistive pulse sensing (described above) or variants thereof [55]. Sikora *et al.* demonstrated that TRPS might be better suited than ELS for measurement of nanoparticles in serum [56]; ELS is an ensemble technique giving an average value across the particle population, whereas TRPS is a single-particle technique. ELS is commonly determined by applying an electric field across the sample and measuring the velocity at which the charged nanoparticles move toward the electrode; this can often be done in the same instrument as is used for DLS size measurements. Recently, zeta particle tracking analysis (zPTA), another single particle technique related to NTA, was introduced; Sikora *et al.* performed a comprehensive comparison for aminated silica of ELS, TRPS, and zPTA in simple and complex media, and found mostly good correlation, although single-particle methods clearly provided additional information as compared to ELS [57].

7.3.2.2 Chemical Surface Functionalization and Targeting

One of the most pronounced promises of nanomedicines has been that of targeted, selective delivery of drugs to the site of pathology. Targeting considerations and strategies are extensively covered elsewhere in this book. As the targeting moieties must be accessible for binding, they have to be exposed on the nanoparticle surface, either incorporated during particle synthesis or chemically postdecorated. Both the total amount of targeting groups and their relative distribution on the surface are important, as both will decide the total surface chemistry and the accessibility to binding sites. A special case of surface functionalization is the attachment of polyethylene glycol (PEGylation) [58]. In order to increase circulation half-life and reduce immunogenicity, this is used extensively not only for nanoparticles but also for, for example, protein drugs.

Considering the undisputed importance of nanoparticle surface functionalization, the scarcity of advanced analytical data published is remarkable. Indirect observations of surface groups are possible through classical affinity assays, interaction column chromatography, or based on apparent nanoparticle size. Many established methods within analytical chemistry, such as optical absorbance, fluorescence, and nuclear magnetic resonance spectroscopy (NMR) will enable the bulk detection of defined chemical groups [59,60], but the spatially resolved analysis, verifying surface localization, is highly demanding on the nanoparticle size scale. Microscale thermogravimetric analysis is useful for quantification of combustible ligands on thermostable nanoparticles [61,62], although this is generally limited to inorganic nanoparticles. Current methods for quantification of PEG, presumed to be located to the surface, on polymeric nanoparticles were reviewed by Rabanel *et al.* [63]. One technique that shows some promise is X-ray photoelectron spectroscopy (XPS) [64,65], although with due caution for artifacts.

An interesting analytical development for analysis of nanoparticles surface groups is that of Secondary Ion Mass Spectrometry (SIMS) [66], where a focused ion beam directed at a surface creates secondary (molecular or polyatomic) ions from the outermost atomic layers of the sample surface, which are subsequently collected and injected into a mass spectrometer. By sputtering away atomic layers during analysis, this can in principle provide 3D data with very high lateral resolution (<100 nm) and with the high analyte specificity of mass spectrometry. SIMS also has the added advantage of being able to analyze with the same technique both the surface molecules and the nanoparticle interior components. A complementary surface MS technique for direct analysis of proteins on nanoparticle surfaces was suggested by Ju and Yeo [67], by performing on-surface proteolysis and subsequent matrix-assisted laser desorption ionization MS (MALDI-TOF-MS) detection of the free proteins.

7.3.3 Composition and Purity

Bulk chemical composition, including the drug loading, of the nanoparticles can arguably be considered to be among the less intricate of the analytical aspects. For most chemical classes of nanoparticle components, well-established methods exist for chemical analysis, including chromatographic separation, optical detection methods, NMR spectroscopy, and elemental or molecular mass spectrometry. Nevertheless, the analysis of composition and purity is fundamental to understand the subsequent studies of nanoparticle interactions with biological systems. As medical nanoparticles evolve toward higher chemical complexity, it should be emphasized that all components, including non-API compounds such as structural lipids or polymers, have the potential to elicit biological effects, and their identity and concentration should be known. Even when the biocompatibility (or intended biological effects) of the single pure components in the nanoformulation has been verified, two important factors remain to quantify: residual manufacturing components, including accidental contaminants, and unintended side products formed during particle synthesis. Two compound groups that are known to have a high potential for unwanted biological effects are residual monomers from polymerization reactions and residual surfactants used during nanoparticle synthesis or functionalization.

One nanoparticle-specific factor to consider in terms of chemical composition and drug loading analysis is that of how to ensure complete accessibility of the analyte in question to the analytical method applied. For most analytes and methods, for example, optical methods or molecular mass spectrometry, this translates into a question of how to ensure complete extraction of the analyte from the nanoparticle. For solid inorganic nanoparticles, this can be done by standard dissolution of the sample in strong acids such as HF, followed by elemental quantification with routine methods such as ICP-OES or ICP-MS. Organic nanoparticles can mostly be disintegrated into selected organic solvents, and by verifying sufficient solubility of the analyte in the chosen solvent, bulk-phase quantification can be performed. Importantly, possible matrix interferences with the analytical technique should be controlled for all complex samples, such as dissolved nanoparticles. Optical methods such as UV absorbance or fluorescence coupled to chromatographic separation will give satisfactory quantification for many drugs and nanoparticle matrix components, provided they contain suitable chromophores. For increased selectivity, and for analytes without optically active groups, mass spectrometry – in particular tandem MS coupled to liquid chromatography – provides high to ultrahigh sensitivity (ng/ml or below) for most small organic molecules. In covalently cross-linked organic nanoparticles, problems could arise with the above methods, as disintegration of the nanoparticle might require very harsh conditions that could chemically degrade the analytes. For the chemical analysis of *intact organic nanoparticles*, NMR is becoming a very interesting option [68]. Besides the direct quantification of encapsulated or embedded molecules, it adds the valuable possibility to investigate the noncovalent chemical environment of the analyte under investigation, thus potentially providing information on the localization of drugs and functional groups in structurally inhomogeneous nanoparticles [69–74]. Another set of technologies that can provide valuable information on internal structure and composition are the scattering techniques, notably Raman scattering, small-angle X-ray scattering (SAXS) or wide-angle X-ray scattering (WAXS), or small-angle neutron scattering (SANS). These techniques have been successfully applied for structural elucidation of a range of nanomedical drug delivery systems [75–77]. The X-ray and neutron scattering techniques are covered in detail elsewhere in this book.

7.4 Characterization of Nanoparticles in the Biological Environment

Nanomedicines are by definition intended to interact with the human body. This means that specific parameters such as immunological and toxicological effects, release of the pharmaceutically active component(s), and biodistribution are of critical importance. The interaction of nanoparticles with cells and organs is covered elsewhere in this book, although sterility and endotoxin is covered in the present chapter as it concerns non-nanoparticle contaminants.

Further building on current state-of-the-art *in vitro* and *in vivo* characterization, *in silico* characterization has emerged as a very interesting research area. By using current knowledge to construct computerized models, and applying detailed physicochemical characterization as input to those models, it might be possible to predict biological effects of novel nanomedicines (and other nanoparticles), thus making the characterization cascade dramatically less resource intensive, and reducing the need for animal experiments significantly. Such modeling of pharmacokinetics is covered elsewhere in this book.

7.4.1
Sterility and Endotoxin

Sterility in the context of medicines manufacturing refers to the process of killing or eliminating all forms of cellular life and other biological pathogens (such as viruses). This is clearly crucial to avoid severe infections upon medicines administration to the patients, and can be achieved by, for example, gamma irradiation or heat treatment. For pharmaceuticals, sterility is generally obtained in the formulation constituents through GMP (good manufacturing practice) conditions. Microbial contamination is mostly measured by growth assays, commonly quantified as colony forming units (cfu) per sample volume applied to general or selective solid growth media. Nucleic acid-based (PCR) methods have found some use, although mainly on the quantification of specific microbial species or classes [78].

Perhaps more challenging than sterility, a critical requirement is the absence of *endotoxins*, which are lipopolysaccharides (LPS) from the membrane of Gram-negative bacteria. Endotoxins will elicit strong toxic/inflammatory effects in humans through the TLR4 signaling pathway; previous research has shown upregulation of inflammatory gene expression in primary human monocytes at levels down to 0.1 Endotoxin Units (EU) per ml [79]; the USP limit for intrathecally administered formulations is 0.2 EU/kg body weight/h, and for all other administrative routes the limit is 5 EU/kg/h [80]. In the preclinical characterization, presence of endotoxins can cause problems by masking biological effects of the pure nanocarrier system. It is notable that endotoxin contamination is found to be very widespread in nanomaterials [81]; the NCL found endotoxin in more than one-third of the nanomedicine samples submitted for preclinical characterization [1]. Methods for endotoxin removal from nanomaterials have been suggested, for example, chromatography techniques or two-phase extraction, but it is currently considered very challenging to remove endotoxin contamination from nanomedicines to an acceptable degree [82], and the recommended action upon endotoxin detection is generally to review and improve the production process to make it endotoxin free.

Common detection methods for endotoxin are the rabbit pyrogen test (RPT) and the Limulus amoebocyte lysate (LAL) assay, and these are both approved by

FDA, EMA, and most regulatory authorities. The LAL test is preferred over RPT for most applications due to cost and turnaround time, and because the RPT requires the use of animals. The LAL assay is based on the endotoxin-specific coagulation of lysate from blood cells of the horseshoe crab, and three formats are commonly available of the LAL assay: gel-clot, chromogenic, and turbidimetric [83]. The LAL assay was originally developed for soluble small-molecule compounds and should be applied with caution for nanomedicines, as significant interferences can occur [79,84]; the strengths and weaknesses of the formats were investigated by Dobrovolskaia *et al.* [85] and reviewed by Li and Boraschi [81]. It should also be observed that the LAL assay detects β-glucans, which could originate from, for example, cellulose-based filters, creating false positives. An alternative LAL method, The Horseshoe Crab factor C assay, has recently been developed that is robust against β-glucans detection [86]. Although there is an immense research interest in the fast, sensitive, and direct detection of endotoxins by physicochemical rather than biological methods [87], the main limitation of these methods is that they detect presence rather than activity of endotoxin and should still be verified by activity assays before *in vivo* experiments.

7.4.2
Surface Adsorption: the Protein Corona

One of the aspects most intensely investigated in nanomedicines recently, is that of the protein corona, recently reviewed in Ref. [88]. Whereas pristine nanoparticles in dispersion generally have a fairly well-defined physical boundary, their high surface free energy leads to rapid, complex, and extensive complexation with biomolecules when they get in contact with biological fluids such as blood plasma. This then effectively masks the synthetic nanoparticle, and dramatically changes what cells "see," thus affecting cellular uptake in a significant way. Therefore, the elucidation of the protein corona is of critical importance to be able to understand and predict toxicological and immunological reactions to nanoparticles, and their pharmacokinetic and pharmacodynamics effect in the body.

A range of methods can be utilized for nonspecific detection and quantification of proteins adsorbed on nanoparticles, including UV absorbance, fluorescence spectroscopy, infrared spectroscopy, surface plasmon resonance, or NMR (e.g., Refs [89,90]). These are techniques that effectively detect the putative presence of protein, but with no information on *which* proteins. Even more general are the sizing techniques such as DLS and FFF-MALS that detect overall change in particle size (by molecular adsorption) rather than chemical groups [91]. Since surface charge plays an important role in nanoparticle–cell interactions, it could be argued that zeta potential is actually a very relevant measurand despite its low specificity in terms of protein identity. Nevertheless, studies indicate a negative zeta potential after corona formation regardless of the surface charge on the pristine nanoparticle [92].

For a more detailed understanding of the formation and effect of the protein corona, a method is required that can quantify individual proteins in a complex mixture. This then approaches a classical proteomics challenge, and the standard proteomics toolbox contains the methods of choice, notably mass spectrometry (MS) mostly coupled online or offline to chromatographic or electrophoretic separation, such as liquid chromatography, size exclusion chromatography, ion chromatography, gel electrophoresis, or capillary electrophoresis [93]. A full review of methods for quantitative proteomics is beyond the scope of this book, but a brief outline is given below. Proteomics is often broadly divided in "top-down" or "bottom-up" [94,95], the former denoting intact proteins as the starting point, whereas the latter implies digestion (usually enzymatic) of the protein sample to peptides. In either case, MS is the detection method of choice, due to its unsurpassed combination of sensitivity, specificity, and selectivity. Rapid improvements in MS instrumentation over the last years mean that when high mass-resolution MS is coupled online to chromatographic or electrophoretic separation, a large fraction of the complete human proteome can now be detected and quantified in a single experiment [96].

Separation of the corona-coated nanoparticles from the protein-containing medium is necessary to get a true quantification of the adsorbed proteins. Common fractionation techniques such as SEC, FFF, or differential centrifugation can be used for this, although the relatively long separation times pose a challenge, as the protein corona is not covalently bound and thus might reorganize in equilibrium with the environment. Also, a fast separation method is desirable for elucidation of the *successive* adsorption of specific proteins. A sucrose cushion-based centrifugation has recently been introduced that resolves some of these challenges [92,97]. Even though the direct measurement of protein organization on the nanoparticle surface is highly challenging, some work is beginning to appear [98] on this, integrating several fractionation and imaging techniques. This is clearly a research area of great relevance to nanomedicine. Finally, it should be mentioned that although the main focus in scientific literature seems to have been on the protein corona, nanoparticle interaction with for example, lipids is of significant interest, for instance in the lung microenvironment [99,100]. MS will generally be the detection method of choice also for lipids.

7.4.3 Drug Release

A key feature of many nanomedicines is their controllable release of the active pharmaceutical component. This may alter the biodistribution of the drug, improve efficacy, and reduce off-target-site toxicity. Thus, the release rate of the drug becomes very important as has been noted by the regulatory authorities EMA and FDA. Analytical methods to measure drug release from nanomedicines have recently been covered extensively by Ambardekar and Stern [101]. The reliable quantification of the free (unbound) and encapsulated fractions of the total drug content in a formulation, as a function of time, would make possible the calculation of release rates. Such dual quantification is not trivial, as the physical separation of the two fractions might influence the release equilibrium from the nanoparticles and thus affect the state to be measured. This becomes a very significant concern in the case of release to complex biological media, where components such as blood cells or protein will generally form reversible drug complexes in equilibrium with the unbound drug, reducing the effective unencapsulated drug concentration. Thus, multiple simultaneous equilibria exist, but only the free drug is biologically active.

Most methods for measuring drug release from nanomedicines are repurposed methods developed for small molecule drugs. These include chromatography methods (size-exclusion chromatography and solid-phase extraction), liquid–liquid extraction, and equilibrium methods (dialysis, ultracentrifugation, and ultrafiltration). All of the above methods have their specific, and often significant, disadvantages, for example, for chromatographic methods, the free drug is not in equilibrium with protein; for dialysis and ultracentrifugation, the long separation times can mask the actual release kinetics; and for dialysis and ultrafiltration, there is the concern of nonspecific binding of drug to the filter. Even though recent data indicate that the SPE-based approach is robust for certain combinations of carriers and drugs [102], the process-induced release of drugs by particle disassembly is a general concern with these methods. Two techniques that have proven useful in *in vivo* studies are based on tracking both the active drug and components of the nanoparticle by using either dual radioisotope labeling, or complementary chemical and biological assays to follow unlabeled components [103]. The use of radioisotopes, however, is generally considered undesirable for most labs, and the detection of unlabeled nanoparticle components is complicated by their potential biochemical entanglement with the native metabolism.

As shown, established drug release methods generally do not address nanoparticle-specific concerns such as selective measurement of the unbound drug or the unintentional drug release during analytical fractionation. Recently, Skoczen *et al.* suggested and validated a novel drug release assay [104] that seems to circumvent most of the problems experienced with traditional methods. This assay is based on ultrafiltration and the use of two distinct stable isotope-labeled analogues of the encapsulated drug, spiked into the release medium. Chemically and biochemically equivalent to the native drug, the first labeled analog will act as an internal reference compound for the equilibria between free, protein-bound, and encapsulated drug, whereas the second labeled analog acts as a process internal standard to correct for drug-specific losses during extraction and sample workup. Importantly, the quantification of drug in the different fractions (retentate, supernatant) is done by mass spectrometry; this enables the simultaneous, specific detection of the native and labeled drugs. The simultaneous detection then helps to eliminate possible concerns of MS-specific matrix effects such as ionization suppression. The use of stable isotope-labeled analogues have long traditions in clinical pharmaceutical analyses of small-molecule drugs and in more general analytical chemistry, and is considered a versatile and robust technique for reliable and sensitive quantification in complex matrices.

Hinna *et al.* [105] describe the use of multilamellar liposomes as biomimetic model sinks for drug release from a liposomal drug carrier, followed by separation of the two populations by FFF. Based on this, they were able to estimate kinetic release parameters for the drug p-THPP (a porphyrin). For optically active drugs, several groups have reported the use of advanced fluorescence methods for monitoring of drug release [106–108]; these methods are, however, not generally applicable to all drug compound classes.

7.5 Conclusions and Future Outlook

The variety and the complexity of nanomedicines have increased dramatically over the recent years, but the translation of new candidate nanomedicines into the clinic has been limited. One bottleneck for such translation has been the lack of established characterization and testing regimes that can provide regulatory authorities with the necessary data to allow novel nanomedicines into clinical testing. This need for nanomaterial-specific characterization is reflected in other regulatory domains as well, such as medical devices, cosmetics and food products [109]. Khorasani *et al.* [3] have proposed a minimum set of standardized techniques for characterization of nanomedicines, that should accelerate their clinical translation, and the NCL has gained invaluable experience with characterization of a large number of real-life candidate nanomedicines [1].

For certain analytical aspects of medical nanoparticles, such as size or bulk chemical composition, both mature and novel technologies exist that can provide reliable data when applied correctly. Other aspects, such as detection and quantification of surface functionalization, protein corona or drug release into biologically relevant systems, are still analytically challenging and will require technology development. One emerging trend in the physicochemical part of the characterization cascade seems to be that of miniaturization and single-particle measurements, often in a high-throughput automated fashion that allows statistical analysis of the data. The widespread adoption of nanoparticle tracking analysis, the application of quartz crystal microbalance [110] and the recent demonstration of single nanoparticle direct mass measurement by MS [111] are examples of this. Microfluidic devices are extensively used for exploratory nanomedicines production [112,113], but recently they have found application also in characterization, notably through the miniaturization of FFF [114,115], or even the miniaturized studies of their biological interactions [116].

Physicochemical characterization of nanomedicines will benefit from the ongoing rapid technology development within general nanotechnology. The implementation of new nanomedicine characterization technologies should be done in close interaction with regulatory authorities to ensure that the data acquired on candidate nanomedicines will actually help increase their clinical translation and contribute to significant improvements in healthcare on the global scale.

References

1 Crist, R.M., Grossman, J.H., Patri, A.K., Stern, S.T., Dobrovolskaia, M.A., Adiseshaiah, P.P., Clogston, J.D., and McNeil, S.E. (2013) Common pitfalls in nanotechnology: lessons learned from NCI's nanotechnology characterization laboratory. *Integr. Biol. (Camb.)*, **5**, 66–73.

2 Cho, E.J., Holback, H., Liu, K.C., Abouelmagd, S.A., Park, J., and Yeo, Y. (2013) Nanoparticle characterization: state of the art, challenges, and emerging technologies. *Mol. Pharm.*, **10**, 2093–2110.

3 Khorasani, A.A., Weaver, J.L., and Salvador-Morales, C. (2014) Closing the gap: accelerating the translational process in nanomedicine by proposing standardized characterization techniques. *Int. J. Nanomedicine*, **9**, 5729–5751.

4 Lin, P.C., Lin, S., Wang, P.C., and Sridhar, R. (2014) Techniques for physicochemical characterization of nanomaterials. *Biotechnol. Adv.*, **32**, 711–726.

5 López-Serrano, A., Olivas, R.M., Landaluze, J.S., and Cámara, C. (2014) Nanoparticles: a global vision. Characterization, separation, and quantification methods. Potential environmental and health impact. *Anal. Methods*, **6**, 38–56.

6 Sapsford, K.E., Tyner, K.M., Dair, B.J., Deschamps, J.R., and Medintz, I.L. (2011) Analyzing nanomaterial bioconjugates: a review of current and emerging purification and characterization techniques. *Anal. Chem.*, **83**, 4453–4488.

7 Gunsolus, I.L. and Haynes, C.L. (2016) Analytical aspects of nanotoxicology. *Anal. Chem.*, **88**, 451–479.

8 Shang, L., Nienhaus, K., and Nienhaus, G.U. (2014) Engineered nanoparticles interacting with cells: size matters. *J. Nanobiotechnol.*, **12**, b26.

9 Varenne, F., Makky, A., Gaucher-Delmas, M., Violleau, F., and Vauthier, C. (2016) Multimodal dispersion of nanoparticles: a comprehensive evaluation of size distribution with 9 size measurement methods. *Pharm. Res.*, **33**, 1220–1234.

10 Fischer, K. and Schmidt, M. (2016) Pitfalls and novel applications of particle sizing by dynamic light scattering. *Biomaterials*, **98**, 79–91.

11 Cao, A. (2003) Light scattering. Recent applications. *Anal. Lett.*, **36**, 3185–3225.

12 Capomaccio, R., Jimenez, I.O., Colpo, P., Gilliland, D., Ceccone, G., Rossi, F., and Calzolai, L. (2015) Determination of the structure and morphology of gold nanoparticle-HSA protein complexes. *Nanoscale*, **7**, 17653–17657.

13 Wyatt, P.J. (2014) Measurement of special nanoparticle structures by light scattering. *Anal. Chem.*, **86**, 7171–7183.

14 Haiss, W., Thanh, N.T., Aveyard, J., and Fernig, D.G. (2007) Determination of size and concentration of gold nanoparticles from UV-vis spectra. *Anal. Chem.*, **79**, 4215–4221.

15 Filipe, V., Hawe, A., and Jiskoot, W. (2010) Critical evaluation of nanoparticle tracking analysis (NTA) by NanoSight for the measurement of nanoparticles and protein aggregates. *Pharm. Res.*, **27**, 796–810.

16 Malloy, A. and Carr, B. (2006) NanoParticle tracking analysis – the Halo™ system. *Part. Part. Syst. Charact.*, **23**, 197–204.

17 Saveyn, H., De Baets, B., Thas, O., Hole, P., and Smith, J., and Van der Meeren, P. (2010) Accurate particle size distribution determination by nanoparticle tracking analysis based on 2-D Brownian dynamics simulation. *J. Colloid Interface Sci.*, **352**, 593–600.

18 Sowerby, S.J., Broom, M.F., and Petersen, G.B. (2007) Dynamically resizable nanometre-scale apertures for molecular sensing. *Sensor Actuators B Chem.*, **123**, 325–330.

19 Weatherall, E. and Willmott, G.R. (2015) Applications of tunable resistive pulse sensing. *Analyst*, **140**, 3318–3334.

20 Luo, L., German, S.R., Lan, W.-J., Holden, D.A., Mega, T.L., and White, H.S. (2014) Resistive-pulse analysis of nanoparticles. *Annu. Rev. Anal. Chem.*, **7**, 513–535.

21 Klang, V., Valenta, C., and Matsko, N.B. (2013) Electron microscopy of pharmaceutical systems. *Micron*, **44**, 45–74.

22 Fox, T.L., Tang, S., Horton, J.M., Holdaway, H.A., Zhao, B., Zhu, L., and Stewart, P.L. (2015) *In situ* characterization of binary mixed polymer brush-grafted silica nanoparticles in aqueous and organic solvents by cryo-electron tomography. *Langmuir*, **31**, 8680–8688.

23 de Jonge, N. and Ross, F.M. (2011) Electron microscopy of specimens in liquid. *Nat. Nanotechnol.*, **6**, 695–704.

24 Ross, F.M. (2015) Opportunities and challenges in liquid cell electron microscopy. *Supramol. Sci.*, **350**, aaa9886.

25 Hoppe, S.M., Sasaki, D.Y., Kinghorn, A.N., and Hattar, K. (2013) *In-situ* transmission electron microscopy of liposomes in an aqueous environment. *Langmuir*, **29**, 9958–9961.

26 Patterson, J.P., Proetto, M.T., and Gianneschi, N.C. (2015) Soft nanomaterials analysed by *in situ* liquid TEM: Towards high resolution characterisation of nanoparticles in motion. *Perspect. Sci.*, **6**, 106–112.

27 Laramy, C.R., Brown, K.A., O'Brien, M.N., and Mirkin, C.A. (2015) High-throughput, algorithmic determination of nanoparticle structure from electron microscopy images. *ACS Nano*, **9**, 12488–12495.

28 Sitterberg, J., Ozcetin, A., Ehrhardt, C., and Bakowsky, U. (2010) Utilising atomic force microscopy for the characterisation of nanoscale drug delivery systems. *Eur. J. Pharm. Biopharm.*, **74**, 2–13.

29 Souza, T.G.F., Ciminelli, V.S.T., and Mohallem, N.D.S. (2015) An assessment of errors in sample preparation and data processing for nanoparticle size analyses by AFM. *Mater. Charact.*, **109**, 198–205.

30 Baalousha, M. and Lead, J.R. (2012) Rationalizing nanomaterial sizes measured by atomic force microscopy, flow field-flow fractionation, and dynamic light scattering: sample preparation, polydispersity, and particle structure. *Environ. Sci. Technol.*, **46**, 6134–6142.

31 Pyrgiotakis, G., Blattmann, C.O., Pratsinis, S., and Demokritou, P. (2013) Nanoparticle-nanoparticle interactions in biological media by atomic force microscopy. *Langmuir*, **29**, 11385–11395.

32 Maver, U., Velnar, T., Gaberšček, M., Planinšek, O., and Finšgar, M. (2016) Recent progressive use of atomic force microscopy in biomedical applications. *Trends Analyt. Chem.*, **80**, 96–111.

33 Garcia, R. and Herruzo, E.T. (2012) The emergence of multifrequency force microscopy. *Nat. Nanotechnol.*, **7**, 217–226.

34 Lee, S., Bi, X., Reed, R.B., Ranville, J.F., Herckes, P., and Westerhoff, P. (2014) Nanoparticle size detection limits by single particle ICP-MS for 40 elements. *Environ. Sci. Technol.*, **48**, 10291–10300.

35 Balcaen, L., Bolea-Fernandez, E., Resano, M., and Vanhaecke, F. (2015) Inductively coupled plasma – tandem mass spectrometry (ICP-MS/MS): a powerful and universal tool for the interference-free determination of (ultra)trace elements – a tutorial review. *Anal. Chim. Acta*, **894**, 7–19.

36 Peters, R., Herrera-Rivera, Z., Undas, A., van der Lee, M., Marvin, H., Bouwmeester, H., and Weigel, S. (2015) Single particle ICP-MS combined with a data evaluation tool as a routine technique for the analysis of nanoparticles in complex matrices. *J. Anal. At. Spectrom.*, **30**, 1274–1285.

37 Elzey, S., Tsai, D.H., Yu, L.L., Winchester, M.R., Kelley, M.E., and Hackley, V.A. (2013) Real-time size discrimination and elemental analysis of gold nanoparticles using ES-DMA coupled to ICP-MS. *Anal. Bioanal. Chem.*, **405**, 2279–2288.

38 Wahlund, K.G. (2013) Flow field-flow fractionation: critical overview. *J. Chromatogr. A*, **1287**, 97–112.

39 Wagner, M., Holzschuh, S., Traeger, A., Fahr, A., and Schubert, U.S. (2014) Asymmetric flow field-flow fractionation in the field of nanomedicine. *Anal. Chem.*, **86**, 5201–5210.

40 Zattoni, A., Roda, B., Borghi, F., Marassi, V., and Reschiglian, P. (2014) Flow field-flow fractionation for the analysis of

nanoparticles used in drug delivery. *J. Pharm. Biomed. Anal.*, **87**, 53–61.

41 Ponyik, C.A., Wu, D.T., and Williams, S.K. (2013) Separation and composition distribution determination of triblock copolymers by thermal field-flow fractionation. *Anal. Bioanal. Chem.*, **405**, 9033–9040.

42 Greyling, G. and Pasch, H. (2016) Multidetector thermal field-flow fractionation: a unique tool for monitoring the structure and dynamics of block copolymer micelles. *Macromolecules*, **49**, 1882–1889.

43 Johann, C., Elsenberg, S., Schuch, H., and Rosch, U. (2015) Instrument and method to determine the electrophoretic mobility of nanoparticles and proteins by combining electrical and flow field-flow fractionation. *Anal. Chem.*, **87**, 4292–4298.

44 Grabielle-Madelmont, C., Lesieur, S., and Ollivon, M. (2003) Characterization of loaded liposomes by size exclusion chromatography. *J. Biochem. Biophys. Methods*, **56**, 189–217.

45 Lespes, G. and Gigault, J. (2011) Hyphenated analytical techniques for multidimensional characterisation of submicron particles: a review. *Anal. Chim. Acta*, **692**, 26–41.

46 Ruysschaert, T., Marque, A., Duteyrat, J.L., Lesieur, S., Winterhalter, M., and Fournier, D. (2005) Liposome retention in size exclusion chromatography. *BMC Biotechnol*, **5**, 11.

47 Lange, H. (1995) Comparative test of methods to determine particle size and particle size distribution in the submicron range. *Part. Part. Syst. Charact.*, **12**, 148–157.

48 Niebel, Y., Buschmann, M.D., Lavertu, M., and De Crescenzo, G. (2014) Combined analysis of polycation/ODN polyplexes by analytical ultracentrifugation and dynamic light scattering reveals their size, refractive index increment, stoichiometry, porosity, and molecular weight. *Biomacromolecules*, **15**, 940–947.

49 Walter, J., Löhr, K., Karabudak, E., Reis, W., Mikhael, J., Peukert, W., Wohlleben, W., and Cölfen, H. (2014) Multidimensional analysis of nanoparticles with highly disperse properties using multiwavelength analytical ultracentrifugation. *ACS Nano*, **8**, 8871–8886.

50 Diaz, L., Peyrot, C., and Wilkinson, K.J. (2015) Characterization of polymeric nanomaterials using analytical ultracentrifugation. *Environ. Sci. Technol.*, **49**, 7302–7309.

51 Benoit, D.N., Zhu, H., Lilierose, M.H., Verm, R.A., Ali, N., Morrison, A.N., Fortner, J.D., Avendano, C., and Colvin, V.L. (2012) Measuring the grafting density of nanoparticles in solution by analytical ultracentrifugation and total organic carbon analysis. *Anal. Chem.*, **84**, 9238–9245.

52 Zhao, H., Ghirlando, R., Alfonso, C., Arisaka, F., Attali, I., Bain, D.L., Bakhtina, M.M., Becker, D.F., Bedwell, G.J., Bekdemir, A. *et al.* (2015) A multilaboratory comparison of calibration accuracy and the performance of external references in analytical ultracentrifugation. *PLoS One*, **10**, e0126420.

53 Dobrovolskaia, M.A., Patri, A.K., Simak, J., Hall, J.B., Semberova, J., De Paoli Lacerda, S.H., and McNeil, S.E. (2012) Nanoparticle size and surface charge determine effects of PAMAM dendrimers on human platelets *in vitro*. *Mol. Pharm.*, **9**, 382–393.

54 Kaszuba, M., Corbett, J., Watson, F.M., and Jones, A. (2010) High-concentration zeta potential measurements using light-scattering techniques. *Philos. Trans A Math Phys. Eng. Sci.*, **368**, 4439–4451.

55 Vogel, R., Anderson, W., Eldridge, J., Glossop, B., and Willmott, G. (2012) A variable pressure method for characterizing nanoparticle surface charge using pore sensors. *Anal. Chem.*, **84**, 3125–3131.

56 Sikora, A., Shard, A.G., and Minelli, C. (2016) Size and zeta-potential measurement of silica nanoparticles in serum using tunable resistive pulse sensing. *Langmuir*, **32**, 2216–2224.

57 Sikora, A., Bartczak, D., Geißler, D., Kestens, V., Roebben, G., Ramaye, Y.,

Varga, Z., Palmai, M., Shard, A.G., Goenaga-Infante, H. *et al.* (2015) A systematic comparison of different techniques to determine the zeta potential of silica nanoparticles in biological medium. *Anal. Methods*, **7**, 9835–9843.

58 Pelaz, B., del Pino, P., Maffre, P., Hartmann, R., Gallego, M., Rivera-Fernández, S., de la Fuente, J.M., and Nienhaus, G.U., and Parak, W.J. (2015) Surface functionalization of nanoparticles with polyethylene glycol: effects on protein adsorption and cellular uptake. *ACS Nano*, **9**, 6996–7008.

59 Tong, L., Lu, E., Pichaandi, J., Cao, P., Nitz, M., and Winnik, M.A. (2015) Quantification of surface ligands on NaYF4 nanoparticles by three independent analytical techniques. *Chem. Mater.*, **27**, 4899–4910.

60 Hennig, A., Borcherding, H., Jaeger, C., Hatami, S., Wurth, C., Hoffmann, A., Hoffmann, K., Thiele, T., Schedler, U., and Resch-Genger, U. (2012) Scope and limitations of surface functional group quantification methods: exploratory study with poly(acrylic acid)-grafted micro- and nanoparticles. *J. Am. Chem. Soc.*, **134**, 8268–8276.

61 Sebby, K.B. and Mansfield, E. (2015) Determination of the surface density of polyethylene glycol on gold nanoparticles by use of microscale thermogravimetric analysis. *Anal. Bioanal. Chem.*, **407**, 2913–2922.

62 Mansfield, E., Tyner, K.M., Poling, C.M., and Blacklock, J.L. (2014) Determination of nanoparticle surface coatings and nanoparticle purity using microscale thermogravimetric analysis. *Anal. Chem.*, **86**, 1478–1484.

63 Rabanel, J.M., Hildgen, P., and Banquy, X. (2014) Assessment of PEG on polymeric particles surface, a key step in drug carrier translation. *J. Control. Release*, **185**, 71–87.

64 Peracchia, M.T., Vauthier, C., Desmaële, D., Gulik, A., Dedieu, J.-C., Demoy, M., d'Angelo, J., and Couvreur, P. (1998) Pegylated nanoparticles from a novel methoxypolyethylene glycol cyanoacrylate-hexadecyl cyanoacrylate amphiphilic copolymer. *Pharm. Res.*, **15**, 550–556.

65 Torelli, M.D., Putans, R.A., Tan, Y., Lohse, S.E., Murphy, C.J., and Hamers, R.J. (2015) Quantitative determination of ligand densities on nanomaterials by X-ray photoelectron spectroscopy. *ACS Appl. Mater. Interfaces*, **7**, 1720–1725.

66 Kim, Y.P., Shon, H.K., Shin, S.K., and Lee, T.G. (2015) Probing nanoparticles and nanoparticle-conjugated biomolecules using time-of-flight secondary ion mass spectrometry. *Mass Spectrom. Rev.*, **34**, 237–247.

67 Ju, S. and Yeo, W.S. (2012) Quantification of proteins on gold nanoparticles by combining MALDI-TOF MS and proteolysis. *Nanotechnology*, **23**, 135701.

68 Lopez-Cebral, R., Martin-Pastor, M., Seijo, B., and Sanchez, A. (2014) Progress in the characterization of bio-functionalized nanoparticles using NMR methods and their applications as MRI contrast agents. *Prog. Nucl. Magn. Reson. Spectrosc.*, **79**, 1–13.

69 Sarker, M., Fraser, R.E., Lumsden, M.D., Anderson, D.J., and Rainey, J.K. (2015) Characterization of variant soft nanoparticle structure and morphology in solution by NMR spectroscopy. *J. Phys. Chem. C*, **119**, 7461–7471.

70 Simeonova, M., Rangel, M., and Ivanova, G. (2013) NMR study of the supramolecular structure of dual drug-loaded poly(butylcyanoacrylate) nanoparticles. *Phys. Chem. Chem. Phys.*, **15**, 16657–16664.

71 Pinto, L.F., Riguera, R., and Fernandez-Megia, E. (2013) Stepwise filtering of the internal layers of dendrimers by transverse-relaxation-edited NMR. *J. Am. Chem. Soc.*, **135**, 11513–11516.

72 Rastrelli, F., Jha, S., and Mancin, F. (2009) Seeing through macromolecules: T2-Filtered NMR for the purity assay of functionalized nanosystems and the screening of biofluids. *J. Am. Chem. Soc.*, **131**, 14222–14224.

73 Orban, D.E., Moretti, A., and Uhrich, K.E. (2016) Spatial location of indomethacin associated with unimeric amphiphilic carrier macromolecules as determined by

nuclear magnetic resonance spectroscopy. *Magn. Reson. Chem.*, **54** (7), 575–583.
74 Pensado, A., Martin-Pastor, M., Zorzi, G.K., Carvalho, E.S., and Sanchez, A. (2016) Structural analysis of nanosystems: solid sorbitan esters nanoparticles (SSN) as a case study. *Eur. J. Pharm. Biopharm.*, **104**, 189–199.
75 Joset, A., Grammenos, A., Hoebeke, M., and Leyh, B. (2015) Investigation of the interaction between a β-cyclodextrin and DMPC liposomes: a small angle neutron scattering study. *J. Incl. Phenom. Macrocycl. Chem.*, **83**, 227–238.
76 Kiselev, M.A., Zemlyanaya, E.V., Zhabitskaya, E.I., and Aksenov, V.L. (2015) Investigation of the structure of unilamellar dimyristoylphosphatidylcholine vesicles in aqueous sucrose solutions by small-angle neutron and X-ray scattering. *Crystallogr. Rep.*, **60**, 143–147.
77 Schilt, Y., Berman, T., Wei, X., Barenholz, Y., and Raviv, U. (2016) Using solution X-ray scattering to determine the high-resolution structure and morphology of PEGylated liposomal doxorubicin nanodrugs. *Biochim. Biophys. Acta*, **1860**, 108–119.
78 Al-Aboody, M. (2015) Review on application of nucleic acid amplification techniques in pharmaceutical products analysis. *J. Appl. Pharm. Sci.*, **5** (12), 154–158.
79 Oostingh, G.J., Casals, E., Italiani, P., Colognato, R., Stritzinger, R., Ponti, J., Pfaller, T., Kohl, Y., Ooms, D., Favilli, F. *et al.* (2011) Problems and challenges in the development and validation of human cell-based assays to determine nanoparticle-induced immunomodulatory effects. *Part. Fibre Toxicol.*, **8**, 1–21.
80 Convention, U.S.P. (2011) In Convention, U. S. P. (ed.): http://www.usp.org/usp-nf/harmonization/stage-6/bacterial-endotoxins-test, pp. 1–5.
81 Li, Y. and Boraschi, D. (2016) Endotoxin contamination: a key element in the interpretation of nanosafety studies. *Nanomedicine*, **11**, 269–287.
82 Vetten, M.A., Yah, C.S., Singh, T., and Gulumian, M. (2014) Challenges facing sterilization and depyrogenation of nanoparticles: effects on structural stability and biomedical applications. *Nanomedicine*, **10**, 1391–1399.
83 Neun, B.W. and Dobrovolskaia, M.A. (2011) *Characterization of Nanoparticles Intended for Drug Delivery* (ed. E.S. McNeil), Humana Press, Totowa, NJ, pp. 121–130.
84 Li, Y., Italiani, P., Casals, E., Tran, N., Puntes, V.F., and Boraschi, D. (2015) Optimising the use of commercial LAL assays for the analysis of endotoxin contamination in metal colloids and metal oxide nanoparticles. *Nanotoxicology*, **9**, 462–473.
85 Dobrovolskaia, M.A., Neun, B.W., Clogston, J.D., Grossman, J.H., and McNeil, S.E. (2013) Choice of method for endotoxin detection depends on nanoformulation. *Nanomedicine*, **9**, 1847–1856.
86 Alwis, K.U. and Milton, D.K. (2006) Recombinant factor C assay for measuring endotoxin in house dust: comparison with LAL, and (1 –> 3)-beta-D-glucans. *Am. J. Ind. Med.*, **49**, 296–300.
87 Das, A.P., Kumar, P.S., and Swain, S. (2014) Recent advances in biosensor based endotoxin detection. *Biosens. Bioelectron.*, **51**, 62–75.
88 Docter, D., Westmeier, D., Markiewicz, M., Stolte, S., Knauer, S.K., and Stauber, R.H. (2015) The nanoparticle biomolecule corona: lessons learned – challenge accepted? *Chem. Soc. Rev.*, **44**, 6094–6121.
89 Shang, L., Wang, Y., Jiang, J., and Dong, S. (2007) pH-dependent protein conformational changes in albumin:gold nanoparticle bioconjugates: a spectroscopic study. *Langmuir*, **23**, 2714–2721.
90 Lundqvist, M., Sethson, I., and Jonsson, B.-H. (2004) Protein adsorption onto silica nanoparticles: conformational changes depend on the particles' curvature and the protein stability. *Langmuir*, **20**, 10639–10647.
91 Jans, H., Liu, X., Austin, L., Maes, G., and Huo, Q. (2009) Dynamic light scattering

as a powerful tool for gold nanoparticle bioconjugation and biomolecular binding studies. *Anal. Chem.*, **81**, 9425–9432.

92 Tenzer, S., Docter, D., Kuharev, J., Musyanovych, A., Fetz, V., Hecht, R., Schlenk, F., Fischer, D., Kiouptsi, K., Reinhardt, C. *et al.* (2013) Rapid formation of plasma protein corona critically affects nanoparticle pathophysiology. *Nat. Nanotechnol.*, **8**, 772–781.

93 Capriotti, A.L., Caracciolo, G., Cavaliere, C., Colapicchioni, V., Piovesana, S., Pozzi, D., and Laganà, A. (2014) Analytical methods for characterizing the nanoparticle–protein corona. *Chromatographia*, **77**, 755–769.

94 Catherman, A.D., Skinner, O.S., and Kelleher, N.L. (2014) Top Down proteomics: facts and perspectives. *Biochem. Biophys. Res. Commun.*, **445**, 683–693.

95 Zhang, Y., Fonslow, B.R., Shan, B., Baek, M.C., and Yates, J.R. 3rd (2013) Protein analysis by shotgun/bottom-up proteomics. *Chem. Rev.*, **113**, 2343–2394.

96 Richards, A.L., Merrill, A.E., and Coon, J.J. (2015) Proteome sequencing goes deep. *Curr. Opin. Chem. Biol.*, **24**, 11–17.

97 Docter, D., Distler, U., Storck, W., Kuharev, J., Wünsch, D., Hahlbrock, A., Knauer, S.K., Tenzer, S., and Stauber, R.H. (2014) Quantitative profiling of the protein coronas that form around nanoparticles. *Nat. Protoc.*, **9**, 2030–2044.

98 Kelly, P.M., Aberg, C., Polo, E., O'Connell, A., Cookman, J., Fallon, J., Krpetic, Z., and Dawson, K.A. (2015) Mapping protein binding sites on the biomolecular corona of nanoparticles. *Nat. Nanotechnol.*, **10**, 472–479.

99 Raesch, S.S., Tenzer, S., Storck, W., Rurainski, A., Selzer, D., Ruge, C.A., Perez-Gil, J., Schaefer, U.F., and Lehr, C.-M. (2015) Proteomic and lipidomic analysis of nanoparticle corona upon contact with lung surfactant reveals differences in protein, but not lipid composition. *ACS Nano*, **9**, 11872–11885.

100 Chhoden, T., Clausen, P.A., Larsen, S.T., Norgaard, A.W., and Lauritsen, F.R. (2015) Interactions between nanoparticles and lung surfactant investigated by matrix-assisted laser desorption/ionization time-of-flight mass spectrometry. *Rapid Commun. Mass Spectrom.*, **29**, 1080–1086.

101 Ambardekar, V.V. and Stern, T.S. (2015) *Non-Biological Complex Drugs: The Science and the Regulatory Landscape* (eds J.A.D. Crommelin and B.J.S. deVlieger), Springer International Publishing, Cham, pp. 261–287.

102 Guillot, A., Couffin, A.C., Sejean, X., Navarro, F., Limberger, M., and Lehr, C.M. (2015) Solid phase extraction as an innovative separation method for measuring free and entrapped drug in lipid nanoparticles. *Pharm. Res.*, **32**, 3999–4009.

103 Stern, S.T., Hall, J.B., Yu, L.L., Wood, L.J., Paciotti, G.F., Tamarkin, L., Long, S.E., and McNeil, S.E. (2010) Translational considerations for cancer nanomedicine. *J. Control. Release*, **146**, 164–174.

104 Skoczen, S., McNeil, S.E., and Stern, S.T. (2015) Stable isotope method to measure drug release from nanomedicines. *J. Control. Release*, **220**, 169–174.

105 Hinna, A.H., Hupfeld, S., Kuntsche, J., Bauer-Brandl, A., and Brandl, M. (2016) Mechanism and kinetics of the loss of poorly soluble drugs from liposomal carriers studied by a novel flow field-flow fractionation-based drug release-/transfer-assay. *J. Control. Release*, **232**, 228–237.

106 Lai, J., Shah, B.P., Zhang, Y., Yang, L., and Lee, K.-B. (2015) Real-time monitoring of ATP-responsive drug release using mesoporous-silica-coated multicolor upconversion nanoparticles. *ACS Nano*, **9**, 5234–5245.

107 Chen, H., Moore, T., Qi, B., Colvin, D.C., Jelen, E.K., Hitchcock, D.A., He, J., Mefford, O.T., Gore, J.C., Alexis, F. *et al.* (2013) Monitoring pH-triggered drug release from radioluminescent nanocapsules with X-ray excited optical luminescence. *ACS Nano*, **7**, 1178–1187.

108 Qiu, F., Wang, D., Zhu, Q., Zhu, L., Tong, G., Lu, Y., Yan, D., and Zhu, X. (2014) Real-time monitoring of anticancer drug release with highly fluorescent star-conjugated copolymer as a drug carrier. *Biomacromolecules*, **15**, 1355–1364.

109 Wacker, M.G., Proykova, A., and Mendes Lima Santos, G. (2016) Dealing with nanosafety around the globe-regulation vs. innovation. *Int. J. Pharm.*, **509** (1–2), 95–106.

110 Olsson, A.L.J., Quevedo, I.R., He, D., Basnet, M., and Tufenkji, N. (2013) Using the quartz crystal microbalance with dissipation monitoring to evaluate the size of nanoparticles deposited on surfaces. *ACS Nano*, **7**, 7833–7843.

111 Zhang, N., Zhu, K., Xiong, C., Jiang, Y., Chang, H.C., and Nie, Z. (2016) Mass measurement of single intact nanoparticles in a cylindrical ion trap. *Anal. Chem.*, **88** (11), 5958–5962.

112 Valencia, P.M., Farokhzad, O.C., Karnik, R., and Langer, R. (2012) Microfluidic technologies for accelerating the clinical translation of nanoparticles. *Nat. Nanotechnol.*, **7**, 623–629.

113 Kim, Y. and Langer, R. (2006) *Reviews in Cell Biology and Molecular Medicine*, Wiley-VCH Verlag GmbH & Co. KGaA.

114 Janča, J. and Sobota, J. (2014) Trends in polymer and particle characterization by microfluidic field-flow fractionation methods: science or business? *Int. J. Polym. Anal. Charact.*, **19**, 296–308.

115 Arosio, P., Muller, T., Mahadevan, L., and Knowles, T.P. (2014) Density-gradient-free microfluidic centrifugation for analytical and preparative separation of nanoparticles. *Nano Lett.*, **14**, 2365–2371.

116 Bjornmalm, M., Yan, Y., and Caruso, F. (2014) Engineering and evaluating drug delivery particles in microfluidic devices. *J. Control. Release*, **190**, 139–149.

8
Nanoparticle Characterization Methods: Applications of Synchrotron and Neutron Radiation

Martha Brennich,[1] Marité Cardenas,[2,3] Hiram Castillo-Michel,[1] Marine Cotte,[1] V. Trevor Forsyth,[4,5] Michael Haertlein,[4] Simon A. J. Kimber,[1] Geraldine Le Duc,[1] Edward P. Mitchell,[1,5] Adam Round,[5,6] Murielle Salome,[1] and Michael Sztucki[1]

[1]European Synchrotron Radiation Facility, Experiments Division, 71 avenue des Martyrs, 38000 Grenoble, France
[2]Malmö University, Biofilm Research Center for Biointerfaces and Department of Biomedical Science, Östra Varvsgatan 11 20506 Malmö Sweden
[3]University of Copenhagen, Department of Chemistry and Nanoscience Center, Universitetsparken 5, DK-2100 Copenhagen, Denmark
[4]Institit Laue Langevin, Life Sciences Group, 71 avenue des Martyrs, 38042 Grenoble, France
[5]Keele University, Faculty of Natural Sciences, Keele, Staffordshire ST5 5BG, UK
[6]European Molecular Biology Laboratory, Grenoble Outstation, 71 avenue des Martyrs, 38000 Grenoble, France

8.1
Advanced Characterization: Synchrotron Light and Neutron Sources

The characterization of materials at the atomic-, nano-, and microscales is of crucial importance in understanding and then tailoring their macroscale properties and function for end-use applications and for effective modern cradle-to-reuse materials cycling. Synchrotron light, as well as the complementary neutron beams, offer exquisite microscopy probes to look into the heart of materials. These techniques, provided by large-scale infrastructure facilities, open the door to advanced characterization for nanoparticles and biologics going far beyond the abilities of conventional analytical techniques.

Today there are around 50 synchrotron light sources operating worldwide, with some 15 or so at "high" electron energy of greater than or equal to 3 GeV, and about 20 neutron sources operating worldwide. These analytical research infrastructures have become *de facto* materials characterization and analytical tools expected and required by scientists, technologists, and engineers serving an incredibly wide range of scientific disciplines in academic research and, increasingly, in industry R&I.

Synchrotron radiation was first practically observed in 1945 at the GE Labs coming from a small cyclotron device (for a history of synchrotron light sources

Pharmaceutical Nanotechnology: Innovation and Production, First Edition. Edited by Jean Cornier, Arno Kwade, Andrew Owen, and Marcel Van de Voorde.

see [1]). At first, this parasitic radiation was considered a nuisance by the physicists seeking insights into the structure and interaction of atomic particles, but later it was realised and then rapidly applied as an analysis tool in its own right. The first storage rings dedicated to producing synchrotron radiation, the so-called second generation of machines, came into operation in the 1970s. This generation of machines was followed by the European Synchrotron Radiation Facility (ESRF, Grenoble), which started operation in 1994 as the first of the third-generation storage rings with "insertion devices" able to generate extremely high intensity laser-like X-ray beams.

Synchrotron sources generate light through the motion of relativistic electrons in magnetic fields. In brief, electrons are first accelerated in a linear accelerator (linac) and then a booster ring to relativistic speeds; they are then injected into the main storage ring where they remain for a period of around a day. As these packets of charged particles circulate, the electron beam is passed through magnetic fields in the form of insertion devices; as they do, they emit intense electromagnetic radiation, which is harvested on beamlines set around the ring. The magnetic field can be tuned to adjust the emitted radiation spectrum, which is typically in the range of 3–30 keV in energy (4.1–0.4 Å in wavelength), but much lower and much higher energies can also be attained according to the characteristics of the storage ring and the needs of the experimental station concerned. As an example, the ESRF operates some 40 experimental stations, or "beamlines" situated around its high-energy 6 GeV storage ring of 844 m circumference. Each station has its own specialty of diffraction, scattering, spectroscopic, or imaging technique. A beamline consists of the X-ray source (the insertion device generating the X-ray beam), an optics hutch where the X-rays are collected and conditioned for the experiment, and an experimental hutch where the sample is positioned.

The resulting synchrotron X-ray sources are intense, hundreds of billions of times that of a conventional hospital source, and with the very low source emittance provide photon beams that allow a very fine spatial resolution and filming of dynamic processes. Key techniques for application are micro- and nanotomography, X-ray fluorescence, pair-distribution function (PDF), and small-angle X-ray scattering (SAXS). The fine resolving ability allows scanning or rastering across samples to provide (for example) elemental (since each element has its own X-ray "fingerprint" from its specific X-ray absorption and fluorescence spectra to which the tunable synchrotron light source can be precisely matched) or structural 2D or 3D information at nanometric levels.

Complementing synchrotron X-rays, neutron beams, produced from research reactors or spallation sources, offer unique insights to structural biology, biomedicine, and soft matter. This results mainly from the fact that the scattering power for neutrons of hydrogen is comparable to the other atoms typically found in biological macromolecules, contrasting strongly with the situation for X-rays where hydrogen atoms scatter very weakly. This is of crucial importance, given that about half of the atoms in the relevant molecules are hydrogen, and are often highly significant to structure/function and structure/property relationships. X-ray scattering lengths increase monotonically as a function of atomic number, reflecting the fact that they are scattered by the atomic electrons. In the case of neutron scattering, where the scattering event is associated with the interaction between the neutron and the atomic nucleus, the variation of scattering length over the periodic table does not follow any such trend and may even vary considerably from isotope to isotope. This means, for example, that hydrogen atoms can be imaged more easily in diffraction studies than in corresponding X-ray work. It also means that contrast variation approaches can be used at low resolution to distinguish particular parts of the system under study. In addition, the ability to exchange hydrogen by its heavier (and more strongly scattering) deuterium (2H or D) isotope offers a completely unique scope to neutron scattering studies of the structure and dynamics of biological systems in essentially all relevant sample habits [2].

Both synchrotron X-ray and neutron beams provide unique, often non-destructive, techniques to probe biological samples and the structure of materials across a wide range of length scales, from atoms to microns to mm and cm. Importantly, both probes are compatible with a large set of sample environments, allowing *in situ*/operando experiments and measurements at high/low temperatures, reactive environments (atmospheres, redox . . .), pressure, and so on. Often these can be set up to mimic the specific conditions of manufacture or end-use of materials, providing industry with key insights into process analysis to tailor materials and production. This is a critical advantage compared to, for example, scanning and transmission electron microscopy.

8.2 Application Examples

Provided below are several, far from exhaustive, examples of pharma-oriented nanoparticle characterization highlighting the possibilities of synchrotron light and neutron beams (Figure 8.1). Figure 8.2 shows schematically the three main families of techniques used at both synchrotron and neutron facilities of diffraction/scattering, microscopy/imaging, and spectroscopy. In most cases, the sample is easily placed and manipulated on a beamline. For example, an active pharmaceutical ingredient (API) is simply sealed in a glass or quartz capillary and attached onto the rotation stages on the beamline using plasticine or specifically designed sample holders with magnets for robotic systems.

Moreover, the techniques themselves are simple to apply for routine measurements looking at API structure and composition, nano-/microstructuration in nanocarriers and amorphous materials, and so on. This is especially the case for comparative studies, looking for example at formulations. Access to facilities is generally rapid for proprietary work, with mail-in services increasingly popular with clients, thereby avoiding costly travel and overnight stays at facilities. There are also a number of companies now providing access to research infrastructures, including light and neutron sources, for proprietary work and adding

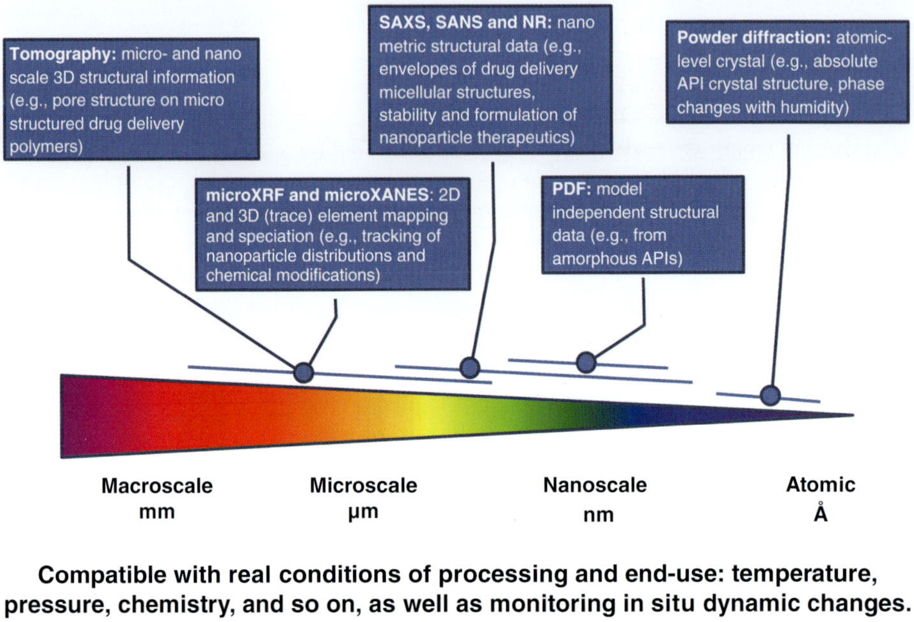

Figure 8.1 Schematic of selected synchrotron X-ray and neutron beam techniques with respect to length scale information provided.

value with full experiment design, support, and ancillary techniques. Even the light sources themselves are developing full service business models, often working with third parties, and going as far as full contract research and per sample pricing to make access as simple and transparent as possible in their work with industry.

8.2.1
Synchrotron Micro-X-ray Fluorescence and Micro-X-ray Absorption Spectroscopy

- Uses the unique X-ray fingerprint of each element to do chemical mapping, even speciation of chemicals, in 2D and 3D at nanometric and micrometric spatial resolution. These techniques can be applied for label-free tracking of nanoparticle distribution/transport and particle compositional studies.

Micro-X-ray fluorescence (μXRF) and Micro-X-ray absorption spectroscopy (μXANES) are techniques that allow the study of nanomaterial properties and/or their interactions with complex (biological) samples using an intense synchrotron X-ray submicron beam with tunable energy (from 2 to 9.2 keV at the ESRF's beamline ID21). These experiments usually aim to obtain 2D maps of elements of interest, but 3D is also possible (complementing the micro- and nanotomography applied at synchrotrons on a huge range of materials, including, for example, nano-/microstructured materials like porous polymers for drug delivery or

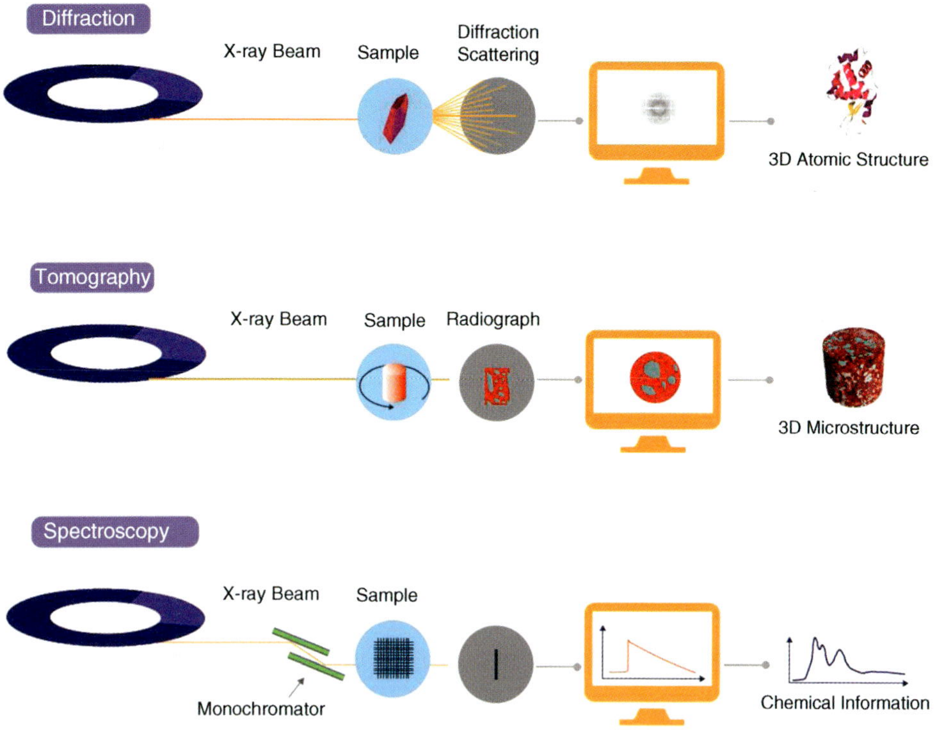

Figure 8.2 Schematic of a synchrotron light source and the three main experiment technique families as applied at both synchrotron and neutron facilities.

real-time dissolution of tablets). Both low-Z elements (e.g., Na, P, S, K, Ca) from the target organic matrix or nanomaterial (often metals, such as Fe, Ag, Si) can be analyzed simultaneously, and importantly, without any staining. For this, the sample is raster scanned under the X-ray microprobe; X-ray absorption promotes electronic transitions that generate element specific X-ray fluorescence (XRF) photons. An energy dispersive detector is used to obtain a fingerprint XRF spectrum for each scanned pixel of the selected region of the sample. After data processing, elemental maps are obtained on which points of interest are selected that can be further investigated by μXANES – providing more detailed information about the chemistry. For this purpose, the synchrotron X-ray incident energy is tuned along the binding energy of a core electron of the element of interest: its chemical state and local geometry can be derived from the absorption variations. The combination of μXRF/μXANES offers a microscopy imaging approach to investigate both the distribution and the potential chemical modifications of elements that are constituents of nanomaterials with promising applications in many areas including pharmaceuticals and medicine.

At the ESRF beamline ID21, [3] this approach has been used to investigate the release of Ag nanoparticles from Acticoat Flex3™ dressings used to treat severe

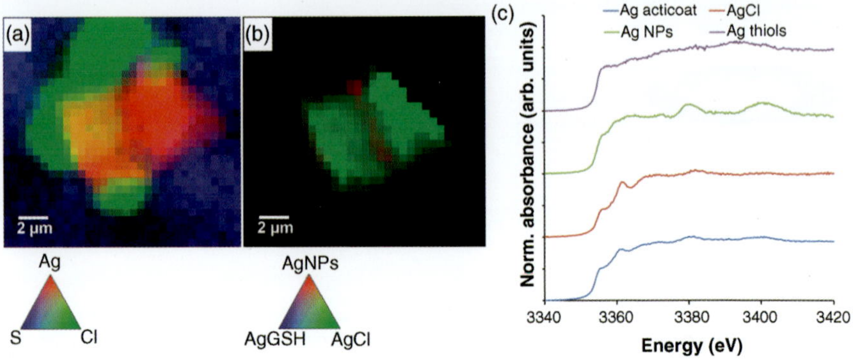

Figure 8.3 (a) μXRF map showing Ag, Cl, and S distribution surrounding a micrometric agglomerate of Acticoat Flex3™ after 2 h of incubation in human plasma. (b) μXANES map of Ag speciation in the same region (AgGSH represents Ag-thiol bonds); NP = nanoparticles. (c) μXANES spectra of Acticoat Flex3™ dressing and references used for linear combination fit Ag^0 NPs (10 nm), AgCl and Ag thiols.

skin burns in hospitals [4]. Ag acts as a multispectral antimicrobial preventing sepsis at the wound; the use of engineered Ag nanoparticles allows modulation of the release of ions from their surface in a controlled way. In order to study the *in vitro* transformation of these Ag particles, a fragment of Acticoat Flex3 was incubated in whole human plasma and freeze dried samples were investigated by μXRF/μXANES. In Figure 8.3, the colocalization of Ag and Cl and the presence of S in the surrounding medium are shown, and the chemical association of Ag and Cl is elucidated by μXANES (Figure 8.3b). The results show a dominant presence of AgCl at the aggregate surface. A linear combination fit of the μXANES data to the references (shown in Figure 8.3c) provides an estimation of the average molar distributions of the species present in the sample: 49% AgCl, 22% Ag nanoparticles, and 20% Ag-thiols (9% unidentified). These types of studies could aid in the optimization of materials that incorporate Ag nanoparticles as the antimicrobial agent, providing insight in the dynamics of dissolution at the micro- and nanoscale.

In another study, the distribution of SiO_2 nanoparticles (often used in biomedical applications such as drug delivery and cancer therapy) was investigated in mice [5]. Liver tissue sections from mice after intravenous exposure to SiO_2 core–shell NPs containing a paramagnetic Fe_3O_4 core were investigated by μXRF/μXANES. The results showed the accumulation of unmodified core–shell nanoparticles in the tissues observed by a high correlation of Fe and Si in μXRF maps and further confirmed by μXANES. This application is part of the development of a new noninvasive MRI protocol to assess the long-term biodistribution of core–shell nanoparticles in organs, which could lead to a safer-by-design approach for developing medical applications of SiO_2 nanoparticles.

8.2.2
Pair Distribution Function

- Complementary to traditional powder diffraction, pair distribution function (PDF) measurements allow amorphous APIs to be characterized with medium-range structural data. This can be important to determine the impact of processing on APIs, and the quantitative determination of polymorphs, phases, and components in APIs. The technique is highly suited to *in situ* measurements as the measuring times can be extremely rapid (millisecond).

Crystalline APIs can be easily screened using standard powder X-ray diffraction techniques. However, the situation is more complex when APIs are nanostructured. As the coherent domain size decreases, the characteristic peaks from a particular polymorph are replaced by broad maxima. Eventually, the diffracted signal is entirely diffused, and hence difficult to analyze. A possible solution is the so-called PDF analysis (the term total scattering is often used synonymously). This exploits the fact that a broad signal in measurement (reciprocal) space corresponds to an extremely sharp one in real (atomic) space. The PDF technique exploits the Fourier relationship between these two quantities to generate a real-space histogram of the bond distances in the sample, which is fully model independent. This includes both intermolecular bond distances and the longer range contacts between molecules that determine which polymorph is formed. The PDF technique has been exploited for neutrons, electrons, and X-rays, although here we concentrate mainly on the latter. The use of high-energy synchrotron X-rays is critical for the success of PDF, allowing a large range of momentum transfer to be sampled and allows good quality PDF data to be recorded.

An example of a pair distribution function is shown in Figure 8.4b for the molecule norbornane, C_7H_{12} (Kimber and Fitch, unpublished). At room temperature, this material exists in a so-called plastic phase, where the globular molecules are freely rotating in relation to each other. Note that the raw diffraction data (Figure 8.4a) only show a single sharp peak and some weak oscillations. In contrast, clear peaks corresponding to intermolecular C—C bond distances can be seen in the PDF, which can easily be matched to the (known) molecular structure. At longer distances in the plastic phase, a crossover to damped density oscillations is seen, showing that no intermolecular order is found.

An example concerning pharmaceutical compounds is provided by a recent study [6] on amorphous forms of paracetamol, and provided direct evidence of polyamorphism. That is, the nanometer structure of amorphous paracetamol uniquely depends upon its processing history, and can be similar to the known crystalline polymorphs. Clearly, this information is crucial for protecting an invention involving amorphous APIs. Other extensions of the method include looking at nanoparticles of APIs in aqueous suspension [7]. The method allows detection and characterization down to concentrations as low as 0.25% in weight. As APIs are usually bound in a matrix of some form, the pair distribution technique thus allows characterization of the final product, or even perhaps during *in situ*

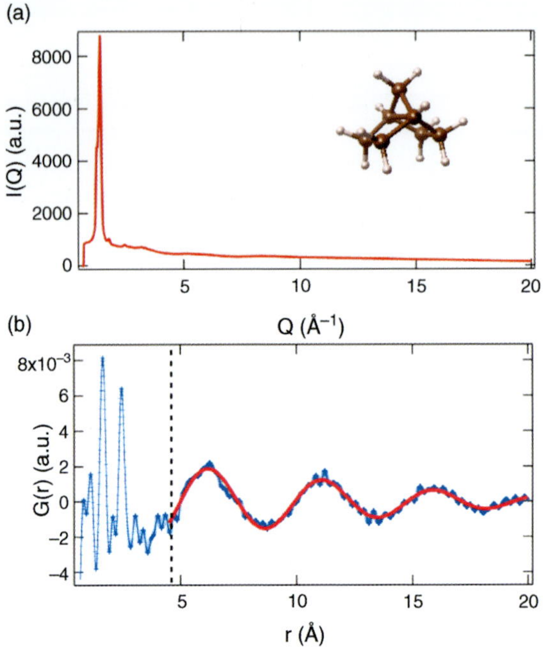

Figure 8.4 (a) Raw X-ray scattering data for norbornane (C_7H_{12}) in the solid plastic form at room temperature. The presence of only one sharp peak precludes standard diffraction techniques like the Rietveld analysis. The molecular structure is shown in the inset. (b) Pair distribution function calculated from (a). Sharp peaks corresponding to C—C distances are observed at length scales corresponding to the size of the molecule (≪5 Å). At longer intermolecular distances, only damped density oscillations are seen, showing that there is no order between neighboring molecules.

processing (e.g., see Ref. [8] where diffraction of high-energy synchrotron X-rays was applied to follow structural changes of ingredients during ball milling).

8.2.3 Small-angle X-ray Scattering

- Providing structural data around the micron- and submicron scale, small-angle X-ray scattering analyses solution and solid states of engineered drug delivery vectors such as nanoholders and phospholipid/micellular structures. It is a high-throughput technique well-suited to qualitative studies on formulation and dynamics (measurement times of milliseconds are possible). It is suited to follow real-time mixing and evolution studies, such as nanoparticle assembly and biodegradation.

Small-angle X-ray scattering (SAXS) is a well-established technique to probe nanoscale structures [9,10]. A (highly) collimated and monochromatic X-ray beam in the order of few hundreds of μm size impinges on a sample and the scattered intensity in the forward direction is collected by a two dimensional detector. SAXS is generally (like light scattering techniques) a noninvasive structural technique. The scattering of X-rays at small angles originate from the spatial fluctuations of the electron density within the material. The transmitted primary beam is absorbed by a beamstop placed in front of the detector, and the flight path before and after the sample is commonly in vacuum, to avoid absorption and scattering by air. Beamline ID02 at the ESRF, for example, uses a 32 m long evacuated flight tube of 400 m^3 volume to facilitate a variation of the sample to detector distance between 0.8 and 31 m [11].

The measured two-dimensional scattering pattern is radially integrated to provide one-dimensional scattering intensity I(q), where q is the length of the scattering vector. Modern synchrotron SAXS instruments cover more than four orders of magnitude in length scales, corresponding to real-space dimension from the μm down to Å range: ultra-small angle (USAXS), small angles (SAXS), and wide angle (WAXS) X-ray scattering. Another advantage of synchrotron sources as compared to lab-based SAXS instruments is the high photon flux and collimation that achieves high angular resolution and allows time-resolved experiments (Tr-SAXS) down to millisecond range, even in dilute samples. The technique can be combined with various sample environments (e.g., varying temperature, humidity, pressure, or rapid mixing) for *in situ* experiments. Submicron beams can also provide high real-space spatial resolution.

Typical samples for pharmaceutical R&D are tablets, suspensions, or freeze-dried powders with a thickness of 1–2 mm. Experiments usually investigate nanoparticles, nanostructures, or molecular ordering/packing on the subnanometer scale. The physical form of API/polymorphs and excipients in drug products can be identified. Small amounts of aggregates or crystalline material can be detected and amorphous, liquid crystalline, and crystalline structures be distinguished. *In situ* studies are able to follow crystallization/dissolution kinetics or follow phase transitions during processing.

SAXS can also deliver valuable information on the structure of self-assembled nanovectors, such as liposomes, which are recognized as efficient platforms for drug delivery [12]. SAXS allows the shape of the drug carrier to be reconstructed alone or loaded with drug in its natural aqueous environment. Structural issues are of primary importance to control the mechanism of action. Overall properties such as mean diameter and surface charge can be obtained by bench instruments (dynamic light scattering and zeta potential). However, it is critical to obtain a full understanding of the kinetic pathways of self-assembly to be able to exploit such systems for controlled drug release that typically occur on a submillisecond timescale [13]. A recent experiment at ID02 used time-resolved (Tr)-SAXS in combination with stopped-flow, which allows rapid mixing of two or more solutions at different ratio and flow rates, to investigate the complexation of small interfering RNA (siRNA) with nonviral synthetic carriers (cationic micelles) for gene delivery [14]. When combined with siRNA, nonviral vectors form complexes with structural features in the nano- to microscale range. The state of the complex used for transfection strongly depends upon the kinetic

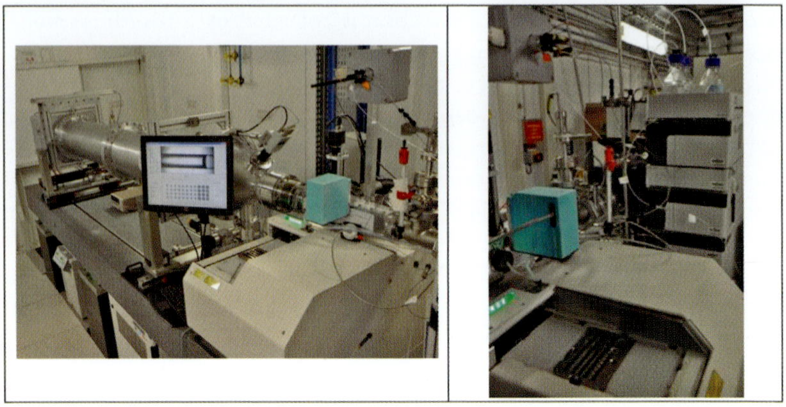

Figure 8.5 Views of the BM29 bioSAXS end-station at the ESRF (Grenoble, France). Left: the robotic liquid handler, sample loading bay and SAXS tube/detector. Right: the associated online SEC system mounted in the experimental hutch.

pathway followed during formation. The Tr-SAXS experiment shows that micelles were formed by two types of divalent cationic surfactants and indicate that complexation occurred within the first 50 ms following a first-order kinetics for the process of complex reorganization. In the new structural arrangement, siRNA and micelles were alternately layered in "sandwiches." Recent interesting applications of small-angle X-ray scattering to solve simple and drug loaded liposome structures under (or not) equilibrium conditions can also be found in [15–17].

Many synchrotron SAXS beamlines are adopting automation and robotics, particularly those specializing in biological samples (e.g., EMBL-Hamburg [18,19], Soleil [20], ALS [21], and ESRF [22,23]) (Figure 8.5). The aim of such systems is to facilitate measurements of many samples under different conditions with speed and reliability. These state-of-the-art sample changers allow full data collection of a complete concentration series (requiring around 100 μl of the highest sample concentration), including background buffer measurements, with cleaning and drying between all measurements, in a little over 5 min – opening the way to qualitative comparison studies across (for example) formulation matrices.

At beamlines with submicrometer beam sizes, microfluidic devices are an alternative approach for studying reaction kinetics, screening buffer solution effects, and so on. Due to their small size they provide controllable flow conditions at low material consumption. In particular, two classes of devices are of interest. First, continuous flow mixers are typically used for mixing two-component systems [24–28]. Temporal resolution is limited by the mixing time, flow rates, and the beam size but not the X-ray flux, and submillisecond resolution can be reached [29]. Second, in droplet microfluidics the reactants are enclosed in small droplets transported by a carrier liquid. This allows a broad range of conditions to be screened individually in well-defined conditions [30] (Pham,

N.V., Radajewski, D., Guillet, P., Round, A., Brennich, M., Pernot, P., Biscans, B., Bonneté, F., and Teychené, S. Coupling digital microfluidics and small-angle X-ray scattering to study the whole crystallization process of proteins in solution. *Acta Cryst. D.*). Another application of microfluidics as sample environment for SAXS is the investigation of shear effects on anisotropic nanoparticles [31].

8.2.4 Small-Angle Neutron Scattering and Neutron Reflectometry

- Like the X-ray equivalent, small-angle neutron studies provide micron to submicron structural data on nano carriers for drug delivery, but are sensitive to hydrogen, opening the way for contrast variation experiments to highlight the, for example, core–shell structures of nanoparticles.

In bionano medicine, neutron scattering finds a wide range of applications. A traditional application is the structural characterization of nano carriers for drug and gene delivery [32–35]. A classical example is the structural characterization of block copolymer micelles in drug delivery [35], where small angle neutron scattering (SANS) is used to probe the internal structure of nanoparticles assembled from poly(lactic acid) (PLA)–poly(ethylene glycol) (PEG) copolymers, with a fully deuterated core-forming PLA(d) block. Contrast variation is typically used in the study of these types of systems and simultaneous analysis of the multiple-contrast SANS datasets using core–shell models enables the construction of volume fraction profiles for the PLA(d)-PEG assemblies. This type of method showed how the mean core radius increased with the molecular weight of the PLA(d) block. Moreover, despite the fact that the shells of all the PLA(d)-PEG assemblies were very solvent (water) rich, the conformation of the stabilizing chains in the shell depended on the length of the PLA(d) block. Lastly, the application of neutron scattering in bionanomedicine has gone beyond that of traditional structural characterization of the nanocontainers. For example, the structural changes occurring at different stages in the human digestive system have been studied using stopped SANS flow [33]. This type of study can now be used to follow (for example) the structural changes that oral drug delivery formulations experience in the human gastrointestinal tract, and use this knowledge to better design drug carriers in the future.

In another approach, the interaction of drug delivery systems with model cell membranes can be studied using neutron reflection [36,37]. Neutron reflection is a powerful technique for studying thin adsorbed layers, since it provides information on the structural features in the direction normal to the interface. In this way, studies of buried interfaces that are otherwise difficult to probe can be carried out. For supported lipid bilayers this means the overall structure; layer thicknesses, lipid composition and potential asymmetry between the leaflets can be characterized through a neutron scattering length density profile [38]. This profile is thus a continuous function of film depth, relating to the chemical composition of the adsorbed layer. The sensitivity of neutron reflection (change in reflectivity profile) depends on the difference in scattering length of the molecules constituting the adsorbed layer and the solvent surrounding them. FIGARO [39], at the ILL, is a unique reflectometer that allows obtaining the reflection at surfaces located above and below the liquid. Using this instrument, the importance of gravity on the transport of bulk aggregates from the bulk to the interface was revealed [40]. In a recent experiment [37], neutron reflection and using the up and down approach at FIGARO it was demonstrated that translocation of a drug (PAMAM dendrimers) across the model cellular membrane and adsorption of the drug carrier occurred only when the membrane (1) was located above the bulk liquid and (2) had sufficient negative charge. These interesting findings suggest that bulk phase separation and gravity could have an impact in drug delivery, and that the drug–membrane interaction can potentially be switched on through tuning the drug carrier charge in order to activate endocytosis pathways on specific cell type.

8.3 Going Beyond Characterization Using Synchrotron X-rays: Nanoparticles for Diagnostic and Therapeutic Approaches

Developments using the ESRF's ID17 Medical Beamline facilities and expertise have shown that gadolinium-based nanohybrid particles (so-called AGuIX®) are excellent candidates as radiosensitisers for treating cancers [41]. This is a rather unique example of the synchrotron X-ray beam being used in combination with nanoparticles to develop a potential therapeutic treatment, rather than a pure characterization of a material. In the medium term, a transfer of the expertise to a startup company is envisaged, allowing the technology to be moved to the clinic. Smaller "compact" light sources are being investigated in various laboratories around the world (see, e.g., the ThomX project, www.equipex-thomx.fr), and which could allow such treatments to be delivered with compact light sources based at hospitals.

In the studies, it was demonstrated that the survival of rats bearing very aggressive brain tumors was multiplied by a factor of five by combining "microbeam radiation therapy" (MRT) technique and the injection of AGuIX nanoparticles. Moreover, half of the rats treated were still alive for more than 100 days after the tumor inoculation. MRT is based on the use of a comb of micro-X-ray beams, illuminating a tumor. The use of microbeams has been shown to assist in healthy tissue healing from the low, but still significant doses. Remarkably, it appears that the delay between the administration of AGuIX nanoparticles and the irradiation is a key parameter, since a beneficial survival effect is observed when the MRT is performed 20 min after injection, while the irradiation performed 5 min after injection is detrimental. The efficacy of the AGuIX has been demonstrated in other tumor models such as lung tumors, pancreas adenocarcinoma, and multiple brain melanoma metastases.

In addition to sensitizing tumors, a key element of the nanoparticles is that they appear well-suited for image-guided therapy (theranostic). Three main reasons lie behind this. First, their size which is sufficiently large to avoid their extravasation from normal vessels while being sufficiently small for loading the tumor. Second, the possibility to monitor biodistribution by MRI is crucial to optimize the radiotherapeutic effectivity. Finally, the significant remanence (24 h) of the AGuIX once trapped in the tumor opens the way to perform MRI followed by the radiotherapy using a unique/single nanoparticle injection with a comfortable delay in between.

Following the success of the initial developments, two Phase 1 clinical trials are planned for 2016 with patients bearing brain metastasis of melanoma and uterus tumors. Within this context a startup enterprise, NH TherAguix, has been created to push forward the clinical trials.

8.4
Looking Ahead and Conclusions

Synchrotron and neutron facilities are now built into the expected set of tools applied by academic scientists to a wide range of techniques – and increasingly in nanopharmaceutical science. Central facilities, such as ESRF and ILL, are building instruments and procedures to optimize access for routine experiments, while still developing novel techniques providing new insights into materials. This former point will be a key area of development for the future, assuring that any scientist from academia or industry can effectively access central synchrotron and neutron facilities without being an expert in the instrument use or technique. Some facilities are starting to apply ISO standard operating methods in selected areas; for example the Australian Light Source operates a quality management system that is ISO9001 compliant, and ELETTRA has recently qualified its infrared facility. Such standard procedures, be they locally managed, formally certified, or self-certified may emerge to support "industrialized" routine access for academia and industry alike.

A large expansion of capacity in such facilities has already taken place and is continuing apace worldwide – particularly with regards to third-generation light sources. In November 2015, the ESRF hosted the first African Light Source Conference and Workshop, which established the basis for a roadmap to move toward an advanced light source for the African continent – the only continent without such a facility.

Looking ahead to new applications of synchrotron light, the ESRF is planning an important upgrade of its storage ring, which will be replaced by a greatly enhanced system. The project called "ESRF-EBS" (Extremely Brilliant Source) will produce a ring in a so-called "multibend achromat lattice" configuration, and will be operational from summer 2020 with a performance increase of up to two orders of magnitude in terms of brilliance and coherence of the X-ray beams produced [42,43]. These enhanced properties are expected to permit unprecedented microscopy probes to study fine details of real materials under real conditions at the level of a few nanometres spatial resolution. Following ESRF, other light sources around the world are planning similar upgrades.

Future developments for neutron characterization will be driven in parallel with instrumental developments at existing sources (ILL, ISIS, NIST, ORNL, and ANSTO) and future facilities such as the European Spallation Source (ESS) being built in Sweden. Fundamental and applied aspects of neutron structural biology and soft condensed matter are being given high priority at these institutes and it can be expected that future instruments will have improved fluxes, optics, and detector systems. At the ILL, for example, order of magnitude improvements are possible for existing instruments and sample preparation developments to maximize the impact of such investments are a continuous priority.

As mentioned above, an ongoing and growing challenge with these central large-scale infrastructures is to ensure their accessibility to nonexpert academic users and industrial clients. As they become exploited as routine and day-to-day tools for science and technology rather than specialized "exotic" facilities, the range of disciplines desiring and requiring access grows. In Europe alone the light source community is some 30 000 scientists strong. This evolution means that the facilities need to adapt from a traditional user base to one that is less specialized and to enable an ease of access from experiment conception, to carrying out the experiment, through to data analysis and data archiving. Within this context, an important but still under-represented community is industry [44,45]. Although academia has realised the power of these large and impressive central facilities to perform top-quality analytical science, a similar growth from industry has not yet been realised. Nonetheless, much of the peer-reviewed academic science does have links to industry. A recent survey performed by the ESRF put this at 30–40% of the academic work. But this is yet to spillover into larger scale proprietary access.

Further investments are being made in new photon and neutron sources. In Europe, the hard X-ray free electron laser XFEL based at Hamburg will soon see first light being generated. In the neutron world, the ESS mentioned above is expected to become operational in the early 2020s. Both of these facilities, together with other similar institutes around the world, are complementing the existing portfolio of photon and neutron science facilities. FELs and spallation sources add further unique techniques to a growing toolbox available for the specialist and nonspecialist alike.

These large-scale multibillion Euro facilities are core instruments for academic science and, increasingly, industrial research and innovation. They act as central knowledge generation hubs, now being made more accessible for all scientists, engineers, and technicians, from academia and industry. Much work remains to provide routine, high-throughput, rapid access, but the future is extremely bright for these large-scale instruments that enable unique characterization for highly relevant materials such as medical nanoparticles and drug systems.

Acknowledgments

Marco Roman, Stijn Smulder, and Peter Hoet are kindly acknowledged for the X-ray fluorescence studies.

References

1 Robinson, A.L. (2015) History of synchrotron radiation. *Synchrotron Radiat. News*, **4**, 4–8.

2 Haertlein, M., Moulin, M., Devos, J., Laux, V., Dunne, O., and Forsyth, V.T. (2016) Biomolecular deuteration for neutron structural biology and dynamics. *Meth. Enzym.*, **566**, 113–157.

3 Salomé, M., Cotte, M., Baker, R., Barrett, R., Benseny-Cases, N., Berruyer, G., Bugnazet, D., Castillo-Michel, H., Cornu, C., Fayard, B., Gagliardini, E., Hino, R., Morse, J., Papillon, E., Pouyet, E., Rivard, C., Solé, V.A., Susini, J., and Veronesi, G. (2013) The ID21 scanning X-ray microscope at ESRF. *J. Phys. Conf. Ser.*, **425**, 182004.

4 Roman, M., Rigo, C., Castillo-Michel, H., Munivrana, I., Vindigni, V., Mičetić, I., Benetti, F., Manodori, L., and Cairns, W.R.L. (2016) Hydrodynamic chromatography coupled to single-particle ICP-MS for the simultaneous characterization of AgNPs and determination of dissolved Ag in plasma and blood of burn patients. *Anal. Bioanal. Chem.*, **408** (19), 5109–5124.

5 Smulders, S., Ketkar-Atre, A., Luyts, K., Vriens, H., De Sousa Nobre, S., Rivard, C., Van Landuyt, K., Baken, S., Smolders, E., Golanski, L., Ghosh, M., Vanoirbeek, J., Himmelreich, U., and Hm Hoet, P. (2016) Body distribution of SiO_2–Fe_3O_4 core–shell nanoparticles after intravenous injection and intratracheal instillation. *Nanotoxicology.*, **10** (5), 567–574.

6 Thi, Y.N., Rademann, K., and Emmerling, F. (2015) Direct evidence of polyamorphism in paracetamol. *CrystEngComm*, **17**, 9029–9036.

7 Terban, M.W., Johnson, M., Di Michiel, M., and Billinge, S.J.L. (2015) Detection and characterization of nanoparticles in suspension at low concentrations using the X-ray total scattering pair distribution function technique. *Nanoscale*, **7**, 5480–5487.

8 Friščić, T., Halasz, I., Beldon, P.J., Belenguer, A.M., Adams, F., Kimber, S.A.J., Honkimäki, V., and Dinnebier, R.E. (2013) Real-time and *in situ* monitoring of mechanochemical milling reactions. *Nat. Chem.*, **5**, 66–73.

9 Narayanan, T. (2008) Synchrotron small-angle X-ray scattering, in *Soft Matter: Characterization*, vol II, Springer, Heidelberg.

10 Narayanan, T. (2009) High brilliance small-angle X-ray scattering applied to soft matter. *Curr. Opin. Colloid Interface Sci.*, **14** (6), 409–415.

11 Van Vaerenbergh, P., Léonardon, J., Sztucki, M., Boesecke, P., Gorini, J., Claustre, L., Sever, F., Morse, J., and Narayanan, T. (2016) *AIP Conf. Proc.*, **1741**, 030034.

12 Pabst, G., Kucerka, N., Nieh, M.-P., Rheinstädter, M.C., and Katsaras, J. (2010) Applications of neutron and X-ray scattering to the study of biologically relevant model membranes. *Chem. Phys. Lipids*, **163**, 460–479.

13 Angelov, B., Angelova, A., Filippov, S., Narayanan, T., Drechsler, M., Štěpánek, P., Couvreur, P., and Lesieur, S. (2013) DNA/fusogenic lipid nanocarrier assembly: millisecond structural dynamics. *J. Phys. Chem. Lett.*, **4**, 1959–1964.

14 Falsini, S., Ristori, S., Ciani, L., Di Cola, E., Supuran, C.T., Arcangeli, A., and In, M. (2014) Time resolved SAXS to study the complexation of siRNA with cationic micelles of divalent surfactants. *Soft Matter*, **10**, 2226–2233.

15 Narayanan, T., Gummel, J., and Gradzielski, M. (2014) Probing the self-assembly of unilamellar vesicles using time-resolved SAXS. *Adv. Planar Lipid Bilayers Liposomes*, **20**, 171–196.

16 Varga, Z., Wacha, A., and Bóta, A. (2014) Osmotic shrinkage of sterically stabilized liposomes as revealed by time-resolved small-angle X-ray scattering. *J. Appl. Crystallogr.*, **47**, 35–40.

17 Pozzi, D., Cardarelli, F., Salomone, F., Marchini, C., Amenitsch, H., La Barbera, G., and Caracciolo, G. (2014) Role of cholesterol on the transfection barriers of cationic lipid/DNA complexes. *Appl. Phys. Lett.*, **105**, 073701.

18 Round, A.R., Franke, D., Moritz, S., Huchler, R., Fritsche, M., Malthan, D.,

Klaering, R., Svergun, D.I., and Roessle, M. (2008) Automated sample-changing robot for solution scattering experiments at the EMBL Hamburg SAXS station X33. *J. Appl. Crystallogr.*, **41**, 913–917.

19 Blanchet, C.E., Zozulya, A.V., Kikhney, A.G., Franke, D., Konarev, P.V., Shang, W., Klaering, R., Robrahn, B., Hermes, C., Cipriani, F., Svergun, D.I., and Roessle, M. (2012) Instrumental setup for high-throughput small- and wide-angle solution scattering at the X33 beamline of EMBL Hamburg. *J. Appl. Crystallogr.*, **45**, 489–495.

20 David, G. and Pérez, J. (2009) Combined sampler robot and high-performance liquid chromatography: a fully automated system for biological small-angle X-ray scattering experiments at the Synchrotron SOLEIL SWING beamline. *J. Appl. Crystallogr.*, **42**, 892–900.

21 Classen, S., Hura, G.L., Holton, J.M., Rambo, R.P., Rodic, I., McGuire, P.J., Dyer, K., Hammel, M., Meigs, G., Frankel, K.A., and Tainer, J.A. (2013) Implementation and performance of SIBYLS: a dual endstation small-angle X-ray scattering and macromolecular crystallography beamline at the Advanced Light Source. *Appl. Crystallogr.*, **46**, 1–13.

22 Pernot, P., Round, A., Barrett, R., De Maria Antolinos, A., Gobbo, A., Gordon, E., Huet, J., Kieffer, J., Lentini, M., Mattenet, M., Morawe, C., Mueller-Dieckmann, C., Ohlsson, S., Schmid, W., Surr, J., Theveneau, P., Zerrad, L., and McSweeney, S. (2013) Upgraded ESRF BM29 beamline for SAXS on macromolecules in solution. *J. Synchrotron Radiat.*, **20**, 660–664.

23 Pernot, P., Theveneau, P., Giraud, T., Nogueira-Fernandes, R., Nurizzo, D., Spruce, D., Surr, J., McSweeney, S., Round, A.S., Felisaz, F., Foedinger, L., Gobbo, A., Huet, J., Villard, C., and Cipriani, F. (2010) New beamline dedicated to solution scattering from biological macromolecules at the ESRF. *J. Phys. Conf. Ser.*, **247**, 012009.

24 Round, A., Brown, E., Marcellin, R., Kapp, U., Westfall, C.S., Jez, J.M., and Zubieta, C. (2013) Determination of the GH3.12 protein conformation through HPLC-integrated SAXS measurements combined with X-ray crystallography. *Acta Cryst.*, **D69**, 2072–2080.

25 Russell, R., Millett, I.S., Tate, M.W., Kwok, L.W., Nakatani, B., Gruner, S.M., Mochrie, S.G., Pande, V., Doniach, S., Herschlag, D., and Pollack, L. (2002) Rapid compaction during RNA folding. *Proc. Natl. Acad. Sci. USA*, **99** (7), 4266–4271.

26 Martel, A., Burghammer, M., Davies, R., DiCola, E., Panine, P., Salmon, J.B., and Riekel, C. (2008) A microfluidic cell for studying the formation of regenerated silk by synchrotron radiation small-and wide-angle X-ray scattering. *Biomicrofluidics*, **2** (2), 024104.

27 Toft, K.N., Vestergaard, B., Nielsen, S.S., Snakenborg, D., Jeppesen, M.G., Jacobsen, J.K., Arleth, L., and Kutter, J.P. (2008) High-throughput small angle X-ray scattering from proteins in solution using a microfluidic front-end. *Anal. Chem.*, **80** (10), 3648–3654.

28 Brennich, M.E., Nolting, J.F., Dammann, C., Nöding, B., Bauch, S., Herrmann, H., and Köster, S. (2011) Dynamics of intermediate filament assembly followed in micro-flow by small angle X-ray scattering. *Lab Chip*, **11** (4), 708–716.

29 Graceffa, R., Nobrega, R.P., Barrea, R.A., Kathuria, S.V., Chakravarthy, S., Bilsel, O., and Irving, T.C. (2013) Sub-millisecond time-resolved SAXS using a continuous-flow mixer and X-ray microbeam. *J. Synchrotron Radiat.*, **20** (6), 820–825.

30 Stehle, R., Goerigk, G., Wallacher, D., Ballauff, M., and Seiffert, S. (2013) Small-angle X-ray scattering in droplet-based microfluidics. *Lab Chip*, **13** (8), 1529–1537.

31 Trebbin, M., Steinhauser, D., Perlich, J., Buffet, A., Roth, S.V., Zimmermann, W., Thiele, J., and Förster, S. (2013) Anisotropic particles align perpendicular to the flow direction in narrow microchannels. *Proc. Natl. Acad. Sci. USA*, **110** (17), 6706–6711.

32 Cárdenas, M., Dreiss, C.A., Nylander, T., Chan, C.P., Cosgrove, T., and Lindman, B. (2005) SANS study of the interaction among DNA, a cationic surfactant, and polystyrene latex particles. *Langmuir*, **21**, 3478–3483.

33 Nawroth, T., Buch, P., Buch, K., Langguth, P., and Schweins, R. (2011) Liposome formation from bile salt–lipid micelles in the digestion and drug delivery model $FaSSIF_{mod}$ estimated by combined time-resolved neutron and dynamic light scattering. *Mol. Pharmaceutics*, **8**, 2162–2172.

34 Bayati, S., Galantini, L., Knudsen, K.D., and Schillén, K. (2015) Effects of bile salt sodium glycodeoxycholate on the self-assembly of PEO–PPO–PEO triblock copolymer P123 in aqueous solution. *Langmuir*, **31**, 13519–13527.

35 Castelletto, V., Hamley, I.W., English, R.J., and Mingvanish, W. (2003) SANS and rheology study of aqueous solutions and gels containing highly swollen diblock copolymer micelles. *Langmuir*, **19**, 3229–3235.

36 Vandoolaeghe, P., Rennie, A.R., Campbell, R.A., and Nylander, T. (2009) Neutron reflectivity studies of the interaction of cubic-phase nanoparticles with phospholipid bilayers of different coverage. *Langmuir*, **25**, 4009–4020.

37 Campbell, R.A., Watkins, E., Jagalski, V., Åkesson-Runnsjo, A., and Cárdenas, M. (2014) Key factors regulating the mass delivery of macromolecules to model cell membranes: gravity and electrostatics. *ACS Macro Lett.*, **3**, 121–125.

38 Fragneto-Cusani, G. (2001) Neutron reflectivity at the solid/liquid interface: examples of applications in biophysics. *J. Phys-Condens Mat.*, **13**, 4973–4989.

39 Campbell, R.A., Wacklin, H.P., Sutton, I., Cubitt, R., and Fragneto, G. (2011) FIGARO: The new horizontal neutron reflectometer at the ILL. *Eur. Phys. J. Plus*, **126**, 107.

40 Campbell, R.A., Yanez Arteta, M., Angus-Smyth, A., Nylander, T., and Varga, I.J. (2012) Multilayers at interfaces of an oppositely charged polyelectrolyte/surfactant system resulting from the transport of bulk aggregates under gravity. *Phys. Chem. B*, **116**, 7981–7990.

41 Le Duc, G., Miladi, I., Alric, C., Mowat, P., Bräuer-Krisch, E., Bouchet, A., Khalil, E., Billotey, C., Janier, M., Lux, F., Epicier, T., Perriat, P., Roux, S., and Tillement, O. (2011) Toward an image-guided microbeam radiation therapy using gadolinium-based nanoparticles. *ACS Nano*, **27;5** (12), 9566–9574.

42 The European Synchrotron Radiation Facility (2007) The Purple Book, Science and Technology Programme 2008–2017.

43 The European Synchrotron Radiation Facility (2014) The Orange Book, ESRF Upgrade Programme Phase II (2015–2022) – Technical Design Study.

44 Mitchell, E., Boller, E., Gordon, E.J., Leonard, G., and Monaco, S. (2011) The industrial research programme at the ESRF: Past, present and challenges for the future. *Synchrotron Radiat. News*, **24**, 18–23.

45 Deblay, P. and Mitchell, E. (2013) Utilisation des lignes de lumière pour des problématiques industrielles. *Reflets de Physiques*, **34–35**, 101–105.

9
Overview of Techniques and Description of Established Processes

Jan Henrik Finke,[1,4] *Michael Juhnke,*[2] *Arno Kwade,*[1,4] *and Heike Bunjes*[3,4]

[1]*TU Braunschweig, Institute for Pharmaceutical Technology and Center of Pharmaceutical Engineering, PVZ, Volkmaroder Str. 5, 38104 Braunschweig, Germany*
[2]*Novartis Pharma AG, Technical R&D, Virchow 6.1.231, PO Box CH-4002 Basel, Switzerland*
[3]*Technische Universität Braunschweig, Institut für Pharmazeutische Technologie, Mendelssohnstraße 1, D-38106 Braunschweig, Germany*
[4]*Technische Universität Braunschweig, Zentrum für Pharmaverfahrenstechnik, Franz-Liszt-Str. 35a, 38106 Braunschweig, Germany*

9.1
Introduction

The production of nanopharmaceuticals requires specialized processes that allow for the controlled preparation of particles in the submicron- and especially in the nanosize range. Often, there are different approaches to reach this goal but usually only a fraction of those have been elaborated from the laboratory scale to large-scale pharmaceutical manufacturing. The general type of production method and the process parameters have to be chosen in dependence on the properties of the materials to be processed (e.g., polar lipids or poorly soluble active ingredients). Thereby, issues of the physiological compatibility of the excipients required to carry out the manufacturing procedure need to be considered. Beyond the necessity to reliably produce the nanoparticles, their physical and chemical stability in the product has to be ensured. This often requires further processing steps, for example, drying, since most of the nanoparticle-generating processes are carried out in a liquid environment and lead to nanoparticulate suspensions as product. Transformation into a solid form is frequently also aspired with regard to patient convenience. On the other hand, quite a few nanopharmaceuticals are intended for injection or infusion, making sterility of the formulation an absolute prerequisite that has to be achieved by adequate processing. Therefore, the preparation of nanopharmaceuticals can add a rather high degree of complexity into pharmaceutical production that may be in certain conflict with the endeavor to keep manufacturing processes as simple as possible. However, processes that are well known from coarser drug particles or from other

Pharmaceutical Nanotechnology: Innovation and Production, First Edition. Edited by Jean Cornier, Arno Kwade, Andrew Owen, and Marcel Van de Voorde.

and closely related industries such as high-pressure homogenization (HPH) and stirred media milling are successfully realized in industry for the production of nanomedicines with, if necessary, subsequent downstream processes like drying.

This chapter describes techniques that can be used for the preparation of pharmaceutical nanoparticles including their processing into the final dosage form. Apart from giving a general overview, a special focus is laid on manufacturing processes already established for the preparation of commercial products. For some nanopharmaceutical products, the respective preparation processes are outlined in more detail to provide an illustration of the considerations that are connected with the preparation of such nanomedicines. While the first part of the chapter deals with nanoparticulate formulations that are most often administered by injection and, thus, in liquid form, the drug nanoparticles covered in the second part of the chapter frequently require transformation into solid dosage forms as they are mostly intended for peroral use.

9.2 Processing of Liquid Drug Carrier Formulations

9.2.1 Colloidal Lipid Emulsions

9.2.1.1 General Aspects and Composition

Colloidal lipid emulsions are the oldest and among the commercially most successful representatives of nanopharmaceuticals. Colloidal fat emulsions for nutrition by intravenous infusion were introduced to the European market in the early 1960s (Table 9.1). They contain droplets of highly purified triglyceride oils (e.g., soybean oil and medium-chain triglycerides) and egg phospholipids as stabilizers against coagulation and coalescence of the droplets [1,2]. Emulsion stability critically depends on the nature of the phospholipid, in particular on the ratio of phosphatidylcholine to phosphatidylethanolamine and the presence of minor components. A small fraction of sodium oleate is often added as it increases stability against flocculation and coalescence by affecting the surface charge of the emulsion droplets. Glycerol is used to adjust tonicity as it does neither interfere with the electrostatic stabilization of the droplets nor does it lead to chemical interactions with the phospholipid [3–5]. In emulsions for parenteral nutrition, the triglyceride oil is to be regarded as the active agent that serves as a source of calories and essential fatty acids for the patient. The oil droplets can, however, also be used as carriers for poorly water soluble, lipophilic drug substances [2,6]. Based on similar basic compositions as found in the emulsions for parenteral nutrition, a variety of drug-containing colloidal lipid emulsions has been made commercially available during the last decades (Table 9.2). In these emulsions, the oil phase often contains a fraction of comparatively polar triglycerides (such as MCT or acetylated monoglycerides) as these increase the solubility of foreign compounds [7].

Table 9.1 Examples for emulsions for parenteral nutrition.

Oil phase	Product
Soybean oil	Lipofundin®, Lipovenös®
Soybean oil + MCT	Lipofundin® MCT, Lipovenös® MCT
Soybean oil + olive oil	Clinoleic®
Soybean oil + MCT + omega-3-fatty acids	Lipidem®
Soybean oil + MCT + olive oil + fish oil	SMOFlipid®
Fish oil	Omegaven® Fresenius

All emulsions are stabilized with egg phospholipids. MCT: medium-chain triglycerides.
Source: Gelbe Liste Pharmindex [8].

Table 9.2 Examples for drug loaded colloidal emulsions for parenteral administration.

Drug	Product examples	Oil phase
Clevidipine	Cleviprex®	Soybean oil
Dexamethasone palmitate	Lipotalon®	Soybean oil
Diazepam	Stesolid®	Soybean oil + acetylated monoglycerides
	Diazepam-®Lipuro	Soybean oil + MCT
Etomidate	Etomidat-®Lipuro	Soybean oil + MCT
Propofol	Disoprivan®	Soybean oil
	Propofol-®Lipuro, Anesia®	Soybean oil + MCT
Lipophilic vitamins	Vitalipid Infant/Adult®	Soybean oil
	Freka Vit Infant/Adult®	Soybean oil

MCT: medium-chain triglycerides.
Source: Gelbe Liste Pharmindex [8].

Colloidal lipid emulsions can also be used as adjuvant to increase the immunogenic response to subunit vaccines. The most prominent representative of this kind of emulsions is the squalene-based emulsion MF59 that is used in the influenza vaccine Fluad®. In this emulsion of about 150 nm mean particle size, the droplets are stabilized by a combination of the nonionic surfactants polysorbate 80 and sorbitan trioleate in an aqueous phase containing a citrate buffer [9].

9.2.1.2 Preparation Process of Intravenous Fat Emulsions

Administration by intravenous infusion or injection calls for strict control of the particle size distribution of lipid emulsions in order to avoid embolism by the lipid droplets. Moreover, a small droplet size and narrow particle size distribution increase the physical stability of the emulsions. The mean particle size in

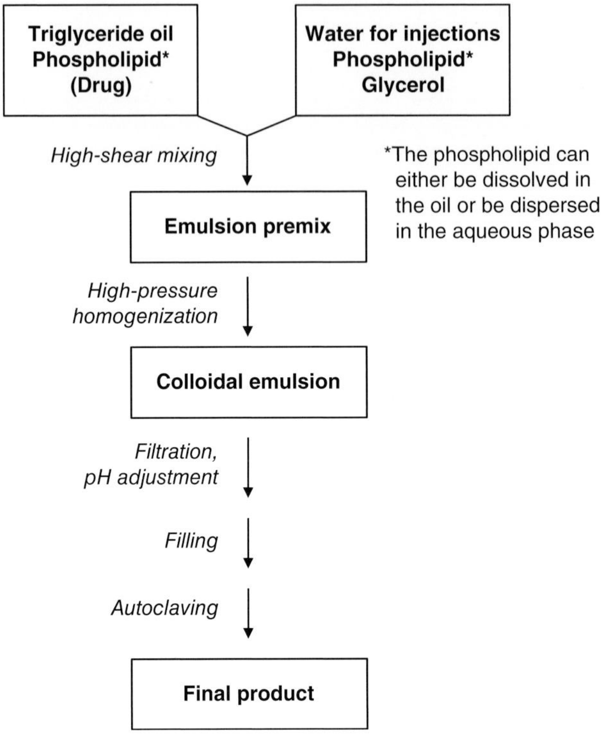

Figure 9.1 Preparation process of colloidal lipid emulsions.

these systems is usually between 200 and 500 nm, and there are tight limitations with regard to the presence of microparticulate contaminants. High-pressure homogenization is the standard technique to obtain emulsions that meet these specifications [10–12].

Details on the production process of triglyceride-based fat emulsions for parenteral administration can be found in several reviews and book chapters, for example, Refs [3,5,10,11]. The general principle of the process is schematically presented in Figure 9.1.

In a first step, the oil and the water phases are prepared for the process typically involving filtration steps to reduce the bioburden. The phospholipid can either be dissolved in the oil or be dispersed in the aqueous phase that also contains the glycerol. For drug-containing emulsions, the drug is added to the oil phase in the so-called "de novo" preparation process. The two phases are combined and the oil phase is dispersed in the water phase by high-shear mixing (e.g., with an Ultra Turrax) to form a crude emulsion for further processing. A sufficiently small particle size of this fine premix (mean size usually below 10 μm) is regarded as advantageous with respect to the formation of an emulsion with narrow droplet size distribution and high physical stability. The formation of droplets with colloidal size is attained by repeated passage through a

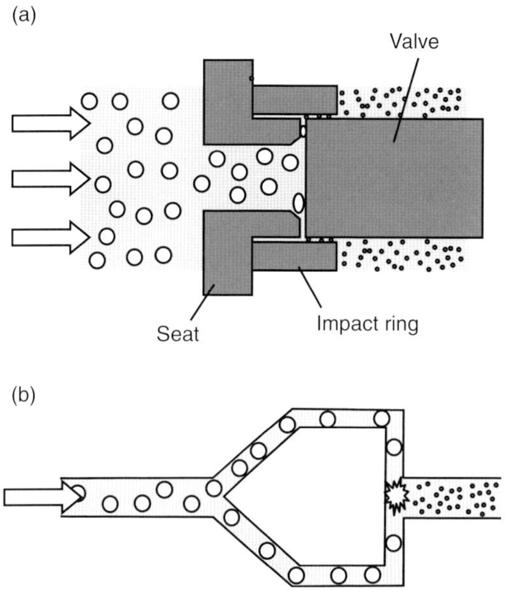

Figure 9.2 Layout of a Gaulin-type homogenization valve (a) and a Y-shaped microfluidizer interaction chamber (b).

two-stage high-pressure homogenizer at elevated temperature, usually employing a Gaulin-type homogenization valve (Figure 9.2). Subsequently, the emulsion is filtered to remove coarser droplets, for example, with a cartridge filter of 1–5 μm pore size, and filled under clean room conditions. In order to protect the unsaturated lipid compounds of the formulation from oxidation, the whole manufacturing process is carried out under nitrogen protection (antioxidants such as vitamin E are also often added for this reason). The emulsions are sterilized by autoclaving under agitation by shaking or rotation [13]. Prior to autoclaving, the pH of the emulsion is adjusted with sodium hydroxide to the slightly alkaline range (e.g., to pH 8–9). This procedure increases the droplet charge (and thus droplet repulsion) as a result of dissociation. Moreover, it induces formation of free fatty acids that act as auxiliary emulsifiers. During autoclaving, the pH drops as a result of hydrolysis stabilizing at a value between 6 and 7 that is most protective with regard to further hydrolysis during storage.

The physical properties and stability of the final product depend on a multiplicity of parameters, including the concentration and chemical composition of raw materials as well as process conditions, for example, temperature and pressure. For example, higher oil concentrations lead to larger droplet sizes, whereas increased process temperature and/or pressure reduce the droplet size as does a higher concentration of emulsifier (at least up to a certain concentration). After a higher number of passes through the homogenizer, a narrower droplet size distribution is obtained [10].

Although the general principles of homogenization have long been under investigation, the exact details of the processes that lead to droplet breakup in the homogenizer valve and affect the particle size distribution obtained remain to be fully clarified [15–17]. The mechanisms of droplet breakup in high-pressure homogenization devices are increasingly being elucidated by means of simulation and modeling [18–20]. Moreover, modern optical methods allow the visualization of the flow patterns in homogenizer valves and provide information on the droplet breakup processes [21–23]. Commercial high-pressure homogenizers (piston-gap homogenizers) are usually based on a spring-loaded valve that forms a gap of adjustable width (radial diffusers). The pressure drop across the valve produces turbulent flow that acts as a main source of droplet disrupting inertial forces [24]. A decrease in gap sizes increases the pressure drop and thus the intensity of droplet disruption. For a given type of homogenizer (and thus flow regime), there is an approximately linear correlation between the logarithm of the homogenization pressure and the logarithm of the resulting droplet size [17]. Besides turbulent flow and inertial forces also laminar shear and cavitation may play a role for droplet disruption [25]. Emulsions for parenteral administration are usually prepared in homogenizers containing two homogenization valves in series ("two-stage" homogenization). Droplet breakup is mainly achieved in the first of the two valves [17]. For orifice-based two-stage high-pressure homogenizers, it has been shown that the back pressure applied by the second stage controls the cavitation pattern observed during homogenization. When no back pressure is applied, cavitation may lead to the formation of vapor-filled pockets leading to inefficient energy transfer resulting in insufficient droplet break up. With increasing back pressure, vapor-pocket formation is suppressed in the favor of single-bubble cavitation until cavitation gets suppressed completely. A back pressure of about 30% of the inlet pressure is considered particularly efficient for such processes [21,23,26–28].

9.2.1.3 Preparation of the Adjuvant Emulsion MF59

The squalene-based emulsion MF59 is not produced in a piston-gap-type homogenizer but in a microfluidizer (thus the designation "MF"). Details about the development and the GMP production process have been published by Ott *et al.* [29,30]. For production of this emulsion, polysorbate 80 is dissolved in sodium citrate buffered (pH 6.5) water for injection, sorbitan trioleate in the squalene oil. High speed mixing of the two phases yields a coarse oil-in-water emulsion that is submitted to several high-pressure homogenization cycles in a microfluidizer to generate a colloidal emulsion with about 150 nm mean particle size. The small particle size allows passing the emulsion through a 0.22 μm filter that is used to remove remaining coarse material and microbiological contaminants. The vaccine formulation is generated by mixing the adjuvant emulsion with an aqueous solution of the antigen. The final formulation is sterilized by another filtration step through a membrane with 0.22 μm pore size.

In a microfluidizer, droplet disruption is achieved in microchannels of fixed geometry located in a so-called interaction chamber. In the typical, Y-shaped microchannel geometry (Figure 9.2, other geometries are also available), the product stream is first split up and later recombined in an impingement area at very high velocities created under high pressure. The interaction of the two streams leads to particularly high turbulence and shear that effectively disrupt the droplets down to small particle sizes [17,24,31]. Microfluidizers are usually considered more efficient in producing small droplets than valve homogenizers [24]. In a direct comparison of the two types of device, similar emulsion droplet sizes were observed after several passes under the same pressure drop. In the microfluidizer, the final droplet size was, however, already achieved after a single pass at high pressures, while processing in a valve homogenizer required several cycles to achieve the same result. This was attributed to a more homogeneous distribution of shear forces created by the microfluidizer as compared to valve homogenizers. Thus, almost all droplets experience the highest shear force already during the first pass of the microfluidizer interaction chamber [31].

9.2.2 Liposomes

9.2.2.1 General Aspects and Composition

Liposomes are phospholipid-based vesicles of different size and lamellarity in aqueous dispersion. One (unilamellar) or more (oligo-/multilamellar) phospholipid bilayers surround an aqueous core in a closed, concentric arrangement resulting in more or less spherical particles. Their size ranges from below 50 nm up to several micrometers [32,33]. Such systems were first described by Bangham and Coworkers in the 1960s [34]. Beyond their importance as model membrane structures, they soon moved into the focus as potential drug delivery systems [35,36] and several formulations have reached the market (Table 9.3). Depending on their physicochemical nature, drugs can be entrapped in the aqueous core of the liposomes or be localized in the phospholipid bilayers.

Liposomes are based on natural and/or (semi)synthetic phospholipids with different headgroups such as phosphatidylcholine (most often) or phosphatidylethanolamine. Depending on the phospholipid chain length and saturation as well as the presence of other membrane ingredients, the fatty acid residues within the hydrated membrane bilayers display different transition (melting) temperatures (T_m). The lipid membranes are rather rigid (gel state) below the T_m, whereas a more flexible (fluid) state of the bilayer is reached above this temperature. Phospholipids with saturated chains can be used to obtain liposomes with a rigid and thus less permeable membrane at body temperature. Cholesterol is often added to stabilize the bilayer; it decreases the fluidity of phospholipid membranes with unsaturated chains. The use of negatively charged phospholipids (e.g., phosphatidylserine and phosphatidylglycerol) in the lipid composition leads to liposomes with negative surface charge; a positive charge can, for example, be achieved by the addition of lipids such as dioleoyloxypropyltrimethylammonium chloride (DOTAP). Surface decoration with polyethyleneglycol (e.g., by incorporation of polyethyleneglyocol-coupled disteaorylphosphatidylethanolamine (PEG-DSPE))

Table 9.3 Examples for liposomal and related products.

Product	Drug	Indications	Form	First approved	Lipid composition
AmBisome®	Amphotericin B	Fungal infections Leishmaniasis	Lyophilized product for intravenous infusion	1990 (Europe) 1997 (USA)	HSPC, DSPG, cholesterol
Amphotec®/ Amphocil®[a)]	Amphotericin B	Fungal infections	Powder for solution for infusion	1993 (EU/UK) 1996 (USA)	Cholesterol sulfate
Abelcet®[a)]	Amphotericin B	Fungal infections	Concentrate for infusion	1995 (USA)	DMPC, DMPG
Depocyt®/ DepoCyte®[a)]	Cytarabine	Cancer	Suspension for injection	1999 (USA) 2001 (EU)	DOPC, DPPG, cholesterol, triolein
DaunoXome®	Daunorubicin	Cancer	Concentrate for solution for infusion	1995 (EU/UK) 1996 (USA)	DSPC, cholesterol
Doxil/Caelyx®	Doxorubicin	Cancer	Concentrate for solution for infusion	1995 (USA) 1996 (EU)	HSPC, mPEG-DSPE, cholesterol
Myocet®	Doxorubicin	Cancer	Powder, dispersion and solvent for concentrate for dispersion for infusion	2000 (EU)	EPC, cholesterol
Visudyne®	Verteporphin	Wet macular degeneration	Powder for solution for infusion	2000 (EU) 2000 (USA)	EPG, DMPC
Marqibo®	Vincristine	Cancer	Kit for the preparation of a liposomal infusion	2012 (USA)	Sphingomyelin, cholesterol

a) Not liposomal products in a strict sense but nanosized lipid complexes (Amphotec, Abelcet) or phospholipid-based nanostructured, foam-like microparticles (Depotcyt).
EPC: egg phosphatidylcholine; EPG: egg phosphatidylglycerol; DMPC: dimyristoylphosphatidylcholine; DMPG: dimyristoylphosphatidylglycerol; DOPC: dioleoylphosphatidylcholine; DPPG: dipalmitoylphosphatidylglycerol; DSPC: distearoylphosphatidylcholine; DSPG: distearoylphosphatidylglycerol; HSPC: fully hydrogenated soy phosphatidylcholine; mPEG-DSPE: PEGylated distearoylphosphatidylethanolamine.
Sources: Approved drug products database of the FDA [37], European Public Assessment Reports of the EMA [38]; additional information from [39] for AmBisome, [40,41] for Amphotec/Amphocil, [76] for Abelcet and [42] for DaunoXome.

or other hydrophilic moieties leads to decreased interaction with the immune system and to longer circulation times after injection [32,33]. The lipid chemistry with regard to liposomes is, for example, outlined in Refs [43,44].

9.2.2.2 Preparation of Liposomal Dispersions

In principle, bilayer structures form spontaneously when phospholipids are hydrated with water. For pharmaceutical applications, however, liposomes with defined size and structure are generally required. Thus, specialized methods leading to different types of liposomes have been established. Comprehensive reviews of classical liposome manufacturing techniques can, for example, be found in Ref. [45] (updated by [46]) and in Ref. [47]. Most of these methods were originally developed for laboratory use and thus without particular attention to large-scale pharmaceutical production. Considerations on the applicability of liposome manufacturing techniques to pharmaceutical production have been published in Refs [48–51]. Most methods either start from a dried lipid mixture or, alternatively, from a lipid solution in an organic solvent.

Lipid Hydration with Subsequent Downsizing

The hydration of a thin lipid film, often called thin lipid film hydration or Bangham method was already used in the very first studies on liposomal structures [52]. The lipids are dissolved in an organic solvent and subsequently brought to dryness as a thin film or deposit, for example, by rotary evaporation of the solvent in a round-bottom flask. Subsequently, the film is rehydrated by shaking with an aqueous medium that usually leads to the formation of large multilamellar vesicles (MLV) with rather broad size distribution. Freeze-drying the lipid solution, for example, from *tert*-butanol, or spray-drying it may enhance dispersion and lead to the formation of less heterogeneous MLV [47,50]. For most pharmaceutical applications, MLV as such are not suitable and they are therefore usually subjected to further mechanical treatment for downsizing. On lab scale, ultrasonication has often been used for this purpose [53]. However, this method bears the risk of local overheating and chemical degradation as well as metal contamination from the ultrasonic probe. Moreover, the very small SUV that may be formed this way are often unstable and fuse upon storage [47,54–56].

For preparation on industrial scale, high-pressure homogenization is much more promising. Starting from the original French press treatment [57] more sophisticated high-shear homogenization methods have been developed to process MLV into SUV. High-pressure homogenizers like those used for the preparation of colloidal lipid emulsions (Figure 9.2) are very efficient in disrupting multilamellar phospholipid structures upon repeated cycling and are able to process lipid dispersions at rather high concentrations and up to very large scale [58–60].

A very prominent method for the preparation of homogeneous liposome dispersions from MLV precursors is repeated extrusion through membrane filters with pore sizes in the nanometer range. This procedure is, for instance, used in the production process of Doxil®/Caelyx® [61]. In most cases, track-etched polycarbonate membranes are used for extrusion since they exhibit a very narrow pore size distribution and are commercially available with many different pore sizes. The method of filter extrusion was introduced by Olson *et al.* in 1979 and later further elaborated using nitrogen or pump-driven extrusion devices [62–64]. A short review of the method is given in Ref. [65]. Usually, MLV dispersions can be extruded directly through the filter of choice resulting in liposomes with sizes in the range of that of the filter pores with a very homogeneous size distribution when an adequate number of cycles (e.g., 10–15) is performed. The use of filters with small pores (e.g., 50–200 nm) leads to the formation of mainly unilamellar vesicles in a highly reproducible manner. A wide range of lipid compositions can be processed if the process is carried out at temperatures above T_m. The lipid concentration of the MLV dispersion to be extruded can be considerably high (e.g., 40% [64]). Although, as also the case with high-pressure homogenization equipment, solvents are generally not required for filter extrusion, the presence of a certain concentration of ethanol may enhance the process [65,66]. Filter extrusion is easily scalable; it can be performed with very small sample volumes (<1 ml) using manual devices as well as on industrial production scale. Compared to other means of MLV disintegration, the method is rather gentle and uses only moderate energy input. Although the exact mechanism of generation of smaller size unilamellar vesicles is still under discussion, it is assumed that disruption and fusion processes take place due to shear stress within the pores and membrane instabilities [65,67–70].

Processing of Dissolved Lipids

Several liposome preparation procedures start with lipid solutions. Traditional techniques are, for example, reverse phase evaporation and detergent depletion [71–73]. Both have their specific advantages but have not been carried forward for the industrial processing of low-molecular-weight compounds so far. In contrast, mixing ethanolic solutions of (phospho)lipids with an aqueous phase is regarded as promising with regard to transfer into the production scale [74]. Injecting lipid solutions in ethanol into a water phase can directly produce small unilamellar vesicles [75]; when the lipid concentration of the solution increases, so does the size of the vesicles obtained [76]. When solutions of very high lipid concentration are mixed with water, this results in the generation of heterogeneous MLV dispersions instead of small unilamellar structures [47]. This phenomenon may be utilized to generate MLV dispersions that can, for example, directly be further processed by filter extrusion as outlined above [66]. The ethanol injection method has been further developed using several new approaches such as hydrodynamic focusing in microchannels or making use of a membrane contactor [77,78]. Like the cross-flow injection method [74] these methods may allow scale up as well as continuous production and could thus bear promise for future process development. After liposome formation, ethanol can be removed by methods such as cross-flow filtration [65]. Absolute removal of ethanol is very difficult but since ethanol is a solvent accepted for parenteral formulations, remaining ethanol traces should usually not pose a significant drawback [50].

9.2.2.3 Drug Incorporation into Liposomes and Other Colloidal Lipid Structures

Direct Incorporation of Lipophilic Substances

Lipophilic drugs are usually processed with the lipids directly during liposome formation leading to their efficient association with the lipid bilayers. Examples for marketed products prepared this way are those containing the antifungal agent amphotericin B and verteporfin for the use in photodynamic therapy.

Amphotericin B The product AmBisome® contains amphotericin B in small (mainly <100 nm) unilamellar liposomes composed of hydrogenated soy phosphatidylcholine (HSPC), cholesterol, and distearoyl phosphatidylglycerol (DSPG) [79]. Starting from a complex between amphotericin B and DSPG in acidified chloroform/methanol, HSPC and cholesterol are added to the organic mixture that is then brought to dryness, for example, by spray-drying. The resulting powder is hydrated with acidic buffer and the mixture submitted to high-pressure homogenization at elevated temperature in a Gaulin-type homogenizer. The resulting unilamellar liposomes can be sterile filtered and lyophilized [79–81]. The marketed product is supplied as freeze-dried powder containing sucrose as cryoprotectant [82].

Beside AmBisome, there are two other amphotericin B products on the market that do not represent liposomes but other types of colloidal lipid structures. Abelcet® contains complexes of amphotericin B with dimyristoyl phosphatidylcholine (DMPC) and dimyristoylphosphatidylglycerol (DMPG) at a high drug-to-lipid ratio; it is supplied as concentrate for suspension for infusion [83]. The complexes are ribbon-like structures [84]. Several possibilities of preparing such complexes have been described. These include hydration of a thin film prepared from organic solutions of amphotericin B with the lipids or combining organic solutions of the drug and the lipids with an aqueous phase, subsequent solvent evaporation, colloid mill treatment, and washing by filtration [85].

The colloidal dispersion of amphotericin B in Amphocil®/Amphotec® contains thin, disk-shaped particles with a mean diameter of about 115 nm [86]. The disks represent about 1:1 molar complexes of the drug with cholesterol sulfate that are thermodynamically stable. Such particles can be prepared by adding a solution of the two compounds in dimethyl sulfoxide to an aqueous medium at elevated temperature [87]. After bringing the solution to room temperature, the solvent can be removed by diafiltration, and tonicity is adjusted by adding lactose. The dispersions can be filtrated through sterile filters with 0.22 μm pore size. Alternatively, amphotericin B and cholesterol sulfate are dried from a methanolic solution in the presence of lactose (which also serves as cryoprotectant for the final formulation). The lipidic film forming on lactose particles is then reconstituted in aqueous medium and resulting particles are subjected to high-energy treatment such as ultrasonication or high-pressure homogenization [88]. The formulation is provided as lyophilized powder to be reconstituted with water for injection [86].

Verteporfin For manufacturing the Visudyne® liposomes, verteporfin is mixed with the phospholipids (egg phosphatidylglycerol and dimyristoyl phosphatidylcholine) and antioxidants (ascorbyl palmitate and butylated hydroxytoluene) as a solution in dichloromethane that is later evaporated. The resulting intermediate product is hydrated with an aqueous lactose solution, and the vesicular structures formed are reduced in size by homogenization. The product is sterile filtered (0.22 μm) and subjected to lyophilization. Lactose is added during the process as a cryo-/lyoprotectant and also serves as isotonizing agent in the final, reconstituted product [89,90].

Remote Loading of Weak Bases

Weak bases can be efficiently entrapped into the aqueous core of liposomes using pH gradients in a process called remote loading [91]. For example, the neutral form of doxorubicin permeates easily through liposome membranes following its concentration gradient. If the liposome interior is acidified, the drug gets trapped inside the liposome in its protonated form. In Caelyx/Doxil, doxorubicin is loaded into liposomes by establishing an ammonium sulfate gradient between the dispersion medium (low ammonium sulfate concentration) and the aqueous core of the liposome (high ammonium sulfate concentration). At sufficiently high pH, the ammonium ion dissociates. The neutral ammonia can leave the liposome leaving behind the proton thus acidifying the liposome core. In a kind of exchange, the neutral form of doxorubicin permeates into the liposome where it is protonated and precipitates as sulfate. Since dissolved doxorubicin is removed from the equilibrium by this process, a doxorubicin gradient is retained and a very high fraction of the doxorubicin present in the system can be encapsulated in a stable, precipitated form [14,92]. The production process of Caelyx/Doxil is outlined in Figure 9.3.

The low pH inside the liposomes (and thus the concentration gradient of neutral doxorubicin) can also be maintained by using a citrate buffer, resulting in encapsulation of close to 100% of the doxorubicin added to the outer phase of the liposome dispersion. Entrapment is enhanced by precipitation of the doxorubicin citrate salt as fiber bundles within the liposomes [66,93]. This procedure is involved in the formation of Myocet®. In contrast to Caelyx/Doxil that is supplied as a concentrated dispersion of loaded liposomes, the loading procedure has to be performed directly prior to administration of Myocet. The product is supplied as a three-vial system containing doxorubicin HCl as a lyophilized powder, an aqueous dispersion of empty liposomes in citric acid buffer (pH 4–5), and a loading buffer. All components are sterile filtered in the course of their respective preparation process. The liposomes are stable, plurilamellar vesicles consisting of egg phosphatidylcholine (EPC) and cholesterol. Prior to loading, the pH of the liposome dispersion medium is adjusted to 7–8 by adding sodium

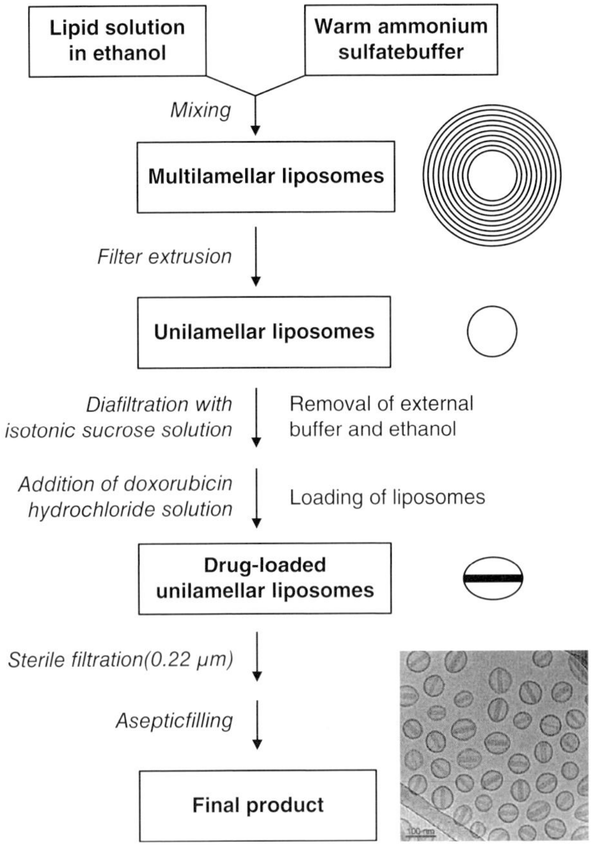

Figure 9.3 Production of Caelyx/Doxil. (Electron micrograph reproduced with permission from Ref. [14]. Copyright 2012, Elsevier Ltd.)

carbonate buffer. The solution of the drug in saline is added and the loading procedure via pH-gradient performed at elevated temperature [94].

A similar procedure is followed for the vincristine-containing product Marqibo®. The liposomal carriers in Marqibo are made from sphingomyelin and cholesterol in an approximate molar ratio of 60:40 and have a nominal mean diameter of 115 nm. The Marqibo kit contains three vials (vincristine sulfate, liposomes, and sodium phosphate injection). Here, the pH of the liposome dispersion medium is altered by adding phosphate buffer before liposome loading by addition of vincristine sulfate solution [95,96].

9.2.2.4 DepotFoam® Technology

A vesicular formulation intended for sustained release of cytarabine (Depocyt/DepoCyte®) was introduced to the pharmaceutical market around the year 2000. This formulation is structurally very different from the products discussed so far since it contains rather large (1–100 μm) multivesicular particles with a foam-like internal structure. The "foam" lamellae consist of phospholipid bilayers. In addition to phospholipids, the formulations contain a small portion of triglyceride oil that is assumed to localize at the contact points of the phospholipid lamellae thus stabilizing the foam-like structure. Without the presence of triglyceride oil, conventional multi- or unilamellar liposomes are formed during the production procedure. The multivesicular particles are manufactured by a double emulsification process. In a first step, an aqueous solution of the drug to be encapsulated is emulsified into a lipohilic phase containing the phospholipids and the triglyceride oil in a water-immiscible, volatile organic solvent. This primary w/o emulsion is emulsified with a second aqueous phase resulting in lipid-containing droplets of organic solvent that incorporate numerous smaller droplets of aqueous drug solution. Upon removal of the organic solvent by evaporation under reduced pressure or in a simple gas flow, the w/o/w emulsion droplets transform into multivesicular particles encapsulating the drug in the multiple vesicular compartments. Aseptic processing is required in order to obtain a sterile product with these large particles [97].

9.2.2.5 **Sterilization of Liposomes**

Most marketed liposomal preparations are intended for parenteral use. Thus, sterility of the formulations has to be ensured. This requirement may pose challenges, since the chemical and physical stability of the liposomal formulations has to be retained. Upon application of energy-inducing terminal sterilization methods such as steam sterilization or γ-irradiation chemical reactions such as oxidation, fragmentation, or hydrolysis of the lipid compounds may occur. Moreover, leakage of encapsulated active compounds may result in particular for substances incorporated into the aqueous core of the liposomes [98–102]. Anyway, autoclaving under standard pharmacopoeial conditions (15 min at 121 °C) has been considered acceptable for some liposomal formulations [101,103]. However, terminal sterilization by heat or irradiation is not an established process in industrial liposome product manufacturing [102] and examples discussed above). Instead, filtration through bacteria-retentive membranes (nominal pore diameter $\leq$0.22 µm) is often applied at some point during the process. Solutions (frequently occurring as intermediates during liposome manufacturing) can easily be treated by membrane filtration as a part of an aseptic production process. Liposome preparation by extrusion through membrane filters automatically includes the bacteria-retention step if sterile filtration equipment with sufficiently narrow pore size is employed [62]. Apart from a certain mechanical impact, filtration can be considered a rather gentle process. It could be applied to filter-extruded liposomes without significant loss of ingredient encapsulated into the aqueous liposome core [104]. The most preferable option of filtration as the final step prior to filling is, however, only possible for liposomes of sufficiently small size and aseptic processing has to be used as last resort in other cases [102].

9.2.2.6 **Drying of Liposomal Dispersions**

With regard to the potential chemical instabilities of liposomal formulation (like oxidation or hydrolysis of the lipids), the availability of adequate stabilization methods would be desirable. Drying is considered particularly promising in this respect. As an established pharmaceutical process that is also applicable to sterile dosage forms when conducted under aseptic conditions lyophilization (or freeze-drying) has hitherto been in the main focus of interest. In brief, the process of lyophilization includes freezing of the aqueous product and subsequent sublimation of frozen water under reduced pressure. All process steps (freezing, primary drying, and secondary drying) have to be conducted under highly controlled conditions, and elaborate process development is required in order to achieve an adequate product quality [105,106]. Usually, the addition of cryo-/lyo-protective excipients such as carbohydrates is required in order to retain the structure of complex ingredients such as proteins or liposomes upon drying and to enhance redispersibility of the lyophilizate. In the area of liposome lyophilization, preserving the particle size distribution of the liposomes as well as their membrane integrity and drug load are of major concern [107,108]. Probably as a result of the corresponding challenges lyophilization is hitherto only been applied in commercial formulations that contain lipophilic drugs intercalated in the lipid membrane as drug leakage does not easily occur in these cases (AmBisome and Visudyne).

9.2.3 Polymeric Nanoparticles

9.2.3.1 General Aspects

There are numerous types of polymeric nanoparticles discussed for pharmaceutical use associated with a broad range of different manufacturing techniques. A comprehensive overview can, for example, be found in the review by Vauthier and Bouchemal [109] that also addresses important issues such as purification, sterilization, and drying of the nanoparticle suspensions. Further surveys of the field are given in Refs [110–112]. Only some essentials are briefly outlined in the following.

Polymeric nanoparticles can either be of the matrix type (nanospheres) resulting from the dispersion of a preformed polymer or direct polymerization of monomers into colloidal particles. Alternatively, they can represent nanocapsules in the usual type of which a polymeric shell surrounds an oil core. The polymeric shell can either be generated by interfacial polymerization or by precipitating the polymer at the particle interface. For most efficient encapsulation into the nanoparticle, drugs are usually processed with the polymer upon nanosphere generation or are incorporated into the core of nanocapsules, respectively.

Polymers employed for the preparation of pharmaceutical nanoparticles must be biocompatible (including their potential degradation products), biodegradable (or small enough for excretion as such), and of high purity. They can be of natural (e.g., albumin and chitosan) or synthetic origin (e.g., polylactide (PLA) and poly(lactide-*co*-glycolide) (PLGA), poly(caprolactone) (PCL), or different types of poly(alkylcyanoacrylates)). Most promising with regard to the translation into nanomedicines are polymeric materials already approved for the intended route of administration by the health authorities such as albumin or PLGA for parenteral use. Surface active agents such as polysorbates, poloxamers, or poly (vinylalcohol) are often required in the formulations to maintain the dispersed state of the nanoparticles. Alternatively, copolymers with hydrophilic moieties (e.g., with polyethyleneglycol or polysaccharides) can be formed that bring about the stabilization of the nanoparticles. The preparation of polymer nanoparticles can start from the monomers (thus involving *in-situ* polymerization) or be based on the processing of preformed polymers. From a perspective of quality control, the latter is usually regarded as more promising since the quality determining parameters of the polymer can be checked prior to processing.

Often, the preparation of polymeric nanoparticles includes the formation of an emulsion as precursor that is followed by precipitation of the polymer from the droplets. The preparation by *emulsification–solvent evaporation* is the classical way of preparing drug-loaded nanospheres from preformed polymers like PL(G)A [113]. Emulsion formation requires the use of a water immiscible solvent to create the disperse phase. Nowadays, ethyl acetate has largely replaced the originally predominating chlorinated solvents such as dichloromethane in this way of preparation. Usually, high-energy emulsification techniques such as high-pressure emulsification are employed to generate sufficiently small droplets of the dispersed phase. Afterward, the solvent is removed under reduced pressure. When a partially water-miscible solvent such as ethyl acetate is used as organic phase, the solvent can be extracted from the emulsion droplets into the aqueous phase by sudden dilution with a large amount of aqueous medium (*emulsification–solvent extraction*). In a variation of this method, a totally water-miscible solvent such as acetone is forced into the emulsified state by addition of a salt or sugar to the aqueous phase resulting in a strong salting-out effect (*emulsification–reverse salting-out*). Emulsions are usually also the starting point when polymeric nanoparticles are prepared by *in-situ* polymerization. In this case, the monomers are emulsified and the polymerization reaction is carried out in the emulsion system. This way of preparation is typical for the processing of poly(alkylcyanoacrylates). Alkylcyanoacrylates are also convenient reagents for interfacial polymerization reactions, usually at the surface of preformed oil droplets leading to nanocapsules; however, nanocapsule formation can also be based on polycondensation reactions (e.g., leading to polyamides or polyurethanes).

An alternative way to form nanoparticles from preformed polymers is nanoprecipitation (also called *solvent displacement*). The polymer is dissolved in a water-miscible organic solvent that is easy to remove by evaporation (e.g., acetone) and the solution is mixed with a nonsolvent (usually an aqueous phase) that may contain a surface-active stabilizer. Upon rapid diffusion of the solvent into the aqueous phase, nanoparticles form by precipitation [114]. Alternatively, dialysis against the nonsolvent can be employed to precipitate the polymer. Nanoparticles from water-soluble polyelectrolytes can be generated by complex formation with oppositely charged macromolecules (e.g., polyplexes between polyamines and nucleic acids or complexes between alginate and polylysine) in a completely aqueous environment. Some polyelectrolytes such as chitosan or alginate can be precipitated into nanoparticles by addition of oppositely charged ions (polyphosphates or calcium, respectively) in a process called ionotropic gelation. Other water-soluble polymers such as albumin or gelatin can precipitated from aqueous solution by simple coacervation, for example, upon the addition of alcohol or salts. Further techniques discussed for the manufacturing of polymeric nanoparticles for pharmaceutical use include supercritical fluid technology, electrospraying, or other means of atomization.

While there is abundant literature concerning lab-scale preparation of polymeric nanoparticles, scale-up approaches have rarely been reported. As one exception, for example, there is a study on the comparative scale-up of nanocapsule manufacturing by three different methods based on either emulsification or precipitation [115]. Continuous processes in microfluidic devices are considered particularly promising with regard to reproducible, scalable manufacturing of pharmaceutical nanocarriers [116].

As nanoparticle preparation often requires the use of additives such as solvents or sometimes relies on the processing of monomers the suspensions frequently have to be purified after nanoparticle generation. Moreover, preparation techniques that yield only low particle concentrations (e.g., nanoprecipitation) need to be followed by adequate concentration steps. Applicable methods include evaporation, centrifugation, and different filtration techniques. When employing such purification/concentration techniques, care has to be taken not to compromise the quality of the nanoparticles (e.g., due to aggregation upon centrifugation or premature drug loss during washing steps).

Nanoparticle dispersions intended for parenteral use have to be sterile. Steam sterilization as the usual method of choice for aqueous systems is, however, often not applicable due to negative effects on the stability of the polymer and/or the nanoparticles. Sterilization by ionizing radiation often leads to alterations in molecular weight, in particular due to chain scissions, albeit the successful application of this method has also been described. Apart from aseptic preparation, sterile filtration often remains as the only promising technique but is only feasible for nanoparticles with sufficiently small size. In order to prevent physical and, in particular, chemical instabilities of the nanoparticle suspensions (e.g., premature hydrolysis of polymers such as PLGA), they are frequently transformed into the dry state after preparation. Freeze-drying is most often employed for this purpose [117]. It usually requires the addition of excipients as cryoprotectants (usually a sugar (e.g., trehalose, sucrose) or mannitol) the type and concentration of which need to be carefully selected as have the process parameters for the drying process. This also applies to spray-drying that is considered an interesting alternative and might particularly be promising for the preparation of products not requiring sterility. Apart from increasing stability, drying can also help to increase the often low concentration of the original nanoparticle suspensions, since the dried products can be reconstituted at much higher concentration.

9.2.3.2 Abraxane®

The only polymer-based nanoparticulate product that has reached the market so far is Abraxane (nab™ (nanoparticle albumin-bound) paclitaxel, ABI-007). In Abraxane, human serum albumin is the only excipient (present in an about ninefold excess (m/m) related to the drug [118]) that serves as stabilizer for the nanoparticles and as drug carrier upon administration. Abraxane is provided as a sterile lyophilized powder. Prior to administration, the powder is reconstituted with 0.9% aqueous sodium chloride solution into a homogeneous, milky suspension with 5 mg/ml albumin-associated paclitaxel [119]. The suspension is based on spherical, rather monodisperse nanoparticles of a mean size around 130 nm that contain the drug in a noncrystalline form [120,121]. The nab™ paclitaxel nanoparticles have been described as consisting of a core of the active substance coated by a layer of human serum albumin that has not been treated by external cross-linkers. The drug is noncovalently associated with the albumin by hydrophobic interaction [122]. While the nanoparticles are stable after reconstitution for several days [122], they dissociate into albumin-paclitaxel complexes of about the size of the native albumin molecule upon intravenous infusion [120].

The details of the formulation and the preparation procedure are considered vital for the product quality [121] but are not available in the public domain. According to the procedure described in the patent, the nanoparticles are prepared by an emulsification–solvent evaporation process. Paclitaxel is dissolved in a water-immiscible organic solvent that is first pre-emulsified in an aqueous solution of human serum albumin. Subsequently, the crude emulsion is treated by high-pressure homogenization. After solvent evaporation under reduced pressure at slightly elevated temperature, the resulting nanoparticles can be sterile filtered and are then submitted to freeze-drying. Addition of a cryoprotectant is not required as the lyophilized cake can readily be reconstituted in water or saline [123].

9.3
Drug Nanoparticles and Process Chains to Solid Formulations

The administration of nanoparticulate drugs first improves the gastrointestinal absorption via an elevated dissolution rate and the possibility to overcome equilibrium saturation solubility by kinetic supersaturation and, by that, a higher concentration gradient over biological membranes leading to enhanced permeation. Second, other biopharmaceutical and safety aspects are improved: quicker onset of action by increased rate of absorption (also for completely, but slowly dissolving APIs), extended dose proportionality, clear reduction of the food effect (differences in bioavailability between fed and fasted state), and reduction of intersubject absorption variation [124,125].

From an engineering point of view, different process steps must be established to successfully implement active pharmaceutical ingredient (API) nanoparticles into "conventional" dosage forms such as tablets and capsules. As a first step, the API itself must be transferred into a nanodisperse state. This is only feasible in liquid-phase processes as dry comminution is limited to approx. 1 μm. As pharmaceutical disperse liquid systems mostly contain water as principal component, stability may be infringed. Chemically, hydrolysis and other reactions based on the presence of water are enabled. Physically, instabilities such as agglomeration, aggregation, and ripening/growth of primary API particles may occur. To reduce these risks, drying of nanosuspensions is necessary. Nonetheless, the depletion of water causes closer contact of the disperse phase compartments, making aggregation and loss of individuality likely to occur. Accordingly, both process steps comminution and drying must be carefully investigated and developed for the drug product of concern.

9.3.1
Drug Particle Size-Determining Processes

Primarily, a differentiation is drawn between top-down and bottom-up processes for the production of drug nanoparticles. Additionally, combined methods, comprising either multiple top-down, bottom-up, or a mixture of both processes, are described.

Around the millennium, different comminution methods for the production of drug nanoparticles were discussed, focusing on media milling and high-pressure homogenization. Although some experts saw homogenization in advantage, stressing the challenge of product contamination in media mills [126], first drug nanoparticle-containing products that entered the market were produced by media milling. Until now, the vast majority of products is produced by media milling for size reduction und subsequent processing to final dosage forms.

9.3.1.1 Comminution Processes (Top-Down Methods)

In principle, it is reported that drug particles can be milled to submicron sizes using media mills or high-pressure homogenizers. However, high-pressure homogenizers cannot deliver the stress intensity necessary to break primary drug particles, only to separate primary particles of agglomerates or soft aggregates [127,128]. Moreover, the stress intensity of high-pressure homogenizers, that is the tensile stress, is independent of particle size or even decreases with decreasing particle size. This hinders even more the usability of high-pressure homogenizers for nanoparticle breakage because the breakage strength of particles increases with decreasing particle size. In contrast to that, in stirred media mills, the more or less constant energy of the beads can be transferred to decreasing particle masses, which increases the stress intensity with increasing product fineness. Therefore, stirred media mills are able to break even very strong primary particles to sizes down to below 20 nm if appropriate operating parameters are applied.

Stirred Media Milling

The outstanding role of stirred media milling in the production of marketable nanoparticulate pharmaceuticals is well demonstrated by the highly successful patent on Nanocrystals® by *Élan* (now Alkermes). It is applied for the production of by far the most marketed formulations (also see Section 9.3.3 and Table 9.4). In order to process poorly water-soluble API particles down to sizes

Table 9.4 Patented processes for the production of API nanoparticles [124,137–142].

Name	Patent	Process type	Company	Year
NanoCrystals®	US5145684 A	wet ball milling	Sterling Drug Company, then Nanosystems, then Élan drug technologies, now Alkermes	1991
Insoluble Drug Delivery-P®	US6682761 B2	HPH	SkyePharma	2000
NanoEdge®	US6884436 B2, US 6869617 B2	Combination:precipitation + high-energy step (e.g., HPH)	Baxter	2001
NanoPure®	US8202540 B1	HPH in nonaqueous solvents or mixtures thereof	PharmaSol	2000
HydroSol®	GB2200048 A, GB2269536 A	HPH	Sandoz, then Novartis	1987
Nanomorph®	DE19637517 A1	HPH	Knoll/BASF, then Soliqs/Abbott	1996
Dissocubes®	US5858410 A, DE4440337 A1	HPH (piston-gap homogenizer)	SkyePharma	1994
Solumatrix®	WO2008000042 A1, WO 2006/069419 A1	Dry milling with matrix material	iCeutica Pty Ltd	2004
SmartCrystals® (Family)		Platform of combinations	Abbott, marketed by Soliqs	
H42	DE102005011786 A1	Spray-drying + HPH	PharmaSol, then Abbott, marketed by Soliqs	2005
H69	DE 102005053862 A1	Precipitation + HPH	PharmaSol, then Abbott, marketed by Soliqs	2005
H96	WO2006108637 A2	Lyophilization + HPH	PharmaSol, then Abbott, marketed by Soliqs	2006
CT	WO2008058755 A1	SMM + HPH	Abbott, marketed by Soliqs	2007

below 1 μm, not only the stress intensity must be sufficiently high, but also the milling process has to provide a very high number of stressing events and must provide the possibility to stabilize the freshly produced particles against agglomeration. Beside the breakage of the API particles, the stabilization of the API particles against agglomeration and recrystallization (particularly Ostwald ripening) is of the same importance [129–132]. In general, media mills such as stirred media mills and planetary ball mills fulfill these requirements [133,134]. For sufficient stabilization, the APIs have to be milled in a carrier fluid that is usually water or another solvent. However, special cases are reported where APIs are dry-milled together with a millable grinding compound like salt, which ideally should be harder than the API itself [135]. Moreover, milling devices can also be used to fulfill a mechanochemical reaction to produce nanosized API particles in dry and wet mode [136].

In general, the development of self-stabilizing nanosuspensions would be highly desirable with regard to reducing formulation complexity, circumventing regulatory hurdles, and avoiding toxicity reasonably originating from stabilizers [143]. Nonetheless, this is not applicable to real drug formulations and stabilization by additives is necessary. Accordingly, for the systematic choice of stabilizing agents for drug nanosuspensions, two main challenges must be overcome. On the one hand, fundamental understanding of stabilization mechanisms, stabilizer adsorption, and differentiation is missing so far. On the other hand, screening approaches for empirical stabilizer identification are not sufficiently automated with regard to high-throughput applications. Nonetheless, miniaturized milling assays guide the way toward quick screening approaches. For conventional stabilizer systems, the combination of anionic surfactants (such as sodium dodecyl sulfate) with cellulose-based polymeric stabilizers (hydroxypropyl methyl cellulose) has proved as most efficient for a broad spectrum of APIs [144,145].

The following explanations concentrate on wet nanogrinding of API using stirred media mills or planetary ball mills (for screening purposes) that are very common also in other industries like (agro)chemical, ceramic, ink, and electronic industry. Stirred media mills, which are available from very small scale of about 20 ml up to several thousand liters, are composed of a stationary grinding chamber with a stirrer inside, which agitates the beads used as grinding media in the mill. For very small quantities of less than 10 ml, usually 1–3 ml, a special setup of planetary ball mill can be applied to investigate the behavior of different formulations [146,147]. Usually up to 80% of the free mill volume is filled with a bulk of grinding beads, which can have sizes from below 100 μm to in extreme cases a few millimeters. However, beads out of yttrium-stabilized zirconium oxide, aluminum oxide, or polystyrene with sizes between 100 and 500 μm are usually applied for nanogrinding of APIs. In general, many different mill and stirrer designs are available on the market [148]. The mill and stirrer design depends on the demanded bead size, throughput and viscosity ranges, and, naturally, on the mill manufacturer. The main differences between the mill designs are the stirrer configuration and the design of the bead separation device. For pharmaceutical applications, usually stirred media mills are applied that can be operated at sufficiently high throughputs in a circuit together with a stirred vessel and that can handle small bead sizes even at higher viscosities. For example, mills with pin stirrer and centrifugal grinding media separation as shown in chapter "Commercial manufacturing of nano-drug delivery systems" are common for nanogrinding of API.

As mentioned before, four conditions have to be fulfilled to achieve product sizes in the nanometer size range: the number of stress events must be extremely high, the stress intensity must be sufficient, and the formulation must avoid high viscosity increases and particle agglomeration. Accordingly, stirred media mills offer the possibility to adjust and tune many different operating parameters and, with this, the stress number and stress intensity [145,149,150]. Beside the milling time and throughput, the main operating parameters are the bead size, bead material, bead filling ratio, and the stirrer tip speed. According to the so-called stressing model of Kwade [151], the specific energy consumption is proportional to the product of stress energy that is the energy available for stressing the particles in one stress event, that is, during one grinding media collision, and stress number that is the number of media contacts during the milling process. In order to ensure a minimum specific energy consumption required to achieve the demanded product fineness (determination see Eq. (9.1) for circuit operation and Eq. (9.2) for continuous operation, i.e., one passage), and with this a high production capacity (see Eq. (9.3)) and a minimum product contamination (product contamination is proportional to specific energy consumption [152,153]), the stress energy, given by Eq. (9.4), should be set to an optimum value [145,154].

Bitterlich *et al.* showed the applicability of the stress model to the fine grinding process of the API cinnarizine. Figure 9.4 depicts the required specific energy as a function of process parameters (grinding media size, density, and stirrer tip speed), which can be described by the stress energy of grinding media (compare Eq. (9.4)). For a constant product formulation, an increase of the required specific energy was observed to reach the target particle size of 267 nm with an increase of the stress energy of grinding media. In general, the applied stress energies are rather low, a clear optimum of stress energy (corresponding to the minimum specific energy input) was not identified yet. It is assumed to be located at even lower stress energies. The low stress energies required for nanogrinding of APIs favor the application of small grinding media sizes that are also linked to high stress numbers. Thus, suitable mill design for the use of grinding media sizes as small as possible becomes more important in order to run API milling processes most efficient. In principle, the stress intensity does not affect the maximum possible product fineness, as long as the product contamination does not affect the stability of the suspension.

$$E_{\mathrm{m}}(t) = \frac{E(t)}{m_{\mathrm{P}}} = \frac{\int_0^t (P(\tau) - P_0)\mathrm{d}\tau}{m_{\mathrm{P}}} \tag{9.1}$$

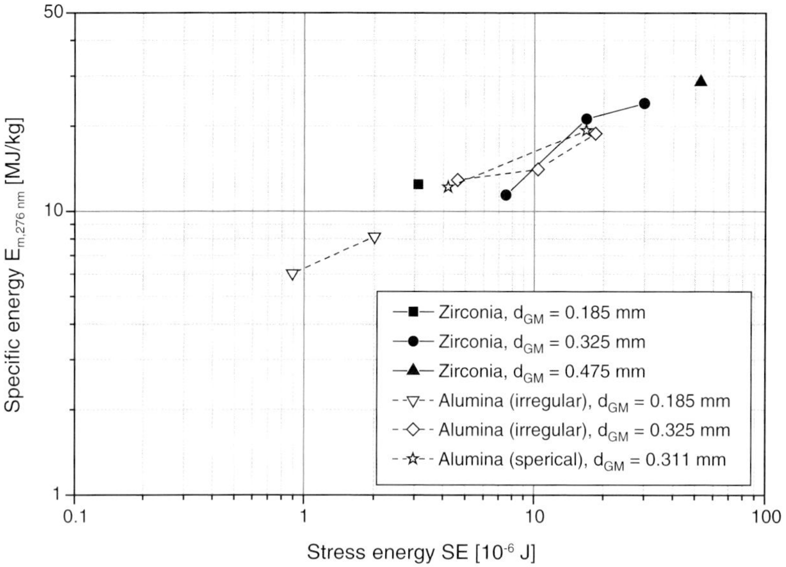

Figure 9.4 Specific energy to obtain a target product particle size of 267 nm (Z-avg) as a function of the applied stress energy for grinding cinnarizine. (Reproduced with permission from Ref. [145], copyright 2014, John Wiley & Sons.)

$$E_{\mathrm{m}} = \frac{P_{\mathrm{stat.}} - P_0}{\dot{m}_{\mathrm{P}}} \tag{9.2}$$

$$\dot{m}_{\mathrm{P}} = \frac{P_{\mathrm{stat.}} - P_0}{E_{\mathrm{m}}} \tag{9.3}$$

$$\mathrm{SE}_{\mathrm{GM}} = d_{\mathrm{GM}}^3 \cdot \rho_{\mathrm{GM}} \cdot v_{\mathrm{t}}^2 \tag{9.4}$$

Here, E_{m} is the specific energy consumption, E is the absolute energy, m_{p} is the mass of solid product, P is the power consumption, P_0 is the no-load power, P_{stat} is the power at stationary operation, $\dot{m}_{\mathrm{P}}$ is the mass flow rate of solid product, $\mathrm{SE}_{\mathrm{GM}}$ is the stress energy of the grinding media, d_{GM} is the size of grinding media, ρ_{GM} is the density of grinding media, and v_{t} is the stirrer tip speed.

As reported in some papers (see, for example, Refs [129,155]), nanogrinding processes show a grinding limit that can be caused by different means: agglomeration of nanosized fragments due to insufficient stabilization, recrystallization of dissolved API, media contact hindering due to a too high viscosity, and real breakage limit due to healing of crystal failures. For milling API, the choice of the right formulation is more critical than the optimum mill parameters. Especially, agglomeration of the very fine API particles, but as discussed above also recrystallization of API substances, can cause a grinding limit that is not determined by the actual breakage behavior of the organic material (Figure 9.5) [129,156].

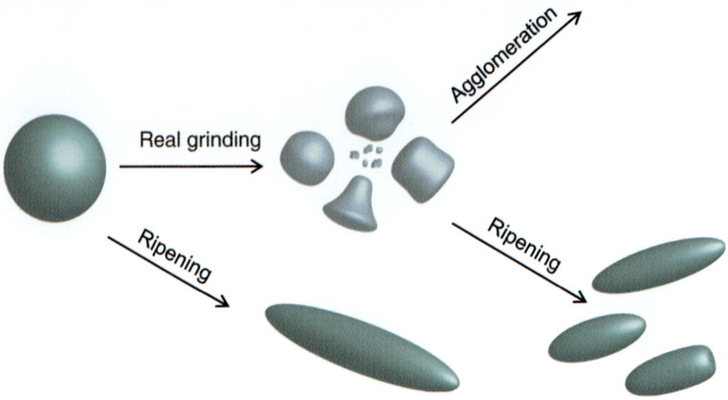

Figure 9.5 Possible mechanisms occurring during the fine grinding of API according to Bitterlich *et al.* (Reproduced with permission from Ref. [145]. Copyright 2014, John Wiley & Sons.)

Usually a combination of surfactant (e.g., SDS) and a polymer (as for example hydroxypropylcellulose) is sufficient to stabilize submicron API particles [157,158]. Eerdenbrugh *et al.* [159,160] give an overview about the stabilizing additives used by before 2008 published top-down processes. However, the maximum possible product fineness very much depends on the choice of the stabilizing additives. Beside agglomeration, the milling process can also be hindered by a high increase in viscosity hindering the intensive contact of the grinding media required to break the API particles. The additives can also change the solubility of the API that can result in different recrystallization even during milling the API. For example, Bitterlich *et al.* [145] showed different particle sizes and morphologies depending on the milling parameters and the choice of stabilization additives.

The minimum particle sizes of cinnarizine and fenofibrate after milling were stongly dependent on the applied particle stabilization that had to be chosen individually for each product. In most cases, the combination of polymer and surfactant matched the quality criteria (Figure 9.6). Similar oberservations were reported by others [144,158,161], the enhanced stability is attributed to a surfactant promoted wetting of particle surfaces favoring polymer adsorption from the liquid phase as well as the formation of a stabilizing complex that forms an electrosteric barrier.

In order to produce narrow particle size distributions of the API particles, the residence time distribution of the overall milling process is very important. Milling API in one passage with very low throughput to achieve the desired fineness causes very broad residence time distributions and by that very wide particle size distributions. Accordingly, for milling API at production scale, stirred media mills are always operated in a circuit or pendulum operation [148]. In a circuit operation, the suspension is pumped from a stirred vessel through the mill back into the same stirred vessel. Against that, in pendulum operation, the suspension is pumped in a second stirred vessel. After the first stirred vessel is empty, the

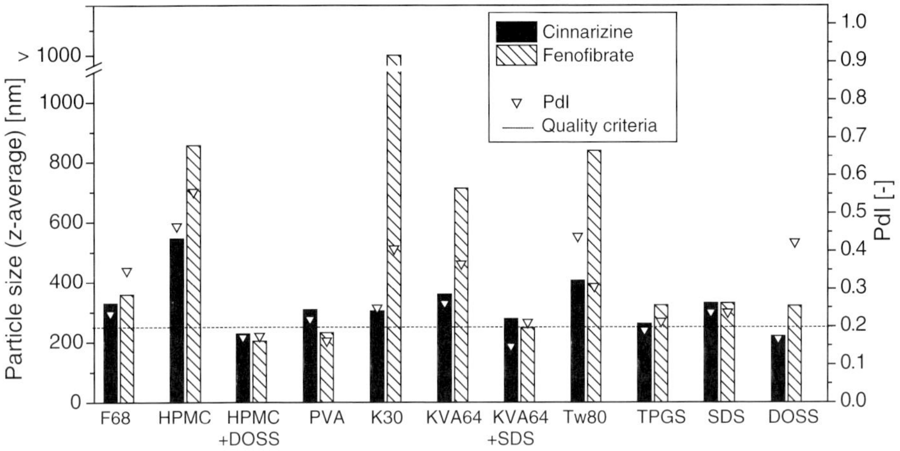

Figure 9.6 Particle size Z-average and PDI of fenofibrate and cinnarizine as a function of the product formulation obtained from planetary ball milling screening study. (Reproduced with permission from Ref. [145]. Copyright 2014, John Wiley & Sons.)

suspension is then pumped from the second stirred vessel through the mill into the first stirred vessel again. Due to less cleaning expenditure usually circuit operations are realized in pharmaceutical industry although the residence time distribution is even at high number of circuits still slightly wider than for pendulum operation. In laboratory scale, also batch milling tests can be carried out. The realization of a narrow residence time distribution is particularly important when the maximum particle size determines the final product quality.

In order to achieve the desired or maximum possible product quality with a minimum of costs, the mill should be efficiently operated. This means to operate the mill with a high power input but low specific energy consumption. Since the production capacity is the quotient of power input and specific energy consumption, this results in a maximum production capacity.

However, the power input is often not only restricted by the installed motor power, but also by the heat generation inside the mill and the wear of grinding media and mill internals. A major point of criticism is the appearance of wear particles during the grinding process causing a contamination of the product that must be taken into account when assessing media milling processes. Hennart *et al.* found that the production of wear is critically linked to the stirrer tip speed in stirred media mills, according to the energy input [162]. An in-depth analysis of contaminants in grinding processes showed that wear production is a function of grinding media quality (chemical composition and structural and mechanical properties) and process parameters (grinding media diameter, stirrer tip speed, and specific energy input) [153,163]. Figure 9.7 depicts on the one hand side the increase of specific energy for reaching the target particle size of 250 nm and on the other hand side the increasing product contamination with increasing stress energy. The smallest stress energy was linked to the smallest

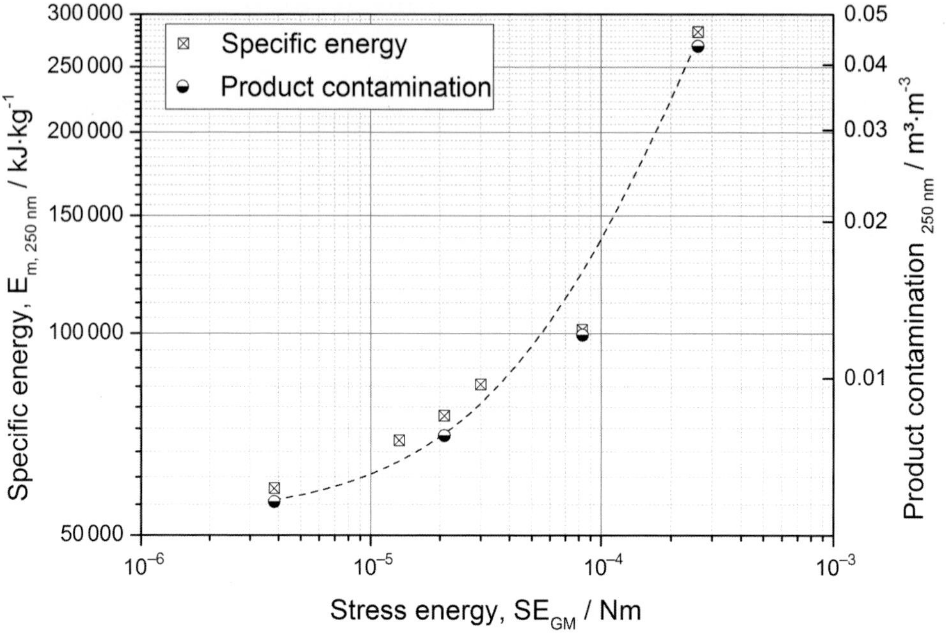

Figure 9.7 Specific energy to obtain a target product particle size of 250 nm ($x_{50,3}$) and product contamination as a function of the applied stress energy of grinding. (Reproduced with permission from Ref. [153]. Copyright 2016, John Wiley & Sons.)

product contamination. They assumed the optimum of stress energy being equal to the minimum of product contamination. During process development, an optimum between particle size reduction, energy efficiency, and avoidance of contamination by wear must be found.

A very important task is the transfer of the milling results from laboratory to production scale. Generally a scale-up of the process using the milling time or the mean residence time is not appropriate, that is, does not give a reasonable result. Instead, based on the consideration of equal cooling behavior and constant specific energy consumption, the following relationship is often applied as a rule of thumb [148,164]:

$$\dot{m}_P \propto P - P_0 \propto A_{GC} \propto V_{GC}^{\frac{2}{3}} \Rightarrow \dot{m}_{P,Prod} = \dot{m}_{P,Lab}\left(\frac{V_{GC,Prod}}{V_{GC,Lab}}\right)^{\frac{2}{3}} \tag{9.5}$$

where A_{GC} is the cooling surface of the grinding chamber, V_{GC} is the volume of the grinding chamber, $\dot{m}_{P,Prod}$ is the mass flow rate of the product at production scale, and $\dot{m}_{P,Lab}$ is the mass flow rate of the product at laboratory scale.

However, in most cases, the milling efficiency and the stress energy distribution as a characteristic of the mills changes with mill size that at least results in different product finesses at same specific energy input. The efficiency of energy transfer from stirrer to the product particles can be described by the so-called energy transfer coefficient ν_E, which can be multiplied with the overall specific energy consumption to get the so-called comminution active specific energy input. Therefore, as a much better scale-up rule, the effective specific energy input as well as the mean stress energy should be identical in laboratory and production scale:

$$\left(E_{m,Lab} \cdot \nu_{E,1,Lab}\right)_{\overline{SE}} = \left(E_{m,Prod} \cdot \nu_{E,1,Prod}\right)_{\overline{SE}}$$

The effective specific energy is the product of the specific energy required to achieve the demanded product quality and the energy transfer coefficient that can differ substantially for different mill sizes. The mean stress energy can be estimated by relatively simple flow considerations inside the stirred media mill [164] or by extensive calculations using coupled CFD (computational fluid dynamics) – DEM (discrete element method) – simulations. Since smaller mills usually have a distinctly higher mean stress energy using the same operating parameters as in production scale, it is very important to operate the lab mills in a manner that the results can be transferred to production scale, that means especially with relatively low stirrer tip speeds. Unfortunately, in case of milling organic substances beside the typical operating parameters important for inorganic materials other parameters such as grinding media wear and temperature can have a further significant influence that has to be considered.

Beside up-scaling, down-scaling for screening purposes is an important issue in pharmaceutical formulation development. Possibilities are described for ball milling in 96-well plates and glass vial [147] (minimum 10 mg) or, more sophisticatedly and closer to scalable and well described stirred media milling processes, in miniaturized ceramic inserts in planetary ball mills (0.7–12.8 mg/batch) [146]. However, these miniaturized milling tests can only be applied for screening formulations, especially stabilizing additives. It has to be noted that the milling results cannot be transferred to real stirred media mills, among others due to different grinding media motion and API solubility.

As stated above, based on the patent of nanosystems/*Élan* and subsequent work, a remarkable number of products have been developed and brought to the market. In chapter "Commercial manufacturing of nano-drug delivery systems" as well as in Section 9.3.3, a table of commercial products, that is, based on nano ground API are given. Moreover, for two APIs and products, respectively, a detailed description of the production and formulation processes is given at the end of this chapter.

Overall it can be concluded, that stirred media milling is a very effective process to decrease particle sizes to the submicron- and nanosize range, even for coarse primary particles, and has several advantages to yield drug nanoparticles as it is applicable even for very poorly soluble compounds (brick dust), appropriate to administration, scale-able from mg- to kg-scale and flexible regarding dosage forms [125]. Important is to use appropriate formulations along the entire process chain especially for stabilization of the very finely ground API particles against agglomeration and recrystallization.

However, main drawback can be agglomeration, product contamination due to wear of grinding media (especially if ceramic grinding media are applied), and recrystallization during milling or, more likely, during storage as a suspension (Ostwald-ripening). Issues regarding wear are to be addressed on two levels, optimizing the process parameters to reduce wear production (as mentioned above) as well as efficient control strategies for wear including suitable analytical methods to safely quantify wear in products.

High-Pressure Homogenization

In general, high-pressure homogenization is a well characterized and scalable process from lab to production scale as described for emulsions in Section 9.2.1.2. It can also be applied for particle deagglomeration and apparent comminution to a certain extent. Other than in emulsification, there is no deducible rule on which properties of the starting material the comminution success of the process relies. Smallest achievable particle sizes reported for HPH in the literature scatter stronger than those reported for wet media milling [137], indicating less reliable process success and worse predictability. In contrast to its extensive use, HPH also brings along the risk of infringing chemical as well as physical stability by high energy input and high local heat that can especially be attributed to cavitation [165].

Regarding the production method, different types of HPH geometries can be applied. Primarily, a differentiation between radial diffusor valves such as piston-gap homogenizers (Section 9.2.1.2) and microfluidic, static channels can be drawn. Comminution efficiency in HPH processes crucially depends on the disruption principle. It was shown that, at least for hard materials, the microfluidization principle with shear as main stressing principle is likely to lead to larger particle sizes compared with piston-gap homogenizers, in which cavitation and impact are supposed to be the main sources of stress [166].

The first patent for HPH in drug comminution was filed in 1994 for a process named Dissocubes® developed by Müller and co-workers, applying a piston-gap homogenizer (Table 9.4, [167]). The trade name of this process is supposed to describe the resulting product as API nanoparticles with a cubic morphology. A further development of piston-gap HPH is the Nanopure® process developed by PharmaSol, now Abbott (Table 9.4, [124]). The process describes the production of API nanoparticles by HPH in nonaqueous media or media with reduced water content. This provides the advantage to extend the working range to lower temperatures to avoid chemical degradation of sensitive APIs. By using media with low vapor pressure, cavitation in homogenization valves can be reduced or completely suppressed. Additionally, it is proposed that the use of other solvents can facilitate subsequent drying processes. Polyethylene glycols of adequate molecular weight are solid under ambient conditions and can be applied as suspension media for HPH in molten state in the Nanopure® process. The resulting suspensions can be filled into capsules or be allowed to solidify and be ground to powder for further processing.

The insoluble drug delivery particles pocess (IDD-P®, owned by SkyePharma, Table 9.4) makes use of the microfluidic HPH principle. In this method, filed in 2000, the Microfluidizer® technology (Microfluidics) is applied as particle size reduction step. In the microfluidic processor, the pressurized product stream is split up into two channels that redirect the flow to collide frontally (Figure 9.2 b) to achieve high energy input by shear forces.

Nearly all marketed products with drug API nanoparticles comprise media milling in their production process. The use of HPH for industrial production of drug nanosuspensions is scarce. Nonetheless, Triglide®, a marketed oral nano formulation of fenofibrate, is produced via high-pressure homogenization using SkyePharma Canada Inc.'s patented IDD-P®. Triglide® entered the market in 2005, 1 year later than its competitive product Tricor®, comminuted by stirred media milling. Both products showed bioequivalence and provide the advantage of food-independent administration [168]. Contrarily, non-nanosized fenofibrate products show a distinct food effect that increases the low bioavailability by 35% in fed state compared with fasted state.

HPH is in general less prone to wear and erosion compared with wet media milling processes. Most parts of pharmaceutically applicable homogenizers are preferably made of steel. Nonetheless, ceramics as well as industrial diamonds are more wear-resistant alternatives for high-throughput processes. In accordance to "Stirred Media Milling," suitable analytical methods must be chosen for each possible contaminant. The main mechanism of wear production in HPH is cavitation. For iron as one likely contaminant it was proved that the concentration of iron in suspension does not exceed 1 ppm, even causing no toxicological risk for parenteral applications [169].

For certain compounds, high-pressure homogenization may cause structural changes of the API. In a case study, the pressure drop dependent polymorphic transition of an anticancer compound was demonstrated. At higher pressure drops, even the formation of a hydrate of the compound was detected [170]. In this case, no adverse toxicity effects were detected for the nanoparticulate hydrate form. In contrary, an improved tolerance was proved and only that enabled pharmacokinetic studies. Nonetheless, such structural changes may interfere with stability for other APIs or cause toxicological issues.

Kocbek *et al.* adapted melt-emulsification, which originates from the production of lipidic drug carriers, for API nanoparticle production [171]. Prerequisite for this method is a low melting temperature of the API below the boiling temperature of water as external phase. In detail, the API is molten and processed as liquid disperse phase in a continuous aqueous phase containing stabilizers/emulsifiers. Droplet disruption is commonly achieved by HPH at elevated temperature. Cooling the hot emulsion is supposed to trigger the crystallization of API droplets to solid API nanoparticles. Melt-emulsification combines the advantages of emulsification (i.e., well characterized, reproducible results, higher efficiency compared to HPH "comminution") with the avoidance of organic solvents (i.e., residues, elevated solubility, and Ostwald ripening).

A hybrid of top-down and buttom-up processes is the emulsion–diffusion method. Herein, the API is solved in an organic solvent that is practically immiscible with water. This phase is emulsified into a commonly stabilizer/emulsifier-containing aqueous solution and homogenized (top-down) to a suitable droplet size. Afterward, the organic solvent diffuses through the water and is evaporated at its liquid–gas interface. Accordingly, the droplets shrink, increasing the concentration of the API that finally precipitates (bottom-up) and remains as a solid API particle in the aqueous phase [171].

9.3.1.2 Bottom-Up Processes

Processes in which the final particle size is reached starting from molecular disperse systems (solutions) are defined as bottom-up processes. Herein, precipitation and crystallization are essential processes that are anyhow necessary to supply the API from its synthesis (mostly in solution) to formulation production in a solid state (as a powder). Accordingly, this interface between synthesis and formulation can be used for particle engineering to meet the criteria necessary for successful drug delivery such as nanoparticulate size. Nonetheless, such methods are not applied in the production of commercialized pharmaceuticals to our knowledge.

Most applied are antisolvent precipitation methods in which the API is dissolved in an organic solvent that is injected into an aqueous stabilizer solution. The use of nonaqueous solvents and their potential residues may, apart from toxicological issues, also infringe the physical and chemical stability of nanosuspensions as they act as cosolvents and may facilitate higher solubility of the API and, by that, Ostwald ripening. In the precipitation processes, nucleation is difficult to be controlled and the products are mostly metastable amorphous nanoparticles that hold the risk of spontaneous crystallization.

The Hydrosol® technology was developed by Sucker and co-workers from Sandoz, later Novartis [172] (Table 9.4). The technique is based on a antisolvent precipitation in static mixers. The resulting particle sizes were 100–200 nm for amorphous particles directly after precipitation. Dependent on the stabilizers used, the amorphous particles are stable over a short period of time (minutes to hours) until crystallization and particle growth occurs. Accordingly, freeze- or spray-drying directly after precipitation are necessary to retain the nanodisperse state. Nanomorph® developed by Knoll/BASF (later Soliqs/Abbott, Table 9.4) is an analogues precipitation method that deliberately concentrates on the production of amorphous API nanoparticles [173].

Other Methods Controlled crystallization during freeze-drying was investigated by de Waard *et al.* [174]. It combines particle generation and drying in a combined process step and directly yields a dry products that can readily be further processed to capsules or tablets. For this method, an aqueous mannitol solution was mixed with a fenofibrate solution in *tert*-butyl alcohol and frozen applying different rates prior to freeze-drying. Higher concentrations of the matrix builder mannitol as well as higher freezing rates resulted in quicker dissolution of the

API from direct compressed tablets (100% release after 10 min compared with less than 30% for physical mixture). Accordingly, it is deduced that with more matrix builder and high freezing rate smaller API particle sizes result and that these remain physically stabilized during the compaction process. The method was further developed and scaled up to better meet industrial needs by mixing the two liquids in a 3-way nozzle directly prior to atomization by compressed air [175]. The resulting droplets were directly sprayed into liquid nitrogen to facilitate very high freezing rates prior to common batch lyophilization. This process allows semicontinuous production and further improves the product by apparently reducing API particle sizes and increasing release rates as compared with the batch process.

Further investigational methods for bottom-up manufacturing of API nanoparticles such as flash nanoprecipitation, microfluidic reaction technologies, emulsion diffusion techniques, rapid expansion of supercritical solution, and other methods are comprehensively compiled in a review of Cheow *et al.* [140]. Nonetheless, these methods do not possess industrial relevance until today.

9.3.1.3 Hybrid/Combinative Methods

If particle size reduction of APIs to a certain fineness, necessary to efficiently improve bioavailability, is not achievable with a single process, the combination of multiple processes to a process chain is often promising. Additionally, the risk of clogging, the need for recirculation, and relatively long process times in HPH as well as WMM can be seen as motivation for the development of combinative processes that comprise methods to alter the initial API structure to a more fragile one [137].

Antisolvent Precipitation and Subsequent HPH The first patented approach for antisolvent precipitation followed by HPH was NanoEdge® developed by Baxter (Table 9.4). After the precipitation, the nanosuspension is treated in a high-energy process (e.g., HPH) as an annealing step to prevent particle growth [124]. Annealing in this case describes the repeated application of energy input to foster the transition of matter from a thermodynamically unstable, amorphous to a stable, crystalline form.

A further developed approach is described by Sinha *et al.* as cavi-precipitation, combining antisolvent precipitation and high-pressure homogenization as a directly subsequent process chain without lag time between the processes [176]. They demonstrate (for ibuprofen in isopropanol into aqueous solution of 0.1%m/V hydroxypropyl methylcellulose and 0.2%m/V sodium dodecyl sulfate) that cavi-precipitation leads to smaller particle sizes compared with the decoupled process combination (separated processes, comparable to NanoEdge®) or high-pressure homogenization only. However, this process chain cannot be applied as a continuous process as the presented results were yielded by 10 cycles of homogenization subsequent to the initial cycle of precipitation/homogenization.

Spray-Drying and Subsequent HPH H42 technology is part of the SmartCrystals® technology family developed by Pharmasol and acquired by Abbott, marketed by Soliqs (Table 9.4, [177]). It describes the process chain of spray-drying the API prior to a particle size reduction step by HPH. Spray-drying is applied in order to improve API processability by yielding fragile API structures that are more prone to deagglomeration and deaggregation processes, achievable by HPH.

Freeze-Drying and Subsequent HPH or Media Milling Another process combination of the SmartCrystals® technology platform is the so-called H69 technology (Table 9.4, [178]). In analogy to H42, the API structure is altered by freeze-drying (instead of spray-drying) to yield a fragile structure, susceptible to deaggregation in subsequent HPH.

The combination of lyophilization of amphotericin B from DMSO solution and subsequent high-pressure homogenization (8 cycles at 1500 bar) led to particle sizes as small as 65 nm [179]. These results demonstrate that pretreatment of the starting API by freeze-drying leads to brittle structures (sponge-like) that can more easily be broken down than the raw material, for example, from crystallization. In tests of the combination of freeze-drying with either HPH or media milling as comminution methods, even a very basic, low-energy milling approach led to clearly smaller particle sizes than HPH (MM: 100–200 nm, HPH: >500 nm). With regard to efficiency, pretreatment/modification of morphology via freeze-drying proved to reduce the milling time from 24 h for untreated to 1 h for modified API [180].

Other Methods The combination of two top-down methods, namely stirred media milling with subsequent HPH, was first described and patented as combination technology (CT) by Abbott (marketed by Soliqs under the SmartCrystals® platform [177], Table 9.4, [181]). Such approaches were scientifically studied by Martena *et al.*, comparing the influence of different sequence orders of stirred media milling and high-pressure homogenization with the sole processes [182]. They showed that for the model API nicergoline, particle sizes smaller than 500 nm were exclusively achieved by stirred media milling. After high-pressure homogenization for 30 cycles at a pressure drop of 1500 bar, particle sizes of approx. 600 nm were reached. Subsequent application of stirred media milling drastically reduced the particle size within 15 min to approx. 300 nm. Interestingly, dissolution experiments showed that the application of HPH is the crucial influence to drastically improve dissolution as high-pressure homogenization (600 nm) clearly demonstrated the quickest and most complete dissolution [182]. However, no appropriate explanations for these phenomena was provided and still in-depth understanding is necessary to create models that predict dissolution success by taking all crucial parameters apart from particle size into account.

9.3.2
Drying Methods and Further Processing

In formulation development, stabilization of the colloidal size of the API particles during drying is of utmost importance to maintain improved dissolution properties in the final product. Accordingly, matrix builders are added to separate the API nanoparticles during and after drying to prevent agglomeration and aggregation due to sintering. Mostly sugars (sucrose, lactose, and mannitol) as well as cellulose derivatives are applied as matrix builders or redispersants. These redispersants can possibly act as stabilizers in preceding milling steps or may be added to the suspension after comminution.

A suitable drying process for API nanosuspensions must primarily fulfill the challenge to not (or to the lowest possible extent) alter the advantages that were adjusted in the comminution step, meaning not to change the particle size after redispersion. Accordingly, redispersibility of drug nanoparticles from solid dosage forms is to be checked in neutral as well as acidic media, mimicking disintegration in liquids outside and in gastric fluid [183].

From the regulatory perspective, it is of utmost importance to conduct in-depth studies regarding the alteration of the biopharmaceutical profile (ADME: absorption, distribution, metabolism, and excretion of API in the human body) compared with solutions as well as to systematically prove the effect of physical properties (i.e. agglomeration, aggregation, and interface/surface) on these [184].

Screening of redispersants/matrix builders and stabilizers (polymeric as well as charged surfactants) can be performed in small-/lab-scale equipment such as fluidized bed processors (e.g., MiniGlatt, Glatt) or spray dryers (Büchi B-190, Büchi) [183].

For the comparison of freeze-drying and spray-drying, it was found that the API properties are more crucial than the drying type and conditions themselves. Especially the surface hydrophobicity as determined by the extent of adsorption of hydrophobic compounds (e.g., D-α-tocopherol polyethylene glycol 1000 succinate) correlated well with the agglomeration and reduced dissolution rates. In addition to that, log P was suggested as fairly correlating and easily accessible parameter during screening, while no correlation was found for other properties such as molecular weight, melting point, solubility, and density [185].

9.3.2.1 Freeze-Drying

Freeze-drying is a highly energy-intensive process that cannot be realized as a continuous process until today. Accordingly, its use in commercial production of pharmaceuticals is kept to a minimum if no other technique is capable of performing equally. There are numerous descriptions of freeze-drying as successful drying method to maintain the colloidal state of nanosuspension in their dried form [159] as well as extensive studies of the influencing factors of successful preservation of the nanodisperse state during freeze-drying [186–188]. Catalent also presented their fast-dissolving tablets platform Zydis®, which applies freeze-drying as key manufacturing step, as successful in maintaining the nanoparticulate state of previously ground APIs after tablet disintegration [189,190]. Nonetheless, no marketed product uses this technology so far. Additionally, freeze-drying can be applied as bottom-up method to initially generate API nanoparticles [174,175], as described in Section 9.3.1.2.

9.3.2.2 **Spray-Drying**

Compared with freeze-drying, spray-drying is a more energy-efficient conversion methods of liquid goods into solids that is also applicable as a continuous process. Nonetheless, the same care must be taken in the formulation and process parameter settings to stabilize the nanodisperse state of the API particles, avoiding agglomeration and aggregation while keeping the final product readily redispersible to overall facilitate a quick dissolution. Typically, sugars and polymers are used as matrix building excipients during the drying process, but also alternative, particulate excipients are investigated.

Spray-drying of cefixime nanosuspensions was successfully performed with mannitol, lactose, and sorbitol as matrix builders. The API:excipient ratio was varied for every excipient from 1:1 to 4:1 and stability was monitored over 6 month storage time. Results showed that stability was improved with higher fractions of excipients. At a ratio of 1:1, all excipients were equally successful in retaining the nanoparticulate state after spray-drying as well as after storage. Regarding the powder properties, spray-dried granules showed a distinctly improved flow behavior compared with untreated cefixime (as judged by Hausner ratio). Sorbitol additionally facilitated the highest supersaturation upon dissolution, making sorbitol the best matrix builder in this study [191].

Chaubal and Popescu showed that the addition of sodium deoxycholate as charged surfactant was crucial to avoid aggregation of API nanoparticles in spray-drying studies of itraconazole nanoparticles with different matrix materials (lactose, sucrose, and mannitol) and stabilizers (Poloxamer 188, Sodium deoxycholate). Additionally, a high enough concentration of matrix builder must be supplied to spatially avoid nanocrystal contact and to retain the nanodisperse form in the dried product [192].

The influence of process parameters of spray-drying on the critical attributes reconstituted particle size and yield was analyzed on a lab-scale spray dryer (Büchi B190). Indomethacin nanosuspension (1% (w/w)) was stabilized with a commercial stabilizer (Dowfax 2A1; 0.5% (w/w)) and no matrix-forming agent was added prior to drying, in this case. It was found that aspiration rate and feed rate of the suspension had a crucial influence on the yield, whereas the inlet temperature was the only significant influence factor on the reconstituted particle size after spray-drying [193].

Nekkanti *et al.* published a complete process chain comprising stirred media milling of a candesartan cilexetil nanosuspension stabilized with HPMC and SDS, spray-drying the resulting nanosuspension in a API:matrix builder ratio of 1:3.5 with mannitol and subsequent tableting in a blend with additional excipients. The spray-drying step yielded hardly increased particle sizes after redispersion. For final tablets, different disintegrants were studied, achieving an acceptable disintegration time as well as a very quick and high dissolution of the API in a discriminating dissolution test [194].

As in most cases a crystalline form of the API with a specific polymorph is favored due to stability issues, an amorphization during all production steps is to be excluded. In a classical process chain, combining stirred media milling with spray-drying, the cause of amorphization must be identified. It is commonly discussed that comminution may cause surface amorphization that may lead to a completely amorphous matter as a function of process time and intensity. This is preferentially true for dry comminution processes. In wet media milling, the dispersion medium, in most cases water, acts as a plasticizer for short-term amorphous matter. By that, the glass transition temperature of the amorphous API is lowered and the relaxation to the crystalline state is favored [195–197]. In contrast to milling, spray-drying – especially of nanoparticle suspensions with polymers as matrix formers – may more probably lead to amorphous fractions of the API. During the drying process, API nanoparticles and polymer get into close contact and realize large contact areas. For many APIs, high solids solubilities in certain polymers exist and facilitates the formation of amorphous regions of solid API solutions around crystalline API cores [198].

This additional amorphization effect based on partial solid solutions may improve dissolution rates in addition to the particle size reduction (surface enlargement), but it may also infringe stability and shelf life of such pharmaceuticals. It challenges stability due to spontaneous recrystallization causing API aggregation and alteration of the dissolution profile. Accordingly, matrix formers and process conditions must carefully be chosen according to API properties to avoid the formation of undesired regions of solid solutions.

In addition to usual polymeric and sugar matrix builders, van Eerdenbrugh *et al.* studied alternative stabilizing principles for different APIs by either particulate excipients, applying hydrophobized silica, microcrystalline cellulose, and dibasic calcium phosphate or a surface-active (soluble) inulin derivative (Inutec® SP1) [199]. They found that a high specific surface area of particulate excipient as well as a uniform distribution of APIs in the spray-dried product, determined by EDX in SEM analysis, lead to quick dissolution profiles. Accordingly, hydrophobic silica were identified most efficient among particulate (insoluble) excipients due to high specific surface area, but the most efficient and robust matrix builder was the surface-active Inulin derivative. This high efficiency, which was also traced back to a highly homogeneous distribution of API in SEM-EDX, is apparently caused by the improvement of wetting of the particle surface as well as partial formation of solid solutions as previously described by van den Mooter *et al.* [200].

Dolenc *et al.* investigated the direct compaction of spray-dried nanosuspensions of celecoxibe admixed with microcrystalline cellulose (1:3; plus 2% magnesium stearate) to tablets [201]. It was found that the same compaction pressures resulted in higher tensile strengths of tablets containing nanofine compared with micronized API. This behavior was attributed to the higher specific surface area and bond number for nanosized API particles. The comparison of tablets with approximately the same tensile strength showed that the dissolution of nanoparticle-loaded tablets was drastically accelerated (approx. 55% in 10 min compared with approx. 10% for micronized API).

Liversidge *et al.* took care of whole process chains from starting material to finished tablets with quicker dissolution and reduced food effect for naproxen [202]. Their process chain comprised nanogrinding in a stirred media mill and spray-drying in all cases. Afterward, alternatively, the spray-dried powder was either directly tableted or roller compacted, granulated, tableted, and the tablets were coated. The new tablets were compared with a marketed formulation and showed, in either case, shorter dissolution and quicker bioavailability in combination with less variability in absorption rate as well as reduced fed-fasted differences.

9.3.2.3 **Spray-Coating, Granulation, and Pelletization**

As an alternative conversion method to solid intermediates, spray-coating of excipient particles can be applied as drying method for API nanosuspensions. This method provides the advantage of using the initial surface of excipient particle as a template for coating nanoparticle suspensions that are dried to layers surrounding a readily soluble core. Nonetheless, the maximum API concentration achievable in such intermediates is distinctly lower than for spray-dried products.

In examples from the literature, sugar beads were coated in a fluidized bed approach layer by layer with hydrocortisone acetate nanoparticles and, subsequently, enteric coating. Accelerated drug release from beads coated with nanosuspension instead of microsuspension was shown [203]. Also a study of binders is provided by Möschwitzer and Müller [204]. They additionally investigate the extrusion of a lactose impregnated with an API nanosuspension. In their case, extruded matrix pellets showed a clearly quicker *in-vitro* release rate than the layered pellets produced by spray-coating.

In process development, the process parameters of the coating apparatus are crucial. In fluidized bed coaters, the establishment and maintenance of a suitable and well-mixed fluidized bed as well as the generation of a homogeneous, fine-droplet spray are important to achieve intra- and interparticulately homogeneous coatings. Decisive process parameters are the drying gas pressure/velocity, temperature, and device geometry as well as the spraying parameters such as type of nozzle, atomization gas flow rate/pressure, and suspension feed rate. Selected process parameters in spray coating of a naproxen and a proprietary compound nanosuspensions were studied by Figueroa *et al.* [205]. They showed that a top spray setup leads to a more porous coating layer (higher porosity, lower specific surface area, and lower bulk density), while a bottom spray setup showed very densely packed coatings, which, however, performed better in *in vivo studies* in beagle dogs (highest AUC). The structural changes were attributed to differences in drying behavior of atomized droplets in cocurrent and counter-current setups regarding the drying gas flow, taking the time before impact on the substrate particles, the drying, and the increase in viscosity into account.

Another example for spray-coating processes is the loading of lactose monohydrate particles with ketoconazole nanosuspension in a fluidized bed processor. A very good redispersibility was shown for these granules as particle size remained virtually unchanged (×10: 63 nm and 65 nm, ×50: 121 nm and 126 nm, and ×90: 242 nm and 239 nm in native and redispersed state, respectively) [206]. This approach in lab scale is comparable to the manufacturing process chain for Emend® described in Section 9.3.3.2. The only exception is that sucrose is additionally used as matrix builder to separate the API nanoparticles in the dried state in Emend®. This is not necessary for the ketoconazole preparation as with only HMPC (1:5 compared to the API) readily redispersible nanoparticulate coatings are yielded [206].

He *et al.* demonstrated that even food proteins (soybean protein isolate, whey protein isolate, and β-lactoglobulin) can be used to stabilize indomethacin nanosuspensions [207]. In combination with additional denatured proteins as well as PVP K30, nanosuspensions were coated onto nonpareil cores by fluid-bed coating. The resulting pellets showed good redispersibility of the nanoparticles and comparable, only slightly delayed (3 min), dissolution of the API compared to the nanosuspensions, which drastically improved as compared with the raw API crystals.

The API nanosuspension can be used as granulation liquid directly after the comminution process. In a model study, a nanosuspension of ibuprofen (stabilized by Tween 80 and PVP K25) yielded by melt emulsification was top-sprayed on a mixture of lactose and microcrystalline cellulose (7:3) [171]. The resulting granules showed a drastically improved *in vitro* release (79% released after 10 min compared with 6% for micronized ibuprofen). Another study applied a nanosuspension of lutein (5% (w/w) stabilized with 2% (w/w) Plantacare® 2000 UP) directly as granulation liquid to form a paste from lactose powder that was subsequently dispersed through a sieve and spheronized [208]. The lutein release from capsules filled with theses pellets was drastically increased compared with coarse lutein powder (75 versus 23% after 30 min).

Bose *et al.* studied the effect of nanonization and conversion to solid dosage form by fluid-bed granulation on all levels from particle size over *in vitro* dissolution up to *in vivo* performance [209]. They found that the substrate for coating (mannitol or lactose) has an influence in dissolution rate and completeness as nanosuspensions coated on lactose only reached a steady state at approx. 70% *in vitro* drug release while coated mannitol provided approx. 100% release. *In vivo* (beagle dogs), the pharmacokinetic parameters were dramatically improved, elevating AUC Sixfold and c_{max} eightfold for the spray-granulated formulation compared with a coarse suspension of the API.

Another option of further processing of nanosuspensions to pellet systems is presented by Vergote *et al.* [210]. In their approach, previously spray-dried ketoprofen nanosuspensions were pelletized to sustained-release pellets by adding starch derivatives and microcrystalline wax in a temperature-controlled high-shear mixer (melt-granulation). Release rate and dissolution completeness were found adjustable by varying starch derivative contents as well as surfactant contents (either added to the nanosuspension or during pelletization). In further studies, such pellets were compressed to tablets and compared to uncompressed pellets in *in vivo* studies [211]. It was found that uncompressed pellets containing nanofine ketoprofen showed a pronounced (in this case undesired) burst release as compared to pellets containing microfine ketoprofen. By compression to tablets, both finenesses of ketoprofen particles showed practically identical plasma curves, reducing the burst release of nanofine particles. Nonetheless, the advantage of nanofine particles is rendered unimportant in specific application.

In summary, there are many applicable ways to convert nanosuspensions into dry powders while retaining the advantages of the nanodisperse state. The decision for a suitable method may be based on characteristics of the API to be formulated (e.g., solubility and hydrophobicity), requirements toward the final dosage form (e.g., dissolution profile, type of dosage form, and spectrum of dose strengths), and also on the availability of process equipment as well as process and energy efficiency.

9.3.2.4 Other Conversion Methods

Nanoextrusion is one promising new approach to yield solid products with incorporated, nanodisperse API. For this approach, a pharmaceutically and procedurally applicable polymer (such as Soluplus) is molten in an extruder. A previously prepared, stabilized, aqueous nanosuspension is added as side feed into the extruder, degassing within the extruder to evaporate the water, extruded, and cooled to yield solid, direct tabletable granules that contain API nanoparticles in a dispersed, deagglomerated state [212]. One-step conversion of nanosuspension to dry product containing dispersed nanoparticles is accordingly feasible. The process was scaled from a lab-scale to an industrial-scale extruder and applied to phenytoin as a relevant API [213]. In that study, a synergetic effect of the nanodispersed state of the API and the solubility improvement of the polymer was show. Nonetheless, only API loading up to 4–5% (w/w) was demonstrated.

9.3.3
Marketed Products Containing Drug Nanoparticles

Nanopharmaceuticals containing API nanoparticles of poorly water-soluble drugs are already commercialized in a number of products since 2000 (Table 9.5). It is apparent that most marketed API nanoparticles are produced by wet ball milling and most of these are based on the Nanocrystals® method patented by Élan, now Alkermes (also see Section "Stirred Media Milling"). In addition to wet media milling, dry milling with excipients also leads to submicron API particle sizes (Solumatrix®) that improve drug dissolution is applied in marketed products (Table 9.5). Only one marketed product is produced by HPH in microsystems, making use of the IDD-P® technique. In contrast to the comminution

Table 9.5 Marketed products containing API nanoparticles [137,139–142,185,214].

Brand name	Drug substance	Drug delivery platform	Comminution process	Company	Dosage form	Year
Rapamune™	Sirolimus	Elan/Alkermes	WBM	Wyet/Pfizer	Tablet	2000
Emend™	Aprepitant	Elan/Alkermes	WBM	Merck & Co	Capsule	2003
Tricor™	Fenofibrat	Abbott	WBM	Abbott	Tablet	2004
Megace™ ES	Megestrol	Elan/Alkermes	WBM	Par Pharmaceuticals	Oral suspension	2005
Triglide™	Fenofibrat	IDD-P®/SkyePharma	HPH	Sciele Pharma Inc.	Tablet	2005
Invega™ Sustenna (US)/Xeplion™ (EU)	Paliperidone palmitate	Elan/Alkermes	WBM	Janssen	i.m. suspension	2009
Invega™ Trinza (US)/Trevicta™ (EU)	Paliperidone palmitate	Elan/Alkermes	WBM	Janssen	i.m. suspension	2015
Zorvolex™	Diclofenac	iCeuticals	Dry milling with matrix	Iroko Pharmaceuticals	Capsule	2013
Tivorbex™	Indomethacin	iCeuticals	Dry milling with matrix	Iroko Pharmaceuticals	Capsule	2014

methods that are known for marketed products, the drying methods for the conversion into solid dosage form mostly remain proprietary knowledge of the manufacturer. Only for few products, information was disclosed and production process chains are described in detail below.

9.3.3.1 **Rapamune®**

In 2000, Rapamune® (former Wyeth, now Pfizer) was the first product in the market to apply pharmaceutical nanotechnology in a solid dosage form. Rapamune® are tablets containing nanoparticles of sirolimus, an immunosuppressant to prevent posttransplantational organ rejection. The manufacturing is based on a multitude of process steps. The nanosuspension is prepared by means of wet media milling in a stirred media mill with highly cross-linked polystyrene beads, applying the NanoCrystals® technology (Table 9.5, detailed discussion in Section "Stirred Media Milling"). Sirolimus is stabilized during this process with an excipient that is not explicitly disclosed. According to the list of inactive ingredients (Table 9.6), glycerol monooleate is likely to act as a stabilizer for these nanoparticles. In parallel, drug-free, inert tablet cores comprising lactose, ethylene glycol 8000, magnesium stearate, and talc are manufactured by direct compression. The API is applied to the tablet core as an active sugar coating. For different marketed strengths of Rapamune®, different multiple coatings are applied. As sirolimus may be degraded by oxidation, especially in the presence of iron ions (iron oxides as colorants), different precautions were taken: In early products, the active layer was coated with a thin sucrose sugar seal layer toward the final colorant layer. In later products, α-tocopherol was added to the active layer as true antioxidant and the sucrose seal layer was spared [215].

Table 9.6 Constituents of Rapamune® tablets [215].

Tablet cores	Coatings
Lactose monohydrate (diluent)	Nanosuspension (API + stabilizer)
Polyethylene glycol 8000 (binder)#	Ethylene glycol 20 000
Magnesium stearate (lubricant)	Glycerol monooleate
Talc (glidant)	Pharmaceutical glace (shellac)
	Calcium sulfate anhydrous
	Microcrystalline cellulose
	Sucrose
	Titanium dioxide
	Brown and yellow iron oxide
	alpha-tocopherol
	Povidone
	Carnauba wax
	Printing ink

Table 9.7 Constituents of Emend® capsules [216].

Capsule filling	Capsule shell
Microcrystalline cellulose (beads)	Gelatin
Hydroxypropyl cellulose	Titanium dioxide
Sucrose	Red and yellow iron oxides
Sodium dodecyl sulfate	Printing ink (shellac, potassium hydroxide, iron oxide)

Table 9.8 Main process steps in Emend® production [216].

Step	Operation
1	Production of a slurry of water, hydroxypropyl cellulose, and aprepitant
2	Premilling
3	Addition of an aqueous sodium lauryl sulfate dispersion
4	Media milling to form a colloidal dispersion
5	Addition of an aqueous sucrose dispersion
6	Spray-coating of microcrystalline cellulose beads with the colloidal dispersion
7	Sieving of the coated beads
8	Blending of coated beads with micronized sodium lauryl sulfate
9	Encapsulation of the blended beads

9.3.3.2 **Emend®**

Emend® was the second marketed product containing drug nanoparticles in 2001. It contains aprepitant as an API indicated to reduce nausea and prevent vomiting, especially under chemotherapy. As in the case of Rapamune®, aprepitant is comminuted by stirred media milling using Nanocrystals® technology. Emend® is provided as capsules filled with beads of microcrystalline cellulose that are active-coated with drug nanoparticles (see excipients in Table 9.7). The coating suspension additionally contains sodium dodecyl sulfate (stabilizer), sucrose (matrix-forming agent), and hydroxypropyl cellulose (stabilizer, matrix-forming agent, and binder). The manufacturing process is described as presented in Table 9.8 [216].

9.4 Industrial Status and Framework

Nanoscience and nanotechnology have already adopted to pharmaceutical research and development with some successfully commercialized nanosized products for applications in therapeutics and diagnosis [142,168,217]. Looking at recent reports and scientific publications as a broader reference, the terminology "nanomedicine" has become more or less established within the above mentioned context, including the evolvement of a patient oriented definition [74,218] considering the complex, interdisciplinary and dynamic area in pharmaceutical research and development.

The development of nanomedicine products for therapeutic and diagnostic applications is often driven by startups, and small- to medium-sized companies, in spite of huge costs for research and development [219,220]. Evidence shows that small- to medium-sized companies are seldom successful in research and development of nanomedicines [219,220], reflected by the limited number of commercialized nanomedicine products [142,168,217,221]. Failure in clinical development and corresponding losses of development costs can be considered as substantial obstacle for the successful commercialization of nanomedicine products by small- to medium-sized companies [219,220]. In general, huge development costs need to be financed over a period of about a decade just like for conventional drug development.

The development and research of nanomedicine products with a commercially profitable lifecycle is considered more challenging, compared to the drug development of conventional drug products, taking into account the following specific aspects:

- Chemical and pharmaceutical profiling at the early stage of drug development regarding safety [221–224] and efficacy [217,225].
- Rational formulation design [226,227].
- Scalability of manufacturing technologies from lab to commercial scale [221,228].
- Investment risks associated with newly required manufacturing technologies.
- Quality control and related strategy for the manufacturing of intermediates and final products [229–231].
- Evolving regulatory framework across the different agencies [121,232–236].
- Limited protection of intellectual property [237–240].
- Limited acceptance by, for example, the public and governmental agencies [241,242].

Nevertheless, several nanomedicine therapeutic products were successfully developed and launched with positive cash flow for the individual companies to provide a positive return on investment over its product lifecycle, such as for Abraxane® (paclitaxel), Doxil® (doxorubicin), Invega® Sustenna®/Xeplion® and Invega® Trinza®/Trevicta® (all paliperidone palmitate), and Tricor® (fenofibrate). Interestingly, nanomedicine products may provide an extended positive cash flow after the expiry of the innovator product patent, due to regulatory challenges to assure patients' benefit and safety of generic "follow-on" products [14,220,233,243].

9.5
Perspectives for Academia, Industry, and Regulatory Authorities

Major effort has been conducted by government programs for a wide variety of countries and continents, despite substantial challenges that impede the technical and clinical development of nanomedicine products [244]. However, the success rate and the number of successful commercialized nanomedicine products are rather limited, compared to conventional drug product applications within the same time frame. Open meetings are continuously organized between academia, industry, and regulatory bodies (e.g., the European Foundation for Clinical Nanomedicine; www.clinam.org) to facilitate the better understanding of the current science and investigative approaches and to identify the key gaps in nanomedicine development programs [245,246]. Governmental programs are now striving from initially more pure science-based research to more applied-based research and development to facilitate the translation into nanomedicine products of commercial and public benefit [244,247–250]. The programs are aiming to address industrial like technical and clinical development processes, decision points, while balancing costs for development, cost of goods and likely income during commercialization with special consideration on the following aspects:

- Focus on unmet medical needs where nanomedicine can make the difference compared to conventional options.
- Collaboration between academia with diverse background, small- to medium-sized companies, industry, clinicians, and regulatory bodies.
- Training, review, and support from industrial partners to ensure professional structures.

In particular, manufacturing technologies for nanomedicine products need to be improved to a technology readiness level to ensure that the product is scalable and ready to meet good manufacturing practice (GMP) standards to properly fulfill the highly regulated area regarding manufacturing and control [244,247–250]. Global healthcare providers should be able to take further the lead to deliver the nanomedicine product to the patient and the market.

References

1 Wretlind, A. (1981) Development of fat emulsions. *JPEN J. Parenter. Enteral. Nutr.*, **5**, 230–235.

2 Hippalgaonkar, K., Majumdar, S., and Kansara, V. (2010) Injectable lipid emulsions – advancements, opportunities and challenges. *AAPS PharmSciTech.*, **11**, 1526–1540.

3 Hansrani, P.K., Davis, S.S., and Grovers, M.J. (1983) The preparation and properties of sterile intravenous emulsions. *J. Parenter. Sci. Technol.*, **37**, 145–150.

4 Yamaguchi, T., Nishizaki, K., Itai, S., Hayashi, H., and Ohshima, H. (1995) Physicochemical characterization of parenteral lipid emulsion: influence of cosurfactants on flocculation and coalescence. *Pharm. Res.*, **12**, 1273–1278.

5 Mikrut, B. (2005) Case study: formulation of an intravenous fat emulsion, in *Injectable Dispersed Systems*, (ed. D.J. Burgess), Taylor & Francis, Boca Raton, pp. 415–425.

6 Klang, S. and Benita, S. (1998) Design and evaluation of submicron emulsions as colloidal drug carriers for intravenous administration, in *Submicron Emulsions in Drug Targeting and Delivery*,

(ed. S. Benita), Harwood Academic Publishers, Amsterdam, pp. 119–152.
7 Alskär, L.C., Porter, C.J.H., and Bergström, C.A.S. (2016) Tools for early prediction of drug loading in lipid-based formulations. *Mol. Pharm.*, **13**, 251–261.
8 Medizinische Medien Informations GmbH (ed.) Gelbe Liste Pharmindex. www.gelbe-liste.de. Accessed April 14, 2016.
9 O'Hagan, D.T. (2007) MF59 is a safe and potent vaccine adjuvant that enhances protection against influenza virus infection. *Expert Rev. Vaccines*, **6**, 699–710.
10 Collins-Gold, L.C., Lyons, R.T., and Bartholow, L.C. (1990) Parenteral emulsions for drug delivery. *Adv. Drug Deliv. Rev.*, **5**, 189–208.
11 Floyd, A.G. (1999) Top ten considerations in the development of parenteral emulsions. *Pharm. Sci. Technolo. Today*, **2**, 134–143.
12 Driscoll, D.F. (2006) Lipid injectable emulsions: pharmacopeial and safety issues. *Pharm. Res.*, **23**, 1959–1969.
13 Berger, T. (2005) Case study: a lipid emulsion – sterilization, in *Injectable Dispersed Systems*, (ed. D.J. Burgess), Taylor & Francis, Boca Raton, pp. 393–413.
14 Barenholz, Y. (2012) Doxil® – the first FDA-approved nano-drug: lessons learned. *J. Control. Release*, **160**, 117–134.
15 Walstra, P. and Smulders, P.E.A. (1998) Chapter 2. Emulsion formation, in *Modern Aspects of Emulsion Science*, (ed. B.P. Binks), Royal Society of Chemistry, Cambridge, pp. 56–99.
16 Santana, R.C., Perrechil, F.A., and Cunha, R.L. (2013) High- and low-energy emulsifications for food applications: a focus on process parameters. *Food Eng. Rev.*, **5**, 107–122.
17 McClements, D.J. (2016) Emulsion formation, in *Food Emulsions: Principles, Practices, and Techniques*, 3rd edn, CRC Press, Boca Raton, pp. 245–288.
18 Floury, J., Bellettre, J., Legrand, J., and Desrumaux, A. (2004) Analysis of a new type of high pressure homogeniser. A study of the flow pattern. *Chem. Eng. Sci.*, **59**, 843–853.
19 Håkansson, A., Trägårdh, C., and Bergenståhl, B. (2009) Dynamic simulation of emulsion formation in a high pressure homogenizer. *Chem. Eng. Sci.*, **64**, 2915–2925.
20 Raikar, N.B., Bhatia, S.R., Malone, M.F., McClements, D.J., Almeida-Rivera, C., Bongers, P., and Henson, M.A. (2010) Prediction of emulsion drop size distributions with population balance equation models of multiple drop breakage. *Colloids Surf. A Physicochem. Eng. Asp.*, **361**, 96–108.
21 Håkansson, A., Fuchs, L., Innings, F., Revstedt, J., Bergenståhl, B., and Trägårdh, C. (2010) Visual observations and acoustic measurements of cavitation in an experimental model of a high-pressure homogenizer. *J. Food Eng.*, **100**, 504–513.
22 Kelemen, K., Gepperth, S., Koch, R., Bauer, H.-J., and Schuchmann, H.P. (2015) On the visualization of droplet deformation and breakup during high-pressure homogenization. *Microfluid. Nanofluidics*, **19**, 1139–1158.
23 Gothsch, T., Schilcher, C., Richter, C., Beinert, S., Dietzel, A., Büttgenbach, S., and Kwade, A. (2015) High-pressure microfluidic systems (HPMS): flow and cavitation measurements in supported silicon microsystems. *Microfluid. Nanofluidics*, **18**, 121–130.
24 Stang, M., Schuchmann, H.P., and Schubert, H. (2001) Emulsification in high-pressure homogenizers. *Eng. Life Sci.*, **1**, 151–157.
25 Floury, J., Legrand, J., and Desrumaux, A. (2004) Analysis of a new type of high pressure homogeniser. Part B. study of droplet break-up and recoalescence phenomena. *Chem. Eng. Sci.*, **59**, 1285–1294.
26 Rooze, J., André, M., van der Gulik, G.-J. S., Fernández-Rivas, D., Gardeniers, J.G.E., Rebrov, E.V., Schouten, J.C., and Keurentjes, J.T.F. (2012) Hydrodynamic cavitation in micro channels with channel sizes of 100 and 750 micrometers. *Microfluid. Nanofluidics*, **12**, 499–508.
27 Finke, J.H., Niemann, S., Richter, C., Gothsch, T., Kwade, A., Büttgenbach, S.,

and Müller-Goymann, C.C. (2014) Multiple orifices in customized microsystem high-pressure emulsification: the impact of design and counter pressure on homogenization efficiency. *Chem. Eng. J.*, **248**, 107–121.

28 Schlender, M., Minke, K., Spiegel, B., and Schuchmann, H.P. (2015) High-pressure double stage homogenization processes: influences of plant setup on oil droplet size. *Chem. Eng. Sci.*, **131**, 162–171.

29 Ott, G., Barchfield, G.L., Chernoff, D., Radhakrishnan, R., van Hoogevest, P., and van Nest, G. (1995) MF59: design and evaluation of a safe and potent adjuvant for human vaccines, in *Vaccine Design*, (eds M.F. Powell and M.J. Newman), Plenum Press, New York, pp. 277–296.

30 Ott, G., Radhakrishnan, R., Fang, J.-H., and Hora, M. (2000) The adjuvant MF59: a 10-year-perspecitve, in *Vaccine Adjuvants*, (ed. D.T. O'Hagan), Humana Press, Totowa, NJ, pp. 211–228.

31 Lee, L. and Norton, I.T. (2013) Comparing droplet breakup for a high-pressure valve homogeniser and a Microfluidizer for the potential production of food-grade nanoemulsions. *J. Food Eng.*, **114**, 158–163.

32 Sharma, A. and Sharma, U.S. (1997) Liposomes in drug delivery: progress and limitations. *Int. J. Pharm.*, **154**, 123–140.

33 Pattni, B.S., Chupin, V.V., and Torchilin, V.P. (2015) New developments in liposomal drug delivery. *Chem. Rev.*, **115**, 10938–10966.

34 Bangham, A.D. (1993) Liposomes: the Babraham connection. *Chem. Phys. Lipids*, **64**, 275–285.

35 Gregoriadis, G. (1976) The carrier potential of liposomes in biology and medicine I. *N. Engl. J. Med.*, **295**, 704–710.

36 Gregoriadis, G. (1976) The carrier potential of liposomes in biology and medicine II. *N. Engl. J. Med.*, **295**, 765–770.

37 Lasic, D.D. (1993) Chemistry of lipids and liposomes, in *Liposomes: From Physics to Applications*, Elsevier Science Ltd, Amsterdam, New York, pp. 9–42.

38 U.S. Food and Drug Administration (ed.) Drugs@FDA. FDA Approved Drug Products. www.accessdata.fda.gov/scripts/cder/drugsatfda/index.cfm. Accessed April 2016.

39 European Medicines Agency (ed.) European public assessment reports. www.ema.europa.eu/ema/index.jsp?curl=/pages/medicines/landing/epar_search.jsp&mid=WC0b01ac058001d124. Accessed April 2016.

40 Gilead. Product approval timeline. www.gilead.com/medicines/product-approval-timeline. Accessed April 2016.

41 Thepharmaletter (1993) First approval for amphocil. www.thepharmaletter.com/article/first-approval-for-amphocil.

42 Hillery, A.M. (1997) Supramolecular lipidic drug delivery systems: From laboratory to clinic. A review of the recently introduced commercial liposomal and lipid-based formulations of amphotericin B. *Adv. Drug Deliv. Rev.*, **24**, 345–363.

43 Datapharm (ed.) electronic Medicines Compendium. DaunoXome Injection 2mg/ml Concentrate for Solution for Infusion. www.medicines.org.uk/emc/medicine/27507. Accessed April 2016.

44 Kohli, A.G., Kierstead, P.H., Venditto, V.J., Walsh, C.L., and Szoka, F.C. (2014) Designer lipids for drug delivery: from heads to tails. *J. Control. Release*, **190**, 274–287.

45 New, R.R.C. (1990) Preparation of liposomes, in *Liposomes*, (ed. R.R.C. New), IRL Press, Oxford University Press, Oxford, New York, pp. 33–104.

46 Lasch, J., Weissig, V., and Brandl, M. (2003) Preparation of liposomes, in *Liposomes*, 2nd edn (eds V.P. Torchilin and V. Weissig), Oxford University Press, Oxford, New York, pp. 3–29.

47 Lasic, D.D. (1993) Industrial manufacturing of liposomes, in *Liposomes: From Physics to Applications*, Elsevier Science Ltd, Amsterdam, NY, pp. 517–542.

48 Lasic, D.D. (1993) Preparation of liposomes, in *Liposomes: From Physics to Applications*, Elsevier Science Ltd, Amsterdam, New York, pp. 63–107.

49 Naeff, R. (1996) Feasibility of topical liposome drugs produced on an industrial scale. *Adv. Drug Deliv. Rev.*, **18**, 343–347.

50 van Winden, E.C.A., Zuidam, N.J., and Crommelin, D.J.A. (1998) Strategies for large scale production and optimized stability of pharmaceutical liposomes developed for parenteral use, in *Medical Applications of Liposomes* (eds D.D. Lasic and D. Papahadjopoulos), Elsevier, Amsterdam, NY, pp. 567–604.

51 Wagner, A. and Vorauer-Uhl, K. (2011) Liposome technology for industrial purposes. *J. Drug Deliv.*, **2011**, 1–9.

52 Bangham, A.D. and Horne, R.W. (1964) Negative staining of phospholipids and their structural modification by surface-active agents as observed in the electron microscope. *J. Mol. Biol.*, **8**, 660–668.

53 Papahadjopoulos, D. and Watkins, J.C. (1967) Phospholipid model membranes. II. Permeability properties of hydrated liquid crystals. *Biochim. Biophys. Acta*, **135**, 639–652.

54 Hauser, H.O. (1971) The effect of ultrasonic irradiation on the chemical structure of egg lecithin. *Biochem. Biophys. Res. Commun.*, **45**, 1049–1055.

55 Freitas, S., Hielscher, G., Merkle, H.P., and Gander, B. (2006) Continuous contact- and contamination-free ultrasonic emulsification – a useful tool for pharmaceutical development and production. *Ultrason. Sonochem.*, **13**, 76–85.

56 Cullis, P.R. (2000) Commentary: liposomes by accident. *J. Lipos. Res.*, **10**, ix–xxiv.

57 Barenholz, Y., Amselem, S., and Lichtenberg, D. (1979) A new method for preparation of phospholipid vesicles (liposomes) – french press. *FEBS Lett.*, **99**, 210–214.

58 Mayhew, E.G., Lazo, R.O., Vail, W.J., King, J., and Green, A.M. (1984) Characterization of liposomes prepared using a microemulsifier. *Biochim. Biophys. Acta*, **775**, 169–174.

59 Brandl, M., Bachmann, D., Drechsler, M., and Bauer, K.H. (1990) Liposome preparation by a new high pressure homogenizer Gaulin Micron Lab 40. *Drug Dev. Ind. Pharm.*, **16**, 2167–2191.

60 Bachmann, D., Brandl, M., and Gregoriadis, G. (1993) Preparation of liposomes using a Mini-Lab 8.30 H high-pressure homogenizer. *Int. J. Pharm.*, **91**, 69–74.

61 Martin, F.J. (2005) Case Study: DOXIL, the development of pegylated liposomal doxorubicin, in *Injectable Dispersed Systems*, (ed. D.J. Burgess), Taylor & Francis, Boca Raton, pp. 427–480.

62 Olson, F.C., Hunt, C.A., Szoka, F.C., Vail, W.J., and Papahadjopoulos, D. (1979) Preparation of liposomes of defined size distribution by extrusion through polycarbonate membranes. *Biochim. Biophys. Acta*, **557**, 9–23.

63 Hope, M.J., Bally, M.B.W.G.J., and Cullis, P.R. (1985) Production of large unilamellar vesicles by a rapid extrusion procedure. Characterization of size distribution, trapped volume and ability to maintain a membrane potential. *Biochim. Biophys. Acta*, **812**, 55–65.

64 Schneider, T., Sachse, A., Röbling, G., and Brandl, M. (1994) Large-scale production of liposomes of defined size by a new continuous high pressure extrusion device. *Drug Dev. Ind. Pharm.*, **20**, 2787–2807.

65 Mui, B. and Hope, M.J. (2007) Formation of large unilamellar vesicles by extrusion, in *Liposome Technology. Volume I*, 3rd edn (ed. G. Gregoriadis), Informa Healthcare, New York, pp. 55–65.

66 Fenske, D.B. and Cullis, P.R. (2007) Encapsulation of drugs within liposomes by pH-gradient techniques, in *Liposome Technology*, 3rd edn (ed. G. Gregoriadis), Informa Healthcare, New York, pp. 27 50.

67 Clerc, S.G. and Thompson, T.E. (1994) A possible mechanism for vesicle formation by extrusion. *Biophys. J.*, **67**, 475–476.

68 Hunter, D.G. and Frisken, B.J. (1998) Effect of extrusion pressure and lipid properties on the size and polydispersity of lipid vesicles. *Biophys. J.*, **74**, 2996–3002.

69 Frisken, B.J., Asman, C., and Patty, P.J. (2000) Studies of vesicle extrusion. *Langmuir*, **16**, 928–933.

70 Bertrand, M. and Joós, B. (2012) Extrusion of small vesicles through nanochannels: a model for experiments

and molecular dynamics simulations. *Phys. Rev. E*, **85**, 051910.

71 Szoka, F. and Papahadjopoulos, D. (1978) Procedure for preparation of liposomes with large internal aqueous space and high capture by reverse-phase evaporation. *Proc. Natl. Acad. Sci. USA*, **75**, 4194–4198.

72 Brunner, J., Skrabal, P., and Hausser, H. (1976) Single bilayer vesicles prepared without sonication. Physico-chemical properties. *Biochim. Biophys. Acta*, **455**, 322–331.

73 Mimms, L.T., Zampighi, G., Nozaki, Y., Tanford, C., and Reynolds, J.A. (1981) Phospholipid vesicle formation and transmembrane protein incorporation using octyl glucoside. *Biochemistry*, **20**, 833–840.

74 Wagner, A., Platzgummer, M., Kreismayr, G., Quendler, H., Stiegler, G., Ferko, B., Vecera, G., Vorauer-Uhl, K., and Katinger, H. (2006) GMP production of liposomes – a new industrial approach. *J. Liposome Res.*, **16**, 311–319.

75 Batzri, S. and Korn, E.D. (1973) Single bilayer liposomes prepared without sonication. *Biochim. Biophys. Acta*, **298**, 1015–1019.

76 Pons, M., Foradada, M., and Estelrich, J. (1993) Liposomes obtained by the ethanol injection method. *Int. J. Pharm.*, **95**, 51–56.

77 Jahn, A., Vreeland, W.N., Gaitan, M., and Locascio, L.E. (2004) Controlled vesicle self-assembly in microfluidic channels with hydrodynamic focusing. *J. Am. Chem. Soc.*, **126**, 2674–2675, filed Feb. 27, 1987 and issued Apr. 18, 1989.

78 Jaafar-Maalej, C., Charcosset, C., and Fessi, H. (2011) A new method for liposome preparation using a membrane contactor. *J. Liposome Res.*, **21**, 213–220.

79 Adler-Moore, J.P. and Proffitt, R.T. (1993) Development, characterization, efficacy and mode of action of Ambisome, a unilamellar liposomal formulation of amphotericin B. *J. Liposome Res.*, **3**, 429–450.

80 Gamble, R.C. (1988) Method for preparing small vesicles using microemulsification. US Patent 4,753,788, field Jan. 31, 1985 and issued June 28, 1988.

81 Proffitt, R.T., Adler-Moore, J.P., and Chiang, S.-M. (1990) Amphotericin B liposome preparation. US Patent 6,770,290, filed Oct. 19, 1990 and issued Aug. 3, 2004.

82 Gilead (2012) AmBisome product information.

83 sigma-tau Pharmaceuticals (2013) Abelcet®: product information.

84 Janoff, A.S., Boni, L.T., Popescu, M.C., Minchey, S.R., Cullis, P.R., Madden, T.D., Taraschi, T.F., Grüner, S.M., Shyamsunder, E., Tate, M., Mendelsohn, R., and Bonner, D.P. (1988) Unusual lipid structures selectively reduce the toxicity of amphotericin B. *Proc. Natl. Acad. Sci. USA*, **85**, 6122–6126.

85 Janoff, A.S., Boni, L., Madden, T.D., Cullis, P.R., Lenk, R.P., Kearns, J.J., Durning, A.G., Klimchak, R., and Portnoff, J. (1997) Low toxicity drug-lipid systems. US Patent 5,616,334, filed Apr. 28, 1995 and issued Apr. 1, 1997.

86 Guo, L.S.S. (2001) Amphotericin B colloidal dispersion: an improved antifungal therapy. *Adv. Drug Deliv. Rev.*, **47**, 149–163.

87 Guo, L.S.S., Fielding, R.M., Lasic, D.D., Hamilton, R.L., and Mufson, D. (1991) Novel antifungal drug delivery: stable amphotericin B-cholesteryl sulfate discs. *Int. J. Pharm.*, **75**, 45–54.

88 Abra, R. (1989) Amphotericin B/cholesterol sulfate composition. US Patent 4,822,777.

89 EMA – European Medicines Agency. Visudyne: European public asessement report (2006) Scientific discussion. http://www.ema.europa.eu/docs/en_GB/document_library/EPAR_-_Scientific_Discussion/human/000305/WC500052403.pdf (accessed December 30, 2015).

90 Desai, N.R., Agha, B.J., and Kale, K.M. (2000) Liposome compositions of porphyrin photosensitizers. US Patent 6,074,666, filed June 13, 1995 and issued June 13, 2000.

91 Madden, T.D., Harrigan, P.R., Tai, L.C.L., Bally, M.B., Mayer, L.D., Redelmeier, T.E., Loughrey, H.C., Tilcock, C.P.S., Reinish,

L.W., and Cullis, P.R. (1990) The accumulation of drugs within large unilamellar vesicles exhibiting a proton gradient: a survey. *Chem. Phys. Lipids*, **53**, 37–46.

92 Barenholz, Y. (2007) Amphiphatic weak base loading into preformed liposomes having a transmembane ammonium ion gradient: from the bench to approved Doxil, in *Liposome Technology*, 3rd edn (ed. G. Gregoriadis), Informa Healthcare, New York, pp. 1–25.

93 Li, X., Hirsh, D.J., Cabral-Lilly, D., Zirkel, A., Gruner, S.M., Janoff, A.S., and Perkins, W.R. (1998) Doxorubicin physical state in solution and inside liposomes loaded via a pH gradient. *Biochim. Biophys. Acta*, **1415**, 23–40.

94 EMA – European Medicines Agency (2015) Myocet: European public asessement report.

95 U.S. Food and Drug Administration. – Marqibo® (vincristine sulfate liposome injection) for intravenous infusion (2012) Label Information. http://www.accessdata.fda.gov/drugsatfda_docs/label/2012/202497s000lbl.pdf (accessed February 27, 2016).

96 U.S. Food and Drug Administration (2012) Sponsor Briefing Document – Marqibo® (vincristine sulfate liposomes injection) for the treatment of advanced relapsed and/or refractory Philadelphoa chromosome negative (ph-) adult acute lymphoblastic leukemia, U.S. Food and Drug Administration.

97 Mantripragada, S. (2002) A lipid based depot (DepoFoam® technology) for sustained release drug delivery. *Prog. Lipid Res.*, **41**, 392–406.

98 Zuidam, N.J., Lee, S.S.L., and Crommelin, D.J.A. (1993) Sterilization of liposomes by heat treatment. *Pharm. Res.*, **10**, 1591–1596.

99 Zuidam, N.J., Lee, S.S.L., and Crommelin, D.J.A. (1995) Gamma-irradiation of non-frozen, frozen, and freeze-dried liposomes. *Pharm. Res.*, **12**, 1761–1768.

100 Zuidam, N.J., Versluis, C., Vernooy, E.A.A.M., and Crommelin, D.J.A. (1996) Gamma-irradiation of liposomes composed of saturated phospholipids. Effect of bilayer composition, size, concentration and absorbed dose on chemical degradation and physical destabilization of liposomes. *Biochim. Biophys. Acta*, **1280**, 135–148.

101 Lukyanov, A.N. and Torchilin, V.P. (1994) Autoclaving of liposomes. *J. Microencapsul.*, **11**, 669–672.

102 Toh, M.-R. and Chiu, G.N.C. (2013) Liposomes as sterile preparations and limitations of sterilisation techniques in liposomal manufacturing. *Asian J. Pharm. Sci.*, **8**, 88–95.

103 Tardi, C., Drechsler, M., Bauer, K.H., and Brandl, M. (2001) Steam sterilisation of vesicular phospholipid gels. *Int. J. Pharm.*, **217**, 161–172.

104 Goldbach, P., Brochart, H., Wehrlé, P., and Stamm, A. (1995) Sterile filtration of liposomes: retention of encapsulated carboxyfluorescein. *Int. J. Pharm.*, **117**, 225–230.

105 Xiaolin, T. and Pikal, M.J. (2004) Design of freeze-drying processes for pharmaceuticals: practical advice. *Pharm. Res.*, **21**, 191–200.

106 Kasper, J.C. and Friess, W. (2011) The freezing step in lyophilization: physico-chemical fundamentals, freezing methods and consequences on process performance and quality attributes of biopharmaceuticals. *Eur. J. Pharm. Biopharm.*, **78**, 248–263.

107 Chen, C., Han, D., Cai, C., and Tang, X. (2010) An overview of liposome lyophilization and its future potential. *J. Control. Release*, **142**, 299–311.

108 Ingvarsson, P.T., Yang, M., Nielsen, H.M., Rantanen, J., and Foged, C. (2011) Stabilization of liposomes during drying. *Expert Opin. Drug Deliv.*, **8**, 375–388.

109 Vauthier, C. and Bouchemal, K. (2009) Methods for the preparation and manufacture of polymeric nanoparticles. *Pharm. Res.*, **26**, 1025–1058.

110 Rao, J.P. and Geckeler, K.E. (2011) Polymer nanoparticles: preparation techniques and size-control parameters. *Prog. Polym. Sci.*, **36**, 887–913.

111 Mora-Huertas, C.E., Fessi, H., and Elaissari, A. (2011) Influence of process and formulation parameters on the formation of submicron particles by solvent displacement and emulsification–

diffusion methods. Critical comparison. *Adv. Colloid Interface Sci.*, **163**, 90–122.
112 Ahlin Grabnar, P. and Kristl, J. (2011) The manufacturing techniques of drug-loaded polymeric nanoparticles from preformed polymers. *J. Microencapsul.*, **28**, 323–335.
113 Allémann, E., Gurny, R., and Doelker, E. (1993) Drug-loaded nanoparticles preparation methods and drug targeting issues. *Eur. J. Pharm. Biopharm.*, **39**, 173–191.
114 Lepeltier, E., Bourgaux, C., and Couvreur, P. (2014) Nanoprecipitation and the "Ouzo effect": application to drug delivery devices. *Adv. Drug Deliv. Rev.*, **71**, 86–97.
115 Galindo-Rodríguez, S.A., Puel, F., Briançonc, S., Allémann, E., Doelker, E., and Fessi, H. (2005) Comparative scale-up of three methods for producing ibuprofen-loaded nanoparticles. *Eur. J. Pharm. Sci.*, **25**, 357–367.
116 Khan, I.U., Serra, C.A., Anton, N., and Vandamme, T.F. (2015) Production of nanoparticle drug delivery systems with microfluidics tools. *Expert Opin. Drug Deliv.*, **12**, 547–562.
117 Abdelwahed, W., Degobert, G., Stainmesse, S., and Fessi, H. (2006) Freeze-drying of nanoparticles: formulation, process and storage considerations. *Adv. Drug Deliv. Rev.*, **58**, 1688–1713.
118 Gradishar, W.J. (2006) Albumin-bound paclitaxel: a next-generation taxane. *Expert Opin. Pharmacother.*, 7, 1041–1053.
119 EMA – European Medicines Agency (2015) Abraxane: European public assessment report – product information.
120 Desai, N., De, T., Ci, S., Louie, L., and Trieu, V. (2008) Characterization and *in vitro*/*in vivo* dissolution of nab-paclitaxel nanoparticles. *Cancer Res.*, **68**, 5624.
121 Desai, N. (2012) Challenges in development of nanoparticle-based therapeutics. *AAPS J.*, **14**, 282–295.
122 Desai, N. (2012) Albumin-drug nanoparticles, in *Drug Delivery in Oncology: From Basic Research to Cancer Therapy*, (eds F. Kratz, P. Senter, and H. Steinhagen), Wiley-VCH, Weinheim, pp. 1133–1161.
123 Desai, N., Tao, C., Yang, A., Louie, L., Zheng, T., Yao, Z., Soon-Shiong, P., and Magdassi, S. (1999) Protein stabilized pharmacologically active agents, methods for the preparation thereof and methods for the use thereof. US Patent 5,916,596, filed Oct. 01, 1996 and issued June 29, 1999.
124 Shegokar, R. and Muller, R.H. (2010) Nanocrystals: industrially feasible multifunctional formulation technology for poorly soluble actives. *Int. J. Pharm.*, **399**, 129–139.
125 Cooper, E.R. (2010) Nanoparticles: a personal experience for formulating poorly water soluble drugs. *J. Control. Release*, **141**, 300–302.
126 Müller, R.H., Jacobs, C., and Kayser, O. (2001) Nanosuspensions as particulate drug formulations in therapy: rationale for development and what we can expect for the future. *Adv. Drug Deliv. Rev.*, **47**, 3–19.
127 Schilde, C., Breitung-Faes, S., and Kwade, A. (2007) Dispersing and grinding of alumina nano particles by different stress mechanisms. *Ceram. Forum. Int.*, **84**, 12–17.
128 Schilde, C., Mages-Sauter, C., Kwade, A., and Schuchmann, H. (2011) Efficiency of different dispersing devices for dispersing nanosized silica and alumina. *Powder Technol.*, **207**, 353–361.
129 Bitterlich, A., Laabs, C., Krautstrunk, I., Dengler, M., Juhnke, M., Grandeury, A., Bunjes, H., and Kwade, A. (2015) Process parameter dependent growth phenomena of naproxen nanosuspension manufactured by wet media milling. *Eur. J. Pharm. Biopharm.*, **92**, 171–179.
130 Verma, S., Kumar, S., Gokhale, R., and Burgess, D.J. (2011) Physical stability of nanosuspensions: investigation of the role of stabilizers on Ostwald ripening. *Int. J. Pharm.*, **406**, 145–152.
131 Knieke, C., Azad, M., Davé, R., and Bilgili, E. (2013) A study of the physical stability of wet media-milled fenofibrate suspensions using dynamic equilibrium curves. *Chem. Eng. Res. Des.*, **91**, 1245–1258.

132 George, M. and Ghosh, I. (2013) Identifying the correlation between drug/stabilizer properties and critical quality attributes (CQAs) of nanosuspension formulation prepared by wet media milling technology. *Eur. J. Pharm. Sci.*, **48**, 142–152.

133 Kondo, N., Iwao, T., Masuda, H., Yamanouchi, K., Ishihara, Y., Yamada, N., Haga, T., Ogawa, Y., and Yokoyama, K. (1993) Improved oral absorption of a poorly water-soluble drug, HO-221, by wet-bead milling producing particles in submicron region. *Chem. Pharm. Bull.*, **41**, 737–740.

134 Merisko-Liversidge, E., Sarpotdar, P., Bruno, J., Hajj, S., Wei, L., Peltier, N., Rake, J., Shaw, J., Pugh, S., and Polin, L. (1996) Formulation and antitumor activity evaluation of nanocrystalline suspensions of poorly soluble anticancer drugs. *Pharm. Res.*, **13**, 272–278.

135 Meiser, F., Cammarano, R., Postma, A., and Caruso, F. (2008) Methods for the preparation of biologically active compounds in nanoparticulate form. WO2008/000042 A1.

136 Payne, T., Meiser, F., Postma, A., Cammarano, R., Caruso, F., Williams, J., Mccormick, P., and Dodd, A. (2006) Nanoparticle composition and methods for synthesis thereof. WO2006069419 A1.

137 Möschwitzer, J.P. (2013) Drug nanocrystals in the commercial pharmaceutical development process. *Int. J. Pharm.*, **453**, 142–156.

138 Keck, C.M. and Muller, R.H. (2006) Drug nanocrystals of poorly soluble drugs produced by high pressure homogenisation. *Eur. J. Pharm. Biopharm.*, **62**, 3–16.

139 Sheth, P., Sandhu, H., Singhal, D., Malick, W., Shah, N., and Kislalioglu, M.S. (2012) Nanoparticles in the pharmaceutical industry and the use of supercritical fluid technologies for nanoparticle production. *Curr. Drug Deliv.*, **9**, 269–284.

140 Cheow, W.S., Xu, R., and Hadinoto, K. (2013) Towards sustainability: new approaches to nano-drug preparation. *Curr. Pharm. Des.*, **19**, 6229–6245.

141 Singh, A., Worku, Z.A., and Van den Mooter, G. (2011) Oral formulation strategies to improve solubility of poorly water-soluble drugs. *Expert Opin. Drug Deliv.*, **8**, 1361–1378.

142 Hafner, A., Lovrić, J., Lakoš, G.P., and Pepić, I. (2014) Nanotherapeutics in the EU: an overview on current state and future directions. *Int. J. Nanomedicine*, **9**, 1005–1023.

143 Wu, L., Zhang, J., and Watanabe, W. (2011) Physical and chemical stability of drug nanoparticles. *Adv. Drug Deliv. Rev.*, **63**, 456–469.

144 Cerdeira, A.M., Mazzotti, M., and Gander, B. (2010) Miconazole nanosuspensions: influence of formulation variables on particle size reduction and physical stability. *Int. J. Pharm.*, **396**, 210–218.

145 Bitterlich, A., Laabs, C., Busmann, E., Grandeury, A., Juhnke, M., Bunjes, H., and Kwade, A. (2014) Challenges in nanogrinding of active pharmaceutical ingredients. *Chem. Eng. Technol.*, **37**, 840–846.

146 Juhnke, M., Berghausen, J., and Timpe, C. (2010) Accelerated formulation development for nanomilled active pharmaceutical ingredients using a screening approach. *Chem. Eng. Technol.*, **33**, 1412–1418.

147 Van Eerdenbrugh, B., Stuyven, B., Froyen, L., Van Humbeeck, J., Martens, J.A., Augustijns, P., and Van den Mooter, G. (2009) Downscaling drug nanosuspension production: processing aspects and physicochemical characterization. *AAPS PharmSciTech.*, **10**, 44–53.

148 Kwade, A. and Schwedes, J. (2007) Wet grinding in stirred media mills. *Handbook Powder Technol.*, **12**, 251–382.

149 Kwade, A. (1999) Wet comminution in stirred media mills – research and its practical application. *Powder Technol.*, **105**, 14–20.

150 Kwade, A. (2004) Mill selection and process optimization using a physical grinding model. *Int. J. Miner. Process.*, **74**, S93–S101.

151 Kwade, A. (2003) A stressing model for the description and optimization of

grinding processes. *Chem. Eng. Technol.*, **26**, 199–205.

152 Breitung-Faes, S. and Kwade, A. (2014) Use of an enhanced stress model for the optimization of wet stirred media milling processes. *Chem. Eng. Technol.*, **37**, 819–826.

153 Flach, F., Breitung-Faes, S., and Kwade, A. (2016) Feinstzerkleinerung organischer Partikeln in Rührwerkskugelmühlen: bestimmung günstiger Formulierungen und Prozessparameter. *Chem. Ing. Tech.*, **88**, 850–856

154 Kwade, A. and Schwedes, J. (2002) Breaking characteristics of different materials and their effect on stress intensity and stress number in stirred media mills. *Powder Technol.*, **122**, 109–121.

155 Knieke, C., Steinborn, C., Romeis, S., Peukert, W., Breitung-Faes, S., and Kwade, A. (2010) Nanoparticle production with stirred-media mills: opportunities and limits. *Chem. Eng. Technol.*, **33**, 1401–1411.

156 Ghosh, I., Bose, S., Vippagunta, R., and Harmon, F. (2011) Nanosuspension for improving the bioavailability of a poorly soluble drug and screening of stabilizing agents to inhibit crystal growth. *Int. J. Pharm.*, **409**, 260–268.

157 Janssens, S. and Van den Mooter, G. (2009) Review: physical chemistry of solid dispersions. *J. Pharm. Pharmacol.*, **61**, 1571–1586.

158 Konnerth, C., Flach, F., Breitung-Faes, S., Damm, C., Schmidt, J., Kwade, A., and Peukert, W. (2016) Impact of stressing conditions and polymer–surfactant interactions on product characteristics of organic nanoparticles produced by media milling. *Powder Technol.*, **294**, 71–79.

159 Van Eerdenbrugh, B., Van den Mooter, G., and Augustijns, P. (2008) Top-down production of drug nanocrystals: nanosuspension stabilization, miniaturization and transformation into solid products. *Int. J. Pharm.*, **364**, 64–75.

160 Van Eerdenbrugh, B., Vermant, J., Martens, J.A., Froyen, L., Van Humbeeck, J., Augustijns, P., and Van den Mooter, G. (2009) A screening study of surface stabilization during the production of drug nanocrystals. *J. Pharm. Sci.*, **98**, 2091–2103.

161 Bilgili, E. and Afolabi, A. (2012) A combined microhydrodynamics–polymer adsorption analysis for elucidation of the roles of stabilizers in wet stirred media milling. *Int. J. Pharm.*, **439**, 193–206.

162 Hennart, S.L.A., Domingues, M.C., Wildeboer, W.J., van Hee, P., and Meesters, G.M.H. (2010) Study of the process of stirred ball milling of poorly water soluble organic products using factorial design. *Powder Technol.*, **198**, 56–60.

163 Juhnke, M., Martin, D., and John, E. (2012) Generation of wear during the production of drug nanosuspensions by wet media milling. *Eur. J. Pharm. Biopharm.*, **81**, 214–222.

164 Stender, H.-H., Kwade, A., and Schwedes, J. (2004) Stress energy distribution in different stirred media mill geometries. *Int. J. Miner. Process.*, **74**, S103–S117.

165 Temtem, M., Neves, F., and Winters, C. (2013) Bridging API manufacturing and formulation through particle design. *Eur. Ind. Pharm.*, **17**, 13–17.

166 Xiong, R., Lu, W., Li, J., Wang, P., Xu, R., and Chen, T. (2008) Preparation and characterization of intravenously injectable nimodipine nanosuspension. *Int. J. Pharm.*, **350**, 338–343.

167 Grau, M.J., Kayser, O., and Müller, R.H. (2000) Nanosuspensions of poorly soluble drugs – reproducibility of small scale production. *Int. J. Pharm.*, **196**, 155–159.

168 Weissig, V., Pettinger, T.K., and Murdock, N. (2014) Nanopharmaceuticals (part 1): products on the market. *Int. J. Nanomedicine*, **9**, 4357–4373.

169 Krause, K.P., Kayser, O., Mäder, K., Gust, R., and Müller, R.H. (2000) Heavy metal contamination of nanosuspensions produced by high-pressure homogenisation. *Int. J. Pharm.*, **196**, 169–172.

170 Sharma, P., Zujovic, Z.D., Bowmaker, G.A., Marshall, A.J., Denny, W.A., and Garg, S. (2011) Evaluation of a crystalline nanosuspension: polymorphism, process induced transformation and *in vivo* studies. *Int. J. Pharm.*, **408**, 138–151.

171 Kocbek, P., Baumgartner, S., and Kristl, J. (2006) Preparation and evaluation of nanosuspensions for enhancing the dissolution of poorly soluble drugs. *Int. J. Pharm.*, **312**, 179–186.

172 Gassmann, P., List, M., Schweitzer, A., and Sucker, H. (1994) Hydrosols – alternatives for the parenteral application of poorly water soluble drugs. *Eur. J. Pharm. Biopharm.*, **40**, 64–72.

173 Shi, Y., Porter, W., Merdan, T., and Li, L.C. (2009) Recent advances in intravenous delivery of poorly water-soluble compounds. *Expert Opin. Drug Deliv.*, **6**, 1261–1282.

174 de Waard, H., Hinrichs, W.L., and Frijlink, H.W. (2008) A novel bottom-up process to produce drug nanocrystals: controlled crystallization during freeze-drying. *J. Control. Release*, **128**, 179–183.

175 de Waard, H., Grasmeijer, N., Hinrichs, W.L., Eissens, A.C., Pfaffenbach, P.P., and Frijlink, H.W. (2009) Preparation of drug nanocrystals by controlled crystallization: application of a 3-way nozzle to prevent premature crystallization for large scale production. *Eur. J. Pharm. Sci.*, **38**, 224–229.

176 Sinha, B., Muller, R.H., and Moschwitzer, J.P. (2013) Systematic investigation of the cavi-precipitation process for the production of ibuprofen nanocrystals. *Int. J. Pharm.*, **458**, 315–323.

177 Salazar, J., Muller, R.H., and Moschwitzer, J.P. (2014) Combinative particle size reduction technologies for the production of drug nanocrystals. *J. Pharm. (Cairo)*, **2014**, 265754.

178 Salazar, J., Heinzerling, O., Muller, R.H., and Moschwitzer, J.P. (2011) Process optimization of a novel production method for nanosuspensions using design of experiments (DoE). *Int. J. Pharm.*, **420**, 395–403.

179 Staedtke, V., Brahler, M., Muller, A., Georgieva, R., Bauer, S., Sternberg, N., Voigt, A., Lemke, A., Keck, C., Moschwitzer, J., and Baumler, H. (2010) *In vitro* inhibition of fungal activity by macrophage-mediated sequestration and release of encapsulated amphotericin B nanosupension in red blood cells. *Small*, **6**, 96–103.

180 Salazar, J., Ghanem, A., Muller, R.H., and Moschwitzer, J.P. (2012) Nanocrystals: comparison of the size reduction effectiveness of a novel combinative method with conventional top-down approaches. *Eur. J. Pharm. Biopharm.*, **81**, 82–90.

181 Petersen, R. (2009) Nanocrystals for use in topical cosmetic formulations and method of production thereof. EP 20099420A1.

182 Martena, V., Shegokar, R., Di Martino, P., and Muller, R.H. (2014) Effect of four different size reduction methods on the particle size, solubility enhancement and physical stability of nicergoline nanocrystals. *Drug Dev. Ind. Pharm.*, **40**, 1199–1205.

183 Kesisoglou, F., Panmai, S., and Wu, Y. (2007) Nanosizing – oral formulation development and biopharmaceutical evaluation. *Adv. Drug Deliv. Rev.*, **59**, 631–644.

184 Zolnik, B.S. and Sadrieh, N. (2009) Regulatory perspective on the importance of ADME assessment of nanoscale material containing drugs. *Adv. Drug Deliv. Rev.*, **61**, 422–427.

185 Van Eerdenbrugh, B., Froyen, L., Van Humbeeck, J., Martens, J.A., Augustijns, P., and Van den Mooter, G. (2008) Drying of crystalline drug nanosuspensions – the importance of surface hydrophobicity on dissolution behavior upon redispersion. *Eur. J. Pharm. Sci.*, **35**, 127–135.

186 Beirowski, J., Inghelbrecht, S., Arien, A., and Gieseler, H. (2011) Freeze drying of nanosuspensions, 2: the role of the critical formulation temperature on stability of drug nanosuspensions and its practical implication on process design. *J. Pharm. Sci.*, **100**, 4471–4481.

187 Beirowski, J., Inghelbrecht, S., Arien, A., and Gieseler, H. (2011) Freeze-drying of nanosuspensions, 1: freezing rate versus formulation design as critical factors to preserve the original particle size distribution. *J. Pharm. Sci.*, **100**, 1958–1968.

188 Beirowski, J., Inghelbrecht, S., Arien, A., and Gieseler, H. (2012) Freeze-drying of

nanosuspensions, part 3: investigation of factors compromising storage stability of highly concentrated drug nanosuspensions. *J. Pharm. Sci.*, **101**, 354–362.

189 Bahl, D. and Crowley, K. (2011) Pharmacokinetics of fenofibrate nanoparticles stabilized and delivered using the Zydis® Technology, In AAPS Annual Meeting and Exposition Washington, D.C.

190 Bahl, D., Vitez, I., and Crowley, K. (2010) Manufacture of nanoparticulate Zydis® fast-dissolve tablets using fish gelatin, In AAPS Annual Meeting and Exposition New Orleans.

191 Alaei, S., Ghasemian, E., and Vatanara, A. (2016) Spray drying of cefixime nanosuspension to form stabilized and fast dissolving powder. *Powder Technol.*, **288**, 241–248.

192 Chaubal, M.V. and Popescu, C. (2008) Conversion of nanosuspensions into dry powders by spray drying: a case study. *Pharm. Res.*, **25**, 2302–2308.

193 Kumar, S., Gokhale, R., and Burgess, D.J. (2014) Quality by design approach to spray drying processing of crystalline nanosuspensions. *Int. J. Pharm.*, **464**, 234–242.

194 Nekkanti, V., Pillai, R., Venkateshwarlu, V., and Harisudhan, T. (2009) Development and characterization of solid oral dosage form incorporating candesartan nanoparticles. *Pharm. Dev. Technol.*, **14**, 290–298.

195 Crowley, K.J. and Zografi, G. (2002) Cryogenic grinding of indomethacin polymorphs and solvates: assessment of amorphous phase formation and amorphous phase physical stability. *J. Pharm. Sci.*, **91**, 492–507.

196 Sharma, P., Denny, W.A., and Garg, S. (2009) Effect of wet milling process on the solid state of indomethacin and simvastatin. *Int. J. Pharm.*, **380**, 40–48.

197 Willart, J.F., Dujardin, N., Dudognon, E., Danede, F., and Descamps, M. (2010) Amorphization of sugar hydrates upon milling. *Carbohydr. Res.*, **345**, 1613–1616.

198 Kayaert, P. and Van den Mooter, G. (2012) Is the amorphous fraction of a dried nanosuspension caused by milling or by drying? A case study with Naproxen and Cinnarizine. *Eur. J. Pharm. Biopharm.*, **81**, 650–656.

199 Van Eerdenbrugh, B., Froyen, L., Van Humbeeck, J., Martens, J.A., Augustijns, P., and Van Den Mooter, G. (2008) Alternative matrix formers for nanosuspension solidification: dissolution performance and X-ray microanalysis as an evaluation tool for powder dispersion. *Eur. J. Pharm. Sci.*, **35**, 344–353.

200 Van den Mooter, G., Weuts, I., De Ridder, T., and Blaton, N. (2006) Evaluation of Inutec SP1 as a new carrier in the formulation of solid dispersions for poorly soluble drugs. *Int. J. Pharm.*, **316**, 1–6.

201 Dolenc, A., Kristl, J., Baumgartner, S., and Planinsek, O. (2009) Advantages of celecoxib nanosuspension formulation and transformation into tablets. *Int. J. Pharm.*, **376**, 204–212.

202 Liversidge, G.G., Eickhoff, W.M., Ruddy, S.B., Mueller, K.R., Roberts, M.E., and Engers, D.A. (1998) Formulations of nanoparticle naproxen tablets. WO 1998035666 A1, filed Feb. 11, 1998 and issued Aug. 20, 1998.

203 Möschwitzer, J. and Muller, R.H. (2006) Spray coated pellets as carrier system for mucoadhesive drug nanocrystals. *Eur. J. Pharm. Biopharm.*, **62**, 282–287.

204 Moschwitzer, J.P. and Muller, R.H. (2013) Factors influencing the release kinetics of drug nanocrystal-loaded pellet formulations. *Drug Dev. Ind. Pharm.*, **39**, 762–769.

205 Figueroa, C.E. and Bose, S. (2013) Spray granulation: importance of process parameters on *in vitro* and *in vivo* behavior of dried nanosuspensions. *Eur. J. Pharm. Biopharm.*, **85**, 1046–1055.

206 Basa, S., Muniyappan, T., Karatgi, P., Prabhu, R., and Pillai, R. (2008) Production and *in vitro* characterization of solid dosage form incorporating drug nanoparticles. *Drug Dev. Ind. Pharm.*, **34**, 1209–1218.

207 He, W., Lu, Y., Qi, J., Chen, L., Yin, L., and Wu, W. (2013) Formulating food protein-stabilized indomethacin nanosuspensions into pellets by fluid-bed coating technology: physical

characterization, redispersibility, and dissolution. *Int. J. Nanomedicine*, **8**, 3119–3128.

208 Mitri, K., Shegokar, R., Gohla, S., Anselmi, C., and Muller, R.H. (2011) Lutein nanocrystals as antioxidant formulation for oral and dermal delivery. *Int. J. Pharm.*, **420**, 141–146.

209 Bose, S., Schenck, D., Ghosh, I., Hollywood, A., Maulit, E., and Ruegger, C. (2012) Application of spray granulation for conversion of a nanosuspension into a dry powder form. *Eur. J. Pharm. Sci.*, **47**, 35–43.

210 Vergote, G.J., Vervaet, C., Van Driessche, I., Hoste, S., De Smedt, S., Demeester, J., Jain, R.A., Ruddy, S., and Remon, J.P. (2001) An oral controlled release matrix pellet formulation containing nanocrystalline ketoprofen. *Int. J. Pharm.*, **219**, 81–87.

211 Vergote, G.J., Vervaet, C., Van Driessche, I., Hoste, S., De Smedt, S., Demeester, J., Jain, R.A., Ruddy, S., and Remon, J.P. (2002) *In vivo* evaluation of matrix pellets containing nanocrystalline ketoprofen. *Int. J. Pharm.*, **240**, 79–84.

212 Khinast, J., Baumgartner, R., and Roblegg, E. (2013) Nano-extrusion: a one-step process for manufacturing of solid nanoparticle formulations directly from the liquid phase. *AAPS PharmSciTech.*, **14**, 601–604.

213 Baumgartner, R., Eitzlmayr, A., Matsko, N., Tetyczka, C., Khinast, J., and Roblegg, E. (2014) Nano-extrusion: a promising tool for continuous manufacturing of solid nano-formulations. *Int. J. Pharm.*, **477**, 1–11.

214 Chen, A., Shi, Y., Yan, Z., Hao, H., Zhang, Y., Zhong, J., and Hou, H. (2015) Dosage form developments of nanosuspension drug delivery system for oral administration route. *Curr. Pharm. Des.*, **21**, 4355–4365.

215 European Medicines Agency (2005) Scientific Discussions – Rapamune – WC500046434.

216 European Medicines Agency (2004) Scientific Discussions – Emend – WC500026534.

217 Duncan, R. and Gaspar, R. (2011) Nanomedicine (s) under the microscope. *Mol. Pharm.*, **8**, 2101–2141.

218 ESF - European Science Foundation (2005) An ESF – European Medical Research Councils (EMRC) Forward Look report; www.esf.org.

219 Alphandéry, E., Grand-Dewyse, P., Lefèvre, R., Mandawala, C., and Durand-Dubief, M. (2015) Cancer therapy using nanoformulated substances: scientific, regulatory and financial aspects. *Expert Rev. Anticancer Ther.*, **15**, 1233–1255.

220 Bosetti, R. and Vereeck, L. (2011) Future of nanomedicine: obstacles and remedies. *Nanomedicine*, **6**, 747–755.

221 Brown, P.D. and Patel, P.R. (2015) Nanomedicine: a pharma perspective. *Wiley Interdiscip. Rev. Nanomed. Nanobiotechnol.*, **7**, 125–130.

222 Mukherjee, B., Maji, R., Roychowdhury, S., and Ghosh, S. (2016) Toxicological concerns of engineered nanosize drug delivery systems. *Am. J. Ther.*, **23**, e139–e150.

223 Duncan, R. (2014) Nanomedicine(s) and their regulation, in *Handbook of Safety Assessment of Nanomaterials*, Pan Stanford, pp. 1–41.

224 Wang, Y., Santos, A., Evdokiou, A., and Losic, D. (2015) An overview of nanotoxicity and nanomedicine research: principles, progress and implications for cancer therapy. *J. Mater. Chem. B*, **3**, 7153–7172.

225 Buckley, S.T., Frank, K.J., Fricker, G., and Brandl, M. (2013) Biopharmaceutical classification of poorly soluble drugs with respect to "enabling formulations". *Eur. J. Pharm. Sci.*, **50**, 8–16.

226 Wacker, M. (2013) Nanocarriers for intravenous injection – the long hard road to the market. *Int. J. Pharm.*, **457**, 50–62.

227 Dawidczyk, C.M., Kim, C., Park, J.H., Russell, L.M., Lee, K.H., Pomper, M.G., and Searson, P.C. (2014) State-of-the-art in design rules for drug delivery platforms: lessons learned from FDA-approved nanomedicines. *J. Control. Release*, **187**, 133–144.

228 Paliwal, R., Babu, R.J., and Palakurthi, S. (2014) Nanomedicine scale-up technologies: feasibilities and challenges. *AAPS PharmSciTech.*, **15**, 1527–1534.

229 Crist, R.M., Grossman, J.H., Patri, A.K., Stern, S.T., Dobrovolskaia, M.A., Adiseshaiah, P.P., Clogston, J.D., and McNeil, S.E. (2013) Common pitfalls in nanotechnology: lessons learned from NCI's Nanotechnology Characterization Laboratory. *Integr. Biol.*, **5**, 66–73.
230 Domingo, C. and Saurina, J. (2012) An overview of the analytical characterization of nanostructured drug delivery systems: towards green and sustainable pharmaceuticals: a review. *Anal. Chim. Acta*, **744**, 8–22.
231 Frater, L., Stokes, E., Lee, R., and Oriola, T. (2006) An overview of the framework of current regulation affecting the development and marketing of nanomaterials, ESRC Centre for Business Relationships Accountability Sustainability and Society (BRASS).
232 Bawa, R. (2011) Regulating nanomedicine – can the FDA handle it? *Curr. Drug Deliv.*, **8**, 227–234.
233 Ehmann, F., Sakai-Kato, K., Duncan, R., Pérez de la Ossa, D.H., Pita, R., Vidal, J.-M., Kohli, A., Tothfalusi, L., Sanh, A., and Tinton, S. (2013) Next-generation nanomedicines and nanosimilars: EU regulators' initiatives relating to the development and evaluation of nanomedicines. *Nanomedicine*, **8**, 849–856.
234 Narang, A.S., Chang, R.K., and Hussain, M.A. (2013) Pharmaceutical development and regulatory considerations for nanoparticles and nanoparticulate drug delivery systems. *J. Pharm. Sci.*, **102**, 3867–3882.
235 Sainz, V., Conniot, J., Matos, A.I., Peres, C., Zupan i , E., Moura, L., Silva, L.C., Florindo, H.F., and Gaspar, R.S. (2015) Regulatory aspects on nanomedicines. *Biochem. Biophys. Res. Commun.*, **468**, 504–510.
236 Hock, S.C., Ying, Y.M., and Wah, C.L. (2011) A review of the current scientific and regulatory status of nanomedicines and the challenges ahead. *PDA J. Pharm. Sci. Technol.*, **65**, 177–195.
237 Bawa, R. (2007) Patents and nanomedicine. *Future Medicine*, **2**, 351–374.
238 Chavhan, S.S., Petkar, K.C., and Sawant, K. (2011) Nanosuspensions in drug delivery: recent advances, patent scenarios, and commercialization aspects. *Crit Rev. Ther. Drug Carrier Syst.*, **28**, 447–488.
239 Chin, W.W.L., Parmentier, J., Widzinski, M., Tan, E.H., and Gokhale, R. (2014) A brief literature and patent review of nanosuspensions to a final drug product. *J. Pharm. Sci.*, **103**, 2980–2999.
240 Kaur, I.P., Kakkar, V., Deol, P.K., Yadav, M., Singh, M., and Sharma, I. (2014) Issues and concerns in nanotech product development and its commercialization. *J. Control. Release*, **193**, 51–62.
241 Kuiken, T. (2011) Nanomedicine and ethics: is there anything new or unique? *Wiley Interdiscip. Rev. Nanomed. Nanobiotechnol.*, **3**, 111–118.
242 Spagnolo, A.G. and Daloiso, V. (2009) Outlining ethical issues in nanotechnologies. *Bioethics*, **23**, 394–402.
243 Mühlebach, S., Borchard, G., and Yildiz, S. (2015) Regulatory challenges and approaches to characterize nanomedicines and their follow-on similars. *Nanomedicine*, **10**, 659–674.
244 Chang, E.H., Harford, J.B., Eaton, M.A., Boisseau, P.M., Dube, A., Hayeshi, R., Swai, H., and Lee, D.S. (2015) Nanomedicine: past, present and future – a global perspective. *Biochem. Biophys. Res. Commun.*, **468**, 511–517.
245 Finch, G., Havel, H., Analoui, M., Barton, R.W., Diwan, A.R., Hennessy, M., Reddy, V., Sadrieh, N., Tamarkin, L., and Wolfgang, M. (2014) Nanomedicine drug development: a scientific symposium entitled "Charting a roadmap to commercialization". *AAPS J.*, **16**, 698–704.
246 Tinkle, S., McNeil, S.E., Mühlebach, S., Bawa, R., Borchard, G., Barenholz, Y.C., Tamarkin, L., and Desai, N. (2014) Nanomedicines: addressing the scientific and regulatory gap. *Ann. N.Y. Acad. Sci.*, **1313**, 35–56.
247 Bremer-Hoffmann, S., Amenta, V., and Rossi, F. (2015) Nanomedicines in the European translational process. *Eur. J. Nanomedicine*, **7**, 191–202.
248 Eaton, M.A., Levy, L., and Fontaine, O.M. (2015) Delivering nanomedicines to

patients: a practical guide. *Nanomedicine*, **11**, 983–992.

249 ETPN – European Technology Platform Nanomedicine (2013) Nanomedicine 2020 – Contribution of nanomedicine to horizon 2020 – White paper to the horizon 2020 framework programme for research and innovation – Recommendations from the nanomedicine community; www.etp-nanomedicine.eu.

250 ETPN – European Technology Platform Nanomedicine (2016) Strategic research and innovation agenda for nanomedicine 2016–2030; www.etp-nanomedicine.eu.

10 Nanopharmacy: Exploratory Methods for Polymeric Materials

Kuldeep Bansal,[1] Luana Sasso,[1] Hiteshri Makwana,[1] Sahar Awwad,[2] Steve Brocchini,[2] and Cameron Alexander[1]

[1]University of Nottingham, School of Pharmacy, University Park, Nottingham NG72RD, UK
[2]University College London, School of Pharmacy, Brunswick Square, London WC2, UK

10.1 Introduction

Polymers are already widely used in pharmaceutical applications as excipients, release modifiers, tablet ingredients, and coatings [1]. Almost every final dosage form and medical device is reliant on the properties and functions of polymers. Polymers are central to the development of new therapies. The pharmaceutical functions of polymers are valuable since they are responsible for key performance attributes of many medicines such as ensuring optimal biodistribution, pharmacokinetics, and pharmacodynamic properties. There is also increasing interest in the use of polymers as "actives," either by direct therapeutic effect or as carriers and conjugates of drug molecules [2–9]. It is also clinically proven that polymers can be used as the active drug ingredient (e.g., Renagel®), and to form extended-release depot (Gliadel®), microsphere (e.g., Zoladex®, Exenatide®) and liposomal (e.g., Doxil®) [10] medicines. Polymers have been conjugated to drug substances to extend their duration of action. Clinically, poly (ethylene glycol) (PEG) has been shown to improve several protein therapeutics that are routinely used. Much clinical development work has also been accomplished with other polymer conjugates (e.g., polymer drug and coblock polymer micelle drug conjugates). Many of these applications involving the conjugation of polymers to other molecules (e.g., low-molecular-weight drugs and proteins), colloids (e.g., gold nanoparticles and liposomes), and other particulates (e.g., microspheres) and in recent years some of these polymeric systems have become considered as members of a "new" class of therapeutic, known as nanomedicines. Many other polymer formulations also fall into the category of nanomedicines, including polymeric micelles, vesicles, and polyelectrolyte complexes. Here, we outline the developing applications for polymeric materials in nanopharmacy and pharmaceutical science, and some of the opportunities for, and also barriers

Pharmaceutical Nanotechnology: Innovation and Production, First Edition. Edited by Jean Cornier, Arno Kwade, Andrew Owen, and Marcel Van de Voorde.

against, the use of macromolecules and conjugates as therapeutics. It is also important to consider some recent routes by which polymers can be made to controlled chain lengths and molar mass distributions, and to evaluate how the physicochemical behavior of polymers and conjugates affect their biological properties and their function as nanomedicines. We focus this chapter on delivery systems in the "nanoscale" size range (5–100 nm), but indicate at this stage that diagnostics, sensors, and implants in the same size ranges have many similar attributes and key features of polymer chemistry. Here, we introduce the most important of these features as reference points for nanopharmacy as a whole.

10.2 Rationale for the Use of Polymers in Nanomedicines

Many potent drugs fail to reach the market because of delivery-related issues. Problems such as poor solubility, lack of absorption, inadequate biodistribution, metabolic modification with loss of therapeutic effect or increased toxicity, and undesirable clearance kinetics all contribute to the failure of candidate drugs to progress through clinical trials [1,2]. Strategies in nanomedicines are being developed and have been clinically shown in several instances to provide localized delivery of drugs. One clinically proven approach in cancer is to conjugate a very potent cytotoxic to an antibody to actively target a molecule. Much work has been done to conjugate cytotoxics to water-soluble polymers to form soluble polymer–drug conjugates and micelles. Upon parenteral administration (i.e., injection), the large size of the polymer will keep these conjugates in the blood compartment. These conjugates will not extravasate easily through healthy blood vessels and because they are large will take longer to clear through the kidney than low-molecular-weight molecules. Hence, polymer conjugates, micelles, and other colloids have the capacity to remain in the blood compartment for extended periods, often by avoiding uptake by the mononuclear phagocyte system (MPS), which is also known at the reticuloendothelial system (RES). This is important because often diseased inflamed tissue is less permeable than healthy tissue. In the case of malignant tissue, this is known as the enhanced permeability and retention effect (EPR) [11,12]. There is a permeability gradient between healthy and diseased tissue where it is possible for a longer circulating drug to preferentially be taken up at the diseased site. Nanomedicines of different types have the capacity to favorably alter pharmacokinetics (increase half-life) and preferentially alter biodistribution (exploit blood vessel permeability).

Polymers are utilized to produce entities that are large enough to be maintained in the blood compartment. Rapid clearance of drug substances (e.g., oligonucleotides and proteins) results in (i) dose dumping, (ii) the lack of a therapeutic dose between each administration, (iii) the need for higher cumulative dosing, and (iv) more frequent dosing. The consequences of too frequent dosing are (i) the increased occurrence of side effects, (ii) there is an increased risk for immunogenicity (in the case of protein therapeutics), and (iii) efficacy is often suboptimal. Clinical need often requires to extend the half-life of a drug substance in the blood to maximize safety and efficacy.

Conjugates and encapsulating systems can serve to compartmentalize a toxic molecule (alter biodistribution) in a way that is not possible otherwise. One of the great promises of nanomedicines is to allow practical use of therapeutics that once administered will have the properties to target specific disease sites where the active drug substance is needed. Nanomedicines are formally defined as medical products that have at least one dimension ranging between 1 and 100 nm[9], and it should be noted that extended circulation half-life is often observed at sizes above ~10–20 nm. However, as discussed elsewhere in this book, the usefulness of definitions in regulation of nanomedicines is currently being debated by regulatory authorities.

However, physiological barriers to drug delivery depend on the route of administration and on the compartmentalization of the target organ [3]. For example, in oral administration, the low pH in the stomach and the adsorption routes through the gut are currently insurmountable obstacles for protein therapeutics. Other examples are the blood–brain barrier of the central nervous system, the multilamellar structure of the skin for topical and transdermal applications, and mucosal barriers against pulmonary, gastric, ocular, or vaginal administration [4]. In the case of proteins, conjugation of PEG is much the same as conjugation of the polymer to a drug. Many protein therapeutics are rapidly degraded and cleared upon injection, but the presence of the conjugated PEG helps to prolong the circulation half-life of a protein without changing its function. There are now several PEG-protein conjugates that are now first-line treatments (e.g., Pegasys® and Neulasta®). In an analogous way, vesicles such as liposomes can be susceptible to rapid clearance upon injection by being taken up by the reticuloendothelial system (RES). While this can be advantageous for the treatment of infections, for example, leishmaniasis with liposomal amphotericin-B (AmBisome®), the conjugation of PEG to liposomal doxorubicin (Doxil®) helps to decrease RES uptake.

Nanomedicines are often considered to be an advanced drug delivery system. These systems offer potential for overcoming some of the barriers that otherwise impede the development of new medicines. Often it is a case that an existing medicine with a large amount of clinical data can be dramatically improved by developing new versions using a nanomedicine approach (e.g., PEGylated proteins).

Advanced drug delivery systems are being particularly actively studied to develop and optimize therapy with the emerging pipeline of the many new drug compounds with properties rather different than those of current small molecule drugs [5–8]. Polymers represent an important category of materials from which nanomedicines can be created and they are an intense focus of current research, owing to the ease by which structures can be designed to perform specific functions. For wholly synthetic polymers, monomer components can be chosen to confer surfactant or amphiphilic properties, that is, with a hydrophobic region to interact with a hydrophobic drug compound and a hydrophilic component to enable dispersion in aqueous media or the bloodstream. For natural polymers, functional group modifications, partial enzymatic degradation, and reformulation can all offer the possibility to make encapsulants or conjugating agents for nanomedicine applications.

However, the explosion of growth in the academic field of nanomedicine has to date not been matched by the clinical adoption of these materials, though it is important to note that there are several pharmaceutical products such as Doxil/Caelyx (polymer-coated liposomal doxorubicin) and Abraxane (albumin–paclitaxel) that are nanomedicines by definition in widespread patient use [13–19]. By far the majority of polymer nanomedicine research has focused on applications in cancer, as this is an area where the unmet medical needs have been most clearly pronounced [11,20]. Nevertheless, the generation of truly effective cancer nanomedicines of any type remains challenging [15], and there are now increasingly important developments in polymers for delivery for antimicrobials [21] and vaccine components [22].

10.3 Polymer Structures and Properties

10.3.1 Polymer Morphology

The structures of polymers can be enormously varied, ranging from single chains of repeating units in a linear arrangement (linear homopolymers), combinations of two or more units without any defined sequence in the chain (statistical copolymers), chains in which blocks of repeat units are joined together (block copolymers), to several chains attached at one or more branching points (branched polymers). Even within some of these arrangements, further variation is possible, for example, depending on how many different monomer sequences are present and how many regions of the polymers can be distinguished, there can be diblock copolymers, triblock-copolymers, and so on. Triblock copolymers can be classified as A + B + A or A + B + C depending on how many different polymers are included in the structure and how they are arranged with respect to each other [23]. Hence, monomers can be covalently linked to each other [24] and can be formed by homopolymer or more polymers with different characteristics and different patterns of assembly (Figure 10.1) [24].

Covalently bound block copolymers can self-assemble and produce micelles, which are formed by a hydrophilic shell and a hydrophobic core, or vesicles (also called polymersomes) with the creation of a hollow compartment surrounded by a double-layer polymer, as depicted in Figure 10.2 [23]. For wholly synthetic polymers, monomer components can be chosen to confer a very wide range of surfactant or amphiphilic properties, that is, with a hydrophobic region to interact with a hydrophobic drug compound and a

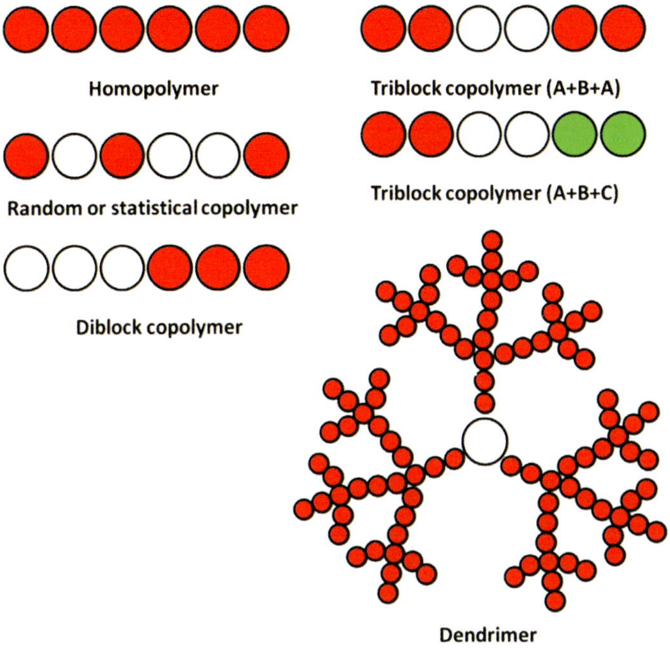

Figure 10.1 Examples of block copolymers are shown the arrangement of a linear homopolymer, a diblock, an A + B + A and A + B + C triblock copolymers, a random or statistical copolymer, and a dendrimer.

hydrophilic component to enable dispersion in aqueous media or the bloodstream. As a consequence, many combinations of different polymers have been investigated for drug delivery [25–29]. While the main focus of this short outline is covalently assembled polymers, it is important to note that

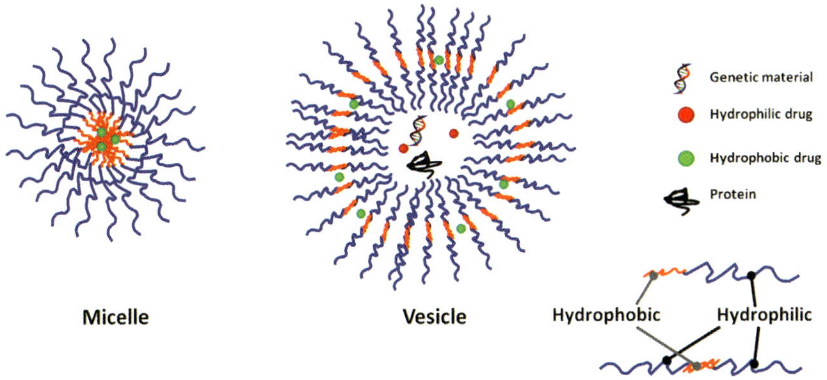

Figure 10.2 Schematic representation of micelles and vesicles with their typical loads. Hydrophobic regions are represented in orange, and hydrophilic regions are represented in blue.

"block copolymers" can also be generated through electrostatic interactions: noncovalently bound electrostatically associated polyion complexes can produce micelles and vesicles, and these have been widely used in investigational drug delivery systems [30–32].

10.3.2
Polymer Structures for Drug Delivery – Micelles and Vesicles

10.4
Formulation of Copolymers into Micelles, Vesicles, and Nanoparticles

Simple block copolymers formed by a hydrophobic segment and a hydrophilic block are surface active materials and rearrange at the solvent–air surface to reduce the contact of the water insoluble part of the copolymer with an aqueous solvent. In this way, they also reduce the surface tension of the solvent at the interphase. Amphiphilic block copolymers self-assemble in aqueous solution above a critical micellar concentration (CMC) that is dependent upon the temperature of the solution and the properties of the hydrophobic block. Above the CMC, the polymers produce aggregates that can be spherical, rod-like (also called worms), or arranged in extended lamellar or curved membranes [33]. The micelle-formation process is reversible, and single block copolymers are present in solution below the CMC of the polymer: this aspect is important in drug delivery where the dilution of micelles in the blood stream to a value below the CMC can cause the micelles to disassemble and release encapsulated drugs before reaching the target [34]. However, polymers can be designed to exhibit low CMC values by changes in hydrophobic block composition, and this process can also be used to change the assembly into worm-like micelles and vesicles dependent on the packing parameters for the block constituents.

In general, the hydrophobic core in self-assembled polymers serves as a reservoir for drugs with low aqueous solubility, while the hydrophilic shell prevents the adsorption of opsonins on the surface, which would otherwise mark the polymers as "foreign bodies." Additionally the size of polymeric micelles (typically 10–200 nm in diameter) serves to help avoidance of renal excretion, while still being small enough to bypass the filtration of interendothelial cells in the spleen. All these factors contribute toward the longer blood circulation time of micelles, which leads to improved accumulation at tissue sites with vascular abnormalities [6,35–37]. Poly(ethylene glycol) or PEG has been the polymer of choice to date for the hydrophilic blocks whereas the hydrophobic block can be chosen based on the required application [6,35–37]. Some of the reasons that make PEG consistently a polymer of choice for fabricating amphiphilic block copolymers are that it is relatively inexpensive, nontoxic, and is already in use in drug products [35]. Additionally, in micellar structures, PEG forms a dense, brush-like shell that imparts steric stability to the formulation [36]. Further, PEG is known to increase the circulatory time of carriers by impeding their

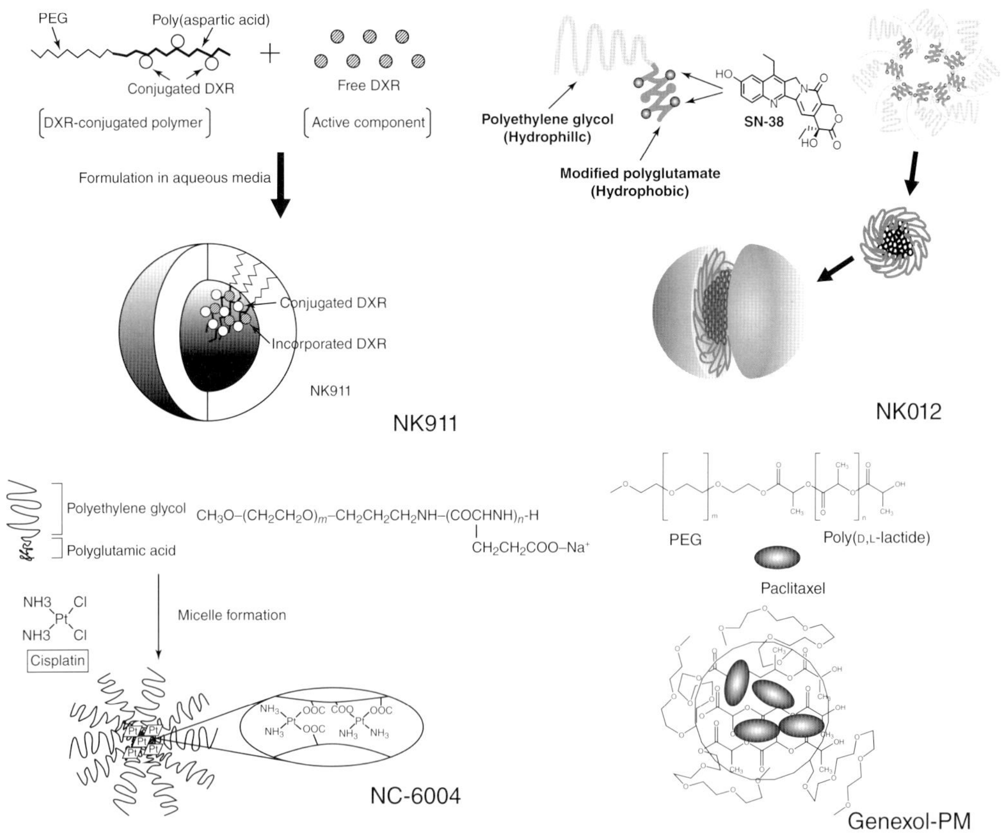

Figure 10.3 Schematic presentation of NK911 [49], NK012 [50], NC-6004 [51], and Genexol-PM [52] micelles. (Reproduced with permission from Refs [49–51]. Copyright 2004 [49] and 2005 [51] Cancer Research UK; Copyright 2010, Elsevier B.V. [50]; and Copyright 2001, Elsevier B.V [52]).

uptake by the cells of the reticulo-endothelial system (RES) [38]. It is also possible to functionalize PEG to attach specific receptor-binding ligands for targeted drug delivery applications [39]. As a consequence, PEG-based polymeric micelles have been widely utilized as solubilizing agents for hydrophobic drugs [35], to increase drug bioavailability, to reduce systemic toxicity, and offer sustained release of loaded drugs, some of which may enhance patient compliance to medication [36,40].

Progress in the field of therapeutic polymer micelles has been considerable [41,42], and a number of examples are in clinical trials, including those based around poly(ethyleneglycol)-block-poly(lactide-*co*-glycolide) (PEG-PLGA) and PEG-block-poly(aspartic acid) micelles (Figure 10.3). A specific formulation of PEG-block-poly(aspartic acid) with doxorubicin (NK911) has reached Phase II clinical trials for metastatic pancreatic cancer [43] and promising human clinical data now exist for Genexol-PM, a PEG-block-polylactide nanoparticle formulation of paclitaxel approved in South Korea for the treatment of breast cancer and non-small cell lung cancer (NSCLC) [44]. A number of other polymer micelles are also in late-stage development or have reached clinical trials, including NK105 (PEG-b-poly(aspartate-4-phenyl-1-butanolate) copolymer [45], Opaxio (paclitaxel-conjugated poly(glutamic acid) for advanced ovarian cancer [46], and SP1049C (Pluronic L61 and F127 co-polymers with doxorubicin) [47]. In the above examples, the drugs are noncovalently retained in the micellar cores, but the use of enzymatically cleavable linkages or redox and acid/base labile systems have also been considered. Conjugation of the topoisomerase I inhibitor irinotecan (SN-38) to PEG-poly(glutamic acid) micelles via labile ester linkages generated the NK012 polymer micelle formulation, which was well-tolerated in Phase 1 trials [48].

In addition to polymeric amphiphiles entering clinical trials, there have been many examples of developmental polymer nanomedicines. Among these there have been elegant studies in which the mode of drug release has been controlled, rather than the simple equilibrium-based diffusion from the original polymer micelles. Although these systems have been investigated more in the lab than in the clinic, notable recent examples include liberation of platinate and ruthenate anticancer drugs by *in-situ* protonation of poly(metal carboxylate) micellar cores [53,54], reductive cleavage of micellar core cross-links by intracellular glutathione [55], changes in coil–coil protein associations induced by molecular switching [56], and organic/inorganic hybrid micelles for combined diagnosis and therapy [57]. A number of comprehensive reviews cover many of the advances in such materials [41,43,58,59]. In all these cases, chemistries have been included in the polymer micelle structures that invoke release of the drug at a disease site. In effect, these materials are able to exploit pathologies or biological anomalies resulting from disease to trigger the delivery response, but there are also other means by which polymers can alter their properties to effect therapy. A whole field of stimuli-responsive polymers now exists [60–62], and we consider some of the general principles underlying the behavior of these materials to offer insights into why they are so intensively investigated but also why there are still some barriers to their clinical applications.

The assembly of block copolymers into micellar and vesicular superstructures can be spontaneous and irreversible or it can be triggered by a reversible stimulus. If the block copolymers are assembled such that drugs are contained in their core (which will be hydrophobic for conventional micelles and hydrophilic for vesicles), a stimulus that disrupts the assembly thus potentially allows for triggered drug release.

10.4.1 Investigational Formulations – Stimuli-Responsive Polymers

Many approaches have been investigated in order to obtain stimuli-responsive or "smart" materials that are able to prolong the release a drug following a specific triggering stimulus. Examples of stimuli resulting in changes in structures of polymer or linkages to drug molecules include variation in pH, temperature, redox status, light, and the utilization of enzyme-mediated catalysis [63–69]. The most widely studied stimuli-responsive polymers are those that change their solution properties with temperature. Thermoresponsive polymers can most easily be classified into two groups: polymers that display a lower critical solution temperature (LCST) and those that display an upper critical solution temperature (UCST). For polymers with LCST behavior, below the critical temperature the polymers are soluble in appropriate solutions, while above the LCST they phase separate from solvent. This effect is driven by the entropy of the system: above the LCST the most energetically favored state is of the polymer and (former) solvent in separate phases. In water, for example this is caused by the release of the bound water from the hydrophilic chains of the polymer to bulk solvent, the entropic gain of which offsets the enthalpic penalty of breaking polymer–water hydrogen bond associations. UCST polymers behave in the opposite way and are insoluble below a given temperature, but above their UCST the enthalpy of the system favors polymer solvation.

Thermoresponsive carriers of drugs have been extensively investigated for applications in diseased or inflammation sites where often a small, but significant, temperature gradient above ambient body temperature is present [70,71]. Certain solid tumors have been reported to be hyperthermic owing to enhanced metabolic and glycolytic activity combined with dysregulated cell homeostasis mechanisms [72]. It is also possible to heat tissues with the external administration of near infrared, ultrasound, or microwave irradiation, with temperatures of ~42 °C being easily attainable at the target region of the body [73].

A number of highly novel synthetic thermoresponsive polymers have been prepared for drug delivery that are based on natural elastin-like polypeptides [26,74]. Precision in synthesis of these polymers was achieved by cloning in genes encoding for specific repeat peptide sequences in expression vectors such that very fine control of LCST in the resultant polypeptides was obtained. Tumor-specific delivery of cytotoxic drugs has been shown in a number of mouse models, with selective accumulation of the polypeptides triggered by a mild thermal gradient induced by focused ultrasound [75,76]. The potential advantage of such systems is that polymer structure can be varied to include pH and temperature response through changes in the peptide repeat sequences, drug loading can be similarly tuned through conjugation at, for example, cysteine residues, and additional functionality such as targeting groups, therapeutic peptide sequences, and so on can all be encoded in the synthetic plasmid design. In the last few years, the synthetic polypeptides have been shown to be highly effective in preclinical evaluations, with higher efficacy than protein-based anticancer drug delivery in several murine tumors [77].

Acid- and base-responsive polymers are also widely studied and well characterized. Their solubility, volume, configuration, or conformation can be reversibly manipulated by pH changes [78]. Methacrylic acid and methyl and ethyl ester copolymers are relatively hydrophobic and water insoluble at low pH values (typically 2–5) and are deprotonated and hydrophilic with increase of pH above 6–7. These polymers (e.g., Eudragits®) have been used to control drug delivery in the gastrointestinal (GI) tract where a pH gradient is present within the stomach (pH ranges between 1 and 3) and the jejunum and ileum (pH between 6 and 7) where the pH gradient can trigger the release of the loaded drug. Other applications of pH-responsive polymers are in cancerous tissues as these sites can be mildly acidic compared to the bloodstream (pH ranges from 6 to 7.2) and at the subcellular level where the pH for endolysosomal compartments has been reported between 4.5 and 6 [79]. Recent examples include the preparation and application of pH-responsive polymersomes, with triggered release of encapsulated DNA and siRNA demonstrated *in vitro* [80] and efficient internalization of polymersomes *in vivo* [81]. Release of nucleic acids occurs due to protonation of basic residues in the polymer backbone when in the acidified intracellular compartments, which in turn leads to destabilization of the vesicle structure and liberation of the entrapped cargo. Similar release mechanisms have been used for nucleic acid delivery from layer-by-layer assembled polymer microparticles [82].

Redox-responsive polymers have been used to exploit the inherent reducing environments in cell interiors that are invoked in cell homeostasis and repair mechanisms. Disulfide groups are often used in these systems as, when they reach the inner cellular environment, they can be reduced by the increased levels of glutathione compared to extracellular environments [83,84]. Polymers have also been prepared that change conformation and solubility due to the salting in and salting out properties of chaotrope (water structure breaker) and kosmotrope (water structure maker) ions [65,85].

In all the above reported cases, the stimulus or trigger induces a nonlinear conformational change in the responsive polymer that can be used to release a physically entrapped drug. However, there are further examples where a covalently linked drug is released from a carrier polymer by acid or base hydrolysis, redox, or enzymatic action, and this can occur either with or without a conformational change of the carrier.

10.5 Conjugation of Polymers to Drugs and Proteins

10.5.1 Polymer–drug Conjugates

The covalent conjugation of polymers to drugs and proteins is widely used and is clinically proven. As proposed by Ringsdorf *et al.* in the 1970s, the concept of a polymer–drug conjugate has inspired much research and these materials can be considered as single-component nanomedicines [86,87]. The model consists of a biocompatible polymeric backbone that can be used to conjugate a number of different components (a) a solubilizing agent, (b) a drug, and (c) a targeting moiety that can enhance binding and uptake. Commonly investigated polymers for drug conjugation include *N*-(2-hydroxypropyl)methacrylamide

(HPMA), poly(ethyleneimine) (PEI), polyglutamic acid (PGA), poly(ethylene glycol) (PEG), chitosan, and dextran [88]. These polymers have been shown to display low levels of *in vivo* cytotoxicity and immunogenicity and are either biodegradable or have not demonstrated unacceptable adverse effects over long periods of administration [89].

Polymer–drug conjugates have been extensively examined for delivery of cytotoxic drugs and highly potent peptides. As large molecules, polymer–drug conjugates can remain in the blood compartment with decreased systemic distribution. Extended circulation times are possible that allow accumulation at diseased tissue sites through passive targeting [90]. Moreover, covalent attachment to a hydrophilic polymer backbone, for example, HPMA, PEG, can overcome the poor aqueous solubility and consequent low bioavailability of many hydrophobic drugs. The nature of the linker by which the drug molecule is conjugated to the polymer can modulate drug release profiles at the intended site. Many acid and proteolytically labile linkers have been studied in efforts to modulate drug release. It is necessary with potent cytotoxic molecules to ensure there is serum stability. Linkers that degrade by proteolysis within the tumor interstitial space or within tumor cells after uptake appear to be the most clinically relevant as evidenced by their use in antibody–drug conjugates. Polymeric conjugates designed to exploit polyvalent interactions have also been extensively explored [91,92]. These conjugates are not necessarily designed to release the drug but exploit cooperative interactions that are possible using polymers.

Many examples now exist employing the concept outlined by Ringsdorf's model for the development of drug–polymer conjugates [93,94]. For example, SMANCS is a conjugate of the copolymer of styrene–maleic acid and neocarzinostatin that is registered for use in Japan for the treatment of hepatocellular carcinoma [95]. PAMAM-based dendrimers have been synthesized from an ethylenediamine (EDA) initiator core conjugated to folic acid and methotrexate (MTX) to form bioactive conjugates [96]. As another representative example, Kihoon *et al.*, have described the development of paclitaxel–PEG and arginine-grafted bioreducible poly(disulfide amine) micelles for gene and drug delivery [97]. In a similar approach, Khan *et al.*, recently developed a targeted, disulfide-cleavable polymer–drug micelle system using camptothecin (CPT) as the therapeutic payload [98]. Encompassing the possibility for drug release within a reducing intracellular environment, the cytotoxic drug CPT was attached to a poly(polyethyleneglycolmethacrylate)-based block copolymer backbone via a cleavable disulfide linker. The CPT-containing block was hydrophobic as a result of the conjugation of multiple CPT residues, while the rest of the copolymer displayed hydrophilic poly(ethyleneglycol) side chains from the polymerized poly(ethylene glycol)methacrylate backbone. The targeting ligand, luteinizing hormone-releasing hormone (LHRH), was end-linked to the hydrophilic block, allowing it to remain accessible on the outside of the resultant self-assembled block copolymer micelles, and thus to interact with overexpressed LHRH receptors on the surfaces of ovarian cancer cells [98].

10.5.2
PEG-Protein Conjugates

Many proteins, peptides, and oligonucleotides [99,100] have been covalently conjugated to PEG. PEGylated proteins have been developed for a wide range of medical indications [99,101]. First described by Frank Davis and co-workers in 1977 [102,103] the first therapeutic PEGylated products (PEG-enzymes) appeared in the early 1990s. There are at least 12 innovator PEGylated biopharmaceuticals registered for clinical use with the most recent being Plegridy® (2014) [104] with some PEGylated proteins now used as first-line treatments (e.g., PEG-interferon alpha-2: Pegasys™ and PegIntron®; and PEG-GCSF: Neulasta® and Lonquex®). PEGylation is a viable strategy for the life cycle management for unmodified proteins to develop biobetter versions. The first PEGylated products are now coming off patent resulting in the development of international standards [105] for biosimilar versions.

10.5.3
Properties of PEGylated Proteins

PEGylated proteins display prolonged circulation times compared to the unmodified proteins. PEG is a random coil and associates with water to increase its hydrodynamic size in solution. This slows the renal clearance of the conjugate. PEG also sterically shields the protein to decrease its proteolytic degradation, opsonization, and uptake by the RES. PEG steric shielding can also help to reduce immunogenicity by shielding potential antigenic sites on the protein [101,106–109] and the propensity for protein aggregation [110].

Once the PEGylated protein is bound to its target, its properties are essentially the same as the unmodified protein [111]. Depending on the site of conjugation, PEG steric shielding can slow the rate of association of the modified protein with its target [112,113], thereby decreasing potency. Disassociation rates for the PEGylated protein are thought to remain the same [112,113] as the unmodified protein. Reduced association due to PEG shielding means that *in vitro* evaluation of PEGylated proteins, and macromolecular drugs generally [114] do not necessarily correlate with *in vivo* efficacy. While a log reduction in protein *in vitro* activity after PEGylation can be observed, most therapeutic proteins are very potent and remain sufficiently potent after PEGylation, enabling them to achieve their clinical benefit.

Although PEG is widely used in consumer and healthcare products, there continues to be concern about the clinical effects of PEG accumulation and immunotoxicity [115,116]. Animals used in accumulation studies are often given much higher bolus and cumulative doses than are given to humans [117,118]. Most therapeutic proteins [119] display immunogenic effects in a proportion of patients, so the metabolism, toxicity, and clearance of PEGylated products can be dependent on the protein [107,108]. If the unmodified protein is safe, then the PEGylated variant is expected to be safe [120]. Products that are hyper-PEGylated with many PEG molecules (liposomes, biomaterials, and nonhuman enzymes) appear most likely to be questioned in terms of PEG immunological safety and impact on clinical efficacy, so it has become important to develop standardized assays for anti-PEG antibodies [109,115,121].

Other natural and synthetic polymers [122] are also being examined for protein and drug conjugation (e.g., polyoxazolines [123], phosphorylcholine methacrylates [124], heparosan polymer [125], and hydroxyethyl starch [126]). Like PEG, these polymers will need to be thoroughly evaluated from a regulatory perspective and polymeric conjugation reagents made reproducibly at scale with narrow polydispersity and with defined chemical functionality.

10.5.4 Preparation of PEGylated Proteins

Many comprehensive reviews have been published that describe the broad spectrum of conjugation reactions that have been used for protein PEGylation [99,127–132]. The conjugation of PEG is also used for a wide range of other applications, such as to PEGylate the surface of particulates [133,134] and to make complex, multifunctional therapeutic proteins (e.g., antibody drug conjugates (ADCs) [135,136]).

PEGylation reagents have been described using both established and recently developed conjugation functional groups [129] to undergo reaction with many different amino acid residues on proteins [99,127,128], including nonnative amino acid side chains (e.g., aldehyde and alkyne) [130–132]. Of the many PEGylation reagents that have been described, those designed to undergo reductive amination with the amine of the *N*-terminal amino acid (PEG-aldehyde), acylation of the lysine side chain amine (PEG-*N*-hydroxysuccinimide (PEG-NHS), and Michael addition of the cysteine thiol (PEG-maleimide and PEG-bis-sulfone) tend to dominate (Figure 10.4). Linear PEGylation reagents are

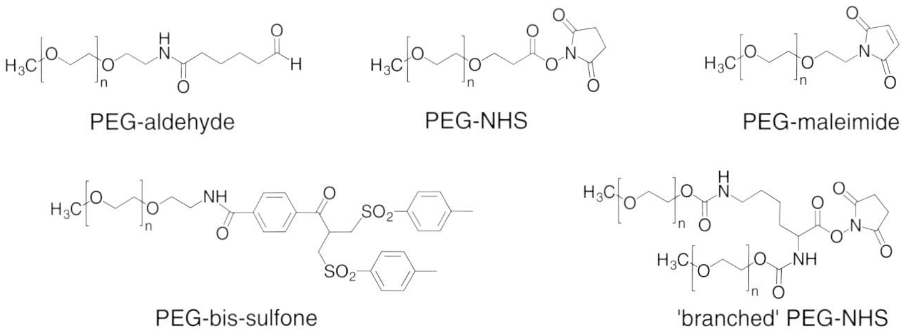

Figure 10.4 Common PEGylation reagents designed to undergo reactions with the terminal amine (PEG-aldehyde), other protein amines (PEG-NHS), protein thiols (PEG-maleimide), and the thiols from protein disulfide bonds (PEG-bis-sulfone). Both linear and branched reagents are often used.

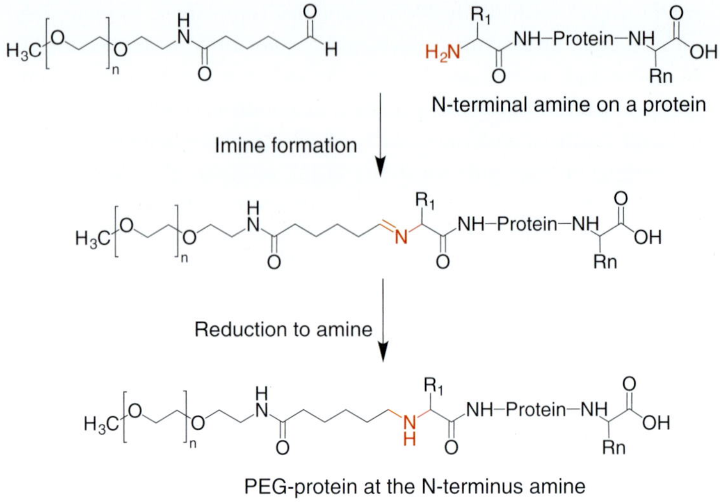

Figure 10.5 Reductive amination used to conjugate PEG to the *N*-termininus of a protein.

generally in the range of 20–30 kDa because the synthesis of narrow molecular weight distribution methoxy-PEGs is more feasible than at higher molecular weights. This has led to the development of “branched” PEGylation reagents [99,127,128] and other reagents with a wide spectrum of PEG morphologies and configurations (e.g., polyPEG [137]).

Narrowly defined reaction conditions using an excess of PEG-aldehyde can sometimes be found to undergo reaction predominantly with the *N*-terminal amine on a protein to give an intermediate imine (Figure 10.5). A borohydride reagent (e.g., $NaBH_4$, $NaCNBH_3$, or $Na(AcO)_3BH$) can then be used to reduce the intermediate imine to give the PEGylated protein. Known as reductive amination, this strategy is used to make PEGylated granulocyte-colony stimulating factor (PEG-GCSF, Neulasta®). Generally, specific conjugate conditions are narrow, conjugation efficiency can be low and *N*-terminal selective difficult to achieve. Other strategies designed to be more efficient and selective for the *N*-terminus (or *C*-terminus) of proteins have recently been described [138,139].

Amine reactive reagents tend to be used in considerable stoichiometric excess to protein. Since there are often several available nucleophilic groups on the protein, nonselective PEG conjugation occurs on the protein to give PEG-protein positional isomers and multiple PEGylated products. PEG NHS esters undergo nonselective acylation with lysine amines, while most accessible nucleophilic groups on the protein (e.g., terminal amine, tyrosine, and serine) also undergo reaction. Reaction with the histidine imidazole side chain results in the formation of a hydrolytically labile carbonyl imidazolide and this along with competitive hydrolysis consumes reagent. When using excess PEGylation reagent that undergoes nonselective conjugation, purification can be challenging [140–142] while giving modest yields of the desired PEGylated protein. In spite of these

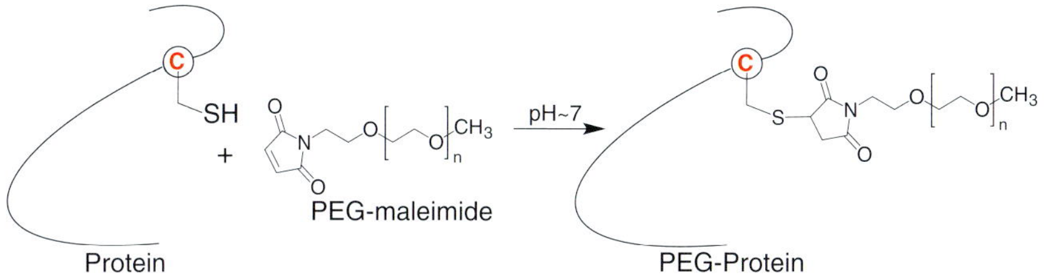

Figure 10.6 PEGylation of a single cysteine thiol with PEG-maleimide.

limitations, PEG-NHS reagents are used in the manufacture of different PEG-interferon medicines (e.g., Pegasys® and PegIntron®).

There are many site-specific approaches that have been described [129,130,132]. Thiol alkylation from a cysteine thiol with an *α,β*-unsaturated carbonyl (Michael addition reaction) is rapid in mild conditions that are conducive to maintain protein tertiary structure and where protein amine nucleophiles tend to be protonated and not reactive (e.g., pH 6–7). PEG-maleimide has been widely used (Figure 10.6). Many maleimide derived PEG-conjugates are often susceptible to deconjugation via a retro-Michael reaction and undergo thiol exchange reactions [143–146]. Efforts to stabilize maleimide conjugates have focused on hydrolysis of the maleimide ring after conjugation [147,148]. Alternative thiol-specific reagents have also been described [149,150]. Some reagents [151] can be reduced in the same way as an imine in reductive aminiation to avoid deconjugation by retro-Michael reaction.

The free cysteine thiol is rare in a protein and is often not available for conjugation because in the majority of proteins there is an even number of cysteines that are paired to form disulfides. The scarcity of free cysteine thiols in therapeutic proteins has resulted in many attempts to engineer a free cysteine to a protein as a site for conjugation. This strategy is viable for proteins without disulfides [152], but for proteins with disulfides, the presence of an unpaired cysteine often results in disulfide scrambling, protein misfolding, and aggregation. Since many therapeutic proteins have disulfides, another way to exploit the selectivity and efficiency of thiol conjugation is by *bis*-alkylation to rebridge disulfides using reagents such as PEG-bis-sulfone [153] (Figure 10.7). Elimination of the sulfinic acid leaving group to give the PEG-mono-sulfone enone allows the PEGylation reaction to proceed by what is thought to be an addition–elimination mechanism. The initially formed conjugate can then be reduced without any loss of protein activity using a borohydride reagent (e.g., $NaBH_4$, $NaCNBH_3$ or $Na(AcO)_3BH$) to prevent deconjugation or exchange reactions via retro-Michael reaction. In practice, this is often not required as the hydrophobic interactions of the protein and the flexibility of the three-carbon bridge prevent deconjugation. Two thiols can also be conjugated using a bis-alkylating maleimide linker [154] that results in a rigid vinylic two-carbon bridge between the thiol cysteines. As with other maleimides, hydrolysis is required to prevent deconjugation and exchange reactions [155]. The bis-sulfone PEGylation

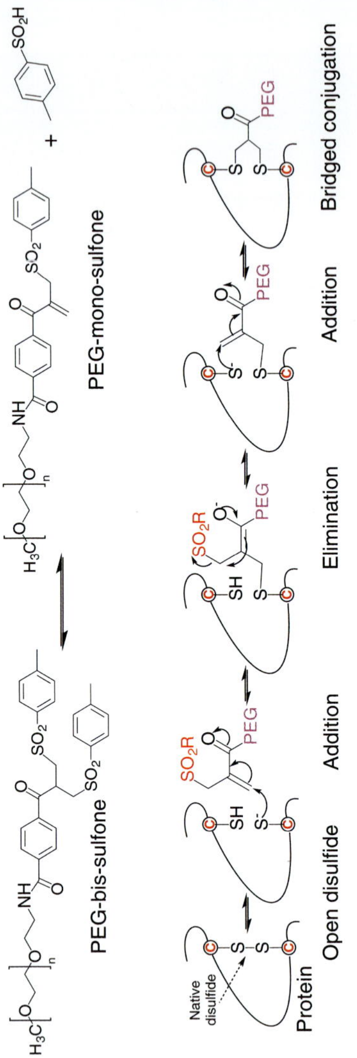

Figure 10.7 Disulfide bridging conjugation.

reagents are also selective for the histidine tag (His–Tag) in proteins [139], which can be placed at either terminus of the protein. His-Tag PEGylation can be accomplished with greater efficiency than is possible with reductive amination [139].

10.5.5 Moving Beyond Protein PEGylation

Many strategies [156] have been examined to optimize the pharmacokinetic properties of proteins (e.g., hyperglycosylation [157], fusion to an antibody Fc or to albumin, non-covalent association to albumin, and encapsulated or association with particulates) [158–160]. Medicines that utilize the properties of macromolecules can provide clinical benefit [161]. Protein PEGylation is a clinically proven approach and it is essentially a recombinant chemical approach where first the protein is made recombinantly and then modified by a conjugation reaction using a PEGylation reagent. Protein engineering and PEGylation are being utilized to modify [130–132,139] existing proteins and to design nonendogeneous proteins (e.g., scaffolds [152,162]) to achieve more efficient PEGylation site-selectivity. These efforts are focused to ensure there will be greater structural homogeneity, activity, and stability [163] in the final PEG-protein product. The combination of protein engineering and chemical synthesis strategies provides a huge range of opportunities for the continued modification of proteins with PEG and other molecules.

Although this chapter is focused on synthetic polymers, it is worth noting that natural polymers such as certain proteins can be considered to have properties that are a hybrid between synthetic and natural materials.

The serum protein albumin has been utilized as a nanoparticulate drug carrier, a long circulating complexation moiety, and a targeting agent [164]. In addition to this, concurrent findings have suggested that plasma proteins such as albumin can accumulate in tumor microenvironments through the EPR effect. Albumin binds to many hydrophobic drugs and also acts as the solubilizing agent for long-chain fatty acids and is essential for the metabolism of lipids. As a result many albumin-based systems have been investigated [93]. Lipid (e.g., myristic and palmitic) functionalized peptides have been developed that noncovalently bind to albumin resulting in extended duration of action. Examples include long-acting insulin (e.g., Levemir® and Tresiba®) and GLP-1 (Victoza®) analogues used to treat type 1 and 2 diabetes, respectively.

Abraxane® [11] is an albumin-bound nanoparticulate (~130 nm) form of paclitaxel. The product entered the market in 2005 for the treatment of breast cancer and has recently also received approval for use in late-stage (metastatic) pancreatic cancer. Paclitaxel formulations have utilized cremophor EL (polyethoxylated castor oil), which carries additional risks of hypersensitivity reactions and motor neuropathies that are sometimes severe and irreversible. The development of Abraxane avoided the need to use cremophor. Albumin is a natural noncovalent carrier of hydrophobic molecules (e.g., vitamins or hormones).

Binding of hydrophobic substances to albumin is reversible. Abraxane exploits endogenous albumin transport pathways, resulting in enhanced transport across endothelial cell monolayers, more rapid tissue distribution, and greater delivery of paclitaxel to tumors, compared to cremophor–paclitaxel. The more rapid and deeper tissue penetration of Abraxane results in slower elimination of paclitaxel and since there is less paclitaxel in the plasma, neutropenia can be less severe. Increased intratumoral accumulation of paclitaxel formulated as Abraxane may also be facilitated through binding of albumin to SPARC (secreted protein acid and rich in cysteine), an extracellular matrix glycoprotein that is overexpressed and associated with poor prognosis in a variety of cancers.

As more academic groups and pharmaceutical companies invest resources in the area of polymer/protein/antibody-based conjugates, increasing levels of emphasis are placed on understanding how the synthetic route (e.g., site of protein modification and strategy of polymer synthesis) can impede the overall generation of novel therapeutics. In addition to bioconjugation strategies, many new routes to synthetic polymers and "hybrid materials" are being developed.

10.6 Recent Advances in Polymer Synthesis for Therapeutic Applications

The wide range of polymers described above shows the diversity of chemical functionality and materials structures that have been used for therapeutic applications. However, recent advances in the synthetic methods for making polymers are now allowing even greater diversity in structures to become accessible [165–169].

Drug delivery materials for clinical use need to be pharmacologically benign or beneficial and either biodegradable or easily eliminated from the body. They should also be chemically well defined, such that any biological activity can be clearly assigned to structure. In practice, obtaining regulatory approval for polymers has been complex, owing to the wide range of molar masses and corresponding property variations in synthetic materials made by traditional free radical and condensation polymerization routes. Even poly(ethylene glycol), which for pharmaceutical applications is made by highly controlled anionic polymerization, is not monodisperse, and so PEG conjugates with proteins are not single molecule entities. Although absolute definition of molecular size is not required currently by regulatory authorities, there is nevertheless a strong driving force for more control in polymerization reactions such that materials properties can be introduced by design, and without batch-to-batch variation. Accordingly, there has been considerable interest in controlled chemistries for polymer nanomedicines.

A selection of these techniques is briefly outlined below, for which we consider both biodegradable polymers for systemic and chronic administration and non-biodegradable polymers for investigational studies.

10.6.1 Biodegradable Polymers for Nanomedicines

Biodegradable polymers have attracted particular attention for drug delivery because they do not accumulate in the body [170,171]. These materials are typically excreted from the body by renal clearance after degradation into small molecules [171,172]. Polymer degradation can take place through chain scission, which can occur by oxidation, thermal activation, radiolysis, photolysis, hydrolysis, and enzymatic activity. However, degradation by hydrolysis and/or enzymes is of the most significance in the context of nanopharmacy because these mechanisms predominate in materials tested in the human body [170–172].

10.6.2 Classification of Biodegradable Polymers

Biodegradable polymers can be divided into two classes based on the source of origin, that is, natural or synthetic. Naturally occurring polymers generally undergo enzymatic degradation, whereas synthetic polymers can be designed to degrade by controllably by hydrolytic reactions as well as by enzymatic routes [172]. Enzymatically degradable polymers can be further defined as materials that possess hydrolytically cleavable bonds but which require catalysts to undergo significant degradation under physiological conditions.

10.6.2.1 Naturally Occurring Biodegradable Polymers for Nanomedicine

Polymers obtained from natural resources are widely available and fulfill most of the properties generally required for a biomaterial, to be used clinically. Natural polymers possess numerous inherent benefits such as natural remodeling, bioactivity, susceptibility to cell-triggered proteolytic degradation, and can also have the ability to present receptor-binding ligands to cells [171]. Many naturally occurring polymers have been reported for drug delivery applications. For instance, micro/nanoparticles prepared from chitosan [173], a modified natural carbohydrate polymer, have been successfully used for the delivery of insulin [174], cyclosporine A [175], and doxorubicin [176] among many others. Several other polymers obtained from natural resources have been reported for various biomedical applications and were reviewed recently [89,171,177–179].

Despite their advantages as biomaterials for drug and/or macromolecule delivery, some restrictions are associated with the natural polymers. For instance, the rate of *in vivo* degradation of such polymers varies considerably with their biological location. Additionally, chemical modification can affect their degradation rate [171], while certain undesirable immunological responses, difficulty in purification and processing, risk of transmitting pathogens (origin related), and batch-to-batch variability can limit their applications [171,180,181].

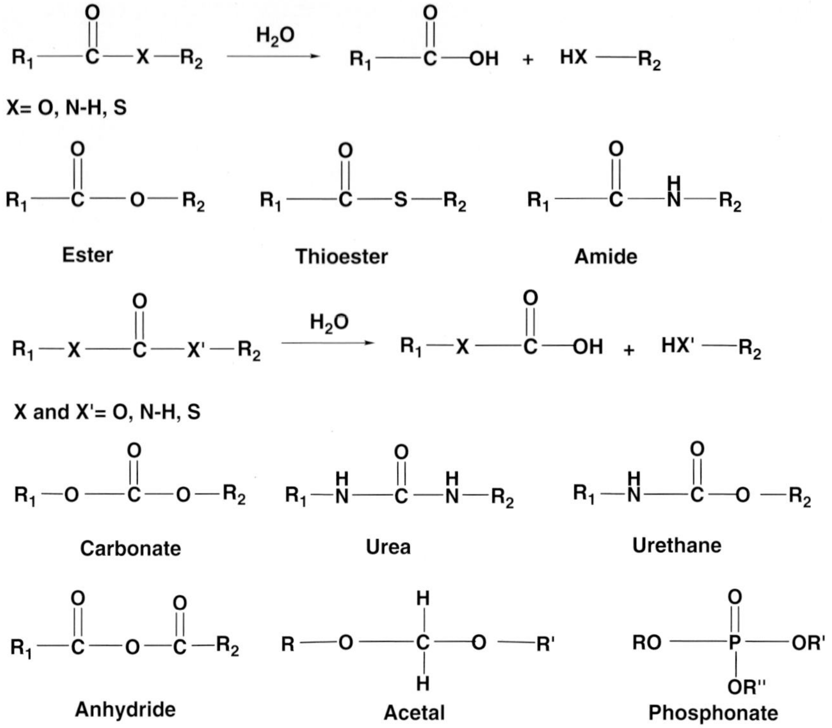

Figure 10.8 Polymers with hydrolytically cleavable functional groups.

10.6.2.2 **Synthetic Biodegradable Polymers for Nanomedicine**

Polymers synthesized for biomedical applications are able to offer certain advantages over naturally occurring counterparts [182,183]. These polymers can be designed to exhibit specific desired properties, such as accelerated or retarded drug release, dependent on the desired application. Furthermore, with synthetic polymers, it is possible to obtain material reproducibly and with better quality control. Polymers with a specific function can be prepared relatively easily by blending or copolymerizing two or more different polymers [171,183,184].

Synthetic biodegradable polymers generally contain a hydrolytically cleavable bond such as esters, thioesters, amides, carbonates, ureas, urethanes, imides, anhydrides, acetals, phosphonates, and so on (Figure 10.8). Among these materials, polyesters are the most studied class of biodegradable polymers due to their easy method of synthesis from commercially available monomers [172,185]. Therefore, in this chapter, we focus primarily on polyester materials.

The two general routes used to synthesize polyesters are step-growth polymerization (i.e., polycondensation) and chain-growth polymerization, which includes ring-opening polymerization (Figure 10.9). Homopolymerization of a single monomer with two different end groups (e.g., lactic acid) or copolymerization of two monomers (e.g., succinic acid and 1,4-butanediol) is the basis of

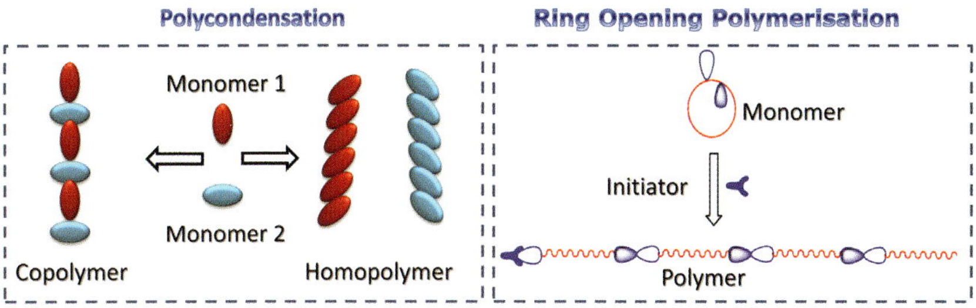

Figure 10.9 Schematics of polycondensation and ring-opening polymerization reactions.

polycondensation reaction. When two functional groups (acid and alcohol) join together during polyester synthesis, a small molecule (condensate), usually water, is liberated as a by-product [186,187].

10.6.3 Mechanisms of Polycondensation Reactions

10.6.3.1 Fischer Esterification

In Fischer esterification, a carboxylic acid reacts with alcohol in the presence of Lewis or Brønsted acid to give esters by releasing a molecule of water [188]. The products and reactants are in equilibrium in this reaction. In order to drive equilibrium for the effective conversion of monomers to polymer, water is removed continuously from the reaction medium [189].

10.6.3.2 Transesterification

Esters can be interconverted by reactions with alcohols in the presence of acid/base catalysts [190]. Efficient conversion to polymer is achieved by use of excess reacting alcohol or, as with Fischer esterification, by continuous removal of low molar mass condensate from the reaction mixture.

These reactions are reversible and additionally, in Fischer esterification reactions, high temperature is often required to generate polyesters in acceptable yield. A milder synthetic method to synthesize esters was developed by Steglich and Neises [191], using dicyclohexyl carbodiimide as a coupling reagent and 4-dimethylaminopyridine acted as a catalyst. Dicyclohexylurea (DHU) is the by-product during the reaction, which can be removed easily by filtration. However, for all polycondensation reactions, broad molar mass distributions are obtained, and high molar masses can only be achieved with rigorous control over stoichiometry of reagents and reaction conditions.

10.6.4 Ring-Opening Polymerization

For biomedical applications, in which good control over molar mass and chain length distribution is often desirable, ring-opening polymerization (ROP) has

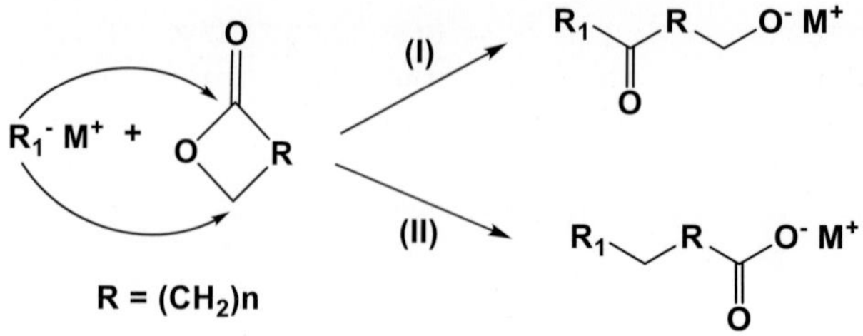

Figure 10.10 Mechanism for ROP of lactone (I) acyl-oxygen scission (II) alkyl-oxygen scission [192].

been widely investigated as a synthetic route to form polyesters. In this method, cyclic esters are ring opened in the presence of a catalyst and the target molecular weight can in theory be predefined, based on the quantity of monomer used. ROP is also advantageous over most polycondensation routes to synthesize polyesters in terms of reaction conditions and time, the absence of by-products as well as the control over the polymer chain lengths. ROP is a form of chain-growth polymerization, where the terminal ends of the chain have a reactive functional group, which repeatedly reacts with another cyclic monomer, opening the next available ring until all monomers are consumed. However, an initiator is always required to open the first ring of the cyclic monomer [192,193]. The three general mechanisms involved in ROP are cationic, anionic, and coordination–insertion. However, it has been reported that high-molecular-weight polyesters are best obtained by either anionic or coordination–insertion mechanisms [192].

10.6.4.1 Anionic ROP

In an anionic ROP, the reaction is started by the nucleophilic attack of a negatively charged initiator on the carbonyl carbon or on the carbon atom present beside the acyl oxygen of the lactone ring, yielding polyester (Figure 10.10). The propagating species in this mechanism is negatively charged that can attack the next available ring [192]. In four-membered rings such as β-butyrolactone, β-propiolactone, either alkyl or acyl-oxygen cleavage has been reported giving a carboxylate or alkoxide, respectively [194]. However, in larger rings such as lactides, only acyl-oxygen scission is generally involved giving an alkoxide as the propagating species [192].

10.6.4.2 Cationic ROP

In this mechanism, a positively charged species of monomer is generated after reacting with a cationic catalyst. The subsequent attack by another monomer leads to ring opening via an S_N2 reaction.

10.6.4.3 Coordination–Insertion ROP

Commonly used initiators that open the lactone ring via this mechanism are metal alkoxides and carboxylates [192]. These initiators have metals with vacant "d" orbitals that can coordinate to ring oxygen atoms: cleavage of the acyl-oxygen bond leads to ring opening of the lactone. The propagation continues by coordination of the monomer to the active species and then insertion of the monomer into the metal-oxygen bond. The coordination of metal with the exocyclic oxygen makes the carbonyl carbon more susceptible for nucleophilic attack. However, in this mechanism, a long reaction time or high temperature can lead to both inter- and intramolecular transesterification reactions [192].

10.6.5 Examples of Synthetic Polyesters as Investigational Nanomedicines

10.6.5.1 Poly(caprolactone)

Poly(caprolactone) (PCL) synthesized by ROP of ε-caprolactone, is one of the most extensively studied biodegradable polymers and its use has been reviewed recently [170,177,195,196]. PCL is relatively stable in the absence of catalytic species and the complete hydrolytic degradation of PCL generally takes 2–3 years [195]. "Capronor" is the regulatory approved formulation of PCL used for the sustained subdermal delivery of contraceptive steroids (levonorgestrel) [195,197]. PCL is a highly versatile material and can be fabricated into a variety of dosage forms, micro and nanostructures (Figures 10.11 and 10.12).

10.6.5.2 Poly(anhydrides)

Poly(anhydrides) have been extensively used for controlled release applications [198,199]. For instance, microspheres of poly(adipic anhydride), synthesized by ROP of oxepan-2,7-dione, have been used to deliver timolol maleate to the eye in a controlled fashion [200]. The key monomer for the synthesis of oxepan-2,7-dione is adipic acid, which is prepared using cyclohexane (hydrocarbon) as starting material [201].

10.6.5.3 Poly(trimethylene Carbonate)

Poly(trimethylene carbonate) (PTMC) has been used in the biomedical field because it degrades into biocompatible 1,3-propanediol and carbonic acid [202]. PTMC is generally synthesized by the ROP of trimethylene carbonate (TMC) which is commercially available. TMC is usually prepared from 1,3-propanediol and ethyl chloroformate or from oxetane and carbon dioxide [203,204]. Nanoparticles [205,206], microparticles [207], and gels [208] have been prepared from PTMC but more often it has been copolymerized with PLA (poly(lactide)) [209] or PCL [210] to improve its drug delivery potential.

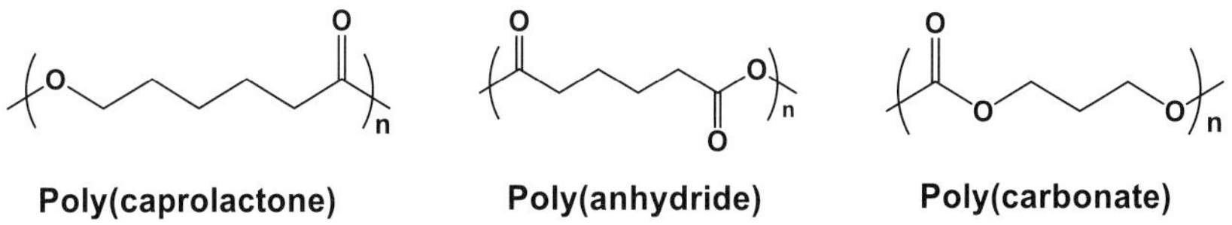

Figure 10.11 Structures of commonly used biodegradable polyesters.

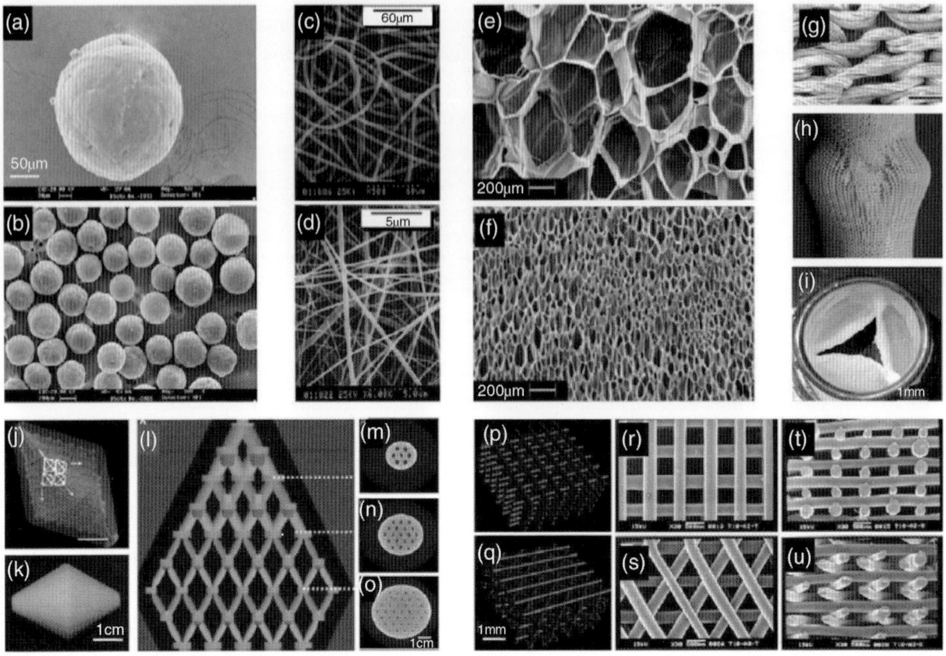

Figure 10.12 Structures made from PCL: nanospheres (a, b), nanofibres (c, d), foams (e, f), knitted textiles (g, h, i). Selective laser sintered scaffold (j–o). Fused deposition modeled scaffolds (p–u) [195]. (Reproduced with permission from Ref. [195], Copyright 2010, Elsevier Ltd.)

10.6.5.4 **Polyesters in Development**

Poly(butylene succinate) (PBSu) is a commercially available polyester but has limited drug delivery applications as a homopolymer because of its poor degradability and functionality [170,211–213]. To address these problems, copolymers of PBSu have been prepared to obtain polymers with suitable properties. For example, a copolymer of PBSu with ω-pentadecalactone, that is, poly(ω-pentadecalactone-*co*-butylene-*co*-succinate) (PPDL-*co*-PBSu) was used for the effective delivery of camptothecin against Lewis lung carcinoma cell lines *in vitro* (Figure 10.13) [214].

10.6.5.5 **Poly(esters) of Lactide and Glycolide**

Poly(lactide) and poly(glycolide) (PGA) (Figure 10.14) are generally prepared by ring-opening polymerization of renewable monomers lactide and glycolide, respectively. PLA and PGA can also be synthesized by polycondensation of lactic acid and glycolic acid, but due to the better control over molecular weight during ROP, cyclic monomers (lactide and glycolide) are generally preferred. Several reviews have been published recently, summarizing their potential for various biomedical applications [172,179,184,215–220].

1

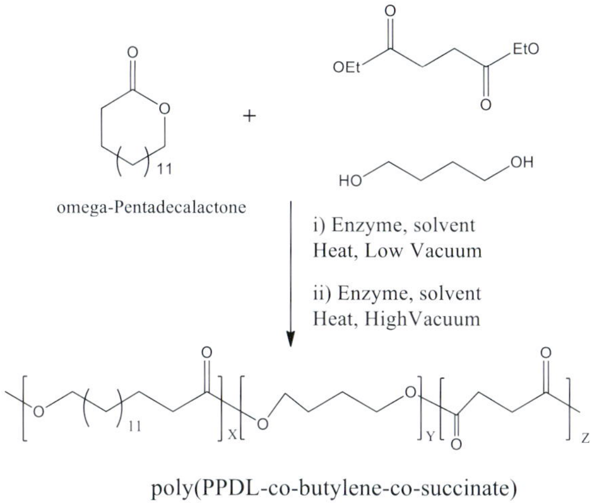

2

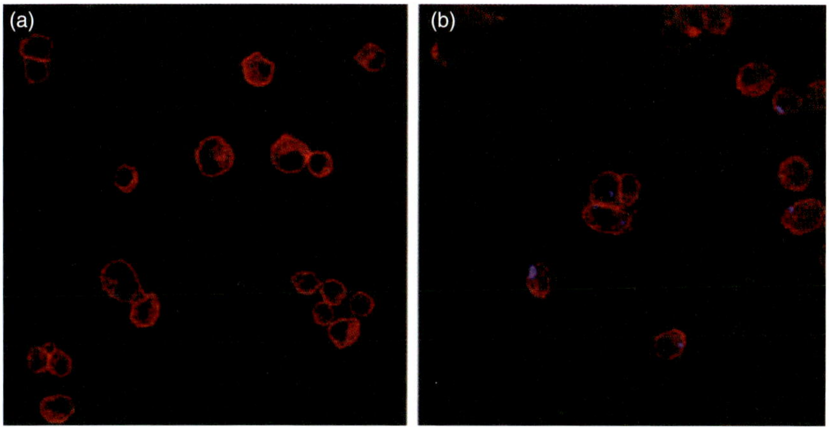

Figure 10.13 (1) Two-stage synthesis method for copolymerization of ω-pentadecalactone, diethyl succinate, and 1,4-butanediol. (2) Confocal microscopic images of Lewis lung carcinoma cells after 2 h incubation with (a) free CPT and (b) CPT-loaded PPDL-*co*-PBSu nanoparticles. Cells and CPT are visualized in the red and blue channels, respectively [214]. (Reproduced with permission from Ref. [214], Copyright 2009, Elsevier Ltd.)

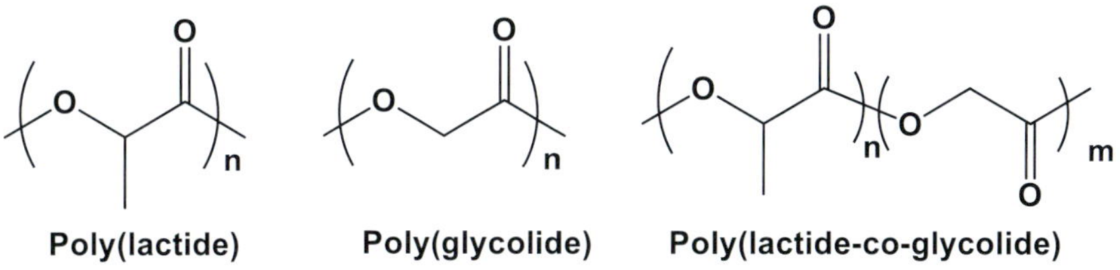

Figure 10.14 Structures of lactide and glycolide-derived polymers.

Table 10.1 Glass transition temperature and degradation time of PLA, PGA, and PLGA [221].

Polymer	Glass transition temperature (T_g) (°C)	Degradation time (months)
PGA	36	2–4
PLA	60–67	18–24
PDLLA	57–59	12–16
50:50 Poly(DLLA-*co*-GA)	46.1	2
85:15 Poly(DLLA-*co*-GA)	45	5

Due to the extent of crystallinity, rapid degradation and limited solubility of PGA in many common organic solvents, the development of this homopolymer for nanopharmacy applications has been restricted. On the other hand, PLA, specifically poly(L-lactic acid) (PLLA) and poly(DL-lactic acid) (PDLLA), has been widely investigated for these applications. PLLA is a semicrystalline polymer owing to the homochiral monomer, whereas PDLLA is an amorphous polymer due to the varying stereochemistries of methyl groups in the polymer chain. The presence of methyl groups in PLA increases its hydrophobicity and hence increases the degradation time [172,217]. Therefore, copolymers of PLA and PGA have been very widely explored to tune the degradation time of the final material (Table 10.1).

PLGA has been fabricated into microspheres [222,223], nanoparticles [224,225], nanofibers [226,227], and micelles [228] (Figure 10.15) for controlled and improved delivery of vaccines [229,230], cytotoxic drugs [231,232], proteins [233,234], antibiotics [235], siRNA [236,237], and so on. PLGA and PLA are authorized by the United States Food and Drug Administration (US-FDA) and European Medicine Agency (EMA) for human use.

Carvone is a natural product found in spearmint (*Mentha spicata*) and caraway oils (*Carum carvi*) that can be used as a precursor to biodegradable polyesters (Figure 10.16). Hydrogenation of carvone produced dihydrocarvone and carvomenthone, which can be easily converted into lactones, that is, dihydrocarvide and carvomenthide by Baeyer–Villiger oxidation [238].

Increasing interest in the use of natural products as polymer precursors has led to the ROP of δ-decalactone catalyzed by 1,5,7-triazabicyclo[4.4.0]dec-5-ene (TBD) to synthesize amorphous poly(δ-decalactone) [239]. The synthesis of high-molecular-weight triblock copolymer, that is, poly (lactide)-b-poly(δ-decalactone)-b-poly(lactide) has also been reported by sequential addition of monomers to reaction media [239].

Macrolactones obtained from naturally occurring musks, such as ω-pentadecalactone and globalide (Gl), have been also explored for the synthesis of poly (ester) by ROP using enzymatic catalysis [240,241]. Poly(ω-pentadecalactone) synthesized from ω-pentadecalactone was found to be well-tolerated in the 3T3

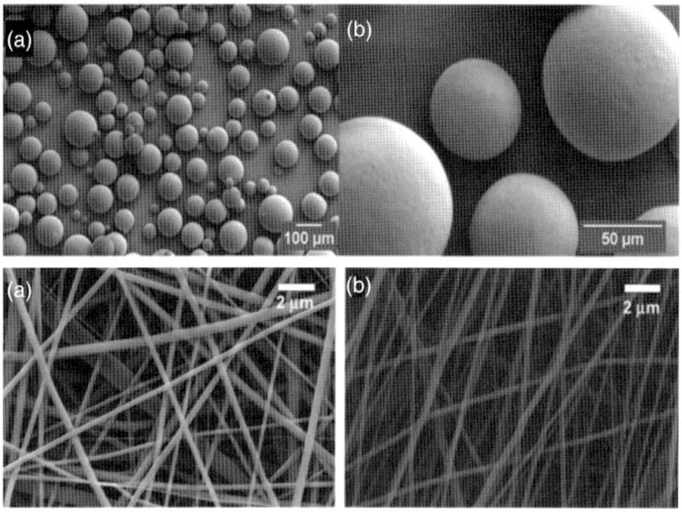

Figure 10.15 SEM pictures of microspheres (a, b) [222] and nanofibers (c, d) [226] from PLGA. (Reproduced with permission from [222,223]. ([222] Copyright 2011, by the authors, [222] Copyright 2009, Elsevier Ltd).

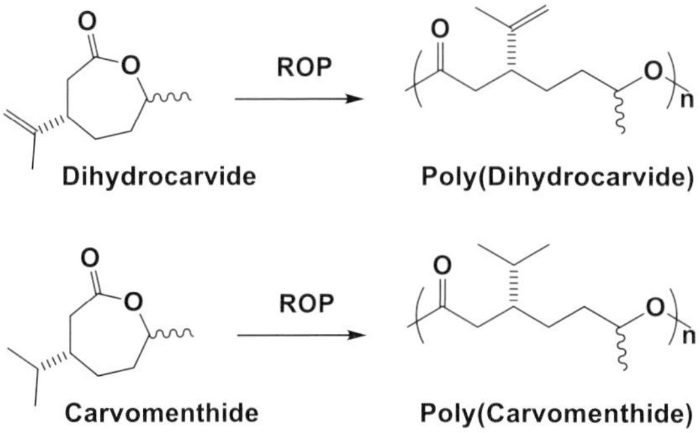

Figure 10.16 Monomers and polymers from carvone analogues.

mouse fibroblast cell line as determined by MTT (3-(4,5-dimethylthiazol-2-yl)-2,5-diphenyltetrazolium bromide) assays. However, due to the high crystallinity and highly hydrophobic nature of the homopolymer, no hydrolytic or enzymatic degradation was observed [241]. To address this problem, a copolymer with *p*-dioxanone (DO) has been synthesized (poly(ω-pentadecalactone-*co*-*p*-dioxanone) (poly(PPDL-*co*-DO)) using different ratios of ω-pentadecalactone and DO. Nanoparticles fabricated using poly(PPDL-*co*-DO) showed hydrolytic degradation at 37 °C (Figure 10.17). Doxorubicin (DOX) and siRNA were successfully encapsulated in the poly(PPDL-*co*-DO) nanoparticles with a maximum encapsulation efficiency of 42 and 33%, respectively. The loaded poly(PPDL-*co*-DO)

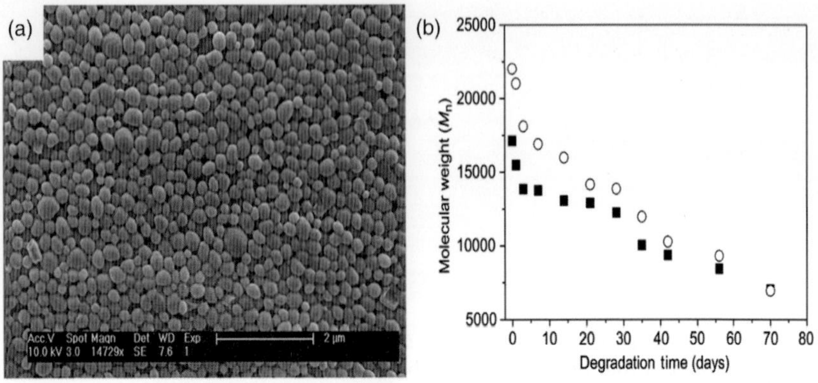

Figure 10.17 (a) SEM image of DOX-loaded nanoparticles prepared from poly(PDL-*co*-DO) copolymers and (b) change in number-average molecular weight with respect to time for blank poly(PDL-*co*-DO) nanoparticles having different concentration of PDL incubated in PBS solution (pH 7.4) at 37 °C [242]. (Reproduced with permission from Ref. [242]. Copyright 2011, Elsevier Ltd.)

nanoparticles demonstrated controlled release of encapsulated molecules *in vitro* for up to 60 days [242].

Domb and Slivniak reported the synthesis of macrolactones using ricinoleic acid (Figure 10.18). Several catalysts were explored to make the polyesters using

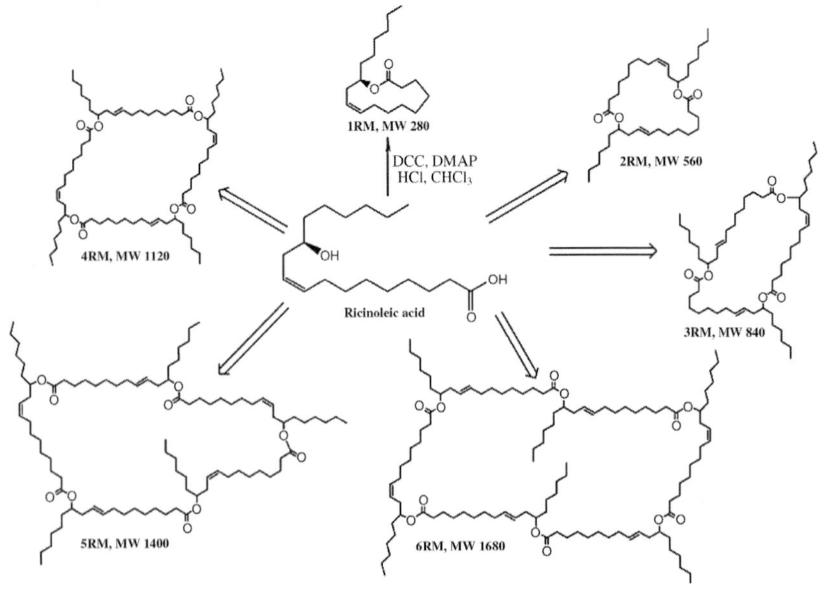

Figure 10.18 Structures of macrolactones synthesized from ricinoleic acid. Abbreviations for cyclic macrolactones: 1RM, monolactone; 2RM, dilactone, 3RM, trilactone; 4RM, tetralactone; 5RM, pentalactone; 6RM, hexalactone [244]. (Reproduced with permission from Ref. [243]. Copyright 2005, American Chemical Society.)

these lactone rings by ROP but only low-molecular-weight homopolymers were obtained. The low reactivity toward ROP of these lactone monomers was suggested to be due to the low ring strain and steric hindrance of the ester bond by the fatty acid side chain [243].

10.7 Controlled Radical Polymerization (CRP)

There is a need for precision and reproducibility with synthetic polymers intended for drug delivery applications, to ensure minimized batch-to-batch variability during synthesis and manufacture, and tight definition of product properties. Most commodity polymers are synthesized through free-radical polymerization techniques, which generate broad product mixtures with a high polydispersity index and corresponding range of properties. For applications such as packaging, a polymer product with a range of molar masses can be advantageous, but for biomedical use a wide spread of chain lengths and thus product heterogeneity can compromise the reproducibility of the product's biological performance.

Recent advances in controlled radical polymerization (CRP) are allowing for the fabrication of polymers with much better characteristics compared to the conventional free radical polymer synthesis routes. CRP has also opened up the vast array of acrylic and vinylic monomers, with a myriad of accessible functional side chains, to nonspecialist polymer chemistry labs [244–246]. Highly optimized CRP routes allow materials with a degree of order analogous to those seen in natural systems [33]. Recent work by the groups of Lutz [247] and Sawamoto [248], among others [249], is pushing toward polymers with truly biomimetic function by refining the concept of sequence control in synthetic materials still further. These groups describe chemistries that enable the stepwise addition of monomers to build up chains of unprecedented complexity. In addition, careful analysis of radical chemistry has enabled the groups of Perrier and Haddleton [169,250] to build block copolymers with up to 10 different constituent monomers, at $> 96\%$ conversion and with active chain ends even after >6 months of storage. Matyjasewski and co-workers have developed metal-catalyzed chemistries to produce arrays of blocks, stars, micelles, and vesicles, with precision control of molecular size while operating in atom-efficient conditions and benign solvents [251].

Polymers with a predetermined molecular weight and architecture can thus be readily synthesized with a narrow molecular weight distribution, and with a wide variety of architectures. The most widely employed CRP techniques are atom transfer radical polymerization (ATRP) and reversible addition fragmentation chain transfer (RAFT). While the mechanisms of these reactions are still subject to some debate and many reviews are available, these routes have nevertheless enabled some very interesting investigational therapeutics to be developed. While there are no CRP polymer therapeutics in late-stage clinical trials at present, some will no doubt reach the clinic for applications where biodegradability and chronic treatment are not requirements.

10.7.1 Atom Transfer Radical Polymerization (ATRP)

Examples of the many investigational therapeutics prepared from ATRP and other metal-catalyzed routes include poly(polyethylene glycol methacrylate)-protein conjugates with enhanced stability and greater retention time *in vivo* than analogous PEG materials [252], degradable polymer nanogels for doxorubicin delivery [253], a hyperbranched polymer found to be highly active in gene delivery [254], and a number of responsive polymers for drug and gene delivery *in vitro* [255–258]. The control inherent in the synthesis has allowed polymer micelles, vesicles, hyperbranched polymers, and star polymers to be synthesized in controlled sizes, ranging from 5–10 nm for micelles and low-molar-mass hyperbranched polymers to 200–300 nm for polymer vesicles. Accordingly, many studies are under way to evaluate how polymer nanomaterials of these sizes behave *in vitro* and *in vivo*.

The use of metal catalysts has been questioned for polymers intended to be used in humans, although the ATRP-variant single-electron transfer-living radical polymerization (SET-LRP) and other routes use very low amounts of copper, and no acute toxicity has been observed. Nevertheless, RAFT chemistries have found increasing favor in drug delivery and nanomedicine studies.

10.7.2 Reversible Addition Fragmentation Chain Transfer (RAFT) Polymerization

The Davis group in Australia pioneered the use of star polymers, produced by RAFT synthesis in the presence of macroinitiators and cross-linkers, in nanopharmacy applications [259,260]. The very fine control in the synthetic routes has allowed the preparation of star polymers with size ranges from 5–6 nm to beyond 40 nm, but with low size dispersity. These particles are thus approaching the dimensions of small viruses, and not surprisingly have been investigated extensively for nucleic acid delivery. In addition, the ease of functionalizing RAFT polymers enables introduction of labeling and diagnostic groups. Combinations of highly active delivery materials with *in situ* detection of drug release or *in vivo* distribution have been generated [261–265]. Again, as with ATRP and other controlled routes, the possibility to make materials of very discrete sizes, with controlled functional group content, block architecture, and self-assembly behavior, is very attractive from a nanomedicine perspective.

10.8 Concluding Remarks

The contributions of polymer science to the developing field of nanopharmacy have been very considerable, and there are many investigations under way, which could contribute still further. However, there are significant remaining challenges to widespread practical implementation of polymer nanomedicines. Scale-up of materials synthesis, processing robustness, cost-of-goods, sustainability of materials, and the economics of nanomedicines are all very important barriers. Even seemingly trivial issues such as sterilization and removal of endotoxins, which are essentially solved problems for small molecule drugs, are problematic for many nanomedicines. Much of the research focus to date has been at the synthesis stage, while characterization, development, and refinement have received much less attention. In part this is because some of the science is still in its infancy. However, there are large parts of the long-established colloid science field that are able to provide pertinent answers to some of the remaining questions on scale-up and processing of polymer nanomedicines. Accordingly, if polymers for nanopharmacy applications are to become a mature commercial and clinical technology, much greater emphasis will be needed on manufacture, regulatory assurance, and health economics.

References

1 Godwin, A., Bolina, K., Clochard, M., Dinand, E., Rankin, S., Simic, S., and Brocchini, S. (2001) *J. Pharm. Pharmacol.*, **53**, 1175–1184.

2 Elsabahy, M. and Wooley, K.L. (2012) *Chem. Soc. Rev.*, **41**, 2545–2561.

3 Vicent, M.J., Ringsdorf, H., and Duncan, R. (2009) *Adv. Drug Deliv. Rev.*, **61**, 1117–1120.

4 Satchi-Fainaro, R., Duncan, R., and Barnes, C.M. (2006) *Polymer Therapeutics Ii: Polymers As Drugs, Conjugates And Gene Delivery Systems*, Springer, Berlin, vol. 193, pp. 1–65.

5 Haag, R. and Kratz, F. (2006) *Angew. Chem., Int. Ed.*, **45**, 1198–1215.

6 Gaucher, G., Dufresne, M.H., Sant, V.P., Kang, N., Maysinger, D., and Leroux, J.C. (2005) *J. Control. Release*, **109**, 169–188.

7 Duncan, R., Vicent, M.J., Greco, F., and Nicholson, R.I. (2005) *Endocr. Relat. Cancer*, **12**, S189–S199.

8 Torchilin, V.P. (2005) *Expert Opin. Ther. Pat.*, **15**, 63–75.

9 Duncan, R. (2003) *Nat. Rev. Drug Discov.*, **2**, 347–360.

10 Perez, A.T., Domenech, G.H., Frankel, C., and Vogel, C.L. (2002) *Cancer Invest.*, **20**, 22–29.

11 Bertrand, N., Wu, J., Xu, X., Kamaly, N., and Farokhzad, O.C. (2014) *Adv. Drug Deliv. Rev.*, **66**, 2–25.

12 Maeda, H., Nakamura, H., and Fang, J. (2013) *Adv. Drug Deliv. Rev.*, **65**, 71–79.

13 Gaspar, R. and Duncan, R. (2009) *Adv. Drug Deliv. Rev.*, **61**, 1220–1231.

14 Duncan, R. and Gaspar, R. (2011) *Mol. Pharm.*, **8**, 2101–2141.

15 Venditto, V.J. and Szoka J Jr., F.C. (2013) *Adv. Drug Deliv. Rev.*, **65**, 80–88.

16 Sun, Q., Radosz, M., and Shen, Y. (2012) *J. Control. Release*, **164**, 156–169.

17 Nyström, A.M. and Fadeel, B. (2012) *J. Control. Release*, **161**, 403–408.

18 Bertrand, N. and Leroux, J.-C. (2012) *J. Control. Release*, **161**, 152–163.

19 Johnston, A.P.R., Such, G.K., Ng, S.L., and Caruso, F. (2011) *Curr. Opin. Colloid Interface*, **16**, 171–181.

20 Baetke, S.C., Lammers, T., and Kiessling, F. (2015) *Brit. J. Radiol.*, **88**, 20150207.

21 Ferguson, E.L., Azzopardi, E., Roberts, J.L., Walsh, T.R., and Thomas, D.W. (2014) *Mol. Pharm.*, **11**, 4437–4447.

22 Rahimian, S., Fransen, M.F., Kleinovink, J.W., Christensen, J.R., Amidi, M., Hennink, W.E., and Ossendorp, F. (2015) *J. Control. Release*, **203**, 16–22.

23 Qiu, L.Y. and Bae, Y.H. (2006) *Pharm. Res.*, **23**, 1–30.

24 van Nostrum, C.F. (2011) *Soft Matter*, **7**, 3246–3259.

25 Zhou, Z., Li, L., Yang, Y., Xu, X., and Huang, Y. (2014) *Biomaterials*, **35**, 6622–6635.

26 MacEwan, S.R. and Chilkoti, A. (2014) *J. Control. Release*, **190**, 314–330.

27 Potta, T., Zhen, Z., Grandhi, T.S.P., Christensen, M.D., Ramos, J., Breneman, C.M., and Rege, K. (2014) *Biomaterials*, **35**, 1977–1988.

28 Chu, T.-W. and Kopecek, J. (2015) *Biomat. Sci.*, **3** (7), 908–922.

29 Kopeček, J. (2013) *Adv. Drug Deliv. Rev.*, **65**, 49–59.

30 Kishimura, A. (2013) *Polym. J.*, **45**, 892–897.

31 Kishimura, A., Liamsuwan, S., Matsuda, H., Dong, W.F., Osada, K., Yamasaki, Y., and Kataoka, K. (2009) *Soft Matter*, **5**, 529–532.

32 Blunden, B.M., Thomas, D.S., and Stenzel, M.H. (2012) *Pol. Chem.*, **3**, 2964–2975.

33 Warren, N.J. and Armes, S.P. (2014) *J. Am. Chem. Soc.*, **136**, 10174–10185.

34 Letchford, K. and Burt, H. (2007) *Eur. J. Pharm. Biopharm.*, **65**, 259–269.

35 Lu, Y. and Park, K. (2013) *Int. J. Pharm.*, **453**, 198–214.

36 Torchilin, V.P. (2007) *Pharm. Res.*, **24**, 1–16.

37 Nishiyama, N. and Kataoka, K. (2006) *Pharmacol. Ther.*, **112**, 630–648.

38 Gref, R., Luck, M., Quellec, P., Marchand, M., Dellacherie, E., Harnisch, S., Blunk, T., and Muller, R.H. (2000) *Colloids Surf. B*, **18**, 301–313.

39 Sutton, D., Nasongkla, N., Blanco, E., and Gao, J. (2007) *Pharm. Res.*, **24**, 1029–1046.

40 Kataoka, K., Harada, A., and Nagasaki, Y. (2001) *Adv. Drug Deliv. Rev.*, **47**, 113–131.

41 Kataoka, K., Harada, A., and Nagasaki, Y. (2012) *Adv. Drug Deliv. Rev.*, **64**, 37–48.

42 Oerlemans, C., Bult, W., Bos, M., Storm, G., Nijsen, J.F.W., and Hennink, W.E. (2010) *Pharm. Res.*, **27**, 2569–2589.

43 Cabral, H. and Kataoka, K. (2014) *J. Control. Release*, **190**, 465–476.

44 Werner, M.E., Cummings, N.D., Sethi, M., Wang, E.C., Sukumar, R., Moore, D.T., and Wang, A.Z. (2013) *Int. J. Radiat. Oncol. Biol. Phys.*, **86**, 463–468.

45 Nakanishi, T., Fukushima, S., Okamoto, K., Suzuki, M., Matsumura, Y., Yokoyama, M., Okano, T., Sakurai, Y., and Kataoka, K. (2001) *J. Control. Release*, **74**, 295–302.

46 Singer, J.W. (2005) *J. Control. Release*, **109**, 120–126.

47 Valle, J.W., Armstrong, A., Newman, C., Alakhov, V., Pietrzynski, G., Brewer, J., Campbell, S., Corrie, P., Rowinsky, E.K., and Ranson, M. (2011) *Invest. New Drugs*, **29**, 1029–1037.

48 Hamaguchi, T., Doi, T., Eguchi-Nakajima, T., Kato, K., Yamada, Y., Shimada, Y., Fuse, N., Ohtsu, A., Matsumoto, S.-i., Takanashi, M., and Matsumura, Y. (2010) *Clin. Cancer Res.*, **16**, 5058–5066.

49 Matsumura, Y., Hamaguchi, T., Ura, T., Muro, K., Yamada, Y., Shimada, Y., Shirao, K., Okusaka, T., Ueno, H., Ikeda, M., and Watanabe, N. (2004) *Br. J. Cancer*, **91**, 1775–1781.

50 Matsumura, Y. (2011) *Adv. Drug Deliv. Rev.*, **63**, 184–192.

51 Uchino, H., Matsumura, Y., Negishi, T., Koizumi, F., Hayashi, T., Honda, T., Nishiyama, N., Kataoka, K., Naito, S., and Kakizoe, T. (2005) *Br. J. Cancer*, **93**, 678–687.

52 Kim, S.C., Kim, D.W., Shim, Y.H., Bang, J.S., Oh, H.S., Kim, S.W., and Seo, M.H. (2001) *J. Control. Release*, **72**, 191–202.

53 Scarano, W., de Souza, P., and Stenzel, M.H. (2015) *Biomater. Sci.*, **3**, 163–174.

54 Kim, Y., Pourgholami, M.H., Morris, D.L., and Stenzel, M.H. (2011) *J. Mater. Chem.*, **21**, 12777–12783.

55 Samarajeewa, S., Shrestha, R., Elsabahy, M., Karwa, A., Li, A., Zentay, R.P., Kostelc, J.G., Dorshow, R.B., and Wooley, K.L. (2013) *Mol. Pharm.*, **10**, 1092–1099.

56 Deacon, S.P.E., Apostolovic, B., Carbajo, R.J., Schott, A.K., Beck, K., Vicent, M.J., Pineda-Lucena, A., Klok, H.A., and Duncan, R. (2011) *Biomacromolecules*, **12**, 19–27.

57 Mi, P., Yanagie, H., Kokuryo, D., Dewi, N., Aoki, I., Nishiyama, N., and Kataoka, K. (2015) *J. Control. Release*, **213**, E88–E88.

58 Binauld, S. and Stenzel, M.H. (2013) *Chem. Commun.*, **49**, 2082–2102.

59 Yang, Z., Gao, D., Cao, Z., Zhang, C., Cheng, D., Liu, J., and Shuai, X. (2015) *Biomat. Sci.*, **3** (7), 1035–1049.

60 de las Heras Alarcon, C., Pennadam, S., and Alexander, C. (2005) *Chem. Soc. Rev.*, **34**, 276–285.

61 Jochum, F.D. and Theato, P. (2013) *Chem. Soc. Rev.*, **42** (17), 7468–7483.

62 Hoffman, A.S. (2013) *Adv. Drug Deliv. Rev.*, **65**, 10–16.

63 Le Meins, J.F., Sandre, O., and Lecommandoux, S. (2011) *Eur. Phys. J. E Soft Matter.*, **34**, 14.

64 LoPresti, C., Lomas, H., Massignani, M., Smart, T., and Battaglia, G. (2009) *J. Mater. Chem.*, **19**, 3576–3590.

65 Magnusson, J.P., Khan, A., Pasparakis, G., Saeed, A.O., Wang, W.X., and Alexander, C. (2008) *J. Am. Chem. Soc.*, **130**, 10852–10853.

66 Kanayama, N., Fukushima, S., Nishiyama, N., Itaka, K., Jang, W.D., Miyata, K., Yamasaki, Y., Chung, U.I., and Kataoka, K. (2006) *ChemMedChem*, **1**, 439–444.

67 Howard, K.A., Dong, M., Oupicky, D., Bisht, H.S., Buss, C., Besenbacher, F., and Kjems, J. (2007) *Small*, **3**, 54–57.

68 Thevenot, J., Oliveira, H., Sandre, O., and Lecommandoux, S. (2013) *Chem. Soc. Rev.*, **42**, 7099–7116.

69 Huo, M., Yuan, J., Tao, L., and Wei, Y. (2014) *Pol. Chem.*, **5**, 1519–1528.

70 Frazier, N. and Ghandehari, H. (2015) *Biotechnol. Bioeng.*, **112**, 1967–1983.

71 McDaniel, J.R., Dewhirst, M.W., and Chilkoti, A. (2013) *Int. J. Hyperthermia*, **29**, 501–510.

72 Sun, X.R., Xing, L.G., Ling, C.C., and Li, G.C. (2010) *Int. J. Hyperthermia*, **26**, 224–231.

73 Paliwal, S. and Mitragotri, S. (2008) *Ultrasonics*, **48**, 271–278.

74 Chen, T.H.H., Bae, Y., and Furgeson, D.Y. (2008) *Pharm. Res.*, **25**, 683–691.

75 Mastria, E.M., Chen, M., McDaniel, J.R., Li, X., Hyun, J., Dewhirst, M.W., and Chilkoti, A. (2015) *J. Control. Release*, **208**, 52–58.

76 McDaniel, J.R., MacEwan, S.R., Li, X., Radford, D.C., Landon, C.D., Dewhirst, M., and Chilkoti, A. (2014) *Nano Lett.*, **14**, 2890–2895.

77 Bhattacharyya, J., Bellucci, J.J., Weitzhandler, I., McDaniel, J.R., Spasojevic, I., Li, X., Lin, C.-C., Chi, J.-T. A., and Chilkoti, A. (2015) *Nat. Commun.*, **6**,-7939.

78 Dai, S., Ravi, P., and Tam, K.C. (2008) *Soft Matter*, **4**, 435–449.

79 Gao, W.W., Chan, J.M., and Farokhzad, O.C. (2010) *Mol. Pharm.*, **7**, 1913–1920.

80 Lomas, H., Canton, I., MacNeil, S., Du, J., Armes, S.P., Ryan, A.J., Lewis, A.L., and Battaglia, G. (2007) *Adv. Mater.*, **19**, 4238–4243.

81 Murdoch, C., Reeves, K.J., Hearnden, V., Colley, H., Massignani, M., Canton, I., Madsen, J., Blanazs, A., Armes, S.P., Lewis, A.L., MacNeil, S., Brown, N.J., Thornhill, M.H., and Battaglia, G. (2010) *Nanomedicine*, **5**, 1025–1036.

82 Lomas, H., Johnston, A.P.R., Such, G.K., Zhu, Z.Y., Liang, K., van Koeverden, M.P., Alongkornchotikul, S., and Caruso, F. (2011) *Small*, **7**, 2109–2119.

83 Luo, Z., Cai, K.Y., Hu, Y., Zhao, L., Liu, P., Duan, L., and Yang, W.H. (2011) *Angew. Chem., Int. Ed.*, **50**, 640–643.

84 Soliman, M., Nasanit, R., Abulateefeh, S.R., Allen, S., Davies, M.C., Briggs, S.S., Seymour, L.W., Preece, J.A., Grabowska, A.M., Watson, S.A., and Alexander, C. (2012) *Mol. Pharm.*, **9**, 1–13.

85 Cho, Y.H., Zhang, Y.J., Christensen, T., Sagle, L.B., Chilkoti, A., and Cremer, P.S. (2008) *J. Phys. Chem. B*, **112**, 13765–13771.

86 Su, H., Koo, J.M., and Cui, H. (2015) *J. Control. Release*, **219**, 383–395.

87 Duncan, R. (2014) *J. Control. Release*, **190**, 371–380.

88 Markovsky, E., Baabur-Cohen, H., Eldar-Boock, A., omer, L., Tiram, G., Ferber, S., Ofek, P., Polyak, D., Scomparin, A., and Satchi-Fainaro, R. (2012) *J. Control. Release*, **161**, 446–460.

89 Vilar, G., Tulla-Puche, J., and Albericio, F. (2012) *Curr. Drug Deliv.*, **9**, 367–394.

90 Canal, F., Sanchis, J., and Vicent, M.J. (2011) *Curr. Opin. Biotechnol.*, **22**, 894–900.

91 Duncan, R. and Vicent, M.J. (2010) *Adv. Drug Deliv. Rev.*, **62**, 272–282.

92 Mammen, M., Choi, S., and Whitesides, G.M. (1998) *Angew. Chem., Int. Ed.*, **37**, 2754–2794.
93 Kratz, F. (2014) *J. Control. Release*, **190**, 331–336.
94 Duncan, R. and Vicent, M.J. (2013) *Adv. Drug Deliv. Rev.*, **65**, 60–70.
95 Maeda, H., Bharate, G.Y., and Daruwalla, J. (2009) *Eur. J. Pharm. Biopharm.*, **71**, 409–419.
96 Medina, S.H. and El-Sayed, M.E.H. (2009) *Chem. Rev.*, **109**, 3141–3157.
97 Kihoon, N., Hye Yeong, N., Kim, P.-H., and Kim, S.W. (2012) *Biomaterials*, **33**, 8122–8130.
98 Magnusson, J.P., Fernandez-Trillo, F., Sicilia, G., Spain, S.G., and Alexander, C. (2014) *Nanoscale*, **6**, 2368–2374.
99 Pasut, G. and Veronese, F.M. (2012) *J. Control. Release*, **161**, 461–472.
100 Li, W., Zhan, P., De Clercq, E., Lou, H., and Liu, X. (2012) *Prog. Polym. Sci.*, **38**, 421–444.
101 Bailon, P. and Won, C. (2009) *Expert Opin. Drug Deliv.*, **6**, 1–16.
102 Abuchowski, A., van Es, T., Palczuk, N.C., and Davis, F.F. (1977) *J. Biol. Chem.*, **252**, 3578–3581.
103 Abuchowski, A., McCoy, J., Palczuk, N.C., and van Es, T., and Davis, F.F. (1977) *J. Biol. Chem.*, **252**, 3582–3586.
104 Annibali, V., Mechelli, R., Romano, S., Buscarinu, M.C., Fornasiero, A., Umeton, R., Ricigliano, V.A.G., Orzi, F., Coccia, E.M., Salvetti, M., and Ristori, G. (2015) *Cytokine Growth Factor Rev.*, **26**, 221–228.
105 Wadhwa, M., Bird, C., Dougall, T., Rigsby, P., Bristow, A., and Thorpe, R. (2015) *J. Immunol. Methods*, **416**, 17–28.
106 Veronese, F., Monfardini, C., and Caliceti, P. (1996) *J. Control. Release*, **40**, 199–209.
107 Zhang, X., Wang, H., Ma, Z., and Wu, B. (2014) *Expert Opin. Drug Metab. Toxicol.*, **10**, 1691–1702.
108 Baumann, A., Tuerck, D., Prabhu, S., Dickmann, L., and Sims, J. (2014) *Drug. Discov. Today*, **19**, 1623–1631.
109 Verhoef, J.J.F., Carpenter, J.F., Anchordoquy, T.J., and Schellekens, H. (2014) *Drug. Discov. Today*, **19**, 1945–1952.
110 Rajan, R.S., Li, T., Aras, M., Sloey, C., Sutherland, W., Arai, H., Briddell, R., Kinstler, O., Lueras, A.M.K., Zhang, Y., Yeghnazar, H., Treuheit, M., and Brems, D.N. (2006) *Protein Sci.*, **15**, 1063–1075.
111 Gonnelli, M. and Strambini, G.B. (2009) *Biochim. Biophys. Acta*, **1794**, 569–576.
112 Kubetzko, S., Sarkar, C.A., and Plückthun, A. (2005) *Mol. Pharmacol.*, **68**, 1439–1454.
113 Khalili, H., Godwin, A., Choi, J., Lever, R., and Brocchini, S. (2012) *Bioconjug. Chem.*, **23**, 2262–2277.
114 Duncan, R. and Gaspar, R. (2011) *Mol. Pharm.*, **8**, 2101–2141.
115 Schellekens, H., Hennink, W.E., and Brinks, V. (2013) *Pharm. Res.*, **30**, 1729–1734.
116 Garay, R.P., El-Gewely, R., Armstrong, J.K., Garratty, G., and Richette, P. (2012) *Expert Opin. Drug Delivery*, **9**, 1319–1323.
117 Rudmann, D.G., Alston, J.T., Hanson, J.C., and Heidel, S. (2013) *Toxicol. Pathol.*, **41**, 970–983.
118 Bendele, A., Seely, J., Richey, C., Sennello, G., and Shopp, G. (1998) *Toxicol. Sci.*, **42**, 152–157.
119 Schellekens, H. (2002) *Clin. Ther.*, **24**, 1720–1740.
120 Webster, R., Didier, E., Harris, P., Siegel, N., Stadler, J., Tilbury, L., and Smith, D. (2007) *Drug Metab. Dispos.*, **35**, 9–16.
121 Gorovits, B., Wakshull, E., Pillutla, R., Xu, Y., Manning, M.S., and Goyal, J. (2014) *J. Immunol. Methods*, **408**, 1–12.
122 Pasut, G. (2014) *React. Funct. Polym.*, **6**, 160–178.
123 Luxenhofer, R., Han, Y., Schulz, A., Tong, J., He, Z., Kabanov, A.V., and Jordan, R. (2012) *Macromol. Rapid Commun.*, **33**, 1613–1631.
124 Lewis, A., Tang, Y., Brocchini, S., Choi, J.-w., and Godwin, A. (2008) *Bioconjug. Chem.*, **19**, 2144–2155.
125 DeAngelis, P.L. (2015) *Expert Opin. Drug Deliv.*, **12**, 349–352.
126 Liebner, R., Mathaes, R., Meyer, M., Hey, T., Winter, G., and Besheer, A. (2014) *Eur. J. Pharm. Biopharm.*, **87**, 378–385.
127 Harris, J.M. and Chess, R.B. (2003) *Nat. Rev. Drug Dis.*, **2**, 214–221.

128 Greenwald, R.B., Choe, Y.H., McGuire, J., and Conover, C.D. (2003) *Adv. Drug Del. Rev.*, **55**, 217–250.

129 Stephanopoulos, N. and Francis, M.B. (2011) *Nat. Chem. Biol.*, **7**, 876–884.

130 Nischan, N. and Hackenberger, C.P.R. (2014) *J. Org. Chem.*, **79**, 10727–10733.

131 Obermeyer, A.C. and Olsen, B.D. (2015) *ACS Macro Lett.*, **4**, 101–110.

132 Boutureira, O. and Bernardes, G.J.L. (2015) *Chem. Rev.*, **115**, 2174–2195.

133 Diethelm, S., Schafroth, M.A., and Carreira, E.M. (2014) *Org. Lett.*, **16**, 3908–3911.

134 Rabanel, J.-M., Hildgen, P., and Banquy, X. (2014) *J. Control. Release*, **185**, 71–87.

135 Agarwal, P. and Bertozzi, C.R. (2015) *Bioconjug. Chem.*, **26**, 176–192.

136 Badescu, G., Bryant, P., Bird, M., Henseleit, K., Swierkosz, J., Parekh, V., Tommasi, R., Pawlisz, E., Jurlewicz, K., Farys, M., Camper, N., Sheng, X., Fisher, M., Grygorash, R., Kyle, A., Abhilash, A., Frigerio, M., Edwards, J., and Godwin, A. (2014) *Bioconjug. Chem.*, **25**, 1124–1136.

137 Podobnik, B., Helk, B., Smilović, V., Škrajnar, Š., Fidler, K., Jevševar, S., Godwin, A., and Williams, P. (2015) *Bioconjug. Chem.*, **26**, 452–459.

138 Soundrarajan, N., Sokalingam, S., Raghunathan, G., Budisa, N., Paik, H.-J., Yoo, T.H., and Lee, S.-G. (2012) *PLoS One*, **7**, e46741–46749.

139 Cong, Y., Pawlisz, E., Bryant, P., Balan, S., Laurine, E., Tommasi, R., Singh, R., Dubey, S., Peciak, K., Bird, M., Sivasankar, A., Swierkosz, J., Muroni, M., Heidelberger, S., Farys, M., Khayrzad, F., Edwards, J., Badescu, G., Hodgson, I., Heise, C., Somavarapu, S., Liddell, J., Powell, K., Zloh, M., Choi, J.-w., Godwin, A., and Brocchini, S. (2012) *Bioconjug. Chem.*, **23**, 248–263.

140 Fee, C. and Van Alstine, J. (2011) *Methods Biochem. Anal.*, **54**, 339–362.

141 Payne, R.W., Murphy, B.M., and Manning, M.C. (2011) *Pharm. Dev. Technol.*, **16**, 423–440.

142 Pfister, D. and Morbidelli, M. (2014) *J. Control. Release*, **180**, 134–149.

143 Alley, S.C., Benjamin, D.R., Jeffrey, S.C., Okeley, N.M., Meyer, D.L., Sanderson, R.J., and Senter, P.D. (2008) *Bioconjug. Chem.*, **19**, 759–765.

144 Baldwin, A.D. and Kiick, K.L. (2012) *Polym. Chem.*, **4**, 133.

145 Zhang, C., Liu, Y., Feng, C., Wang, Q., Shi, H., Zhao, D., Yu, R., and Su, Z. (2014) *Electrophoresis*, **36**, 371–374.

146 Shen, B.-Q., Xu, K., Liu, L., Raab, H., Bhakta, S., Kenrick, M., Parsons-Reponte, K.L., Tien, J., Yu, S.-F., Mai, E., Li, D., Tibbitts, J., Baudys, J., Saad, O.M., Scales, S.J., McDonald, P.J., Hass, P.E., Eigenbrot, C., Nguyen, T., Solis, W.A., Fuji, R.N., Flagella, K.M., Patel, D., Spencer, S.D., Khawli, L.A., Ebens, A., Wong, W.L., Vandlen, R., Kaur, S., Sliwkowski, M.X., Scheller, R.H., Polakis, P., and Junutula, J.R. (2012) *Nat. Biotechnol.*, **30**, 184–189.

147 Lyon, R.P., Setter, J.R., Bovee, T.D., Doronina, S.O., Hunter, J.H., Anderson, M.E., Balasubramanian, C.L., Duniho, S.M., Leiske, C.I., Li, F., and Senter, P.D. (2014) *Nat. Biotechnol.*, **32**, 1059–1062.

148 Fontaine, S.D., Reid, R., Robinson, L., Ashley, G.W., and Santi, D.V. (2015) *Bioconjug. Chem.*, **26**, 145–152.

149 Toda, N., Asano, S., and Barbas, C.F. (2013) *Angew. Chem., Int. Ed.*, **25**, 12592–12596.

150 Patterson, J.T., Asano, S., Li, X., Rader, C., and Barbas J III, C.F. (2014) *Bioconjug. Chem.*, **25**, 1402–1407.

151 Badescu, G., Bryant, P., Swierkosz, J., Khayrzad, F., Pawlisz, E., Farys, M., Cong, Y., Muroni, M., Rumpf, N., Brocchini, S., and Godwin, A. (2014) *Bioconjug. Chem.*, **25**, 460–469.

152 Mitchell, T., Chao, G., Sitkoff, D., Lo, F., Monshizadegan, H., Meyers, D., Low, S., Russo, K., DiBella, R., Denhez, F., Gao, M., Myers, J., Duke, G., Witmer, M., Miao, B., Ho, S.P., Khan, J., and Parker, R.A. (2014) *J. Pharmacol. Exp. Ther.*, **350** 412–424.

153 Shaunak, S., Godwin, A., Choi, J.W., Balan, S., Pedone, E., Vijayarangam, D., Heidelberger, S., Teo, I., Zloh, M., and Brocchini, S. (2006) *Nat. Chem. Bio.*, **2** (6), 312–313.

154 Jones, M.W., Strickland, R.A., Schumacher, F.F., Caddick, S., Baker, J.R., Gibson, M.I., and Haddleton, D.M. (2012) *J. Am. Chem. Soc.*, **134**, 1847–1852.

155 Nunes, J.P.M., Morais, M., Vassileva, V., Robinson, E., Rajkumar, V.S., Smith, M.E.B., Pedley, R.B., Caddick, S., Baker, J.R., and Chudasama, V. (2015) *Chem. Commun.*, **51**, 10624–10627.

156 Kontermann, R.E. (2011) *Curr. Opin. Biotechnol.*, **22**, 868–876.

157 Elliott, S., Lorenzini, T., Asher, S., Aoki, K., Brankow, D., Buck, L., Busse, L., Chang, D., Fuller, J., and Grant, J. (2003) *Nat. Biotechnol.*, **21**, 414–421.

158 Ezan, E., Becher, F., and Fenaille, F. (2014) *Expert Opin. Drug Metab. Toxicol.*, **10**, 1079–1091.

159 Ezan, E. (2013) *Adv. Drug Del. Rev.*, **65**, 1065–1073.

160 Mitragotri, S., Burke, P.A., and Langer, R. (2014) *Nat. Rev. Drug Discov.*, **13**, 655–672.

161 Duncan, R. (2014) *J. Control. Release*, **190**, 371–380.

162 Borchmann, D.E., Carberry, T.P., and Weck, M. (2013) *Macromol. Rapid Commun.*, **35**, 27–43.

163 Lawrence, P.B., Gavrilov, Y., Matthews, S.S., Langlois, M.I., Shental-Bechor, D., Greenblatt, H.M., Pandey, B.K., Smith, M.S., Paxman, R., Torgerson, C.D., Merrell, J.P., Ritz, C.C., Prigozhin, M.B., Levy, Y., and Price, J.L. (2014) *J. Am. Chem. Soc.*, **136**, 17547–17560.

164 Kratz, F. and Elsadek, B. (2012) *J. Control. Release*, **161**, 429–445.

165 Roy, R.K., Meszynska, A., Laure, C., Charles, L., Verchin, C., and Lutz, J.-F. (2015) *Nat. Commun.*, **6**, 7237.

166 Lutz, J.-F., Sumerlin, B., and Matyjaszewski, K. (2014) *Macromol. Rapid Commun.*, **35**, 122.

167 Lutz, J.-F., Ouchi, M., Liu, D.R., and Sawamoto, M. (2013) *Supramol. Sci.*, **341**, 628.

168 Gody, G., Maschmeyer, T., Zetterlund, P.B., and Perrier, S. (2014) *Macromolecules*, **47**, 3451–3460.

169 Anastasaki, A., Nikolaou, V., Pappas, G.S., Zhang, Q., Wan, C., Wilson, P., Davis, T.P., Whittaker, M.R., and Haddleton, D.M. (2014) *Chem. Sci.*, **5**, 3536–3542.

170 Ikada, Y. and Tsuji, H. (2000) *Macromol. Rapid Commun.*, **21**, 117–132.

171 Nair, L.S. and Laurencin, C.T. (2007) *Prog. Polym. Sci.*, **32**, 762–798.

172 Ulery, B.D., Nair, L.S., and Laurencin, C.T. (2011) *J. Polym. Sci. Pol. Phys.*, **49**, 832–864.

173 Agnihotri, S.A., Mallikarjuna, N.N., and Aminabhavi, T.M. (2004) *J. Control. Release*, **100**, 5–28.

174 Sarmento, B., Ribeiro, A., Veiga, F., Sampaio, P., Neufeld, R., and Ferreira, D. (2007) *Pharm. Res.*, **24**, 2198–2206.

175 De Campos, A.M., Sanchez, A., and Alonso, M.J. (2001) *Int. J. Pharm.*, **224**, 159–168.

176 Janes, K.A., Fresneau, M.P., Marazuela, A., Fabra, A., and Alonso, M.J. (2001) *J. Control. Release*, **73**, 255–267.

177 Kumari, A., Yadav, S.K., and Yadav, S.C. (2010) *Colloids Surf. B*, **75**, 1–18.

178 Kaul, G. and Amiji, M. (2005) *Pharm. Res.*, **22**, 951–961.

179 Gombotz, W.R. and Pettit, D.K. (1995) *Bioconjug. Chem.*, **6**, 332–351.

180 Malafaya, P.B., Silva, G.A., and Reis, R.L. (2007) *Adv. Drug Deliv. Rev.*, **59**, 207–233.

181 Lee, S.-H. and Shin, H. (2007) *Adv. Drug Deliv. Rev.*, **59**, 339–359.

182 Tian, H., Tang, Z., Zhuang, X., Chen, X., and Jing, X. (2012) *Prog. Polym. Sci.*, **37**, 237–280.

183 Middleton, J.C. and Tipton, A.J. (2000) *Biomaterials*, **21**, 2335–2346.

184 Gunatillake, P., Mayadunne, R., and Adhikari, R. (2006) *Biotechnol. Annu. Rev.*, **12**, 301–347.

185 Okada, M. (2002) *Prog. Polym. Sci.*, **27**, 87–133.

186 Jikei, M. and Kakimoto, M. (2001) *Prog. Polym. Sci.*, **26**, 1233–1285.

187 Kuchanov, S., Slot, H., and Stroeks, A. (2004) *Prog. Polym. Sci.*, **29**, 563–633.

188 Forbes, D.C. and Weaver, K.J. (2004) *J. Mol. Catal. A Chem.*, **214**, 129–132.

189 Fischer, E. and Speier, A. (1895) *Ber. Dtsch. Chem. Ges.*, **28**, 3252–3258.

190 Remme, N., Koschek, K., and Schneider, C. (2007) *Synlett*, 491–493.

191 Neises, B. and Steglich, W. (1978) *Angew. Chem., Int. Ed.*, **17**, 522–524.

192 Albertsson, A.C. and Varma, I.K. (2003) *Biomacromolecules*, **4**, 1466–1486.

193 Nuyken, O. and Pask, S.D. (2013) *React. Funct. Polym.*, **5**, 361–403.
194 Kurcok, P., Kowalczuk, M., Hennek, K., and Jedlinski, Z. (1992) *Macromolecules*, **25**, 2017–2020.
195 Woodruff, M.A. and Hutmacher, D.W. (2010) *Prog. Polym. Sci.*, **35**, 1217–1256.
196 Shuai, X.T., Ai, H., Nasongkla, N., Kim, S., and Gao, J.M. (2004) *J. Control. Release*, **98**, 415–426.
197 Darney, P.D., Klaisle, C.M., Monroe, S.E., Cook, C.E., Phillips, N.R., and Schindler, A. (1992) *Fertil. Steril.*, **58**, 137–143.
198 Tamada, J. and Langer, R. (1992) *J. Biomater. Sci. Polym. Ed.*, **3**, 315–353.
199 Kumar, N., Langer, R.S., and Domb, A.J. (2002) *Adv. Drug Deliv. Rev.*, **54**, 889–910.
200 Albertsson, A.C., Carlfors, J., and Sturesson, C. (1996) *J. Appl. Polym. Sci.*, **62**, 695–705.
201 Albertsson, A.C. and Eklund, M. (1995) *J. Appl. Polym. Sci.*, **57**, 87–103.
202 Zhang, Z., Kuijer, R., Bulstra, S.K., Grijpma, D.W., and Feijen, J. (2006) *Biomaterials*, **27**, 1741–1748.
203 Gabriele, B., Mancuso, R., Salerno, G., Ruffolo, G., Costa, M., and Dibenedetto, A. (2009) *Tetrahedron Lett.*, **50**, 7330–7332.
204 Darensbourg, D.J., Moncada, A.I., Choi, W., and Reibenspies, J.H. (2008) *J. Am. Chem. Soc.*, **130**, 6523–6533.
205 Zhang, Y. and Zhuo, R.X. (2005) *Biomaterials*, **26**, 2089–2094.
206 Jiang, X., Sha, X., Xin, H., Chen, L., Gao, X., Wang, X., Law, K., Gu, J., Chen, Y., Jiang, Y., Ren, X., Ren, Q., and Fang, X. (2011) *Biomaterials*, **32**, 9457–9469.
207 Habraken, W.J.E.M., Zhang, Z., Wolke, J.G.C., Grijpma, D.W., Mikos, A.G., Feijen, J., and Jansen, J.A. (2008) *Biomaterials*, **29**, 2464–2476.
208 Amsden, B.G., Timbart, L., Marecak, D., Chapanian, R., Tse, M.Y., and Pang, S.C. (2010) *J. Control. Release*, **145**, 109–115.
209 Danquah, M., Fujiwara, T., and Mahato, R.I. (2010) *Biomaterials*, **31**, 2358–2370.
210 Park, S.H., Choi, B.G., Joo, M.K., Han, D.K., Sohn, Y.S., and Jeong, B. (2008) *Macromolecules*, **41**, 6486–6492.
211 Papadimitriou, S., Papageorgiou, G.Z., Kanaze, F.I., Georgarakis, M., and Bikiaris, D.N. (2009) *J. Nanomater.*, **2009**, 1–11.
212 Zhang, S.P., Yang, J., Liu, X.Y., Chang, J.H., and Cao, A.M. (2003) *Biomacromolecules*, **4**, 437–445.
213 Ba, C.Y., Yang, J., Hao, Q.H., Liu, X.Y., and Cao, A. (2003) *Biomacromolecules*, **4**, 1827–1834.
214 Liu, J., Jiang, Z., Zhang, S., and Saltzman, W.M. (2009) *Biomaterials*, **30**, 5707–5719.
215 Makadia, H.K. and Siegel, S.J. (2011) *React. Funct. Polym.*, **3**, 1377–1397.
216 Wu, X.S. (1995) *Encyclopedic Handbook of Biomaterials and Bioengineering, Part A: Materials*, CRC, vol. 2, pp. 1015–1054.
217 Jain, R.A. (2000) *Biomaterials*, **21**, 2475–2490.
218 Tsuji, H. (2005) *Macromol. Biosci.*, **5**, 569–597.
219 Nicolas, J., Mura, S., Brambilla, D., Mackiewicz, N., and Couvreur, P. (2013) *Chem. Soc. Rev.*, **42**, 1147–1235.
220 Avgoustakis, K. (2004) *Curr. Drug Deliv.*, **1**, 321–333.
221 Park, T.G. (1995) *Biomaterials*, **16**, 1123–1130.
222 Kirby, G.T.S., White, L.J., Rahman, C.V., Cox, H.C., Qutachi, O., Rose, F.R.A.J., Hutmacher, D.W., Shakesheff, K.M., and Woodruff, M.A. (2011) *React. Funct. Polym.*, **3**, 571–586.
223 Jhunjhunwala, S., Raimondi, G., Thomson, A.W., and Little, S.R. (2009) *J. Control. Release*, **133**, 191–197.
224 Danhier, F., Ansorena, E., Silva, J.M., Coco, R., Le Breton, A., and Préat, V. (2012) *J. Control. Release*, **161**, 505–522.
225 Cheng, J., Teply, B.A., Sherifi, I., Sung, J., Luther, G., Gu, F.X., Levy-Nissenbaum, E., Radovic-Moreno, A.F., Langer, R., and Farokhzad, O.C. (2007) *Biomaterials*, **28**, 869–876.
226 Lee, J.Y., Bashur, C.A., Goldstein, A.S., and Schmidt, C.E. (2009) *Biomaterials*, **30**, 4325–4335.
227 Jiang, H.L., Hu, Y.Q., Li, Y., Zhao, P.C., Zhu, K.J., and Chen, W.L. (2005) *J. Control. Release*, **108**, 237–243.

228 Song, Z., Feng, R., Sun, M., Guo, C., Gao, Y., Li, L., and Zhai, G. (2011) *J. Colloid Interface Sci.*, **354**, 116–123.
229 Johansen, P., Men, Y., Audran, R., Corradin, G., Merkle, H.P., and Gander, B. (1998) *Pharm. Res.*, **15**, 1103–1110.
230 Thomas, C., Gupta, V., and Ahsan, F. (2010) *Pharm. Res.*, **27**, 905–919.
231 Fonseca, C., Simoes, S., and Gaspar, R. (2002) *J. Control. Release*, **83**, 273–286.
232 Avgoustakis, K., Beletsi, A., Panagi, Z., Klepetsanis, P., Karydas, A.G., and Ithakissios, D.S. (2002) *J. Control. Release*, **79**, 123–135.
233 Van De Weert, M., Hennink, W.E., and Jiskoot, W. (2000) *Pharm. Res.*, **17**, 1159–1167.
234 Zhu, G.Z., Mallery, S.R., and Schwendeman, S.P. (2000) *Nat. Biotechnol.*, **18**, 52–57.
235 Jeong, Y.-I., Na, H.-S., Seo, D.-H., Kim, D.-G., Lee, H.-C., Jang, M.-K., Na, S.-K., Roh, S.-H., Kim, S.-i., and Nah, J.-w. (2008) *Int. J. Pharm.*, **352**, 317–323.
236 Murata, N., Takashima, Y., Toyoshima, K., Yamamoto, M., and Okada, H. (2008) *J. Control. Release*, **126**, 246–254.
237 Patil, Y. and Panyam, J. (2009) *Int. J. Pharm.*, **367**, 195–203.
238 Lowe, J.R., Martello, M.T., Tolman, W.B., and Hillmyer, M.A. (2011) *Pol. Chem.*, **2**, 702–708.
239 Martello, M.T., Burns, A., and Hillmyer, M. (2012) *Acs Macro Lett.*, **1**, 131–135.
240 Kumar, A., Kalra, B., Dekhterman, A., and Gross, R.A. (2000) *Macromolecules*, **33**, 6303–6309.
241 van der Meulen, I., de Geus, M., Antheunis, H., Deumens, R., Joosten, E.A.J., Koning, C.E., and Heise, A. (2008) *Biomacromolecules*, **9**, 3404–3410.
242 Liu, J., Jiang, Z., Zhang, S., Liu, C., Gross, R.A., Kyriakides, T.R., and Saltzman, W.M. (2011) *Biomaterials*, **32**, 6646–6654.
243 Slivniak, R. and Domb, A.J. (2005) *Biomacromolecules*, **6**, 1679–1688.
244 Moad, G., Rizzardo, E., and Thang, S.H. (2008) *Acc. Chem. Res.*, **41**, 1133–1142.
245 Matyjaszewski, K. and Tsarevsky, N.V. (2009) *Nat. Chem.*, **1**, 276–288.
246 Kamigaito, M., Ando, T., and Sawamoto, M. (2001) *Chem. Rev.*, **101**, 3689–3746.
247 Zamfir, M. and Lutz, J.-F. (2012) *Nat. Commun.*, **3**, 1138.
248 Nakatani, K., Ogura, Y., Koda, Y., Terashima, T., and Sawamoto, M. (2012) *J. Am. Chem. Soc.*, **134**, 4373–4383.
249 Chuang, Y.-M., Ethirajan, A., and Junkers, T. (2014) *ACS Macro Lett.*, **3**, 732–737.
250 Gody, G., Maschmeyer, T., Zetterlund, P.B., and Perrier, S. (2013) *Nat. Commun.*, **4**, 3505.
251 Simakova, A., Averick, S.E., Konkolewicz, D., and Matyjaszewski, K. (2012) *Macromolecules*, **45**, 6371–6379.
252 Gao, W., Liu, W., Mackay, J.A., Zalutsky, M.R., Toone, E.J., and Chilkoti, A. (2009) *Proc. Natl. Acad. Sci.*, **106**, 15231–15236.
253 Oh, J.K., Siegwart, D.J., Lee, H.I., Sherwood, G., Peteanu, L., Hollinger, J.O., Kataoka, K., and Matyjaszewski, K. (2007) *J. Am. Chem. Soc.*, **129**, 5939–5945.
254 Newland, B., Tai, H.Y., Zheng, Y., Velasco, D., Luca, A.Di., Howdle, S.M., Alexander, C., Wang, W.X., and Pandit, A. (2010) *Chem. Commun.*, **46**, 4698–4700.
255 Averick, S.E., Paredes, E., Irastorza, A., Shrivats, A.R., Srinivasan, A., Siegwart, D.J., Magenau, A.J., Cho, H.Y., Hsu, E., Averick, A.A., Kim, J., Liu, S., Hollinger, J.O., Das, S.R., and Matyjaszewski, K. (2012) *Biomacromolecules*, **13**, 3445–3449.
256 Gallon, E., Matini, T., Sasso, L., Mantovani, G., Armiñan de Benito, A., Sanchis, J., Caliceti, P., Alexander, C., and Vicent, M.J., and Salmaso, S. (2015) *Biomacromolecules*, **16**, 1924–1937.
257 Mastrotto, F., Salmaso, S., Lee, Y.L., Alexander, C., Caliceti, P., and Mantovani, G. (2013) *Pol. Chem.*, **4**, 4375–4385.
258 Abulateefeh, S.R., Spain, S.G., Thurecht, K.J., Aylott, J.W., Chan, W.C., Garnett, M.C., and Alexander, C. (2013) *Biomat. Sci.*, **1**, 434–442.
259 Boyer, C., Teo, J., Phillips, P., Erlich, R.B., Sagnella, S., Sharbeen, G., Dwarte, T., Duong, H.T.T., Goldstein, D., Davis, T.P.,

Kavallaris, M., and McCarroll, J. (2013) *Mol. Pharm.*, **10**, 2435–2444.

260 Valade, D., Boyer, C., Davis, T.P., and Bulmus, V. (2009) *Aust. J. Chem.*, **62**, 1344–1350.

261 Fuchs, A.V., Gemmell, A.C., and Thurecht, K.J. (2015) *Pol. Chem.*, **6**, 868–880.

262 Eliezar, J., Scarano, W., Boase, N.R.B., Thurecht, K.J., and Stenzel, M.H. (2015) *Biomacromolecules*, **16**, 515–523.

263 Wang, K., Peng, H., Thurecht, K.J., Puttick, S., and Whittaker, A.K. (2014) *Pol. Chem.*, **5**, 1760–1771.

264 Rolfe, B.E., Blakey, I., Squires, O., Peng, H., Boase, N.R.B., Alexander, C., Parsons, P.G., Boyle, G.M., Whittaker, A.K., and Thurecht, K.J. (2014) *J. Am. Chem. Soc.*, **136**, 2413–2419.

265 Tan, J.H., McMillan, N.A.J., Payne, E., Alexander, C., Heath, F., Whittaker, A.K., and Thurecht, K.J. (2012) *J. Polym. Sci. Pol. Chem.*, **50**, 2585–2595.

11
Overview and Presentation of Exploratory Methods for Manufacturing Nanoparticles/"Inorganic Materials"

Xavier Le Guevel

Institute for Advanced Biosciences (IAB), University Grenoble-Alpes (UGA), INSERM-U1209, CNRS-UMR 5309, Rond-point de la Chantourne, 38706 La Tronche, France

11.1 Introduction

Inorganic materials, nanoparticles (NPs) in particular, have gained a growing interest over the last 20 years for therapy and imaging in the field of cancer, autoimmune, and infectious diseases [1]. The fine tuning of their physicochemical properties (size, shape, surface charge, pore size, etc.) by top-down and bottom-up approaches combining to their intrinsic properties such as magnetism, luminescence, scattering, plasmonic offer a versatile platform to design a myriad of new delivery nanosystems. Several strategies have been reported to attach drugs or genetic materials to the inorganic NPs with additional stabilizing agents and/or targeted molecules on their surface. It leads to the formulation of new complex nanosystems with drastic change of their intrinsic properties, colloidal stability, diffusion, and surface chemistry compared to the bare inorganic NPs. This critical aspect needs to be carefully evaluated in different media (water, buffer, and complete medium) before moving forward to *in vitro* and *in vivo* investigation.

The progress in inorganic NPs-based delivery system has often been represented following three major chronological steps: (1) the first generation of NPs composed of one single material with the attachment of therapeutics, (2) the second generation of NPs with the "interconnection" of organic, biological, and inorganic moieties exhibiting multifunctional properties accompanied with high colloidal stability and active targeting, and (3) the third generation of NPs since the last 5–10 years with the emergence of stimuli-responsive-hybrid nanosystems enable to release therapeutics remotely by endogenous (redox, enzyme, and pH) and exogenous (temperature, light, and magnetic field) triggering [2,3]. The most investigated inorganic NPs applied in nanomedicine could be classified in the following list: metal, metal oxide, semiconductors, and lanthanides. It will be impossible to summarize all the advances in synthesis and biomedical

Pharmaceutical Nanotechnology: Innovation and Production, First Edition. Edited by Jean Cornier, Arno Kwade, Andrew Owen, and Marcel Van de Voorde.

applications of those hybrid organic/inorganic nanosystems, so we will present in this chapter, the main strategies and breakthroughs in the synthesis of each type of inorganic NPs highlighting the benefit for imaging and therapy through concrete examples (see Table 11.1). Regarding the aspect of their biocompatibility and toxicity, an important parameter for clinical transfer considering the poor biodegradability of most of those materials, it will be addressed in another chapter.

11.2 Gold NPs

From the large library of metal nanoparticles developed for drug and gene delivery applications, gold nanoparticles (Au NPs) are probably the most investigated and reported ones in the literature [4,86–88] with few examples currently in clinical trials for rheumatoid arthritis and cancer therapy [89]. The success of Au NPs relies on the ability to tailor size, shape, and surface chemistry with a high monodispersity and reasonably good colloidal stability. The ease to decorate Au NP surface with organic or biological molecules make them excellent candidates for active targeting and delivery system. Au NPs has the ability to absorb a relatively high amount of X-ray that can be used for radiotherapy [5]. In addition, the unique optical properties of Au NPs have shown also a huge potential for imaging allowing to track them in *in vitro/in vivo* model and to study the biodistribution and the toxicity of the therapeutic agents carried by those particles [26].

11.2.1 Different Shapes and Optical Properties

Since the simple and robust method reported by Turkevitch in the 1950s to prepare 10–20 nm diameter spherical Au NPs stabilized by citrate, tremendous effort has been pursued in this direction to produce gold particles with various size and high monodispersity. The range of the particle size synthesized encompasses from very few atoms also called “nanoclusters” [6,90–92] to 100 nm diameter or more. The second breakthrough came in the early 1990s initiated by Brust–Schiffrin where controlling finely the growth of alkane-thiolated gold particles (particle size below 10 nm) in biphasic polar/apolar solvent led to monodisperse and size tunable Au NPs [93]. The Brust–Schiffrin method has been adapted and improved by many research groups over the past 20 years, enabling to obtain stable particles protected by a single thiolate monolayer that could be isolated and redissolve in various solvents. In addition, the choice of large library of thiol organic linkers allows the preparation of Au NPs with various surface functionalities. Other robust methods have been described in the literature using surfactant or polyelectrolyte, notably the seeded-mediated route to produce spherical Au NPs in the range 50–200 nm with a very high reproducibility [94].

Table 11.1 Overview of inorganic nanoparticles for pharmaceutical applications.

NP class	Surface coating	NP size	Stimulus	Applications	Diagnostic modalities	Refs
Gold spheres	PEG, polymers, small organic molecules	2–50 nm	X-ray	Radiotherapy	CT	[4–6]
Gold spheres	Polymers, polyelectrolytes	2–50 nm		Drug delivery	TPM	[7–14]
Gold spheres, nanorods	Nucleic acids, DNA, siRNA	2–50 nm		Gene delivery	TPM, fluorescence	[15–22]
Gold spheres, nanorods	PEG, polymers, small organic molecules	2–50 nm	pH, redox, temperature	Drug, peptide, protein, gene delivery	PAT, TPM	[16,23–25]
Gold nanorods, nanoshells, nanocages	PEG, polymers, small organic molecules	30–100 nm	NIR laser	Photochemotherapy	TPM, SERS, PAT	[26–32]
Gold spheres, nanorods, stars	Liposomes	10–100 nm	NIR laser, pH	Drug delivery, photochemotherapy	SERS, TPM, PAT	[33,34]
Gold spheres, nanorods, nanocages	Silica	10–100 nm		Drug delivery, photochemotherapy	TPM, SERS	[35–39]
MFe_2O_4, M = Mn, Fe, Co		15 nm	Magnetic field	Hyperthermia	MRI	[40]
Iron oxide	Polyelectrolytes	200–400 nm	Magnetic field	Gene delivery		[41]
Iron oxide	Silica	200 nm			MRI	[42–44]
Gd	Protein	50–120 nm	Magnetic field	Radiotherapy	TPM, MRI	[45,46]
Manganese oxide		200 nm	Magnetic field, pH	Drug delivery	MRI	[47]
Iron oxide	Carbon	7–9 nm	Radio frequency	Drug delivery	MRI	[48]

(*continued*)

Table 11.1 *(Continued)*

NP class	Surface coating	NP size	Stimulus	Applications	Diagnostic modalities	Refs
Iron oxide, cobalt	Gold	9 nm		Gene delivery	MRI	[49]
Mesoporous silica		100–500 nm		Drug delivery	Fluorescence	[50–52]
Mesoporous silica	Polymer, polyelectrolytes		pH, temperature, photoirradiation	Drug delivery	Fluorescence	[53–55]
Mesoporous silica		100 nm	Magnetic field	Drug delivery, hyperthermia	Fluorescence	[56]
Porous silicon	Small organic molecules, carbonization, oxidation	150–350 nm		Drug delivery	Fluorescence	[57–62]
Calcium Phosphate	Small organic molecules, polyelectrolytes	20–150 nm		Gene delivery	Fluorescence	[63–69]
Calcium phosphate	Polymers, lipids	20–150 nm	Magnetic field	Drug delivery	MRI, Fluorescence	[63,70,71]
Aluminum oxide		30–80 nm		Adjuvant		[72]
Silver		5–50 nm		Antibacterial		[73,74]
Quantum Dots, lanthanides	Small organic molecules, polyelectrolytes, polymers, liposomes, silica	5–30 nm	pH, temperatures	Drug delivery	Fluorescence	[75–85]

CT: computer tomography; SERS: surface enhanced Raman scattering; TPM: two photon microscopy; PAT: photoacoustic tomography; MRI: magnetic resonance imaging.

We can also cite the emergence of green chemistry to prepare Au NPs of different sizes using natural products such as tea leaves [95–97].

Variety of one-, two-, and three-dimensional gold nanocrystals has been attempted over the last 20 years using physical and chemical routes [27,98]. The bottom-up approach is reckoned to be the most dominant method to produce anisotropic Au NPs with various shapes (rods [99], prisms [100], stars [101], hexapods [102], etc.) and hollows Au NPs (shells [103] and cages [104]). El-Sayed and Murphy's teams were the pioneers to develop seed-mediated synthesis of anisotropic gold and silver particle with a high yield and good reproducibility using highly concentrated surfactant (cetyltriammonium bromide, CTAB) solution. For instance synthesis of Au nanorods with a very fine control of the aspect ratio length over diameter could be achieved and the seeding-growth method is now widely used by many research labs from different disciplines [99,105]. The other popular approach to obtain 3D and more complex nanostructures is based on the modified polyol process in presence of PVP acting as reducing agents [104,106]. Galvanic replacement has shown quite recently great success to design in very fast and reproducible way Au nanocages with single and multiple walls [98,107] and Au nanoshells [108]. In the same time, the mechanistic aspect of anisotropic Au NPs growth is till under investigation helping to define the critical parameters to construct precisely gold nano-object [109].

The unique and strong interaction of metal nanoparticles, especially gold and silver, with light in the visible and in the near-infrared region (NIR) offer a formidable advantage to use them for biosensing and as contrast agents. This effect called localized plasmon resonance (LSPR) is originated to the electric field of the light-inducing waves of collective electron oscillations confined to the surface of the nanoparticle [110]. LSPR of metal NPs is highly dependent on their composition, size, and shape and reveals to be highly sensitive to the environmental change. Thus, the presence of molecules of interest could be detected close to the NP surface at very low concentration by looking at the plasmon shift. The strong enhancement of the Raman (surface-enhanced Raman scattering, SERs) or fluorescence signals of species close to Au NP surface of various shapes are also intensively exploited for diagnostic applications [111,112]. The localization of the plasmon band in the red-NIR region for anisotropic Au NPs also found a particular interest in the field of medicine where tissue scattering and blood absorption is reduced and light penetration is increased in this spectral range [4]. For instance, Halas' team developed targeted gold nanoshells for cancer therapy and gene therapy vectors using a NIR illumination to trigger thermal damages and gene release, respectively [28,103].

Gold NPs could be visualized in cellular environment and in animal models by multiple imaging techniques such as dark-field microscopy, two-photon microscopy, photoacoustic (PA) imaging, photothermal (PT) imaging, optical coherence tomography, and X-ray imaging thanks to their optical properties (i.e., absorption, scattering, and fluorescence enhancement), high electronic density, and good photostability [29]. For example, the strong absorption of Au NPs such as nanorods, nanoshells, or nanocages in the NIR region allow to improve the imaging detection using PA and PT to study several disease processes in mice and in rats [113]. The ability to combine X-ray computed imaging and other optical imaging techniques to detect Au NPs offers a great advantage to detect tumors in live animal [114].

11.2.2 Conjugated (Covalent and Noncovalent)

A large variety of organic ligand containing phosphine, amine, or thiol groups could be conjugated on Au NPs surface creating a monolayer or bilayer preventing particle aggregation. Au NPs protected by mono and bidentate thiol linkers [115,116] are the most commonly used to design Au NPs-based delivery systems. Rotello's team have reported a considerable number of custom-made thiolated ligands able to release anticancer drugs and biomolecules in *in vitro* and *in vivo* models using external and endogenous stimuli [15,16].

Two main approaches based on covalent and noncovalent binding are generally described to load molecule of interests (drug, oligonucleotides, RNA, peptide, aptamers, etc.) on Au NPs. The noncovalent approach is based on the weak interaction (electrostatic, hydrophobic, hydrogen bindings, and steric immobilization) between the loaded compounds and the capping agent. This approach has been classified previously in two distinct classes: the surface mediated and the encapsulation strategy [23]. The noncovalent strategy offers the advantage to release unmodified drugs or biomolecules to the targeted sites. For instance, DNA, RNA, peptides, and proteins have been conjugated noncovalently to Au NPs surface coated with cationic polymers or amino acids and those delivery systems have demonstrated a very high cell transfection efficiency (>10-fold compared to polyethylenimine transfection agent) preventing enzymatic digestion [17]. We can cite for example the synthesis of Au NPs coated with tunable amino acid density that could deliver efficiently DNA in mammalian cells by glutathione regulation present at the intracellular level [24]. Using the encapsulation route, Caruso *et al.* described a Layer-by Layer technique to coat Au NPs sequentially with cationic and then anionic material polymer incorporating drug such as Doxorubicin between the organic layer [7]. This method has shown significant improvement of drug delivery in different cell types compared to the free drugs [8].

Drugs and biomolecules (oligonucleotides, DNA, RNA, antibodies, proteins, and peptides) could be also covalently conjugated directly to Au NP surface via thiol groups or to the monolayer surface by amino, alkyl, and carboxyl coupling. Mirkin's lab and other research groups have developed various nanosystems based on antisense oligonucleotides and silencing RNA (siRNA) conjugated to Au NPs for gene regulation [15,18,19]. The high performance of "oligoantisense nanoparticles" has been attributed to the synergy of the high genetic transfection by the NPs into the cells, and to the binding of complementary DNA on the grafted oligonucleotides, which are densely packed on gold surface. Anticancer drugs, such as doxorubicin (DOX) [25], cisplatin [22], paclitaxel [9], or tamoxifen [10], have been covalently conjugated to Au NPs by either modifying the drugs or the NP surface. The esterification of paclitaxel and doxorubicin enable to design stable anticancer drugs–gold conjugates exhibiting an enhanced toxicity in *in vitro* and *in vivo studies* compared to the free drugs [11,12]. Another promising approach consists in the coupling the drug to the NPs using photocleavable molecules, which could lead to the drug release under light irradiation. Thus, Rotello's team incorporate a UV-photocleavable *ortho*-nitrobenzyl (ONB) compound between Au NP and 5-fluorouracil to control the drug release under UV irradiation leading to cell death [30].

11.2.3 Polymer/Polyelectrolyte Coating

The advances on the synthesis of functional polymeric nanoparticles and the ability to graft organic groups on Au NP surface enable to design new hybrid nanosystems for theranostic applications [13]. Natural and synthetic polymeric materials, such as poly(lactic-*co*-glycolic acid), dextran, and chitosan among others, have been coated on Au NPs of various size and shape. Those nanosystems present the advantages to combine the high drug payload in the polymer moiety and the intrinsic properties of gold for imaging and photochemo therapy [31,117]. Polyelectrolyte material is another interesting candidate for drug delivery applications forming nanogels in solution. Those nanogels have high biocompatibility with controlled and sustained drug release under various stimuli such as pH, ionic strength, or temperature [2,3]. The synthesis of the core/shell structure gold/nanogel could be achieved by seed polymerization on Au NPs or by the *in situ* Au NP growth in the polyelectrolyte network [14]. As an example, poly(NIPAM-*co*-acrylamide), a thermoresponsive polymer, was coated on Au nanorods and the anticancer drug DOX was loaded (24%) in those hybrid gold-nanogels (Figure 11.1a and b). A NIR laser irradiation of tumor-bearing mice where the smart nanosystems strongly accumulated after intravenous injection induced a thermal effect leading to the DOX release and stopped almost completely the tumor growth (Figure 11.1c and d) [32].

11.2.4 Lipids

Hybrid nanosystems composed of Au NPs and phospholipids, essentially liposomes, are mainly prepared following three main approaches incorporating the metal NPs in (i) the inner phase of the liposomes, (ii) in the liposome membrane, and (iii) on the liposome surface [33]. By incorporating Au NPs with star and rod shapes inside liposomes sensitive to pH, it was possible to release efficiently by NIR light irradiation a model drug calcein into the cytosol of human retinal pigment epithelial cells (ARPE-19) [34].

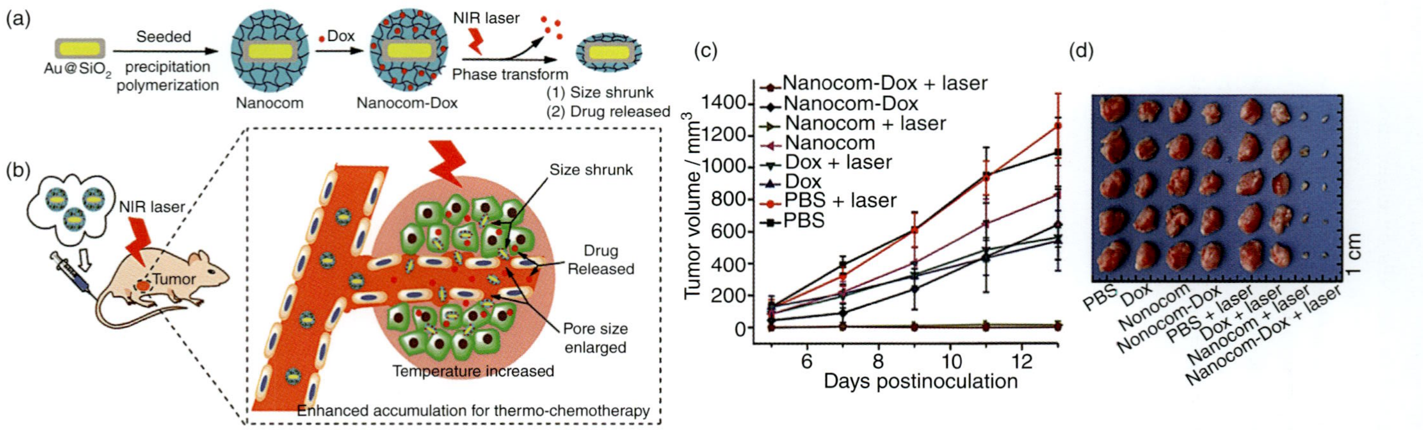

Figure 11.1 (a) Scheme of nanocomposite formulation process, and (b) NIR laser-induced targeted thermochemotherapy using the nanocomposite. (c and d) *In vivo* antitumor activity against murine 4T1 breast tumor after systematic administration or intratumoural injection. (c) The antitumor activity including PBS, Dox, Nanocom, and Nanocom-Dox groups (with or without laser irradiation) through tail vein by measuring the tumor volume. (d) Tumor dissection photographs through systematic administration. (Reproduced with permission from Ref. [117]. Copyright 2014, American Chemical Society.)

11.2.5 Composite

Mesoporous metal oxide coating on Au NPs could be considered as relative simple strategy to improve drug-loading capacity per NPs by loading drug inside pores of tunable size and geometry [118]. The choice of a large selection of organosilanes enables also to functionalize the metal oxide shell to improve the colloidal stability of the NPs and for targeting purpose. Different techniques by selective etching strategy and using self-template method showed very efficient results to grow Au NPs or incorporate previously synthesized Au NPs in hollow, rattle, and core/shell types of mesoporous silica NPs (MSNs) [119]. Gold could be also coated on MSNs to form gold nanoshell with tunable thickness, which prevent leakage from the particle until the drug release triggered by NIR laser irradiation. Using both nanosystems: Au core/mSi shell and MSNs core/Au shell loaded with anticancer drugs, several research groups showed promising results in *in vitro* and *in vivo* studies to kill cancer cells using NIR laser irradiation without damaging drastically healthy tissues [35–39].

11.3 Magnetic NPs

Magnetic NPs have gained a tremendous interest for biomedical applications such as contrast agents for magnetic resonance imaging (MRI), hyperthermia for cancer therapy [40], magnetic transfection for gene delivery [41], tissue engineering [120], and as a platform for drug delivery [121]. Iron oxide so-called super paramagnetic iron oxide NPs (SPIONs) and others ferrites doped with metal cations (Mn^{2+}, Co^{2+}, Zn^{2+}, etc.) are the most studied magnetic NPs with few translation in preclinical and clinical studies [3]. Nevertheless, there are other magnetic NPs from alloys such as $CoPt_3$ [122] or FePt [123], janus NPs [42,43], and self-assembled gadolinium complexes [45,46] that exhibit also remarkable magnetic properties with high potential as theranostic agents [124].

11.3.1 Synthesis

The ultrasmall SPIONs magnetite (Fe_3O_4) and maghemite (Fe_2O_3) with diameter smaller than 20 nm were usually prepared from Fe^{2+}/Fe^{3+} aqueous salt solution by coprecipitation method [125]. However, even in presence of stabilizing agents to control NP growth, this synthesis leads to a high polydispersity in size and in shape. Therefore, the high-temperature reductive decomposition of metal salt or organometallic precursors in organic solutions containing stabilizing surfactants is nowadays preferred to obtain monodisperse SPIONs [126,127]. Since then, intensive works reported in excellent reviews are dedicated to understand the correlation between the growing process of those NPs and their magnetic properties [121,128–130]. In parallel, other techniques have been developed to produce magnetic NPs by microemulsion [131] and hydrothermal synthesis [132] and show promising results despite a still lack of monodispersity and a low yield.

11.3.2
Stabilization/Protection of Magnetic NPs

After synthesis, metal magnetic NPs have a strong tendency to aggregate and oxidize in solution leading to particle precipitation and the loss of their superparamagnetic behavior. To answer this issue, several strategies have been proposed to protect the NP surface by oxidized passivation and by coating with organic or inorganic material [133]. For instance, a wide library of polymers and surfactants can be anchored and physisorbed on magnetic NPs. It allows to improve the colloidal stability, biocompatibility, and to bring additional features such as swelling property, temperature and pH responses, hydrophobic cavities to incorporate poorly soluble drug, and terminal chemical groups for further postfunctionalization [128]. Inorganic shell protecting the magnetic NPs could be performed by chemical grafting of silica or titanium precursors controlling the sol/gel reaction to tailor the thickness and the porosity of the metal oxide layer [44,47,134]. Carbon [48] and noble metal coatings on magnetic NPs, mainly gold [49] and silver [135], have been achieved by different chemical methods from solvent replacement to reverse microemulsion or reduction reaction. Gold nanoshell on magnetic NPs can be considered as a very interesting hybrid nanosystem for theranostic applications offering new features such as optical properties (imaging and photothermo reactivity) and particle surface easy to modify with thiol and aminated molecules. The important aspect after the stabilization/protection of the magnetic NPs is to ensure the relatively small size, high colloidal stability, and monodispersity of the NPs avoiding any significant loss of their magnetization.

11.3.3
Hybrid Magnetic Nanosystem for Delivery

Nanoconstructs containing magnetic nanoparticles find their application in nanomedicine to undergo physical change under an external magnetic field triggering local heat (hyperthermia) and the release of drugs entrapped physically or chemically into/onto the nanoformulation. Additional surface biofunctionalization with specific molecules (peptides, antibody, carbohydrate, etc.) could also enhance the therapeutic benefit by active targeting. There are plethora of new hybrid magnetic NPs for therapy and imaging described in the literature [136]. We can cite the smart nanosystem design by Zink's group based on DOX-loaded mesoporous silica containing Zinc-doped-SPIONs, and the nanovalves (cucurbit [6]uril), which could prevent drug leakage from the pores (Figure 11.2). Due to

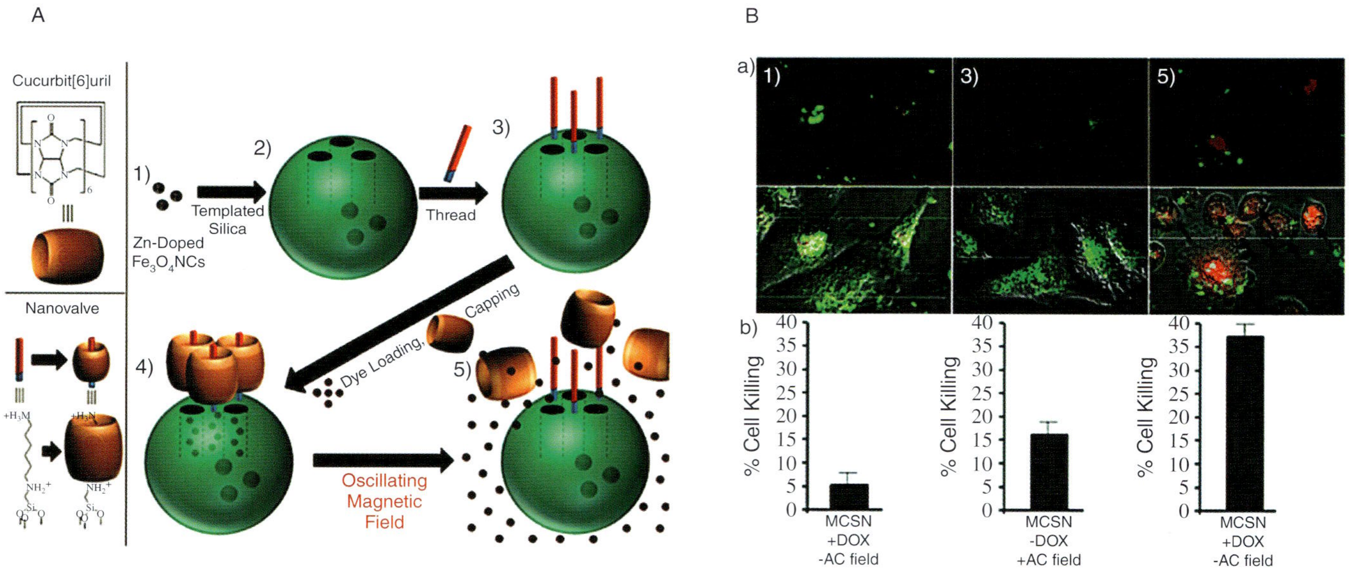

Figure 11.2 (A) Scheme of Sketch of nanoparticles, machines, and assembly. A ZnNCs (1) are synthetically positioned at the core of the mesoporous silica nanoparticles (2). The base of the molecular machine is then attached to the nanoparticle surface (3). Drug is loaded into the particle and capped (4) to complete the system. Release can be realized using remote heating via the introduction of an oscillating magnetic field (5). The particles and machines are not drawn to scale. (B) Results of MDA-MB-231 exposure to the MARS. Panel (a) shows fluorescent microscope images (1, 3, and 5) and fluorescent images with differential interference contrast (2, 4, and 6). Color scheme: green, fluorescently labeled MARS; red, doxorubicin (DOX); yellow, merged green, and red. MARS nanoparticles containing DOX were taken up into the cells, but before the AC field was applied, no drug release (images 1 and 2) and negligible cell death [~5%; panel (b), left bar] occurred. Images 3 and 4 show the effects of the magnetic field on MARS nanoparticles without DOX in the pores. Heating from the particles accounted for 16% of the cell killing [panel (b), middle bar]. Images 5 and 6 demonstrate DOX release after a 5 min AC field exposure, which caused 37% of the cell death [panel b, right bar]. The arrows in image 6 indicate the location of apoptotic cells. (Reproduced with permission from Ref. [135]. Copyright 2010, American Chemical Society.)

the presence of the magnetic nanocrystals, an external magnetic field induced a hyperthermic effect leading to the cleavage of the nanovalves. DOX could be then released from the hybrid nanosystem inside breast cancer cells promoting cell death [56].

11.4
Metal Oxide NPs

11.4.1
Silica/Silicon

Nonporous and mesoporous silica NPs are viewed as one of the most promising and flexible platform in the field of nanobiomedicine [137]. In particular, mesoporous silica particles (MSNs) are extensively investigated as drug delivery carriers thanks to their size and shape tunable, high drug payload, and the ability to functionalize the surface with a large library of organosilanes [50–52]. Mesostructures, morphologies, and size of MSNs could be finely tailored by controlling parameters such as pH value, nature of the silica precursors, and of the surfactants, concentration, counterions, salts, and temperature. The progress in synthesis to tune the pore size from 1.5 to 30 nm and to selectively functionalize the inner pore and the external NP surface has led to the production of many drug-loaded MSNs exhibiting good stability and high drug loading combine with targeting features. In addition, a careful surface functionalization of MSNs with polyethylene groups or lipid bilayers may prevent particle aggregation and rapid dissolution to produce acid silicic species. In order to even increase the payload in the MSNs, hollow mesoporous silica NPs (HSNs) have been achieved through different strategies from soft templating (single micelle, vesicle, or microemulsion) to hard templating (polymer beads, metal, or metal oxide NPs). More complexes MSNs have been designed to release drug under external (light, external magnetic field, and temperature) and endogeneous (pH, redox reaction, and enzyme) stimuli so-called gatekeeper nanosystem [50,51,53,54,56,138]. For this, pores are blocked with selected agents such as NPs [55], organic or biologic molecules, and are then opened under specific conditions in order to release drug or biomolecules from the nanocarriers to the targeted cells, tissues, or organs. As one of the many examples of stimuli-responsive MSNs developed over the last 10 years, Bein, Braüchle, and his colleagues incorporated drug models (rhodamine derivative and calcein) inside MSNs following by the grafting of a red light photosensitizer (aluminum phthalocyanine disulfonate) on the surface. NPs were then coated with a lipid bilayer that was decorated with targeted ligands such as folic acid or epidermal growth factor. Under red laser irradiation, this nanosystem could remotely release the model drugs in HeLA cells by activating the photosensitizer, which generated reactive oxygen species inducing the disruption of the lipid bilayer [50].

Porous silicon NPs (pSi), a subtype of silica nanomaterial combining high porosity and hydrophobic property, have gained particular interest as delivery systems allowing the insertion of high content of poorly soluble drugs. The standard methods to produce pSi rely on electrochemical anodization [57] and etching of native oxide present on silicon wafer. Pore size (2–50 nm) could be finely tuned by adjusting experimental parameters (doping type, HF concentration, and applied voltage) and the particle surface by oxidation or chemical modifications [57–59]. Drug molecules have been loaded in pSi by covalent attachment, physical trapping, and spontaneous adsorption. In order to prevent fast drug release, pSi can be coated using polymer, lipids, protein, or metal oxide layers. Santos' team have extensively investigated pSi for therapeutic applications demonstrating the release of drugs and biomolecules in targeted cells and in organs accompanied with a very low toxicity [60–62,139].

11.4.2
Calcium Phosphate, Hydroxyapatite

The biocompatibility and biodegradability of calcium phosphate (CaP) present in human bone and teeth make this inorganic material an attractive candidate as cargo to deliver molecules of interest in the body. Another advantage of CaP for delivery action refers to his dissolution in acidic environment (pH 4), which can be used to selectively deliver therapeutics in cells, tissues, and organs. The pH solubility allows the complete degradation of CaP in lysosomes preventing accumulation of material in cells and the efficient release of payload for cancer therapy in acidic tumor environment. CaP NPs and crystalline forms such as hydroxyapatite (HA) NPs with control size and shape are commonly prepared by coprecipitation or microemulsion methods. In case of the amorphous CaP NPs, a protective layer using HA, polymers, or lipids is required to prevent a fast burst and to achieve an efficient release of the payload at the targeted sites. Consequently, many efforts have been dedicated to load dyes, drugs, and biomolecules in CaP and HA NPs with an improved colloidal stability [63,70,71]. The most successful results for therapy have been obtained in gene transfection (DNA and siRNA) both in *in vitro* and *in vivo* studies [64–69]. It should be noted that the incorporation of drugs and photosensitizers, which are mainly hydrophobic and poorly soluble, in CaP and HA NPs still remains challenging due to the high degree of hydrophilicity of the scaffold.

11.4.3
Others: Titanium Oxide and Aluminum Oxide

Other nonporous and mesoporous metal oxide NPs have been used as therapeutic delivery systems exploiting their intrinsic properties. Notably, we can cite the photocatalytic properties of titanium oxide NPs for skin delivery applications [140] or the immunogenicity of aluminum oxide NPs in the design of nanovaccines for immunotherapeutic treatments [72,141].

11.5 Others (Silver, Quantum Dots, and Lanthanides)

Silver (Ag) NPs are mainly developed for antibacterial applications due to the strong reactivity of Ag ions etched from the NPs, which could pass through biofilms and kill bacteria. There are few examples of hybrid nanosystems incorporating Ag NPs notably for implants to prevent infections [73] but the risk of long-term accumulation in the body and the well-known acute toxicity of silver [74] make this strategy still questionable.

Quantum dots (QDs) are fluorescent semiconductors nanocrystals that gained tremendous interest for diagnostic and therapy thanks to remarkable optical properties (high sensitivity, multiplexing, high resolution, and high photostability) combined to their small size and the ease to functionalize their surface with molecule of interests such as anticancer drugs, DNA, or siRNA [75]. A high effort has been pursued over the last 15 years to produce bright QDs with tunable fluorescence from the UV to the NIR region with high colloidal stability and various surface (bio)functionalities. In the same time, new nanocrystalline forms of QDs have emerged to replace the first generation of QDs such as Cadmium-based QDs, which exhibit strong toxicity [142]. QDs reveal to be an excellent platform to evaluate the interaction between NPs with biological environment. For instance, QDs were employed extensively to study how physicochemical parameters of NPs influence the intracellular uptake [143,144], the biodistribution in animals [145], or to quantify passive and active targeting for cancer therapy [76]. Therefore, QDs represent excellent contrast agents to (a) track drug or genetic material grafted on their surface or (b) to study the fate and the cargo release kinetic of bigger drug-loaded nanocarriers such as liposomes or polymeric NPs with QDs loaded inside or coated on the surface of the NPs [77–79].

Lanthanide complexes are a class of rare-earth metals protected by organic ligands exhibiting luminescence with a very sharp emission and remarkable optical properties suitable for bioimaging (upconversion, high Stokes-shift, and long luminescence lifetime) [80]. An intense work is dedicated to the chemical coordination of the metal core selecting organic molecules called "antenna" to tune the fluorescence emission and to boost the quantum yield efficiency [80]. As a sub-type of the lanthanide complexes, lanthanide-doped upconverting luminescent nanoparticles (UCNPs) possess features, which make them promising as theranostic agents with the ability to attach molecules covalently or noncovalently on the outer layer and to track them by fluorescence imaging using NIR laser irradiation ($\lambda = 980$ nm) [81]. UCNPs are synthesized by thermal decomposition or hydro(solvo)thermal techniques, and various strategies have been applied to modify UCNP surface with polymers, lipids, silica to attach drugs, and nonspecific and targeting ligands [82]. Like for QDs, UCNPs-based delivery systems are prepared following two distinct approaches: incorporation of UCNPs in bigger NPs with a high payload capacity or by linking molecules to the UCNP surface. UCNPs-based delivery systems were investigated for therapeutic applications notably to study release siRNA in live cells [83] and to target tumor overexpressing cRGD [84] or folic acid [85] receptors and deliver DOX [146].

11.6 Conclusion and Perspective

In summary, the fast progress during the last two decades to design inorganic NPs with various shape, size, and surface chemistry with the understanding of their physical properties have opened the door to a multitude of drug delivery systems acting both as contrast and therapeutic agent (i.e., theranostics). The rational design of smart nanosystems that could overcome biological barriers and trigger remotely drugs or biomolecules to targeted sites by various stimuli offers a promising strategy to move nanomedicine forward. With a few examples of gold and magnetic based-delivery systems currently in preclinical and clinical phases, the inorganic NPs seem to have a bright future for personalized medicine.

Nevertheless, compared to biodegradable NPs such as liposomes or natural polymeric NPs, inorganic NPs have lower drug loading efficiency and low biodegradability. The unknown long-term toxicity for most of the new hybrid drug delivery systems still represents a huge obstacle for therapeutic applications. Coming back to more fundamental questions, there are still lacks of understanding on the NP interaction with the biological environment from the cell interaction with the protein corona contribution to the NP effect on the immune response. Those points need to be carefully investigated for each new delivery nanosystems proposed in order to select the most suitable particles to treat diseases.

Acknowledgment

This work was supported by the Instituto de Salud Carlos III (ISCII) on the project No. CP12/03310 cofinanced by European Regional Development Fund (ERDF).

References

1 Nie, Z., Petukhova, A., and Kumacheva, E. (2010) Properties and emerging applications of self-assembled structures made from inorganic nanoparticles. *Nat. Nanotechnol.*, **5**, 15–25.

2 Mura, S., Nicolas, J., and Couvreur, P. (2013) Stimuli-responsive nanocarriers for drug delivery. *Nat. Mater.*, **12**, 991–1003.

3 Molina, M., Asadian-Birjand, M., Balach, J., Bergueiro, J., Miceli, E., and Calderón, M. (2015) Stimuli-responsive nanogel composites and their application in nanomedicine. *Chem. Soc. Rev.*, **44**, 6161–6186.

4 Jain, S., Hirst, D.G., and O'Sullivan, J.M. (2012) Gold nanoparticles as novel agents for cancer therapy. *Br. J. Radiol.*, **85**, 101–113.

5 Hainfeld, J.F., Dilmanian, F.A., Slatkin, D.N., and Smilowitz, H.M. (2008) Radiotherapy enhancement with gold

nanoparticles. *J. Pharm. Pharmacol.*, **60**, 977–985.

6 Zhang, X.D., Luo, Z., Chen, J., Shen, X., Song, S., Sun, Y., Fan, S., Fan, F., Leong, D.T., and Xie, J. (2014) Ultrasmall Au10-12(SG)10-12 nanomolecules for high tumor specificity and cancer radiotherapy. *Adv. Mater.*, **26**, 4565–4568.

7 Becker, A.L., Johnston, A.P.R., and Caruso, F. (2010) Layer-by-layer-assembled capsules and films for therapeutic delivery. *Small*, **6**, 1836–1852.

8 Yan, Y., Such, G.K., Johnston, A.P.R., Lomas, H., and Caruso, F. (2011) Toward therapeutic delivery with layer-by-layer engineered particles. *ACS Nano*, **5**, 4252–4257.

9 Gibson, J.D., Khanal, B.P., and Zubarev, E.R. (2007) Paclitaxel-functionalized gold nanoparticles. *J. Am. Chem. Soc.*, **129**, 11653–11661.

10 Dreaden, E.C., Mwakwari, S.C., Sodji, Q.H., Oyelere, A.K., and El-Sayed, M.A. (2009) Tamoxifen-poly(ethylene glycol)-thiol gold nanoparticle conjugates: enhanced potency and selective delivery for breast cancer treatment. *Bioconjug. Chem.*, **20**, 2247–2253.

11 Sun, T.M., Wang, Y.C., Wang, F., Du, J.Z., Mao, C.Q., Sun, C.Y., Tang, R.Z., Liu, Y., Zhu, J., Zhu, Y.H., Yang, X.Z., and Wang, J. (2014) Cancer stem cell therapy using doxorubicin conjugated to gold nanoparticles via hydrazone bonds. *Biomaterials*, **35** 836–845.

12 Heo, D.N., Yang, D.H., Moon, H.J., Lee, J.B., Bae, M.S., Lee, S.C., Lee, W.J., Sun, I.C., and Kwon, I.K. (2012) Gold nanoparticles surface-functionalized with paclitaxel drug and biotin receptor as theranostic agents for cancer therapy. *Biomaterials*, **33**, 856–866.

13 Muddineti, O.S., Ghosh, B., and Biswas, S. (2015) Current trends in using polymer coated gold nanoparticles for cancer therapy. *Int. J. Pharm.*, **484**, 252–267.

14 Sierra-Martin, B. and Fernandez-Barbero, A. (2015) Multifunctional hybrid nanogels for theranostic applications. *Soft Matter*, **11**, 8205–8216.

15 Ding, Y., Jiang, Z., Saha, K., Kim, C.S., Kim, S.T., Landis, R.F., and Rotello, V.M. (2014) Gold nanoparticles for nucleic acid delivery. *Mol. Ther.*, **22**, 1075–1083.

16 Rana, S., Bajaj, A., Mout, R., and Rotello, V.M. (2012) Monolayer coated gold nanoparticles for delivery applications. *Adv. Drug Deliv. Rev.*, **64**, 200–216.

17 Han, G., Martin, C.T., and Rotello, V.M. (2006) Stability of gold nanoparticle-bound DNA toward biological, physical, and chemical agents. *Chem. Biol. Drug Des.*, **67**, 78–82.

18 Rosi, N.L., Giljohann, D.A., Thaxton, C.S., Lytton-Jean, A.K.R., Han, M.S., and Mirkin, C.A. (2006) Oligonucleotide-modified gold nanoparticles for infracellular gene regulation. *Science*, **312**, 1027–1030.

19 Giljohann, D.A., Seferos, D.S., Prigodich, A.E., Patel, P.C., and Mirkin, C.A. (2009) Gene regulation with polyvalent siRNA-nanoparticle conjugates. *J. Am. Chem. Soc.*, **131**, 2072–2073.

20 Oishi, M., Nakaogami, J., Ishii, T., and Nagasaki, Y. (2006) Smart PEGylated gold nanoparticles for the cytoplasmic delivery of siRNA to induce enhanced gene silencing. *Chem. Lett.*, **35**, 1046–1047.

21 Seferos, D.S., Giljohann, D.A., Rosi, N.L., and Mirkin, C.A. (2007) Locked nucleic acid-nanoparticle conjugates. *Chembiochem*, **8**, 1230–1232.

22 Dhar, S., Daniel, W.L., Giljohann, D.A., Mirkin, C.A., and Lippard, S.J. (2009) Polyvalent oligonucleotide gold nanoparticle conjugates as delivery vehicles for platinum(IV) warheads. *J. Am. Chem. Soc.*, **131**, 14652–14653.

23 Doane, T. and Burda, C. (2013) Nanoparticle mediated non-covalent drug delivery. *Adv. Drug Deliv. Rev.*, **65**, 607–621.

24 Ghosh, P.S., Kim, C.K., Han, G., Forbes, N.S., and Rotello, V.M. (2008) Efficient gene delivery vectors by tuning the surface charge density of amino acid-functionalized gold nanoparticles. *ACS Nano*, **2**, 2213–2218.

25 Wang, F., Wang, Y.C., Dou, S., Xiong, M.H., Sun, T.M., and Wang, J. (2011) Doxorubicin-tethered responsive gold

nanoparticles facilitate intracellular drug delivery for overcoming multidrug resistance in cancer cells. *ACS Nano*, **5**, 3679–3692.

26 Dreaden, E.C., Alkilany, A.M., Huang, X., Murphy, C.J., and El-Sayed, M.A. (2012) The golden age: gold nanoparticles for biomedicine. *Chem. Soc. Rev.*, **41**, 2740–2779.

27 Li, N., Zhao, P., and Astruc, D. (2014) Anisotropic gold nanoparticles: synthesis, properties, applications, and toxicity. *Angew. Chem., Int. Ed.*, **53**, 1756–1789.

28 Bardhan, R., Lal, S., Joshi, A., and Halas, N.J. (2011) Theranostic nanoshells: from probe design to imaging and treatment of cancer. *Acc. Chem. Res.*, **44**, 936–946.

29 Webb, J.A. and Bardhan, R. (2014) Emerging advances in nanomedicine with engineered gold nanostructures. *Nanoscale*, **6**, 2502–2530.

30 Agasti, S.S., Chompoosor, A., You, C.C., Ghosh, P., Kim, C.K., and Rotello, V.M. (2009) Photoregulated release of caged anticancer drugs from gold nanoparticles. *J. Am. Chem. Soc.*, **131**, 5728–5729.

31 Xiao, Z., Ji, C., Shi, J., Pridgen, E.M., Frieder, J., Wu, J., and Farokhzad, O.C. (2012) DNA self-assembly of targeted near-infrared-responsive gold nanoparticles for cancer thermo-chemotherapy. *Angew. Chem., Int. Ed.*, **51**, 11853–11857.

32 Zhang, Z., Wang, J., Nie, X., Wen, T., Ji, Y., Wu, X., Zhao, Y., and Chen, C. (2014) Near infrared laser-induced targeted cancer therapy using thermoresponsive polymer encapsulated gold nanorods. *J. Am. Chem. Soc.*, **136**, 7317–7326.

33 Kojima, C., Hirano, Y., and Kono, K. (2009) Preparation of complexes of liposomes with gold nanoparticles. *Methods Enzymol.*, **464**, 131–145.

34 Lajunen, T., Viitala, L., Kontturi, L.S., Laaksonen, T., Liang, H., Vuorimaa-Laukkanen, E., Viitala, T.;Le., Guével, X., Yliperttula, M., Murtomäki, L., and Urtti, A. (2015) Light induced cytosolic drug delivery from liposomes with gold nanoparticles. *J. Control. Release*, **203** 85–98.

35 Liu, H., Chen, D., Li, L., Liu, T., Tan, L., Wu, X., and Tang, F. (2011) Multifunctional gold nanoshells on silica nanorattles: a platform for the combination of photothermal therapy and chemotherapy with low systemic toxicity. *Angew. Chem., Int. Ed.*, **50**, 891–895.

36 Zhang, Z., Wang, L., Wang, J., Jiang, X., Li, X., Hu, Z., Ji, Y., Wu, X., and Chen, C. (2012) Mesoporous silica-coated gold nanorods as a light-mediated multifunctional theranostic platform for cancer treatment. *Adv. Mater.*, **24**, 1418–1423.

37 Shen, S., Tang, H., Zhang, X., Ren, J., Pang, Z., Wang, D., Gao, H., Qian, Y., Jiang, X., and Yang, W. (2013) Targeting mesoporous silica-encapsulated gold nanorods for chemo-photothermal therapy with near-infrared radiation. *Biomaterials*, **34**, 3150–3158.

38 Wu, X., Li, L., Zhang, L., Wang, T., Wang, C., and Su, Z. (2015) Multifunctional spherical gold nanocluster aggregate@polyacrylic acid@mesoporous silica nanoparticles for combined cancer dual-modal imaging and chemo-therapy. *J. Mater. Chem. B*, **3**, 2421–2425.

39 Yang, J., Shen, D., Zhou, L., Li, W., Li, X., Yao, C., Wang, R., El-Toni, A.M., Zhang, F., and Zhao, D. (2013) Spatially confined fabrication of core-shell gold nanocages@mesoporous silica for near-infrared controlled photothermal drug release. *Chem. Mater.*, **25**, 3030–3037.

40 Lee, J.H., Jang, J.T., Choi, J.S., Moon, S.H., Noh, S.H., Kim, J.W., Kim, J.G., Kim, I.S., Park, K.I., and Cheon, J. (2011) Exchange-coupled magnetic nanoparticles for efficient heat induction. *Nat. Nanotechnol.*, **6**, 418–422.

41 Prijic, S., Prosen, L., Cemazar, M., Scancar, J., Romih, R., Lavrencak, J., Bregar, V.B., Coer, A., Krzan, M., Znidarsic, A., and Sersa, G. (2012) Surface modified magnetic nanoparticles for immuno-gene therapy of murine mammary adenocarcinoma. *Biomaterials*, **33**, 4379–4391.

42 Zhang, L., Zhang, F., Dong, W.F., Song, J.F., Huo, Q.S., and Sun, H.B. (2011) Magnetic-mesoporous Janus

nanoparticles. *Chem. Commun.*, **47**, 1225–1227.

43 Yan, J., Chaudhary, K., Chul, B.S., Lewis, J.A., and Granick, S. (2013) Colloidal ribbons and rings from Janus magnetic rods. *Nat. Commun.*, **4**, 1516.

44 Vogt, C., Toprak, M.S., Muhammed, M., Laurent, S., Bridot, J.L., and Müller, R.N. (2010) High quality and tuneable silica shell-magnetic core nanoparticles. *J. Nanopart. Res.*, **12**, 1137–1147.

45 Cao, C.Y., Shen, Y.Y., Wang, J.D., Li, L., and Liang, G.L. (2013) Controlled intracellular self-assembly of gadolinium nanoparticles as smart molecular MR contrast agents. *Scientific Reports*, **3**, 1024.

46 Rima, W., Sancey, L., Aloy, M.T., Armandy, E., Alcantara, G.B., Epicier, T., Malchère, A., Joly-Pottuz, L., Mowat, P., Lux, F., Tillement, O., Burdin, B., Rivoire, A., Boulé, C., Anselme-Bertrand, I., Pourchez, J., Cottier, M., Roux, S., Rodriguez-Lafrasse, C., and Perriat, P. (2013) Internalization pathways into cancer cells of gadolinium-based radiosensitizing nanoparticles. *Biomaterials*, **34** 181–195.

47 Chen, Y., Yin, Q., Ji, X., Zhang, S., Chen, H., Zheng, Y., Sun, Y., Qu, H., Wang, Z., Li, Y., Wang, X., Zhang, K., Zhang, L., and Shi, J. (2012) Manganese oxide-based multifunctionalized mesoporous silica nanoparticles for pH-responsive MRI, ultrasonography and circumvention of MDR in cancer cells. *Biomaterials*, **33** 7126–7137.

48 Xu, Y., Karmakar, A., Heberlein, W.E., Mustafa, T., Biris, A.R., and Biris, A.S. (2012) Multifunctional magnetic nanoparticles for synergistic enhancement of cancer treatment by combinatorial radio frequency thermolysis and drug delivery. *Adv. Healthc. Mater.*, **1**, 493–501.

49 Robinson, I., Tung, L.D., Maenosono, S., Wälti, C., and Thanh, N.T.K. (2010) Synthesis of core-shell gold coated magnetic nanoparticles and their interaction with thiolated DNA. *Nanoscale*, **2**, 2624–2630.

50 Argyo, C., Weiss, V., Bräuchle, C., and Bein, T. (2014) Multifunctional mesoporous silica nanoparticles as a universal platform for drug delivery. *Chem. Mater.*, **26**, 435–451.

51 Li, Z., Barnes, J.C., Bosoy, A., Stoddart, J.F., and Zink, J.I. (2012) Mesoporous silica nanoparticles in biomedical applications. *Chem. Soc. Rev.*, **41**, 2590–2605.

52 Mamaeva, V., Sahlgren, C., and Lindén, M. (2013) Mesoporous silica nanoparticles in medicine – recent advances. *Adv. Drug Deliv. Rev.*, **65**, 689–702.

53 Park, C., Oh, K., Lee, S.C., and Kim, C. (2007) Controlled release of guest molecules from mesoporous silica particles based on a pH-responsive polypseudorotaxane motif. *Angew. Chem., Int. Ed.*, **46**, 1455–1457.

54 Yan, H., Teh, C., Sreejith, S., Zhu, L., Kwok, A., Fang, W., Ma, X., Nguyen, K.T., Korzh, V., and Zhao, Y. (2012) Functional mesoporous silica nanoparticles for photothermal-controlled drug delivery *in vivo*. *Angew. Chem., Int. Ed.*, **51**, 8373–8377.

55 Lai, C.Y., Trewyn, B.G., Jeftinija, D.M., Jeftinija, K., Xu, S., Jeftinija, S., and Lin, V.S.Y. (2003) A mesoporous silica nanosphere-based carrier system with chemically removable CdS nanoparticle caps for stimuli-responsive controlled release of neurotransmitters and drug molecules. *J. Am. Chem. Soc.*, **125**, 4451–4459.

56 Thomas, C.R., Ferris, D.P., Lee, J.H., Choi, E., Cho, M.H., Kim, E.S., Stoddart, J.F., Shin, J.S., Cheon, J., and Zink, J.I. (2010) Noninvasive remote-controlled release of drug molecules in vitro using magnetic actuation of mechanized nanoparticles. *J. Am. Chem. Soc.*, **132**, 10623–10625.

57 Salonen, J. and Lehto, V.P. (2008) Fabrication and chemical surface modification of mesoporous silicon for biomedical applications. *Chem. Eng. J.*, **137**, 162–172.

58 Buriak, J.M., Stewart, M.P., Geders, T.W., Allen, M.J., Choi, H.C., Smith, J., Raftery, D., and Canham, L.T. (1999) Lewis acid mediated hydrosilylation on porous silicon surfaces. *J. Am. Chem. Soc.*, **121**, 11491–11502.

59 Wojtyk, J.T.C., Morin, K.A., Boukherroub, R., and Wayner, D.D.M. (2002) Modification of porous silicon surfaces with activated ester monolayers. *Langmuir*, **18**, 6081–6087.
60 Bimbo, L.M., Mäkilä, E., Laaksonen, T., Lehto, V.P., Salonen, J., Hirvonen, J., and Santos, H.A. (2011) Drug permeation across intestinal epithelial cells using porous silicon nanoparticles. *Biomaterials*, **32**, 2625–2633.
61 Bimbo, L.M., Sarparanta, M., Santos, H.A., Airaksinen, A.J., Mäkilä, E., Laaksonen, T., Peltonen, L., Lehto, V.P., Hirvonen, J., and Salonen, J. (2010) Biocompatibility of thermally hydrocarbonized porous silicon nanoparticles and their biodistribution in rats. *ACS Nano*, **4**, 3023–3032.
62 Shahbazi, M.A., Fernández, T.D., Mäkilä, E.M., Le Guével, X., Mayorga, C., Kaasalainen, M.H., Salonen, J.J., Hirvonen, J.T., and Santos, H.A. (2014) Surface chemistry dependent immunostimulative potential of porous silicon nanoplatforms. *Biomaterials*, **35**, 9224–9235.
63 Tabaković, A., Kester, M., and Adair, J.H. (2012) Calcium phosphate-based composite nanoparticles in bioimaging and therapeutic delivery applications. *Wiley Interdiscip. Rev. Nanomed. Nanobiotechnol.*, **4**, 96–112.
64 Mostaghaci, B., Loretz, B., Haberkorn, R., Kickelbick, G., and Lehr, C.M. (2013) One-step synthesis of nanosized and stable amino-functionalized calcium phosphate particles for DNA transfection. *Chem. Mater.*, **25**, 3667–3674.
65 Sokolova, V.V., Radtke, I., Heumann, R., and Epple, M. (2006) Effective transfection of cells with multi-shell calcium phosphate-DNA nanoparticles. *Biomaterials*, **27**, 3147–3153.
66 Pittella, F., Cabral, H., Maeda, Y., Mi, P., Watanabe, S., Takemoto, H., Kim, H.J., Nishiyama, N., Miyata, K., and Kataoka, K. (2014) Systemic siRNA delivery to a spontaneous pancreatic tumor model in transgenic mice by PEGylated calcium phosphate hybrid micelles. *J. Control. Release*, **178**, 18–24.
67 Giger, E.V., Castagner, B., Räikkönen, J., Mönkkönen, J., and Leroux, J.C. (2013) siRNA transfection with calcium phosphate nanoparticles stabilized with PEGylated chelators. *Adv. Healthcare Mater.*, **2**, 134–144.
68 Lee, M.S., Lee, J.E., Byun, E., Kim, N.W., Lee, K., Lee, H., Sim, S.J., Lee, D.S., and Jeong, J.H. (2014) Target-specific delivery of siRNA by stabilized calcium phosphate nanoparticles using dopa-hyaluronic acid conjugate. *J. Control. Release*, **192**, 122–130.
69 Cao, X., Deng, W., Wei, Y., Su, W., Yang, Y., Wei, Y., Yu, J., and Xu, X. (2011) Encapsulation of plasmid DNA in calcium phosphate nanoparticles: stem cell uptake and gene transfer efficiency. *Int. J. Nanomedicine*, **6**, 3335–3349.
70 Sokolova, V., Kozlova, D., Knuschke, T., Buer, J., Westendorf, A.M., and Epple, M. (2013) Mechanism of the uptake of cationic and anionic calcium phosphate nanoparticles by cells. *Acta Biomater.*, **9**, 7527–7535.
71 Zhao, X.Y., Zhu, Y.J., Chen, F., Lu, B.Q., Qi, C., Zhao, J., and Wu, J. (2013) Calcium phosphate hybrid nanoparticles: self-assembly formation, characterization, and application as an anticancer drug nanocarrier. *Chem. Asian J.*, **8**, 1306–1312.
72 Maquieira, A., Brun, E.M., Garcés-García, M., and Puchades, R. (2012) Aluminum oxide nanoparticles as carriers and adjuvants for eliciting antibodies from non-immunogenic haptens. *Anal. Chem.*, **84**, 9340–9348.
73 Zhao, L., Wang, H., Huo, K., Cui, L., Zhang, W., Ni, H., Zhang, Y., Wu, Z., and Chu, P.K. (2011) Antibacterial nano-structured titania coating incorporated with silver nanoparticles. *Biomaterials*, **32**, 5706–5716.
74 Ahamed, M., AlSalhi, M.S., and Siddiqui, M.K.J. (2010) Silver nanoparticle applications and human health. *Clin. Chim. Acta*, **411**, 1841–1848.
75 Probst, C.E., Zrazhevskiy, P., Bagalkot, V., and Gao, X. (2013) Quantum dots as a platform for nanoparticle drug delivery vehicle design. *Adv. Drug Deliv. Rev.*, **65**, 703–718.

76 Cai, W., Shin, D.W., Chen, K., Gheysens, O., Cao, Q., Wang, S.X., Gambhir, S.S., and Chen, X. (2006) Peptide-labeled near-infrared quantum dots for imaging tumor vasculature in living subjects. *Nano Lett.*, **6**, 669–676.

77 Weng, K.C., Noble, C.O., Papahadjopoulos-Sternberg, B., Chen, F.F., Drummond, D.C., Kirpotin, D.B., Wang, D., Horn, Y.K., Hann, B., and Park, J.W. (2008) Targeted tumor cell internalization and imaging of multifunctional quantum dot-conjugated immunoliposomes *in vitro* and *in vivo*. *Nano Lett.*, **8**, 2851–2857.

78 Al-Jamal, W.T., Al-Jamal, K.T., Bomans, P.H., Frederik, P.M., and Kostarelos, K. (2008) Functionalized-quantum-dot-liposome hybrids as multimodal nanopartides for cancer. *Small*, **4**, 1406–1415.

79 Zintchenko, A., Susha, A.S., Concia, M., Feldmann, J., Wagner, E., Rogach, A.L., and Ogris, M. (2009) Drug nanocarriers labeled with near-infrared-emitting quantum dots (quantoplexes): imaging fast dynamics of distribution in living animals. *Mol. Ther.*, **17**, 1849–1856.

80 Armelao, L., Quici, S., Barigelletti, F., Accorsi, G., Bottaro, G., Cavazzini, M., Tondello, E. (2010) Design of luminescent lanthanide complexes: from molecules to highly efficient photo-emitting materials. *Coord. Chem. Rev.* **254**, 487–505.

81 Shen, J., Zhao, L., and Han, G. (2013) Lanthanide-doped upconverting luminescent nanoparticle platforms for optical imaging-guided drug delivery and therapy. *Adv. Drug Deliv. Rev.*, **65**, 744–755.

82 Haase, M. and Schäfer, H. (2011) Upconverting nanoparticles. *Angew. Chem., Int. Ed.*, **50**, 5808–5829.

83 Li, Z., Tao, Y., Huang, S., Gao, N., Ren, J., and Qu, X. (2013) Lanthanide-based hollow mesoporous nanoparticles: a novel multifunctional platform for simultaneous gene delivery and cell imaging. *Chem. Commun.*, **49**, 7129–7131.

84 Xiong, L., Chen, Z., Tian, Q., Cao, T., Xu, C., and Li, F. (2009) High contrast upconversion luminescence targeted imaging in vivo using peptide-labeled nanophosphors. *Anal. Chem.*, **81**, 8687–8694.

85 Xiong, L.Q., Chen, Z.G., Yu, M.X., Li, F.Y., Liu, C., and Huang, C.H. (2009) Synthesis, characterization, and in vivo targeted imaging of amine-functionalized rare-earth up-converting nanophosphors. *Biomaterials*, **30**, 5592–5600.

86 Conde, J., Ambrosone, A., Hernandez, Y., Tian, F., McCully, M., Berry, C.C., Baptista, P.V., Tortiglione, C., and De La Fuente, J.M. (2015) 15 years on siRNA delivery: beyond the state-of-the-art on inorganic nanoparticles for RNAi therapeutics. *Nano Today*, **10**, 421–450.

87 Sardar, R., Funston, A.M., Mulvaney, P., and Murray, R.W. (2009) Gold nanoparticles: past, present, and future. *Langmuir*, **25**, 13840–13851.

88 Saha, K., Agasti, S.S., Kim, C., Li, X., and Rotello, V.M. (2012) Gold nanoparticles in chemical and biological sensing. *Chem. Rev.*, **112**, 2739–2779.

89 Pedrosa, P., Vinhas, R., Fernandes, A., and Baptista, P.V. (2015) Gold nanotheranostics: proof-of-concept or clinical tool? *Nanomaterials*, **5**, 1853–1879.

90 Le Guével, X., Tagit, O., Rodríguez, C.E., Trouillet, V.;Pernia., Leal, M., and Hildebrandt, N. (2014) Ligand effect on the size, valence state and red/near infrared photoluminescence of bidentate thiol gold nanoclusters. *Nanoscale*, **6**, 8091–8099.

91 Jin, R. (2010) Quantum sized, thiolate-protected gold nanoclusters. *Nanoscale*, **2**, 343–362.

92 Zhu, M., Aikens, C.M., Hollander, F.J., Schatz, G.C., and Jin, R. (2008) Correlating the crystal structure of A thiol-protected Au25 cluster and optical properties. *J. Am. Chem. Soc.*, **130**, 5883–5885.

93 Brust, M., Walker, M., Bethell, D., Schiffrin, D.J., and Whyman, R. (1994) Synthesis of thiol-derivatised gold nanoparticles in a two-phase liquid-liquid system. *J. Chem. Soc., Chem. Commun.*, 801–802.

94 Perrault, S.D. and Chan, W.C.W. (2009) Synthesis and surface modification of highly monodispersed, spherical gold nanoparticles of 50–200 nm. *J. Am. Chem. Soc.*, **131**, 17042–17043.
95 Mittal, A.K., Chisti, Y., and Banerjee, U.C. (2013) Synthesis of metallic nanoparticles using plant extracts. *Biotechnol. Adv.*, **31**, 346–356.
96 Elia, P., Zach, R., Hazan, S., Kolusheva, S., Porat, Z., and Zeiri, Y. (2014) Green synthesis of gold nanoparticles using plant extracts as reducing agents. *Int. J. Nanomedicine*, **9**, 4007–4021.
97 Sharma, R.K., Gulati, S., and Mehta, S. (2012) Preparation of gold nanoparticles using tea: A green chemistry experiment. *J. Chem. Educ.*, **89**, 1316–1318.
98 González, E., Arbiol, J., and Puntes, V.F. (2011) Carving at the nanoscale: sequential galvanic exchange and Kirkendall growth at room temperature. *Science*, **334**, 1377–1380.
99 Jana, N.R., Gearheart, L., and Murphy, C.J. (2001) Wet chemical synthesis of high aspect ratio cylindrical gold nanorods. *J. Phys. Chem. B*, **105**, 4065–4067.
100 Shankar, S.S., Rai, A., Ankamwar, B., Singh, A., Ahmad, A., and Sastry, M. (2004) Biological synthesis of triangular gold nanoprisms. *Nat. Mater.*, **3**, 482–488.
101 Senthil Kumar, P., Pastoriza-Santos, I., Rodríguez-González, B., Javier García De Abajo, F., and Liz-Marzán, L.M. (2008) High-yield synthesis and optical response of gold nanostars. *Nanotechnology*, **19** (1), 015606.
102 Kim, D.Y., Yu, T., Cho, E.C., Ma, Y., Park, O.O., and Xia, Y. (2011) Synthesis of gold nano-hexapods with controllable arm lengths and their tunable optical properties. *Angew. Chem., Int. Ed.*, **50**, 6328–6331.
103 Prodan, E., Nordlander, P., and Halas, N.J. (2003) Electronic structure and optical properties of gold nanoshells. *Nano Lett.*, **3**, 1411–1415.
104 Skrabalak, S.E., Chen, J., Sun, Y., Lu, X., Au, L., Cobley, C.M., and Xia, Y. (2008) Gold nanocages: synthesis, properties, and applications. *Acc. Chem. Res.*, **41**, 1587–1595.
105 Nikoobakht, B. and El-Sayed, M.A. (2003) Preparation and growth mechanism of gold nanorods (NRs) using seed-mediated growth method. *Chem. Mater.*, **15**, 1957–1962.
106 Kim, F., Connor, S., Song, H., Kuykendall, T., and Yang, P. (2004) Platonic gold nanocrystals. *Angew. Chem., Int. Ed.*, **43**, 3673–3677.
107 Xia, X., Wang, Y., Ruditskiy, A., and Xia, Y. (2013) 25th anniversary article: galvanic replacement: a simple and versatile route to hollow nanostructures with tunable and well-controlled properties. *Adv. Mater.*, **25**, 6313–6332.
108 Prevo, B.G., Esakoff, S.A., Mikhailovsky, A., and Zasadzinski, J.A. (2008) Scalable routes to gold nanoshells with tunable sizes and response to near-infrared pulsed-laser irradiation. *Small*, **4**, 1183–1195.
109 Personick, M.L. and Mirkin, C.A. (2013) Making sense of the mayhem behind shape control in the synthesis of gold nanoparticles. *J. Am. Chem. Soc.*, **135**, 18238–18247.
110 Jain, P.K. and El-Sayed, M.A. (2010) Plasmonic coupling in noble metal nanostructures. *Chem. Phys. Lett.*, **487**, 153–164.
111 Chen, H., Shao, L., Li, Q., and Wang, J. (2013) Gold nanorods and their plasmonic properties. *Chem. Soc. Rev.*, **42**, 2679–2724.
112 Wang, Y., Polavarapu, L., and Liz-Marzán, L.M. (2014) Reduced graphene oxide-supported gold nanostars for improved SERS sensing and drug delivery. *ACS Appl. Mater. Interfaces*, **6**, 21798–21805.
113 Wang, L.V. and Hu, S. (2012) Photoacoustic tomography: *in vivo* imaging from organelles to organs. *Science*, **335**, 1458–1462.
114 Dykman, L. and Khlebtsov, N. (2012) Gold nanoparticles in biomedical applications: recent advances and perspectives. *Chem. Soc. Rev.*, **41**, 2256–2282.
115 Mei, B.C., Susumu, K., Medintz, I.L., and Mattoussi, H. (2009) Polyethylene

glycol-based bidentate ligands to enhance quantum dot and gold nanoparticle stability in biological media. *Nat. Protoc.*, **4**, 412–423.

116 Zhang, S., Leem, G., Srisombat, L.O., and Lee, T.R. (2008) Rationally designed ligands that inhibit the aggregation of large gold nanoparticles in solution. *J. Am. Chem. Soc.*, **130**, 113–120.

117 Kumari, A., Yadav, S.K., and Yadav, S.C. (2010) Biodegradable polymeric nanoparticles based drug delivery systems. *Colloids Surf. B*, **75**, 1–18.

118 Tang, F., Li, L., and Chen, D. (2012) Mesoporous silica nanoparticles: synthesis, biocompatibility and drug delivery. *Adv. Mater.*, **24**, 1504–1534.

119 Wong, Y.J., Zhu, L., Teo, W.S., Tan, Y.W., Yang, Y., Wang, C., and Chen, H. (2011) Revisiting the Stöber method: Inhomogeneity in silica shells. *J. Am. Chem. Soc.*, **133**, 11422–11425.

120 Singh, D., McMillan, J.M., Kabanov, A.V., Sokolsky-Papkov, M., and Gendelman, H.E. (2014) Bench-to-bedside translation of magnetic nanoparticles. *Nanomedicine (Lond)*, **9**, 501–516.

121 Reddy, L.H., Arias, J.L., Nicolas, J., and Couvreur, P. (2012) Magnetic nanoparticles: design and characterization, toxicity and biocompatibility, pharmaceutical and biomedical applications. *Chem. Rev.*, **112**, 5818–5878.

122 Shevchenko, E.V., Talapin, D.V., Schnablegger, H., Kornowski, A., Festin, Ö., Svedlindh, P., Haase, M., and Weller, H. (2003) Study of nucleation and growth in the organometallic synthesis of magnetic alloy nanocrystals: the role of nucleation rate in size control of $CoPt_3$ nanocrystals. *J. Am. Chem. Soc.*, **125**, 9090–9101.

123 Sun, S. (2006) Recent advances in chemical synthesis, self-assembly, and applications of FePt nanoparticles. *Adv. Mater.*, **18**, 393–403.

124 Yamada, Y., Suzuki, T., and Abarra, E.N. (1998) Magnetic properties of electron beam evaporated CoPt alloy thin films. *IEEE Trans. Magn.*, **34**, 343–345.

125 Shen, T., Weissleder, R., Papisov, M., Bogdanov, A. Jr., and Brady, T.J. (1993) Monocrystalline iron oxide nanocompounds (MION): physicochemical properties. *Magn. Reson. Med.*, **29**, 599–604.

126 Zeng, H. and Sun, S. (2008) Syntheses, properties, and potential applications of multicomponent magnetic nanoparticles. *Adv. Funct. Mater.*, **18**, 391–400.

127 Jana, N.R., Chen, Y., and Peng, X. (2004) Size- and shape-controlled magnetic (Cr, Mn, Fe, Co, Ni) oxide nanocrystals via a simple and general approach. *Chem. Mater.*, **16**, 3931–3935.

128 Lu, A.H., Salabas, E.L., and Schüth, F. (2007) Magnetic nanoparticles: synthesis, protection, functionalization, and application. *Angew. Chem., Int. Ed.*, **46**, 1222–1244.

129 Xu, C. and Sun, S. (2013) New forms of superparamagnetic nanoparticles for biomedical applications. *Adv. Drug Deliv. Rev.*, **65**, 732–743.

130 Lee, N. and Hyeon, T. (2012) Designed synthesis of uniformly sized iron oxide nanoparticles for efficient magnetic resonance imaging contrast agents. *Chem. Soc. Rev.*, **41**, 2575–2589.

131 Okoli, C., Sanchez-Dominguez, M., Boutonnet, M., Järås, S., Civera, C., Solans, C., and Kuttuva, G.R. (2012) Comparison and functionalization study of microemulsion-prepared magnetic iron oxide nanoparticles. *Langmuir*, **28**, 8479–8485.

132 Zhang, H. and Zhu, G. (2012) One-step hydrothermal synthesis of magnetic Fe_3O_4 nanoparticles immobilized on polyamide fabric. *Appl. Surf. Sci.*, **258**, 4952–4959.

133 Mahdavi, M., Ahmad, M.B., Haron, M.J., Namvar, F., Nadi, B.;Ab., Rahman, M.Z., and Amin, J. (2013) Synthesis, surface modification and characterisation of biocompatible magnetic iron oxide nanoparticles for biomedical applications. *Molecules*, **18**, 7533–7548.

134 Hasanpour, A., Niyaifar, M., Mohammadpour, H., and Amighian, J. (2012) A novel non-thermal process of TiO_2-shell coating on Fe_3O_4-core nanoparticles. *J. Phys. Chem. Solids*, **73**, 1066–1070.

135 Mahmoudi, M. and Serpooshan, V. (2012) Silver-coated engineered magnetic nanoparticles are promising for the success in the fight against antibacterial resistance threat. *ACS Nano*, **6**, 2656–2664.

136 Singh, A. and Sahoo, S.K. (2014) Magnetic nanoparticles: a novel platform for cancer theranostics. *Drug Discov. Today*, **19**, 474–481.

137 Shahbazi, M.A., Herranz, B., and Santos, H.A. (2012) Nanostructured porous Si-based nanoparticles for targeted drug delivery. *Biomatter*, **2**, 296–312.

138 Zhang, L., Li, Y., and Yu, J.C. (2014) Chemical modification of inorganic nanostructures for targeted and controlled drug delivery in cancer treatment. *J. Mater. Chem. B*, **2**, 452–470.

139 Sarparanta, M.P., Bimbo, L.M., Mäkilä, E.M., Salonen, J.J., Laaksonen, P.H., Helariutta, A.M.K., Linder, M.B., Hirvonen, J.T., Laaksonen, T.J., Santos, H.A., and Airaksinen, A.J. (2012) The mucoadhesive and gastroretentive properties of hydrophobin-coated porous silicon nanoparticle oral drug delivery systems. *Biomaterials*, **33**, 3353–3362.

140 Monteiro-Riviere, N.A., Wiench, K., Landsiedel, R., Schulte, S., Inman, A.O., and Riviere, J.E. (2011) Safety evaluation of sunscreen formulations containing titanium dioxide and zinc oxide nanoparticles in UVB sunburned skin: an *in vitro* and *in vivo* study. *Toxicol. Sci.*, **123**, 264–280.

141 Sun, B., Ji, Z., Liao, Y.P., Wang, M., Wang, X., Dong, J., Chang, C.H., Li, R., Zhang, H., Nel, A.E., and Xia, T. (2013) Engineering an effective immune adjuvant by designed control of shape and crystallinity of aluminum oxyhydroxide nanoparticles. *ACS Nano*, **7**, 10834–10849.

142 Chen, N., He, Y., Su, Y., Li, X., Huang, Q., Wang, H., Zhang, X., Tai, R., and Fan, C. (2012) The cytotoxicity of cadmium-based quantum dots. *Biomaterials*, **33**, 1238–1244.

143 Barua, S. and Rege, K. (2009) Cancer-cell-phenotype-dependent differential intracellular trafficking of unconjugated quantum dots. *Small*, **5**, 370–376.

144 Al-Hajaj, N.A., Moquin, A., Neibert, K.D., Soliman, G.M., Winnik, F.M., and Maysinger, D. (2011) Short ligands affect modes of QD uptake and elimination in human cells. *ACS Nano*, **5**, 4909–4918.

145 Bakalova, R., Zhelev, Z., Kokuryo, D., Spasov, L., Aoki, I., and Saga, T. (2011) Chemical nature and structure of organic coating of quantum dots is crucial for their application in imaging diagnostics. *Int. J. Nanomedicine*, **6**, 1719–1732.

146 Dai, Y., Yang, D., Ma, P., Kang, X., Zhang, X., Li, C., Hou, Z., Cheng, Z., and Lin, J. (2012) Doxorubicin conjugated NaYF4: Yb^{3+}/Tm^{3+} nanoparticles for therapy and sensing of drug delivery by luminescence resonance energy transfer. *Biomaterials*, **33**, 8704–8713.

12
Scale-Up and cGMP Manufacturing of Nanodrug Delivery Systems for Clinical Investigations

Mostafa Nakach and Jean-René Authelin

Pharmaceutical Engineering, Pharmaceutical Sciences Opérations, Phramceutical Development Platform, Impasse des ateliers, 94403 Vitry/Seine, France

12.1
Introduction

Nanodrug delivery systems include a variety of objects: nanocrystals, nanoemulsions, liposomes, polymeric nanoparticles, and other nanosystems aimed to be administered either by oral or parenteral route [1]. In the latter case, they must be sterile. The prefix "nano" also implies a wide range of sizes from few tens of nanometers to several hundreds of nanometers.

Depending on the particle characteristics and sterility requirements, different processing techniques are used. This chapter summarizes the manufacturing processes involved in nanodrug delivery systems. In Section 12.2, an overview of the different processes will be provided, roughly classified into two families [2]:

- Processes where the particles are created from the molecular level up to nanoparticle scale. In the case of solid nanoparticles, these processes are usually named "bottom-up."
- Processes where objects initially of the millimeter or micrometer size are reduced to the nano-objects scale by an energetic comminution process. In the case of solid nanoparticles, these processes are usually named "top-down."

Processes involving a size reduction step by bead milling or by high-pressure homogenization are by far the commercially most applied technologies [1]. Therefore, detailed information on these technologies will be provided in Section 12.4.

In Section 12.5, scale-up and scale-down strategies are reviewed. A case study is presented to illustrate the issues related to scale-up and commercial process development, followed by details of scale-up/scale-down rules and general development methodology.

In Section 12.6 an example of a GMP unit is reviewed in terms of technology configuration, unit design, and its functionalities.

Pharmaceutical Nanotechnology: Innovation and Production, First Edition. Edited by Jean Cornier, Arno Kwade, Andrew Owen, and Marcel Van de Voorde.

12.2 Presentation of Major Manufacturing Processes of Different Nanodrug Delivery Systems

12.2.1 Process Including a Precipitation Step: The So-Called Bottom-Up Process

The bottom-up technology is usually used for the manufacture of nanocrystalline, nanoamorphous, or nanopolymeric suspension [3,4]. The process starts from the molecules that are dissolved and precipitated by adding a solvent (generally organic) to a nonsolvent (generally water). In this case, the preparation of the nanoparticles is done by condensation methods (formation of particles by nucleation and crystal growth).

In the case of nanocrystalline or nanoamorphous suspension, the API and lipophilic stabilizer are dissolved in an organic solvent that is miscible with water. In the case of nanopolymeric suspension, the hydrophilic stabilizer and polymer (biocompatible and biodegradable: polylactides, polyglycolides, and poly (lactide-*co*-glycolides) are dissolved in water. The two solutions are mixed together in order to form a precipitate by organic solvent diffusion in water. The organic solvent is then removed by extraction or evaporation. This process category is illustrated by the flowchart provided in Figure 12.1.

The control of the particle growth/crystal growth using this technique is often very challenging. Furthermore, the scaling up of the process is difficult [6].

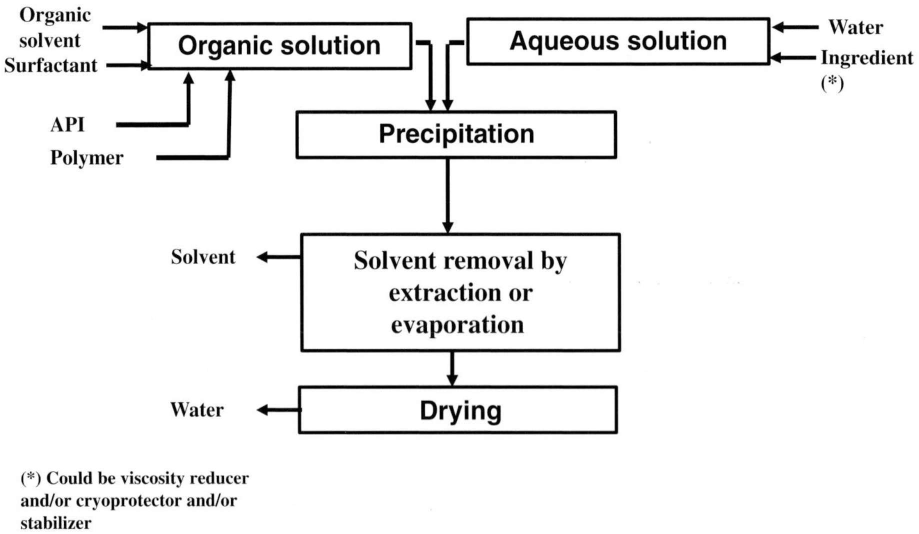

Figure 12.1 Flowchart of manufacturing of nanocrystalline, nanoamorphous, or nanopolymeric suspension using solvent diffusion method [5].

12.2.2
Process Including a Comminution Step: The So-Called Top-Down Process

The common point of these processes is the use of a comminution technology, usually a bead mill or a high-pressure homogenizer. High-pressure homogenizers may often be used for different purposes, for instance, to manufacture emulsions [7], solid nanoparticles [1], or liposomes [8]. However, the bead mill is mostly applied only for the production of solid nanoparticles.

12.2.2.1 Manufacturing of Nanocrystalline Suspension Using Direct Comminution

The top-down process (comminution) is the most widely used method for the preparation of the nanocrystalline suspensions. Indeed, the particle size can be controlled by judicious selection of stabilizer as well as by application of optimal process conditions [9]. The top-down process consists of dispersing the API in the vehicle (usually aqueous stabilizer solution). This step is followed by particle size reduction. The role of the stabilizer agent is to protect the suspension against flocculation and crystal growth (Ostwald ripening) [10]. The obtained suspension can be kept "as is" if it is chemically and physically stable. If the suspension is not stable, further processing is required such as spray- or freeze-drying or fluid bed granulation. The process principle and its flowchart are illustrated in Figures 12.2 and 12.3.

The top-down process has several advantages compared to the bottom-up process. In the case where the selected crystalline form of the API is stable in the milling vehicle (generally water), the top-down process has the following advantages:

i) It is free from organic solvent
ii) APIs that are poorly soluble in organic and aqueous media can be processed.

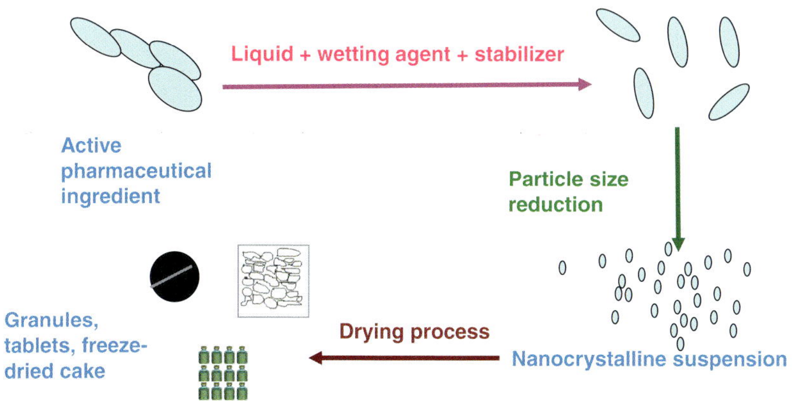

Figure 12.2 Principle of manufacturing of nanocrystalline suspension [5].

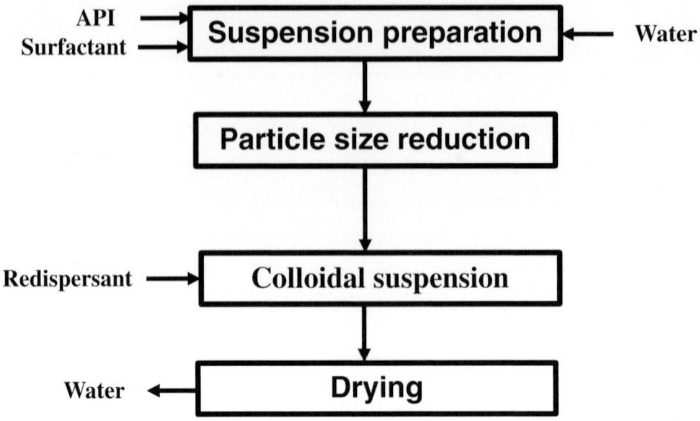

Figure 12.3 Process flowchart of top-down process [5].

iii) The number of manufacturing steps is significantly reduced (four versus six).
iv) The risk to generate amorphous state or polymorphic transition is reduced to negligible. In fact, contrary to dry milling processes, during wet milling of crystalline drugs, the water may behave as an inhibitor of the formation of amorphous material due to the reduced glass transition temperature [11].
v) The target particle size of the suspension is more easily obtained and controlled.
vi) It is possible to process highly concentrated suspensions (up to 40 wt%).
vii) The scaling up of the process is feasible and well established.

However, wear of grinding media is by far the most important disadvantage of the top-down process, mainly when stirred bead mills are used [12].

12.2.2.2 Manufacturing of Nanocrystalline, Nanoamorphous, or Nanopolymeric Suspension Using Emulsification Technique

Achieving solid nanoparticles by the emulsification method consists of manufacturing an organic solution where the API or API polymer and surfactant are dissolved in an organic solvent (which is nonmiscible with water). Afterward, the organic phase is dispersed in continuous aqueous phase containing a stabilizer to form a coarse emulsion. The vesicle size of the emulsion is then reduced by high-pressure homogenization. This step is followed by solvent removal (by evaporation) in order to form the solid nanoparticles. The evaporation step can be fulfilled using an agitated thin film evaporator where the residence time is generally below 1 s (diffusion coefficient around $10^{-12}\,m^2/s$ for droplets having size about 10^{-6} m [13]). This process is illustrated by the flowchart provided in Figure 12.4.

12.2.2.3 Manufacturing of Lipid Emulsions

For lipid emulsions, the dispersed phase is made of oil and stabilizer. The continuous phase consists of water and surfactant. The two phases are mixed

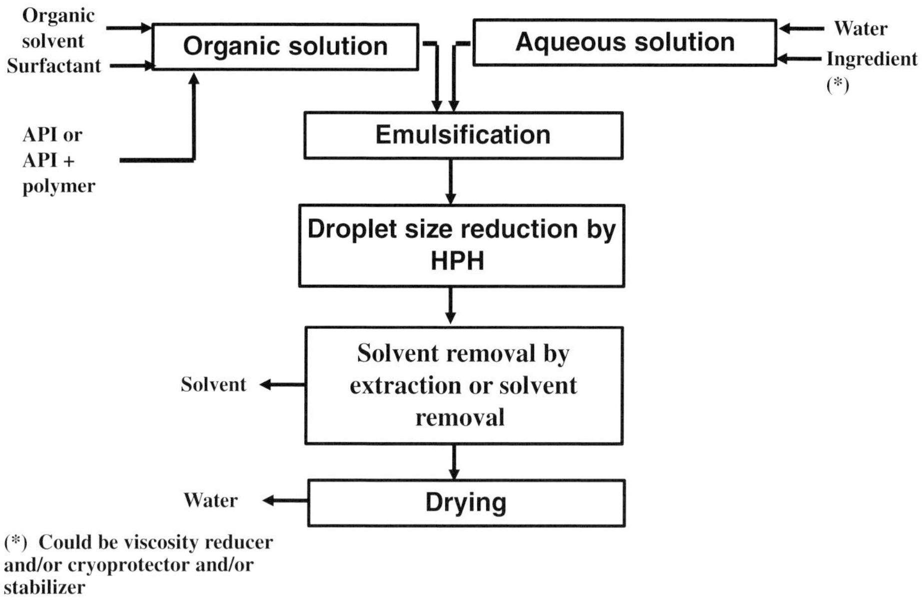

Figure 12.4 Flowchart of the manufacturing of nanocrystalline, nanoamorphous, or nanopolymeric suspension by emulsification method [5].

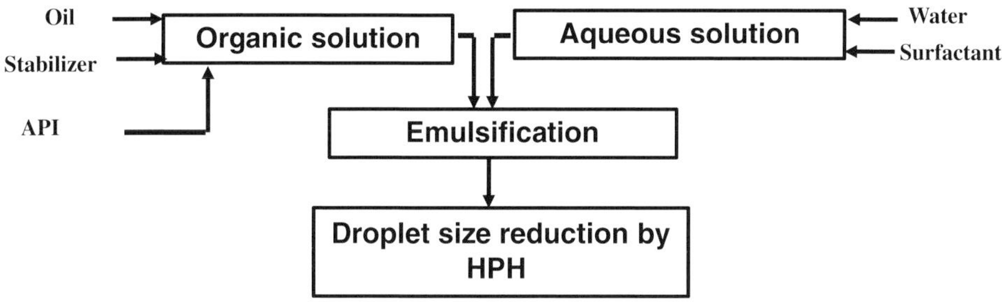

Figure 12.5 Flowchart of the manufacturing of nanoemulsion [14].

together to form a coarse emulsion. The droplet size is then reduced using high-pressure homogenization. A typical flowchart manufacturing process is illustrated in Figure 12.5.

12.2.3 Manufacturing of Liposomes

Liposomes are made of a membranous lipid bilayer and a core of aqueous solution. Membranes are usually made of phospholipids, which are molecules that have a hydrophilic head group and a hydrophobic tail group. The head is attracted to water, and the tail, which is made of a long hydrocarbon chain, is repelled by water.

Liposomes can be produced according to the following two different manufacturing processes [8]:

i) The Bangham method is the first liposome manufacturing technique described by British hematologist Dr. Alec D. Bangham FRS in 1961 and is widely used at laboratory scale. The method is usually the first choice at the preclinical stage. The method is based on lipid film hydration. The lipids and API are first dissolved in an organic solvent. The solvent is then removed by rotary evaporation yielding a thin lipid film. The obtained film is rehydrated by adding an aqueous medium at a temperature above the transition temperature (T_c or T_m) of the lipid. The obtained dispersion is treated to reduce the particle size using sonication, colloidal milling, or high-pressure homogenization.
ii) *Direct injection:* In this manufacturing technique, the organic solution of lipids and API is injected into an aqueous solution at temperature above the transition temperature of the lipid. The particle size of the obtained dispersion is reduced using sonication, colloidal milling, or high-pressure homogenization. The organic solvent is removed by *in situ* evaporation under vacuum or using agitated thin film evaporator or during freeze-drying.

A variant of these two options is to prepare liposomes API-free using one of the techniques described above. The API is then loaded into liposomes simply by agitation or by pH gradient [15].

Typical manufacturing processes are illustrated in Figures 12.6–12.8.

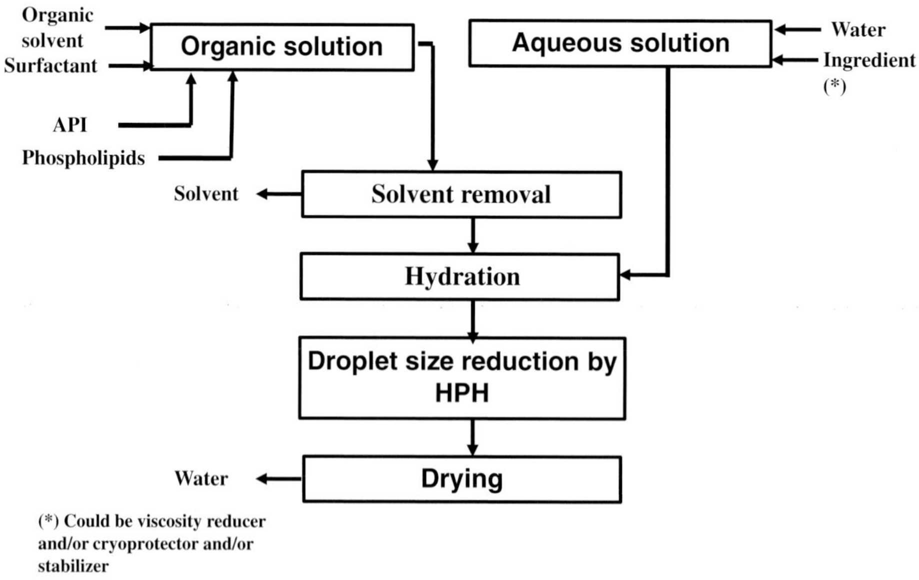

Figure 12.6 Flowchart of the manufacturing of liposomes using Bangham method [8].

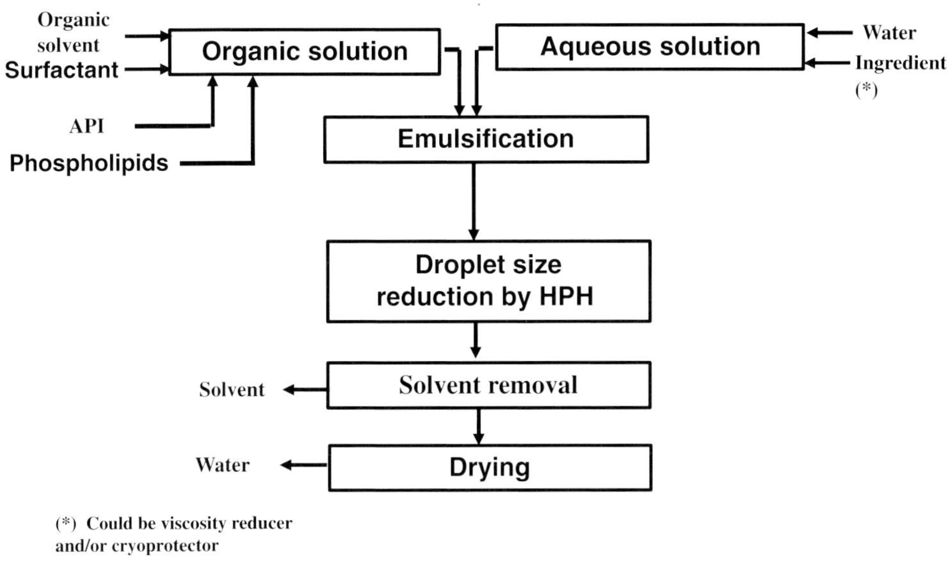

Figure 12.7 Flowchart of the manufacturing of liposomes using direct injection method [8].

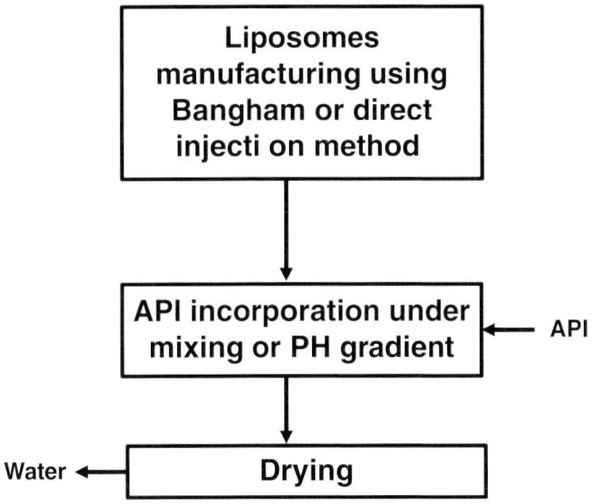

Figure 12.8 Flowchart of the manufacturing of liposomes using direct loading method [8].

12.2.4 Conversion of Nanosuspensions into Solid Intermediate for Downstream Processing into Final Drug Product

So far we have discussed processes that deliver nanosuspensions or nanoemulsions. However, in general, some more processing, typically to manufacture an acceptable pharmaceutical form, is necessary. As these processes (e.g., freeze-drying, spray-drying, and granulation) are not specific to

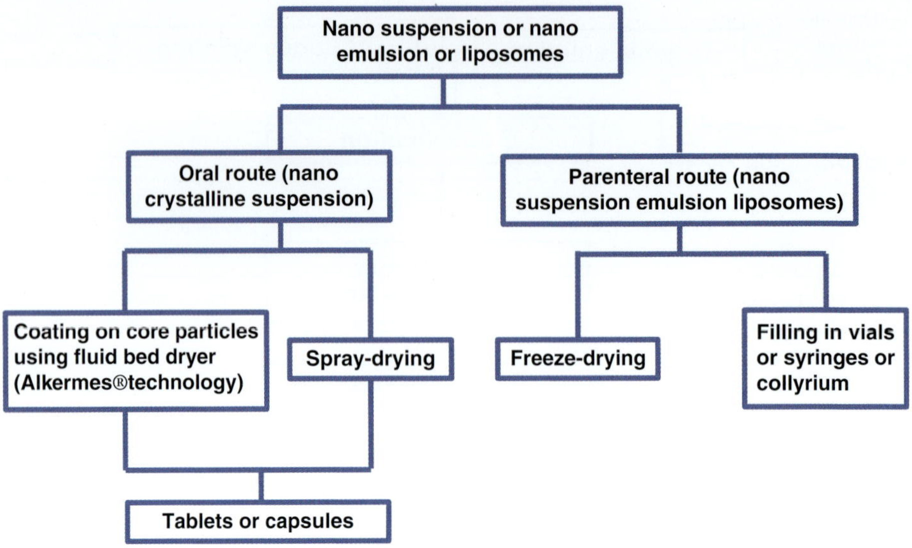

Figure 12.9 Downstream processing of nanodrug delivery systems.

nanomedicines, they will not be described in detail here. Figure 12.9 provides an overview of the main options.

12.3 Nanodrug Delivery Systems as Marketed Products

The marketed nanodrug delivery systems are compiled in Table 12.1 [16,17].

12.4 Particle/Vesicle Size Reduction Technologies

There are two main ways in which particle/vesicle size reduction is performed: high-pressure homogenization and bead milling. In this section, both technologies will be described in terms of milling principles and configurations available on the market.

12.4.1 High-Pressure Homogenization

The first high-pressure homogenizer was developed by Auguste Gaulin in 1899. He introduced his machine for "treating milk" at the Paris World's Fair in 1900 [18]. The technology was then used in different industries such as pharmaceutical, food, cosmetic, biotechnology, and environmental. It is used for the

Table 12.1 List of marketed product based on nanoparticles.

Product (broad name)	Used API	Manufacturing process	Route of administration	Manufacturer
Avinza	Morphine sulfate	Nanocrystalline suspension	Oral	Alkermes/Pfizer
Emend	Aprepitant	Nanocrystalline suspension	Oral	Alkermes/Merck
Focalin XR	Dexmethylphenidate Hcl	Nanocrystalline suspension	Oral	Alkermes/Novartis
Rapamune	Sirolimus	Nanocrystalline suspension	Oral	Alkermes/Wyeth
Megace ES	Megestrol acetate	Nanocrystalline suspension	Oral	Alkermes/Par/BMS
Naprelan	Naproxen	Nanocrystalline suspension	Oral	Alkermes
Ritalin LA	Methylphenidate Hcl	Nanocrystalline suspension	Oral	Alkermes/Novartis
Tricor	Fenofibrate	Nanocrystalline suspension	Oral	Alkermes/Abott
Triglide	Fenofibrate	Nanocrystalline suspension	Oral	SkyePharma/First Horizon Pharmaceuticals/Sciele Pharma
Invega Sustenna	Paliperidone	Nanocrystalline suspension	Intamuscular	Janssen
Marqibo	Vincristine sulfate	Liposomes	Intravenous	Talon Therapeutics Inc.
DepoCyt	Cytarabine	Liposomes	Intravenous	Sigma-Tau Pharmaceuticals, Inc.
Ambisome	Amphotericin B	Liposomes	Intravenous	Gilead Sciences, Inc./Astellas Pharma US, Inc.
Doxil/Caelyx	Doxorubicin HCl	Liposomes	Intravenous	Janssen
DaunoXome	Daunorubicin	Liposomes	Intravenous	Galen Limited
Myocet	Doxorubicin citrate	Liposomes	Intravenous	Teva B.V.
Diprivan	Propofol	Emulsion	Intravenous	AstraZeneca

preparation and/or stabilization of emulsions, liposomes, and suspensions. It is also used for cell disruption of yeasts or bacteria in order to release intracellular products such as recombinant proteins [19].

The mechanism of particle or vesicle size reduction is based on cavitation (which will be detailed when piston gap technology is discussed) [1], high shear forces, and collision of the vesicles or particles against each other.

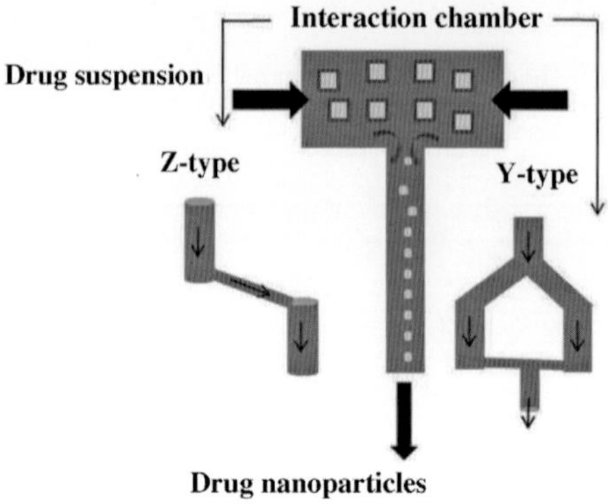

Figure 12.10 Microfluidization technology [21].

12.4.1.1 Different High-Pressure Homogenizer Design

Nowadays, two technologies are used in the industry: microfluidization and piston gap technologies.

Microfluidics Technology

Microfluidization works on a jet stream principle where the suspension is accelerated and passed at a high velocity through specially designed interaction chambers. Frontal collision of fluid streams under high pressures (up to 1700 bar) inside the interaction chamber (Y shape) generates shear forces, particle collision, and cavitation forces necessary for particle size reduction. The interaction chamber can be made of stainless steel, polycrystalline diamond (PCD), or aluminum oxide. There are two types of interaction chambers: Y-chamber is useful for liquid–liquid emulsions and finds application in preparing liposomes, while Z-chamber is typically used for cell disruption and nanodispersion. A schematic representation of both chambers is shown in Figure 12.10 [20].

Piston Gap Technology

The high-pressure homogenizer consists of the combination of a high-pressure plunger pump and a homogenization valve (see Figure 12.11). The role of the plunger pump is to provide the specific energy level required for the homogenization valve. The homogenization valve consists of a fixed valve seat and an adjustable valve. These parts form an adjustable radial precision gap. The gap conditions, the resistance, and thus the homogenization pressure vary as a function of the force acting on the valve. An external impact ring forms a defined outlet cross section and prevents the valve from being damaged (see Figure 12.12) [2].

The dispersion or suspension passes through the high-pressure homogenization device with a very high velocity. According to Bernoulli's equation, the dynamic pressure of the fluid increases, and at the same time the static pressure decreases below the pressure of saturation of the dispersion medium (generally

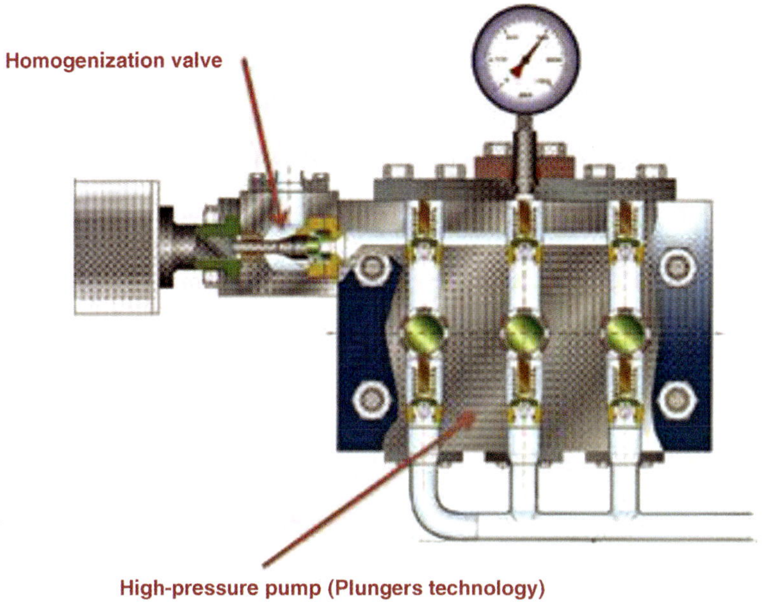

Figure 12.11 High-pressure homogenizer piston gap technology [22,23].

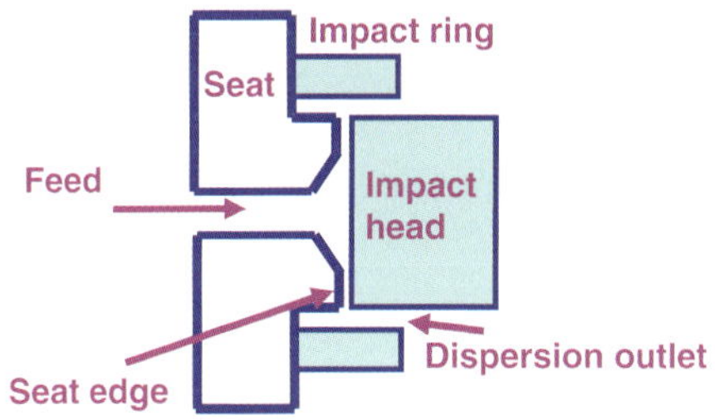

Figure 12.12 Homogenization [2].

water). This leads to the boiling of the milling medium and formation of vapor bubbles that implode when the dispersion or suspension leaves the gap. Considering the schematic representation described in Figure 12.13, if p_1 is the inlet pressure and p_2 is the outlet pressure, at the entrance, the velocity increases rapidly in the convergence zone and, therefore, the pressure decreases and can eventually reach the vapor pressure p_v of the liquid causing formation of vapor bubbles (cavities in the liquid). When the cavitation bubbles implode (collapse of the cavities), shock waves are generated in the liquid. These shock waves break apart the dispersion.

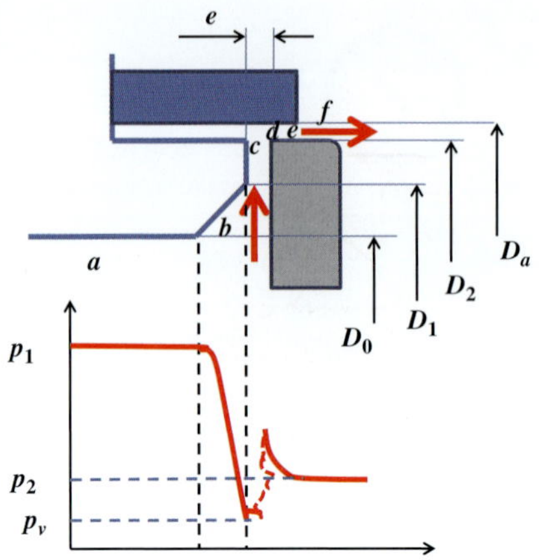

Figure 12.13 Pressure evolution within the valve (piston gap technology) [24].

Thus, the mechanisms that can lead to breakage of the particles are as follows:

i) The effects of laminar and turbulent shear in the convergence zone, which are sensitive to the viscosity of the fluid,
ii) The implosion of vapor bubbles when cavitation takes place,
iii) The impact of particles on the impact ring is more or less reduced by the fluid viscosity.

High-pressure homogenization for the production of crystalline suspensions was developed by R.H. Müller in 1998 [25] by using Disso Cubes technology. The patent rights of Disso Cubes were initially owned by Drug Delivery Services GmbH (DDS) and are currently owned by SkyePharma PLC. Disso Cubes uses piston-gap-type high-pressure homogenizers [2].

12.4.2 Stirred Bead Milling

Stirred bead mills are increasingly used for fine and ultrafine grinding of minerals, ceramic materials, paint, pigments, chemical products, microorganisms, pharmaceutical products, and other materials. The stirred bead milling process has led to successful launch of a number of products (see Section 12.3). The proprietary technology is owned by Elan Company. It was developed in 1990 by Nanosystems (Kodak group affiliate). Their applications have been widely described in patents and literature [9].

The mill consists of a milling chamber, a milling shaft, milling media, and very often a recirculation vessel. The milling chamber is charged with the milling media, water, product to be milled (i.e., drug), and stabilizer. The milling media or pearls are then agitated by the stirrer at a certain circumferential velocity. The process can be performed in either batch or recirculation mode. Once the formulation and the process are optimized, very little batch-to-batch variation in the quality of the dispersion is observed. The principle of milling is based on the high energy and shear forces generated as a result of the impact between the milling media. This energy input breaks the microparticulate drug between the milling media into nanosized particles. Due to the high energy used during milling, the process needs to be performed under controlled temperature.

The milling media plays a major role in suspension quality to be used in pharmaceutical industry. Beads are available in different sizes and different materials. They can be made of ceramic (zirconium oxide, alumina oxide, silicon nitride, zirconium silicate, steatite, mullite, etc.) or polymeric (cross-linked polystyrene). The bead material is a critical factor as it can contaminate or interact with the active drug substance. Elan technology uses cross-linked polystyrene beads that are known to be considered as noncontaminating whatever the milling process conditions. However, zirconium oxide or alumina oxide beads are known to contaminate.

12.4.2.1 Different Mill Designs

A large number of different types of closed stirred media mills were developed by the industry, especially in the last 20 years. Various mill designs differ mostly in their chamber and stirrer geometry as well as in the separation device, which allows free discharge of the product, but prevents the grinding media from leaving the mill. In general, three different mill designs are used for producing nanocrystalline suspension (see Figures 12.14–12.16):

i) Disks mill
ii) Pin stirred bead mill
iii) Annular mill

12.4.2.2 Conclusions: Size Reduction

It is noteworthy that the high-pressure homogenization is a versatile technology that can be used for the production of nanocrystalline suspension, nanoamorphous suspension, polymeric nanoparticles, emulsion, and liposomes. However,

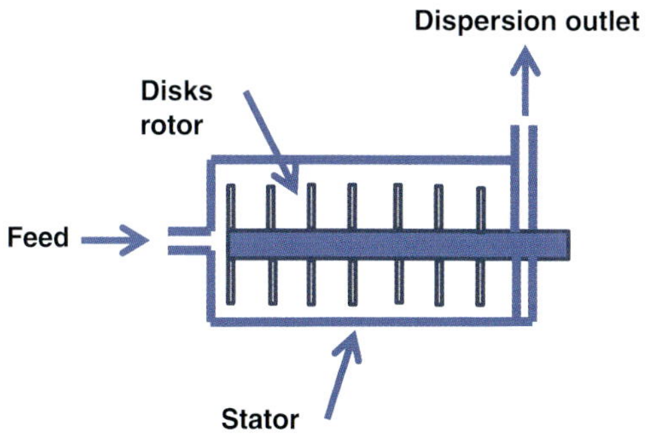

Figure 12.14 Disks mill design [26].

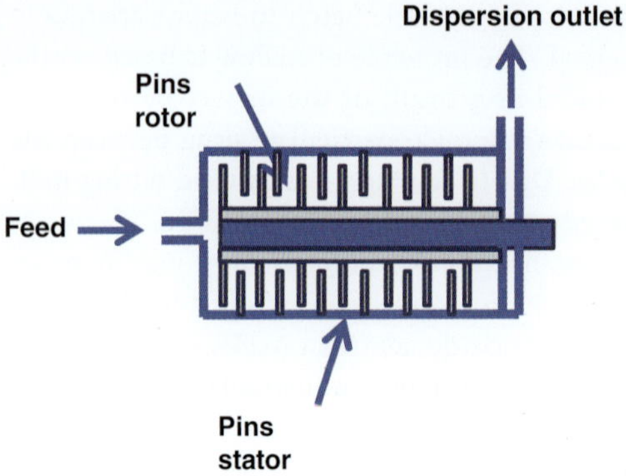

Figure 12.15 Pin stirred bead mill [26].

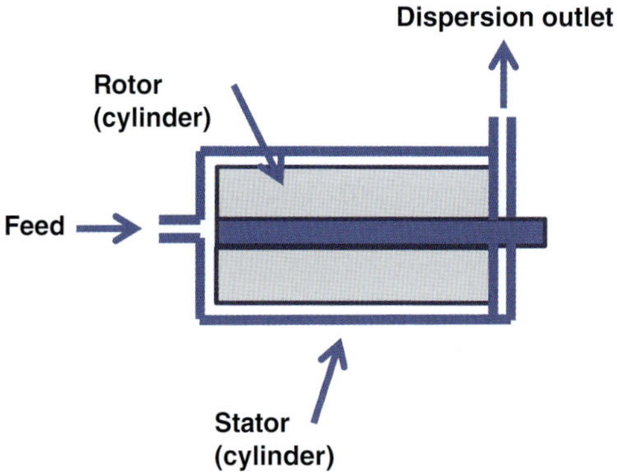

Figure 12.16 Annular mill [26].

bead milling is mainly used only for the manufacturing of nanocrystalline suspensions for which it is more powerful than the HPH. Indeed, the particle size of nanocrystalline suspension produced by bead milling is lower than that produced by HPH (100 versus 200 nm).

12.5
Process Development and Scale-Down/Scale-Up Strategy

This section has two parts. In the first part, a case study will be presented to illustrate the pitfalls and risks associated with process development in which scale-down rules have not been considered resulting in inconsistent product quality attributes. The second part will focus on scale-up rules of particle/vesicle size reduction technology, which is the core of manufacturing techniques applied to nanodrug delivery systems.

12.5.1
API x Case Study

The academic literature of nanodrug delivery systems is focused more on laboratory-scale processes than on industrial manufacturing process. Pharmaceutical companies are faced, quite rapidly in the course of development, with necessity of increasing batch scale to produce larger quantities of nanodrug delivery systems for clinical trials. At this stage, the adaptation of the laboratory process to large scale may lead to inconsistent product quality. In the present case study, we will discuss the problems associated with the industrialization of highly promising liposome dispersion from laboratory scale to 200 l scale.

In this section, after presenting the drug product definition, the laboratory process and the issues related to its scale-up will be discussed. Finally, the adaptations that were needed to make the process scalable and to get the same quality attribute as the laboratory process will be provided.

12.5.1.1 Drug Product Definition

The drug product is a liposomal formulation of API that is poorly water soluble (solubility in water <100 μg/ml at 20 °C) and highly soluble in purified and injectable lecithin (100 mg/ml). The API is incorporated within the phospholipid bilayer of liposomes. It is a freeze-dried injectable formulation. The product is then reconstituted with water for injection and gives a liposomal dispersion of API. The dispersion is diluted in glucose 5% exclusively – for intravenous infusion.

12.5.1.2 Study Context of the Laboratory-Scale Process

The process was developed at 1 l scale using the Bangham technique, that is, by a rot-evaporator for lipid film formation and hydration using water for injection (WFI) (see Figure 12.17). The dispersion obtained (multilamellar vesicles (MLVs)) was then downsized to small unilamellar vesicles (SUVs) using a microfluidics homogenizer. Then, the cryoprotector was added to the homogenized dispersion. At the end, the dispersion was filtered successively at 0.22 and 0.1 μm, filled in vials, and freeze-dried. The residual organic solvent within the dispersion was found to be below 0.4 wt%. The liposomes produced were used in clinical study and resulted in an acceptable clinical profile. Based on the high promise of the product, it was decided to study the scaling up of the process with a view to its industrialization at 200 l scale.

12.5.1.3 Scaling Up of the Bangham Manufacturing Technique

The rot-evaporator could be operated at maximum volume of 50 l, which did not fit with the industrial package of 200 l. Consequently, four subbatches would need to be manufactured and pooled. The transfer of subbatches during pooling would require a hazardous handling step, which could have led to environmental, hygiene, and safety issues. Furthermore, heat transfer within the rot-evaporator is extremely slow, and therefore evaporation time at 50 l scale would be long.

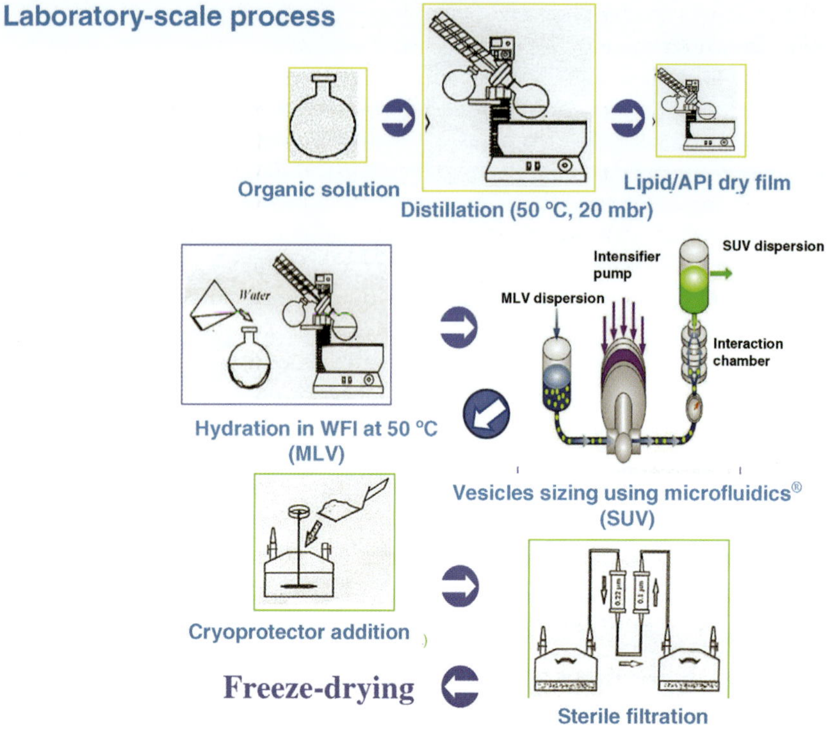

Figure 12.17 Schematic Bangham method used for API As' liposomes manufacturing.

Based on this risks analysis, it was decided to scale up the process using a stainless steel vessel.

As illustrated in Figure 12.18a and b, respectively, the stainless steel vessels used at 3 and 70 l scales for the evaporation step lead to API/lipids in paste form instead of a film. The residual solvent (ethanol) within the paste was found heterogeneous. In addition, as illustrated in Figure 12.18c, the hydration step was found to be incomplete after 2 h of mixing at high shear rate (mixer rotated at tip speed of 2.5 m/s combined with colloidal milling operated at shear rate (tip speed divided by gap between rotor and stator) of $50\,000\,s^{-1}$). By comparison,

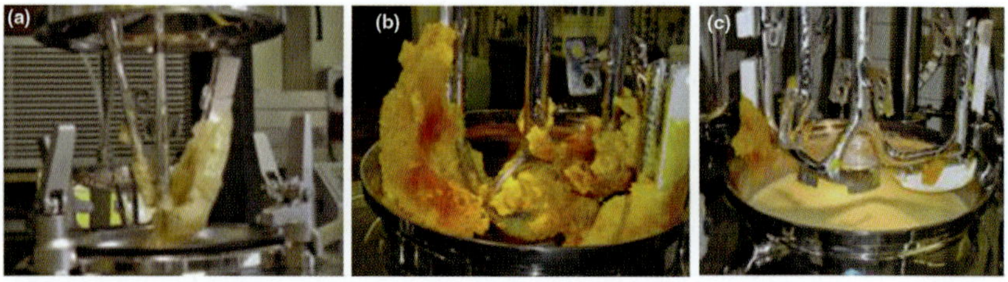

Figure 12.18 Paste formation and hydration at 3 and 70 l scale.

hydration was completed in 20 min when using the Bangham technique at the 1 l scale. Based on these difficulties, the probability of success of the scale-up was considered as uncertain. Then, it was decided to adapt the manufacturing process by switching from Bangham to direct injection method.

12.5.1.4 Development and Scaling Up of Direct Injection Method

The method is based on direct emulsification of organic phase in aqueous phase (see Figure 12.7). The method required ethanol content optimization in order to dissolve the different ingredients (API, inactive ingredient), to handle organic phase (transfer to emulsification vessel and filtration), to form liposomes during emulsification, and to allow vesicle size reduction. The ethanol can be removed

i) during freeze drying,
ii) after emulsification, or
iii) after dispersion sizing.

Ethanol Amount Optimization

As it can be seen in Figure 12.19, the kinetic of vesicle size reduction was driven by the ethanol content in the dispersion. One can observe that as long as the amount of organic solvent in the dispersion is reduced to at least 3.2 wt% (corresponding to 24.8% in the organic phase), the direct injection method leads to the same vesicle size (measurement using dynamic light scattering) reduction kinetic as the Bangham method (see Figure 12.20).

Note: The recycling number is expressed by the equation described in Section 12.5.2.2.

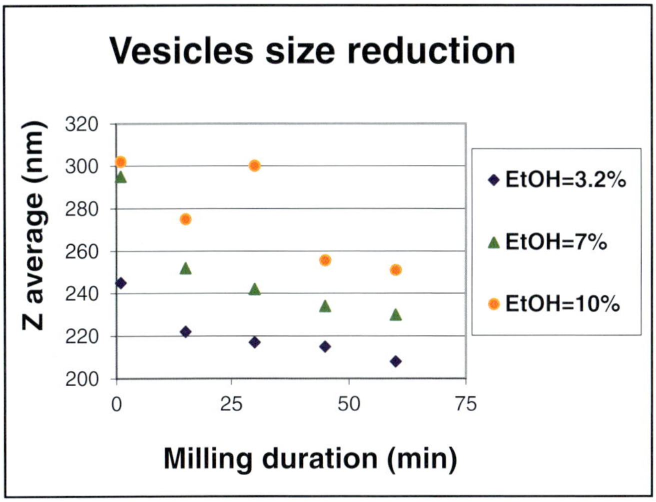

Figure 12.19 Vesicle size reduction as function of ethanol content in dispersion.

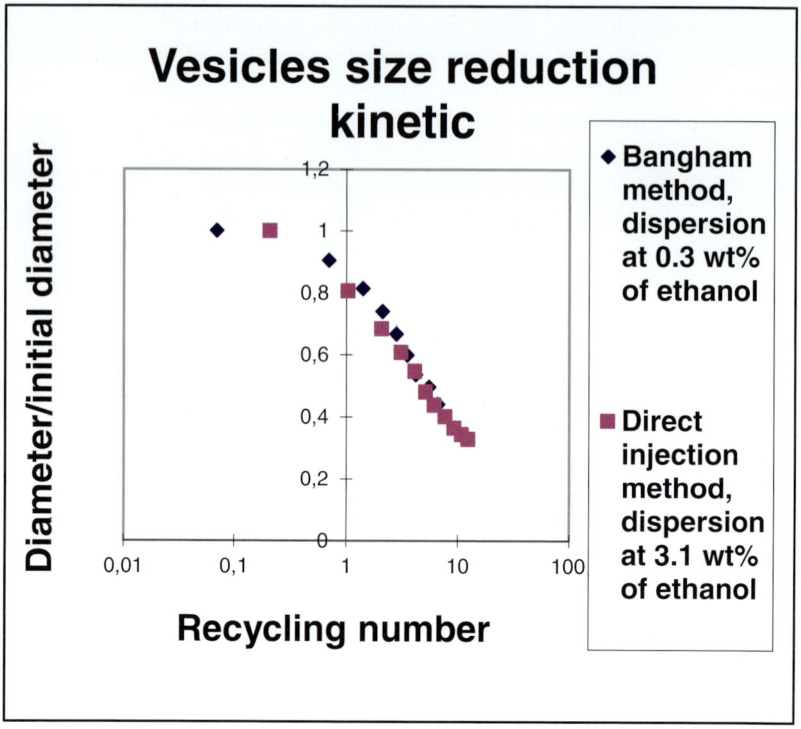

Figure 12.20 Comparison of vesicle size reduction kinetic of Bangham and direct injection methods.

Based on the low amount of ethanol to be used during manufacturing of liposomes and in order to keep the manufacturing process simple, the most straightforward way to remove ethanol seemed to be during freeze-drying step.

Solvent Removal during Freeze-Drying Step

Different trials were carried out with liposomal dispersion having ethanol residual content in the range of 3.2–0.3%. This range represents the typical ethanol residual content of liposomal dispersions obtained by direct injection method (≤3.2 wt%) and Bangham method (≤0.4 wt%) It was found that the ethanol residual content within the dispersion has a dramatic impact on freeze-dried material. In fact, when the residual solvent within the dispersion is higher than 1.5 wt%, the cake was raised in the vial by the solvent vapors (see Figure 12.21) and its reconstitution time was prolonged significantly. This result suggested that the ethanol residual content within the dispersion obtained using direct injection methods needs to be lower than 1.5 wt%. For this purpose, reconstituted freeze-dried products obtained using direct injection method and Bangham method and having ethanol residual content at 1.2 wt% have been analytically compared. The results did not show any significant difference in

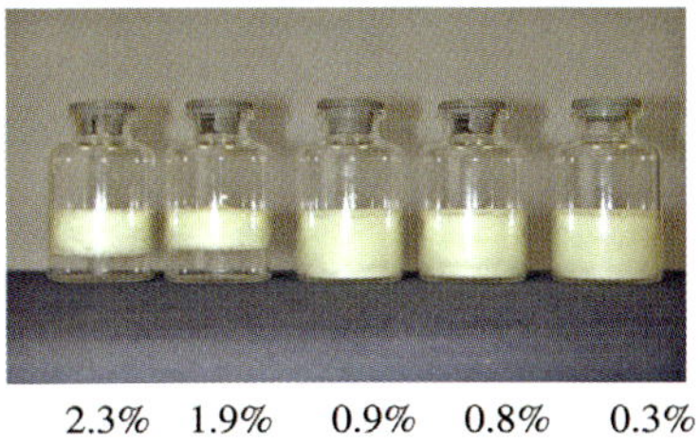

Figure 12.21 Aspect of freeze-dried cake as function of residual ethanol content.

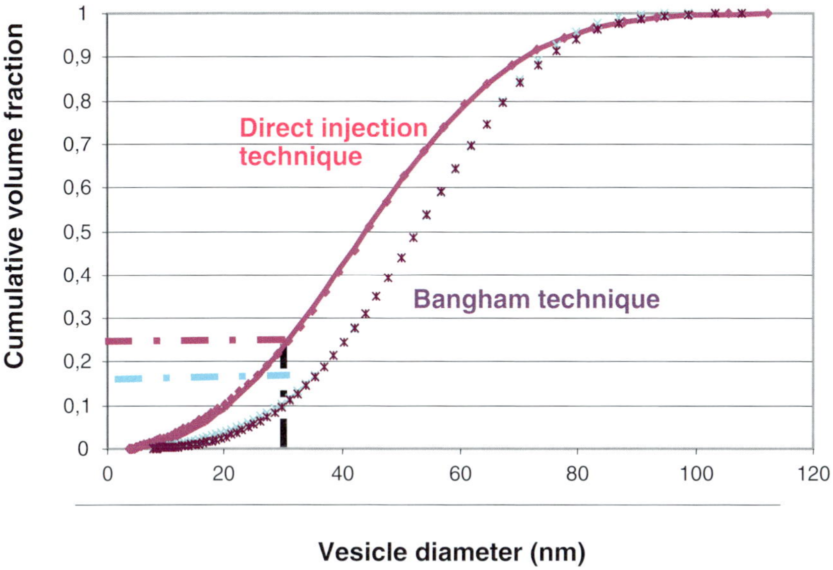

Figure 12.22 Vesicle distribution of liposomes produced by Bangham and direct inject methods.

terms of appearance, color, assay, impurities profile, and *in vitro* behavior. However, as it can be seen in Figure 12.22, a significant difference was observed in terms of average size and size distribution. Indeed, the average size (measurement using multiangle light scattering) of material produced using Bangham technique was found to be higher than that produced using direct injection method (15 nm difference). In addition, the measurement of the size distribution using size exclusion chromatography confirmed that the material produced using direct injection technique exhibited high fraction of small liposomes (quantity below 30 nm more than doubled from Bangham technique to direct injection). Based on these results (aspect of freeze-dried product and vesicle size after reconstitution), it was decided to discard removal of ethanol during freeze-drying step.

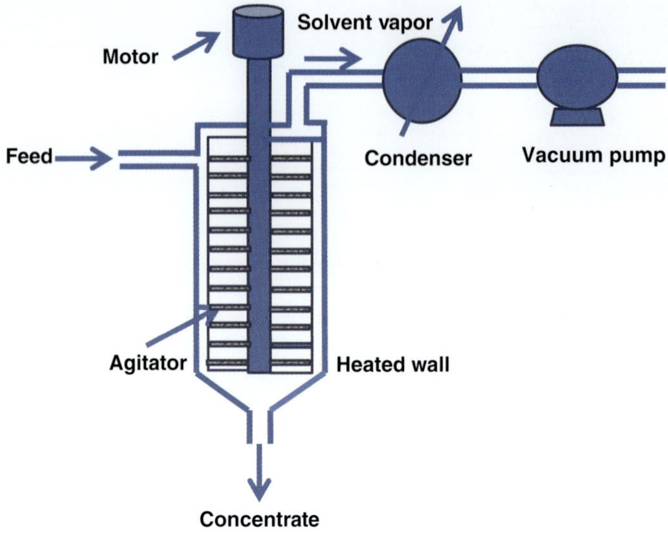

Figure 12.23 Schematic of agitated thin film evaporator [27].

Solvent Removal after Emulsification

An agitated thin film evaporator is used for evaporation of highly viscous and sticky products. This type of evaporators has been specially designed to provide high degree of agitation, effecting heat transfer as well as scraping the walls of the evaporator to prevent deposition of the product (see Figure 12.23).

Due to high viscosity of the native dispersion (50 mPa s), the evaluation of a solvent removal using agitated thin film evaporator was not conclusive. In fact, vesicle growth was observed during evaporation (see Figure 12.24). Moreover, a high buildup of material on the equipment walls as well as vesicle transportation within vacuum circuit was observed. This option was abandoned.

$$\textit{Note}: \text{ The removed fraction of dispersion} = \frac{\text{mass of distillate}}{\text{initial mass of dispersion}}.$$

Solvent Removal after Dispersion Sizing

Osmotic distillation is a nonthermal membrane separation process in which a liquid mixture containing a volatile component is placed in contact with a microporous, non-liquid-wettable membrane whose opposite surface is exposed to a second liquid phase capable of absorbing the volatile component on the opposite side of the membrane (see Figure 12.25). The process was used to extract ethanol from liposome dispersion (after size reduction) using water as the extracting solvent (permeate). The driving force of the process is based on the difference in vapor pressure (chemical potential or osmotic pressure) between the ethanol of the sized dispersion and the permeate.

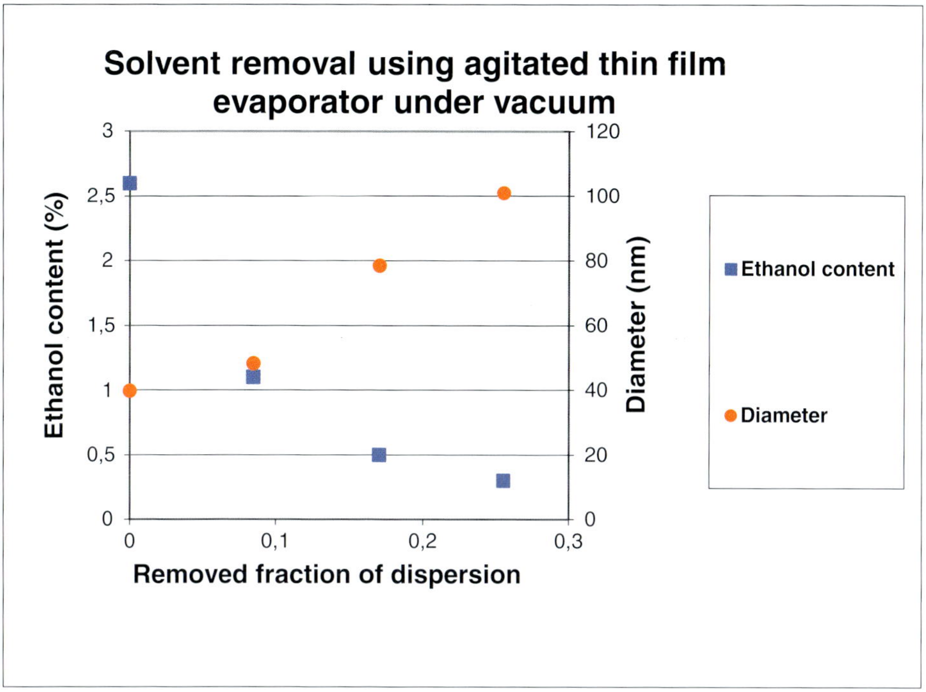

Figure 12.24 Removal of ethanol and vesicle size change during evaporation using agitated thin film evaporator.

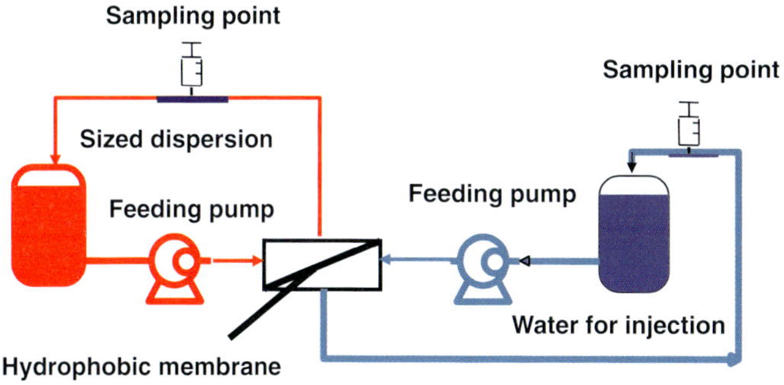

Figure 12.25 Schematic of osmotic distillation [28].

The use of this technique was found very effective in removing ethanol from sized dispersion without altering the quality of liposomes (see Figure 12.26). These findings indicate that the final residual ethanol can be managed by controlling the residence time of dispersion and permeate on the membrane. In addition, the analytical comparison of reconstituted freeze-dried liposomes obtained using direct injection method at 0.15% of ethanol and Bangham

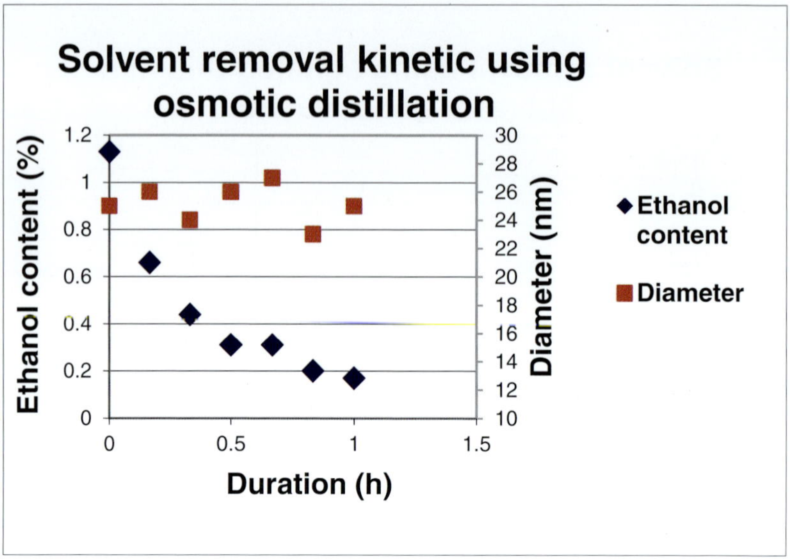

Figure 12.26 Solvent removal kinetic and vesicle size change using osmotic distillation.

Table 12.2 Characteristic diameters (d_{10}, d_{50}, and d_{90}) of vesicle size distribution of liposomes obtained using Bangham and direct injection techniques.

	Residual ethanol in sized dispersion (%)	Number of analyzed samples	d_{10} (nm)	d_{50} (nm)	d_{90} (nm)
Bangham	0.3	6	31.2 ± 1.0	53.2 ± 0.7	75.1 ± 0.8
Direct injection	0.2	5	31.5 ± 0.4	56.7 ± 0.6	82.5 ± 1.2

method does not show any drastic difference by means of appearance, color, identification, assay, impurities content, *in vitro* behavior, and vesicle size distribution (see Table 12.2).

Impact of the Process on the Vesicle Size of the Final Product

Different trials were performed using direct loading technique (free of ethanol – see Figure 12.8), direct injection technique (at different ethanol residual content), and Bangham technique. As illustrated in Figure 12.27, it was found that the ethanol residual content before freeze-drying was identified as the critical parameter to control the liposome size distribution of the final product.

Scaling Up of Vesicle Size Reduction Technique

Based on geometric configuration similarity of high-pressure homogenization valve and scale-up/scale-down rules (keeping the power density (see equation in

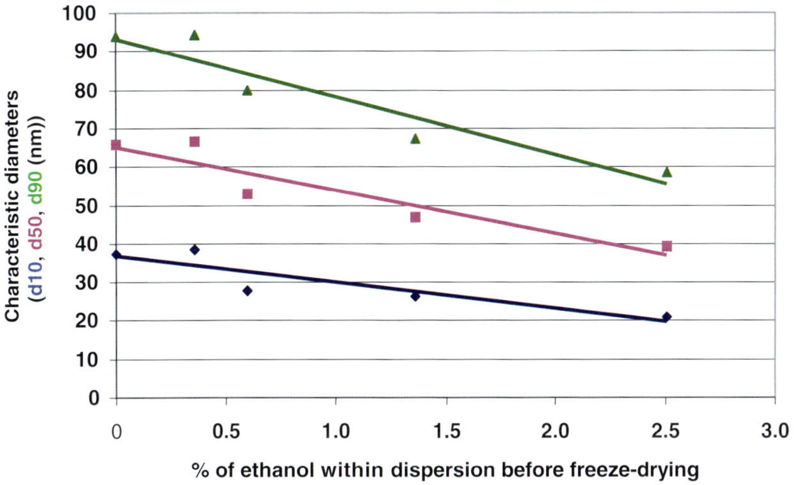

Figure 12.27 Characteristic diameters (d_{10}, d_{50}, and d_{90}) of vesicle size distribution of liposomes as function of residual ethanol content in dispersion before freeze-drying.

Section 12.5.2.2) and recycling number constant between different scales), it was found that the vesicle size reduction kinetic is accurately reproducible from one batch to another and from one scale to another (see Figures 12.28 and 12.29).

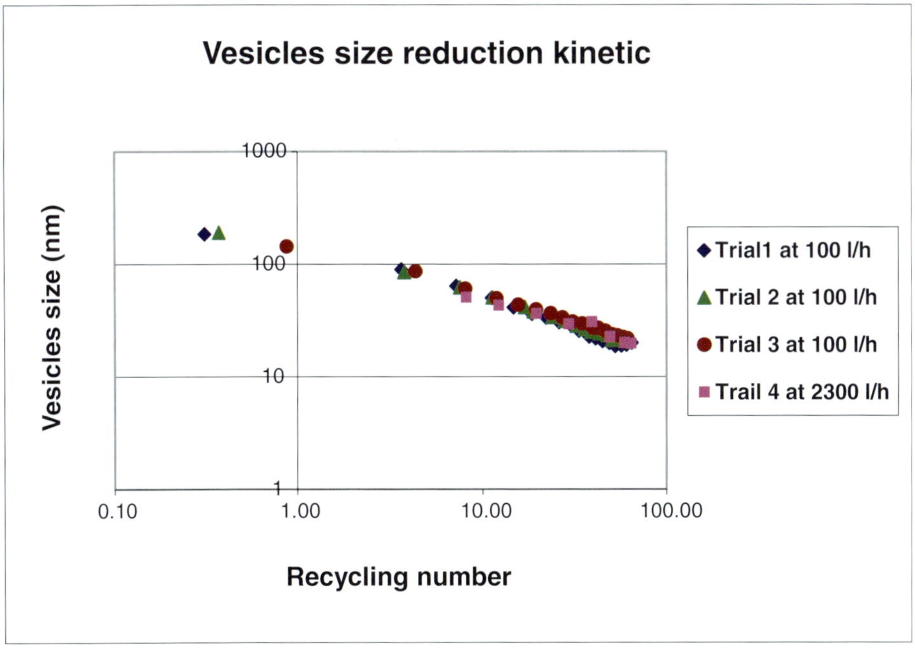

Figure 12.28 Vesicle size reduction kinetic obtained at two different scales (100 and 2300 l/h).

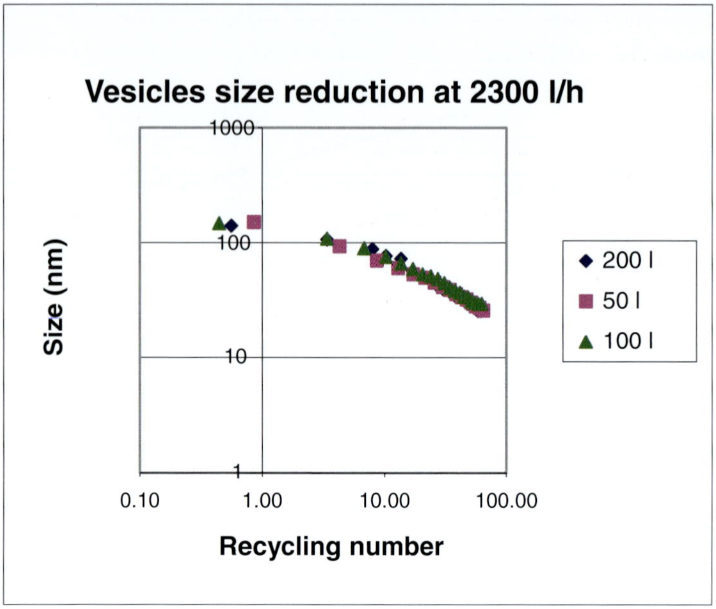

Figure 12.29 Vesicle size reduction kinetics obtained in three different batches (50, 100, and 200 l) using HPH at 2300 l/h.

12.5.1.5 Lessons Learned

This case study illustrates that when industrial considerations are not anticipated in early stage, the quality attributes of the product may be affected during scaling-up activities. Solving this issue may involve costly additional process development. Therefore, in early stage, laboratory processes should be applied that are scalable to industrial size by using a relevant scale-down approach.

12.5.2 Scale-Up and Scale-Down Strategies

The manufacturing process of nanodrug delivery systems can be profoundly impacted by the formulation design. Indeed, during manufacturing, the dispersion or suspension undergo high temperature, high shear rate, and a long duration of manufacturing. A prerequest for any scale-up is to ensure that the formulation is correctly designed and sufficiently robust with regard to the manufacturing process conditions. The literature includes a large number of publications dealing with the formulation engineering of nanodrug delivery systems that can help the identification of a robust formulation design [29].

The manufacturing processes of nanodrug delivery systems that have been described cover a wide variety of unit operation for which the scale-up cannot be exhaustively described within the limited scope of this chapter. Moreover, many steps are not specific to nanodrug delivery systems (mixing, filtration, solvent removal, etc.). Only scaling up of particle/vesicle size reduction (bead milling and high-pressure homogenization) will be discussed as it is the core of the manufacturing process.

12.5.2.1 Scaling Up of Bead Milling Technology

Given the case where the geometric similarity (shape and dimension) of the grinding chamber and stirrer is ensured, the rough scale-up rule is to keep constant the specific energy (SEC) of milling [30]:

$$\text{SEC} = \frac{P_{\text{t}} \cdot t}{m},$$

$\text{SEC} = \frac{\int_0^t (P_{(t)} - P_{(0)})\text{d}t}{m}$,where P_{t} is the total power consumed inside the grinding chamber decreased by the nonloaded power $P_{(0)}$, $P_{(\text{t})}$ is the power at time of milling t and m is the solid mass inside the chamber.

The specific energy depends on stirrer tip speed, solid concentration, bead size, bead filling ratio, and mean residence time of milling. If stirrer tip speed, solid concentration, bead size, and bead filling ratio are kept constant between small and large scale, it is important to keep the mean residence time constant between both scales in order to guarantee the same particle size of the milled suspension. The mean residence time can be defined as

$$\text{mean residence time} = \text{real milling time} \times \frac{\text{Active volume}}{\text{Bathc volume}}.$$

The active volume is defined as

$$\begin{aligned}\text{Active volume} = &\ (\text{volume of the milling chamber}) \\ &- (\text{real volume of beads}).\end{aligned}$$

The real volume of beads is defined as

$$\text{Real volume of beads} = (\text{apparent volume of beads}) \times \frac{d_{app}}{d_{rea}},$$

where d_{app} and d_{real} are the apparent and real density of beads, respectively.

12.5.2.2 Scaling Up of High-Pressure Homogenization

Given the case where the geometric similarity (shape and dimensions) of the homogenization valve (piston gap technology) or interaction chamber shape (microfluidization technology) is ensured, the scale-up rule is to keep constant recycling number and power density;

$$\text{RN} = \frac{Q_{\text{v}}}{V} \times t,$$

where RN is the recycling number, Q_V is the volume flow rate (m^3/s) of homogenization, V is the batch volume (m^3), and t is the time of homogenization (s).

$$P_V = \frac{Q_V \cdot P}{v},$$

where P_V is the power density (w/m^3), P is the homogenization pressure (Pa), and v is the volume (m^3) of the gap within homogenization valve (piston gap technology) or volume (m^3) of the interaction chamber (microfluidization technology).

12.5.2.3 Generic Development Methodology

Previously, two important topics have been highlighted: the necessity to design a robust formulation and to use scalable process equipment throughout development to ensure continuity of product quality attributes.

In order to illustrate the industrial implementation, which guarantees the quality attributes of nanodrug delivery systems during the stages of process development, examples of high-pressure homogenization and bead milling manufacturing chains at different scales are presented. The positioning of each scale according to the development stage of the product is shown. The same concept can be established for other unit operations.

The manufacturing chains are presented in Figures 12.30 and 12.31 and described in Table 12.3.

Note: A miniaturized high-pressure homogenizer or bead mill that can process few milligrams of material is not commercially available. It can be replaced by planetary stirred bead mill (for nanocrystalline suspension) or by sonication probe (for emulsion or liposome).

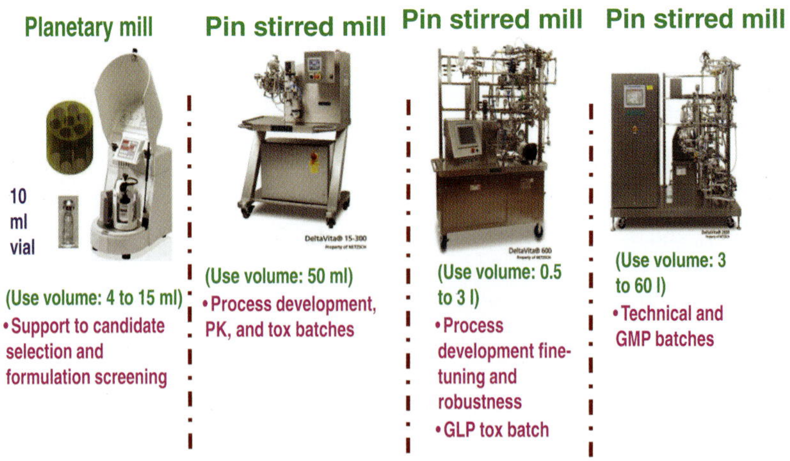

Figure 12.30 Bead milling used as value chain for manufacturing of nanocrystalline suspension from early to late or commercial stage [31]. (With courtesy of Netzsch.)

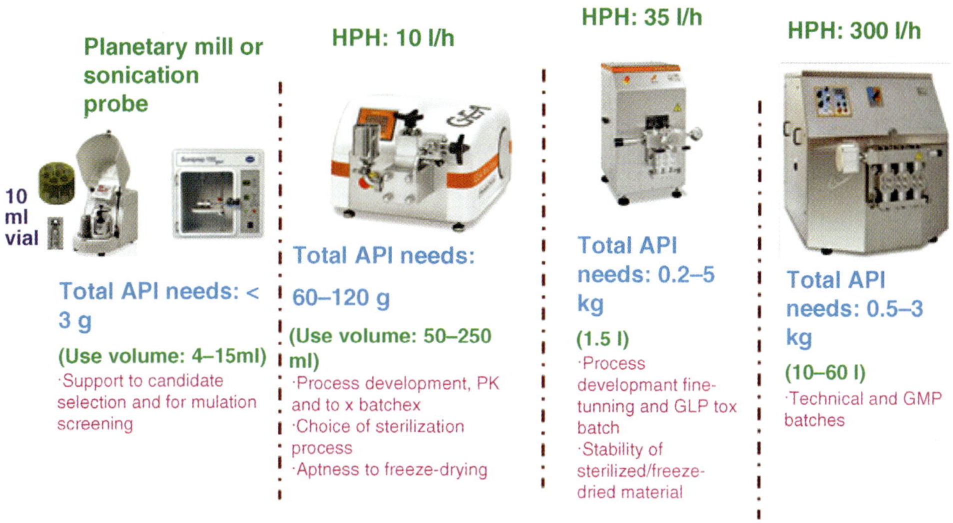

Figure 12.31 High-pressure homogenization used as value chain for manufacturing of nanocrystalline suspension, nanoamorphous suspension, polymeric nanosuspension, emulsion, and liposomes from early to late or commercial stage [22] (With courtesy of GEA-Niro-Soavi.).

Table 12.3 Value chains for the production of nanodrug delivery systems.

Nanodrug delivery systems	Equipment			
	Support to discovery and formulation design	Process development and preclinical batches manufacturing	Process development fine-tuning, robustness study, and GLP batches manufacturing	Technical, GMP, and commercial batches manufacturing
Nanocrystalline suspension	Planetary stirred bead mill	Laboratory-scale bead mill or laboratory-scale HPH	Pilot-scale bead mill or pilot-scale HPH	Industrial scale bead mill or industrial scale HPH
Nanoamorphous suspension, polymeric nano-suspension, emulsion, and liposomes	Sonication probe	Laboratory-scale HPH	Pilot-scale HPH	Industrial scale HPH

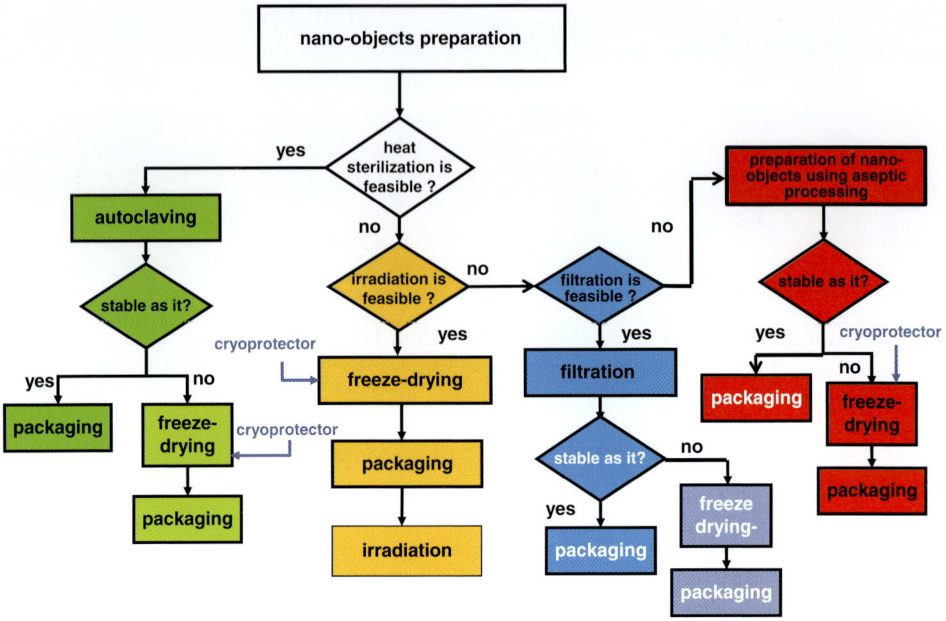

Figure 12.32 Decision tree of nanodrug delivery systems sterilization.

12.6 Technological Concept for Manufacture of Drug Product for Human Use (GMP Unit)

In this section, only sterile processing will be described as it is the most critical process in pharmaceutical manufacturing. Indeed, the inherent risk of microbiological contamination associated with the process is critical to ensure patient safety.

The manufacturing unit should be able to manufacture nanodrug delivery systems having a particle/vesicle size distribution compatible with parenteral administration, specifically with intravenous administration for which it is necessary to eliminate the risk of capillary embolism (lumen diameter of about 6 μm) [32,33]. The GMP unit should be able to manufacture sterile nanodrug delivery systems that can be classified into three categories, as illustrated in Figure 12.32:

i) Those that can be sterilized in final container (terminally sterilized).
ii) Those that cannot be terminally sterilized but can be sterilized by filtration and filled aseptically in the final container. It should be noted that the sterile filtration of nanosuspension is rarely feasible due to fouling of filter membranes by particles. Moreover, it is noteworthy that the filtration of liposomes may require 0.1 μm filter to ensure the dispersion sterility (health authority's requirement).

iii) Those that cannot be terminally sterilized or sterilized by filtration and must be aseptically prepared. It has to be considered that in the case of preparation of nanosuspension by milling, a sterile API is needed.

Furthermore, the manufacturing unit should be compliant with pharmaceutical regulations such as current good manufacturing practices (cGMPs), in particular with regard to qualification and validation, 21 CFR part 11, American and European Pharmacopoeia. The unit should also be compliant with current safety regulations.

Later in this section the following topics will be reviewed:

i) Description of process technology configuration for the manufacturing of nanocrystalline suspension using top-down process
ii) Description of process technology configuration for the manufacturing of nanocrystalline suspension using bottom-up process, nanoemulsion, liposomes, or polymeric nanoparticles
iii) Equipment design requirements in terms of concept, sterilization, cleaning, drying, and pressurization
iv) Facility and utility requirements

12.6.1 Process Technology Configuration for Manufacturing of Nanocrystalline Suspension Using Top-Down Process

The process technology is described in Figure 12.33. Such a unit requires a variety of vessels, mill, piping, and auxiliary equipment for API incorporation, filtration, and transfer. The unit is composed of the following:

- V1 vessel used for the preparation of stabilizer solution. It is connected to a double 0.22 μm filter to ensure sterilization of stabilizer solution.
- V2 vessel used for the preparation of suspension. It is equipped with recirculation loop made of feeding pump to feed suspension within the mill and cooling exchanger to remove dissipated heat during milling.
- A micrometer-range filtration used for removing any big particles.
- An isolator used for the incorporation of API. It can be configured to operate under two different conditions:
  - Negative pressure in case of handling of highly active API and terminal sterilization of the final suspension. In this case, the isolator is used as a barrier for protecting operators from API toxicity;
  - Positive pressure in case of handling of sterile API. In this case, the isolator is used as a barrier for protecting API from any microbial contamination.
- A stirred media mill or high-pressure homogenizer.
- V3 vessel used for the preparation of cryoprotector solution in case of freeze-drying of nanosuspension. It is connected to a double 0.22 μm filter to ensure sterilization of cryoprotector solution.
- V4 vessel used for mixing of the cryoprotector solution and the nanosuspension.

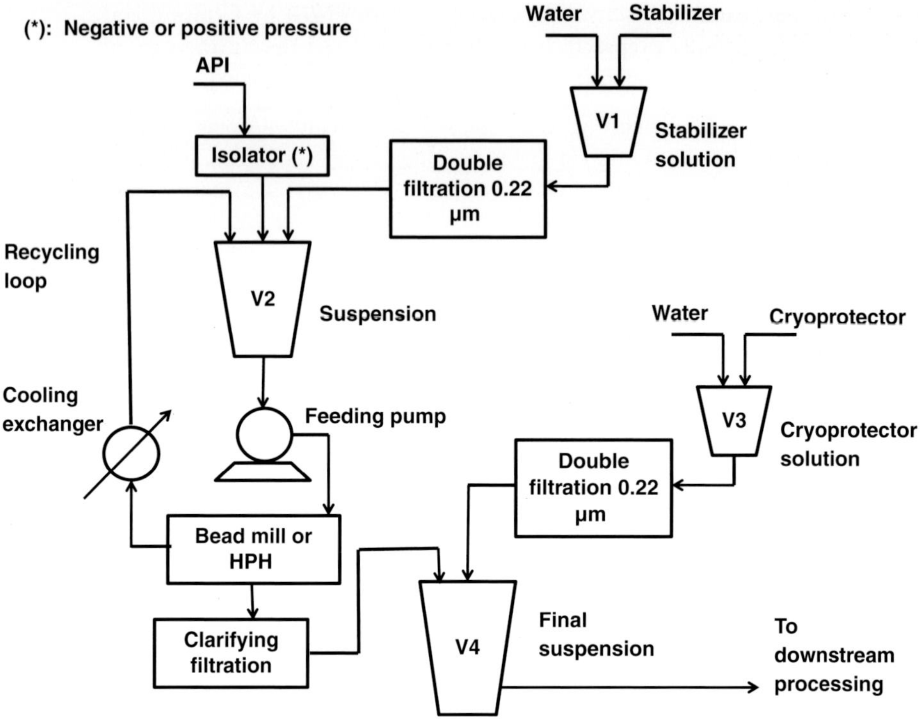

Figure 12.33 Process technology configuration of intravenously injectable nanoparticles using top-down process.

12.6.2 Process Technology Configuration for Manufacturing of Nanocrystalline Suspension Using Bottom-Up Process or for Nanoemulsion, Liposomes, or Polymeric Nanoparticles

The process technology is described in Figure 12.34. The unit can be composed of the following:

- V1 vessel used for the preparation of organic or oil solution. It is connected to a double 0.22 μm filter to ensure sterilization of solution.
- An isolator used for the incorporation of API. It is generally operated under negative pressure. The isolator is used in case of handling of high-toxic API as barrier for protecting operators from API toxicity.
- V2 vessel used for the preparation of suspension, emulsion, or liposomes. It is equipped with recirculation loop made of feeding pump to feed suspension within the mill and cooling exchanger to remove dissipated heat during milling.
- A mill used for vesicles or particle size reduction. Generally, high-pressure homogenization is the most applied technology for this application.

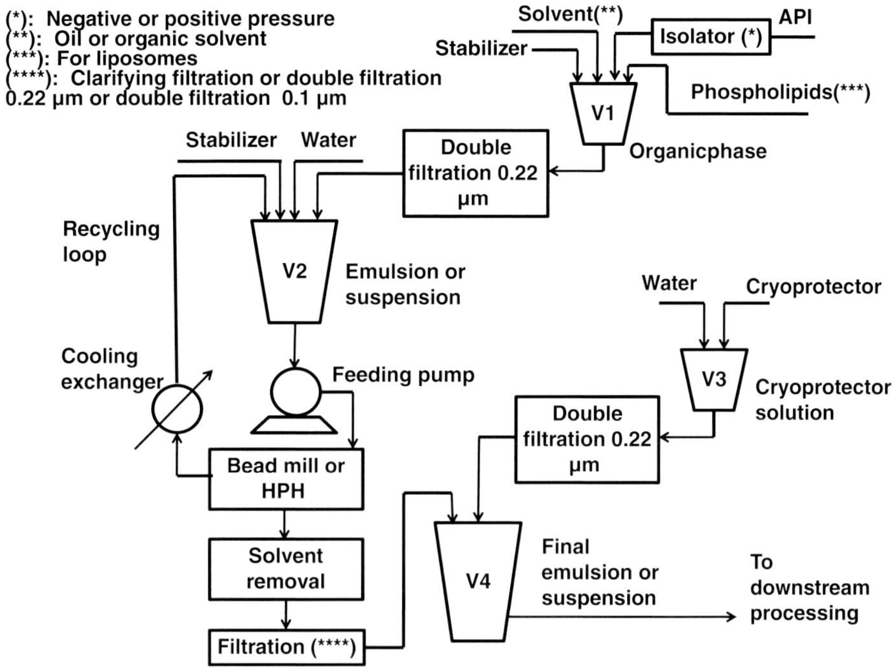

Figure 12.34 Process technology configuration of intravenously injectable nanoemulsion liposomes.

- Solvent removal equipment used in case of polymeric nanosuspension or liposomes manufacturing. It can be an agitated thin evaporator or an osmotic distillation.
- A double sterile filtration (0.22 or 0.1 μm) to ensure sterilization of dispersion if it is feasible.
- V3 vessel used for the preparation of cryoprotector solution in case of freeze-drying of nano-objects. The vessel is connected to a double 0.22 μm filter to ensure sterilization of cryoprotector solution.
- V4 vessel used for mixing of the cryoprotector solution and the nano-objects dispersion.

12.6.3 Equipment Design Requirements

Two options of design are possible depending upon development stage or batch size. For early development and batch sizes below 10 l, some parts (vessels, filters, and piping) of the unit can be made of disposable equipment as far as the nanodrug delivery systems are compatible with the unit materials. In this case the mill, feeding pump, and cooling exchanger have to be sterilized using an autoclave. Alternatively, the unit can be as fixed platform made of stainless steel and correctly designed for the following unit steps:

i) Equipment sterilization in place (SIP)
ii) Manufacturing of nanodrug delivery systems
iii) Equipment cleaning in place (CIP)
iv) Equipment drying in place
v) Equipment pressurization during storage period between sterilization and use

The platform should be equipped to perform purges and designed to avoid split routes, dead ends, and T-junctions. The unit may be equipped with temperature and pressure measurement instruments in order to perform thermal mapping and monitoring of sterilization parameters. It may also be equipped with instrumentation for measuring mass and volume of liquid and solid materials (weighing cells, flow meters, etc.). The vessels may be connected to required utilities (water for injection, purified water, air, nitrogen, clean steam, steam, liquid for heating or cooling, etc.). Any utility in direct product contact should be equipped with point of use filters.

12.6.3.1 Equipment Sterilization

The objective is to ensure that product contact surfaces are sufficiently sterile to achieve the required product bio-burden. All equipment should be sterilized using validated cycles. Vessels and the mill should be sterilized using clean steam or overheated water. The filters (for liquid and gas) should be sterilized using clean steam and the isolator should be sterilized using vapors of hydrogen peroxide. At the end of the sterilization step, the unit needs to be carefully cooled, dried, and pressurized. The sterilization process should be validated by simulating the manufacturing process using microbiological growth medium (media fill).

12.6.3.2 Equipment Cleaning

The objective is to clean the product contact surfaces of vessels, equipment, and pipes in place without dismantling the platform. For this purpose, the unit should be designed to ensure a turbulent flow ($Re > 3000$) during cleaning with velocity >1.5 m/s. Cleaning can be done at high temperatures of 70–90 °C using detergents such as caustics, acids, or surfactant. At the end of cleaning, the unit has to be rinsed using water for injection.

12.6.3.3 Equipment Drying

Drying is an important step to perform after cleaning and after sterilization that prevents residual water within the unit avoiding any microbial growth. Drying should be done by draining of water using hot air. The drying efficiency of the unit can be monitored using relative humidity probe that can be placed in the air exhaust line.

12.6.4
Facility Requirements

During production, it is necessary to control the environment from any microbial, pyrogen, and particle contamination. The manufacturing of parenteral nanodrug delivery systems is generally performed in C-grade room (class 10 000: ISO 14644-1 Cleanroom Standards) in which a laminar flow hood can be used during material addition (e.g., stabilizer). A D-grade room (class 100 000: ISO 14644-1 Cleanroom Standards) can be used if the unit can be operated as a closed barrier system.

It is important to note that such a unit should be designed simply and specifically for the parenteral route in order to not compromise sterility assurance and facilitate supervision of the platform.

12.7
Conclusion

In this chapter it was shown that a variety of processes are used for the production of nanodrug delivery systems. For a large number of applications, two technologies can be used: high-pressure homogenization (HPH) and bead milling. The HPH is a versatile technology. It allows manufacturing of nanocrystalline suspension, nanoamorphous suspension, polymeric nanoparticles, emulsion, and liposomes, whereas bead milling can be used only for the manufacturing of nanocrystalline suspension, although providing smaller particle sizes. For process development, it has been shown that it is important to anticipate the industrial manufacturability at earlier stages in order to avoid any inconsistency of product quality. The latter part of the discussion has been dedicated to the design of a manufacturing unit for product for human parenteral administration and its specificity according the nanodrug delivery system to be manufactured.

References

1 Müller, R.H., Jacobs, C., and Kayser, O. (2001) Nanosuspensions as particulate drug formulations in therapy: rationale for development and what we can expect for the future. *Adv. Drug. Deliv. Rev.*, **47**, 3–19.

2 Nagaraju, P., Krishnachaithanya, K., Srinivas, V.D., and Padma, S.V. (2010) Nanosuspensions: a promising drug delivery systems. *Int. J. Pharm. Sci. Nano*, **2**, 679–684.

3 Nagavarma, B., Hemant, K.S.Y., Ayaz, A., Vasudha, L., and Shivakumar, H.G. (2012) Different techniques for preparation of polymeric nanoparticles: a review. *Asian J. Pharm. Clin. Res.*, **5**, 16–23.

4 Singh Chahal, A., Madgulkar, A., Kshirsagar, S., Bhalekar, M., Dikpati, A., and Gawli, P. (2012) Amorphous nanoparticles for solubility enhancement. *J. Adv. Pharm. Sci.*, **2**, 167–178.

5 Tadros, T. (2009) *Nanodispersion*, Walter de Gruyter GmbH, Berlin.

6 Shah, D.A., Murdande, S.B., and Dave, R.H (2015) A review: pharmaceutical and pharmacokinetic aspect of nanocrystalline suspensions. *J. Pharm. Sci.*, **105**, 10–24.
7 Panagiotou, T. and Fisher, R. (2012) Improving product quality with entrapped stable emulsions: from theory to industrial application. *Challenges*, **3**, 84–113.
8 Dua, J., Rana, A.C., and Bhandari, A. (2012) Liposome: methods of preparation and applications. *Int. J. Pharma. Stud. Res.*, **3**, 14–20.
9 Peltonen, L. and Hirvonen, J. (2010) Pharmaceutical nanocrystals by nanomilling: critical process parameters, particle fracturing and stabilization methods. *J. Pharm. Pharmacol.*, **62**, 1569–1579.
10 Ostwald, W. (1901) Uber die vemeintliche Isomerie des roten und gelben Queck-silberoxyds und die Oberflachen-spannung Fester Korper. *Z. Phys. Chem.*, **34**, 495–512.
11 Puneet, S., William, A.D., and Sanjay, G. (2009) Effect of wet milling process on the solid state of indomethacin and simvastatin. *Int. J. Pharm.*, **380**, 40–48.
12 Becker, M. and Schwedes, J. (1999) Comminution of ceramics in stirred media mills and wear of grinding beads. *Powder Technol.*, **105**, 374–381.
13 Duda, J. (1985) Molecular diffusion in polymeric system. *Pure Appl. Chem.*, **57**, 1681–1690.
14 Benita, S. and Levy, M. (1993) Submicron emulsions as colloidal drug carriers for intravenous administration: comprehensive physicochemical characterization. *J. Pharm. Sci.*, **82**, 1069–1079.
15 Haran, G., Cohen, R., Bar, L.K., and Barenholz, L. (1993) Transmembrane ammonium sulfate gradients in liposomes produce efficient and stable entrapment of amphipathic weak bases. *Biochim. Biophys. Acta*, **1151**, 201–215.
16 Shegokar, R. and Müller, R.H. (2010) Nanocrystals: industrially feasible multifunctional formulation technology for poorly soluble actives. *Int. J. Pharm.*, **399**, 129–139.
17 Aula, S., Lakkireddy, S., Jamil, K., Kapley, A., Swamy, A., and Lakkireddy, H. (2015) Biophysical, biopharmaceutical and toxicological significance of biomedical nanoparticles. *RSC Adv.*, **5**, 47830–47859.
18 Innings, F. (2015) High-pressure homogenizer design, in *Engineering Aspects of Food Emulsification and Homogenization* (eds M. Rayner and P. Dejmek), CRC Press, p. 149.
19 Wuytack, E.Y., Diels, A., and Michiels, C. (2002) Bacterial inactivation by high-pressure homogenisation and high hydrostatic pressure. *Int. J. Food Microbiol.*, **77**, 205–212.
20 Nekkanti, V., Vabalaboina, V., and Pillai, R. (2012) Drug nanoparticles: an overview, in *The Delivery of Nanoparticles*, InTech, pp. 111–132.
21 Sharma, R., Jain, S., and Tiwari, R. (2015) Nanoparticle technology: formulating poorly water-soluble compounds – a review. *Int. J. Pharm. Sci. Res.*, **6**, 57.
22 Niro-Soavi, G. (2015) Technical document. www.niro-soavi.com/.
23 Soavi, G.-N. (2004) High-pressure pumps and homogenizers. Available at WWW. Niroinc.com.
24 Midoux, N. and Nakach, M. (2011) High pressure homogenisation. Sanofi internal document.
25 Timpe, C. (2010) Drug solubilization strategies applying nanoparticulate formulation and solid dispersion approaches in drug development. *Pharm. Rev.*, **13**, 12–21.
26 Kwade, A. (1999) Wet comminution in stirred media mills: research and its practical application. *Powder Technol.*, **105**, 14–20.
27 Satoru, K., Kazutaka, T., and Yasuhiro, M. (1988) Flow structure and mixing mechanism in an agitated thin-film evaporator. *J. Chem. Eng. Jpn.*, **21**, 639–644.
28 Deshmukh, S., Sapkal, V., and Sapkal, R. (2012) Performance enhancement of membrane distillation process of fruit juice. *J. Membr. Sci. Techol.*, **1**, 104.
29 Nakach, M., Authelin, J.R., Tadros, T., Galet, L., and Chamayou, A. (2014) Engineering of nano-crystalline drug suspension: employing a physico-chemistry based stabilizer selection methodology or approach. *Int. J. Pharm.*, **476**, 277–288.

30 Stenger, F., Mende, S., Schwedes, J., and Peukert, W. (2005) The influence of suspension properties on the grinding behavior of alumina particles in the submicron size range in stirred media mills. *Powder Technol.*, **156**, 103–110.
31 Netzsch (2015) Technical document. Available at www.netzsch-grinding.com/.
32 Douglas, F., Kafilmout, K., and Patt, N. (1971) Foreign particle embolism in drug addicts: respiratory pathophysiology. *Ann. Intern. Med.*, **75**, 865–872.
33 Ward, S., Heyneman, L.E., Reittner, P., Kazerooni, E.A., Godwin, J.D., and Müller, N. (2000) Talcosis associated with IV abuse of oral medications CT findings. *Am. J. Roentgenol.*, **174**, 789–793.

13
Occupational Safety and Health

Thomas H. Brock

Berufsgenossenschaft Rohstoffe und Chemische Industrie, FR Gefahrstoffe, Biologische Arbeitsstoffe und Analytik, Kurfürsten-Anlage 62, 69115 Heidelberg, Germany

13.1
Nanomaterials at the Workplace

The development of nanotechnology – due to the variety of disciplines involved and their methods, it would perhaps even be more appropriate to use the plural nanotechnologies – has led to the creation of a large variety of materials in laboratories in recent years. Many of these have also been applied in practice, often not even being recognized as a nanotechnological application by the downstream user, end user, or consumer.

There is a general consensus that nanotechnologies are those using structures within the range of approximately 1–100 nm. There have been numerous attempts to clearly define this complex field, all of which more or less attempt to impose precise classifications [1]. The definition of the National Nanotechnology Initiative in the USA is given here as an example: "Nanotechnology is the understanding and control of matter at the nanoscale, at dimensions between approximately 1 and 100 nm, where unique phenomena enable novel applications. Encompassing nanoscale science, engineering, and technology, nanotechnology involves imaging, measuring, modeling, and manipulating matter at this length scale [2]." The European Commission defines nanotechnology as follows: "Nanotechnology is the study of phenomena and fine-tuning of materials at atomic, molecular, and macromolecular scales, where properties differ significantly from those at a larger scale. Commission Recommendation of 18 October 2011 on the definition of nanomaterial [. . .] are materials that often have specific properties due to their small particle size" [3].

There are basically two types of material with nanoscale structures occurring at the workplace. Ultrafine aerosols are differentiated from the nanomaterials that are generally understood to be nanomaterials and are consciously and intentionally manufactured or used as such, as although they can share the same

Pharmaceutical Nanotechnology: Innovation and Production, First Edition. Edited by Jean Cornier, Arno Kwade, Andrew Owen, and Marcel Van de Voorde.

properties in principle, they can also be created unintentionally and cause exposure. Both types are to be considered equally for occupational health and safety measures. The ultrafine aerosols can be released by nanomaterials, although these are often created through processing steps on coarser materials. In the following we will mainly discuss nanomaterials; however, the statements made can mostly be applied to ultrafine aerosols, too.

The large number of such nanomaterials means that the risks and potential hazards with regard to the nanomaterials produced or used can only be determined and quantified to a limited extent. The emergent properties of many nanomaterials also make this task very difficult. The gaps in the basic understanding of their effects have not been sufficiently closed to date, and as such other protective strategies will have to be taken.

When assessing the risks and deriving corresponding protective measures for employees at the workplace, it is helpful to use the categorization of the incredibly varied materials with nanoscale structures in line with the definition of the ISO Technical Committee 229 [4].

At first, a differentiation is made between free, unbound *nano-objects* (with the exception of the very frequently observed aggregates and agglomerates of the respective nano-objects, as well as solutions or suspensions of such nano-objects or their aggregates or agglomerates) and bound nanostructures in the form of composite nanomaterials embedded in various kinds of matrices or as surface structures of these. Both together form nanomaterials, comprising all materials that occur at the workplace and that use nanotechnologies in any way, and that possess structures within the range of 1–100 nm in at least one spatial dimension. For the purposes of occupational health and safety, it has proved necessary not to restrict this observation to the 100 nm limit, but also to take into account larger objects such as agglomerates and aggregates up to the micrometer range (at least 600 nm).

Such nano-objects are initially *nanoparticles* that fall into the relevant range in all three spatial dimensions. These include partially spherical particles (Figure 13.1) that often have a quite irregular form as well as highly symmetrical molecules such as fullerenes. Many metal atom clusters and metal oxides are examples of these. The widely used term “nanoparticle” is therefore limited to the above. It may take time to get used to this terminology, but it is very helpful when evaluating nanomaterials at the workplace as it enables better categorizations.

Fibrous nano-objects are in the nanoscale range in two spatial dimensions and can be very long. High aspect ratio nanomaterials (HARN) can provide particular cause for concern, especially in the case of highly rigid structures. Fibrous nano-objects include fibers, wires, and rods. Single- or multiwalled nanotubes are examples of these. In addition to carbon, they can also be manufactured from other elements such as silicon or titanium.

Plate-shaped nano-objects are only in the nanoscale in one spatial dimension and can be very broad. The most famous example of this kind of nano-object is graphene with its unusual mechanical and electrical properties.

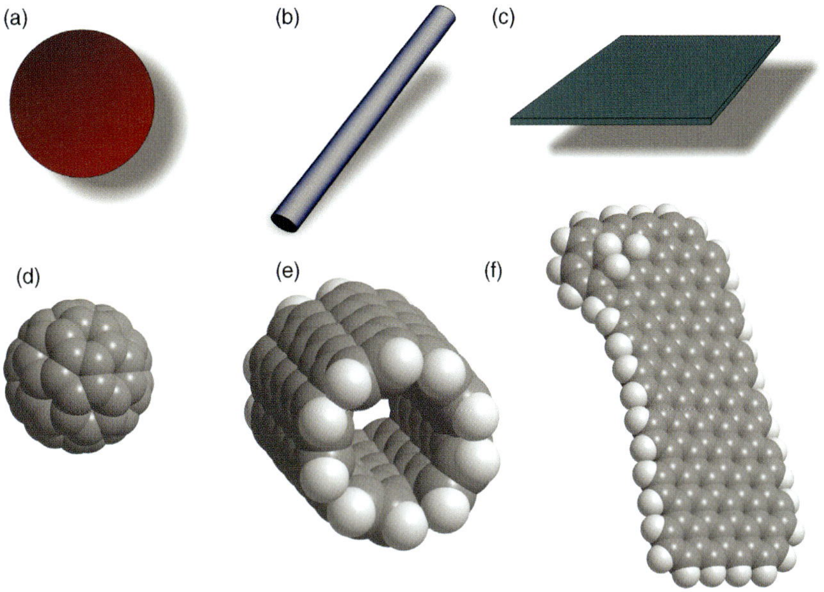

Figure 13.1 Forms of nanoobjects: (a): particle; (b): fibrous; (c): plate-shaped nano-objects; (d): example of a C_{60} molecule; (e) a short section of an SWCNT[1]; and (f) a graphene platelet (with H-atoms at the edge valences).

Composite nanomaterials contain nano-objects (and occasionally also their agglomerates or aggregates) or possess nanoscale structural elements. These nanomaterials are encountered very often in the field, for example, many of them are construction materials or coating materials. Examples of these are shown in Figure 13.2.

The European Commission concretizes the observance of nanoscale proportions, which frequently exist in bulk materials, in a recommendation from 2011: "A natural, incidental, or manufactured material containing particles, in an unbound state or as an aggregate or as an agglomerate and where, for 50% or more of the particles in the number size distribution, one or more external dimensions is in the size range 1–100 nm. In specific cases and where warranted by concerns for the environment, health, safety, or competitiveness, the number size distribution threshold of 50% may be replaced by a threshold between 1 and 50%. By derogation from the above, fullerenes, graphene flakes, and single-wall carbon nanotubes with one or more external dimensions below 1 nm should be considered as nanomaterials" [5]. It will certainly be necessary to also consider other large molecules that fall into this sub-1 nm range.

The primary particles have a tendency to congregate quickly to the less tightly bound agglomerates or the polyvalent and very firmly bound aggregates (Figure 13.3).

1) SWCNT: single-walled carbon nanotube

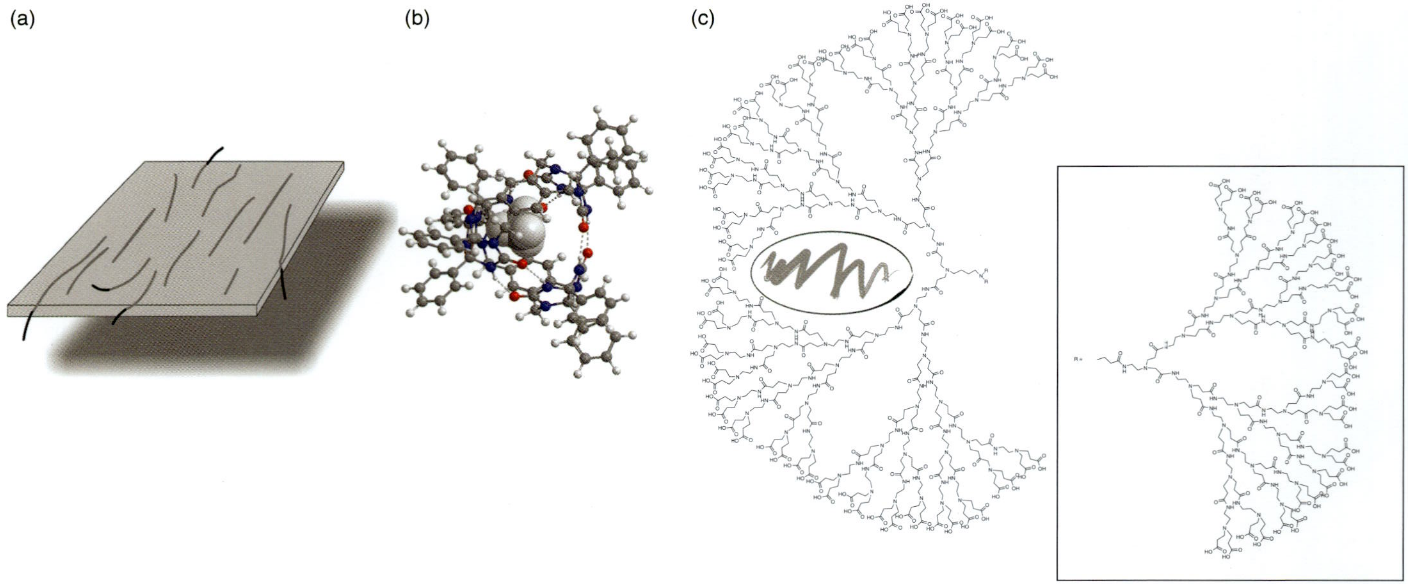

Figure 13.2 Composite nanomaterials. (a) A plate-shaped material containing nanotubes integrated in the matrix and in some cases protruding outwards. (b) A methane molecule in a molecular cage. (c) A dendritic material offering space for accommodating guest molecules in its voids within the molecule, for example, active substances (for reasons of clarity only the left half of the molecule is shown in detail, and only one of the voids is marked).

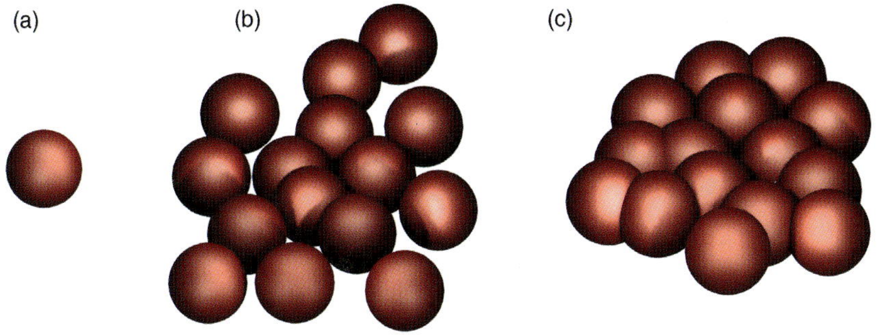

Figure 13.3 (a) Primary particle. (b) Agglomerate. (c) Aggregate in ideal shape.

13.2 Legal Aspects

In the European Union, substances, preparations and their products may only be brought to market within the scope of the REACH legislation (Registration, Evaluation, Authorization and Restriction of Chemicals) of 2007. This legislation is in the process of being updated. Regulation in the United States is based on ToSCA (Toxic Substances Control Act) of 1976. Work on a revision of this law commenced in 2015 with the TSCA Modernization Act. Corresponding regulations also exist in other states such as Japan, Australia, or Switzerland. Because nanomaterials are not explicitly mentioned in these regulations, there are constant discussions as to the necessity of specific regulations for nanomaterials, as it is argued that quantities below the threshold (this is 1 t/year according to REACH) require an additional regulation due to the large number of particles (nano-objects). The stipulated tests are also not specifically devised for nanomaterials. However, according to REACH, nanomaterials that belong to substances produced in a quantity of at least 1 t/year are to be taken into account when assessing hazards and safe conduct [6,7]. Further help on REACH can be obtained from the national REACH helpdesks.

There is a harmonized European Union law for occupational health and safety with regard to substances and materials, supplemented by national implementations and additions. These contain more specific details on working safely with nanomaterials and protection from ultrafine aerosols, for example, in the German Ordinance on Hazardous Substances (GefStoffV) with its corresponding technical rules and announcements as well as the rules and informative publications of the statutory accident insurance institutions. These include the Announcement on Hazardous Substances 527 [8] or the laboratory guidelines "Working Safely in Laboratories" [9] with the complementary publication on "Nanomaterials in the Laboratory" [10]. The corresponding NIOSH publications are "Safe Nanotechnology in the Workplace" [11] and "General Safe Practices for Working with Engineered Nanomaterials in Research Laboratories" [12]. The procedures described here are similar, with occasional differences in the detail. The resulting measures are described in more detail in Section 13.5.3. Further publications are available in various countries [13–21].

13.3 Management of Uncertainty

Performing a risk assessment is a common and proven method for determining any potential risks associated with manufacturing and utilizing hazardous substances – or at least for making a realistic assessment of them. This requires the compilation of various kinds of information in order to at least make a qualitative assessment of the risks or, better still, perform a reliable estimation of the risks. Appropriate measures can then be derived from this and established.

The information about parameters required for this can be obtained or determined more or less easily. When handling active substances and the pharmaceuticals manufactured out of them, the raw and auxiliary materials, solvents and reagents also have to be assessed. This includes in particular information and data on the following:

- Size distribution and shape
- Toxicology
- Pharmacological effect
- Fire and explosion behavior, autoignitability
- Additions, coatings, soiling
- Chemical and physical–chemical properties, such as catalytic effects, reactivities, radical formation, surface activity, specific surface, ζ potential, absorptivity, kinetics of the agglomeration or aggregation, dustiness behavior, solubilities, aging, and stability
- Exposure possibilities and levels (inhalation, dermal, and oral).

A risk can now be described as the product of the probability of damage occurring and the severity of the damage. While the levels of exposure are correlated with the probability of occurrence, the determined severity of damage resulting from the effect is linked to the required ability to assess or determine these sufficiently. For the most part, this will be feasible for the aforementioned points with a greater or lesser degree of effort, even though materials such as fibrous nano-objects or composite nanomaterials can pose significant difficulties regarding the selection of measurement system and methods. On the other hand, even after years of intensive research not enough is known about toxicology to make generally valid statements.

13.4 Risks of Nanomaterials for Researchers and Workers

In the pharmaceutical industry, it is common to use internal reference values as OELs (occupational exposure limits). This is also possible for nanomaterials handled as active substances or medicinal products within certain limits. The special translocation routes that can be taken by (e.g., the penetration through the alveoli into the blood stream or the penetration through cytoplasmic membranes) such nanomaterials should be taken into account; for targeted drug delivery these effects should be viewed in combination.

One possible procedure with regard to the toxicological properties of nanomaterials is categorization according to Announcement on Hazardous Substances 527 (BekGS 527) [8]. This divides nanomaterials into four categories with regard to their toxic properties.

- Category I — Soluble nanomaterials without specific toxic properties (solubility at least 100 mg/l water at room temperature)
- Category II — Soluble nanomaterials with specific toxic properties
- Category III — Granular biopersistent dusts without specific toxic properties
- Category IV — Fibrous nanomaterials

If no conclusive data about a material are provided by a manufacturer or supplier, it can be allocated to one of the categories with some expert knowledge. The associated measures are categorized according to time and effort involved. Category I materials do not require special measures above and beyond the general protective and hygienic measures. Materials from categories II and III often have threshold values that must be adhered to. Category IV materials can be handled in the same manner as materials from one of the three previous categories if it has been proven – for instance by the manufacturer – that these do not possess any asbestos-like properties. HARN belong to category IV.[2)] Nanomaterials with active agents will often belong to category II; the properties of the active substance are to be taken into consideration.

The physical and chemical properties are often not sufficiently perceived as causes of possible risks. The large specific surface areas of nanomaterials often cause higher reactivities and reaction speeds, meaning that flammable materials in the nanoscale range can have significantly lower minimum ignition energies than coarser material or can even take on self-igniting properties [22].

It is therefore necessary for the society to agree on how to balance the risks and benefits for the environment, for users, and of course also for the world of work, although the benefits must not be limited to an economic perspective. Questions relating to the more efficient utilization of our energy resources, the provision of drinkable water for those parts of humanity in need and not least medicinal benefits are equally important arguments here.

The decision mainly falls between the so-called "strong" and the – perhaps unfortunately named – "weak" precautionary principle. In the former, this would mean that an application of nanotechnologies – at least beyond basic research – would not be permitted. As a consequence, this would also affect a range of long-established and indispensable technologies such as electronics and information technology that use a considerable number of nanotechnological methods. In this case, all the positive effects of nanomaterials could not be utilized, although the risks of nanomaterials would be eliminated, so

2) HARN: high aspect ratio nanomaterial: WHO fiber with at least one dimension between 1 and 100 nm

would the collection of knowledge. There would be significantly less motivation to invest intensively in the necessary research due to this moratorium. As a result, the risks posed by ultrafine aerosols, which can still persist, would also be understood less. In the case of the "weak" precautionary principle, on the other hand, the aim is to proceed in the most rational way possible in order to keep any risks as low as possible without being able to quantify them. There is a residual risk of effects that could not be detected or expected according to the current state of knowledge; however, this approach allows benefitting from the advantages of the application.

This second principle based on a rational approach to uncertainty has often been chosen, as even if gaps in data do not allow uncertainty to be eliminated, effective measures for minimizing any risks can be taken.

13.5 Prudent Practices and Proven Concepts for Controlling Risks

13.5.1 Risk Assessment

One problem with the manufacturing and use of nanomaterials as well as the production of ultrafine aerosols is the often insufficient data situation for assessing the risks. Filling these data gaps is generally most difficult with regard to toxic effects.

It is important to obtain or generate data at an early stage, where possible. Extensive data often already exists for nanomaterials that are manufactured and used on a larger scale. Measurements can be performed easily for some properties, but can be difficult for others.

The source of knowledge for operational use is primarily the product information material provided by the manufacturer or supplier, that is, the safety data sheets and technical information sheets. Enquiries to the manufacturer or supplier can help to close information gaps in the documentation. Sometimes, it is necessary to show some perseverance when making enquiries to this end. All available information is not always provided immediately, but the reminder of a possible partial legal responsibility or at least a voluntary obligation within the scope of responsible care can be very helpful here. Manufacturers have to gather information elsewhere, as of course they cannot simply refer to safety data sheets, but rather have to draw these up in full themselves. After all, it should be possible to determine the level of risk for internal use.

It is absolutely vital to perform a risk assessment before commencing work. This is often necessary even before setting up production equipment and perhaps even laboratory and technical rooms with the required infrastructure in order to determine the technical and organizational prerequisites for safe working in the first place. In a laboratory that was set up for a specific purpose and where, for example, supply and exhaust air capacities were reduced for cost-related or other operational reasons, work on manufacturing nanomaterials will often not be possible. Now the renewed risk analysis would require costly and difficult retrofitting of the ventilation technology. It may even be discerned that it is not possible to perform this retrofitting as, for example, no further supply or exhaust air capacity is available in the building and cannot be expanded, and procedures cannot be adapted to the extent that supply and exhaust air technology can be dispensed with. As a result, the planned work – at least in this room or building – cannot be performed. If the organization nonetheless insists on the work being carried out, serious – and even legal – consequences may be the result. The careful and thorough compilation of the risk assessment and, where required, the immediate adaptation to changed operational conditions such as the use of new chemicals with a risk potential that was previously not existent in this form and therefore not taken into account, therefore sit at the heart of occupational health and safety. Of course, regulatory provisions also have to be observed.

The typical sequence of such a risk assessment is shown in Figure 13.4.

All exposure routes are to be taken into account for determining the exposure situation and checking the effectiveness of the measures taken.

The work procedure and the dustiness behavior of the material are significant for assessing *skin contact.* Nanomaterials that are chemically very similar can differ greatly in terms of their dustiness behavior. For example, in the case of two iron oxides with similarly sized primary particles, one of them released large amounts of nanoscale particles when decanting and the other very little. If the documentation contains no details on the dustiness behavior and enquiries to the manufacturer or supplier do not yield the desired information, it is recommended to identify this data prior to entry into production at the latest. Standardized procedures are available for this.

With the data obtained in this manner and the exact knowledge of the work procedure and equipment to be used, it can be determined whether a relevant release of nano-objects will occur at all during the (intended) processes. Even if a nanomaterial does not release relevant amounts of nano-objects, this can still take place as a result of the work procedure, for example, through mechanical or thermal influences that destroy the matrix or segregate aggregates and agglomerates again. Even the drying of a solution or suspension can lead to nano-objects being released into the air from the dry residues. For some work procedures, the exposure situation is clear and further investigation is superfluous, for example, if a high-performance mill, which creates nano-objects out of larger material through intensive milling within the scope of a top-down process, is opened in a room after the milling process without any additional protective measures having been taken, one would generally determine that enormous quantities of nano-objects have been released.

As well as defining the technical (and other) measures, knowledge of the dust formation also allows the contamination risk to the skin presented by the deposit of released nano-objects to be assessed. Although in line with current knowledge, it is believed that human skin provides a reliable barrier to nanomaterials

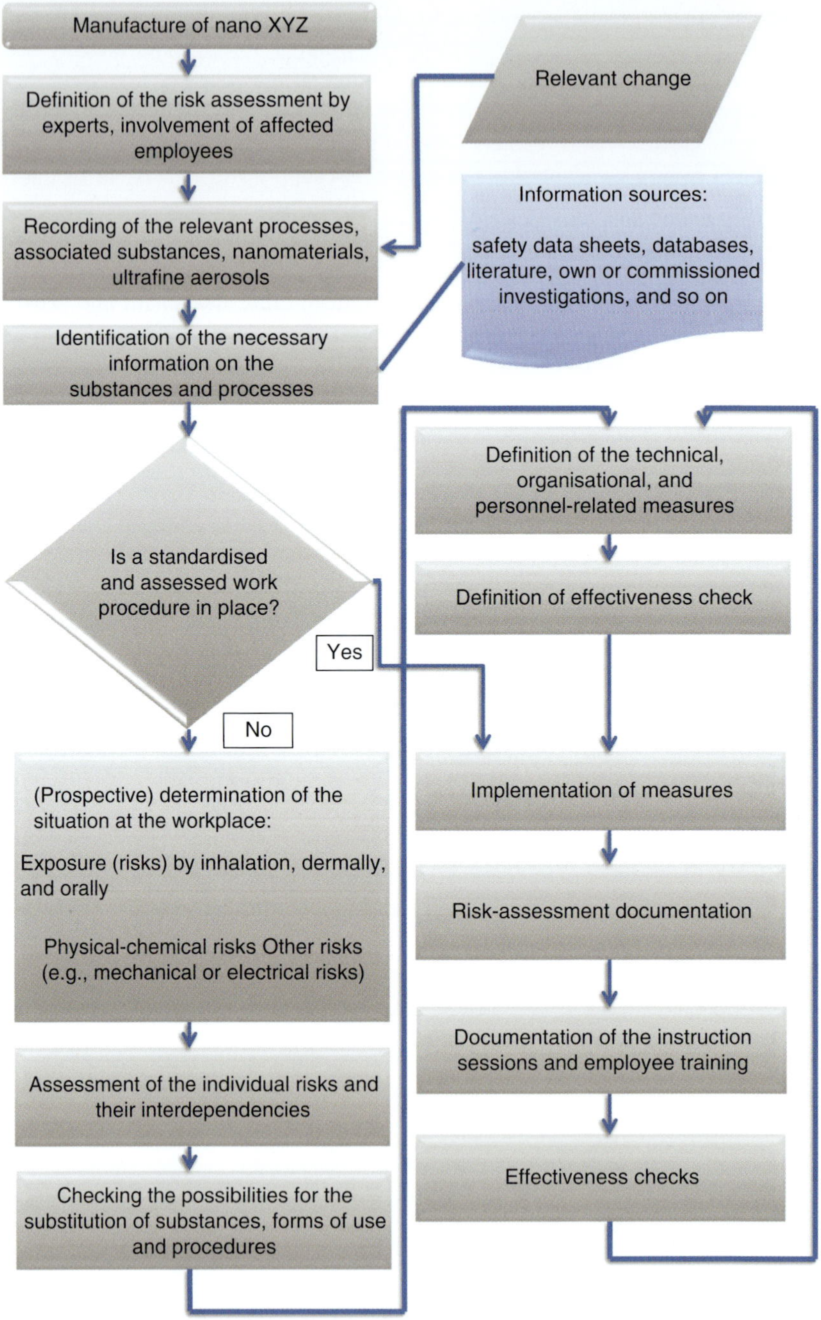

Figure 13.4 Flowchart of a risk assessment (the end is only reached upon completion of the entire work process).

when in good condition, this must not result in work being performed with unprotected hands, arms, or even unprotected facial skin due to the existing data gaps in this area, unless this has already been proven for the specific nanomaterial processed. It is necessary to wear protective gloves (in the case of disposable gloves it is generally recommended to wear two pairs on top of each other as a precaution), regularly check them for contamination and damage, and change them regularly.

The release of dust can also lead to deposits on the surfaces of work equipment and devices, surfaces in the room and on clothing. These deposits can then be released back into the air in an uncontrolled manner at a later stage and cause exposure by inhalation, which can occur at a different place and time to the release of material that caused it. Because it is particularly difficult to detect such exposure, it is essential that this dispersal of contamination is avoided by taking technical measures. Swipe samples or direct reading measurements of manually swirled up dust can provide clarity here.

Oral exposure that can result from the dispersal of such contamination through hand movements or even sweat is therefore associated with such contamination.

Particular attention has to be paid to *exposure by inhalation*, as in this case the effect on the organism can be especially intensive. As it often cannot be ruled out that in particular the less tightly bound aggregates of primary particles or fibrous nano-objects can be segregated again in the organism, the scale of dimensions to be considered should not be limited to 1–100 nm, but rather also extend into the higher range, that is, up to the micrometer range. Many measuring devices automatically detect these sizes.

13.5.2 Workplace Measurements

A tiered approach has proven useful for assessing *exposure by inhalation*. Because several measuring methods require a great deal of time, effort, and expense, an attempt should first be made to determine whether a relevant exposure has occurred or can even be hypothesized. In an enclosed system operated in a vacuum, discharges would not be expected as long as the system is sealed and this is also monitored. The critical operating states in this case would be the extraction of the products, depending on how the filling process takes place and in particular leaks and accidents as well as cleaning and maintenance work. For these, the exposure would have to be assessed separately across all exposure routes.

The measuring strategy consists on the one hand of the basic exposure assessment, which can be performed at all workplaces using measuring equipment and the assessment with limited basic skills and with limited effort and expenditure. Handheld measured devices are used here that allow measurement errors to be kept to a minimum relatively easily provided that the user has a sufficient level of

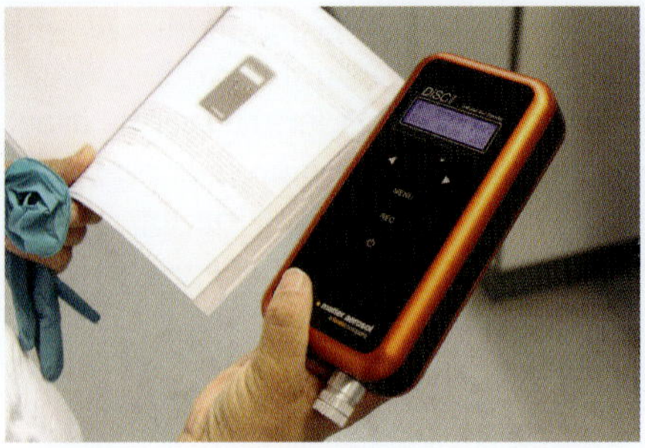

Figure 13.5 Handheld measuring device for particle concentration and the mean diameter (determined internally and calculated as an idealized spherical particle).

basic knowledge. If the nano-objects deviate too significantly from the spherical form, meaningful measuring results may be very difficult to be obtained. Figure 13.5 shows an example of a handheld device.

The technical expenditure is disproportionately higher within the scope of the expert exposure judgment, and is therefore accompanied by high requirements on the people carrying out the measurements. This approach should be employed if it was not possible to achieve a sufficient level of certainty in the first stage. Figure 13.6 shows a diagram with the sequence of this tiered approach, which is based on an OECD document [23].

There are very few limits for exposure to nanomaterials, and none based on health. However, several assessment values can be used as an aid for the assessment (for further information on these values, see Refs [24, 25]):

NIOSH: nanoscale titanium dioxide $0.3\,mg/m^3$, carbon nanotubes $0.007\,mg/m^3$; NIOSH/BSI: $\lambda_s \cdot c_0$ (λ_s: safety factor 0.066, c_0: concentration of the nanoscale material); manufacturers: $0.05\,mg/m^3$ for MWCNT;[3] DGUV: $2 \cdot 10^5\,cm^{-3}$ for biopersistent granular NM,[4] $\rho > 6\,g/cm^3$, $4 \cdot 10^5\,cm^{-3}$ for biopersistent granular NM, $\rho < 6\,g/cm^3$; BMAS: category I: general risk assessment and exposure control, category I II: typically $<0.1\,mg/m^3$, category I III: $c = \lambda_s \cdot c_0$, $\lambda_s = 0.5$, $c < 0.5\,mg/m^3$, category I IV: $10^5\,cm^{-3}$

Although mass concentrations are traditionally used for assessment, number concentrations and surface concentration are probably more meaningful for nanomaterials.

The mostly limited resources for carrying out such measurements can be better adapted to the level of difficulty of the inquiry and the scale of the problem in this way. These measurements allow reliable documentation of conditions at the workplace in accordance with present knowledge, and it is possible to define measures appropriate to the scale of the problem.

3) multiwalled carbon nanotubes
4) NM: Nanomaterials

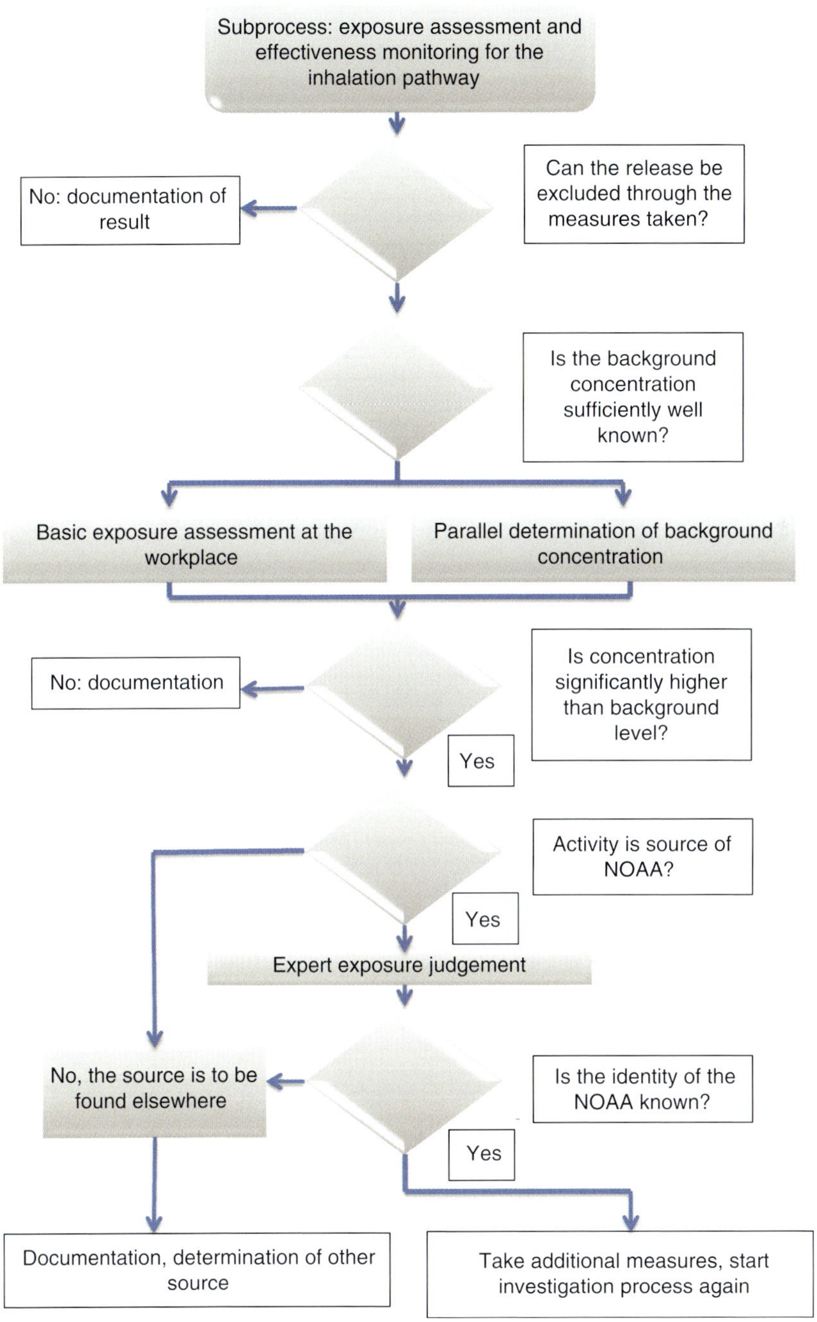

Figure 13.6 Tiered approach for determining the situation regarding exposure by inhalation (NOAA: nano objects and their agglomerates).

13.5.3 Protective Measures

Typical work procedures that can lead to exposure to nanomaterials are as follows:

- Manufacturing and refurbishment.
- Manufacturing of preparations and medications.
- Processing of coarser nanomaterials while releasing nano-objects (aggregates or agglomerates of nano-objects or nano-objects that have been extracted from the matrix during processing, for example, nanodroplets from polymers) or compound structures made up of nano-objects and matrix (e.g., carbon nanotubes that protrude from such polymer nanodroplets).
- Waste disposal.
- Cleaning of devices and equipment (e.g., a work surface in a laboratory fume hood).
- Exposure to nanomedicines (e.g., through stab wounds).
- Analyses and examinations of material samples and human material (if nanomedicines have been administered).
- Accidents and leaks.

The protective measures are typically taken in the following order:

- Substitution of hazardous substances, use of applications or processes that lead to less exposure.
- Technical measures.
- Organizational measures.
- Personal protective measures.

Experience shows that the protective measures already established for handling other (hazardous) substances also ensure a high level of protection when dealing with nanomaterials. Therefore, it is usually not necessary to develop completely new protective measures, but rather to search the existing toolbox for the appropriate measures and apply these properly. As such, technical ventilation measures not only help against toxic gases and dusts, but also with nanomaterials, and their effectiveness always depends on whether they have been designed, built, and applied correctly. A range of simple questions allows a check to be carried out as to whether the most common risks are present and which protective measures need to be taken (see Refs [26,27]).

- Are the containers labeled in a meaningful way? In particular, exact designation of the nanomaterial, pictograms, H-phrases, and P-phrases as per the GHS are necessary, simplified labeling for own storage bottles in the laboratory is possible.
- Is the safety data sheet available? Up-to-date safety data sheet for the exact same nanomaterial in question, not for similar products from other manufacturers or suppliers.

- Does the safety data sheet contain all details necessary for the risk assessment? A complete safety data sheet must be present.
- Has the nanomaterial been examined sufficiently? Check the information on toxicity, as well as on fire and explosion behavior and dangerous reactions (is data missing?).
- Does the nanomaterial belong to one of the following groups: granular biopersistent dusts, substances with intrinsic toxicity, rigid fibers according to the WHO? In this case, increased protective measures against simple dusts are necessary, in particular for rigid fibers according to the WHO or higher substance toxicity.
- Is the nanomaterial flammable or self-igniting? Even small quantities can lead to incipient fires or cause a violent explosion in combination with air: take explosion protection measures (e.g., inertisation or working in a vacuum).
- Is the minimum ignition energy lower than for coarser dusts of the material? With metals, in particular, the minimum ignition energy can be lowered significantly; special care is therefore required in avoiding ignition sources (e.g., electrostatics).
- Is there a risk of explosion when mixed with air? Swirling up dust or nebulization (after vaporization of volatile matter) can cause explosive aerosols.
- Is there a risk of a violent reaction or explosion when mixed with other substances? Large surfaces and, if applicable, catalytic activities can lead to an accelerated reaction.
- Is the dustiness behavior of the nanomaterial known or can it be determined by the material itself? If necessary, this can be measured using a handheld particle counter when decanting; otherwise, perform a measurement or request data.
- Are nanomaterials handled openly during the activity? Substance release and contamination of the work area are possible; there may be a risk of ignition.
- Can apparatuses and systems be designed in such a way that they have to be opened as little and as rarely as possible? This can be achieved using automatic metering equipment, for example, see Figure 13.7.
- Can the nanomaterial be released during the activities? This can result in dust formation, nebulization, or dried leaks. Depending on the risk, additional technical protective measures are to be taken.
- Are there airflows (from supply or exhaust air units, or unintentional flows caused by draughts in the room)? These should not carry the nanomaterials away and distribute or deposit them in air exhaust ducts or in the room. Some nanomaterials give off dust so easily that they need to be protected from airflows (e.g., in a glove box or with a decanting pipe, Figure 13.9) during handling. Flow conditions can be determined and assessed using battery-operated fog generators or larger mains-operated equipment for larger rooms, or test setups in fume hoods or systems in ventilated rooms (Figure 13.8). Apparatuses and systems can block airflows or cause vortexes, and as a result unexpected exposure can occur.

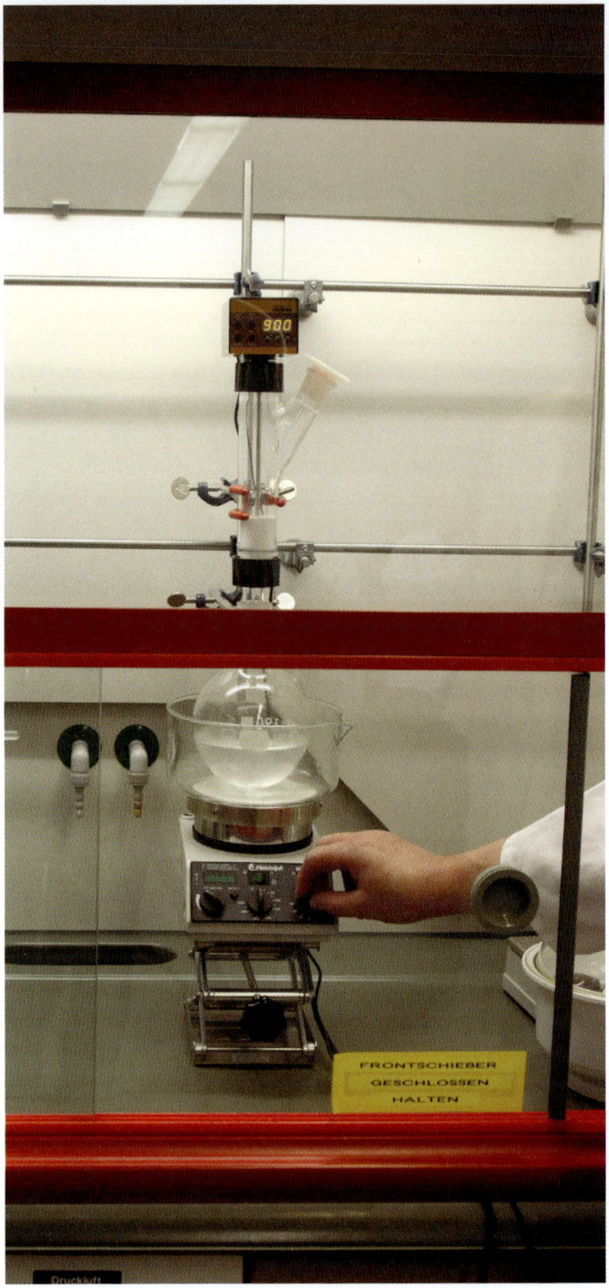

Figure 13.7 Automatic metering with controlled powder dosing funnel on a laboratory device.

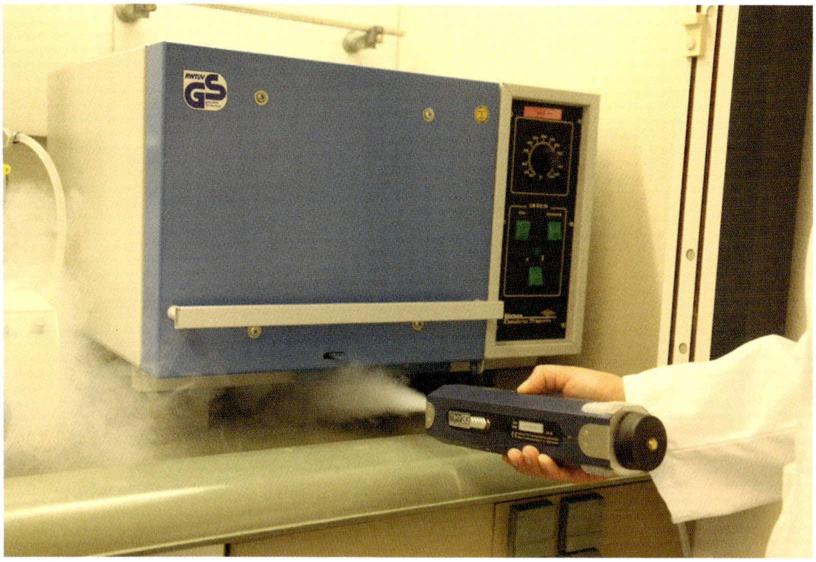

Figure 13.8 Checking unhindered airflow under an oven in the fume hood using a battery-operated fog generator.

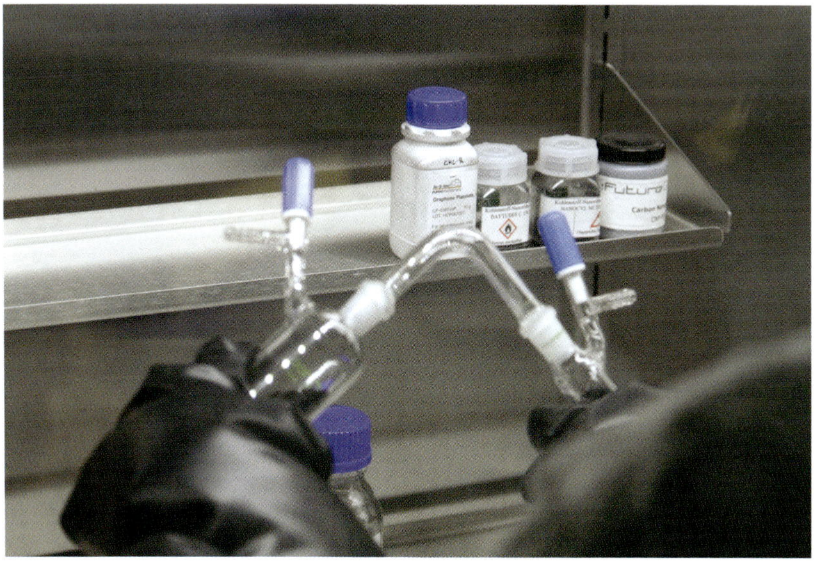

Figure 13.9 Dust-free decanting using a decanting pipe (to protect the product, it is also possible to work under inert gas).

- Is the nanomaterial in powder form, or is it a suspension or solution? If it is in a solution or suspension, a release is only possible through nebulization or spraying. Contact with skin must always be avoided.
- Can a suspension or solution dry out and release nanomaterial? Solid materials that give off dust may be created after drying.
- Does nanomaterial accumulate as powder during manufacture or processing? Powders can give off dust more or less easily and can be blown away easily. If necessary, weighing processes can be performed in turbulence-free ventilated weighing enclosures, in enclosed automatic scales or through reweighing of closed containers that are only opened in the fume hood (glove box, etc.). Grinding bowls of mills can be brought into the fume hood while closed and opened there.
- Are powdery nanomaterials created from coarser materials through milling, grinding, cutting, laser ablation, and so on? Nanoscale aerosols may be created, coarser dusts can contain nanomaterials (possibly only partially).
- Can nanomaterial escape from unstable containers such as bags in the form of dust? When compressed, air escapes with dust (this may even escape in the vacuum lock). Use solid containers; these should not be too large.
- Is contaminated equipment precleaned so that it can be cleaned by auxiliary staff without any danger? Adhering nanomaterials can contaminate the laboratory and other rooms and can result in people becoming exposed.
- Is a release of dusts from contaminated equipment avoided until it is cleaned? Equipment must be cleaned without delay. Until then, it must be sealed, enclosed or at least stored in the fume hood.
- Are hygienic measures implemented for avoiding dispersal of contamination? Contaminated equipment and work tools, for example, writing equipment or contaminated gloves must not be removed from the possibly contaminated area (e.g., the fume hood) before being cleaned (or being packed ready for disposal). Sleeve guards can prevent nanomaterials clinging to the arms when working in the fume hood.
- Are machines that can release nanomaterials (e.g., tablet presses) enclosed and ventilated?
- Is the extracted air sufficiently filtered? High-performance filters also hold back nanomaterials efficiently.
- Do further reagents, products, solvents, and other auxiliary materials need to be used? The risks associated with these materials must also be taken into account, for example, handling in particle-filtered circulation operation is critical if gases or vapors also occur, or when an ductless hood with absorption or adsorption filters is used and a breakthrough cannot be detected in time (due to desorption caused by a stronger absorbing substance or an used up absorbent).
- Are suitable auxiliary materials used to remove spills that in turn release nanomaterials themselves, for example, damp cloths when drying? Pack contaminated auxiliary material as hazardous waste so that it is fully sealed before it can release nanomaterials.

- Is the dispersal of contamination prevented by the appropriate design of workplaces, processes, and experiments? Interrupt work in the contaminated area (fume hood) as little as possible, do not remove contaminated objects (e.g., gloves) from the area, ensure that special attention is paid to hygiene.
- Is waste collected in suitable sealed containers and is it disposed of often enough? The larger the container, the more dust can be released, the potential risk increases with the amount of waste stored, in addition, dangerous mixtures or aging processes can lead to gases and vapors being released, which in turn can cause fires or explosions.
- Is the necessary personal protective equipment used? Alongside protective goggles and suitable shoes, this also includes clothing. If there is a risk that the face, head, or body can become contaminated with nanomaterials, a protective screen, hood, or disposable suit (preferably made of closed textiles without seams or hollows) must be worn (define hygiene measures and disposal procedures).
- Are the employees instructed and trained? The properties of and risks posed by nanomaterials are not universally known and must be explained, staff must be familiarized with and trained in safe work processes and protective measures.

Further properties are to be taken into account in order to assess the risk, in particular the ignition and burning behavior, aging and decay, and the catalytic effect.

The following guidelines assign protective measures to the nanomaterials for orientation purposes; the risk assessment can provide a different result in specific cases. Measures are, of course, also related to other hazardous substances used in the process (e.g., reactants, solvents, auxiliary materials) and equipment.

- Category I: basic protective and hygiene measures, avoidance of all unnecessary releases and exposures.
- Category II: see measures of category IV.
- Category III: in contrast to group I, protective measures against exposure by inhalation are to be taken in particular (dust-free handling in fume hood, safety cabinet;[5)] glove box or closed apparatus also possible).
- Category IV (if no deviating properties are proven), also group II: compared to group I, additional measures are to be taken in order to avoid exposure by inhalation, dermally and orally (dust-free handling in a tested fume hood, safety cabinet,[4] glove box, closed apparatus or system, preferably *clean-in-place* or *wash-in-place* in the case of a closed apparatus or system).

Measures for avoiding unwanted contamination of work areas may also be necessary without a risk being established.

Particle-filtering respiratory masks offer high filtration efficiency for nano-objects and are particularly effective in the range below approx. 200 nm.

5) if no protection from gases and vapours or from fragments or splashes propelled around the room, is required

However, respiratory protection measures should be used with caution. The wearing of additional equipment can be a burden for employees, and it should be considered that, in contrast to volatile gases and vapors, a long-lasting contamination in the area of the workplace is possible, even at greater distances depending on the airflow conditions. Deposits can occur along the entire length of exhaust ducts, particularly in places with little flow or where vortexes can form. Although this can be prevented through design measures, channels are repeatedly designed incorrectly. In normal breathable air, nano-objects usually occur in close proximity to the place from which they were released and are almost exclusively gathered in aggregates or agglomerates having been attracted toward other coarser dust particles or droplets [28]. In a low-particle atmosphere, on the other hand, the nano-objects primarily agglomerate together due to a lack of other bodies to collide with.

The use of nanomaterials in healthcare comprises a whole spectrum of various types [29]. Classification into categories as per the Announcement on Hazardous Substances 527 (BekGS 527) is suggested here:

- Metallic particles (e.g., iron oxides, silver, or gold cluster) for cancer treatment, magnetic resonance imaging or used as antimicrobial agents, for example, – cat. I, II, or III
- Gold shell nanoparticles or fullerenes for the transportation of drugs, for example, – cat. II
- Carbon nanotubes for coupling to DNA in gene therapy or lab on a chip applications, for example, – cat. IV
- Quantum dots (often containing cadmium) for tagging biomolecules, for example, – cat. II
- Dendrimers as a carrier for drugs, for example, – cat. II
- Lipid-based nanoparticles for drug delivery – cat. I.

Transported active substances, coatings, or soiling are to be taken into account in all categories. Nanomaterials that only display additional effects under specific conditions must be assessed on the basis of these effects, and not on their inherent nature. For example, when assessing radiosensitive nanoparticles that release nitrogen monoxide in an organism when irradiated with X-rays, this effect should certainly also be taken into consideration [30].

Special care should be taken when handling nanotubes. These can also have a carcinogenic effect on humans if they have certain geometries and length–diameter ratios and a rigid structure [31]. They often form entangled structures with individual nanotube ends protruding from them and can also cause inflammatory reactions. When handled, these sometimes release no nanotubes at all, although it is unclear whether this is also the case under physiological conditions. In this case, safe work can be performed using closed apparatuses, tested enclosures and extractions, tested laboratory fume cupboards or glove boxes. The exhaust air can only be released into the work area after special cleaning. Overviews of this can be found, for example, in Refs [32,33].

Mihail Roco divided nanotechnologies into the following four generations [34]:

- First: Passive nanostructures: for example, coatings, nanoparticles, nanostructured metals, polymers, ceramics
- Second: Active nanostructures: for example, 3D transistors, amplifiers, targeted drugs, actuators, adaptive structures
- Third: Nanosystems: for example, guided assembling; 3D networking and new hierarchical architectures, robotics, evolutionary
- Fourth: Molecular nanosystems: for example, molecular devices "by design," atomic design, emerging functions.

Until now, the measures and effectiveness checks focused on nanomaterials of the first two generations, and also on the third generation to a limited extent. Many nanotechnological applications in the pharmaceutical industry are to be classified as passive (first generation) or active (second generation) structures. These are characterized by the fact that they behave like normal substances with regard to quantities, concentration, and dose. But the systems begin to show a resemblance to biological systems to the extent that a multiplication that is no longer actively controlled from outside can occur. Up to a point, this is already the case with the self-organizing processes of the third generation; whether multiplication mechanisms of the fourth generation can establish themselves outside of real biological systems is the subject of much debate, at least it is not unthinkable. In these cases one would expect an independent increase in particle numbers, quantities, concentrations, and doses, as is usual in nature. However, concepts for protective measures against such substances already exist; indeed, the methods are also available for safe handling of organisms and DNA. And like every self-reproducing system, unlimited multiplication is inconceivable as all systems of this kind reach the boundaries regarding available space, nourishment, and room for waste. With technological adjustments, this should therefore also make it possible to safely control nanomaterials of future developments.

13.6 Instruction and Training

A system of training consisting of instruction briefings, training sessions, and if necessary also practical exercises suitable for sufficiently training and motivating the employees is of great importance to the success of occupational health and safety. This should not only convey the correct uses of the work tools and how to work safely with the substances in question, but also nurture safety-consciousness and practice the appropriate patterns of behavior. In the ideal scenario, the employees will act in a safe manner as a matter of conviction.

Classic frontal instruction is usually no longer viewed as up-to-date and is less efficient than more modern forms of knowledge conveyance. Trainers welcome work means that allow them to implement the concepts more easily. Brochures and placards are available alongside relevant literature, while well-devised presentations can increase the attentiveness of the audience. Modern interactive media such as computer programs or Internet-based learning packages can provide new impulses here. An example of this is the "Nanorama Laboratory" [35] of the German Social Accident Insurance Institution for the Raw Materials and Chemical Industry (BG RCI), German Social Accident Insurance (DGUV) and The Innovation Society, St. Gallen, which shows how the basics of working safely with nanomaterials in the laboratory can be learned by virtually exploring a real laboratory. Its twin "Nanorama Production of Nanomaterials" is to be launched soon. At the same time, however, further information and support can also be requested. Similar Nanoramas for production and processing are also available [36].

13.7 Summary

Nanomaterials can possess very different properties. Nanopharmaceuticals are designed to interact with the organism and may show involuntary pharmacological effects on the workers as well as toxic effects. In the absence of information to the contrary this requires a higher level of precautionary measures. In accordance with the current level of knowledge, the materials can be handled in a manner appropriate to their properties and while ensuring a relative high level of safety, even with the current gaps in knowledge. Any national legal provisions must always be adhered to. In addition, the development of the state of knowledge must be carefully observed in order to make any necessary amendments. Preventive occupational health and safety must therefore be used; after all, it is "better safe than sorry."

References

1 Shatkin, J.A. (2013) *Nanotechnology – Health and Environmental Risks*, 2nd edn, CRC Press, Boca Raton, FL.

2 National Nanotechnology Initiative (NNI) (2015) What is nanotechnology? Available at http://www.nano.gov/nanotech-101/hat/definition (accessed November 20, 2015).

3 European Commission (2015) Nanotechnologies – policy issues. Available at https://ec.europa.eu/research/industrial_technologies/policy_en.html (accessed November 20, 2015).

4 ISO (2015) Nanotechnologies – vocabulary – part 1: core terms, ISO/TS 80004-1.

5 European Commission (2011) Commission recommendation of 18 October on the definition of nanomaterial. Available at http://eur-lex.europa.eu/legal-content/EN/TXT/?uri=CELEX:32011H0696 (accessed November 20, 2015).

6 European Commission (2012) Communication from the Commission to the European Parliament, the Council and the European Economic and Social Committee – second regulatory review on nanomaterials, Brussels. Available at http://eur-lex.europa.eu/LexUriServ/LexUriServ.do?uri=COM:2012:0572:FIN:DE:PDF (accessed November 20, 2015).

7 Murashov, V., Schulte, P., Geraci, C., and Howard, J. (2011) Regulatory approaches to worker protection in nanotechnology industry in the USA and European Union. *Ind. Health*, **49**, 280.
8 Committee on Hazardous Substances of the German Federal Ministry of Labour and Social Affairs (2015) Announcement 527 "Manufactured Nanomaterials." Available at http://www.baua.de/en/Topics-from-A-to-Z/Hazardous-Substances/TRGS/Announcement-527.html;jsessionid=C4F5BF7EE5E373563E80E35FA8461BC0.1_cid323 (accessed November 20, 2015).
9 German Social Accident Insurance (DGUV) (2015) DGUV Information 213–851 Working Safely in Laboratories – Basic Principles and Guidelines. Available at http:www.guidelinesforlaboratories.de (accessed November 20, 2015).
10 German Social Accident Insurance (DGUV), (2015) DGUV Information 213–854 Nanomaterials in the Laboratory. Available at http://www.dguv.de/medien/fb-rci/dokumente/info_zu_213_854.pdf (accessed November 20, 2015).
11 Centers for Disease Control and Prevention – National Institute for Occupational Safety and Health (2008) Safe nanotechnology in the workplace. Available at http://www.cdc.gov/niosh/docs/2008-112/pdfs/2006-112.pdf (accessed November 20, 2015).
12 Centers for Disease Control and Prevention – National Institute for Occupational Safety and Health (2012) General safe practices for working with engineered nanomaterials in research laboratories. Available at http://www.cdc.gov/niosh/docs/2012-147/pdfs/2012-147.pdf (accessed November 20, 2015).
13 U. S., Food and Drug Administration (2014) Considering whether an FDA-regulated product involves the application of nanotechnology. Available at http://www.fda.gov/RegulatoryInformation/Guidances/ucm257698.htm#intro (accessed December 5, 2015).
14 Italian Workers' Compensation Authority (INAIL) (2011) *White Book, Exposure to Engineered Nanomaterials and Occupational Health and Safety Effects*, Italian Workers' Compensation Authority, Department of Occupational Medicine, formerly ISPESL, Rome, pp. 1–211.
15 Australian Government Department of Health (2015) Nanotechnology and therapeutic products. Available at www.tga.gov.au/nanotechnology-and-therapeutic-products (accessed December 5, 2015).
16 REACHnano consortium (2015) Guidance on available methods for risk assessment of nanomaterials, Valencia. Available at http://www.invassat.gva.es/documents/161660384/162311778/01+Guidance+on+available+methods+for+risk+assesment+of+nanomaterials/8cae41ad-d38a-42f7-90f3-9549a9c13fa0 (accessed December 2, 2015).
17 Austrian Workers' Compensation Board (AUVA) (2010) Nanotechnologien, Vienna (German language only). Available at http://www.auva.at/portal27/portal/auvaportal/content/contentWindow?viewmode=content&action=2&contentid=10007.672853 (accessed December 2, 2015) .
18 Ministry of Health, Labour and Welfare (Japan) (2009) Notification on precautionary measures for prevention of exposure etc. to nanomaterials. Available at http://www.jniosh.go.jp/publication/doc/houkoku/nano/files/mhlw/Notification_0331013_en.pdf.
19 Institut national de recherche et de sécurité (INSR) (2012) Les nanomatériaux. Définitions, risques toxicologiques, caractérisation de l'exposition professionnelle et mesures de prevention, Paris. Available at http://www.inrs.fr/dms/inrs/CataloguePapier/ED/TI-ED-6050/ed6050.pdf (accessed December 2, 2015).
20 Health and Safety Executive (HSE) (2013) Using nanomaterials at work. Available at http://www.hse.gov.uk/pubns/books/hsg272.pdf (accessed December 2, 2015).
21 European Medicines Agency (2015) Scientific guidelines: nanomedicines. Available at http://www.ema.europa.eu/ema/index.jsp?curl=pages/regulation/general/general_content_000564.jsp&mid=WC0b01ac05806403e0 (accessed December 5, 2015).

22 Bouillard, J.X. (2015) Fire and explosion of nanopowders, in *Nanoengineering: Global Approaches to Health and Safety Issues* (ed. P.I. Dolez), Elsevier, Amsterdam.

23 Organisation for Economic Co-operation and Development (2015) Harmonized tiered approach to measure and assess the potential exposure to airborne emissions of engineered nano-objects and their agglomerates and aggregates at workplaces, ENV/JM/MONO 19.

24 Institute for Occupational Safety and Health of the German Social Accident Insurance organisation (DGUV), (2015) Criteria for assessment of the effectiveness of protective measures. Available at http://www.dguv.de/ifa/Fachinfos/Nanopartikel-am-Arbeitsplatz/Beurteilung-von-Schutzma%C3%9Fnahmen/index.jsp (accessed December 2, 2015).

25 van Broekhuizen, P., van Veelen, W., Streekstra, W.-H., Schulte, P., and Reunderss, L. (2012) Exposure limits for nanoparticles: report of an international workshop on nano reference values. *Ann. Occup. Hyg.*, **56**, 515.

26 Brock, T.H. (2014) Safe handling of nanomaterials in the laboratory, in *Handbook of Nanosafety* (eds U. Vogel, K. Savolainen, Q. Wu, M. van Tongeren, D. Brouwer, and M. Berges), Academic Press, Amsterdam, p. 296.

27 German Social Accident Insurance (DGUV) (2012) *Sicheres Arbeiten in der pharmazeutischen Industrie* (German language only), Heidelberg.

28 Seipenbusch, M., Binder, A., and Kasper, G. (2008) Temporal evolution of nanoparticle aerosols in workplace exposure. *Ann. Occup. Hyg.*, **52**, 707.

29 European Agency for Safety and Health at Work, (2015) E-fact 73: Nanomaterials in the Healthcare Sector: Occupational Risks and Prevention. Available at http://osha.europa.eu/en/tools-and-publications/publications/e-facts/e-fact-73-nanomaterials-in-the-healthcare-sector-occupational-risks-and-prevention/view (accessed November 28, 2015).

30 Fan, W., Bu, W., He, Q., Ni, D., Cui, Z., Liu, J., and Shi, J. (2015) X-ray radiation-controlled no-release for on-demand depth-independent hypoxic radiosensitization. *Angew. Chem.*, **127**, 14232.

31 Donaldson, K., Poland, C.A., Murphy, F.A., MacFarlane, M., Chernova, T., and Schinwald, A. (2013) Pulmonary toxicity of carbon nanotubes and asbestos – similarities and differences. *Adv. Drug Deliv. Rev.*, **65**, 2078.

32 Centers for Disease Control and Prevention – National Institute for Occupational Safety and Health (2015) Current intelligence bulletin 65: occupational exposure to carbon nanotubes and nanofibers. Available at http://www.cdc.gov/niosh/docs/2013-145/ (accessed November 29, 2015).

33 Lotz, G. (2015) Arbeitsmedizinisch-toxikologische Beratung bei Tätigkeiten mit Kohlenstoffnanoröhren (CNT), Dortmund (German language only).

34 Roco, M.C. (2004) Nanoscale science and engineering: unifying and transforming tools. *AIChE J.*, **50**, 890.

35 Brock, T.H. and Wiedler, T. (2014). Available at http://nano.dguv.de/nanorama/bgrci (accessed November 27, 2015).

36 Brock, T.H. and Wiedler, T. (2015). Available at http://nano.dguv.de/nanoramen/ (accessed December 4, 2015).

Edited by Jean Cornier,
Andrew Owen, Arno Kwade,
and Marcel Van de Voorde

Pharmaceutical Nanotechnology

Further Volumes of the Series "Nanotechnology Innovation & Applications"

Axelos, M. A. V. and Van de Voorde, M. (eds.)

Nanotechnology in Agriculture and Food Science

2017

Print ISBN: 9783527339891

Fermon, C. and Van de Voorde, M. (eds.)

Nanomagnetism

Applications and Perspectives

2017

Print ISBN: 9783527339853

Mansfield, E., Kaiser, D. L., Fujita, D., Van de Voorde, M. (eds.)

Metrology and Standardization for Nanotechnology

Protocols and Industrial Innovations

2017

Print ISBN: 9783527340392

Meyrueis, P., Sakoda, K., Van de Voorde, M. (eds.)

Micro- and Nanophotonic Technologies

2017

Print ISBN: 9783527340378

Müller, B. and Van de Voorde, M. (eds.)

Nanoscience and Nanotechnology for Human Health

2017

Print ISBN: 9783527338603

Puers, R., Baldi, L., van Nooten, S. E., Van de Voorde, M. (eds.)

Nanoelectronics

Materials, Devices, Applications

2017

Print ISBN: 9783527340538

Raj, B., Van de Voorde, M., Mahajan, Y. (eds.)

Nanotechnology for Energy Sustainability

2017

Print ISBN: 9783527340149

Sels, B. and Van de Voorde, M. (eds.)

Nanotechnology in Catalysis

Applications in the Chemical Industry, Energy Development, and Environment Protection

2017

Print ISBN: 9783527339143

Edited by Jean Cornier, Andrew Owen,
Arno Kwade, and Marcel Van de Voorde

Pharmaceutical Nanotechnology

Innovation and Production

WILEY-VCH
Verlag GmbH & Co. KGaA

Volume Editors

Dr. Jean Cornier
vdlconsult
Seumestr. 7
81379 München
Germany

Prof. Andrew Owen
University of Liverpool
Department of Molecular & Clinical Pharmacology
Ashton Street
Liverpool, L69 3GE
UK

Prof. Arno Kwade
TU Braunschweig
Partikeltechnik
Volkmaroder Str. 5
38104 Braunschweig
Germany

Prof. Dr. Dr. h.c. Marcel H. Van de Voorde
Member of the Science Council
of the French Senate and National Assembly, Paris
Rue du Rhodania, 5
BRISTOL A, Appartement 31
3963 Crans-Montana
Switzerland

Series Editor

Prof. Dr. Dr. h.c. Marcel H. Van de Voorde
Member of the Science Council
of the French Senate and National Assembly, Paris
Rue du Rhodania, 5
BRISTOL A, Appartement 31
3963 Crans-Montana
Switzerland

Cover credits: Pills bottom and background: fotolia_© Sven Bähren
3D pill top right with nanostructure inside: © mauritius-images

Library of Congress Card No.: applied for

British Library Cataloguing-in-Publication Data
A catalogue record for this book is available from the British Library.

Bibliographic information published by the Deutsche Nationalbibliothek
The Deutsche Nationalbibliothek lists this publication in the Deutsche Nationalbibliografie; detailed bibliographic data are available on the Internet at http://dnb.d-nb.de.

Print ISBN: 978-3-527-34054-5
ePDF ISBN: 978-3-527-80067-4
ePub ISBN: 978-3-527-80069-8
Mobi ISBN: 978-3-527-80070-4
oBook ISBN: 978-3-527-80068-1

Cover Design Adam Design
Typesetting Thomson Digital, Noida, India
Printing and Binding Markono Print Media Pte Ltd, Singapore
Printed on acid-free paper

Thanks to my wife for her patience with me spending
many hours working on the book series through
the nights and over weekends.
The assistance of my son Marc Philip related to the complex
and large computer files with many sophisticated scientific
figures is also greatly appreciated.

Marcel Van de Voorde

Series Editor Preface

Since years, nanoscience and nanotechnology have become particularly an important technology areas worldwide. As a result, there are many universities that offer courses as well as degrees in nanotechnology. Many governments including European institutions and research agencies have vast nanotechnology programmes and many companies file nanotechnology-related patents to protect their innovations. In short, nanoscience is a hot topic!

Nanoscience started in the physics field with electronics as a forerunner, quickly followed by the chemical and pharmacy industries. Today, nanotechnology finds interests in all branches of research and industry worldwide. In addition, governments and consumers are also keen to follow the developments, particularly from a safety and security point of view.

This books series fills the gap between books that are available on various specific topics and the encyclopedias on nanoscience. This well-selected series of books consists of volumes that are all edited by experts in the field from all over the world and assemble top-class contributions. The topical scope of the book is broad, ranging from nanoelectronics and nanocatalysis to nanometrology. Common to all the books in the series is that they represent top-notch research and are highly application-oriented, innovative, and relevant for industry. Finally they collect a valuable source of information on safety aspects for governments, consumer agencies and the society.

The titles of the volumes in the series are as follows:

Human-related nanoscience and nanotechnology

- *Nanoscience and Nanotechnology for Human Health*
- *Pharmaceutical Nanotechnology*
- *Nanotechnology in Agriculture and Food Science*

Nanoscience and nanotechnology in information and communication

- *Nanoelectronics*
- *Micro- and Nanophotonic Technologies*
- *Nanomagnetism: Perspectives and Applications*

Nanoscience and nanotechnology in industry

- Nanotechnology for Energy Sustainability
- Metrology and Standardization of Nanomaterials
- Nanotechnology in Catalysis: Applications in the Chemical Industry, Energy Development, and Environmental Protection

The book series appeals to a wide range of readers with backgrounds in physics, chemistry, biology, and medicine, from students at universities to scientists at institutes, in industrial companies and government agencies and ministries.

Ever since nanoscience was introduced many years ago, it has greatly changed our lives – and will continue to do so!

March 2016 *Marcel Van de Voorde*

About the Series Editor

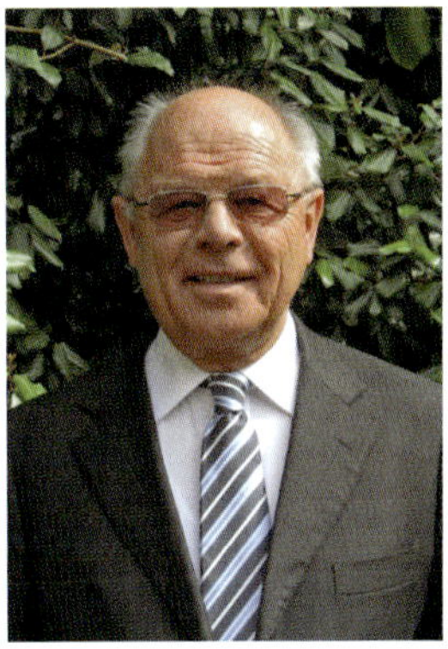

Marcel Van de Voorde, Prof. Dr. ir. Ing. Dr. h.c., has 40 years' experience in European Research Organisations, including CERN-Geneva and the European Commission, with 10 years at the Max Planck Institute for Metals Research, Stuttgart. For many years, he was involved in research and research strategies, policy, and management, especially in European research institutions.

He has been a member of many Research Councils and Governing Boards of research institutions across Europe, the United States, and Japan. In addition to his Professorship at the University of Technology in Delft, the Netherlands, he holds multiple visiting professorships in Europe and worldwide. He holds a doctor honoris causa and various honorary professorships.

He is a senator of the European Academy for Sciences and Arts, Salzburg, and Fellow of the World Academy for Sciences. He is a member of the Science Council of the French Senate/National Assembly in Paris. He has also provided executive advisory services to presidents, ministers of science policy, rectors of Universities, and CEOs of technology institutions, for example, to the president and CEO of IMEC, Technology Centre in Leuven, Belgium. He is also a Fellow of various scientific societies. He has been honored by the Belgian King and European authorities, for example, he received an award for European merits in Luxemburg given by the former President of the European Commission. He is author of multiple scientific and technical publications and has coedited multiple books, especially in the field of nanoscience and nanotechnology.

Contents

Foreword

Albert Einstein once remarked: "Look deep into nature, and then you will understand everything better." Beginning with the idea that most people would not believe in, nanotechnology has allowed us – literally – to look deep into the functioning of biological mechanisms at molecular level and thereby define new pathways for diagnosis and treatment of human disease. The nanotechnology-based production of pharmaceuticals therefore has the potential to revolutionize the treatment of human disease, facilitate changes in future healthcare systems by enabling more personalized, predictive, preventive, regenerative, and even remote (tele)medicine, and has a major impact on the survival of the human race.

The book gives a thorough overview of the science and technology in the nanopharmacy spectrum worldwide, and it also clearly highlights the research requirements that Europe needs to undertake during the next decade if it is to achieve invaluable breakthroughs in this fascinating field of nanopharmacy – breakthroughs that will enable Europe to place itself among the top-ranking competitive industrial regions in the world.

This is because nanotechnologies provide the tools for analysis and manipulation of biological processes at the nanoscale, which is where diseases take root and progress. The result is an increasingly better understanding of the molecular biology of disease leading to new targets for more specific and earlier diagnostic and therapeutic strategies.

This publication – which gives me genuine pleasure to introduce to you – is perhaps the first time that Europe and the wider world have a unique opportunity. This is both to assess the current state of the art and to provide the larger nanomedicine community with new resources and strategies. It will make the best of European and international innovation so as to generate a highly competitive industrial sector. At the forefront is the very latest thinking in fundamental research, characterization and safety issues of nanotechnology as applied to the development of new drugs and treatments for medicine. This will help to meet the enormous challenge of bringing new innovative, safe, and cost-effective products to the patient in as short a time frame as possible. There is strong emphasis on patient needs and concerns, including personalized approaches that will make for new, efficient, and effective solutions for healthcare.

Applications of nanotechnology for healthcare perhaps best exemplify how interdisciplinary research is vital for future success. This is because all disciplines and their stakeholders are represented in this work: beginning with the laboratory-based scientists and including regulators, representatives from industry, and most important of all representatives from society at large. All play an equal part in delivering the appropriate benefits at the right time at the right price to the right patient.

Only collaborations, such as those represented in this publication, will bring new discoveries from science into products that generate greater economic value through more rapid societal use. It is literally the attention to such small details that can make this happen, for Albert Einstein also remarked: "Whoever is careless with the truth in small matters cannot be trusted with important matters."[1)]

This publication is a great initiative and will give an impetus to the entire nanopharmacy community in Europe. For this reason, I believe that this book should find a large distribution facilitating a broad debate between all policy-making bodies and research institutes in Europe.

Director-General, Publications Office,
European Commission, Luxembourg

Rudolf Walter Strohmeier

1) 2010, The Ultimate Quotable Einstein, Edited by Alice Calaprice, Section: On Humankind, Quote Page 187 and 188, Princeton University Press, Princeton, New Jersey.

Industrial Requirement on Nanopharmacy Research

Information on "nanotechnology" is proliferating within the scientific literature and media. In the field of pharmacy and medicine alone, the number of publications on nanotechnology has increased substantially over the past two decades. Searching the chemical database on CAS controlled terms for entries on "nano" in combination with medicine, pharmaceuticals, therapeutics, or formulations resulted in only eight publications in 1995. Since then the number of publications has jumped to 173 in 2005 and over 1400 in 2015. Therefore, nanotechnology in pharmacy became a very important field for academic and industrial research and development.

Nano-relevant techniques and applications are very diverse; they range from nanosized crystals of pharmaceutical drug substances to lipid carriers of submicrometer range, to functionalized particles for targeting, to particles for nucleotide or peptide delivery, among others. The abundance of technological options and possible applications appears to be overwhelming, and sometimes confusing. In this "gold rush" for an emerging key technology of the twenty-first century, it seems to be the right time to pause, take stock of the scientific basis for nanotechnology-enabled progress, and take a systematic and holistic view of emerging applications.

For these reasons, *Pharmaceutical Nanotechnology* starts by providing the reader with an understanding of the fundamental basic and applied sciences of nanotechnology in the context of pharmaceutical applications. This includes challenges associated with GMP manufacturing, scale-up, methods for characterization, and potential occupational and environmental safety issues. It is recognized that current and future applications of nanotechnology are at very different stages of maturity. Consequently, the book also provides the course of pharmaceutical drug development in a systematic manner. Opportunities and challenges are also addressed from the perspective of early discovery, preclinical and clinical development, to regulation and commercialization.

Throughout this journey, the reader will realize that nanotechnology is not a vague vision of a miracle technology that might come up in some distant future, but is already a reality in a substantial number of commercial products, including oral, dermatological, and parenteral treatments. On the other hand, the potential utility of nanotechnology in pharmacy is by far not fully exploited.

New findings and concepts continue to emerge as is illustrated by over 320 new patent applications in the field of pharmaceutical and medical applications of nanotechnology in 2015 alone. Nanotechnology may play a crucial role in drug targeting and cellular delivery, oral and intravenous delivery of insoluble compounds, topical delivery to the lung, eye, and skin, diagnostic applications, and many other areas. The key to these new applications still lies in new research and sound science is still needed to elucidate mechanisms that underpin observed benefits. Despite the large number of publications, we still need a better and deeper understanding of the principles for preparation, characterization, and fate of nanoparticles in the body as well as in the environment.

Pharmaceutical nanotechnology still has the opportunity to avoid mistakes that have been made in the development and introduction of previous groundbreaking technologies. Researchers have previously been very enthusiastic about new opportunities, but the public were not brought on the journey, and sometimes unfounded worries about adverse effects are common. Therefore, *Pharmaceutical Nanotechnology* also addresses nanotoxicology and safety and ethical and societal aspects as integrated components of research and development of nanopharmaceutical products.

As demonstrated by the impressive list of contributors to this book, the challenges will hardly be met by a single inventor or institution. The topics are so diverse that they require multifunctional capabilities and collaborations in early laboratory research, pharmaceutical formulation, process engineering, material characterization, clinical evaluation and implementation, and regulatory and intellectual property considerations. *Pharmaceutical Nanotechnology* brings all these disciplines together to give a cross-cutting and in-depth review of this stimulating new field and is a very helpful basis for students and a base for academic research as well as provides industry with excellent innovation ideas. I wish the readers inspiring insights into the exciting field of the smallest particles.

Chief Scientist of Chemical & Pharmaceutical Development, Bayer Pharma AG, Berlin — *Peter Serno*

Head of Chemical & Pharmaceutical Development, Bayer Pharma AG, Wuppertal — *Olaf Queckenberg*

Introduction

Pharmaceutical Nanotechnology aims at applying nanotechnology to drug therapy of diseases and medical diagnostics. More exactly it involves the preparation and delivery of therapeutic substances in the molecular and nanometer size range to the expected site of action in the human body, reaching maximum efficacy while alleviating undesirable side effects at healthy organs and tissues. The importance of this emerging field of research and developments relies on the fact that nearly all present medicines exhibit poor pharmacokinetics and bioavailability characteristics, and instead of specifically concentrating and acting at their target sites they widely distribute within the body. Pharmaceutical Nanotechnology requires very specific knowledge on many topics such as drug formulation, drug delivery, route of administration, specific targeting, imaging, and diagnosis, and so on. Research in this field requires a multidisciplinary approach, involving pharmacists, material and chemical engineers, cellular biologists, and biophysicists as well as ICT specialists and medical specialists.

The goal of this unique book is to present an overall picture of the use of nanotechnology in pharmacy. It is designed to be a reference textbook on the application of nanotechnology in the development of nanostructures for therapeutic use. Focus is placed on the manufacturing and researching of candidate nanostructures as well as their translation into marketable medicines by industry. We also review the most interesting and promising developments in this emerging but fast developing field.

Following this brief introduction, Part One consists of Chapters 1–5 that give an *entry to the Nanopharmacy revolution* by addressing the history, potential, challenges, and most recent developments and applications of nanotechnology in pharmacy.

In Part Two, *a systematic review of the fundamentals of nanopharmacy* is performed with a description of the used nanostructures, their characterization methods, and a detailed overview of the preparation and manufacturing methods and issues. Established processes as well as new exploratory methods are separately reviewed and concrete actual examples of utilization given. All relevant aspects are being addressed including scale-up and occupational health.

Part Three reviews *the various steps in the development of a new nanodrug*. It includes the use of nanotools and models in drug discovery, drug targeting and design strategies, and nonclinical and clinical studies. Emphasis is laid on nanotoxicology and nanosafety aspects as well as regulatory issues for translation to the clinic of the most promising nanostructures. As the introduction of these new medicines may be controversial, ethical and societal aspects are also addressed in a specific chapter.

In Part Four, *key medical applications of nanodrugs* are reviewed. Diagnostics and imaging use and physical methods for treatment are first described. In the several following chapters and through the description of the various delivery routes in the body, main treatment areas such as cancer or infectious and neurodegenerative diseases are explained.

Finally, Part Five describes *market prospects and industrial commercialization aspects* with special focus on the commercial translation and its bottlenecks like the protection of intellectual property. Actual information about current commercialized products and market figures are also provided.

The chapters are written by leading researchers in pharmacy, biology, chemistry, physics, engineering, and medicine as well as law and social science from academia, industry, national/international laboratories, and government agencies in Europe, Israel, and the United States.

It is expected that this book will become a standard work for pharmacists and the pharmaceutical industry but also a database and a reference for scientists, researchers, and students, as well as for agencies, government, and regulatory authorities.

This book may bring inspiration for scientists, new ideas for drug developers, innovation in industry, and guidelines for toxicologists and finally will result in the establishment of guidelines for agencies and government authorities to establish safe rules in using this new promising technology. The book may result in breakthroughs in the pharmaceutical nanotechnology in such a way that medical doctors may cure life-threatening diseases such as cancer or infections with nanotechnology-based medicines, and thus in the welfare of the society.

Jean Cornier
Andrew Owen
Arno Kwade
Marcel Van de Voorde

Part Three
Development of Nanopharmaceuticals

14
Micro- and Nano-Tools in Drug Discovery

Andreas Dietzel,[1] Monika Leester-Schädel,[1] and Stephan Reichl[2]

[1]TU Braunschweig, Institute of Microtechnology, Alte Salzdahlumer Str. 203, 38124 Braunschweig, Germany
[2]TU Braunschweig, Department of Pharmaceutics, Mendelssohnstr. 1, 38106 Braunschweig, Germany

14.1
Introduction

The development of new drugs is complex, scientifically demanding, and time- and cost-intensive. New prospects and perspectives open up from the enormous developments in micro- and nanofabrication and the emerging research field of micro- or nanofluidics. The central theme of this field is to design, build, and operate devices that can manipulate fluids, particles, and biological materials such as proteins and cells in miniaturized volumes. Such devices are also known as lab-on-a-chip systems (LOC), bio-microelectromechanical systems (BioMEMS), or miniaturized total analysis systems (μTAS). They allow us bridging the gap between volumes that are typical in classical laboratories or pilot factories and the microscale volumes common in biology. These micro- and nano-tools can be the key to automated drug discovery, drug formulation, fast screening, protein crystallization, drug delivery, microbioreactors, organ-on-a-chip (OOC), and many other applications. Their applications in pharmaceutical research and technology are numerous [1] and cannot be completely covered in this chapter. In the following, general concepts of micro- and nanofluidics and typical processes for their fabrication shall be explained before two application fields, nanoformulation and OOC, are introduced.

14.2
General Concepts of Miniaturization

In microfluidic devices, convectional flow and diffusion, both being mass transport processes, are in competition. While diffusional transport follows concentration gradients, convection moves matter in a flow direction. Systems

Pharmaceutical Nanotechnology: Innovation and Production, First Edition. Edited by Jean Cornier, Arno Kwade, Andrew Owen, and Marcel Van de Voorde.

can be characterized by comparing the time required to pass a characteristic length by diffusive transport with the time to pass the same distance by convective transport. The time for diffusive transport and mixing scales with the square of the characteristic length in a fluid volume. In other words, heat and mass transport are intensified in miniaturized systems. However, many microfluidic systems are characterized by not only low Reynolds numbers (laminar flow) but also slow diffusive transport over the characteristic distance. This regime allows establishing chemical gradients in microdevices remaining practically constant over time. However, the same situation also leads to challenges when species need to be mixed in the absence of turbulent mixing. But in many cases it is desired that a reagent get into intense contact with a functionalized surface or with another fluid reagent, meaning that the reagents in the system need to be well mixed. If reaction kinetics are to be studied, a characteristic volume has to be mixed much faster than the timescale of reaction kinetics.

Interfacial tension force scales only linearly with length dimension and therefore becomes the largest force at very small scales. This force has to be considered in particular when a second phase (another liquid or gas) is also present in the microgeometries or in cases where the walls of microchannels are facing changing wetting situations. A second phase can, for instance, form independent compartments in which chemical processes can proceed. Water droplets can be created within a microfluidic oil stream forming tiny reaction chambers with dimensions down to a few micrometers in which the time required for diffusional mixing becomes extremely short.

Cells in culture flasks and Petri dishes hardly resemble *in vivo* conditions, and investigations demanding large numbers of experiments under varying conditions are often not feasible with these. However, micro- and nano-tools offer new perspectives not only for the manipulation and analysis of cells enabling parallelization, high-throughput experiments, and integration of more functionality but also for realizing *in vivo* similar situations. Patterned substrates, fluidic elements for medium exchange, and elements for stimuli and for measurements of different physical nature, such as mechanical, optical, or electrical, can be integrated in microfabricated fluidic devices. Moreover, not only single cells but also larger populations and 3D tissues can be cultivated in microgeometries. The concept of organ-on-a-chip offers new approaches to quantitative and systems biology, screening of pharmaceutical materials, and bioprocessing at small scales. In nanoliter-sized assay chambers, the cell environment can be defined and controlled very precisely, while consumption of expensive reagents during experiments becomes very low [2]. The intensified transport of heat and mass in small volumes allows dynamic control of conditions and therefore new types of experiments in which transient states also become observable. Microenvironments define the local chemical, thermal, and mechanical parameters in the direct surrounding of the cell. Temperature, dissolved molecules, and suspended (nano) particles are regulated with the cell medium. The mechanical environment includes influences not only from the culture substrate but also from shear forces exerted by the surrounding flow. In conventional culturing, environmental parameters can only be globally controlled for a larger population of cells, but locally addressing parameters of the cell microenvironment and dynamically changing these parameters become possible with microfluidic devices. In monitoring single cells or small cell clusters, the statistical noise originating from population heterogeneity is suppressed. Adherent cells can be studied using patterned adhesive patches, whereas nonadherent cells can be localized by hydrodynamic traps to perform experiments.

14.3
Micro- and Nanofabrication

Micro- and nano-tools could not be considered without advances in micro- and nanofabrication. Following an approach initially developed for microelectronics, such tools are fabricated in a cleanroom environment using monocrystalline silicon as base material. It typically involves mask-based photolithography, dry and wet etching, and thin film deposition. Glass can be used as an alternative or in combination with silicon and allows optical access to the fluid in the microdevices. A different approach using the so-called soft lithography and PDMS (polydimethylsiloxane) material has found widespread applications because it is relatively cheap and easy to use. In most cases, the manipulation of fluids at microscales takes place in closed volumes or channels. Several bonding techniques were developed allowing closure by a lid, which in many cases can be transparent. Recently, maskless techniques such as inkjet or 3D printing, laser micromachining, and microelectrical discharge machining have received more and more attention.

14.3.1.1 Photolithography
Photolithography is one of the most essential process steps in micro- and nanofabrication. It allows transferring the CAD-designed micro- and nanostructures onto the substrate surface using UV radiation. Therefore, the substrate surface is coated with a UV-light-sensitive polymer, the resist. The micro- and nanostructures can either be directly written into the resist with a focused UV beam or transferred by exposing the resist through a mask carrying the micro- and nanostructures as opaque features. The first mentioned method is currently becoming more and more popular, because the process speed has already been strongly enhanced, the design of micro- and nanostructures can quickly be modified, and the costly fabrication of masks can be spared. In a subsequent developing step, the exposed resist areas either become insoluble (negative tone resist) or soluble (positive tone resist). The resist layer thus patterned can be used as masking layer in a subsequent etch process, protecting the resist-deposited areas against the etch attack on one hand and generating the etch openings on the other. Another application for resist structures is the lift-off process, where, in addition, a thin metal layer is deposited onto the resist. Afterward, the resist is removed together with the overlying metal. The metal only remains in the resistless areas.

14.3.1.2 Depth Lithography

In the early 1980s, a microfabrication method combining lithography, electroplating, and molding was established to create high-aspect ratio structures. This method is called LIGA, which is a German acronym for **Li**thography, **G**alvanoformung, and **A**bformung. The initial LIGA process is the depth lithography. The first resists usable for layer thicknesses of up to some hundred micrometers were X-rays-sensitive requiring an equipment and cost-intensive generation of X-ray radiation. Today UV-sensitive polymer resists such as SU-8 are available making depth lithography and LIGA quite attractive for a broad application area. The exposed and subsequently developed resist can either be used as final device, for example, for micromechanical structures, or as lost mold for a following electroplating process. The electroplated device can again be used as ready-made metallic microdevice, for example, a microcoil or other electromagnetic components, or it serves as (negative) mold to reproduce the original SU-8 microstructure.

14.3.1.3 Soft Lithography

Soft lithography can be seen as a shortened variant of the LIGA technology, enabling the low-cost fabrication of high-aspect micro- and nanostructures mainly used for fluidic components. The term is derived from elastomeric (= soft) materials such as PDMS, of which the microstructures are made. As for the LIGA technology, at first a rigid mold (or master structure) has to be fabricated. Here again, SU-8 is a suitable and commonly used mold material. Then, the PDMS prepolymer is poured over the SU-8 mold and subsequently heated to 70 °C for 60 min to enhance the cross-linking. Afterward, the PDMS replica can be peeled off the mold (Figure 14.1).

14.3.1.4 Wet Chemical and Dry Etching

In microfabrication, etch techniques are equivalents to machining processes such as drilling, milling, and grinding in precision engineering and mechanics.

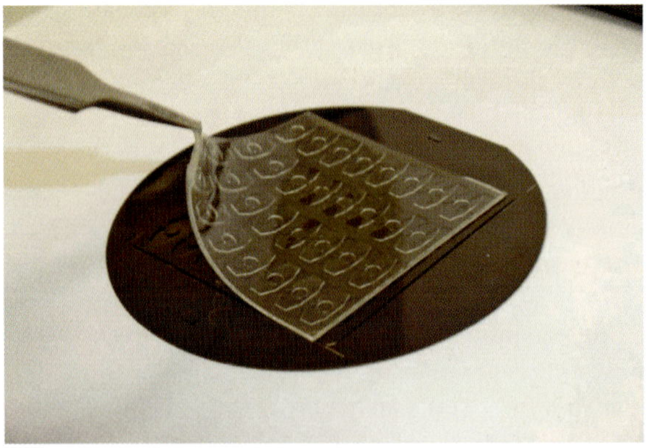

Figure 14.1 Peeling off a PDMS layer. The mold is made of SU-8.

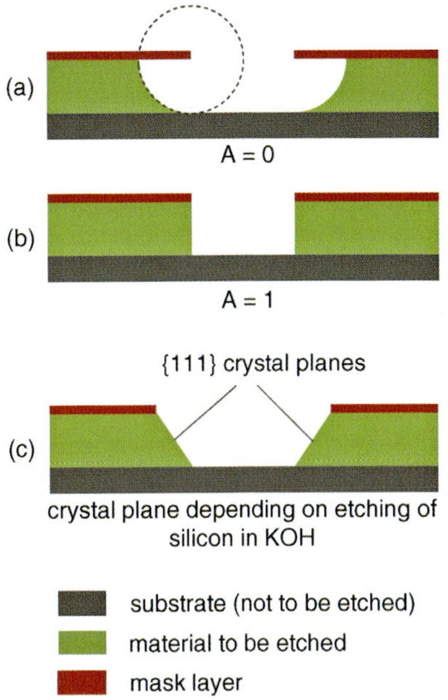

Figure 14.2 Isotropic etching (a), anisotropic etching (b), and anisotropic etching of silicon in KOH (c).

With etch techniques, very small structure widths and high etch depths, resulting in high aspect ratios, can be performed. Nevertheless, restrictions concerning the microstructure design are adverse.

The etch rate can be direction-independent (isotropic) or direction-specific (anisotropic), depending upon the etch technique, the etchants, and the material to be etched (Figure 14.2).

Another important influencing factor is the selectivity, which describes the relation between the etch rate of the mask layer (which should ideally be zero) and the layer or substrate material to be etched. For example, silicon oxide (SiO_2) film on top of a silicon substrate is usually wet chemical etched with buffered hydrofluoric acid ($NH_4F + HF + H_2O$) with an average etch rate of 200 nm/min. The etch rate of the silicon substrate is about 2 nm/min, so the selectivity of this double etch system is approximately 100.

Etch techniques are mainly divided into wet chemical and dry etching (Figure 14.3). Wet etching uses different chemical solutions and is normally isotropic. The substrate is either dipped into an etch bath with controlled temperature and wetted by flow or sprayed with the etch solution. An exception is the wet etching of bulk silicon with potassium hydroxide solution ($KOH + H_2O$) or EDP solution (ethylenediamine + pyrocatechol + H_2O). In these cases, the etching rate is anisotropic and related to the silicon crystal planes. The result is pyramidal etch flanks, which are formed by the {111} crystal planes having a very low etch rate. The anisotropic etching with KOH solution is a well-

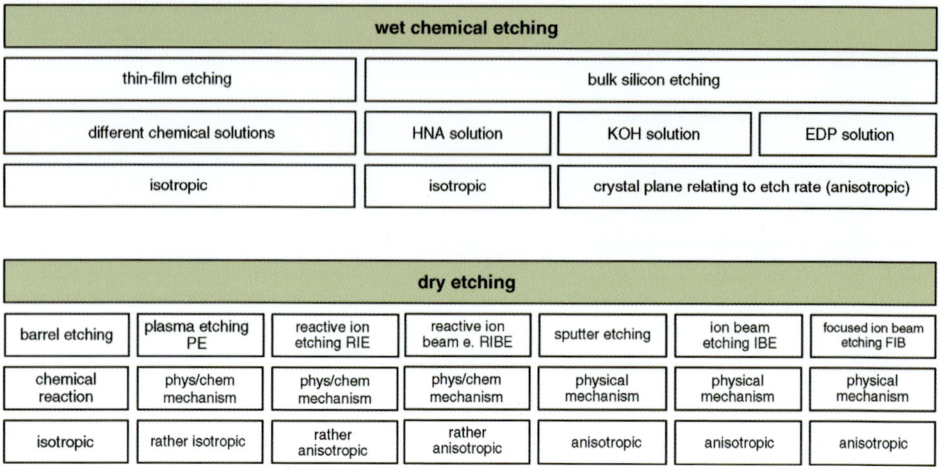

Figure 14.3 Overview of wet chemical and dry etch techniques.

controllable and straightforward silicon bulk fabrication process. However, the design freedom is limited, among other things, to rectangular cavities and tilted sidewalls.

Dry etch techniques can also be anisotropic, isotropic, and combinations of both. "Dry" in this context means that the etchants are gaseous. Purely physical dry etch techniques such as sputter etching and ion beam etching generate nearly vertical sidewalls with any structural design, but the selectivity of mask layer and material to be etched is quite low. Dry etch techniques that are based on chemical reactions are isotropic and, therefore, also design limiting, but the selectivity is high. Accordingly, they are used to etch micro- and nanostructures with low etching depth as well as thin films. Other dry etch techniques such as plasma etching and reactive ion etching combine chemical and physical mechanisms (Figure 14.3). The decision whether a wet or a dry etch technique is used depends on many different influencing factors. These are, for example, the inevitable process temperature, the etch rate, as already mentioned the selectivity, the health risk of the etchants and/or the chemical products, and, of course, the equipment and process costs.

14.3.1.5 **Thin Film Deposition**

The method of thin film deposition mostly depends on the material to be deposited (Figure 14.4). In case of silicon bulk micromachining, silicon oxide (SiO_2) and silicon nitride (Si_3N_4) are used as insulating or mask layers with a thickness of some 100 nm. SiO_2 can be formed by thermal oxidation, resulting in a high-quality layer but demanding a pure silicon substrate. If the requirements concerning dielectric strength and defect density are relatively low, the plasma-enhanced chemical vapor deposition (PE CVD) offers the advantages of lower process temperature, a variety of substrate materials, and a more than 10 times

	thin film deposition											
method	thermal oxidation		chemical vapor deposition (CVD)					physical vapor deposition (PVD)		other	
sub-division	wet	dry	atmospheric pressure CVD	low-pressure CVD	plasma-enhanced CVD	epitaxy	metal-organic CVD	thermal evaporation	sputtering	electro-plating	spin on
film material	SiO_2		SiO_2	SiO_2, Si_3N_4,	SiO_2, Si_3N_4,	silicon	metals, semi-conductors	metals	conducting and non-conducting materials	metals (Cu, Fe, Ni, NiFe, Au etc.)	polymers
charac-teristics	high film quality, high process temperature		thermal activation at atmospheric pressure; suitable for surface planarization	pressure = 10–100pa; high film quality	low process temperature (<100°C) lower film quality	same crystal struc-true as teh sub-strate	moderate process temperature, large material variety	material limitation concerning boiling point	good film adhesion, large material variety	large film thickness possible	viscosity and rotational speed determine the film thickness

Figure 14.4 Overview of the most usable thin film deposition methods.

higher deposition rate. Similarly, Si_3N_4 films are fabricated by low-pressure chemical vapor deposition (LP CVD) and PE CVD as well. Thin metal layer being used as conducting elements, mask, and adhesion layers are fabricated by thermal evaporation, metal–organic chemical vapor deposition (MO CVD), sputtering, or electroplating. Thermal evaporation is the oldest and the most simple physical vapor deposition (PVD) technique based on sublimating of the heated metal. The layer subsequently grows by condensation. The disadvantages of thermal evaporation are varying deposition rates, inhomogeneous films, and a limited material selection. Sputtered thin metal films are more homogeneous and usually better adhesive to the substrate, steps can be reliably covered, and more different materials are available. The sputtering mechanism is based on the bombardment of a solid target material with positive ions. Due to impulse repeating, target atoms are released and accelerated to the substrate. Electroplating takes place in an electrolytic cell and is based on reduction–oxidation reaction of the metallic coating material (e.g., copper, nickel, and gold). The substrate works as cathode, where the dissolved metal cations are reduced to generate the coating. Current density, temperature, and solution of the electrolyte are to be controlled carefully.

14.3.1.6 Bonding Techniques

Bonding of micro- and nanostructures, usually on wafer level, becomes necessary if monolithic fabrication is impossible or uneconomic. In order to ensure a reliable and long-term stable bond result, the material combination, the previous alignment, and the process control have to be well determined and tested. Current bonding techniques are the silicon direct bonding (SDB), the anodic bonding, the thermal bonding, the plasma-activated bonding, and the bonding with intermediate layers. Silicon direct bonding, as the name implies, only works with pure silicon wafers without any intermediate layer. The result is a reliable connection and, because of the absence of other materials, an excellent biocompatibility of the device. Limitations result from high process temperatures and high demands concerning cleanliness and flatness of the bond surfaces. Anodic bonding is an electric field-assisted technique involving no intermediate layers and, in contrast to the SDB, with relatively low process temperatures. Suitable bond materials are borosilicate glass combined with silicon or metals. The bond mechanism is based on the displacement of electrical charges within the borosilicate glass resulting in a permanent high electric field force between both bond surfaces and hence an interatomic bonding. Two glass substrates are commonly bonded due to thermal activation. The process takes place in a vacuum furnace at about 600 °C. The result is a fully transparent, chemical, and temperature stable micro- or nanosystem usable for medical and biological applications. Direct bonding of PDMS to itself and to materials such as glass, silicon, SU-8, and so on requires prior activation of the bond surfaces, which can be done due to plasma treatment within, for example, a barrel etcher. Thus, PDMS and glass surfaces become hydrophilic. In case of other materials, the plasma activation affects intensive surface cleaning and the introduction of polar functional groups, enabling a homogeneous bond. Bonding with intermediate layer in turn can be divided into solid–liquid interdiffusion bonding (SLID), which is based on the formation of intermetallic compounds between a low-temperature and a high-temperature melting metal, the adhesive bonding with glues, epoxies, or various plastic agents, and the glass frit bonding with low-temperature melting glass as intermediate layer.

14.3.1.7 3D Printing

Nowadays, several additive manufacturing technologies are understood as 3D printing (Figure 14.5). The most common one is the fused deposition modeling (FDM) – also named fused filament fabrication FFF). FDM uses plastic filaments or metal wires, which are melted and deposited layer for layer to form the entire object. This technology is excellently usable for low-cost rapid prototyping and rapid manufacturing, especially of lightweight constructions. Its disadvantages are however a low surface quality and a limited potential for miniaturization. Selective laser printing (SLP) uses metal powder, which is sintered layer-by-layer due to laser radiation. The remaining loose powder is blown away afterward. Compared to machining processes, SLP enables the fabrication of complex

	3D printing				
designation	fused deposition modeling FDA	selective laser printing SLP	laminated object manufacturing LOM	stereo-lithography SL	powder-based 3D printing
object material	plastic filment or metal wires	metal powder	paper, plastic or metal laminates	UV-sensitive resin	different powder materials
design method	CAD				
technology	melting and layer-wise deposition	layer-wise sintering by laser radiation	laser-cutting and gluing	layered laser-cutting	powder particles are interlinked with printed fluids

Figure 14.5 Three-dimensional printing technologies.

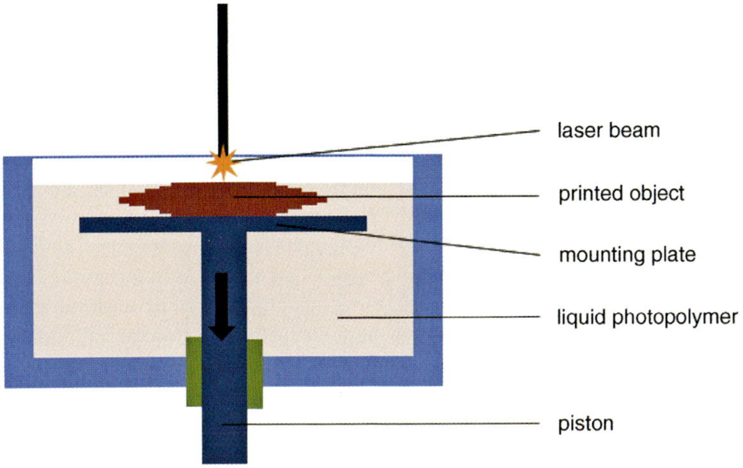

Figure 14.6 Schematic buildup of an SL printer.

three-dimensional devices with, for example, internal support structures, but the production time for each device is still rather long. Another 3D printing technology is the laminated object manufacturing (LOM). Here adhesive-coated paper, plastic, or metal laminates are tailored by laser cutting and glued together. The 3D printing technology with the highest potential for miniaturization is stereolithography (SL). The printing process starts with a vat of liquid UV-sensitive resin (photopolymer). Inside the vat, a piston with a platform serves as mounting plate for the final printed object. At the beginning, the platform is located directly at the resin surface, where an UV laser is focused on. The laser cures the resin layer-wise, as the platform moves downward bit-by-bit (Figure 14.6).

Similar to SLP are 3D printing technologies using nonmetal powder materials. To interlink the particles, a binder in the form of an appropriate liquid, which can also serve as active ingredient, is printed onto the surface of the powder bulk. Remaining loose powder is blown away. This procedure is repeated several times to fabricate a solid 3D object. An innovative powder-based method is the so-called powder–liquid 3D printing. This technology was developed at the Massachusetts Institute of Technology (MIT) together with a pharmaceutical US company to print highly dosed drugs. The powdered medication is applied as thin layer and stitched together due to an aqueous fluid. The result is a porous, water-soluble matrix that rapidly disintegrates with a sip of liquid.

14.3.1.8 Microelectrical Discharge Machining (μEDM)

Electrical discharge machining (EDM) is a well-established method to process primarily hard metals. The material is removed from the metallic workpiece due to electrical discharges (sparks) generated between the tool electrode and the workpiece, both in close distance. The tool electrode can (a) be a permanently fed wire (wire-cut EDM), (b) a sinker (die-sink EDM), which represents the negative form of the finished component, or (c) a rod for milling and drilling. The use of EDM in microsystem technologies is not yet very widespread. It offers the promising advantage of fabricating three-dimensional micro- and nanostructures made of, for example, stainless steel or other wear-resistant and unconventional materials. This opens among others the possibility to develop and fabricate microfluidic systems for the dispersion and emulsification of solid lipid nanoparticles, working at pressures in the range of 500–2000 bar.

14.3.1.9 **Laser Fabrication**

Laser fabrication is an innovative and exciting opportunity to produce micro- and nanodevices made of a large variety of materials. Many different laser types, such as excimer lasers, CO_2 lasers, and short or ultrashort pulsed solid-state lasers, are available to ablate material due to thermal energy. The laser fabrication reflects as well the trend toward maskless micro- and nanopatterning and its main advantage is the ability to quickly respond to customer's change requests concerning the device design. With femtosecond lasers, even temperature-sensitive materials such as polymers or organic substances can be patterned because of the nearly nonexistent heat input into the material. Furthermore, femtosecond lasers generate multiphoton absorption processes, which can be used to locally expose material and thereby write latent 3D structures into the volume of transparent materials. Multiphoton absorption even allows structuring with submicrometer resolution.

14.3.1.10 **Surface Functionalization**

Surface functionalization means the individual tailoring or adapting of physical, chemical, or biological surface properties due to coating or modification processes. For micro- and nanodevices, predominantly for fluidic applications, the following surface properties are often relevant:

- Hydrophilic – hydrophobic
- Adhesive – nonsticky/self-cleaning
- Rough – smooth
- Reactive – nonreactive
- Reflective – nonreflective
- Wear/corrosion-resistant – lubricating
- Black/white – colored
- Conducting – insulating.

Furthermore, biocompatibility, surface energy, and the protection against biofilms are particularly important for some applications. The technologies to change surface characteristics range from electroplating, CVD/PVD, and diffusion to plasma, laser, ion, electron, microwave, and solar beams based processes. A particular overview of the most common surface engineering technologies can be found in Ref. [3]. Surface functionalization also includes the biochemical activation of surfaces with receptor molecules selectively reacting with target molecules such as antibody/antigen reactions.

14.4 Nanoformulation

The nanoformulation of drugs can extremely improve their bioavailability. However, a precise control of particle size and drug loading remains a challenge in conventional batch mode processing. On the other hand, formation and manipulation of solid particles in microscopic devices are more susceptible to fouling, and partial or full blockage with agglomerated particles can disrupt the flow and render the device unusable. In general, adding an extra phase of solid, liquid, or gaseous material that does not mix with the other will add extra complexity to a microfluidic device, but it also offers advantageous new concepts [4,5]. In particular, nanoformulation using novel miniaturized systems benefits from the unique advantages of good control of local application of energy and intensification of mass and heat transfer at small scales. Moreover, for screening of formulations, only small amounts of the active pharmaceutical ingredient (API) are often available in the early stages of the development and methods for small volume production are highly desired. In this context, there are two distinct approaches for application of miniaturized systems for nanoformulation: (i) In the top-down approach, an existing formulation with suspended droplets or particles pass through a microchannel structure under high pressure to become homogenized and to display smaller droplets or particle sizes and more narrow size distributions. (ii) In the bottom-up process, the nanoparticles are created in miniaturized systems by solidification or precipitation processes.

14.4.1 High-Pressure Nanonization Systems

High-pressure emulsification at conventional scales is an established, industrial top-down process. However, in the development of pharmaceutical emulsions or nanoscale lipid dispersions, microsystems for high-pressure emulsification offer capabilities of small volume production along with narrow particle size distribution and high physicochemical stability [6]. A modular high-pressure microchannel system was designed and built from μEDM-structured stainless steel sheets that are stacked and clamped together to obtain a leak-proof complete system [7] (see Figures 14.7 and 14.8). Due to high-pressure drops across the microchannels, the system operates in a high Reynolds number regime and high inertial forces are acting on the fluid that is somewhat untypical for microfluidic systems. Robustness and leak tightness at elevated temperatures beyond the melting temperature of solid lipids and at high pressures up to 2000 bar are enabled by the clamping mechanism and by choosing stainless steel as base material for the microfluidic sheets [8]. The structuring of the sheets was accomplished by a microelectrical discharge machining (μEDM) process in combination with a final electrochemical polishing process [9,10]. For cleaning or removing blockage, the device can be easily disassembled and reassembled.

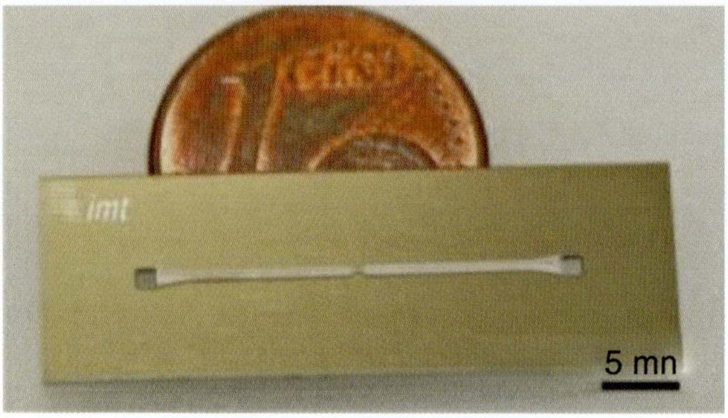

Figure 14.7 Microchannel emulsification sheet fabricated from stainless steel at the Institute of Microtechnology (TU Braunschweig) by μEDM [10].

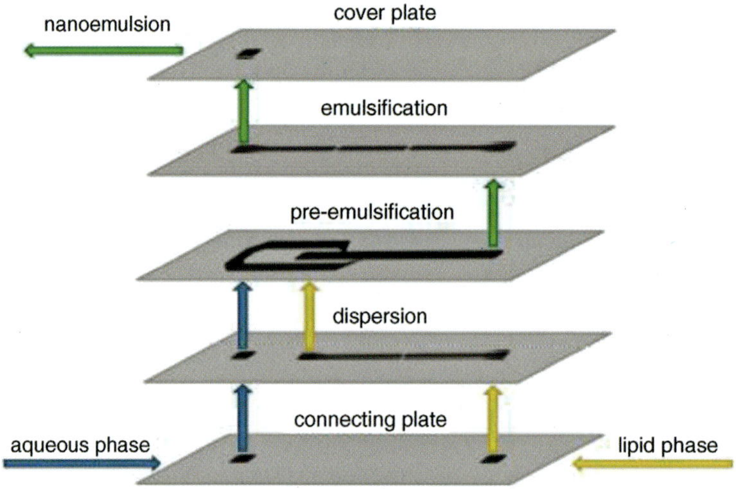

Figure 14.8 Sketch of the modular high-pressure microfluidic system illustrating the assembling principle and flow-through path. (From Ref. [7].)

In the pre-emulsification module, a high-velocity jet of an aqueous surfactant solution splits the flow of the viscous oil into small separate droplets to form a coarse emulsion [11]. In the subsequent emulsification module, the coarse emulsion with a not necessarily narrow size distribution flows through the microchannel with local constrictions in which flow velocities increase. As droplets pass the constrictions, they elongate due to shear stress and turbulent flow characteristics and tiny droplets of nanoscale dimensions rip off. A variety of different microchannels were designed: straight, z-shaped, y-shaped, and orifice channels as well as combinations thereof. The final droplet size inversely correlates with the driving pressure drop as shown in Figure 14.9. However, formulation-dependent parameters also affect the efficiency of dispersion. A large

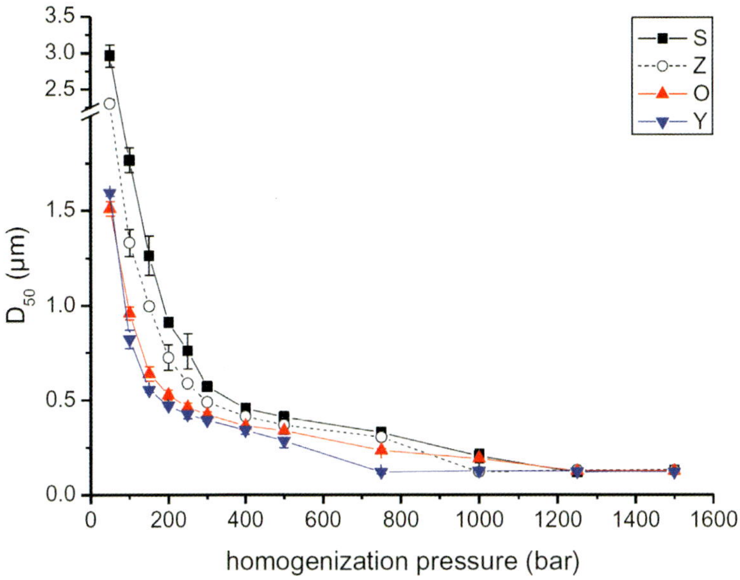

Figure 14.9 Droplet sizes obtained with different microsystem geometries. (Adapted with permission from Ref. [14]. Copyright 2012, Elsevier B.V.).

volume fraction of the phase to be dispersed is a challenge and the droplet's oil viscosity strongly influences the outcome of the process. If viscosities of both phases are similar, fluid dynamic stresses are better transferred from the continuous to the disperse phase and the most efficient emulsification is obtained [12]. Different designs of microchannels were tested and the highest droplet breakup efficiency was obtained with double orifices of 80 μm and, subsequently, 120 μm. Although cavitation occurs, it is not likely to be the dominating mechanism in droplet breakup [13].

For producing solid lipid nanoparticle (SLN) dispersions, this device including the tubing has to be heated to elevated temperatures to keep the lipid in a molten stage. A conventionally prepared hot pre-emulsion was passed through the emulsification module under a pressure of around 1250 bar once or several times before being cooled to room temperature, enabling solidification of SLN with a mean particle size of around 120 nm [10,14], which is comparable to results with conventional processes at large scales requiring more passages. SLN were also loaded with different APIs or model compounds [15–17].

14.4.2
Low-Pressure Nanonization Systems

Nanoparticle formation is influenced by a large number of control parameters. High-throughput and low-volume methods such as microfluidic flows, in which even plugs or droplets are created, provide excellent possibilities of crystallization

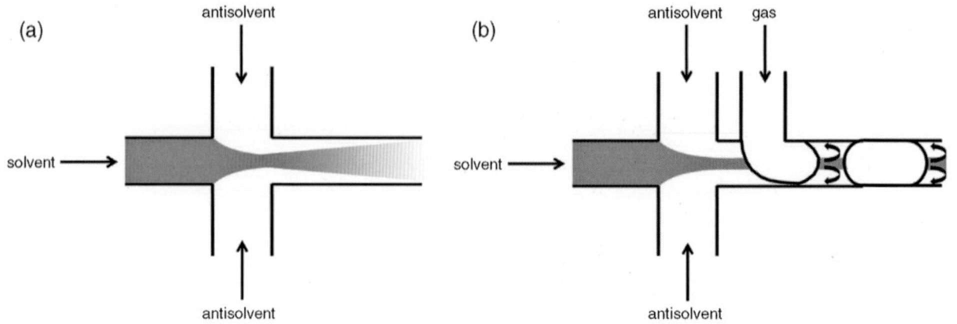

Figure 14.10 Basic principle of nanoparticle fabrication in a flow focusing device based on a solvent–antisolvent approach (a). To intensify the mixing, gas can be injected breaking up the liquid into plugs (b).

experiments consuming little of the precious materials. Microfluidic systems operating under typical conditions are characterized by lower pressure drops, lower flow velocities, and low Reynolds numbers. Microfluidic behavior is strongly influenced by the interplay of viscous and interface tension forces, in particular for multiphase flow phenomena involving bubbles and droplets. Nanoparticle fabrication can be observed in a simple microchannel configuration called flow focusing (see Figure 14.10). Under completely laminar flow conditions, a lipid solution is injected that subsequently meets an antisolvent fluid that squeezes the lipid solution into a narrow stripe. Then the lipid solution comes in intimate contact with the antisolvent and diffusion smears out the initially sharp interface when proceeding along the outlet channel. Thereafter, solubility progressively decreases and nanoparticles precipitate [18].

A somewhat different approach was first reported by Yen *et al.* where flow was segmented by gas bubbles for high-temperature synthesis of quantum dots [19]. Later Yun *et al.* reported about the continuous production of solid lipid nanoparticles in a stream formed by flow focusing and subsequently separated into plugs by gas injection [20]. In this approach, the formation of plugs is controlled by constant pressure inflow of an inert gas such as N_2 that periodically disrupts the flow (see schematic in Figure 14.10 and real device in Figure 14.11). Very regular droplets are formed through the interplay between interfacial tensions and viscous forces. They can act as independent compartments in which precipitation occurs; however, compared to flow without gas, inflow is accelerated through intensified mixing in compartments. Within the fluid plug compartments, not only diffusion but also vortices resulting from interactions with the channel walls promote the mixing. By controlling the inflows of fluids and gas, the plug size and as a consequence also the time required for complete mixing can be influenced. This in turn controls the precipitation and determines size and size distribution of obtained nanoparticles.

In a yet another approach, lipid droplets are formed as a disperse phase after flow focusing in a sheath flow of a continuous phase when the focused lipid

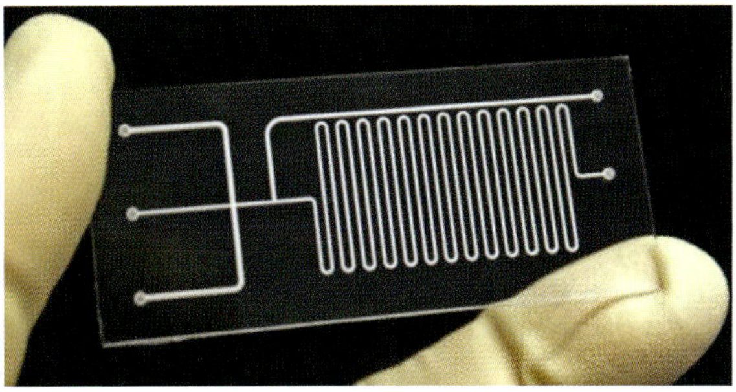

Figure 14.11 Microfluidic nanoparticle fabrication device fabricated from glass by femtosecond laser ablation at the Institute of Microtechnology (TU Braunschweig). Inlets for solvent and antisolvent are placed at the left-hand side of the chip, whereas inlet for gas and the outlet are placed on the right-hand side.

stream passes a constriction area. This approach is shown in Figure 14.12 and images from a droplet microfluidics device are shown in Figure 14.13. The use of droplet reactors was first demonstrated by Shestopalov *et al.* for nanocrystal synthesis [21]. The droplets form one after the other, each being produced at practically identical situations given by the balance of interfacial tension and viscous friction forces [22]. These droplets as a whole can solidify to form lipid particles. But droplets can also act as independent compartments in which precipitation can proceed if supersaturation is reached. The continuous phase can be chosen to resemble an inert environment, but in a permeable environment supersaturation may be reached by loss of the solvent into the droplet environment where the time required for diffusion scales with the square of size. Complete diffusion in femtoliter droplet volumes becomes extremely fast and can occur in times that can drop to few milliseconds or even below. Also, the

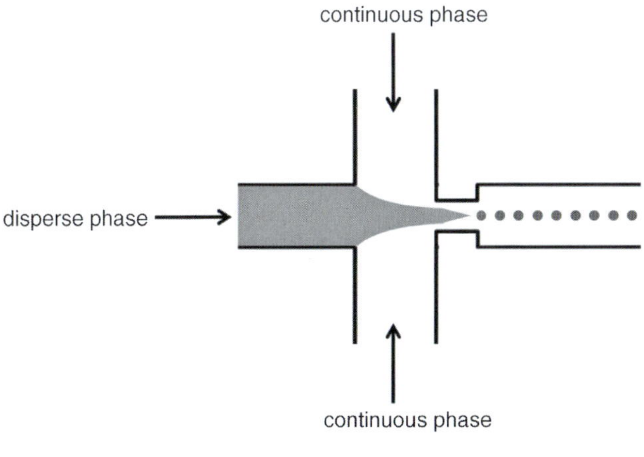

Figure 14.12 Principle of microfluidic droplet flow reactor.

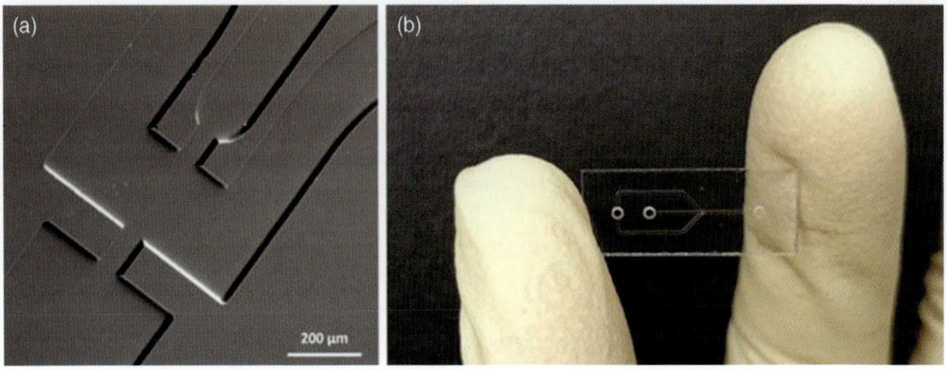

Figure 14.13 Flow focusing system for droplet formation fabricated from glass by lithographic and wet etching techniques at the Institute of Microtechnology (TU Braunschweig). (a) Electron microscopic micrograph of the constriction area for droplet formation. (b) Complete droplet microfluidic system made from glass.

temperature equalizes very fast in these droplet compartments and temperature gradients disappear.

When studying protein crystallization, it is desired to find conditions allowing the formation of nuclei in supersaturated solutions with subsequent growth of high-quality crystals.

A protein solution can in this way be mixed with precipitants and captured in nanoliter droplets. If the solution is supersaturated, nucleation and crystallization will eventually occur and high-quality crystals are obtained [23]. As long as droplets are embedded in a continuous phase that is impermeable to the solutes in the droplet, this process can be considered as a microbatch method. Only when the kinetics of crystallization is sufficiently fast, particles can be formed in the microsystem without requiring separate aging containers [24]. Three-dimensional microfluidics can provide flow focusing with improved symmetry. This reduces the tendency of droplet channel wall interactions even when energetically favored by interfacial tensions. The current status of microscale methods for nanocrystal synthesis and the role microreactors might ultimately play in laboratory-scale research and industrial production is discussed by Philips *et al.* [25].

14.5 Organ-on-a-Chip

During the preclinical phase of drug development, decisions regarding the further development of a new drug substance are extremely critical since failure of substances during the clinical phase causes high costs and even may create adjournments in the development pipeline of a pharmaceutical company. To minimize the risk of late failure, results from preclinical investigations and tests regarding the activity, toxicity, and pharmacokinetics should be as meaningful as possible.

Preclinical studies are traditionally performed in animal experiments and, more recently, two-dimensional cell culture models, allowing reducing animal testing in sense of the 3R principle (reduction, refinement, and replacement of animal experiments). Animal experiments are associated with ethical concerns, high variability of data, and difficulties in extrapolation of clinical effects to humans because of interspecies differences. However, 2D cell culture models are not able to reflect the complex cell–cell interactions of the human body and extracellular environments. Tremendous advances in micro- and nanofabrication and in chip-based cell cultivation recently led to rapidly intensifying research on three-dimensional cell culture models, the so-called organ-on-a-chip systems. Such OOC systems allow improved cell–cell and cell–matrix interactions and support the expression of organotypic properties by creating *in vivo* like microenvironments. These systems combine the benefits of engineered, physiological-like microenvironments with the advantages of well-characterized, human cell lines. They are not reconstructs of entire organs, but resemble units with relevant tissue- or organ-level functions. Design principles and fabrication methods are based on MEMS technology and include elements such as multiple channels with splitting and merging branches, pumps, valves, and integrated electrical and biochemical sensors [26]. Human-based tissue-like systems to be used in the field of drug development that can mimic the natural complexity of tissues are an emerging field of research. Moreover, microsystems give the operator the opportunity to fully control the biological microenvironment and to induce physiological forces or gradients. Dynamic flow conditions in many cases stimulate cell morphologies and metabolism similar to the *in vivo* situation as well as an increased lifespan for primary cells [27,28]. With the small dimensions of OOCs, it is possible to work with very low consumption of drugs, to allow automation and high-throughput, and to parallelize experiments, which are important for drug screening [26]. Furthermore, OOCs including biosensors allow online measurements of the viability and functionality of the cells in real time. Due to the complexity of such systems, extensive manufacturing techniques and wisely chosen materials are needed [29]. The basic concept underlying the establishment of an OOC for drug testing is shown in Figure 14.14.

During the last 5 years, most progress in the field of OOCs for drug screening was achieved for so-called single-organ systems focusing on just one tissue/organ. These OOCs are primarily used for determining drug toxicity or pharmacokinetic processes as drug absorption (gut-on-a-chip) [31], drug metabolization (liver-on-a-chip) [32], or drug excretion (kidney-on-a-chip) [33]. Furthermore, OOCs representing drug transport barriers, such as the blood–brain barrier (BBB), became more and more important for drug screening processes of preclinical phase. Figure 14.15 illustrates structure and design of one of the first BBB on chip systems. The cocultivation of astrocytes and microvascular endothelial cells under dynamic flow conditions leads to expression of organotypic barrier properties of the BBB that can be determined online via integrated sensor

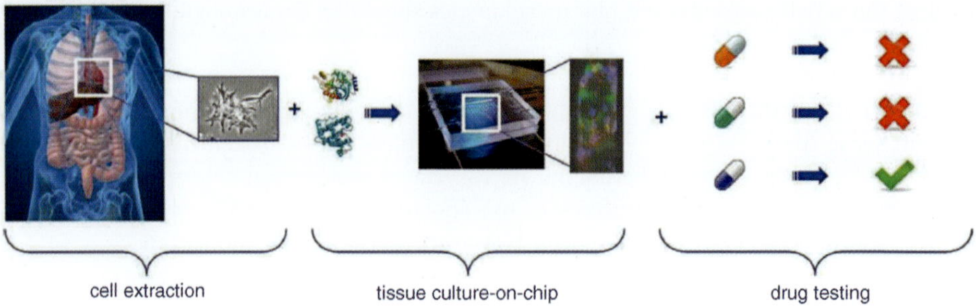

Figure 14.14 Concept underlying the development and use of an OOC for pharmaceutical applications. The developments of OOC systems always start with the establishment of primary cultures or stem cells from a living organism (left). In many cases, immortalized cell lines are also used. After design and manufacturing, process cells are transferred into the microfluidic chip and cultivated under organ-adapted cultivation conditions, consisting of a suitable medium composition containing growth factors as well as matrix and mechanical stimuli. The organ-related chip design in combination with selective cultivation conditions forms a specific microenvironment that supports the expression of organotypic features. Quality assurance of OOC in terms of the organotypic state of the tissue is performed by using suitable analytical methods, such as immunostaining (center) or biosensor-based testing. Further analytical tools are also needed for subsequent drug testing. Typically, the tissue is exposed to drug candidates or formulations, and the response of the tissue is measured in various ways, depending on the functionality of the organ. Such studies often include test regimes concerning cell viability, toxicity, or metabolism of the drug substance, pharmacological effects, drug absorption, and transport processes (b). (Reproduced with permission from Ref. [30]. Copyright 2013, Elsevier B.V.)

technology, for example, the transepithelial electrical resistance (TEER) in this case.

In a next step approximating animal models even better, OOCs containing tissues from different origins of the human body can be connected by microfluidic networks to form multiple OOCs or even "human-on-a-chip" systems [35]. Besides the replacement and improvement of established animal- or cell-based preclinical test strategies, OOCs will offer several new opportunities in pharmaceutical research and development such as the simulation of diseased organisms or the generation of personalized chips. It can be assumed that future steps in the development process toward marketable next-generation OOCs will include standardization of design principles, improvement of analytics, and integrable biosensors. Furthermore, the identification of new biocompatible materials for OOCs with improved properties compared with the previously used materials could be a challenging task for the next years. Especially, with view on rational use and widespread application of OOC in drug discovery, next-generation OOCs have to be user-friendly, reproducible, cost-effective, and available in high quantities for high-throughput screening. In the next 5–10 years, many efforts are therefore needed to transfer current laboratory-based prototyping to commercial manufacturing of OOCs and bring these OOCs from the laboratory

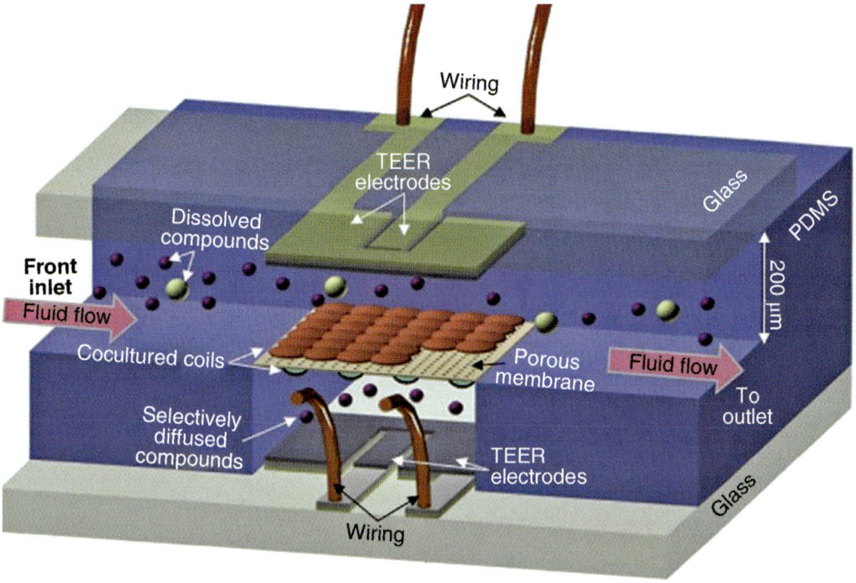

Figure 14.15 Structure and design of a chip system for the reconstruction of the blood–brain barrier (BBB), as described by Booth and Kim [34]. The OOC is formed by cocultivation of endothelial cells and astrocytes on a polycarbonate membrane, which is integrated between two PDMS layers containing fluid channels. The chip also contains electrodes that are deposited and structured on glass slides to allow transepithelial electrical resistance (TEER) measurement. The TEER value is routinely determined as surrogate parameter for endothelial barrier integrity. (Reproduced with permission from Ref. [34]. Copyright 2012, The Royal Society of Chemistry.)

scale to the industrial scale as a useful micro-tool in preclinical phase of drug discovery.

References

1 Dietzel, A. (ed.) (2016) *Microsystems for Pharmatechnology: Manipulation of Fluids, Particles, Droplets, and Cells*, Springer, New York.

2 Beißner, N., Lorenz, T., and Reichl, S. (2016) Organ on chip, in *Microsystems for Pharmatechnology: Manipulation of Fluids, Particles, Droplets, and Cells* (ed. A. Dietzel), Springer, New York, pp. 299–339.

3 Eichler, M., Klages, C.P., and Lachmann, K. (2016) Surface functionalization of microfluidic devices, in *Microsystems for Pharmatechnology* (ed. A. Dietzel), Springer.

4 Bunjes, H. and Mueller-Goymann, C.C. (2016) Microsystems for emulsification, in *Microsystems for Pharmaceutical Engineering* (ed. A. Dietzel), Springer, New York, pp. 153–179.

5 Windbergs, M. (2016) On-chip fabrication of drug delivery systems, in *Microsystems for Pharmaceutical Engineering* (ed. A. Dietzel), Springer, New York, pp. 181–196.

6 Schilde, C., Gothsch, T., Beinert, S., and Kwade, A. (2016) Microsystems for

dispersing nanoparticles, in *Microsystems for Pharmatechnology: Manipulation of Fluids, Particles, Droplets, and Cells* (ed. A. Dietzel), Springer, New York, pp. 197–219.

7 Finke, J.H., Gothsch, T., Richter, C., Beinert, S., Thies, J.-W., Dietzel, A., Büttgenbach, S., Müller-Goymann, C.C., and Kwade, A. (2014) Modular overall microsystem for the integrated production and loading of solid lipid nanoparticles. Concluding results of the research group mikroPART – FOR 856: Microsystems for Particulate Life Science Products, funded by the Deutsche Forschungsgemeinschaft (DFG) (Applicants A. Kwade, I. Kampen, and J.H. Finke), Braunschweig.

8 Gothsch, T., Finke, J.H., Beinert, S., Lesche, C., Schur, J., Buettgenbach, S., Mueller-Goymann, C., and Kwade, A. (2011) Effect of microchannel geometry on high-pressure dispersion and emulsification. *Chem. Eng. Technol.*, **34** (3), 335–343.

9 Richter, C., Krah, T., and Buettgenbach, S. (2012) Novel 3D manufacturing method combining microelectrical discharge machining and electrochemical polishing. *Microsyst. Technol.*, **18** (7–8), 1109–1118.

10 Richter, C., Stegemann, D., Vierheller, A., Gothsch, T., Finke, J.H., Kwade, A., Mueller-Goymann, C.C., Dietzel, A., and Buettgenbach, S. (2013) Innovative process chain for the development of wear resistant 3D metal microsystems. *Microelectron. Eng.*, **110**, 392–397.

11 Richter, C., Demming, S., Lorenz, T., Al-Halhouli, A.T., Vierheller, A., Thies, J.-W., Dietzel, A., and Büttgenbach, S. (2014) Design and fabrication of micro systems for particulate life science products, in *Concluding results of the research group mikroPART. Microsystems for Particulate Life Science Products, FOR 856, funded by the Deutsche Forschungsgemeinschaft* (eds A. Kwade, I. Kampen, and J.H. Finke), DFG, Braunschweig.

12 Finke, J.H., Niemann, S., Richter, C., Gothsch, T., Kwade, A., Büttgenbach, S., and Müller-Goymann, C.C. (2014) Multiple orifices in customized microsystem high-pressure emulsification: the impact of design and counter pressure on homogenization efficiency. *Chem. Eng. J.*, **248**, 107–121.

13 Gothsch, T., Schilcher, C., Richter, C., Beinert, S., Dietzel, A., Büttgenbach, S., and Kwade, A. (2015) High-pressure microfluidic systems (HPMS): flow and cavitation measurements in supported silicon microsystems. *Microfluid. Nanofluidics*, **18**, 121–130.

14 Finke, J., Schur, J., Richter, C., Gothsch, T., Kwade, A., Büttgenbach, S., and Müller-Goymann, C.C. (2012) The influence of customized geometries and process parameters on nanoemulsion and solid lipid nanoparticle production in microsystems. *Chem. Eng. J.*, **209**, 126–137.

15 Finke, J.H., Richter, C., Gothsch, T., Kwade, A., Büttgenbach, S., and Müller-Goymann, C.C. (2014) Coumarin 6 as a fluorescent model drug: how to identify properties of lipid colloidal drug delivery systems via fluorescence spectroscopy? *Eur. J. Lipid. Sci. Technol.*, **116** (9), 1234–1246.

16 Paranjpe, M., Finke, J., Richter, C., Gothsch, T., Kwade, A., Büttgenbach, S., and Müller-Goymann, C.C. (2014) Physicochemical characterization of sildenafil loaded solid lipid nanoparticle dispersions (SLN) for pulmonary application. *Int. J. Pharm.*, **476** (1–2), 41–49.

17 Pretor, S., Bartels, J., Lorenz, T., Dahl, K., Finke, J.H., Peterat, G., Krull, R., Al-Halhouli, A.T., Dietzel, A., Büttgenbach, S., Behrends, S., Reichl, S., and und Müller-Goymann, C.C. (2015) Cellular uptake of coumarin-6 under microfluidic conditions into HCE-T cells from nanoscale formulations. *Mol. Pharm.*, **12** (1), 34–45.

18 Karnik, R., Gu, F., Basto, P., Cannizzaro, C., Dean, L., Kyei-Manu, W., Langer, R., and Farokhzad, O.C. (2008) Microfluidic platform for controlled synthesis of polymeric nanoparticles. *Nano. Lett.*, **8** (9), 2906–2912.

19 Yen, B.K.H., Günter, A., Schmidt, M.A., Jensen, K.F., and Bawendi, M.G. (2005) A microfabricated gas–liquid segmented flow reactor for high-temperature

synthesis: the case of CdSe quantum dots. *Angew. Chem., Int. Ed.*, **44**, 5447–5451.

20 Yun, J., Zhang, S., Shen, S., Chen, Z., Yao, K., and Chen, J. (2009) Continuous production of solid lipid nanoparticles by liquid flow-focusing and gas displacing method in microchannels. *Chem. Eng. Sci.*, **64**, 4115–4122.

21 Shestopalov, I., Tice, J.D., and Ismagilov, R.F. (2004) Multi-step synthesis of nanoparticles performed on millisecond time scale in a microfluidic droplet-based system. *Lab Chip*, **4**, 316–321.

22 Seemann, R., Brinkmann, M., Pfohl, T., and Herminghaus, S. (2012) Droplet based microfluidics. *Rep. Prog. Phys.*, **75**, 016601.

23 Zheng, B., Tice, J.D., Roach, L.S., and Ismagilov, R.F. (2004) A droplet-based, composite PDMS/glass capillary microfluidic system for evaluating protein crystallization conditions by microbatch and vapor-diffusion methods with on-chip X-ray diffraction. *Angew. Chem., Int. Ed.*, **43** (19), 2508–2511.

24 Moschou, P., de Croon, M.H.J.M., van der Schaaf, J., and Schouten, J.C. (2014) Advances in continuous crystallization: toward microfluidic systems. *Rev. Chem. Eng.*, **30** (2), 127–138.

25 Phillips, T.W., Lignos, I.G., Maceiczyk, R.M., deMello, A.J., and deMello, J.C. (2014) Nanocrystal synthesis in microfluidic reactors: where next? *Lab Chip*, **14**, 3172–3180.

26 van der Meer, A.D. and van den Berg, A. (2012) Organs-on-chips: breaking the *in vitro* impasse. *Integr. Biol.*, **4** (5), 461–470.

27 Van Midwoud, P.M., Groothuis, G., Merema, M.T., and Verpoorte, E. (2010) Microfluidic biochip for the perifusion of precision-cut rat liver slices for metabolism and toxicology studies. *Biotechnol. Bioeng.*, **105** (1), 184–194.

28 Wagner, I., Materne, E., Brincker, S., Sueßbier, U., Fraedrich, C., Busek, M., Sonntag, F., Sakharov, D.A., Trushkin, E.V., Tonevitsky, A.G., Lauster, R., and Marx, U. (2013) A dynamic multi-organ-chip for long-term cultivation and substance testing proven by 3D human liver and skin tissue co-culture. *Lab Chip*, **13** (18), 3538–3547.

29 Capulli, A.K., Tian, K., Mehandru, N., Bukhta, A., Choudhury, S.F., Suchyta, M., and Parker, K.K. (2014) Approaching the *in vitro* clinical trial: engineering organs on chips. *Lab Chip*, **14** (17), 3181–3186.

30 Selimović, Š., Dokmeci, M.R., and Khademhosseini, A. (2013) Organs-on-a-chip for drug discovery. *Curr. Opin. Pharmacol.*, **13** (5), 829–833.

31 Kim, H.J., Huh, D., Hamilton, G., and Ingber, D.E. (2012) Human gut-on-a-chip inhabited by microbial flora that experiences intestinal peristalsis-like motions and flow. *Lab Chip*, **12** (12), 2165–2174.

32 Dash, A., Inman, W., Hoffmaster, K., Sevidal, S., Kelly, J., Obach, R.S., Griffith, L.G., and Tannenbaum, S.R. (2009) Liver tissue engineering in the evaluation of drug safety. *Expert Opin. Drug Metab. Toxicol.*, **5** (10), 1159–1174.

33 Jang, K., Mehr, A.P., Hamilton, G.A., McPartlin, L.A., Chung, S., Suh, K., and Ingber, D.E. (2013) Human kidney proximal tubule-on-a-chip for drug transport and nephrotoxicity assessment. *Integr. Biol. (UK)*, **5** (9), 1119–1129.

34 Booth, R. and Kim, H. (2012) Characterization of a microfluidic *in vitro* model of the blood–brain, barrier (μBBB). *Lab Chip*, **12** (10), 1784–1792.

35 Maschmeyer, I., Lorenz, A.K., Schimek, K., Hasenberg, T., Ramme, A.P., Hubner, J., Lindner, M., Drewell, C., Bauer, S., Thomas, A., Sambo, N.S., Sonntag, F., Lauster, R., and Marx, U. (2015) A four-organ-chip for interconnected long-term co-culture of human intestine, liver, skin and kidney equivalents. *Lab Chip*, **15** (12), 2688–2699.

15
Computational Predictive Models for Nanomedicine

Marco Siccardi, Alessandro Schipani, and Andrew Owen

University of Liverpool, Institute of Translational Medicine, Department of Molecular and Clinical Pharmacology, 70 Pembroke Place, L69 3GE, Liverpool, UK

15.1
Introduction

The application of nanotechnology in medicine continues to proliferate, and impact in the pharmaceutical sector is expected to increase as future opportunities progress to the clinic. Numerous nanomedicine strategies have emerged as advanced approaches to enhance drug delivery and revolutionize the treatment of numerous diseases. Nanomaterials can be applied to gradually release drugs in biological fluids in order to favor drug absorption, protect drugs from degradation, and increasing the length of time for which drugs can be present in the blood circulation and tissues. Additionally, nanomaterials can be coupled with ligands for targeting their accumulation, along with the associated pharmacophore, to where they are mostly needed.

The processes that underpin nanomedicine pharmacokinetics and pharmacodynamics are not as fully characterized as conventional medicines and consequently the development of novel nanomaterials is complicated by extensive development and optimization processes based on experimental and preclinical models. The broad variety of materials used for synthesis and their potential combinations define an almost inexhaustive list of delivery strategies available for research and medical use. Polymers can be used as carriers for drug molecules either by forming solid polymer matrix nanoparticles to encapsulate drugs or through the construction of vehicles such as block copolymer liposomes/vesicles, micelles, and nanoemulsions [1]. Noncovalent or covalent conjugation of polymers to small molecules has been successfully used to increase circulatory times and favor the delivery of therapeutic agents through triggered and controlled release [2]. A wide variety of inorganic oxides have been used to create nanoparticles, such as gold [3], silver [4], silica [5], and iron [6]. However, the influence that these

Pharmaceutical Nanotechnology: Innovation and Production, First Edition. Edited by Jean Cornier, Arno Kwade, Andrew Owen, and Marcel Van de Voorde.

formulations and their characteristics have on distribution patterns, efficiency and toxicity are only partially understood.

Powerful pharmacological and toxicological tools to simulate the potential effects of small and macromolecules on biological systems are represented by computational models. These approaches constitute mathematical representations of biological processes to simulate and predict the behavior of complex systems using computer simulation and analysis. Such models can find application in the simulation of molecular, cellular, physiological, and anatomical biological processes, integrating existing knowledge with *in vitro* and preclinical data with the overall objective of generating novel hypotheses and translational predictions. Computational models have gained much traction in recent years as *in silico* tools for predicting efficacy, toxicity, and distribution for small molecules and have already been successfully used for traditional formulations during novel product development and to answer clinical questions post-licensing. Computational platforms offer the possibility to predict relevant endpoints and simulate various scenarios, providing rational selection of promising candidates. Therefore, the development process can be simplified or augmented by using *in silico* approaches that provide quantitative predictions. Additionally, post-licensing clinical scenarios can be simulated through computational models in order to optimize dosing for populations that are not commonly included in clinical trials (e.g., paediatrics), or to inform or identify improved therapeutic strategies (e.g., to overcome drug–drug interactions or aid implementation of pharmacogenetics testing). As such, *in silico* methods can facilitate development and optimization across a range of scenarios relevant to nanopharmacy (Figure 15.1).

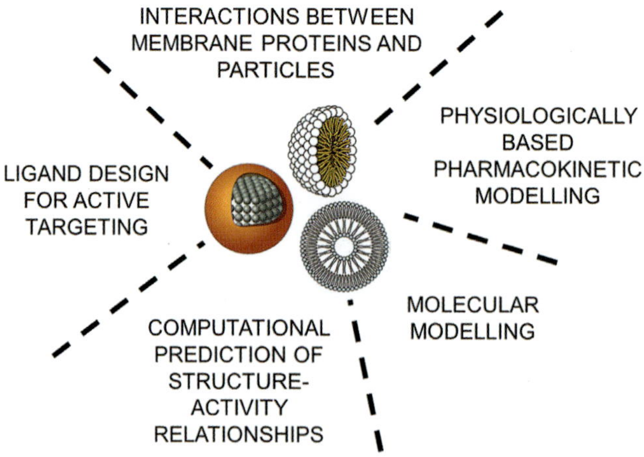

Figure 15.1 Applications of computational predictive models in the nanomedicine field.

15.2
Molecular Modeling in Nanomedicine

The use of ligands on nanoparticle surfaces can support the active targeting of therapeutic agents to specific sites of the human body, increasing the efficacy of drug delivery, and ameliorating toxicity. The selection of appropriate ligands that can effectively bind on the nanoparticle surface and determine effective targeting specificity is a complex process. Membrane proteins can be exclusively expressed on diseased cells and therefore nanoparticles can be fictionalized with ligands with high affinity targets. This approach has been explored for several pathologies such as cancer, arthritis, multiple sclerosis, and infectious diseases. As for many other types of nanomedicine studies, the design of actively targeted nanoparticles cannot be only based in traditional experimental assay but has to rely on the integration of different types of data in a predictive mathematical framework. Computer simulation and predictive models have been applied to clarify the influence of parameters of nanoparticles tethered with ligands on the targeting efficiency to identify optimal design.

The affinity of binding between ligands and target membrane proteins can be quantified with a variety of experimental approaches such as fluorescence resonance energy transfer (FRET), nuclear magnetic resonance (NMR), and surface plasmon resonance (SPR), to name a few. Design parameters such as ligand density, ligand length, ligand binding affinity, and nanoparticle shape, size, and cell surface rigidity have been recognized to influence targeting efficiency [7–10].

Monte Carlo computer simulations have been used to measure the interaction between actively targeted nanoparticles and ligands and proteins on surfaces of healthy and diseased cells. In many cases, target proteins can be also expressed at a lower level in healthy cells complicating the delivery of nanoparticles to where they are mostly needed. Targeting selectivity can be maintained through lower targeting affinity and multivalent binding that can only occur in cells with extremely high expression of the target protein. With such computational models, the design of active targeting strategies can be defined for specific applications and optimal density of targeting ligands can be informed based on the characteristics of the target cells [11]. Additionally, Monte Carlo simulations support a better understanding of the interactions between a ligand-coated nanoparticle and surface targets, informing the rational design.

Over recent decades, molecular modeling has become a fundamental component for drug discovery programmes and has the potential of finding relevant application in nanopharmacy. The molecular modeling approach is based on defining the relative positions of the atoms by a set of Cartesian coordinates. The representative 3D structure of molecules of interest is an essential element to build a rational interpretation of the relationship between the molecular structure and its biological activity and to establishquantitative structure–activity relationships (QSAR). This approach represents the starting point for the application of molecular modeling for small molecules, but can also be used to investigate more complex molecular structures such as nanoparticles and their ligands [12]. The 3D molecular structure of nanoparticles is based on the intrinsic characteristics of the nanostructure, which can be parameterized using a set of mathematical statistical models. Interactions between different molecules and structures can be simulated using molecular mechanic methods to determine bond lengths, angles, and torsions as well as nonbonded interactions [13]. The core assumption underpinning the molecular mechanic methods is that the bonds have "natural" lengths and angles. The equilibrium values of these bond lengths and bond angles and the corresponding force constants are defined in the force field.

In general, molecules are not rigid but they do have differing degrees of "rigidity," which depends upon the complexity of their structure (number of atoms, number of rotatable bonds, and intermolecular interactions). Consequently, a molecule can exist in several conformations, and the low-energy conformers (local minimums) predominate. The geometric optimization calculation is used to identify a low potential energy conformation considering the appropriate force field. This method is based on minimization algorithms with the objective of finding the conformations with the lowest potential energy, or present to the greatest extent. Some nanostructures, such as nanotubes have a comparatively rigid structure, which make them more geometrically predictable, resulting in a less computationally intense geometrical optimization. However, more flexible structures such as liposomes present greater conformational challenges. For these types of nanostructures, molecular dynamics simulation methods can be applied to identify the energetically most favored 3D structure. Molecular dynamics simulations are performed by integrating the equation of motion over a period of time for the molecular system. This method adds an essential contribution to the understanding of dynamic processes in large molecules with high degrees of freedom, at the atomic level.

The computational time required to run this type of analysis can be lengthy, thus some simplifications need to be introduced, which can perpetrate inaccuracy. Molecular mechanics calculations are often carried out under vacuum conditions, and in some cases, the explicit effect of solvent inclusion can be neglected (e.g., unipolar hydrocarbons). However, for molecules containing charge and dipoles, the effect of solvent should be considered to prevent overestimation of the electrostatic interaction by the force field. This could potentially result in imperfect molecule geometry during the energy minimization calculation due to bias toward unrealistic low-energy conformations. Most of the force fields used in molecular dynamics simulations use united atom potential energy functions, omitting the nonpolar hydrogens from the molecule, which reduce the numbers of atoms and therefore the computational time [14]. The conformational flexibility of, for example, a liposome is strongly affected by the surrounding environment, especially at the surface. Therefore, the accuracy of molecular dynamics simulations may increase when explicitly considering solvent. The effect of the solvents is a historical issue [15], and the solvent molecule can be substituted by the neutral spherical atoms, thus significantly reducing the computational effort [16].

Computational models for the investigation of interactions between drugs, nanoparticles, and molecular targets may improve the design of materials for nanopharmacy applications. Molecular docking methods can predict the predominant binding mode(s) of a small molecule with a protein, but can also be used to characterize nanoparticle binding to a ligand (Figure 15.2). Docking methods analyze high-dimensional spaces and use a scoring function that ranks candidate dockings. Molecular docking can be used to perform virtual screening on large libraries of compounds and propose structural hypotheses of how the ligands interact with the target, providing a rational approach in nanoparticle optimization [17].

Given the large number of nanoparticles that are being developed for biomedical applications, the use of computational methods in the assessment of their properties is of key importance. High-throughput biochemical screening of either diverse nanoparticle libraries or focused libraries tailored for specific

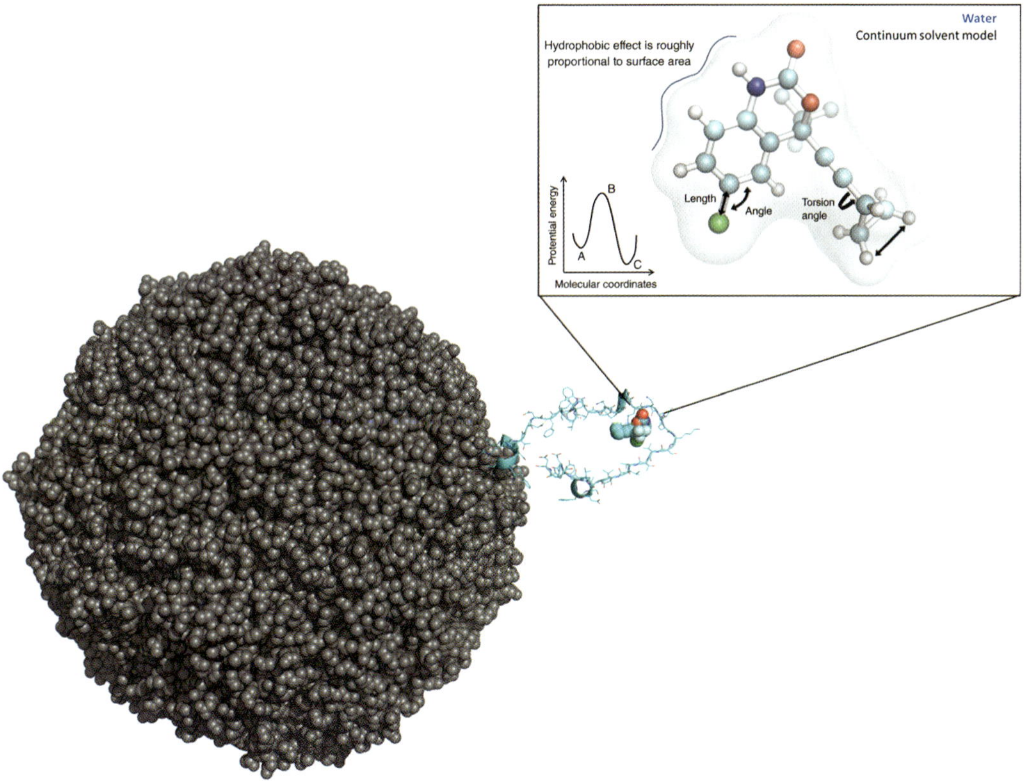

Figure 15.2 Prediction of the nanoparticle ligand–target interaction affinity using molecular docking technique.

targets can be achieved using computational modeling techniques. Among these predictive approaches, structure–activity relationship (SAR) and quantitative structure–activity relationship studies are theoretical models that relate the structure of molecules to their properties. SARs are qualitative relationships between molecular structure or substructure and the presence or absence of a biological activity. SARs can also be based on the ensemble of steric and electronic features of a molecule that define the intermolecular interaction with a target molecule. QSARs are quantitative relationships based on data analysis approaches such as multivariate linear regression, and aim to identify molecular descriptors predicting biological activity. The molecular descriptors can be the structural or physicochemical properties of the whole molecule or a functional group. For nanoparticles, this is limited by the lack of available biological data and the low number of descriptors that are optimized for representing the structural and chemical characteristics of nanoparticles [18]. An additional computational approach is presented by 3D-QSARs, which correlate the variation in biological or chemical activity with information on the 3D structure for a series of molecules. Quantum mechanical methods may also be valid tools in molecular modeling of nanoparticles. When force field parameters for a certain structure are not available, quantum chemical methods can be used for geometry optimization. The calculation of transitional states or reaction path as well as the determination of geometries influenced by polarization or unusual electron distribution in a molecule is the domain of quantum mechanical calculations, and it can be used to predict nanoparticle properties at a more mechanistic level [19].

15.3 Computational Approaches for Predicting Nanotoxicology

The large number of nanotechnologies that are being explored provides a major task in terms of toxicological characterization. As such, computational models for the rationalization of nanotoxicology may reduce the burden on time-consuming toxicological studies that require complex *in vitro* and *in vivo* experimental approaches. It should however be recognized that ultimate ratification of a medicines safety will always require empirical evaluation.

Nanotoxicological studies are complex and holistic predictors of toxicity for nanoparticles have not been identified. However, the role of specific structures in the definition and modulation of adverse effects is increasingly clear [20]. Multiple nanoparticle characteristics can interplay in the definition of toxicity and define multifactorial scenarios that can complicate safety investigations. Size and shape of nanomaterials have been correlated with toxicity and different types of molecular mechanisms can be involved in the generation of side effects. Nanomaterials are intrinsically characterized by the high surface area to mass ratio that profoundly increases the area of the material that is in contact with the surrounding biological environment. The increased surface area has been investigated in the context of inflammatory processes and significant proinflammatory effects have been correlated with surface area for a variety of nanomaterials [21]. Carbon nanotubules structured as long fibers can induce inflammation more effectively that nanotubes with different shapes, such as nonfibrous bundled aggregates [22]. Surface charge can influence the electrostatic interaction between nanomaterials and the molecular and cellular targets for toxicological and other pharmacodynamic effects. This is additionally modulated by surface coating of nanomaterials or biological endogenous molecules that adhere to their surface during or following absorption. The structure–toxicity relationships are highly multifactorial and can vary between different materials. Therefore, the generation of predictive computational models such as quantitative nanostructure–toxicity relationship (QNTR) requires the integration of various types of data and collaborative interdisciplinary efforts involving chemists, pharmacologists, and toxicologists.

For QNTR, physicochemical and structural characteristics of nanomaterials are initially described mathematically to obtained descriptors, including shape, size, surface area, functional groups, zeta potential, polydispersity index, lipophilicity, and stability. To acquire essential information for the development of QNTR models, effective *in vitro* high-throughput screening methods are required. These experimental methods provide a quantitative measure of dose- and time-dependent cellular injury that underpins adverse reaction *in vivo*. It should be noted therefore that a prerequisite for this and other types of modeling is the presence of robust *in vitro* methods for prediction of *in vivo* behavior. Moreover, a quantitative description of the toxicity is required to establish potential relationships, which can be identified using statistical models (e.g., linear or nonlinear regression analysis) or machine learning methods (i.e., neural networks) [23]. The final step in model development is a validation, through which the robustness of the QNTR and its ability to predict toxicity is evaluated by statistical cross-validation techniques (i.e., use of the model to accurately predict behavior of other nanomaterials).

Such methodological approaches have been traditionally used for small molecules but QNTR methods have only recently been applied to nanomaterials. Recent studies have highlighted the possibility to identify predictors or toxicity across different types of nanomaterials as well as different organisms [24]. A rational evaluation of the mechanisms regulating the various types of toxicity can favor an optimized development of predictive models. Mechanism-based high-throughput experimental screening strategies have been applied to inform prediction of the nanomaterial properties that are associated with potentially negative outcomes *in vivo* [25]. This approach was based on a well-characterized library of nanomaterials, including metals, metal oxides, carbon and nanotubes, and various silica-based nanoparticles. The large library allowed the introduction of characteristics in combination and the variation of specific properties to better characterize their potential effect. High-throughput screening methods were then applied to describe cellular toxicities such as mitochondrial damage, reactive oxygen species (ROS) generation, cellular apoptosis, red blood cell

(RBC) lysis, cell growth/proliferation, and various assessments of inflammation. Limited but critical validation studies were then carried out in animals to validate the high-throughput screening. The combination of *in vitro* and *in vivo* data was subsequently used to identify structure–toxicity relationships, establishing predictive toxicology paradigms [25].

Although QNTR approaches can effectively be used to identify nanomaterial characteristics associated with side effects, safety in humans (and other organisms) is strictly influenced by exposure and distribution, and this cannot always be robustly captured within the *in vitro* environment. Nanomaterial distribution into key organs is extremely relevant in this context (see Section 15.4.2) and has not to date been incorporated into such predictive toxicological studies. Nanomaterials can accumulate in specific tissues and cell populations, therefore exacerbating their potential to cause toxicity in a cell- or tissue-specific manner. Additionally, chronic exposure to nanomaterials has the potential to generate negative outcomes *in vivo* that are not effectively captured by assays or animal studies based on a single-step toxicological exposure. This is particularly important in the context that certain nanomaterials are known to accumulate during multiple dosing [26]. More refined experimental *in vitro* assays combined with comprehensive systems biology approaches could help to improve characterization of toxicological effects supporting the development of QNTR models in the future.

15.4 Simulation of Nanoparticle Pharmacokinetics

As discussed above, toxicity and efficacy are profoundly affected by nanoparticle distribution and the appropriateness of existing regulation for nanomedicines has been the subject of significant recent debate, as discussed elsewhere in this book. Consequently, understanding the interactions between nanomaterials and the human body is of great importance for efficient development of safe and effective new drug delivery systems.

Numerous processes define the disposition of nanoparticles and the absorption, distribution, metabolism, and elimination (ADME) of nanomaterials can differ substantially from traditional small-molecule medicines. In most cases, nanomaterial ADME is not fully characterized and can vary based on the characteristics of the nanoparticles (Figure 15.3).

15.4.1 Nanoparticle Absorption

Some nanomedicines aim to favor the absorption of drugs through release in the intestinal lumen in a controlled manner, which reduces solubility issues through enhanced dissolution. The intestinal wall acts as a selective barrier to pathogens and macromolecules, and consequently direct absorption of nanoparticulates

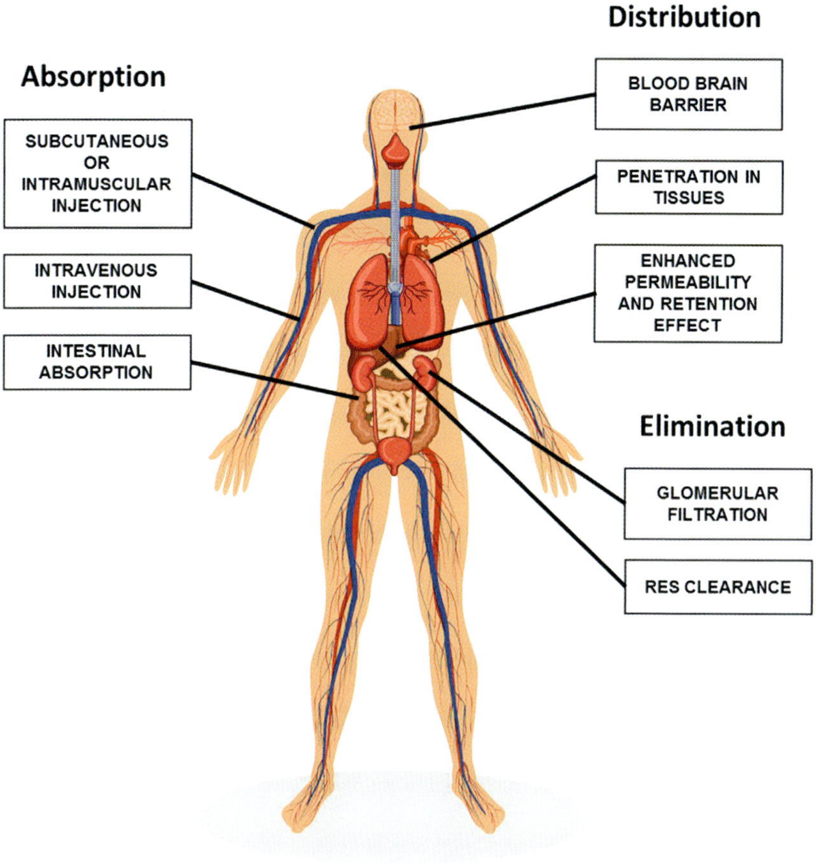

Figure 15.3 Molecular and physiological processes defining nanoparticle distribution in the human body.

can be complicated. Small molecules can be absorbed by partitioning into the lipid bilayers and crossing the intestinal epithelial cells by passive diffusion or actively via transporters. However, nanomaterial absorption may be more complicated due to the intrinsic anatomy and physiology of the intestinal barrier. The transport of nanomaterials across the intestine can be mediated by numerous processes, including binding to the cell surface, endocytosis, phagocytosis, intracellular trafficking, and exocytosis, resulting in transcytosis with the involvement of multiple subcellular structures. An additional relevant process is paracytosis, during which nanomaterials move between cells through opened tight junctions [27,28]. Certain lipid-based nanomedicines have been demonstrated to deliver drugs via the lymph after oral administration [29,30]), potentially enabling circumvention of the hepatic portal vein with resultant avoidance of first-pass metabolism in the liver. Clathrin- and caveolae-mediated endocytosis and macropinocytosis are common mechanisms of nanomaterial absorption through the intestinal wall, although heterogeneity in the efficiency of absorption processes has been described for different nanomaterials. Consequently, it is difficult to identify a predominant process determining permeation of nanomaterials [31–33] and, for many materials, multiple processes are likely to play a role.

Several nanomaterials are not efficiently absorbed through the oral route, and other strategies have been explored to deliver nanoparticles, providing specific benefits such as direct targeting to the desired site of action [34] or an extended period of drug action [35]. Although the administration through the skin is complicated by its impermeable nature [36,37], transdermal administration has been explored for nanomaterials such as solid lipid nanoparticles and nanoemulsions. These materials are characterized by good biocompatibility, lower cytotoxicity, and desirable drug release modulation [38–40]. Ocular nanomedicine delivery provides a useful route of administration for the treatment of morbidities of the eye, but multiple anatomical barriers can limit the application of this route of administration [41]. Nasal administration represents a valuable option to favor penetration of drugs and nanoparticles into the CNS and brain as described for chitosan nanoparticles of tizanidine [34]. An additional route of administration is presented by inhalation into the lungs due to the large surface area, ease of access and the thinness of the air–blood barrier. Particle size is a major factor determining the diffusion of nanomaterials in the bronchial tree, with particles in the nanosized region more likely to reach the alveolar region and particles with diameters between 1 and 5 μm expected to deposit in the bronchial alveoli [42,43]. Particles can gradually release drug, which can subsequently distribute systemically, or alternatively the particles can be phagocyted by alveolar macrophages [44]. Different types of nanomaterials are characterized by limited permeation through biological membranes and anatomical barriers. Consequently, in order to reach the systemic or local circulation, intravenous administration can be the preferred route [45].

15.4.2 Nanoparticle Distribution

Following absorption, the distribution of nanomaterials can vary widely depending on the delivery system used, the characteristics of the nanomaterial, and potentially the variability between individuals (organ size, body-fat index, etc.). The stability of the nanoparticles can influence the distribution patterns, as the physicochemical characteristics of the free drug and the nanomaterial differ greatly. Several nanotechnologies remain structurally stable during the absorption process, therefore presenting intact nanoparticles in the systemic circulation and therefore altering the distribution and clearance of the drug payload. Once the nanomaterials reach the systemic circulation, numerous proteins can adhere on the surface of the nanoparticles defining a dynamic protein corona [46,47]. Size and physicochemical properties of the nanomaterials are influenced by the protein corona, affecting processes such as nanomaterial degradation, cellular uptake [48], accumulation, and penetration through the capillary fenestrations [49]. Nanoparticles can accumulate in defined cell populations and diffuse into tissues and organs through specific processes, such as the enhanced permeability and retention effect. Biological barriers can limit the penetration of nanoparticles in organs, and the blood–brain barrier (BBB) represents an obstacle for many therapeutic agents and nanomaterials [50].

15.4.3 Nanoparticle Elimination

The elimination of nanoparticles is also mediated by a broad range of mechanisms in different tissues, from chemical and enzymatic degradation to renal and biliary elimination. Nanomaterials can be degraded in tissues or blood, gradually releasing their components. The immune system plays a pivotal role in the elimination of foreign elements from the body, including not only pathogens but also nanomaterials. Cells with phagocytic activities (e.g., macrophages) frequently define nanoparticle uptake, accumulation, and clearance. Macrophages in the liver (Kupffer cells), spleen, and lungs are a major pool of the total macrophages in the body and can effectively phagocytose nanomaterials, mediating their accumulation in these organs [51,52]. Renal elimination is another relevant mechanism defining nanomaterial excretion, considering that the glomerular endothelium is characterized by fenestrations of 50–100 nm, with capillaries having a basement membrane (300 nm thickness) as well as podocytes with phagocytic function.

15.4.4 Physiologically Based Pharmacokinetic Models (PBPK)

Physiologically based pharmacokinetic (PBPK) modeling is emerging as a powerful pharmacological tool to simulate the distribution of drugs and nanomaterials. This approach has gained much traction in recent years as an *in silico* platform for predicting pharmacokinetics *in vivo* and has already been successfully used for traditional formulations and small molecules during drug development, or to answer clinical questions postlicensing. PBPK modeling combines mathematical equations to describe the anatomical, physiological, and molecular processes regulating pharmacokinetics, with *in vitro* data to simulate and predict ADME of conventional and nanoenabled medicines (Figure 15.4).

In PBPK models, anatomically meaningful compartments are defined, which integrate specific properties of a given organ or tissue (i.e., blood flow, mass, and permeation limits) with medicine characteristics, to create a mathematical representation of the human body. Mathematical equations are applied to describe the processes defining pharmacokinetics, such as tablet dissolution rate following administration, renal clearance, actions of drug transporters, gastrointestinal pH, phase I and phase II metabolism, and numerous other biological mechanisms. In addition, mathematical equations are being used to describe ADME by taking into account the physicochemical properties,

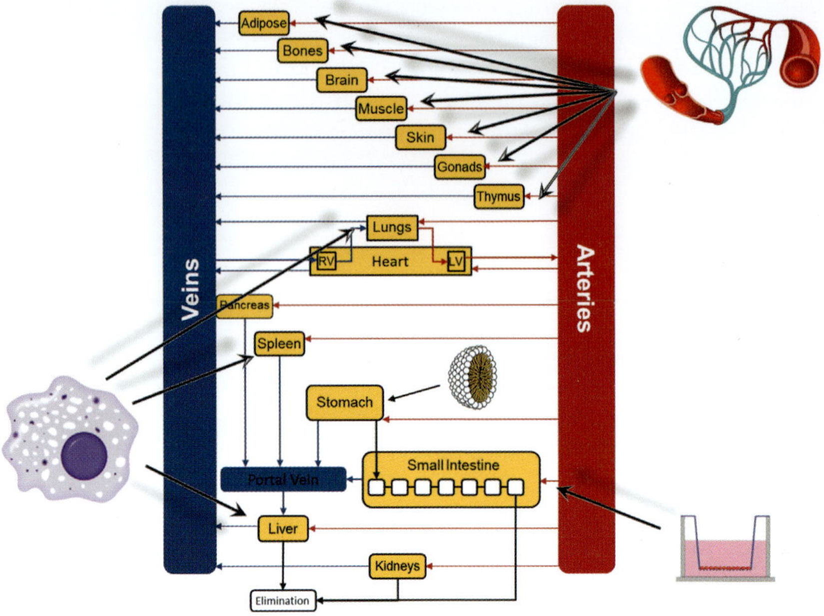

Figure 15.4 Graphical representation of a PBPK model for the simulation and prediction of nanoparticles. Each arrow represents a differential equation describing the movement of nanoparticles through compartments. Experimental data from *in vitro* assay can be integrated to simulate key ADME processes.

transmembrane permeability, metabolizing, and transporting substrate specificity of the investigated drug.

Nanomaterials can have dramatically different ADME properties to small molecules and traditional formulations, drug elimination in PBPK models for small molecules is simulated taking into account the role of the liver, kidneys, and gut metabolism. However, the clearance of nanomedicines can be more complicated, where multiple and parallel alternative tissues are also capable of elimination. The elimination of nanomedicines can mean the excretion of intact nanomaterials from the body but also the degradation of nanomaterials (and subsequent release of drug) in plasma, tissues, and organs. Potential elimination sites may include the reticuloendothelial system [53], tissues with specific pH [54], and compartments within cells [55] as well as other sites. New elimination mechanisms may become important in traditional organs of clearance, for example, the destruction of nanoparticles by Kupffer cells in the liver [56]. For nanomedicines that ultimately release their therapeutic payload, the conventional mechanisms for small-molecule ADME need to be considered in parallel for the released drug. Consequently, the design of PBPK models for nanomedicines should include specific algorithms and novel modeling strategies that describe these processes in a technology-specific manner. A better mechanistic understanding of the molecular, anatomical, and physiological events that define nanoparticle distribution is required, and will serve to have a beneficial impact on development of novel nanoparticle assessment strategies.

Importantly, all ADME processes are highly variable between individuals and a major strength of PBPK modeling is that virtual patients can be simulated considering known population variability in specific anatomical and physiological factors. Variability in organ size and other anatomical factors have been correlated with demographic and anthropometric variables [57–59], and multifactorial equations have been developed to generate anatomical and physiological parameters and their interindividual variability. This set of equations constitutes an essential component of PBPK approaches and serves to correctly capture the variability present in a predefined population. Through this approach it is possible to generate a virtual (but realistic) description of anatomical characteristics of patients and therefore obtain a representative evaluation of the variability in populations. This characteristic, as well as numerous others, makes PBPK modeling particularly suitable for the discovery and optimization of therapeutic agents, which often show tissue-specific activity and nonlinear concentration–efficacy relationships.

15.4.5
Integration of Experimental Data in PBPK Models

All the aforementioned biological mechanisms defining nanoparticle disposition have been described through experimental approaches *in vitro* or *in vivo*. These findings represent useful resources to evaluate the disposition process and can be integrated in computational predictive approaches to simulate pharmacokinetics of nanomedicines in virtual patients (or preclinical species). To describe the drug release from the nanomaterial, *in vitro* assays can be used to analyze nanomaterial breakdown dynamics in biological fluids using dialysis [60]. The absorption of nanomaterials through skin or other barriers can be clarified through different experimental approaches [61]. Phagocytic and endocytic uptake by populations of cells can be experimentally investigated using primary cells or optimized cell lines, providing a quantitative evaluation of nanoparticle uptake and accumulation.

15.4.6
Examples of PBPK Models

The authors have been directly involved in development and optimization of PBPK modeling approaches for small molecules, simulating relevant clinical scenarios such as drug–drug interactions, dose personalization, and adjustment for special populations [62–66], and have also recently developed models for predicting the pharmacokinetics or distribution of nanomedicine candidates [67–69]. Recently, we described innovative PBPK models to inform the development of long-acting injectable nanomedicines for antiretroviral drugs, providing a quantitative prediction of optimal dose and formulation characteristics across a panel of commonly prescribed drugs [69]. Additionally, we described a PBPK model for predicting distribution of superparamagnetic iron oxide nanoparticles (SPIONs) in animals and humans, providing a quantitative estimate of nanoparticle diffusion and accumulation in tissues and organs [68].

Although a limited number of PBPK models for nanoparticles have so far been developed (Table 15.1), this computational technique may have an important beneficial impact on the development of novel technologies. The studies to date for different types of nanomaterials and their main characteristics are summarized below. The first publication describing a PBPK model for a nanomaterial was published in 2008, aiming to predict the distribution of quantum dots, considering a distribution coefficient to simulate the diffusion of nanoparticles into tissues. The PBPK model was subsequently compared against preclinical data to evaluate the precision of the predictions [70]. An additional PBPK model for quantum dot pharmacokinetics was subsequently developed, integrating experimental *in vitro* and *in vivo* data from multiple sources [71]. Tissue-to-plasma coefficient values were extrapolated from experimental rat data and pharmacokinetics was simulated with a simplified PBPK model. Prediction of nanoparticle penetration into tissues was suboptimal (especially in the first hours) potentially due to the low number of compartments included in the simulation and a limited description of quantum dot metabolism and elimination. Inhaled carbon nanoparticle distribution has also been simulated through PBPK modeling, integrating imaging data collected in humans using 99m-technetium-labeled nanoparticles [72]. Twenty-four tissue compartments were included in the model, although the lymphatic circulatory system was absent. This publication successfully included several factors that are likely to be relevant to nanomedicine pharmacokinetics, such as particle size-related effects on tissue distribution and postdose degradation of nanoparticles.

The pharmacokinetics of silver nanoparticles has been simulated considering the correlation between particle sizes, accumulation in tissue, and potential health risks for humans. Animal experimental data could not be accurately simulated, possibly due to the effect of other uncaptured nanoparticle characteristics such as surface charge and coating [73]. Five PLGA nanomaterials were also investigated through PBPK modeling, characterizing the relationship between nanoparticle properties (size, zeta potential, and density of PEG molecules per unit surface area) and distribution parameters. Subsequently, this semimechanistic model was successfully utilized to predict the distribution of a sixth nanoparticle (PLGA-mPEG 495) in mice [74], emphasizing the predictive potential of PBPK modeling. The pharmacokinetics of gold dendrimer composite nanomaterials in mice with melanoma was also simulated, describing how charge and size influenced their distribution [75]. Additionally, a PBPK model for ionic silver and nanoencaspulated silver was used to reproduce exposure conditions (dermal, oral, and inhalation) of *in vivo* experiments and compared simulated with real pharmacokinetic data for plasma and tissues. The PBPK model was also used to assess relevant routes of exposure, such as dietary intake, use of three

Table 15.1 Relevant example of PBPK models or nanomaterials.

Material composition	Size	Validation	Key findings	Refs
Quantum dots	20 nm	mice (single dose)	Key PBPK parameters are derived from animal data. Predictive capability for the time-dependent kinetic and distributional changes of QD705 in tissues.	[69]
Quantum dots	7–80 nm	Mice and rats (different doses)	Partition coefficients estimated from quantum dot biodistribution. The PBPK model predicted the experimentally observed persistence of QDs in tissues but not early time profiles.	[70]
Technetium-labeled carbon nanoparticles	5–10 nm	Human clinical data previously published	The PBPK model is the first model able to use imaging data to describe the absorption and distribution of nanoparticles.	[71]
Silver nanoparticles	20, 80, and 110 nm	Rats, both single and repeated injection	Model parameters were derived by fitting to animal data. No clear relation between parameter values and corresponding particle diameters became apparent.	[72]
Five poly(lactic-*co*-glycolic) acid (PLGA) nanoparticles	57–133 nm	Mice (single dose)	The developed model adequately simulates the experimental data indicating that the model is suitable for description of PLGA-mPEG nanoparticle biodistribution.	[73]
Five gold/dendrimer composite nanodevices (CNDs)	5–22 nm	Mice (single dose)	Model parameter values were fitted to the animal data. size and charge of nanodevices could explain the observed variability.	[74]
Solid drug nanoparticle (SDN)	n/a	Existing traditional formulation distribution data in humans	Simulation of the pharmacokinetics resulting from the intramuscular injection of SDN of antiretrovirals	[68]
Ionic silver and nanoencaspulated silver	15–150 nm	Experimentally assessed organ concentrations from previous publications	Various exposure conditions were simulated to provide a estimation of silver accumulation in different organs.	[75]
Superparamagnetic iron oxide nanoparticles (SPIONs)	21 nm	Mice (different doses)	Key input paramenters are derived from novel experimental approaches. The PBPK model provided a quantitative prediction of SPIONs in organs in mice and humans.	[67]
Dexamethasone fluorescently labeled nanoparticles	n/a	Mice (single dose)	Decrease of nanoparticles from plasma with concomitant increase in the liver, spleen, and kidneys before decaying at longer timepoints.	[76]

separate consumer products, and occupational contact [76]. Finally, fluorescently labeled nanoparticles for the controlled delivery of dexamethasone were investigated using PBPK and the simulated data showed concentrations in plasma decreased rapidly with a spike in nanoparticle concentration in the liver, spleen, and kidneys [77].

15.4.7 Limitations of the PBPK Approach

Several limitations related to PBPK model design have the potential of reducing the precision and accuracy of prediction. The mechanisms defining the distribution of nanoparticles are only partially characterized and a better understanding of the nanoparticle ADME is essential to define computational strategies for robust PBPK models. PBPK model development should consider specific nanomaterial characteristics, and novel modeling strategies are essential. Additionally, data generated through experimental investigations need to be integrated into the mathematical framework representing distribution, and novel algorithms are therefore required to correctly integrate experimental data within the simulations. The distribution of small molecules is traditionally integrated by deriving blood-to-tissue ratios of free drug from physicochemical properties [78], but this strategy is not suitable for nanomaterials. Permeability through capillary fenestration and active mechanisms such as endo and phagocytosis need to be implemented as mechanistic structures within models to define a quantitative evaluation of nanoparticle accumulation in tissues. Due to the propensity of traditional formulations and small molecules to distribute through the blood circulation, PBPK models do not routinely consider the lymphatic system. Conversely, the disposition of numerous nanomaterials has been described to be mediated by the lymphatic system [79,80] and a better evaluation is therefore highly desirable. The metabolism and elimination of small molecules is usually simulated considering enzymatic reactions, involving the phase I phase II enzymes in the liver or other tissues in conjunction with renal excretion. For nanomaterials, multiple alternative mechanisms in numerous tissues can be involved in the elimination process defining a more complicated scenario. Nanoparticles can be removed as intact structures or be gradually degraded with subsequent release of drugs in plasma, tissues, and organs, and the mechanism that prevails is highly composition-dependent requiring empirical determination. Sites of elimination include the reticuloendothelial system [53], tissues with specific pH [54], the kidney, and compartments within cells [55,81].

15.4.8 Future Perspective of PBPK Modeling

By providing an estimation of the expected pharmacokinetics and distribution in humans or in preclinical species, PBPK models can support the optimization of the development process, identifying nanomaterials with pharmacological potential. However, modeling approaches for nanopharmacy applications are currently in their infancy and the processes regulating pharmacokinetics and distribution of nanoparticles are known to be different. PBPK models can assist in answering questions that cannot otherwise be examined using only experimental and preclinical models. They provide the opportunity for rational design of nanomedicines, identifying strategies to maximize the efficacy and safety of novel technologies. A mechanistic understanding of the molecular and physiological events that define nanoparticle distribution can have a beneficial impact on development of novel nanoparticle assessment strategies.

Polymers, surfactants, or other excipients used in the synthesis of nanomaterials can have a potential effect on expression and activity of key proteins regulating the disposition of drugs or nanoparticles [82]. Current PBPK strategies do not include a mechanistic description of excipient distribution and their effect on such processes. The inclusion of these elements is particularly relevant when the pharmacokinetics of the nanoparticles and the encapsulated drug is influenced by the effected enzymes. Such computational strategies have been applied for small molecules where inhibition and induction mechanisms for metabolism enzymes [83–85] and drug transporters [86] are included in the models. Existing PBPK models for nanomaterials are based upon data obtained from animals as surrogates for mechanistic descriptions of nanoparticle distribution, and therefore a quantitative platform to derive key variables. This approach can be complicated by the poor understanding of how nanomedicine distribution data differ between animals and humans. Membrane pore sizes as well as endocytic and phagocytic activity in key tissues can differ between species and it is therefore essential that the predictive models are not only based on animal data but take into account species differences.

The successful application of PBPK approaches for nanopharmacy is strictly dependent on the integration of a wide range of data from various scientific disciplines. Information from polymer synthesis, materials chemistry, molecular and clinical pharmacology, and mathematical modeling should be combined to define a comprehensive understanding of nanomaterial distribution and, derisk the design of novel nanomedicines.

15.5 Conclusion

Computational approaches aim to provide reliable and quantitative predictions for relevant pharmacological properties of novel and existing therapeutic agents, including nanoparticle-based medicines. Traditional pharmacological and biological approaches can find successful application for the description and quantification of specific pharmacological and biological mechanisms but lack predictive power. Through a rational integration of existing knowledge and experimental data, computational approaches can offer the possibility to not only describe key mechanisms regulating relevant pharmacokinetics and pharmacodynamics of nanomedicines but also provide quantitative predictions, and thereby place individual mechanisms in whole-body context.

However, more work is required to realize the potential of computational approaches in nanopharmacy, and the authors are playing an active role in two initiatives that should help address some of the current gaps in knowledge. First, the U.S. National Institutes of Health (NIH) recently funded the Long Acting/Extended Release Resource Program (LEAP; www.longactinghiv.org), which has a PBPK modeling core at the heart of its ambition. The LEAP modeling core will be available as a resource to stake holders actively involved in the development of long-acting nanomaterials for infectious diseases. Second, the European Commission recently funded the European Nanomedicine Characterization Laboratory (EU-NCL; www.euncl.eu) to provide a trans-European infrastructure, providing materials characterization to developers to help facilitate nanomedicine translation. The EU-NCL will address structure–activity relationships for nanomaterials that will help fill some of the knowledge gaps relating to nanoparticle–biological interactions.

The accuracy and precision of models can often be limited and comprehensive strategies of validation should be implemented to have a better understanding of model limitations. Poor modeling performance is usually caused by incorrect underlying assumptions or poor underpinning experimental data. As well as simplifying the drug development process, allowing the accelerated design and prediction of nanoparticle distribution, efficacy and toxicity in humans or in preclinical species, computational modeling has the potential to dramatically reduce the number of animals needed during preclinical development [87]. Thus, validated nanospecific computational modeling approaches represent a pivotal advancement for refining, replacing and reducing the use of preclinical species during development programmes, as has been achieved for conventional medicines.

The integration of different computational techniques in future nanopharmacy programmes could greatly simplify the selection of valuable candidates. This process can allow multiple models to be adopted to address the needs of investigators, considering data from different fields in a holistic vision of the development process. As described, computational models have been successfully applied in the optimization of ligands, evaluation of distribution, prediction of toxicity, and clarification of molecular structure. These tools can support a more detailed understanding of mechanisms regulating nanoparticle disposition, toxicity, and efficacy to favor a rational development process. By ensuring iteration between manufacturing, *in vitro* and *in vivo* approaches toward the selection of optimal drug delivery candidates, computational models can accelerate new material platforms toward therapeutic benefits in a more efficient manner than conventional experimental approaches alone. Moreover, the developed mathematical models can find application in regulatory science, to address clinical pharmacology regulatory questions for the approval of novel nanomaterials. Thus, computational modeling has a wide spectrum of potential impact for nanopharmacy, with expected benefits for academia to industry, clinician to patient and manufacturer to regulatory agency.

References

1 Wischke, C. and Schwendeman, S.P. (2008) Principles of encapsulating hydrophobic drugs in PLA/PLGA microparticles. *Int. J. Pharm.*, **364** (2), 298–327.

2 Joralemon, M.J., McRae, S., and Emrick, T. (2010) PEGylated polymers for medicine: from conjugation to self-assembled systems. *Chem. Commun. (Camb.)*, **46** (9), 1377–1393.

3 Thakor, A.S., Jokerst, J., Zavaleta, C., Massoud, T.F., and Gambhir, S.S. (2011) Gold nanoparticles: a revival in precious metal administration to patients. *Nano Lett.*, **11** (10), 4029–4036.

4 Ong, C., Lim, J.Z., Ng, C.T., Li, J.J., Yung, L.Y., and Bay, B.H. (2013) Silver nanoparticles in cancer: therapeutic efficacy and toxicity. *Curr. Med. Chem.*, **20** (6), 772–781.

5 Wu, X., Wu, M., and Zhao, J.X. (2014) Recent development of silica nanoparticles as delivery vectors for cancer imaging and therapy. *Nanomedicine*, **10** (2), 297–312.

6 Ittrich, H., Peldschus, K., Raabe, N., Kaul, M., and Adam, G. (2013) Superparamagnetic iron oxide nanoparticles in biomedicine: applications and developments in diagnostics and therapy. *Rofo*, **185** (12), 1149–1166.

7 Moore, N.W. and Kuhl, T.L. (2006) The role of flexible tethers in multiple ligand-receptor bond formation between curved surfaces. *Biophys. J.*, **91** (5), 1675–1687.

8 Hagy, M.C., Wang, S., and Dormidontova, E.E. (2008) Optimization of functionalized polymer layers for specific targeting of mobile receptors on cell surfaces. *Langmuir*, **24** (22), 13037–13047.

9 Liu, J., Weller, G.E., Zern, B., Ayyaswamy, P.S., Eckmann, D.M., Muzykantov, V.R., and Radhakrishnan, R. (2010) Computational model for nanocarrier binding to endothelium validated using *in vivo*, *in vitro*, and atomic force microscopy experiments. *Proc. Natl. Acad. Sci. USA*, **107** (38), 16530–16535.

10 Wang, S. and Dormidontova, E.E. (2010) Nanoparticle design optimization for enhanced targeting: Monte Carlo simulations. *Biomacromolecules*, **11** (7), 1785–1795.

11 Duncan, G.A. and Bevan, M.A. (2015) Computational design of nanoparticle drug delivery systems for selective targeting. *Nanoscale*, **7** (37), 15332–15340.

12 Kumar, P., Khan, R.A., Choonara, Y.E., and Pillay, V. (2013) A prospective overview of the essential requirements in molecular modeling for nanomedicine design. *Future Med. Chem.*, **5** (8), 929–946.

13 Wu, J.S., Lin, S.Y., Liao, F.Y., Hsiao, W.C., Lee, L.C., Peng, Y.H., Hsieh, C.L., Wu, M.H., Song, J.S., Yueh, A., Chen, C.H., Yeh, S.H., Liu, C.Y., Lin, S.Y., Yeh, T.K., Hsu, J.T., Shih, C., Ueng, S.H., Hung, M.S., and Wu, S.Y. (2015) Identification of substituted naphthotriazolediones as novel tryptophan 2,3-Dioxygenase (TDO) inhibitors through structure-based virtual screening. *J. Med. Chem.*, **58** (19), 7807–7819.

14 Jorgensen, W.L. and Schyman, P. (2012) Treatment of halogen bonding in the OPLS-AA force field: application to potent anti-HIV agents. *J. Chem. Theory Comput.*, **8** (10), 3895–3801.

15 Lee, B. and Richards, F.M. (1971) The interpretation of protein structures: estimation of static accessibility. *J. Mol. Biol.*, **55** (3), 379–400.

16 Connolly, M.L. (1983) Solvent-accessible surfaces of proteins and nucleic acids. *Science*, **221** (4612), 709–713.

17 Javkhlantugs, N., Bayar, H., Ganzorig, C., and Ueda, K. (2013) Computational study on the interactions and orientation of monoclonal human immunoglobulin G on a polystyrene surface. *Int. J. Nanomedicine.*, **8**, 2487–2496.

18 Poater, A., Saliner, A.G., Carbo-Dorca, R., Poater, J., Sola, M., Cavallo, L., and Worth, A.P. (2009) Modeling the structure-property relationships of nanoneedles: a journey toward nanomedicine. *J. Comput. Chem.*, **30** (2), 275–284.

19 Jayabharathi, J., Ramanathan, P., Karunakaran, C., and Thanikachalam, V. (2015) Site specific interaction between TiO_2 nanoparticles and phenanthrimidazole – a first principles quantum mechanical study. *J. Fluoresc.*, **25** (4), 1063–1083.

20 Shvedova, A.A., Kagan, V.E., and Fadeel, B. (2010) Close encounters of the small kind: adverse effects of man-made materials interfacing with the nano-cosmos of biological systems. *Annu. Rev. Pharmacol. Toxicol.*, **50**, 63–88.

21 Monteiller, C., Tran, L., MacNee, W., Faux, S., Jones, A., Miller, B., and Donaldson, K. (2007) The pro-inflammatory effects of low-toxicity low-solubility particles, nanoparticles and fine particles, on epithelial cells *in vitro*: the role of surface area. *Occup. Environ. Med.*, **64** (9), 609–615.

22 Osmond-McLeod, M.J., Poland, C.A., Murphy, F., Waddington, L., Morris, H., Hawkins, S.C., Clark, S., Aitken, R., McCall, M.J., and Donaldson, K. (2011) Durability and inflammogenic impact of carbon nanotubes compared with asbestos fibres. *Part. Fibre Toxicol.*, **8**, 15.

23 Burden, F.R. and Winkler, D.A. (1999) Robust QSAR models using Bayesian regularized neural networks. *J. Med. Chem.*, **42** (16), 3183–3187.

24 Kleandrova, V.V., Luan, F., Gonzalez-Diaz, H., Ruso, J.M., Speck-Planche, A., and Cordeiro, M.N. (2014) Computational tool for risk assessment of nanomaterials: novel QSTR-perturbation model for simultaneous prediction of ecotoxicity and cytotoxicity of uncoated and coated nanoparticles under multiple experimental conditions. *Environ. Sci. Technol.*, **48** (24), 14686–14694.

25 Nel, A., Xia, T., Meng, H., Wang, X., Lin, S., Ji, Z., and Zhang, H. (2013) Nanomaterial toxicity testing in the 21st century: use of a predictive toxicological approach and high-throughput screening. *Acc. Chem. Res.*, **46** (3), 607–621.

26 Puvanakrishnan, P., Park, J., Chatterjee, D., Krishnan, S., and Tunnell, J.W. (2012) *In vivo* tumor targeting of gold nanoparticles: effect of particle type and dosing strategy. *Int. J. Nanomed.*, **7**, 1251–1258.

27 Tuma, P. and Hubbard, A.L. (2003) Transcytosis: crossing cellular barriers. *Physiol. Rev.*, **83** (3), 871–932.

28 Tatham, L.M., Rannard, S.P., and Owen, A. (2015) Nanoformulation strategies for the enhanced oral bioavailability of antiretroviral therapeutics. *Ther. Deliv.*, **6** (4), 469–490.

29 Ling, S.S., Magosso, E., Khan, N.A., Yuen, K.H., and Barker, S.A. (2006) Enhanced oral bioavailability and intestinal lymphatic transport of a hydrophilic drug using liposomes. *Drug Dev. Ind. Pharm.*, **32** (3), 335–345.

30 Paliwal, R., Paliwal, S.R., Mishra, N., Mehta, A., and Vyas, S.P. (2009) Engineered chylomicron mimicking carrier emulsome for lymph targeted oral delivery of methotrexate. *Int. J. Pharm.*, **380** (1–2), 181–188.

31 Hillaireau, H. and Couvreur, P. (2009) Nanocarriers' entry into the cell: relevance to drug delivery. *Cell Mol. Life Sci.*, **66** (17), 2873–2896.

32 Smith, P.J., Giroud, M., Wiggins, H.L., Gower, F., Thorley, J.A., Stolpe, B., Mazzolini, J., Dyson, R.J., and Rappoport, J.Z. (2012) Cellular entry of nanoparticles via serum sensitive clathrin-mediated endocytosis, and plasma membrane permeabilization. *Int. J. Nanomed.*, **7**, 2045–2055.

33 He, B., Lin, P., Jia, Z.R., Du, W.W., Qu, W., Yuan, L., Dai, W.B., Zhang, H., Wang, X.Q., Wang, J.C., Zhang, X., and Zhang, Q. (2013) The transport mechanisms of polymer nanoparticles in Caco-2 epithelial cells. *Biomaterials*, **34** (25), 6082–6098.

34 Patel, D., Naik, S., and Misra, A. (2012) Improved transnasal transport and brain uptake of tizanidine HCl-loaded thiolated chitosan nanoparticles for alleviation of pain. *J. Pharm. Sci.*, **101** (2), 690–706.

35 van't Klooster, G., Hoeben, E., Borghys, H., Looszova, A., Bouche, M.P., van Velsen, F., and Baert, L. (2010) Pharmacokinetics and

disposition of rilpivirine (TMC278) nanosuspension as a long-acting injectable antiretroviral formulation. *Antimicrob. Agents Chemother.*, **54** (5), 2042–2050.

36 Menon, G.K., Cleary, G.W., and Lane, M.E. (2012) The structure and function of the stratum corneum. *Int. J. Pharm.*, **435** (1), 3–9.

37 Rehman, K. and Zulfakar, M.H. (2013) Recent advances in gel technologies for topical and transdermal drug delivery. *Drug Dev. Ind. Pharm.*, **40** (4), 433–440.

38 Cappel, M.J. and Kreuter, J. (1991) Effect of nanoparticles on transdermal drug delivery. *J. Microencapsul.*, **8** (3), 369–374.

39 Gide, P.S., Gidwani, S.K., and Kothule, K.U. (2013) Enhancement of transdermal penetration and bioavailability of poorly soluble acyclovir using solid lipid nanoparticles incorporated in gel cream. *Indian J. Pharm. Sci.*, **75** (2), 138–142.

40 Khurana, S., Jain, N.K., and Bedi, P.M. (2013) Nanoemulsion based gel for transdermal delivery of meloxicam: physico-chemical, mechanistic investigation. *Life Sci.*, **92** (6–7), 383–392.

41 de Salamanca, A.E., Diebold, Y., Calonge, M., Garcia-Vazquez, C., Callejo, S., Vila, A., and Alonso, M.J. (2006) Chitosan nanoparticles as a potential drug delivery system for the ocular surface: toxicity, uptake mechanism and *in vivo* tolerance. *Invest. Ophthalmol. Vis. Sci.*, **47** (4), 1416–1425.

42 Musante, C.J., Schroeter, J.D., Rosati, J.A., Crowder, T.M., Hickey, A.J., and Martonen, T.B. (2002) Factors affecting the deposition of inhaled porous drug particles. *J. Pharm. Sci.*, **91** (7), 1590–1600.

43 Patton, J.S. and Byron, P.R. (2007) Inhaling medicines: delivering drugs to the body through the lungs. *Nat. Rev. Drug Discov.*, **6** (1), 67–74.

44 Bailey, M.M. and Berkland, C.J. (2009) Nanoparticle formulations in pulmonary drug delivery. *Med. Res. Rev.*, **29** (1), 196–212.

45 Wacker, M. (2013) Nanocarriers for intravenous injection – the long hard road to the market. *Int. J. Pharm.*, **457** (1), 50–62.

46 Tenzer, S., Docter, D., Kuharev, J., Musyanovych, A., Fetz, V., Hecht, R., Schlenk, F., Fischer, D., Kiouptsi, K., Reinhardt, C., Landfester, K., Schild, H., Maskos, M., Knauer, S.K., and Stauber, R.H. (2013) Rapid formation of plasma protein corona critically affects nanoparticle pathophysiology. *Nat. Nanotechnol.*, **8** (10), 772–781.

47 Liptrott, N.J., Giardiello, M., Hunter, J.W., Tatham, L., Tidbury, L.R., Siccardi, M., Rannard, S., and Owen, A. (2015) Flow cytometric analysis of the physical and protein-binding characteristics of solid drug nanoparticle suspensions. *Nanomedicine (Lond.)*, **10** (9), 1407–1421.

48 Paula, A.J., Araujo Junior, R.T., Martinez, D.S., Paredes-Gamero, E.J., Nader, H.B., Duran, N., Justo, G.Z., and Alves, O.L. (2013) Influence of protein corona on the transport of molecules into cells by mesoporous silica nanoparticles. *ACS Appl. Mater. Interfaces*, **5** (17), 8387–8393.

49 Peng, Q., Zhang, S., Yang, Q., Zhang, T., Wei, X.Q., Jiang, L., Zhang, C.L., Chen, Q.M., Zhang, Z.R., and Lin, Y.F. (2013) Preformed albumin corona, a protective coating for nanoparticles based drug delivery system. *Biomaterials*, **34** (33), 8521–8530.

50 Varatharajan, L. and Thomas, S.A. (2009) The transport of anti-HIV drugs across blood-CNS interfaces: summary of current knowledge and recommendations for further research. *Antiviral Res.*, **82** (2), A99–A109.

51 Arnida, Janat-Amsbury, M.M., Ray, A., Peterson, C.M., and Ghandehari, H. (2011) Geometry and surface characteristics of gold nanoparticles influence their biodistribution and uptake by macrophages. *Eur. J. Pharm. Biopharm.*, **77** (3), 417–423.

52 Geraets, L., Oomen, A.G., Krystek, P., Jacobsen, N.R., Wallin, H., Laurentie, M., Verharen, H.W., Brandon, E.F., and de Jong, W.H. (2014) Tissue distribution and elimination after oral and intravenous administration of different titanium dioxide nanoparticles in rats. *Part. Fibre Toxicol.*, **11**, 30.

53 Owens, D.E. 3rd and Peppas, N.A. (2006) Opsonization, biodistribution, and pharmacokinetics of polymeric

nanoparticles. *Int. J. Pharm.*, **307** (1), 93–102.

54 Kim, D., Lee, E.S., Park, K., Kwon, I.C., and Bae, Y.H. (2008) Doxorubicin loaded pH-sensitive micelle: antitumoral efficacy against ovarian A2780/DOXR tumor. *Pharm. Res.*, **25** (9), 2074–2082.

55 Mkandawire, M., Pohl, A., Gubarevich, T., Lapina, V., Appelhans, D., Rodel, G., Pompe, W., Schreiber, J., and Opitz, J. (2009) Selective targeting of green fluorescent nanodiamond conjugates to mitochondria in HeLa cells. *J. Biophotonics*, **2** (10), 596–606.

56 Sadauskas, E., Wallin, H., Stoltenberg, M., Vogel, U., Doering, P., Larsen, A., and Danscher, G. (2007) Kupffer cells are central in the removal of nanoparticles from the organism. *Part. Fibre Toxicol.*, **4**, 10.

57 Price, P.S., Conolly, R.B., Chaisson, C.F., Gross, E.A., Young, J.S., Mathis, E.T., and Tedder, D.R. (2003) Modeling interindividual variation in physiological factors used in PBPK models of humans. *Crit. Rev. Toxicol.*, **33** (5), 469–503.

58 Willmann, S., Hohn, K., Edginton, A., Sevestre, M., Solodenko, J., Weiss, W., Lippert, J., and Schmitt, W. (2007) Development of a physiology-based whole-body population model for assessing the influence of individual variability on the pharmacokinetics of drugs. *J. Pharmacokinet. Pharmacodyn.*, **34** (3), 401–431.

59 Bosgra, S., van Eijkeren, J., Bos, P., Zeilmaker, M., and Slob, W. (2012) An improved model to predict physiologically based model parameters and their inter-individual variability from anthropometry. *Crit. Rev. Toxicol.*, **42** (9), 751–767.

60 Lazzari, S., Moscatelli, D., Codari, F., Salmona, M., Morbidelli, M., and Diomede, L. (2012) Colloidal stability of polymeric nanoparticles in biological fluids. *J. Nanopart. Res.*, **14** (6), 920.

61 Saraceno, R., Chiricozzi, A., Gabellini, M., and Chimenti S. (2013) Emerging applications of nanomedicine in dermatology. *Skin Res. Technol.*, **19** (1), e13-9.

62 de Roche, M., Siccardi, M., Stoeckle, M., Livio, F., Back, D., Battegay, M., and Marzolini, C. (2012) Efavirenz in an obese HIV-infected patient – a report and an *in vitro-in vivo* extrapolation model indicate risk of underdosing. *Antivir. Ther.*, **17** (7), 1381–1384.

63 Siccardi, M., Almond, L., Schipani, A., Csajka, C., Marzolini, C., Wyen, C., Brockmeyer, N.H., Boffito, M., Owen, A., and Back, D. (2012) Pharmacokinetic and pharmacodynamic analysis of efavirenz dose reduction using an *in vitro-in vivo* extrapolation model. *Clin. Pharmacol. Ther.*, **92** (4), 494–502.

64 Moss, D.M., Siccardi, M., Back, D.J., and Owen, A. (2013) Predicting intestinal absorption of raltegravir using a population-based ADME simulation. *J. Antimicrob. Chemother*, **68** (7), 1627–1634.

65 Siccardi, M., Marzolini, C., Seden, K., Almond, L., Kirov, A., Khoo, S., Owen, A., and Back, D. (2013) Prediction of drug-drug interactions between various antidepressants and efavirenz or boosted protease inhibitors using a physiologically based pharmacokinetic modelling approach. *Clin. Pharmacokinet.*, **52** (7), 583–592.

66 Siccardi, M., Olagunju, A., Seden, K., Ebrahimjee, F., Rannard, S., Back, D., and Owen, A. (2013) Use of a physiologically-based pharmacokinetic model to simulate artemether dose adjustment for overcoming the drug-drug interaction with efavirenz. *In Silico Pharmacology*, **1** (4), doi: 10.1186/2193-9616-1-4.

67 McDonald, T.O., Giardiello, M., Martin, P., Siccardi, M., Liptrott, N.J., Smith, D., Roberts, P., Curley, P., Schipani, A., Khoo, S.H., Long, J., Foster, A.J., Rannard, S.P., and Owen, A. (2013) Antiretroviral solid drug nanoparticles with enhanced oral bioavailability: production, characterization, and *in vitro-in vivo* correlation. *Adv. Healthc. Mater.* **3** (3), 400–411.

68 Henrique Silva, A., Vasquez Mansilla, M., Zysler, R.D., Pisciotti, M.L.M., Locatelli, C., Rajoli, R.K.R., Owen, A., Creczynski-Pasa, T.B., and Siccardi, M. (2015) A physiologically based pharmacokinetic model to predict the superparamagnetic iron oxide nanoparticles (SPIONs)

accumulation *in vivo*. 8th CLINAM, Basel, Switzerland.

69 Rajoli, R.K., Back, D.J., Rannard, S., Freel Meyers, C.L., Flexner, C., Owen, A., and Siccardi, M. (2015) Physiologically based pharmacokinetic modelling to inform development of intramuscular long-acting nanoformulations for HIV. *Clin. Pharmacokinet.*, **54** (6), 639–650.

70 Lin, P., Chen, J.W., Chang, L.W., Wu, J.P., Redding, L., Chang, H., Yeh, T.K., Yang, C.S., Tsai, M.H., Wang, H.J., Kuo, Y.C., and Yang, R.S. (2008) Computational and ultrastructural toxicology of a nanoparticle, quantum dot 705, in mice. *Environ. Sci. Technol.*, **42** (16), 6264–6270.

71 Lee, H.A., Leavens, T.L., Mason, S.E., Monteiro-Riviere, N.A., and Riviere, J.E. (2009) Comparison of quantum dot biodistribution with a blood-flow-limited physiologically based pharmacokinetic model. *Nano Lett.*, **9** (2), 794–799.

72 Pery, A.R., Brochot, C., Hoet, P.H., Nemmar, A., and Bois, F.Y. (2009) Development of a physiologically based kinetic model for 99m-technetium-labelled carbon nanoparticles inhaled by humans. *Inhal. Toxicol.*, **21** (13), 1099–1107.

73 Lankveld, D.P., Oomen, A.G., Krystek, P., Neigh, A., Troost-de Jong, A., Noorlander, C.W., Van Eijkeren, J.C., Geertsma, R.E., and De Jong, W.H. (2010) The kinetics of the tissue distribution of silver nanoparticles of different sizes. *Biomaterials*, **31** (32), 8350–8361.

74 Li, M., Panagi, Z., Avgoustakis, K., and Reineke, J. (2012) Physiologically based pharmacokinetic modeling of PLGA nanoparticles with varied mPEG content. *Int. J. Nanomedicine*, **7**, 1345–1356.

75 Mager, D.E., Mody, V., Xu, C., Forrest, A., Lesniak, W.G., Nigavekar, S.S., Kariapper, M.T., Minc, L., Khan, M.K., and Balogh, L.P. (2012) Physiologically based pharmacokinetic model for composite nanodevices: effect of charge and size on *in vivo* disposition. *Pharm. Res.*, **29** (9), 2534–2542.

76 Bachler, G., von Goetz, N., and Hungerbuhler, K. (2013) A physiologically based pharmacokinetic model for ionic silver and silver nanoparticles. *Int. J. Nanomedicine*, **8**, 3365–3382.

77 Gilkey, M.J., Krishnan, V., Scheetz, L., Jia, X., Rajasekaran, A.K., and Dhurjati, P.S. (2015) Physiologically based pharmacokinetic modeling of fluorescently labeled block copolymer nanoparticles for controlled drug delivery in leukemia therapy. *CPT Pharmacometrics Syst. Pharmacol.*, **4** (3), e00013.

78 Poulin, P. and Theil, F.P. (2002) Prediction of pharmacokinetics prior to *in vivo* studies. 1. Mechanism-based prediction of volume of distribution. *J. Pharm. Sci.*, **91** (1), 129–156.

79 Aji Alex, M.R., Chacko, A.J., Jose, S., and Souto, E.B. (2011) Lopinavir loaded solid lipid nanoparticles (SLN) for intestinal lymphatic targeting. *Eur. J. Pharm. Sci.*, **42** (1–2), 11–18.

80 Abuqayyas, L. and Balthasar, J.P. (2012) Application of PBPK modeling to predict monoclonal antibody disposition in plasma and tissues in mouse models of human colorectal cancer. *J. Pharmacokinet. Pharmacodyn.*, **39** (6), 683–710.

81 Misra, R. and Sahoo, S.K. (2010) Intracellular trafficking of nuclear localization signal conjugated nanoparticles for cancer therapy. *Eur. J. Pharm. Sci.*, **39** (1–3), 152–163.

82 Martin, P., Giardiello, M., McDonald, T.O., Rannard, S.P., and Owen, A. (2013) Mediation of *in vitro* cytochrome P450 activity by common pharmaceutical excipients. *Mol. Pharm.* **10** (7), 2739–2748.

83 Fenneteau, F., Poulin, P., and Nekka, F. (2010) Physiologically based predictions of the impact of inhibition of intestinal and hepatic metabolism on human pharmacokinetics of CYP3A substrates. *J. Pharm. Sci.*, **99** (1), 486–514.

84 Ke, A.B., Nallani, S.C., Zhao, P., Rostami-Hodjegan, A., and Unadkat, J.D. (2012) A PBPK model to predict disposition of CYP3A-metabolized drugs in pregnant women: verification and discerning the site of CYP3A induction. *CPT Pharmacometrics Syst. Pharmacol.*, **1**, e3.

85 Yamashita, F., Sasa, Y., Yoshida, S., Hisaka, A., Asai, Y., Kitano, H., Hashida, M., and

Suzuki, H. (2013) Modeling of rifampicin-induced CYP3A4 activation dynamics for the prediction of clinical drug-drug interactions from *in vitro* data. *PLoS One,* **8** (9), e70330.

86 Gertz, M., Cartwright, C.M., Hobbs, M.J., Kenworthy, K.E., Rowland, M., Houston, J.B., and Galetin, A. (2013) Cyclosporine inhibition of hepatic and intestinal CYP3A4, uptake and efflux transporters: application of PBPK modeling in the assessment of drug-drug interaction potential. *Pharm. Res.*, **30** (3), 761–780.

87 Thomas, S. (2009) Physiologically-based simulation modelling for the reduction of animal use in the discovery of novel pharmaceuticals. *Altern. Lab. Anim.*, **37** (5), 497–511.

16
Drug Targeting in Nanomedicine and Nanopharmacy: A Systems Approach*)

Jingwei Shao,[1,2] *Lisa McConnachie,*[2] *and Rodney J.Y. Ho*[1,2]

[1]*Fuzhou University, Cancer Metastasis Alert and Prevention Center, College of Chemistry, 523 Gongye Rd, Gulou, Fuzhou, Fujian 350002, PR China*
[2]*University of Washington, Departments of Pharmaceutics and Bioengineering, H272 Health Science Building, Seattle, WA 98195-7610, USA*

16.1
Introduction

The goal of drug targeting is to improve the therapeutic index of a given drug, making a medicine more effective, safer, or both. In return, it is hoped that therapeutic index improvements could translate into patient acceptance, compliance, and elevate life quality. In the context of pharmaceutical sciences, drug targeting is within the broader scope of drug formulation and delivery research to aid medicinal product development. However, drug formulation research typically focuses on transformation of a chemical or biological entity into an appropriate dosage form suitable for injection or other less invasive routes of administration, such as oral, rectal, vaginal, or topical. In other words, formulation scientists concern themselves predominantly with developing drugs in dosage forms that are practical, stable, reproducible, and provide sufficient bioavailability. Bioavailability or the fraction of the total administered dose of the drug that is absorbed has typical assessment criteria based on overall time-course of drug concentrations in blood. While targeted drug designs require consideration of route and appropriate dosage form, these issues are integrated, and are secondary to issues related to the extent of drug exposure in target tissues and cells, compared to exposure in by stander and off target cells. To accomplish this, scientists must have sufficient knowledge on tissue and cells expressing the drug-target within the body for which the drug is intended.

*) This work is supported in part by NIH grants UM1 AI120176, UL1TR000423, and AI-077390. JS is supported in part by a visiting scholar grant from Fujian province.

Pharmaceutical Nanotechnology: Innovation and Production, First Edition. Edited by Jean Cornier, Arno Kwade, Andrew Owen, and Marcel Van de Voorde.

The effectiveness of drug delivery design depends heavily on the validated, detailed, and integrated knowledge about the drug-target localization within the body, specific tissue, cells, and their kinetics and dynamics between healthy and disease states. Drug targeting is more than just having the administered drug delivered and a majority of the fraction available in the blood. Without the understanding of drug-target tissues and cell distribution profiles, assessment of success in drug targeting defined as the fraction of the drug found in the target tissues and cells may be rather ineffective.

Drug targeting research requires consideration of tissue and cell targets within the body that the drug compound is intended to modulate. Thus, it requires one to integrate systems knowledge about the relationship between the disease state and drug effects as it relates to the drug target. The details of drug target distribution in the body, as well as drug (molecular) distribution after dosing are essential elements for design consideration. The systems' understanding allows definition of the gap or problem that drug targeting could impact. With technological innovations in drug particles that are small, or nanodrug particles, increasing appreciation of their physiochemical properties on differential localization in tissues and cells, these technologies could be used to address specific drug delivery gaps. The nano(carrier)drug particles, instead of the molecular characteristics of the active drug, with their specific surface properties as well as differential particulate and cell interactions at the sites of absorption, distribution, metabolism, and elimination often determine the overall disposition profile in the body. By providing appropriate design through a systems approach, a nanodrug containing more potent (and perhaps even toxic) compounds could be delivered with high selectivity to target tissues and cells. The ability to quantify the target cells and tissues within the body may improve not only apparent potency, but also safety. As a result, the overall therapeutic index, a ratio of toxicity over drug potency, could be improved significantly.

While there are many nano materials being reported in the literature as potential candidates for nanomedicine, due to a number of challenges, including formulation complexity, safety, *in vivo* stability, scalability, and reproducibility, progress has been limited in translating them into pharmaceutical development plans. Other challenges, such as business viability and additional time requirements for drug-targeting research in the context of focusing on financial reward related to the first to market for specific disease indication, have also contributed to limiting research investments in drug targeting research as a part of an early phase in a new drug development. However, the concern on time delay and the need for additional capital investment in drug targeting research could be overcome with a successful demonstration of the product intended for drug targets that conventional formulation approaches are unable to solve. We will provide some nanodrug targeting examples and highlight how a system's understanding and definition have aided in the process. While nanoproduct examples are drawn from lipid-based systems where most of the information is available, the general principles outlined are broadly applicable across nanocarrier systems.

In the following, we will first discuss the concept of the Systems Approach to Drug Targeting, with an overall goal to improve on-target drug distribution into tissues and cells that modulate clinical impacts. This will be followed by discussion of [1] existing nanoformulated drug products [2], the process of transforming nanoformulations into a drug [3], the role of nanoformulations and a systems approach in product development with specific examples. This chapter concludes with the current status and future prospects for targeted nanopharmacy research and development.

16.2 A Systems Approach to Drug Delivery and Drug Targeting

Innovations in drug delivery systems hold promising business opportunities and attract significant research interest. Drug delivery encompasses physical dosage form, molecular design optimization and engineering, and other physiochemical approaches built on the understanding of drug metabolism and pharmacokinetics (DMPK) as well as therapeutic outcomes (generally referred to as pharmacodynamics (PD)) [2–4]. With a narrower definition – covering drug dosage forms, carriers, and formulations. Annual drug delivery business captures about US$50–82 billion revenue in the United States. Even with a tremendous growth in the knowledge of disease and proven drug targets, it is well documented that clinical translation of advances in medical sciences and drug discovery, and late stage clinical failure due to unforeseen toxicity or lack of efficacy is a frequent drug development challenge. We have previously proposed a concept called a Systems Approach to Drug Delivery and Targeting [5]. This Systems Approach (presented in Figure 16.1) has been used to address drug insufficiency and the residual virus in lymphoid tissues of HIV patients on chronic drug therapies [6]. As some of these details are discussed in recent reviews and commentary, we will only introduce the rationale and concept below.

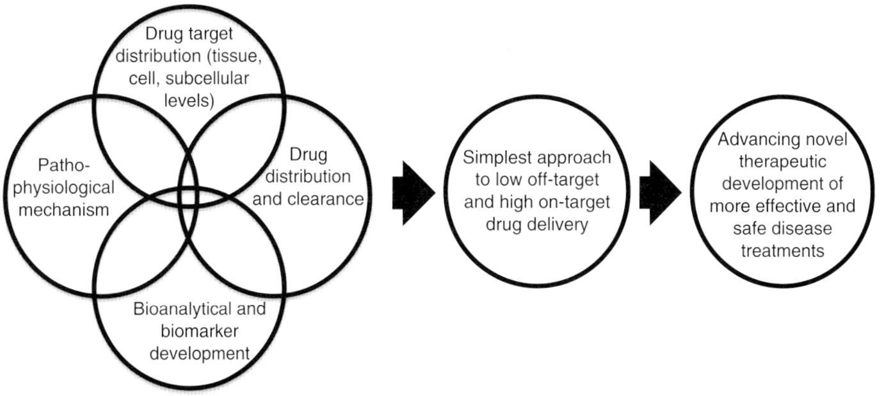

Figure 16.1 A graphical representation of the Systems Approach to Drug Delivery and Targeting.

The Systems Approach incorporates an integrated approach to drug development that includes the biological and physiological context, drug distribution, drug action, and validated measures or surrogate markers of disease outcomes. The increasing molecular, cellular understanding of drug targets associated with a disease symptom allows better definition of key or rate-limiting steps to targeted drug exposure. A more accurate definition of rate limiting steps to targeted drug delivery allows setting the target profile of a drug delivery system to best deliver the drug to target tissues. This could be achieved by maximizing overlap between the distribution of drug molecule (and exposure) and that of drug targets (cells and tissues) throughout the body. Thus, based on the integration of molecular, cellular, and physiological knowledge, and an understanding of pharmacology and pharmacokinetics of drug–drug target interactions; the Systems Approach for drug delivery could be specifically designed to reduce off-target effects and improve on-target drug exposure *in vivo*. The time-course of drug concentrations and the extent of drug exposure to target cells and tissues in the body in relation to blood levels, which are typically monitored by the classical pharmacokinetic parameters, are all parts of the overall model of the Systems Approach.

The emphasis of most drug delivery systems is on developing sustained drug release polymers or smart particles, and demonstrating their capabilities *in vitro* as proof of concepts. In contrast, the Systems Approach provides guidance and specification on *in vivo* tissues and cell targets prior to initiating the engineering aspect of nanoparticles such as surface decoration with targeting moieties. Within the Systems Approach, the simplest tissue and cell localization strategy would be favored. This minimalist approach is beneficial to develop a scalable drug delivery system requiring fewer steps and ensuring a stable pharmaceutical dosage or particulate form to reach the target site of action. The overall strategy of the Systems Approach should include the drug formulation with a cost-effective and scalable preparation method to accelerate product development.

A major goal of the Systems Approach to Drug Delivery and Targeting is to accelerate product development through reducing risks and improving success rates by considering the following issues early in the course of product development. A visual representation can be seen in Figure 16.1.

- The definition and characteristics of drug targets at molecular, intra/extra-cellular, and tissues levels as they are related to clinical outcomes.
- The distribution, uptake, metabolism, and elimination of a drug or drug candidate (with unique properties) in the tissues and cells within the body.
- Finding an opportunity to integrate the physiochemical properties of a drug and the physiologic/biologic systems limitation to design the simplest and best drug delivery system.
- Designing a simple and effective means to influence drug distribution and exposure in cells and tissues expressing high levels of drug-targets.
- Validating the surrogate marker that represents disease outcome to assist in early decisions on drug development.

The Systems Approach integrates the knowledge intercepts among four areas of biomedical research. (1) Drug target localization information from an intracellular context to cells and tissues as well as organs in the body, (2) knowledge about the biodistribution and clearance of drug candidates in the body over time, (3) the physiological and pathological consequences of the aberration in drug targets that reflects disease symptoms, and (4) quantitative or bioanalytical markers that could be measured in blood or other samples for predicting drug levels and disease outcome. These overlapping themes and conditions should be taken into consideration when implementing the Systems Approach to Drug Delivery and Targeting.

16.3
Current Nanomedicine Products

The application of pharmaceuticals of small size is a proven and important area of pharmaceutical research and development. Pharmaceuticals of small size include colloids, drug crystals and co-crystals, drug particles, drug-lipid particles, drugs encapsulated in lipid vesicles or liposomes, biopolymers or associated with protein, and protein aggregates [7–10]. When these drug-carrier particles or complexes are small and in the range of 10–1000 nm, they are often referred to as nanoparticles or nanomedicine, and the process or method to produce the dosage form is generally known as the nanoformulation of drugs. These nanoformulations are generally intended to improve pharmaceutical properties and drug response by improving drug solubility, stability, and to some extent, modifying biodistribution of a given compound to improve pharmacokinetics, safety, and efficacy profile. While the examples are discussed in the context of overall product design for dispensing in outpatient and hospital settings, it should be noted that some of these could be amenable for adaptation through innovative compounding in local pharmacy. Thus, both pharmacists working in the pharmaceutical research and development as well as those in clinical practice could play a significant role in development and use of nanopharmacy knowledge. Some examples of nanomedicine in clinical use are summarized in Table 16.1.

The nanoformulations in clinical application presented in Table 16.1 exemplify the use of (1) nanodrug crystals designed to address drug solubility and enhance oral absorption of hydrophobic compounds, (2) protein-bound paclitaxel designed to improve safety, (3) lipid bound amphotericin intended to improve safety plus drug accumulation in spleen cells where invading organisms localize, (4) lipid-associated doxorubicin engineered to reduce cardiotoxicity (safety) and improving the pharmacokinetic profile, and (5) antibody IgG molecules and derivatives intended to provide targeting and prolonged circulation time in plasma. What is less well appreciated in nanomedicine is that an antibody (immunoglobulin), with a molecular weight of 150 000 Da, has a diameter of about 10 nm and is thus a nanoglobular protein particle (*albeit* with unique

Table 16.1 Some nanomedicine products and drug delivery objectives.

Nanomedicine platform	Product	Particle size (diameter)	Objective
Liposomes	Doxil (Doxorubicin)	~90–100 nm	Minimize cardiac drug binding; drug accumulation in tumor
	Daunoxome (Daunorubicin)	~45 nm	Same as above
	Ambisome (Amphotericin B)	~100 nm	Reduce nephrotoxicity and increase potency against fungal infection in spleen
Lipidic colloid	Amphotec (Amphotericin B)	~115 nm (Elongated disk)	Same as above
Flattened liposome vesicles	Abelcet (Amphotericin B)	~1600 nm	Same as above
Nanocrystal	Rapamune (Sirolimus)	20–1000	Improve solubility and bioavailability
	Emend (Aprepitant)		Same as above
	Tricor (Fenofibrate)		Same as above
Protein and protein bound drug	Immunoglobulin IgG and monoclonal IgG	20	Intrinsic property that provide long-acting up to 30 d
	Gama globulin	20	Same as above
	Abraxane-Albumin-paclitaxel	130	Increase solubility and injection site tolerability

long-circulating properties with an approximate 30 day half-life in blood; for a review, please see Ref. [1]).

Nanoformulations have been utilized in the pharmaceutical industry to also produce commercial products that have higher efficacy than their traditional formulation counterparts. The commercial success of Doxil (a liposomal nanoformulation of doxorubicin) and Abraxane (a protein bound paclitaxel), for example, show the value of applying nanotechnology to drug delivery [11]. Liposomal doxorubicin is able to reduce the cardiotoxicity seen with doxorubicin and other anthracyclines, but not completely mitigate it. Liposomal doxorubicin was also thought to have a reduced distribution in off-target cells such as cardiomyocytes (which overexpresses the cardiolipin that binds to doxorubicin and other anthracycline) and an increased distribution in malignant cells relative to conventional doxorubicin [12]. This effect has been attributed to (1) preventing doxorubicin from binding to cardiolipin lipids on cardiomyocyte and related cardiotoxicity and (2) enhanced permeation and retention (EPR) of doxorubicin nanoparticles in tumor cells through the leaky tumor neo vasculature supplying oxygen and nutrients to the rapidly growing tumor cells. The extended circulation time of liposomal doxorubicin, Doxil allows time to penetrate through leaky neovasculature. Collectively, the EPR effects and long-circulation time of the nanoparticulate doxorubicin resulted in preferential distribution and accumulation in the tumor. As a result, without having any ligand or receptor recognizing the tumor, these liposome nanoparticles provide apparent target selective accumulation of the liposome encapsulated drug doxorubicin [13]. As no other preferential tumor accumulation requires target tumor cell-selective molecules expressed on liposomes, such a drug delivery system is generally referred to as a passive drug targeting system. The strategy to improve tumor accumulation by EPR requires tumors that exhibit neovasculature; unfortunately, not all tumors exhibit neovasculature or need one for supporting their growth and thus the EPR approach to drug targeting may be ineffective. It is likely that the same leaky vasculature accumulation mechanisms of Doxil may contribute treatment-limiting toxicity reported in some cancer patients reported with redness, swelling, and pain on palms of the hands or soles of the feet (generally referred to as Palmar-Plantar Erythrodysesthesia or PPE). Whether it is limited to doxorubicin or in patients with cancer related leaky peripheral vasculature is not clear. Regardless, particulate-dependent preferential drug accumulation, based on a systems understanding is a viable and proven nanoparticle drug targeting approach.

In the case of abraxane (albumin bound paclitaxel), the initial formulation of paclitaxel involved the use of Cremophor EL, dehydrated ethanol, and Tween 80 to formulate insoluble paclitaxel into an injectable dosage form. This approach limited the dose-dependent efficacy of paclitaxel, because the cosolvents were poorly tolerated by patients. By binding to albumin and the complex paclitaxel assumes water soluble profile of albumin, this nanoformulation circumvented the need for the surfactant/ethanol for paclitaxel suspension and the related adverse drug (formulation) reactions. In addition to improving the overall solubility of paclitaxel, albumin has been demonstrated, after product approval, to serve as a drug carrier in binding to a cell-surface receptor (gp60) on malignant endothelial cells [14]. In this case of albumin-bound paclitaxel, abraxane improves the therapeutic index by significantly reducing the local injection site reaction and improving patient compliance while maintaining the potency of the parent drug.

16.4
Transformation of a Discovery of Disease Target to a Therapeutic Product

The discovery of a gene, a gene product, or a protein linked directly to a human disease often makes new headlines and raises public expectation that a therapeutic treatment or vaccine will be available soon. In reality, however, it may take years and significant public and private investments to transform the initial discovery of a purported drug target to validation and drugging the target with a therapeutic compound. As shown in Figure 16.2, significant public and private funds must be invested in basic, translational, and applied research. After the initial discovery, expanded basic research is required to generate detailed knowledge about the disease etiology, mechanisms, and potential therapeutic target validation before initiating translational research in earnest. Detailed understanding about the drug target at cellular, subcellular, or molecular levels is needed to initiate a molecule design that likely modulates the functions of the drug target. Even if one discovers molecules or compounds that affect drug target functions such as inhibiting binding or enzymatic activity *in vitro* or at cellular levels, these compounds are not considered as a drug candidate at this stage. Additional key considerations, which describe the characteristics of compound time-course of compound distribution and elimination – generally referred to as pharmacokinetic – profile within the body, are needed to determine whether the compound has promising functions to be a drug candidate. Poor pharmacokinetic properties could prevent these compounds from being able to reach the drug target in biology systems.

Having an inhibitor or receptor binding with high potency would require consideration of whether these compounds have characteristics that would match the drug target distribution profile with that of the compound safety, tissue distribution, and metabolic profile. For example, if the drug is exclusively localized within the blood, and if the drug target is located in tissue and cells are inaccessible or has limited access to blood (e.g., brain tissue), even with the most potent compounds, it would have no effect on the drug target or related function. Thus, the systems' knowledge on drug target distribution, the requirement of pharmacokinetic profile of drug candidate, and the ability of the compounds in question to match these requirements are important parameters for success of clinical translation for a new discovery to a therapeutic product.

The journey for a therapeutic product starts from exploratory and hypothesis-driven basic research, commonly supported by government (public) entities and

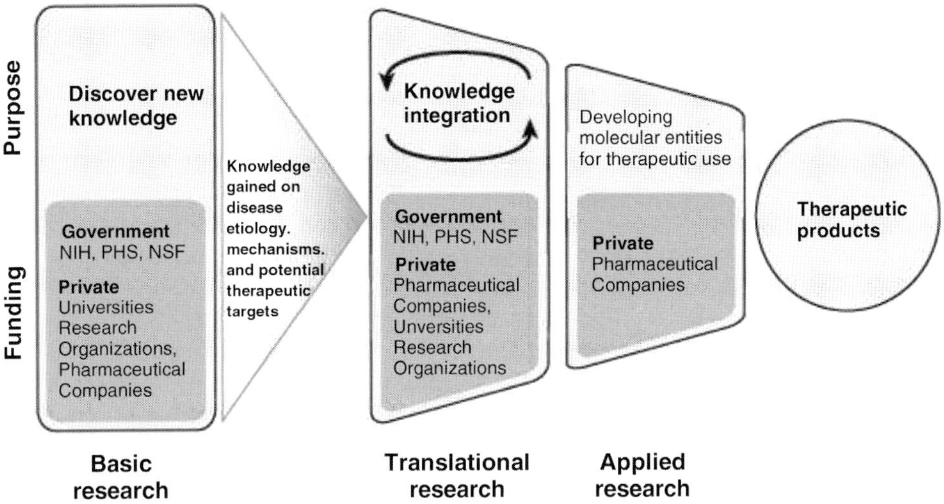

Figure 16.2 The process of pharmaceutical drug discovery and development – an integrated science that leverages on the collective knowledge and resources from both government and private sectors. The transformation of a therapeutic concept or molecule to a therapeutic product begins from basic research discovery to translational research, followed by preclinical and clinical applied research. Successful therapeutic molecules that are effective and safe for human disease symptoms are then made available to benefit a patients' health. Governments and private entities for generating and integrating knowledge about disease etiology and molecular and cellular mechanisms typically support the exploratory and hypothesis-driven basic research efforts. This integrated disease knowledge is leveraged to develop potential therapeutic solutions. The process requires collaboration between government, universities, and pharmaceutical companies, and is often referred to as clinical or preclinical translational research. Promising therapeutic molecules undergo clinical drug development through applied research, which is often the most capital intensive and is primarily funded by pharmaceutical companies. The entire drug development process requires funding and support from multiple agencies and contributions of expertise across several different health disciplines. The successful interactions and choice of drug candidates leads to therapeutic drug and vaccine products. Abbreviations: NIH, National Institutes of Health; NSF, National Science Foundation; PHS, Public Health Service. Adapted from Ref. [1].

private entities, to generate and integrate molecular, cellular, and systems knowledge on disease etiology (Figure 16.2). This integrated disease knowledge is leveraged to develop potential therapeutic solutions. Collaboration among universities, government, and pharmaceutical companies is often needed to support preclinical, clinical, and translational research. This translational research allows scientists, investors, and product development sponsors to assess the overall merit of a therapeutic concept. Translational studies are often considered by investors as a way to determine the odds of success and derive a commercial value. Promising therapeutic candidates undergo clinical drug development through applied research. Applied or clinical research is often the most capital intensive and is funded primarily by pharmaceutical companies. The entire drug development process requires funding and support from multiple agencies and contributions of expertize across different health disciplines. When successful, these interactions lead to the development of drugs and vaccines that impact health through cures, treatments, or prevention of disease. (While it is not discussed, readers are advised to learn from other chapters in this book (and a recent publication [1] regarding the process – regulatory and funding model – in clinical development to gain approval of a product for clinical use and pharmacy dispensing)).

16.5 The Role of Targeted Nanoformulations and a Systems Approach in Drug Development

Developing targeting strategies to preferentially localize drugs at key sites and produce maximum pharmacologic effects has long been the ultimate goal of pharmaceutical scientists. In theory, preferential localization of drugs to target tissues and cells can be achieved with drug carriers and target recognition molecules such as ligands, receptors, or antibodies [15–17]. However in practice, identification of target tissues and cells of interest can be complex.

Often effector cells and tissues are either not well defined or are distributed widely throughout the body. In addition, specific carriers, or targeting molecules capable of providing differential distribution to target sites, are not always available. It is now established that drug molecules distribution in the body to different tissues and cells to a varying degree is due to a number of physical and chemical characteristics. The physical–chemical properties and interactions with the biological milieu in the body are now referred to as drug-like properties. While a number of improvement and variations have been proposed, drug-like properties for compounds intended for oral dosing could be predicted based on a set of predictive factors referred to as the rule of five. From an analysis of compounds that have been successfully translated into drugs, Lipinski *et al.* [18] have proposed a set of predictive parameters including – (1) molecular weight, (2) hydrophobicity (octanol/water partition measured as Log P), and (3) hydrogen bonding. For most small-molecule drugs, the rule of five predicts poor absorption or permeation across cell membrane barriers when the molecule has more than 5 hydrogen bond donors (or 10 hydrogen bond acceptors), hydrophobicity greater than 5 Log P, and a molecular weight greater than 500 Da. As a majority of protein drugs, even small peptides with 5–6 amino acids and that have a molecular weight greater than 500 Da, are held together by many hydrogen bonds with surrounding water and other molecules with different amino acid sequences. These are not good drug candidates with optimal membrane permeability across the blood vessels or gut wall. However, development of these rules and tools for measurement have provided investigators with a better understanding of how each molecule is unique as observed through their specific distribution, localization, and clearance properties that require crossing different permeability barriers within the body's system. Depending on the route of administration, the barriers include gut to blood, blood to tissues, blood to brain, tissues to cells, and others. During the drug development process, drug-like properties are characterized. These pharmaceutical properties (sometimes referred to as physiochemical properties) for small and large molecules have provided a fuller understanding of the role of physical and chemical characteristics of the molecule with respect to a drug-like desirable property. They have also provided the information gap on barriers to specific tissues and cells key to potentiating therapeutic and toxic effects. The physiochemical properties and time-course of drug distribution in the body of a drug candidate can provide systems-wide data on its exposure and impact on the biologic system.

Cell-specific drug delivery systems must provide a significant degree of target-tissue accumulation *in vivo* to be clinically useful. Typically, target cells and tissues are evaluated *in vitro* during early drug development. The *in vitro* information on drug sensitivity in target cells and tissues cannot be directly translated without knowing the location of these drug targets in the body's system. Tissue distribution of drug targets as well as drug localization must be considered early in the course of drug development to understand the overall performance of the delivery system or drug carrier.

16.6
Targeting Drugs to Sites of Action

Liposome and lipid vesicles composed of natural or synthetic endogenous lipids and lipid derivatives have a long history of human experience and research. We will draw examples from liposome targeting research to discuss some of the drug targeting principles and keys to success in clinical translations. While many biomaterials, such as biodegradable polymers and biocompatible dendrimers, as well as carbon, gold, and silica are in their early stages of laboratory study to demonstrate feasibility for drug targeting; their safety and scalability are also being evaluated with earnest. For more information on drug targeting using these platforms, refer to other chapters in this book and other published articles.

With respect to the requirement of a systems understanding for clinical transition, nanosize drug carriers, such as liposomes expressing specific ligands, were designed and shown to produce target-selective delivery to cancer cells *in vitro*. The *in vitro* results, however, could not be directly correlated with the degree of *in vivo* tumor suppression in the extravascular space because of the poor nanoparticle permeability across the endothelial lining to tumors with intact vasculature. Only with demonstration of enhanced liposome-encapsulated drug doxorubicin accumulation in Kaposi sarcoma (tumor), the apparent selective drug accumulation in some tumors was due to leaky neovasculature that supply blood to tumor, along with the longer blood circulation time afforded by surface modified liposomes. These liposomes, as discussed earlier, are designed without the need of ligand for cell and tissue selection. Although the targeted liposome decorated with a ligand, such as an antibody or receptor-seeking molecule on the surface, had an avid affinity for the target cells, it could not penetrate across the vasculature to reach the target after IV administration. As a result, after many years of research target-specific delivery to tumor cells has still not been realized [19,20]. Such a limitation was only recognized late in the development of the first few products based on liposome delivery systems. Early consideration of physiological barriers and *in vivo* physiological context could have significantly reduce developmental time and cost of lipid-based nanomedicine. It is now much more appreciated that targeting to tissues and cells can be accomplished not only by a ligand–receptor-mediated process, but also be based on a number of endogenous mechanisms including particle size-dependent uptake and clearance. In the following, we will discuss a systems-wide approach to improve the fraction of a drug delivered to tissues and cells in an effort to maximize therapeutic actions at respective target sites, and in the process, minimize exposure to off-target sites that may elicit untoward effects.

16.7
A Size-Dependent Targeting to Tissues and Cells

Most proteins in a solution assume an overall hydrodynamic size of only a few nanometers (nm) in diameter. Upon hydration, immunoglobulin G (IgG), for example, exhibits a diameter of about 5 nm. In the absence of receptor-mediated uptake, protein and peptide particles are too small to be recognized by mononuclear phagocyte or MPS cells. Systematic studies with lipid particles of varying diameters indicate that spherical particles greater than 50–70 nm are taken up by phagocytes in the MPS and cleared readily into the liver for degradation and excretion, while particles smaller than 30 nm in general appear to be less susceptible to elimination through the MPS. Similar observations were made with efficient phagocytic uptake of bacterial and fungal infection, which was cleared to the spleen and liver. Clearance of particulate drugs in the spleen and liver are mostly inactivated and eliminated. In some cases, however, the drug accumulation in these eliminating organs and tissue could induce untoward effects.

The idea of exploiting differential particle size for drug targeting is not completely new and we could learn much from physiological processes in nature. As summarized in Figure 16.3, the ability of macrophages and phagocytes of the MPS to clear a substance increases significantly with increasing sizes of nanoparticulate matter. Mononuclear phagocytes that have naturally taken up particles are found in the liver and spleen. Many of these phagocytes circulate in and out of these and other tissues such as lymph nodes throughout the body. However, a majority of the particulate matter taken up by MPS would eventually clear and be transferred by cells into the spleen and liver, the eliminating organs. For many drugs, these organs are often associated with undesirable or toxicological consequences. Other than drugs targeted to the spleen and liver, for many drugs, clearing the drug particles into these sites also prevents the nanodrug

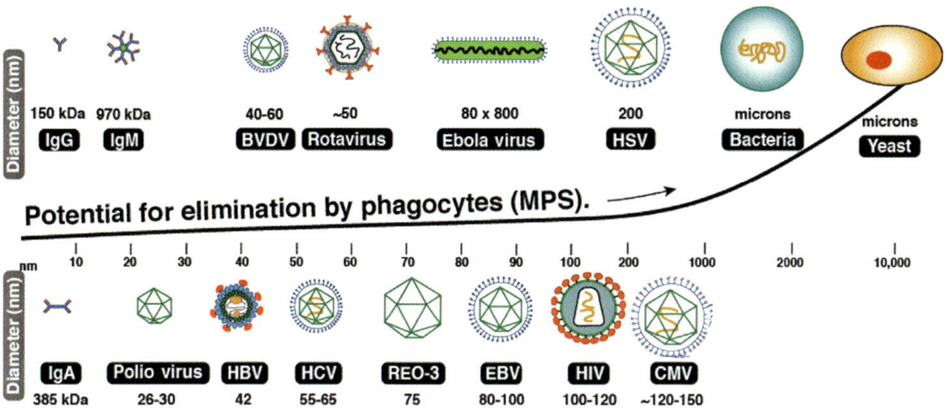

Figure 16.3 Particle size and an increase in potential for phagocytic recognition by cells of mononuclear phagocyte system (MPS). Proteins and peptides, including antibody molecules such as immunoglobulin G (IgG), A (IgA), or multimeric M (IgM) exhibit a hydrodynamic diameter of ~10–20 nm, while various viruses with or without a member coat range from 20 to 200 nm. Some of these viruses, such as the Ebola virus, have an overall elongated structure. In the absence of receptor-mediated binding, phagocytic cells in the human's mononuclear phagocyte system recognize particles with increasing affinity as the size of particle increases. Particle sizes less than 20–50 nm are not readily recognizable by phagocytes, while particles larger than 1–2000 are taken up quickly by these cells. Particles and viruses that are within 100–200 nm are often not subjected to exhibit lower potential for macrophage and phagocyte-mediated clearance. Abbreviations: HBV, hepatitis B virus; HCV, hepatitis C virus; EBV, Epstein–Barr virus; HIV, human immunodeficiency virus; CMV, cytomegalovirus; bovine viral diarrhea virus; HSV, herpes simplex virus. Adapted from Ref. [1].

formulations to reach intended targeted tumor and viral infected tissues. On the other hand, this size-dependent mechanism serves to clear invading microbes or drug carriers in the absence of antibody or receptor recognition to prevent opportunistic infection.

Based on the understanding of particulate uptake and clearance mechanisms, drug carriers in the range of nano- or micrometer diameters can be developed for respective drug target applications. For example, avoidance of phagocytosis would be useful to design a carrier intended to increase the plasma residence time of proteins. On the other hand, if a drug is required to accumulate in phagocytic target cells (e.g., cells affected by yeast infection) for therapeutic action, an increase in the apparent size of the molecule may be beneficial. Encapsulation of proteins and peptides in liposome carriers of 100 nm or larger has been shown to greatly improve protein localization in phagocytically active MPS cells, leading to a therapeutic drug in lymphoid organs such as the spleen and lymph nodes.

Taking advantage of particle size-dependent accumulation, soluble recombinant viral protein antigens could be formulated into their particulate forms to enhance MPS uptake. As a result, antigen-presenting cells within the MPS provide an immune response necessary for vaccines to be effective. *In vivo* liposome disposition studies indicate that large liposomes are taken up efficiently by macrophages in blood and tissues, including the liver and spleen. Since macrophages are thought to be predominantly responsible for processing and presenting liposome-associated or encapsulated antigens, the liposome formulation provides an excellent way to enhance antigen delivery and presentation for both humoral and cellular immune responses to vaccines. Mechanisms of liposome-mediated immune enhancement have been reviewed previously [21]. Antigens taken up by macrophages are presented in the major histocompatibility (MHC, self- versus nonself-recognition transplantation marker) class II antigens. Antigens delivered to other phagocytic cells such as Langerhans and dendritic cells may also enhance the presence of antigens in MHC class I antigens [22]. Thus, both antibody and cell-mediated immune responses can be enhanced by particulate forms of recombinant antigens.

The influence of physicochemical properties of liposomes such as charge density, membrane fluidity, and epitope density on the immune response elicited by antigens has been extensively studied [23]. In addition to antigens, other immune stimulators that are amphoteric muramyl peptides or lipid-soluble compounds, such as monophosphoryl lipid A or muramyl tripeptidyl-phosphatidylethanolamine, can also be incorporated into liposomes to increase their adjuvant effect in eliciting an immune responses [24]. A liposome-based hepatitis A vaccine (*Epaxal*), developed by the Swiss Serum and Vaccine Institute, has been tested in humans [25]. This vaccine contains formalin-inactivated hepatitis A virus particles attached to liposomes together expressing the influenza virus hemagglutinin. The advantage of the vaccine is that it not only induces antibodies to the hepatitis A antigen but also elicits an immune response against the influenza virus protein on the liposome surface [26]. The inclusion of influenza hemagglutinin in the preparation also enhances the binding and fusion of hepatitis A liposomes to target cells.

Particle size-dependent targeting of drugs to the spleen and lymph nodes can also be achieved with other lipid–drug complexes. An example is amphotericin B bound to either a lipid mixture as a lipid–drug complex or to liposomes that direct this otherwise effective drug of choice with serious side effects to the spleen, MPS, and the site of fungal accumulation. Amphotericin is a drug of choice to treat serious fungal infection despite a high risk of nephrotoxicity and infusion-related reactions. Incorporation of amphotericin B in a liposome formulation has provided a size amenable for an MPS uptake. It also reduces amphotericin B precipitation at the site of injection. An amphotericin B in a liposome formulation called *Ambisome* has greatly improved the drug's accumulation in the spleen (~200 mg/g of tissue) for antifungal action. Binding of poorly soluble amphotericin B to lipid in *Ambisome* also prevents precipitations of amphotericin in host cell membranes in the kidney, thus reduce the renal toxicity observed with free amphotericin B antifungal therapy. In a multicenter clinical trial (MSG-032) that enrolled 687 patients, a much higher dose was administered with improved safety and reduced infusion site reactions as well as nephrotoxicity detected by an increase in the measured serum creatinine amount. More importantly, at the recommended dose, the breakthrough infection rate due to fungal infection was reduced by 2.4-fold (7.8 versus 11%) [27]. The amphotericin B-lipid complex accumulates preferentially in MPS cells *in vivo*, thereby improving delivery of amphotericin B to fungal-infected phagocytes in the spleen [28,29]. As a consequence of this distribution, the kidney is exposed to less free amphotericin B and nephrotoxicity is reduced, thereby improving the therapeutic index of the parent drug. At least three lipid-associated amphotericin formulations – *Ambisome*, *Abelcet*, and *Amphotec* – have been developed to exploit this mechanism. At 0.6 mg/kg of the *Abelcet* form of lipid-associated amphotericin B, data from pharmacokinetic studies point to about a fourfold increase (34.1 versus 132.7 mL/min) in plasma clearance likely due to rapid uptake of lipid-bound drug particles by macrophages that accumulated in the spleen (the site of microbe accumulation) in patients with leishmaniasis [27]. In theory, amphotericin B can be replaced with other hydrophobic antibiotics or peptide derivatives to provide similar degrees of success in reaching fungal accumulation in the spleen and MPS.

16.8 Ligand–Receptor-Based Targeting: Active Drug Targeting

The quantitative detail of tissue and cell localization of drug targets is one of the most challenging aspects of drug development. Most contemporary drug molecules are developed based on either receptor, effector, or enzyme binding and inhibition at the molecular level. However, these drug target molecules may be distributed in many tissues and cells at varying degrees. In most cases, very few drug targets specific to diseased cells exist, with the exception of virus-infected cells that express viral-directed proteins, such as HIV specific protease. Most drug targets, such as cancer-associated phenotype markers or receptors, are expressed in many cell types and tissues. However, their expression levels may be lower in control or healthy cells. Even in the case of viral protein targets distinctly expressed in infected cells, a drug's design to inhibit the enzyme may also cross-react with human protease enzymes. Nevertheless, integrating a better understanding of drug and drug target-tissue distribution in the various biological systems – systems approach – in drug delivery would allow one to take full advantage of developing the most effective targeted drug delivery strategies.

Ligand–receptor-based targeting is intended to leverage the knowledge of the target tissues that mediate pharmacologic, biologic, and toxicologic responses. Some of the challenges and complexities are driven from an incomplete understanding of the target-specific ligand–receptor interaction and the degree of receptor expression on target cells versus bystander cells. Exclusive or predominant expression of these receptors on target cells and tissues rarely occur. The same thinking can be applied to antigen–antibody interactions; either a ligand or a receptor could be used as an antigen to produce a selective monoclonal antibody for targeting. Recall that a typical immunoglobulin or monoclonal IgG molecule, when hydrated fully in a solution, exhibits a hydrodynamic diameter of about 10 nm. In theory, ligand–receptor-based targeting to tissues and cells is only limited by our ability to identify target-specific antigens or ligands and develop antibodies against them. These antibodies or targeting molecules can be conjugated to cytotoxic agents such as toxins or drugs, or expressed on drug carriers loaded with therapeutic agents.

Based on these principles, cell-associated ligands, receptors (i.e., galactose receptors on hepatocytes or folate receptors in actively growing cells and tumors), or antigens, such as carcinoembryonic antigen (CEA), can be used for targeting. Tumor antigens identified so far are also expressed on nontarget healthy cells, albeit in low densities. In fact, *tumor-specific antigens* – the term used to describe antigens isolated from certain tumor cells and tissues (e.g., prostate antigen) – are now referred to as *tumor-associated antigens*, which are expressed at much higher levels in tumor cells than in normal cells. Therefore, knowledge of the receptor's density or degree of overexpression in target tissues compared to nontarget sites, and the ability of the particle to perfuse target tissues, allows one to refine the design of targeted drug delivery system.

Scientists are making progress in understanding tumor-associated antigens and their distribution and expression in normal versus different types of tumor cells. Knowledge about the differential expression of galactose, glucose, and mannose sugar receptor density in hepatocytes and mononuclear phagocytes are integrated in the design of intracellular enzyme replacement therapies. Some therapeutic proteins carry glycosyl group or glycosylated as a part of post-translational protein synthesis. These glycosyl group attached to proteins are sugar polymers with varying sequences, including galactose, glucose, and mannose but are ended with a terminal sialic acid cap. A number of intracellular enzymes active within the lysosome compartment, including β-glucuronidase and β-agalsidase, are glycoproteins with a terminal N-acetylmuramic acid (or sialic acid cap) in its native form. The terminal sialic acid on a glycoprotein is known to prevent exposure of the internal sugar residues such as galactose and mannose. It has been known for quite some time that hepatocytes in the liver exhibit a high density of galactose receptors; macrophages of the MPS express the mannose receptor. Based on this knowledge and the understanding that metabolic enzyme deficiency of β-glucuronidase and β-agalsidase is related to enzyme deficiency within the lysosomes of MPS cells, the clinical product is targeted to these intracellular sites with recombinant enzymes that are modified to expose mannose. The availability of mannose on the glycoprotein enzyme (β-glucuronidase (*Ceredase*) and β-agalsidase (*Fabrazyme*)) allows target localization of *Ceredase* and *Fabrazyme* as effective therapy for the reversal of a genetic disorder due to progressive accumulation of glycolipid in patients.

16.8.1
Target Selected Delivery of a Toxin with an Antibody

While antibody molecules, particularly IgG ($d \sim 10$ nm), exhibit intrinsic biologic activities such as neutralizing pathogens, binding to receptors, and receptor-mediated consequences, these effects may not be sufficiently potent for therapeutic applications. To increase antibody potency against tumor cells, highly potent bacterial toxins are conjugated to an antibody. In this case, the antibody provides binding selectivity to the toxin molecules. Antibody–toxin conjugates, which can be produced chemically or by a recombinant approach as a fusion protein, are generally known as *immunotoxins*.

Most of the toxins used to construct immunotoxins interfere with protein synthesis by either catalytic inactivation of the elongation factor through ADP-ribosylation or by directly inactivating ribosomes [30]. It has been estimated that only one to five toxin molecules per cell are required to completely abrogate intracellular protein synthesis and elicit cytotoxicity. Very often, bacterial toxins contain two domains. Typically, the A subunit contains cytotoxic sequences, and the B subunit contains binding activity. The two subunits can be separated to retain only the cytotoxic component, thereby eliminating the potential for toxins being directed toward nonspecific targets. Toxins studied in immunotoxin development include diphtheria toxin (derived from *Corynebacterium diphtheriae*), ricin, abrin, mistletoe lectin, and modeccin. Some toxins that are expressed as a single chain protein do not contain binding domains (e.g., saporin and gelonin). Pseudomonas exotoxin A (derived from *Pseudomonas aeruginosa*) contains a binding domain but it can be muted to prevent it from binding to intrinsic targets. These cytotoxic subunits are then chemically linked to an antibody selective for a target antigen (e.g., Erb-2 breast cancer-associated antigen).

A newer class of immunotoxins, recombinant immunotoxins, contains the variable minimum antigen binding domain of an antibody (Fv) fused with a toxin gene and expressed by recombinant DNA technology. The use of Fv 25 kDa, as supposed to IgG 150 kDa, for targeting provides sixfold molecular size reduction. These recombinant toxins, like conventional immunotoxins, can be directed to target antigens or receptors. Anti-Tac-PE38 (targeted to CD25 antigen and designated as LMB-2) and RFB4-PE38 (targeted to CD22 antigen and designated as BL22) are recombinant immunotoxins containing truncated Pseudomonas exotoxin (PE) that have been shown to exhibit clinical activity in patients with hematologic malignancies. BL22 and LMB-2 also show a lower degree of vascular leak syndrome and are thought to be less immunogenic than conventional immunotoxin conjugates. Several other recombinant immunotoxins with major responses have been reported, particularly in hematological malignancies [31]. In 36 patients with drug resistant hairy cell leukemia (HCL), the above mentioned BL22 (RFB4-PE38) immunotoxin was tested in a Phase II clinical trial. The results showed that BL22 is active in HCL and appeared to be tolerable in two treatment cycles that led to nearly a threefold improvement in the complete response rate [32].

Recombinant immunotoxins based on the Fv domain typically have a molecular weight of 60–65 kDa, compared with a molecular weight of 200 kDa for conventional immunotoxins. The overall molecular weight reduction by about threefold could increase tumor penetration and also host immune response against immunotoxin.

A close relative of immunotoxins is the growth factor fusion toxin, in which the antibody is replaced with a ligand or a growth factor to provide selectivity of the toxin domain in an immunotoxin. One such molecule containing human interleukin-2 (IL-2) fused to truncated diphtheria toxin (denileukin diftitox or *Ontak*) has been approved by the FDA for treating lymphoma.

The progress made in the identification and characterization of target receptors, increasing the potency while reducing toxin molecule premature release, and the more compact size of recombinant immunotoxin molecules suggest that the immunotoxin field is poised to make a major impact on cancer treatment. A more compact protein should allow a higher degree of penetration into solid tumor masses; also, the increased differentiation power due to improvement in tumor-associated antigen recognition should yield improved safety. If the smaller and more compact immunotoxins are proven to have less immunogenic potential, repeated dosing could become feasible, which could extend clinical impact.

In addition to the use of a toxin as an effector, radionuclides have also been shown to be very effective agents to improve the therapeutic response of an antibody. With the progress made in conjugate chemistry, stability of a radionuclide either directly conjugated or chelated to antibody derivatives has improved. As a result, a number of high-energy radionuclides such as In-111 and Y-90 are prepared by a specialized pharmacy and facility for therapeutic use. For many years the impact of radionuclide attachment on a parent therapeutic antibody was not fully understood. With the availability of the same therapeutic antibody molecule with and without a radionuclide conjugate, it was clearly shown that a significant gain in both overall response and complete response rate is seen with the radiolabeled anti-CD20 antibody used to treat patients with transformed B-cell non-Hodgkin's lymphoma (NHL). In clinical studies, the nonradiolabeled version of the anti-CD20 antibody (*Rituxan*) was compared with the radiolabeled version (*Zevalin*) that uses the In-111 and Y-90 isotopes. The overall response rates and complete response rates for *Rituxan* and *Zevalin* were 56 versus 74–80% and 16 versus 30%, respectively. This indicates that there is approximately a twofold increase in complete response rate in NHL when the radiolabeled antibody is used for therapy. Another anti-CD20 antibody labeled with radioiodine (the I-131 isotope) also showed added benefits over that of native antibody. In a pivotal study for regulatory approval involving the I-131-labeled antiCD20 antibody *Bexxar*, the overall response rate over 26 months was 68% and the complete response rate was 33%.

16.8.2 Targeting of Drug in Lipid Nanoparticles Based on Ligand–Receptor Interactions

Active targeting of liposomes, lipid, and other nanoparticles usually involves chemically-coupled ligands expressed on a particle surface. A number of ligands or receptors, such as antibodies, growth factors, cytokines, hormones, and toxins, have been anchored and expressed on liposome surfaces so that drugs, proteins, and nucleic acids may be introduced into target cells. *In vitro*, liposomes coated with monoclonal antibodies (immunoliposomes) can provide target-specific binding to cells in *in vitro* experimental systems [33,34]. However, *in vivo*, a number of pharmaceutical properties – stability and the appropriate disposition profile – must be met before active targeting of liposomes using ligand–receptor interactions can be realized. Some of these properties include (1) stability of liposomes expressing specific targeting molecules and availability for target cell binding, (2) sufficient circulation time of the lipid–drug carrier in plasma and blood for it to perfuse target organs or tissues, and eventually interact with and bind to the target cells, and (3) a sufficient fraction of the drug-bound carrier to localize in the target tissue to allow a sufficient carrier with drugs to selectively bind to target cells. Without sufficient residence time in the blood circulation, most of the liposomes will be cleared without making contact with cell targets. Other important factors include the ligand and receptor interactions on the target cells with sufficient specificity. The targeting molecule(s) expressed on the liposome surface must also be sufficiently stable *in vivo* and exhibit minimum potential of being extracted from the particles by serum proteins found in blood.

16.9 Conclusions and Future Prospects

Advances in the knowledge of the distinctions in drug disposition, barriers to absorption, and the mechanisms of distribution and elimination have led to the development of novel drug delivery strategies. Advanced drug delivery and drug research has yielded products with an improved therapeutic index and other improvements in safety and efficacy. For example, some drug formulations can reduce dosing frequency yet provide better therapeutic response. Research to discover sites of drug action through proteomic modeling and high-throughput screening has yielded targets that have been used to construct fusion proteins with added effector function to enhance pharmacologic activity. As the efficiency of identifying drug targets has improved, combinatorial chemistry and high-throughput synthesis and drug screening technology has matured and pharmaceutical formulation and delivery strategies have become the rate-limiting steps in bringing new molecular entities to market. The growing knowledge of these properties collectively referred to as biopharmaceutical characteristics and drug target distribution and pharmacokinetics as they are linked to therapeutic responses, has allowed development of novel drug delivery strategies. These strategies can now be considered in the context of human physiological interactions – referred to as a "systems approach" to drug delivery. Clinical examples exist on a passive or active drug targeting strategy; using nanomaterials that are biocompatible or biodegradable improves the therapeutic index that leads to dose reduction or minimizing untoward effects at extended doses. The best results are often achieved with strategies that influence drug localization and exposure to target tissues and cells but keep that drug away from organs linked to toxicity. The biodistribution of all drug targets in cells and tissues within the body is not yet fully understood. However, virus- or bacteria-laden cell distribution, and by extension their protein target localization in cells and tissues, are now mapped, elucidated, and validated for defined organs within the body. Such knowledge has and will continue to influence nanodrug-targeting design for successful development of targeted drug delivery systems to improve the therapeutic index. Some of these practices could be implemented also in pharmacy and clinical setting for compounding and reformulation of drug dosage forms.

References

1 Ho, R.J.Y. (2013) *Biotechnology and Biopharmaceuticals: Transforing Proteins and Genes into Drugs*, 2nd edn, John Wiley & Sons, Inc., Hoboken, NJ.
2 Weinberg, B.D., Blanc, E., and Ga, J.M. (2008) Polymer implants for intratumoral drug delivery and cancer therapy. *J. Pharm. Sci.*, **97** (5), 1681–1702.
3 Ortwine, D.F. and Aliagas, I. (2013) Physicochemical and DMPK *in silico* models: facilitating their use by medicinal chemists. *Mol. Pharm.*, **10** (4), 1153–1161.
4 Rodrigues, S. and Grenha, A. (2015) Activation of macrophages: establishing a role for polysaccharides in drug delivery strategies envisaging antibacterial therapy. *Curr. Pharm. Des.*, **21** (33), 4869–4887.
5 Ho, R.J.Y., Yu, J., Li, B., Kraft, J.C., Freeling, J.P., Koehn, J. *et al.* (2015) Systems approach to targeted and long-acting HIV/AIDS therapy. *Drug Deliv. Transl. Res.*, **5** (6), 531–539.
6 Freeling, J.P. and Ho, R.J.Y. (2014) Anti-HIV drug particles may overcome lymphatic drug insufficiency and associated HIV persistence. *Proc. Natl. Acad. Sci. USA.*, **111** (25), E2512–E2513.
7 Hurler, J., Zakelj, S., Mravljak, J., Pajk, S., Kristl, A., Schubert, R. *et al.* (2013) The effect of lipid composition and liposome size on the release properties of liposomes-in-hydrogel. *Int. J. Pharm.*, **456** (1), 49–57.
8 Al Zaki, A., Hui, J.Z., Higbee, E., and Tsourkas, A. (2015) Biodistribution, clearance, and toxicology of polymeric micelles loaded with 0.9 or 5 nm gold nanoparticles. *J. Biomed. Nanotechnol.*, **11** (10), 1836–1846.
9 Mekaru, H., Lu, J., and Tamanoi, F. (2015) Development of mesoporous silica-based nanoparticles with controlled release capability for cancer therapy. *Adv. Drug Deliv. Rev.*, **95**, 40–49.
10 Xu, H.Y., Fan, M.M., Elhissi, A.M.A., Zhang, Z.R., Wan, K.W., Ahmed, W. *et al.* (2015) PEGylated graphene oxide for tumor-targeted delivery of paclitaxel. *Nanomedicine*, **10** (8), 1247–1262.
11 Chan, J.M., Zhang, L., Yuet, K.P., Liao, G., Rhee, J.W., Langer, R. *et al.* (2009) PLGA-lecithin-PEG core–shell nanoparticles for controlled drug delivery. *Biomaterials*, **30** (8), 1627–1634.
12 Barrett-Lee, P.J., Dixon, J.M., Farrell, C., Jones, A., Leonard, R., Murray, N. *et al.* (2009) Expert opinion on the use of anthracyclines in patients with advanced breast cancer at cardiac risk. *Ann. Oncol.*, **20** (5), 816–827.
13 Greish, K. (2010) Enhanced permeability and retention (EPR) effect for anticancer nanomedicine drug targeting. *Methods Mol. Biol.*, **624**, 25–37.
14 Bashour, S.I. and Ibrahim, N.K. (2015) CCR 20th anniversary commentary: setting the stage for nanoparticle albumin-bound paclitaxel-how far science has come. *Clin. Cancer Res.*, **21** (9), 1975–1977.
15 Dengl, S., Hoffmann, E., Grote, M., Wagner, C., Mundigl, O., Georges, G. *et al.* (2015) Hapten-directed spontaneous disulfide shuffling: a universal technology for site-directed covalent coupling of payloads to antibodies. *Faseb J.*, **29** (5), 1763–1779.
16 Shi, J.F. and Xu, B. (2015) Nanoscale assemblies of small molecules control the fate of cells. *Nano Today*, **10** (5), 615–630.

17 Yu, L.J., Wall, B.A., Wangari-Talbot, J., and Chen, S. (2016) Metabotropic glutamate receptors in cancer. *Neuropharmacology*, doi: 10.1016/j.neuropharm.2016.02.011.
18 Lipinski, C.A., Lombardo, F., Dominy, B.W., and Feeney, P.J. (2001) Experimental and computational approaches to estimate solubility and permeability in drug discovery and development settings. *Adv. Drug Deliv. Rev.*, **46** (1–3), 3–26.
19 Cornelis, M.C., Byrne, E.M., Esko, T., Nalls, M.A., Ganna, A., Paynter, N. *et al.* (2015) Genome-wide meta-analysis identifies six novel loci associated with habitual coffee consumption. *Mol. Psychiatry*, **20** (5), 647–656.
20 Lian, T. and Ho, R.J.Y. (2001) Trends and developments in liposome drug delivery systems. *J. Pharm. Sci.*, **90** (6), 667–680.
21 Alving, C.R. and Rao, M. (2008) Lipid A and liposomes containing lipid A as antigens and adjuvants. *Vaccine*, **26** (24), 3036–3045.
22 Lian, T., Bui, T., and Ho, R.J.Y. (1999) Formulation of HIV-envelope protein with lipid vesicles expressing ganglioside GM1 associated to cholera toxin B enhances mucosal immune responses. *Vaccine*, **18** (7–8), 604–611.
23 Kersten, G.F. and Crommelin, D.J. (1995) Liposomes and ISCOMS as vaccine formulations. *Biochim. Biophys. Acta*, **1241** (2), 117–138.
24 Bui, T., Dykers, T., Hu, S.L., Faltynek, C.R., and Ho, R.J.Y. (1994) Effect of MTP-PE liposomes and interleukin-7 on induction of antibody and cell-mediated immune responses to a recombinant HIV-envelope protein. *J. Acquir. Immune Defic. Syndr.*, **7** (8), 799–806.
25 Ambrosch, F., Wiedermann, G., Jonas, S., Althaus, B., Finkel, B., Gluck, R. *et al.* (1997) Immunogenicity and protectivity of a new liposomal hepatitis A vaccine. *Vaccine*, **15** (11), 1209–1213.
26 Gluck, R., Mischler, R., Finkel, B., Que, J.U., Scarpa, B., and Cryz, S.J. Jr. (1994) Immunogenicity of new virosome influenza vaccine in elderly people. *Lancet*, **344** (8916), 160–163.
27 Walsh, T.J., Finberg, R.W., Arndt, C., Hiemenz, J., Schwartz, C., Bodensteiner, D. *et al.* (1999) Liposomal amphotericin B for empirical therapy in patients with persistent fever and neutropenia. National Institute of Allergy and Infectious Diseases Mycoses Study Group. *N. Engl. J. Med.*, **340** (10), 764–771.
28 Adedoyin, A., Swenson, C.E., Bolcsak, L.E., Hellmann, A., Radowska, D., Horwith, G. *et al.* (2000) A pharmacokinetic study of amphotericin B lipid complex injection (Abelcet) in patients with definite or probable systemic fungal infections. *Antimicrob. Agents Chemother.*, **44** (10), 2900–2902.
29 Chopra, R. (2002) AmBisome in the treatment of fungal infections: the UK experience. *J. Antimicrob. Chemother.*, (49 Suppl 1), 43–47.
30 Pastan, I.I. and Kreitman, R.J. (1998) Immunotoxins for targeted cancer therapy. *Adv. Drug Deliv. Rev.*, **31** (1–2), 53–88.
31 Kreitman, R.J., Wilson, W.H., Bergeron, K., Raggio, M., Stetler-Stevenson, M., FitzGerald, D.J. *et al.* (2001) Efficacy of the anti-CD22 recombinant immunotoxin BL22 in chemotherapy-resistant hairy-cell leukemia. *N. Engl. J. Med.*, **345** (4), 241–247.
32 Kreitman, R.J., Stetler-Stevenson, M., Margulies, I., Noel, P., Fitzgerald, D.J., Wilson, W.H. *et al.* (2009) Phase II trial of recombinant immunotoxin RFB4(dsFv)-PE38 (BL22) in patients with hairy cell leukemia. *J. Clin. Oncol.*, **27** (18), 2983–2990.
33 Ho, S.C. and Huang, L. (1983) A novel cytochemical marker for liposome decomposition in lysosomes. *J. Histochem. Cytochem.*, **31** (3), 404–410.
34 Huang, A., Huang, L., and Kennel, S.J. (1980) Monoclonal antibody covalently coupled with fatty acid. A reagent for *in vitro* liposome targeting. *J. Biol. Chem.*, **255** (17), 8015–8018.

17
Nanoparticle Toxicity: General Overview and Insights Into Immunological Compatibility

Marina A. Dobrovolskaia

Nanotechnology Characterization Laboratory, Cancer Research Technology Program, NCI at Frederick, Frederick National Laboratory for Cancer Research, Leidos Biomedical Research, Inc., 1050 Boyles Street, Frederick, MD 21702-1201, USA

17.1
Introduction

Nanoparticles include a broad spectrum of materials with different chemical compositions, architectures, and physicochemical properties. Industrial applications of nanomaterials include among others, materials for coloration, radiation protection, membranes and filters, imaging and molecular diagnostics, magnetic chemistry, flow through reactors, and fuel cells [1]. The benefits of using nanoparticles in the industry usually include reduced cost and better efficiency. For example, using nanoparticles as solar battery constituents allows decreasing the cost of photochemical electricity generation, significantly [1]. Also, nanoparticles are not uncommon in consumer products and cosmetics [2,3]. For example, certain clothing, wound dressings, washing machine liners, sunglasses, and sporting equipments contain nanomaterials for improving durability and increasing resistance to water and microbial growth [2]. Nanosized titanium and zinc oxides are common components of sunscreens while liposomes and nanoemulsions are ingredients in various cosmetic products [3]. The unique physicochemical properties of nanosized particles make them promising candidate drugs and drug carriers because nanoparticles help improving solubility, pharmacokinetics, biodistribution and decreasing the toxicity of traditional small molecules, and biotechnology-derived pharmaceuticals. Many nanotechnology-based formulations of existing drugs are already commercially available while others are in various stages of preclinical and clinical development [4].

Along with the increasing use of nanomaterials come the concerns regarding their safety. Two factors are used to evaluate the risk of using nanomaterials in terms of human health. They are exposure and hazard. Consequently, the risk assessment paradigm evaluates the risk as the exposure multiplied by the hazard.

Pharmaceutical Nanotechnology: Innovation and Production, First Edition. Edited by Jean Cornier, Arno Kwade, Andrew Owen, and Marcel Van de Voorde.

In the absence of exposure, the risk is also absent regardless of the toxicity. For example, even a highly toxic compound provides no exposure if sealed in a closed container and is therefore considered as safe. In contrast, a material with significantly lower toxicity but higher exposure may not be safe. The risk management mitigates adverse effects by controlling the probability of release during the intended use (low exposure) and the composition (low hazard).

Nanoparticles are considered as chemicals and are regulated under Registration, Evaluation, Authorization, and Restriction of Chemicals (REACH) in the European Union [5], and under the Toxic Substances Control Act (TSCA) in the United States [6]. Several international initiatives are also underway to ensure safe production and low environmental impact of nanotechnology-based products. For example, the International Organization for Standardization (ISO) and the Organization for Economic Cooperation and Development (OECD), are engaged in nanotechnology safety issues by providing standard development for nanomaterial characterization [7,8]. OECD has founded a Working Party on Manufactured Nanomaterials (WPMN) [9]. WPMN runs several projects aimed at the understanding of the properties and potential risks of nanomaterials. The United States and Canada have collaborative initiatives operated by the Regulatory Cooperation Council (RCC) [10]. The RCC efforts go beyond the environmental safety of nanomaterials, and among other areas cover the medicinal application of nanotechnology products. Nanoparticles intended for medical applications or used as components of medical devices are regulated according to the regulatory framework established by the US Food and Drug Administration (FDA) and European Medicines Agency (EMA) for traditional low molecular weight drugs, and biotechnology products. Formulations containing both a nanocarrier and a low molecular weight drug or biological (e.g., therapeutic antibody or protein), are considered as combination products and are reviewed by the Office of Combination Products in the United States [11,12]. Collectively, international organizations and country-specific regulatory agencies (e.g., US FDA, US Environmental Protection Agency, EMA, ISO, OECD, Health Canada, and RCC) focus their efforts on several areas. These focus areas include testing and assessment, risk assessment and regulatory programs, exposure evaluation and mitigation, control over safety, and cooperation on the environmentally sustainable use of nanotechnology.

Toxicology of nanomaterials is a broad subject, and many comprehensive reviews and books are available to the reader who is interested in a detailed overview of a particular aspect of this rapidly growing area of research [13–21]. The purpose of this chapter is to provide a general summary of the field and highlight the most prominent findings. Several types of nanomaterial toxicity resulting from the common exposure routes such as dermal, inhalation, gastrointestinal, and systemic delivery are reviewed here. While the focus of this book is nanopharmacy, examples of both incidental and biomedical nanoparticles will be reviewed, because of the unprecedented need for interdisciplinarity and the importance of learning from research conducted across applications.

17.2 Systemic Toxicity

Nanoparticles can enter the body intentionally (e.g., following intravenous injection for medical applications) or accidently (e.g., through environmental exposure). Irrespective of exposure route, nanoparticles must enter the systemic circulation in order to distribute throughout the body and accumulate in the target tissue. Organs of the mononuclear phagocytic system (MPS) are commonly named as targets for engineered nanomaterials. For example, cationic dendrimers with different core structures including melamine and polyamidoamine were shown to be hepatotoxic due to sequestration by Kupffer cells [22,23]. Since uptake by the MPS organs depends on opsonization, which in turn is determined by the particle size and surface functionality, modification of nanoparticle surface with hydrophilic polymer coatings (e.g., polyethylene glycol or PEG) is a common approach to reducing the toxicity of nanoparticle to liver, spleen, and bone marrow. The liver and spleen are common target organs for lipid-based nanoparticles due to their higher tropism for phagocytic cells [24–26]. The kidney is often a target organ for nanomaterials that clear through the urinary excretion route. Such materials include small particles with hydrodynamic size less than 10 nm. For example, low generation dendrimers, water-soluble fullerene derivatives and certain types of carbon nanotubes were shown to be toxic to kidneys [27–29]. Mechanisms of nanoparticle systemic toxicity commonly include oxidative stress and lysosomal dysfunction. For example, neodymium oxide particles, quantum dots, and fullerenes induce autophagic activation *in vitro* [30–32]. CNT-induced oxidative stress activates cell signaling pathways, which stimulate expression of proinflammatory and fibrotic cytokines [33]. Accumulation in and activation of macrophages and neutrophils were also described as the source of ROS in response to metallic nanomaterials [34–36]. Metal oxides, such as titanium dioxide (TiO_2), cerium oxide (CeO_2), and zinc oxide (ZnO) have been shown to induce oxidative stress [37]. Generation of ROS in response to nanomaterials may have a different mechanism, which is determined by the nanoparticle physicochemical properties. For example, most of the metal-based nanoparticles trigger free radical formation and toxicity related to them through Fenton-type reactions [38,39]. In contrast, carbon nanotubes induce ROS via mitochondrial damage [40]. Lipid-based nanoparticles activate oxidative stress pathways through mechanisms independent of mitochondria and peroxisomes [41], and thus a consideration of the material-basis for adverse effects is needed.

When nanoparticles are used for drug delivery, both the toxicity of nanoparticle carrier and that of the drug have to be considered. Due to their unique physicochemical properties, nanoparticle-based carriers may change the distribution of the drug and as such result in an altered toxicity profile (Figure 17.1). For example, the anticancer drug doxorubicin distributes to bone marrow and cardiomyocytes, resulting in myelosuppression and cardiotoxicity [42]. However, when the same drug is encapsulated in a PEGylated liposome, the carrier protects the drug from distribution to the bone marrow and heart tissue, thus

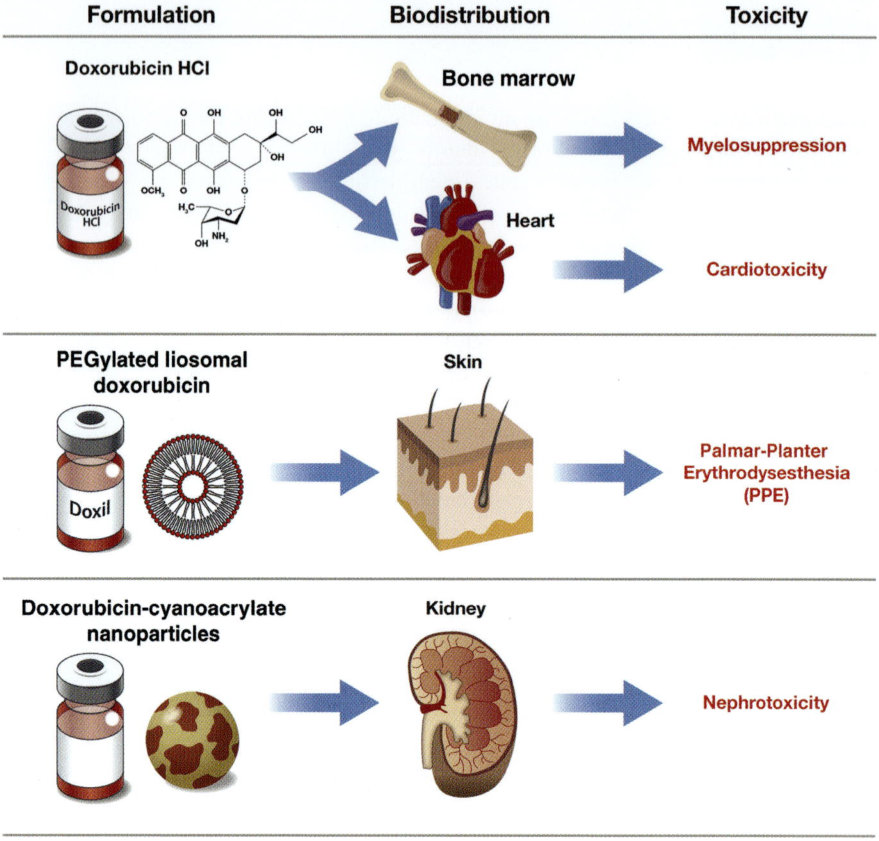

Figure 17.1 *The role of nanoparticle distribution in drug toxicity.* Nanoparticles may change biodistribution of the drug. Altered distribution results in altered toxicity.

reducing myelosuppression and cardiotoxicity. Conversely, the PEGylated liposome results in drug accumulation in the skin and resulting in a different toxicity known as palmar-plantar erythrodysesthesia (PPE) [43]. When the cyanoacrylate-based nanoparticle is used as a carrier for doxorubicin the drug and the toxicity associated with it relocates to the kidney [44]. Therefore, it is critical to consider the tissue distribution of the carrier to monitor the toxicity of the drug associated with it.

17.3 Pulmonary Toxicity

Nanoparticles can travel in the air by Brownian diffusion, and as such, they may be inhaled and deposit within alveolar regions of the lungs [45–47]. Particle translocation from the lungs to other organs depends on many factors such as composition, size, shape, and surface properties of the inhaled nanoparticles [45–47]. When investigating the distribution of inhaled nanomaterials it is also important to recognize that study design may contribute significantly to test results and may explain some discrepancies between studies. For example, some studies reported the distribution of iridium nanoparticles, administered through tracheal instillation, from the lungs to liver, spleen, brain, and heart of experimental rats [48,49]. In contrast to these studies, another report showed a lack of carbon nanoparticle distribution to the secondary organs [50]. Since inhalation cannot exclude ingestion, particle accumulation in the liver following inhalation may also include gastrointestinal absorption, which is responsible for subsequent distribution of nanoparticles to the liver, spleen and other organs. Based on these points Oberdorster *et al.* concluded that considering study design is necessary for data interpretation [49]. The same group later suggested to include several end-points (reactive oxygen species, lactate dehydrogenase leakage, protein oxidation induction, number of polymorphonuclear neutrophils in bronchoalveolar fluid) in the study design to correlate *in vitro* and *in vivo* toxicology data [51].

Another challenge in conducting pulmonary toxicity studies on engineered nanomaterials is related to the presence of incidental particulates in the air. For example, a study investigating occupational exposure in an engine machining plant reported that concentration of incidental nanoparticles from natural furnace exhaust was greater than that produced by the engine machining [52]. When incidental nanoparticulate background was accounted for, the airborne exposure of nanoparticles was found to be relatively low. For example, an early study by Maynard *et al.* reported that airborne mass concentration of carbon nanotubes does not exceed fifty micrograms per cubic meter, and many of these materials are present in a form of aggregates with size exceeding one micrometer [53]. Similarly, the low airborne level of carbon black nanoparticles was found in the carbon black production facility [54]. These studies suggest that occupational exposure to nanosized particulates in the industry producing nanoparticles is low and can be effectively controlled by using personal protective equipment (e.g., masks, respirators) and installing air filters in the manufacturing facilities. However, the situation is quite different depending on the environmental settings. Several studies investigating the quality of air in urban areas reported the presence of carbon-based particulates, and attributed higher rates of inflammatory lung disorders to the nanoparticles, showing that the presence of certain particles promoted lung inflammation [55–62]. Since the dominant clearance mechanism of inhaled nanoparticles includes phagocytosis by alveolar macrophages, oxidative stress and cytokine production resulting in the inflammation are common toxicities reported with engineered nanomaterials [56,61,62]. While these studies emphasize the importance of the quality of air, it would be inaccurate to ascribe irritation and inflammation in lungs only to the nano size of the airborne particulate contaminants. It is also important to recognize that the increased inflammation in lungs reported in these studies is a cumulative result of the particle aggregation to larger micron sized materials, and the presence of other environmental factors contributing to the inflammation such as endotoxins. Inoue *et al.* reported that certain airborne particulates are not inflammatory on their own, but exaggerate inflammatory properties of endotoxins [63–66]. Therefore, mitigation of the inhalation toxicity of nanoparticles should include control over contributing contaminants such as endotoxins.

Nanoparticle pulmonary toxicity is not greater than that of the larger particles with the same composition [67,68]. Studies by Warheit *et al.* suggest that nanoparticle surface properties are more important factors determining pulmonary toxicity than the particle size [67,68]. In one such study, the authors compared quartz particles with a size range from 12 to 500 nm after intratracheal instillation in rats [67]. Pulmonary inflammation was assessed by estimating enzyme profile and detecting inflammatory cells in bronchoalveolar fluid of the animals [67]. The inflammatory potential of nanoparticles in this study correlated with surface reactivity, which the authors measured by the particles' ability to damage red blood cells. By using this measure, the authors demonstrated that toxicity of 12 nm particles was lower than that of 500 nm particles. Interestingly, another study also showed that hemolysis correlated with inflammation *in vivo* [69]. *In vitro–in vivo* correlation of the hemolysis tests has been suggested by several studies (reviewed by Brown and coworkers [70]). Collectively, these data indicate that estimation of erythrocyte damage by nanomaterials can be used not only to assess their hematocompatibility but also to predict potential pulmonary inflammation for particles administered by the inhalation route.

Since inhaled asbestos mineral fibers are known to cause inflammation in lungs and to increase the risk of pulmonary diseases including fibrosis and cancer, many studies have been conducted to estimate the pulmonary toxicity of fibrous nanomaterials. Carbon nanotubes were the main focus of these studies. The studies demonstrated that surface properties and aspect ratio of carbon nanotubes are the primary determinants of their pulmonary toxicity, not their nanosize *per se* [71–74]. A recent comprehensive report by Kayat J *et al.* presents more details about the pulmonary toxicity of carbon nanotubes [75]. Lessons learned from inhalation toxicity of carbon nanotubes in the environmental setting are relevant to the pharmaceutical use of nanotubes as drug carriers and can also benefit the safer development of fibrous nanocarriers (e.g., nanobelts and nanoribbons) with other elemental composition.

The majority of data regarding nanoparticle-mediated pulmonary toxicity are generated in rats and based on intratracheal instillation. NCL toxicologist, Dr. Steve Stern, has argued that this study design may not be the most predictive of human toxicity due to interspecies differences and a propensity of the model to lead to lung overload in rats [76]. Therefore, it is important to consider this point when attempting to extrapolate data obtained in the rat model to make meaningful conclusions about human toxicity.

The factors described above largely apply to the occupational exposure to nanopharmaceuticals during the production cycle. These factors are important to consider in the safety assessment of nanomedicines administered via inhalation routes. However, additional factors (e.g., dose, dosing schedule, metabolism) need consideration when determining the pulmonary toxicity of nanotechnology-based pharmaceuticals.

17.4 Cutaneous Toxicity

Since one of the common routes of exposure to nanomaterials includes contact with the external body surface, cutaneous toxicity is often a safety consideration. This type of toxicity is commonly applicable to nanomaterials used in sunscreens (e.g., titanium and zinc oxides) and cosmetics (e.g., liposomes and emulsions) and lessons learned may be important for nanopharmacy in terms of dermally administered medicines. The dermal route of exposure attracts safety concerns due to the tendency of airborne particles to agglomerate and settle of the skin surface. Many studies have utilized TiO_2 nanoparticles ranging in size from 10 to 60 nm as well as their larger aggregates [77–83]. Nanoparticles did not appear to penetrate through stratum corneum of the epidermis. However, accumulation in hair follicles was reported in some cases (reviewed in details by Nohynek *et al.* [84,85]). In contrast to nanomaterials used in sunscreens, smaller particles such as quantum dots were shown to have limited dermal penetration [86]. Investigation of the structure–activity relationships between size, shape, and surface properties of quantum dots and their ability to penetrate the skin demonstrated that smaller spherical particles have greater tendency to cross the intact skin barrier [86]. Another confirmation of this observation comes from the study utilizing maghemite and iron nanoparticles *in vitro* in a human skin model, and showing that penetration of the barrier is attributed to particle sizes below 10 nm [87]. In contrast to the intact skin, which serves as a reliable barrier preventing particle penetration, damaged skin allows dermal penetration to even micron-sized particles [88,89].

Available studies demonstrated mild irritation and potential for phototoxicity in response to topically applied metal oxide nanomaterials [90–92]. Similarly, carbon nanotubes, fullerenes and carbon-based nanoparticles were not irritating or sensitizing in clinical patch test and rabbit ocular toxicity studies [93,94]. Despite low toxicity upon topical application, many of these nanomaterials were found to be toxic to keratinocytes and other dermal cell lines *in vitro* [95,96]. The explanation for this discrepancy between *in vivo* topical toxicity tests and *in vitro* experiments comes from studies demonstrating that nanoparticles do not cross the intact skin barrier. The limited dermal penetration was the reason for modifying standard skin sensitization test called the local lymph node assay to include subcutaneous injection of the tested nanoparticles instead of applying them topically [97]. Indeed, subcutaneous injection of carbon nanotubes and carbon nanofibers in rats resulted in a granuloma-like response [98,99].

The take-home message from these studies is that a robust safety evaluation should include relevant routes of exposure and that understanding of the full toxicity potential requires the use of the most sensitive models, which may require adding additional routes of exposure. Lessons learned from studies utilizing incidental nanoparticles can inform toxicity studies of topically applied nanotechnology-based pharmaceuticals.

17.5 Immunotoxicity

Nanoparticle toxicity to the immune system depends on particle interactions with plasma proteins and cells in blood as well as at the sites of particle accumulation. Particle size, surface charge, architecture, and composition are the key factors determining immunotoxicity. However, it is important to consider that an effect on the immune system can be either beneficial or deleterious depending on whether its manifestation is desirable or not. Nanoparticles can be engineered to either avoid the immune system or to specifically target its components. Nanoparticles engineered for specific targeting of the immune system benefit the therapy of cancer, HIV/AIDS, inflammatory and autoimmune disorders, as well as vaccine efficacy. In contrast, nanoparticles designed to avoid immune interactions are used as drug carriers for a variety of other applications. Comprehensive coverage of this subject is available in the "Handbook of Immunological Properties of Engineered Nanomaterials" [100] and a recent review [101]. Therefore, this section provides several examples for the purpose of demonstrating the structure–activity relationship between most prominent nanoparticle physicochemical properties and their effects on the immune system (Figure 17.2). Nanoparticles with a cationic surface or carrying cationic ligands interact with biological membranes electrostatically and lead to a variety of cellular damages leading to hemolysis, platelet activation, and aggregation, induction of leukocyte procoagulant activity and disseminated intravascular coagulation (DIC) [102–105]. For example, cationic dendrimers of different architecture and size (G5 and G4 PPI dendrimers [106,107], G4 PAMAM dendrimers [108,109], G3 PAMAM and G3 PPI dendrimers [110], and G4 PLL dendrimers [111]) were shown to be hemolytic both *in vitro* and *in vivo*. The percent hemolysis varied from 14 to 86% *in vitro* in whole blood from human donors and various animal species, and was dependent on the density of surface groups. Likewise, cationic PAMAM dendrimers but not their anionic and neutral counterparts altered key platelet functions and perturbed plasma coagulation, which culminated in DIC [102–104]. Particle size, surface charge and conformation of polymer coatings are important determinants of particle clearance by the MPS. Small particles (100–200 nm) with unprotected surfaces and surface coated with a hydrophilic polymer in a "mushroom" configuration are primarily cleared by Kupffer cells in the liver. Red pulp macrophages in the spleen eliminate particles of larger size. The addition of hydrophilic polymer coatings in a "brush" configuration protects particles from immune recognition while the increase in particle size above 300 nm provides no protection, regardless of polymer conformation [112]. High aspect ratio particles, as well as certain

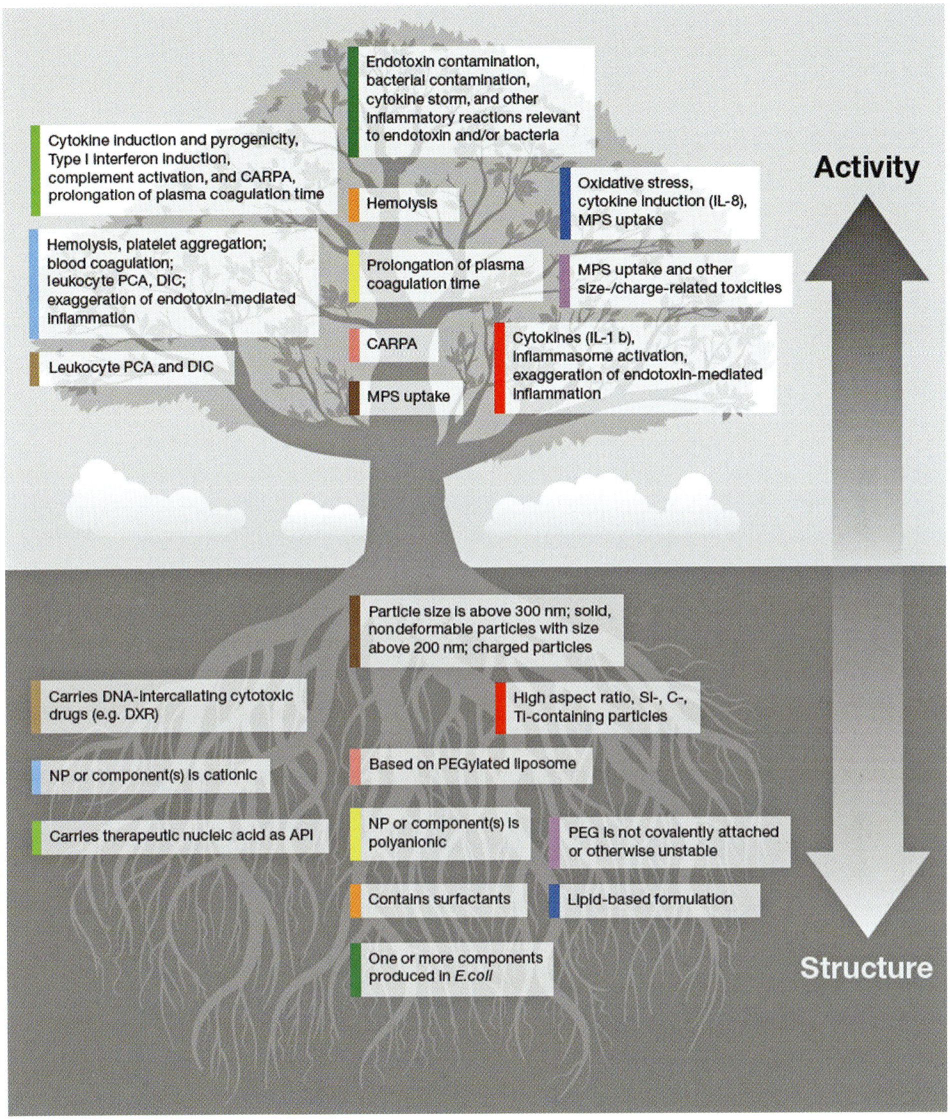

Figure 17.2 *Structure–activity relationship summary.* Shown is the structure–activity relationship between nanoparticles and their effects on the immune system. Each block listed in the bottom (structure) part of the figure is color coded. To find what toxicity is related to the given "structure" block, please find a block in the top (activity) part of the figure marked with the color matching that of the structure "block." PCA – procoagulant activity; DIC – disseminated intravascular coagulation; CARPA – complement activation-related pseudoallergy; MPS – mononuclear phagocytic system; IL – interleukin; PEG – poly (ethylene glycol); NP – nanoparticle; DXR – doxorubicin; API – active pharmaceutical ingredient; DNA – deoxyribonucleic acid. Reproduced with permission from Ref. [101].

metallic particles (e.g., Si), result in inflammasome activation and induction of proinflammatory cytokine IL-1 β. These particles, as well as certain cationic and carbon-based particles, can exaggerate endotoxin-mediated inflammation [113]. The therapeutic payload also influences immunotoxicity and is a key conisderation for nanopharmacy. For example, induction of cytokines, type I interferons, fever-like reaction, prolongation of plasma coagulation time, and complement activation are common dose-limiting toxicities of therapeutic nucleic acids [114]. These toxicities are also commonly observed with nanoformulated nucleic acids, which limit their translation into the clinic [115,116]. Cytotoxic oncology DNA-intercalating drugs (e.g., doxorubicin, daunorubicin, vincristine) are known to induce leukocyte PCA and DIC [117–119]. It is critical to distinguish nanoparticle-mediated immunotoxicity from that triggered by chemical and biological impurities. The presence of traces of CTAB used as a stabilizing agent in the synthesis of gold nanorods was implicated in cytotoxicity of these particles [120]. Iron and nickel used to catalyze reactions involved in the synthesis of carbon nanotubes were also shown to trigger inflammatory reactions in response to nanotubes [121]. A common biological impurity affecting over 30% of preclinical grade nanomaterials is bacterial endotoxin [122,123]. If not properly identified in and eliminated from nanoformulations, these contaminants can confound the results of nanoparticle immunotoxicity studies, and their assessment is therefore critical to interpretation of immunological safety data.

17.6 Unintended Presence of Nanosized Materials in Pharmaceutical Formulations

When nanoparticles are used for drug delivery, toxicity of both the drug and the nanocarrier is monitored. It has also become a common practice in pharmaceutical product development to investigate the toxicity of the final product containing a particle and a drug, as well as to evaluate the toxicity of the nanocarrier and the drug separately. Often for immunological toxicity, a mixture of the drug and the carrier is also used to estimate the benefit of drug conjugation to (or encapsulation within) the nanoparticle platform. The review of preclinical challenges with pharmaceutical products in which a drug is intentionally formulated using a nanocarrier is available elsewhere [123,124].

This section of the chapter will review another, rather unique and in my opinion underappreciated challenge. The challenge is related to the presence of unintended, undesirable, uncontrolled nano-sized particulate materials in pharmaceutical products containing traditionally formulated pharmaceuticals. These particulate contaminants result from rubber stopping, metal switches, plastic filler lines, syringe lubricants, and Tyvek gowns worn by personnel in drug manufacturing facilities [125]. Rubber, tungsten, silicon, and cellulose fibers have all been named among common contaminants [125]. While the role of these materials in toxicity of low molecular weight drugs is not very critical, their presence in biologics is crucial due to the contribution to the immunogenicity of these materials (i.e., a contaminant may exacerbate or mitigate antibody response to a therapeutic protein). It is believed that particles contribute to the immunogenicity of therapeutic proteins and antibodies by promoting protein aggregation (a factor critical in breaking tolerance to the protein) and by exaggerating inflammatory properties of low doses of endotoxin (a factor common in recombinant therapeutics due to their generation in *E. coli*) [125–129]. The US FDA requires manufacturers of therapeutic proteins and antibodies to monitor the presence and to characterize contaminating particulate regarding their contribution to the product immunogenicity [125,130]. A more detailed overview of this subject is available elsewhere [131]. It should be noted that the role of nanosized particulate contaminants in the immunogenicity of nucleic acid-based therapeutics is unknown. One may speculate that similar concerns will apply to this category of therapeutic products relevant to nanopharmacy.

17.7
Conclusion

Nanoparticle toxicity is a broad subject covering environmental, occupational, and health safety concerns. Evaluation of nanoparticle toxicity is based on several key factors, which include (1) intended application, (2) intended route of administration or exposure, (3) relevant dose and dose metrics, (4) considering systemic distribution and evaluating systemic toxicity even when the intended route is not intravenous, (5) using the most relevant and most sensitive models, (6) considering nanoparticle metabolism, and (7) recognizing both long-term and acute toxicities. Such an integrated assessment of multidimensional features of nanomaterials will guide their subsequent applications in medicine, and glean insight into the mechanistic foundation of their toxicologic signatures in a variety of applications. Recognition of the safety of therapeutic nanomaterials to patients should coevolve with appreciating facets of environmental and occupational safety. Cooperation between these areas will ascertain the minimal detrimental impact on the patients' health, the environment and the health of professionals involved in the production and handling of nanomaterials.

Acknowledgments

This study was supported by federal funds from the National Cancer Institute, National Institutes of Health, under contract HHSN261200800001E. The content of this publication does not necessarily reflect the views or policies of the Department of Health and Human Services nor does mention of trade names, commercial products, or organizations imply endorsement by the US Government. Information presented in Section 17.5 and Figure 17.2 are reproduced with permission from Ref. [101].

References

1 Stark, W.J., Stoessel, P.R., Wohleben, W., and Hafner, A. (2015) Industrial applications of nanoparticles. *Chem. Soc. Rev.*, **44**, 5793–5805.

2 Kessler, R. (2011) Engineered nanoparticles in consumer products: understanding a new ingredient. *Environ. Health Perspect.*, **119** (3), a120–a125.

3 Raj, S., Jose, S., Sumod, U.S., and Sabitha, M. (2012) Nanotechnology in cosmetics: opportunities and challenges. *J. Pharm. Bioall. Sci.*, **4** (3), 186–193.

4 Powers, M. (2006) Nanomedicine, Device & Diagnostics Report. Nanomedicine and nano device pipeline surges 68%. *NanoBiotech. News*, **2006**, 1–69.

5 Commission E. (2016). Available at http://ec.europa.eu/environment/chemicals/nanotech/reach-clp/index_en.htm (accessed March 24, 2016).

6 EPA (2016). Available at http://www.epa.gov/reviewing-new-chemicals-under-toxic-substances-control-act-tsca/control-nanoscale-materials-under (accessed March 20, 2016).

7 ISO (2016). Available at http://www.iso.org/iso/iso_technical_committee?commid=381983 (accessed March 20, 2016).

8 OECD (2016). Available at http://www.oecd.org/science/nanosafety/ (accessed March 20,2016).

9 WPMN (2016). Available at http://www.oecd.org/sti/sci-tech/oecdworkingpartyonnanotechnology.htm (accessed March 20,2016).

10 RCC (2016). Available at http://www.trade.gov/rcc/ (accessed March 20,2016).

11 Cruz, C.N., Tyner, K.M., Velazquez, L., Hyams, K.C., Jacobs, A., Shaw, A.B. *et al.* (2013) CDER risk assessment exercise to evaluate potential risks from the use of nanomaterials in drug products. *AAPS J.*, **15** (3), 623–628.

12 Tyner, K.M., Zou, P., Yang, X., Zhang, H., Cruz, C.N., and Lee, S.L. (2015) Product quality for nanomaterials: current U.S. experience and perspective. *Wiley Interdiscip. Rev. Nanomed. Nanobiotechnol.*, **7** (5), 640–654.

13 Azhdarzadeh, M., Saei, A.A., Sharifi, S., Hajipour, M.J., Alkilany, A.M., Sharifzadeh, M. *et al.* (2015) Nanotoxicology: advances and pitfalls in research methodology. *Nanomedicine (Lond.)*, **10** (18), 2931–2952.

14 Bahadar, H., Maqbool, F., Niaz, K., and Abdollahi, M. (2016) Toxicity of nanoparticles and an overview of current experimental models. *Iran Biomed. J.*, **20** (1), 1–11.

15 Ema, M., Hougaard, KS., Kishimoto, A., and Honda, K. (2016) Reproductive and developmental toxicity of carbon-based nanomaterials: a literature review. *Nanotoxicology*, **10** (4), 391–412.

16 Kang, H., Mintri, S., Menon, A.V., Lee, H.Y., Choi, H.S., and Kim, J. (2015) Pharmacokinetics, pharmacodynamics and toxicology of theranostic nanoparticles. *Nanoscale*, **7** (45), 18848–18862.

17 Khalili Fard, J., Jafari, S., and Eghbal, M.A. (2015) A review of molecular mechanisms involved in toxicity of nanoparticles. *Adv. Pharm. Bull.*, **5** (4), 447–454.

18 Leite, P.E., Pereira, M.R., and Granjeiro, J.M. (2015) Hazard effects of nanoparticles in central nervous system: searching for biocompatible nanomaterials for drug delivery. *Toxicol. In Vitro*, **29** (7), 1653–1660.

19 Liu, J., Feng, X., Wei, L., Chen, L., Song, B., and Shao, L. (2016) The toxicology of ion-shedding zinc oxide nanoparticles. *Crit. Rev. Toxicol.*, **46** (4), 348–384.

20 Ojer, P., Iglesias, T., Azqueta, A., Irache, J.M., and Lopez de Cerain, A. (2015) Toxicity evaluation of nanocarriers for the oral delivery of macromolecular drugs. *Eur. J. Pharm. Biopharm.*, **97** (Pt A), 206–217.

21 Sutariya, VB. and Pathak, Y. (2014) *Biointeractions of Nanomaterials*, CRC Press.

22 Neerman, M.F., Zhang, W., Parrish, A.R., and Simanek, E.E. (2004) *In vitro* and *in vivo* evaluation of a melamine dendrimer as a vehicle for drug delivery. *Int. J. Pharm.*, **281** (1–2), 129–132.

23 Roberts, J.C., Bhalgat, M.K., and Zera, R.T. (1996) Preliminary biological evaluation of polyamidoamine (PAMAM) Starburst dendrimers. *J. Biomed. Mater. Res.*, **30** (1), 53–65.
24 Caron, W.P., Lay, J.C., Fong, A.M., La-Beck, N.M., Kumar, P., Newman, S.E. *et al.* (2013) Translational studies of phenotypic probes for the mononuclear phagocyte system and liposomal pharmacology. *J. Pharmacol. Exp. Ther.*, **347** (3), 599–606.
25 Song, G., Petschauer, J.S., Madden, A.J., and Zamboni, W.C. (2014) Nanoparticles and the mononuclear phagocyte system: pharmacokinetics and applications for inflammatory diseases. *Curr. Rheumatol. Rev.*, **10** (1), 22–34.
26 Suk, J.S., Xu, Q., Kim, N., Hanes, J., and Ensign, L.M. (2016) PEGylation as a strategy for improving nanoparticle-based drug and gene delivery. *Adv. Drug Deliv. Rev.*, **99** (Pt A), 28–51.
27 Chen, H.H., Yu, C., Ueng, T.H., Chen, S., Chen, B.J., Huang, K.J. *et al.* (1998) Acute and subacute toxicity study of water-soluble polyalkylsulfonated C60 in rats. *Toxicol. Pathol.*, **26** (1), 143–151.
28 Lee, C.C., MacKay, J.A., Frechet, J.M., and Szoka, F.C. (2005) Designing dendrimers for biological applications. *Nat. Biotechnol.*, **23** (12), 1517–1526.
29 Wang, H., Wang, J., Deng, X., Sun, H., Shi, Z., Gu, Z. *et al.* (2004) Biodistribution of carbon single-wall carbon nanotubes in mice. *J. Nanosci. Nanotechnol.*, **4** (8), 1019–1024.
30 Chen, Y., Yang, L., Feng, C., and Wen, L.P. (2005) Nano neodymium oxide induces massive vacuolization and autophagic cell death in non-small cell lung cancer NCI-H460 cells. *Biochem. Biophys. Res. Commun.*, **337** (1), 52–60.
31 Seleverstov, O., Zabirnyk, O., Zscharnack, M., Bulavina, L., Nowicki, M., Heinrich, J.M. *et al.* (2006) Quantum dots for human mesenchymal stem cells labeling. A size-dependent autophagy activation. *Nano. Lett.*, **6** (12), 2826–2832.
32 Yamawaki, H. and Iwai, N. (2006) Cytotoxicity of water-soluble fullerene in vascular endothelial cells. *Am. J. Physiol. Cell Physiol.*, **290** (6), C1495–C1502.
33 Li, J.J., Muralikrishnan, S., Ng, C.T., Yung, L.Y., and Bay, B.H. (2010) Nanoparticle-induced pulmonary toxicity. *Exp. Biol. Med. (Maywood)*, **235** (9), 1025–1033.
34 Kennedy, I.M., Wilson, D., and Barakat, A.I. (2009) Uptake and inflammatory effects of nanoparticles in a human vascular endothelial cell line. *Res. Rep. Health Eff. Inst.*, **136**, 3–32.
35 Lee, H.M., Shin, D.M., Song, H.M., Yuk, J.M., Lee, Z.W., Lee, S.H. *et al.* (2009) Nanoparticles up-regulate tumor necrosis factor-alpha and CXCL8 via reactive oxygen species and mitogen-activated protein kinase activation. *Toxicol. Appl. Pharmacol.*, **238** (2), 160–169.
36 Zhang, Z., Berg, A., Levanon, H., Fessenden, R.W., and Meisel, D. (2003) On the interactions of free radicals with gold nanoparticles. *J. Am. Chem. Soc.*, **125** (26), 7959–7963.
37 Buzea, C., Pacheco, I.I., and Robbie, K. (2007) Nanomaterials and nanoparticles: sources and toxicity. *Biointerphases*, **2** (4), MR17–MR21.
38 Huang, Y., Wu, C., and Aronstam, R. (2010) Toxicity of transition metal oxide nanoparticles: recent insights from *in vitro* studies. *Materials*, **3** (10), 4842–4859.
39 Fubini, B. and Hubbard, A. (2003) Reactive oxygen species (ROS) and reactive nitrogen species (RNS) generation by silica in inflammation and fibrosis. *Free Radic. Biol. Med.*, **34** (12), 1507–1516.
40 He, X., Young, S.H., Schwegler-Berry, D., Chisholm, W.P., Fernback, J.E., and Ma, Q. (2011) Multiwalled carbon nanotubes induce a fibrogenic response by stimulating reactive oxygen species production, activating NF-kappaB signaling, and promoting fibroblast-to-myofibroblast transformation. *Chem. Res. Toxicol.*, **24** (12), 2237–2248.
41 Ilinskaya, A.N., Clogston, J.D., McNeil, S.E., and Dobrovolskaia, M.A. (2015) Induction of oxidative stress by Taxol(R) vehicle Cremophor-EL triggers production of interleukin-8 by peripheral blood mononuclear cells through the mechanism not requiring de novo

synthesis of mRNA. *Nanomedicine*, **11** (8), 1925–1938.

42 Chatterjee, K., Zhang, J., Honbo, N., and Karliner, J.S. (2010) Doxorubicin cardiomyopathy. *Cardiology*, **115** (2), 155–162.

43 Lorusso, D., Di Stefano, A., Carone, V., Fagotti, A., Pisconti, S., and Scambia, G. (2007) Pegylated liposomal doxorubicin-related palmar-plantar erythrodysesthesia ('hand-foot' syndrome). *Ann. Oncol.*, **18** (7), 1159–1164.

44 Manil, L., Couvreur, P., and Mahieu, P. (1995) Acute renal toxicity of doxorubicin (adriamycin)-loaded cyanoacrylate nanoparticles. *Pharm. Res.*, **12** (1), 85–87.

45 Bailey, M.R., Ansoborlo, E., Guilmette, R.A., and Paquet, F. (2003) Practical application of the ICRP human respiratory tract model. *Radiat. Prot. Dosimetry.*, **105** (1–4), 71–76.

46 Bailey, M.R., Ansoborlo, E., Guilmette, R.A., and Paquet, F. (2007) Updating the ICRP human respiratory tract model. *Radiat. Prot. Dosimetry.*, **127** (1–4), 31–34.

47 Gregoratto, D., Bailey, M.R., and Marsh, J.W. (2011) Particle clearance in the alveolar-interstitial region of the human lungs: model validation. *Radiat. Prot. Dosimetry.*, **144** (1–4), 353–356.

48 Kreyling, WG., Semmler, M., Erbe, F., Mayer, P., Takenaka, S., Schulz, H. *et al.* (2002) Translocation of ultrafine insoluble iridium particles from lung epithelium to extrapulmonary organs is size dependent but very low. *J. Toxicol. Environ. Health A.*, **65** (20), 1513–1530.

49 Oberdorster, G., Sharp, Z., Atudorei, V., Elder, A., Gelein, R., Lunts, A. *et al.* (2002) Extrapulmonary translocation of ultrafine carbon particles following whole-body inhalation exposure of rats. *J. Toxicol. Environ. Health A.*, **65** (20), 1531–1543.

50 Brown, J.S., Zeman, K.L., and Bennett, W.D. (2002) Ultrafine particle deposition and clearance in the healthy and obstructed lung. *Am. J. Respir. Crit. Care Med.*, **166** (9), 1240–1247.

51 Han, X., Corson, N., Wade-Mercer, P., Gelein, R., Jiang, J., Sahu, M. *et al.* (2012) Assessing the relevance of *in vitro* studies in nanotoxicology by examining correlations between *in vitro* and *in vivo* data. *Toxicology*, **297** (1–3), 1–9.

52 Peters, T.M., Heitbrink, W.A., Evans, D.E., Slavin, T.J., and Maynard, A.D. (2006) The mapping of fine and ultrafine particle concentrations in an engine machining and assembly facility. *Ann. Occup. Hyg.*, **50** (3), 249–257.

53 Maynard, A.D., Baron, P.A., Foley, M., Shvedova, A.A., Kisin, E.R., and Castranova, V. (2004) Exposure to carbon nanotube material: aerosol release during the handling of unrefined single-walled carbon nanotube material. *J. Toxicol. Environ. Health A*, **67** (1), 87–107.

54 Kuhlbusch, T.A., Neumann, S., and Fissan, H. (2004) Number size distribution, mass concentration, and particle composition of PM1, PM2.5, and PM10 in bag filling areas of carbon black production. *J. Occup. Environ. Hyg.*, **1** (10), 660–671.

55 Blum, J.L., Rosenblum, L.K., Grunig, G., Beasley, M.B., Xiong, J.Q., and Zelikoff, J.T. (2014) Short-term inhalation of cadmium oxide nanoparticles alters pulmonary dynamics associated with lung injury, inflammation, and repair in a mouse model. *Inhal. Toxicol.*, **26** (1), 48–58.

56 Brown, D.M., Kanase, N., Gaiser, B., Johnston, H., and Stone, V. (2014) Inflammation and gene expression in the rat lung after instillation of silica nanoparticles: effect of size, dispersion medium and particle surface charge. *Toxicol. Lett.*, **224** (1), 147–156.

57 Kodali, V., Littke, M.H., Tilton, S.C., Teeguarden, J.G., Shi, L., Frevert, C.W. *et al.* (2013) Dysregulation of macrophage activation profiles by engineered nanoparticles. *ACS Nano.*, **7** (8), 6997–7010.

58 Murr, L.E., Soto, K.F., Garza, K.M., Guerrero, P.A., Martinez, F., Esquivel, E.V. *et al.* (2006) Combustion-generated nanoparticulates in the El Paso, TX, USA/Juarez, Mexico Metroplex: their comparative characterization and potential for adverse health effects. *Int. J. Environ. Res. Public Health*, **3** (1), 48–66.

59 Nemmar, A., Holme, J.A., Rosas, I., Schwarze, P.E., and Alfaro-Moreno, E. (2013) Recent advances in particulate matter and nanoparticle toxicology: a review of the in vivo and in vitro studies. *Biomed. Res. Int.*, **2013**, 279371.

60 Park, H.J., Sohn, J.H., Kim, Y.J., Park, Y.H., Han, H., Park, K.H. *et al.* (2015) Acute exposure to silica nanoparticles aggravate airway inflammation: different effects according to surface characteristics. *Exp. Mol. Med.*, **47**, e173.

61 Park, J.W., Lee, I.C., Shin, N.R., Jeon, C.M., Kwon, O.K., Ko, J.W. *et al.* (2016) Copper oxide nanoparticles aggravate airway inflammation and mucus production in asthmatic mice via MAPK signaling. *Nanotoxicology*, **10** (4), 445–452.

62 Thompson, E.A., Sayers, B.C., Glista-Baker, E.E., Shipkowski, K.A., Taylor, A.J., and Bonner, J.C. (2014) Innate immune responses to nanoparticle exposure in the lung. *J. Environ. Immunol. Toxicol.*, **1** (3), 150–156.

63 Inoue, K. and Takano, H. (2011) Aggravating impact of nanoparticles on immune-mediated pulmonary inflammation. *Sci. World J.*, **11**, 382–390.

64 Inoue, K., Takano, H., Yanagisawa, R., Hirano, S., Sakurai, M., Shimada, A. *et al.* (2006) Effects of airway exposure to nanoparticles on lung inflammation induced by bacterial endotoxin in mice. *Environ. Health Perspect.*, **114** (9), 1325–1330.

65 Inoue, K., Takano, H., Yanagisawa, R., Hirano, S., Kobayashi, T., Fujitani, Y. *et al.* (2007) Effects of inhaled nanoparticles on acute lung injury induced by lipopolysaccharide in mice. *Toxicology*, **238** (2–3), 99–110.

66 Inoue, K. (2011) Promoting effects of nanoparticles/materials on sensitive lung inflammatory diseases. *Environ. Health Prev. Med.*, **16** (3), 139–143.

67 Warheit, D.B., Webb, T.R., Colvin, V.L., Reed, K.L., and Sayes, C.M. (2007) Pulmonary bioassay studies with nanoscale and fine-quartz particles in rats: toxicity is not dependent upon particle size but on surface characteristics. *Toxicol. Sci.*, **95** (1), 270–280.

68 Warheit, D.B., Webb, T.R., Sayes, C.M., Colvin, V.L., and Reed, K.L. (2006) Pulmonary instillation studies with nanoscale TiO2 rods and dots in rats: toxicity is not dependent upon particle size and surface area. *Toxicol. Sci.*, **91** (1), 227–236.

69 Clouter, A., Brown, D., Hohr, D., Borm, P., and Donaldson, K. (2001) Inflammatory effects of respirable quartz collected in workplaces versus standard DQ12 quartz: particle surface correlates. *Toxicol. Sci.*, **63** (1), 90–98.

70 Wildt, B., Malinauskas, R.A., and Brown, R.P. (2013) The effects of engineered nanomaterials on erythrocytes, in *Handbook of Immunological Properties of Nanomaterials* (eds M.A. Dobrovolskaia and S.E. McNeil), World Scientific Publishing, Singapore.

71 Thess, A., Lee, R., Nikolaev, P., Dai, H., Petit, P., Robert, J. *et al.* (1996) Crystalline ropes of metallic carbon nanotubes. *Science*, **273** (5274), 483–487.

72 Donaldson, K. and Tran, C.L. (2004) An introduction to the short-term toxicology of respirable industrial fibres. *Mutat. Res.*, **553** (1–2), 5–9.

73 Lam, C.W., James, J.T., McCluskey, R., and Hunter, R.L. (2004) Pulmonary toxicity of single-wall carbon nanotubes in mice 7 and 90 days after intratracheal instillation. *Toxicol. Sci.*, **77** (1), 126–134.

74 Shvedova, A.A., Kisin, E.R., Mercer, R., Murray, A.R., Johnson, V.J., Potapovich, A.I. *et al.* (2005) Unusual inflammatory and fibrogenic pulmonary responses to single-walled carbon nanotubes in mice. *Am. J. Physiol. Lung Cell Mol. Physiol.*, **289** (5), L698–L708.

75 Kayat, J., Gajbhiye, V., Tekade, R.K., and Jain, N.K. (2011) Pulmonary toxicity of carbon nanotubes: a systematic report. *Nanomedicine*, **7** (1), 40–49.

76 Stern, S.T. and McNeil, S.E. (2008) Nanotechnology safety concerns revisited. *Toxicol. Sci.*, **101** (1), 4–21.

77 Schulz, J., Hohenberg, H., Pflucker, F., Gartner, E., Will, T., Pfeiffer, S. *et al.* (2002) Distribution of sunscreens on skin. *Adv. Drug Deliv. Rev.*, (54 Suppl 1), S157–S163.

78 Pflucker, F., Wendel, V., Hohenberg, H., Gartner, E., Will, T., Pfeiffer, S. *et al.*

(2001) The human stratum corneum layer: an effective barrier against dermal uptake of different forms of topically applied micronised titanium dioxide. *Skin Pharmacol. Appl. Skin. Physiol.*, (14 Suppl 1), 92–97.

79 Gamer, A.O., Leibold, E., and van Ravenzwaay, B. (2006) The *in vitro* absorption of microfine zinc oxide and titanium dioxide through porcine skin. *Toxicol In Vitro*, **20** (3), 301–307.

80 Mavon, A., Miquel, C., Lejeune, O., Payre, B., and Moretto, P. (2007) *In vitro* percutaneous absorption and in vivo stratum corneum distribution of an organic and a mineral sunscreen. *Skin Pharmacol. Physiol.*, **20** (1), 10–20.

81 Sadrieh, N., Wokovich, A.M., Gopee, N.V., Zheng, J., Haines, D., Parmiter, D. *et al.* (2010) Lack of significant dermal penetration of titanium dioxide from sunscreen formulations containing nano- and submicron-size TiO_2 particles. *Toxicol. Sci.*, **115** (1), 156–166.

82 Lademann, J., Weigmann, H., Rickmeyer, C., Barthelmes, H., Schaefer, H., Mueller, G. *et al.* (1999) Penetration of titanium dioxide microparticles in a sunscreen formulation into the horny layer and the follicular orifice. *Skin Pharmacol. Appl. Skin Physiol.*, **12** (5), 247–256.

83 Coelho, S.G., Patri, A.K., Wokovich, A.M., McNeil, S.E., Howard, P.C., and Miller, S.A. (2016) Repetitive application of sunscreen containing titanium dioxide nanoparticles on human skin. *JAMA Dermatol.*, **152** (4), 470–472.

84 Nohynek, G.J., Lademann, J., Ribaud, C., and Roberts, M.S. (2007) Grey goo on the skin? Nanotechnology, cosmetic and sunscreen safety. *Crit. Rev. Toxicol.*, **37** (3), 251–277.

85 Nohynek, G.J., Dufour, E.K., and Roberts, M.S. (2008) Nanotechnology, cosmetics and the skin: is there a health risk? *Skin Pharmacol. Physiol.*, **21** (3), 136–149.

86 Ryman-Rasmussen, J.P., Riviere, J.E., and Monteiro-Riviere, N.A. (2006) Penetration of intact skin by quantum dots with diverse physicochemical properties. *Toxicol. Sci.*, **91** (1), 159–165.

87 Baroli, B., Ennas, M.G., Loffredo, F., Isola, M., Pinna, R., and Lopez-Quintela, M.A. (2007) Penetration of metallic nanoparticles in human full-thickness skin. *J. Invest. Dermatol.*, **127** (7), 1701–1712.

88 Rouse, J.G., Yang, J., Ryman-Rasmussen, J.P., Barron, A.R., and Monteiro-Riviere, N.A. (2007) Effects of mechanical flexion on the penetration of fullerene amino acid-derivatized peptide nanoparticles through skin. *Nano. Lett.*, **7** (1), 155–160.

89 Tinkle, S.S., Antonini, J.M., Rich, B.A., Roberts, J.R., Salmen, R., DePree, K. *et al.* (2003) Skin as a route of exposure and sensitization in chronic beryllium disease. *Environ. Health Perspect*, **111** (9), 1202–1208.

90 Wang, S.Q. and Tooley, I.R. (2011) Photoprotection in the era of nanotechnology. *Semin Cutan. Med. Surg.*, **30** (4), 210–213.

91 Wang, C.C., Wang, S., Xia, Q., He, W., Yin, J.J., Fu, P.P. *et al.* (2013) Phototoxicity of zinc oxide nanoparticles in HaCaT keratinocytes-generation of oxidative DNA damage during UVA and visible light irradiation. *J. Nanosci. Nanotechnol.*, **13** (6), 3880–3888.

92 He, W., Wu, H., Wamer, W.G., Kim, H.K., Zheng, J., Jia, H. *et al.* (2014) Unraveling the enhanced photocatalytic activity and phototoxicity of ZnO/metal hybrid nanostructures from generation of reactive oxygen species and charge carriers. *ACS Appl. Mater. Interfaces*, **6** (17), 15527–15535.

93 Huczko, A. and Lange, H. (2001) Carbon nanotubes: experimental evidence for a null risk of skin irritation and allergy. *Fullerene Sci. Technol.*, **9**, 247–250.

94 Huczko, A., Lange, H., and Calko, E. (1999) Fullerenes: experimental evidence for a null risk of skin irritation and allergy. *Fullerene Sci. Technol.*, **7**, 935–939.

95 Shvedova, A.A., Castranova, V., Kisin, E.R., Schwegler-Berry, D., Murray, A.R., Gandelsman, V.Z. *et al.* (2003) Exposure to carbon nanotube material: assessment of nanotube cytotoxicity using human keratinocyte cells. *J. Toxicol. Environ. Health A.*, **66** (20), 1909–1926.

96 Sayes, C.M., Gobin, A.M., Ausman, K.D., Mendez, J., West, J.L., and Colvin, V.L.

(2005) Nano-C60 cytotoxicity is due to lipid peroxidation. *Biomaterials*, **26** (36), 7587–7595.
97 Dobrovolskaia, M.A., Germolec, D.R., and Weaver, J.L. (2009) Evaluation of nanoparticle immunotoxicity. *Nat. Nanotechnol.*, **4** (7), 411–414.
98 Yokoyama, A., Sato, Y., Nodasaka, Y., Yamamoto, S., Kawasaki, T., Shindoh, M. *et al.* (2005) Biological behavior of hat-stacked carbon nanofibers in the subcutaneous tissue in rats. *Nano. Lett.*, **5** (1), 157–161.
99 Sato, Y., Yokoyama, A., Shibata, K., Akimoto, Y., Ogino, S., Nodasaka, Y. *et al.* (2005) Influence of length on cytotoxicity of multi-walled carbon nanotubes against human acute monocytic leukemia cell line THP-1 *in vitro* and subcutaneous tissue of rats *in vivo*. *Mol. Biosyst.*, **1** (2), 176–182.
100 Dobrovolskaia, M.A. and McNeil, S.E. (eds) (2013) *Handbook of Immunological Properties of Engineered Nanomaterials*, 1st edn, World Scientific Publishing Ltd., Singapore.
101 Dobrovolskaia, M.A., Shurin, M., and Shvedova, A.A. (2015) Current understanding of interactions between nanoparticles and the immune system. *Toxicol. Appl. Pharmacol.* **299**, 78–89.
102 Greish, K., Thiagarajan, G., Herd, H., Price, R., Bauer, H., Hubbard, D. *et al.* (2012) Size and surface charge significantly influence the toxicity of silica and dendritic nanoparticles. *Nanotoxicology.*, **6** (7), 713–723.
103 Jones, C.F., Campbell, R.A., Brooks, A.E., Assemi, S., Tadjiki, S., Thiagarajan, G. *et al.* (2012) Cationic PAMAM dendrimers aggressively initiate blood clot formation. *ACS Nano.*, **6** (11), 9900–9910.
104 Jones, C.F., Campbell, R.A., Franks, Z., Gibson, C.C., Thiagarajan, G., Vieira-de-Abreu, A. *et al.* (2012) Cationic PAMAM dendrimers disrupt key platelet functions. *Mol. Pharm.*, **9** (6), 1599–1611.
105 Ziemba, B., Halets, I., Shcharbin, D., Appelhans, D., Voit, B., Pieszynski, I. *et al.* (2012) Influence of fourth generation poly(propyleneimine) dendrimers on blood cells. *J. Biomed. Mater. Res. A*, **100** (11), 2870–2880.
106 Agashe, H.B., Dutta, T., Garg, M., and Jain, N.K. (2006) Investigations on the toxicological profile of functionalized fifth-generation poly (propylene imine) dendrimer. *J. Pharm. Pharmacol.*, **58** (11), 1491–1498.
107 Bhadra, D., Yadav, A.K., Bhadra, S., and Jain, N.K. (2005) Glycodendrimeric nanoparticulate carriers of primaquine phosphate for liver targeting. *Int. J. Pharm.*, **295** (1–2), 221–233.
108 Asthana, A., Chauhan, A.S., Diwan, P.V., and Jain, N.K. (2005) Poly(amidoamine) (PAMAM) dendritic nanostructures for controlled site-specific delivery of acidic anti-inflammatory active ingredient. *AAPS PharmSciTech*, **6** (3), E536–E542.
109 Bhadra, D., Bhadra, S., Jain, S., and Jain, N.K. (2003) A PEGylated dendritic nanoparticulate carrier of fluorouracil. *Int. J. Pharm.*, **257** (1–2), 111–124.
110 Malik, N., Wiwattanapatapee, R., Klopsch, R., Lorenz, K., Frey, H., and Weener, J.W. (2000) *et al.* Dendrimers: relationship between structure and biocompatibility in vitro, and preliminary studies on the biodistribution of 125I-labelled polyamidoamine dendrimers *in vivo*. *J. Control. Release*, **65** (1–2), 133–148.
111 Agrawal, P., Gupta, U., and Jain, N.K. (2007) Glycoconjugated peptide dendrimers-based nanoparticulate system for the delivery of chloroquine phosphate. *Biomaterials*, **28** (22), 3349–3359.
112 Gbadamosi, J.K., Hunter, A.C., and Moghimi, S.M. (2002) PEGylation of microspheres generates a heterogeneous population of particles with differential surface characteristics and biological performance. *FEBS Lett.*, **532** (3), 338–344.
113 Baron, L., Gombault, A., Fanny, M., Villeret, B., Savigny, F., Guillou, N. *et al.* (2015) The NLRP3 inflammasome is activated by nanoparticles through ATP, ADP and adenosine. *Cell Death Dis.*, **6**, e1629.
114 Levin, A.A. (1999) A review of the issues in the pharmacokinetics and toxicology of phosphorothioate antisense oligonucleotides. *Biochim. Biophys. Acta.*, **1489** (1), 69–84.

115 Dobrovolskaia, M.A. and McNeil, S.E. (2015) Immunological and hematological toxicities challenging clinical translation of nucleic acid-based therapeutics. *Expert Opin. Biol. Ther.*, **15** (7), 1023–1048.

116 Dobrovolskaia, M.A. and McNeil, S.E. (2015) Strategy for selecting nanotechnology carriers to overcome immunological and hematological toxicities challenging clinical translation of nucleic acid-based therapeutics. *Expert Opin. Drug Deliv.*, **12** (7), 1163–1175.

117 Kim, S.H., Lim, K.M., Noh, J.Y., Kim, K., Kang, S., Chang, Y.K. *et al.* (2011) Doxorubicin-induced platelet procoagulant activities: an important clue for chemotherapy-associated thrombosis. *Toxicol. Sci.*, **124** (1), 215–224.

118 Swystun, L.L., Shin, L.Y., Beaudin, S., and Liaw, P.C. (2009) Chemotherapeutic agents doxorubicin and epirubicin induce a procoagulant phenotype on endothelial cells and blood monocytes. *J. Thromb. Haemost.*, **7** (4), 619–626.

119 Wheeler, H.R. and Geczy, C.L. (1990) Induction of macrophage procoagulant expression by cisplatin, daunorubicin and doxorubicin. *Int. J. Cancer*, **46** (4), 626–632.

120 Leonov, A.P., Zheng, J., Clogston, J.D., Stern, S.T., Patri, A.K., and Wei, A. (2008) Detoxification of gold nanorods by treatment with polystyrenesulfonate. *ACS Nano.*, **2** (12), 2481–2488.

121 Madani, S.Y., Mandel, A., and Seifalian, A.M. (2013) A concise review of carbon nanotube's toxicology. *Nano. Rev.*, doi: 10.3402/nano.v4i0.21521.

122 Dobrovolskaia, M.A. and McNeil, S.E. (2013) Nanoparticles and endotoxin, in *Handbook of Immunological Properties of Engineered Nanomaperials* (eds M.A. Dobrovolskaia and S.E. McNeil), World Scientific Publishing Ltd., Singapore, pp. 77–115.

123 Crist, R.M., Grossman, J.H., Patri, A.K., Stern, S.T., Dobrovolskaia, M.A., Adiseshaiah, P.P. *et al.* (2013) Common pitfalls in nanotechnology: lessons learned from NCI's Nanotechnology Characterization Laboratory. *Integr. Biol. (Camb.)*, **5** (1), 66–73.

124 Dobrovolskaia, M.A. (2015) Pre-clinical immunotoxicity studies of nanotechnology-formulated drugs: challenges, considerations and strategy. *J. Control. Release*, **220** (Pt B), 571–583.

125 Carpenter, J., Cherney, B., Lubinecki, A., Ma, S., Marszal, E., Mire-Sluis, A. *et al.* (2010) Meeting report on protein particles and immunogenicity of therapeutic proteins: filling in the gaps in risk evaluation and mitigation. *Biologicals*, **38** (5), 602–611.

126 Rosenberg, A.S. (2003) Immunogenicity of biological therapeutics: a hierarchy of concerns. *Dev. Biol. (Basel)*, **112**, 15–21.

127 Rosenberg, A.S. (2006) Effects of protein aggregates: an immunologic perspective. *AAPS J.*, **8** (3), E501–E507.

128 Rosenberg, A.S., Verthelyi, D., and Cherney, B.W. (2012) Managing uncertainty: a perspective on risk pertaining to product quality attributes as they bear on immunogenicity of therapeutic proteins. *J. Pharm. Sci.*, **101** (10), 3560–3567.

129 Christie, M., Torres, R.M., Kedl, R.M., Randolph, T.W., and Carpenter, J.F. (2014) Recombinant murine growth hormone particles are more immunogenic with intravenous than subcutaneous administration. *J. Pharm. Sci.*, **103** (1), 128–139.

130 Parenky, A., Myler, H., Amaravadi, L., Bechtold-Peters, K., Rosenberg, A., Kirshner, S. *et al.* (2014) New FDA draft guidance on immunogenicity. *AAPS J.*, **16** (3), 499–503.

131 Dobrovolskaia, M.A. (2016) Nanoparticles and antigenicity, in *Handbook of Immunological Properties of Engineered Nanomaterials* (eds M.A. Dobrovolskaia and S.E. McNeil), World Scientific Publishing Ltd., Singapore.

18
An Overview of Nanoparticle Biocompatibility for Their Use in Nanomedicine

Matthew S.P. Boyles,[1] Leagh G. Powell,[1] Ali Kermanizadeh,[2] Helinor J. Johnston,[1] Barbara Rothen-Rutishauser,[3] Vicki Stone,[1] and Martin J.D. Clift[4]

[1]Heriot Watt University, Nano Safety Research Group, School of Engineering and Physical Sciences, Institute of Biological Chemistry, Biophysics and Bioengineering, Edinburgh EH14 4AS, UK
[2]University of Copenhagen, Department of Public Health, Section of Environmental Health, Copenhagen, Oster Farimsagsgade 5 DK-1014, Denmark
[3]University of Fribourg, BioNanomaterials, Adolphe Merkle Institute, Fribourg, CH-1700, Switzerland
[4]Swansea University Medical School, In Vitro Toxicology Group, Institute of Life Sciences, Singleton Park Campus, Swansea SA2 8PP, UK

18.1
Introduction

The field of nanotechnology promises to provide countless advantages to consumer, industrial, and technology sectors. Such advantages have been proposed to improve applications used within our daily lives (i.e., sporting equipment, cosmetics, food packaging), but most notably the medical field has received significant attention as to the ability for nanoparticles (NPs) to act in beneficial new forms of globally effective clinical applications [1]. Despite such heightened focus on the proposed advantages of nanotechnology, owing to its rapid global advancement and development, there has been significant concern as to the potential adverse effects that NPs may have on human health and the environment. This is especially prudent considering the potential clinical use of NPs [1].

In principle, NPs may enter the human body through four major exposure routes: intravenous injection, ingestion, epidermal application, or inhalation [2–4]. In respect to each of these exposure routes to the human body, there is increased possibilities for NPs to enter the bloodstream and subsequently translocate to distal organs (e.g., liver, kidneys), where they may accumulate (as well as potentially be eliminated, e.g., through the urine or feces) [5–7]. While

The authors declare no conflict of interest. The authors are completely responsible for the context of the chapter and the views portrayed within.

Pharmaceutical Nanotechnology: Innovation and Production, First Edition. Edited by Jean Cornier, Arno Kwade, Andrew Owen, and Marcel Van de Voorde.

there is the need to assess the short-term biological response (i.e., biocompatibility) following exposure and their potential translocation, there is an even greater need to study how the potential for NPs to accumulate in primary as well as in distal organs may relate to adverse biological responses over time (i.e., chronic effects and their mechanisms), especially considering their potential use within a medical setting [2].

The purpose of this chapter is therefore to provide an overview of the current knowledge regarding the safety concerns related to nanomedicine, focusing upon specific, common materials that are being used to create NP-based medical applications. Further to this, the manipulation of these materials prior to their clinical use, to aid biocompatibility, is also discussed.

18.2
Nanomedicine

Nanomedicine is defined as the application and utilization of nanotechnology to medicine and human health, and in most cases is applied to the diagnosis and treatment of disease. The market for nanomedicine was estimated as having a market value of $4.8 billion in 2012 [8]. Over the last two decades a wide range of NPs have been developed, including liposomes, polymeric materials, quantum dots (QD), carbon nanotubes (CNTs), and various inorganic NPs with the size, shape, charge, and other physico-chemical characteristics tailored to provide the opportunity for specific functionality, and thus accommodating many different medical applications. This has resulted in a range of NPs being made available for potential medical use with desirable optical, electronic, magnetic, and biological attributes.

The concepts within nanomedicine include theranostics (therapeutics and diagnostics, as well as drug delivery), preventive, and individualized medicine. For these applications to be successful, multifunctional platforms and machinery are needed, including high sensitivity, specificity, resolution, and accuracy [9]. The current nanomedicine-based applications mainly include vehicles for targeted drug delivery, diagnostic NP platforms for biomedical imaging, and therapeutic platforms for the treatment of disease [10,11]. The physicochemical properties of NPs are crucial for successful execution of these approaches [12–14]. The size of NPs is a fundamental variation from their bulk counterparts, and it is this small size which substantially contributes to how these materials can behave in biological systems. This is exemplified for iron oxide NPs, which have a significantly enhanced magnetic [15]. The small size of iron oxide NPs allows effective penetration into human tissue and cells allowing for the detection of histopathological, cellular, and molecular changes during treatment or diagnosis [9]. Furthermore, the small size results in a large surface-to-volume ratio and increased surface activity making the NPs desirable for surface chemical modifications for improved biocompatibility and enhanced targeting and conjugation of specific biomarkers [16]. Finally, the utilization of nanostructures allows for the construction of the materials in layers to allow incorporation of different payloads for realization of multifunctionality, that is, multimodal nanoprobes have been advocated for simultaneous imaging to improve efficiency. A number of NPs have been proposed as potential candidates for multifunctionality including gold (Au), QDs, and iron oxide NPs [17].

Despite these promising new medical functions, the safety concern for NPs is a key determinant factor in their clinical applications. It is imperative to establish structure–activity relationships (SARs) and implement risk reduction strategies for all materials proposed for medical applications. As the same physicochemical characteristics that make NPs desirable for medical applications might contribute to their potential adverse effects; this includes their size and surface properties which can significantly influence their bioavailability, transport, biotransformation, cellular uptake, and overall biological response [18,19].

18.3 Biocompatibility of Nanoparticles for Medical Application

To date, numerous NPs selected for biomedical applications have undergone rigorous toxicological evaluation both *in vitro* and *in vivo* (i.e. animal experimentation) (see below). However, due to a number of "nano" specific complications their pharmacokinetics, namely, systematic absorption, distribution, metabolism, and excretion, are poorly understood [2]. After the administration of NPs into the human body, irrespective of their route of entry, interactions between NPs and non-cellular biological environments immediately occur. This interaction (i.e., interaction of the NP surface with proteins and lipids) can affect the NP physicochemical characteristics [20–22]. Therefore, it is critical that these interactions are carefully investigated and understood when conducting any toxicity assessment. In some tissues (i.e., liver and spleen), NPs enter the tissue by size-dependent cellular uptake or endocytosis, or phagocytosis by macrophages so that they are selectively and specifically removed from the blood [23]. This cellular internalization offers the basis for diagnostic or therapeutic applications of NPs *in vivo*. Thus, for toxicological evaluation, cellular uptake and intracellular trafficking are also extremely important [24]. The extravasation of the NPs may be restricted by the existence of natural barriers formed by the tight junctions between endothelial and epithelial cells. This being said, a number of studies have demonstrated that certain materials may bypass these barriers (highlighted by the blood–brain barrier or the placenta) with adverse effects noted in terms of neurotoxicity, and reproductive and developmental toxicity amongst others [2]. It is also important to note that following bodily distribution NPs may undergo metabolic processes [25]. Finally, it is understood that the principal proportion of NPs are excreted from the body via urine and/or feces [26]. However, certain materials are retained in the body for extended periods of time [27] and consequently may contribute to NP-induced chronic toxicity. Therefore, to minimize or even abolish the potential toxicity and possible health risks of NPs the assessment of NP biodurability is absolutely crucial [2].

As touched upon, a number of underlying questions remain to be addressed: (1) The specific properties of NPs that should be characterized for nanomedical applications and how this may relate to their potential toxicity. (2) A thorough understanding of both the available data and the current knowledge gaps that exist on nanomedicine toxicity, exposure route and bio-persistence, and clearance. (3) The specific NP characteristics that contribute to toxicity in relation to medical applications. (4) Specific delivery mechanisms influencing nanomedicine toxicity. (5) Role of concurrent multiple exposure/dose in application of nanomedicines and pharmaceuticals.

Currently, the majority of the research in the field of nanomedicine is predominately focused on the NP applications. Therefore, the systematic toxicological evaluation of NPs is often not considered during the product development process. A number of important points require special attention for future research. First, the unique exposure routes in nanomedicine that intentionally bypass the normal absorption process might be a great concern with regards to material toxicity. It is also important to remember that biopersistent materials might accumulate within organs or tissue and hence require special attention with regards to their toxicological potential [2,24]. Finally, it is imperative that acute and chronic toxicity and suitable end-points with appropriate doses are investigated for safe design and utilization of NPs for medical applications.

18.3.1
Metal-Based Nanoparticles

Of metal-based NPs used in nanomedicine, metal oxides and noble metals are well studied, of which iron oxide NPs and AuNPs, respectively, have arguably received the most focus. Iron oxide NPs in medical applications, with considerations of toxicity, have been the focus of a recent extensive review [28], therefore, focus here is instead given to AuNPs. The use of noble metal NPs, particularly AuNPs, stems from their quantum size effects [29] and unique photophysical and photochemical properties, which has driven their use in photochemical reactions, or as photocatalysts and biological sensors [30]. Moreover, with their assumed low level of biological activity, easy functionalization [29] enabling considerable surface loading capacity of proteins [31], and increased stability compared to other metal NPs [29], AuNPs are often the foremost choice for carrier molecules allowing their use for disease diagnosis, such as cancer [32], for general whole body imaging via computed tomography (CT) scans [32,33], or as drug or gene delivery systems [30,34–38].

There is a certain level of contention concerning the use of AuNPs in medicine, based on the toxicity that some studies have observed in response to what is usually considered an inert material. Based on the current scientific literature, there are a number of characteristics such as size and surface chemistry that can influence the response of biological systems to AuNPs. It is these characteristics that can induce toxicity in response to AuNPs, but likewise, it is these characteristics that make these particles suitable "carrier" molecules. The cytotoxicity of this carrier molecule can be almost non-existent, such as in polyethylene glycolylated (PEG) AuNP exposure of lung and colon cell lines [34], lysine-capped AuNPs of 3–8 nm in mouse macrophages *in vitro* [39], and 15 nm citrate-coated AuNPs in numerous cell types [40]. In these cases internalization of AuNPs occurred, as it also did when HeLa cells were exposed with 4 nm PEGylated AuNPs [41]. Gu *et al.* [41] observed that their particularly small PEGylated AuNPs would enter and localize within the cells' nucleus. However, the larger PEGylated AuNPs used by Brown *et al.* [34] did not localize within the nucleus of A549 epithelial cells, this could only be achieved when their AuNPs were additionally tethered to platinum. These interactions of AuNPs with cells and cell nuclei are important and beneficial events for nanomedicines, and would imply that in these cases the "carrier" molecule is an effective one. However, the additional functionalization with platinum used by Brown *et al.* [34] also carried with it additional cytotoxicity. The authors reported this level of cytotoxicity to be greater than that induced by oxaliplatin, a platinum-based anticancer drug and therefore a beneficial trait of these proposed anti-cancer treatments. This may be true, but without demonstrating selectivity of cancer cells over normal healthy cells, these findings should be considered with caution.

Other AuNP constructs exhibit relatively high toxicity, and examination of these may indicate the origin of such responses. Although the small (3–8 nm) PEGylated AuNPs used by Gu *et al.* [41] and Brandenberger *et al.* [40] displayed limited toxicity, decreasing the size of Au-phenylphosphine NPs from 15 to 2 nm, actually increased cytotoxicity in numerous cell types [42]. This is of particular importance, as characteristics such as small size are considered vital in delivery of therapeutic genes into a cells nucleus [36]. Inversely, while spherical AuNPs between 25 and 50 nm induced cell death in a breast cancer cell type *in vitro*, no cell death was apparent for AuNPs of lesser (down to 2 nm) or greater (up to 100 nm) size [43]. These studies indicate that surface chemistry may principally be responsible for the induced cytotoxicity, and to a lesser extent cell type. This is corroborated when considering that increased cytotoxicity is associated with a change from negative to positive surface charge [44]. This raises the question of suitable functionalization, but also functional group specificity, as Au nanorods coated with polyelectrolyte (PE) are internalized by human cervical cancer cells *in vitro*, with no observable cell death or changes to cell stress genes, while PE alone is toxic [45]. CTAB-AuNPs are cytotoxic to the immortalized K562 leukemia cell line *in vitro*, but only when conjugated; citrate-AuNPs with CTAB removed show no such toxicity [46]. AuNPs of 10 nm induce cell death, (pro-)inflammatory responses, and increase the potential for oxidative stress in macrophages [47] and lung epithelial cells [48,49] *in vitro* when functionalized with chitosan, a polysaccharide derivative of chitin. This is of some concern as prospective nanomedicines formed of AuNP-chitosan conjugates are often reported [37,38,50]. With intravenous administration, it is likely that these materials are able to enter macrophages and subsequently accumulate in the liver and spleen [51], so responses of macrophages to Au-chitosan conjugates would be implicit in the acceptance of these materials. Likewise, with inhalation the contact with lung epithelial cells would be immediate, and, moreover, primary normal epithelial cells can be more susceptible to toxicity induced by AuNP-chitosan conjugates than cancer cell lines [48]. The positive charge of Au-chitosan NPs appears responsible for their toxicity, as citrate-coated anionic AuNPs do not elicit these same responses [47,48]. However, it is this cationic nature that make charged NPs attractive for medical applications, as a link between positive charge and increased cellular uptake has been reported, where cationic AuNPs mediate interactions with negatively charged lipid bilayer of cells [47,52,53]. It is therefore important to subtly modify NP constructs to account for this. This concept was achieved by Regiel-Futyra *et al.* [49], who reported that any adverse biochemical effects noted were alleviated through the addition of chitosan at different molecular weights to the NP surface exhibiting.

These studies clearly highlight the need for suitable functionalization to reduce unwanted effects and to retain colloidal stability of the NPs, but also to attain cellular responses necessary for therapeutic success. However, they also identify that functionalization and/or NP size may be responsible for unwanted toxicity. In both cases, mechanisms to avoid cells that are not of the target tissue, or to specifically target cells, such as those of malignancies, would aid in potentially reducing unwanted toxicity to any healthy tissue. This places greater emphasis on avoidance or targeting methods, usually achieved by functionalization or novel synthesis methods.

18.3.1.1 **Methods of Targeting Metal NPs**

The majority of prospective applications for AuNP therapeutics are based on intravenous injection. In imaging and diagnosis of cancers, for example, the standard methods currently used rely upon CT scanning. CT scanning is efficient, though is restricted to the size of lesions, where particularly small growths can go undetected [33]. One application of AuNPs is as contrast agents for CT scanning, enabling detection of small tumors [33,54], while hybridization of Au and iron oxide NPs can allow combination imaging utilizing CT and magnetic resonance imaging (MRI) [55]. With this intravenous application, there is often a reliance on targeting, to reduce non-target tissue exposure and to reduce the dose needed. Targeting of AuNPs can be passive [54,55] or specific, with the use of conjugated antibodies [33,56,57] or peptides [51]. For specific molecular targeting, 30 nm citrate-AuNPs were conjugated with anti-epidermal growth factor receptor (EGFR) antibodies, aiding the delivery of AuNPs to target cancer cells due to the high surface expression of EGFR on cancer cells [33]. While passive targeting with AuNPs alone improved the detection on CT scans, EGFR conjugation greatly increased image resolution [33]. These methods also reduce secondary exposure scenarios, as EGFR-targeting NPs accumulate less in secondary organs such as the liver, when compared to non-specific antibody-conjugated AuNPs [33]. These findings were reflected in a study by Hainfeld *et al.* [57]; as passive targeting of 15 nm AuNPs alone improved tumor detection compared to traditional CT scanning, whereas when using AuNPs conjugated with anti-Her2 antibodies, lesion detection was again improved. In terms of drug delivery, complex functionalization of AuNPs can enable multifunctional materials. PEG coating of AuNPs is thought to increase the retention time within the circulatory system by improving water solubility and limiting protein adsorption to the particle surface [58]. Secondary functions can then be achieved with further functionalization, such as enhanced anchoring and uptake of thioctic acid by tumor tissue[59]. In this fashion, AuNPs may cross the blood–brain barrier to deliver treatments such as phthalocyanine 4, a photodynamic therapy agent, to brain tumors, with delivery and uptake further enhanced by tumor specificity aided by EGF peptides to target the EGFR-overexpressing cells [35]. However, it should be noted that targeting mechanisms are not always widely applicable, as although targeting of many cancer cells can be through moieties for the EGFR [33,35], EGFR mutations are not found in all cancers, in fact a frequency of as low as 20% has been reported [60]. Therefore, broader tumor targeting has been investigated and can be achieved by functionalization with peptide ligands for broad-spectrum or specific tumors [51,61–63].

There is clearly much to gain in using these targeted delivery, multifunctional materials. However, the size-dependent cytotoxicity previously described is not the only influence AuNPs size has; NP size can also play crucial roles in treatment efficacy. AuNPs of 20 nm permeate deeper into the tumor interstitial space compared to 40–100 nm NPs [58]. While particularly small AuNPs (2 and 6 nm) enter the nucleus of a breast cancer cell-line, which was prevented by an increase in size to 10 and 15 nm, respectively; leading the authors to surmise that this small size can play an important role in gene delivery-based systems [36]. These properties, and the aforementioned attributes of AuNP functionalization, can result in high localized concentrations, or conversely, high retention rate and circulation in blood, which necessitates that caution is needed and toxicity at the site of administration and upon biodistribution needs considering. Non-selective and even selective targeting can result in a build up of AuNPs in untargeted organs, such as the liver and spleen [57,58]. AuNPs of 40 nm will predominately accumulate in macrophages of the liver (referred to as Kupffer cells) after intravenous injection with some present in the spleen, while, interestingly, with intraperitoneal injection, AuNPs accumulate, still in macrophages, and predominantly in the liver, but also the lymph nodes, spleen, and small intestine [64]. However, using conjugated AuNPs to detect and target gastrin-releasing peptide receptors, highly expressed in pancreatic tumors, Chanda *et al.* [51] demonstrated a high level of targeting and low accumulation of ~20 nm AuNPs in the reticuloendothelial system (RES). AuNPs with specific sizes of 40–80 nm allow accumulation in numerous organs to a greater extent than AuNPs of a smaller or larger size [58]. This raises the question of targeting specificity. For example, AuNP complexes containing a popular cancer drug doxorubicin (DOX), and coated with tumor-specific targeting motifs, iRGD peptides, encourage uptake and controlled intracellular release of DOX. The cytotoxicity of these complexes was comparable to exposure of DOX alone *in vitro*. However, the tumor cell targeting was not specific, as cancer cell-line B16 and primary normal cell-line

HUVEC were shown to internalize these conjugates at almost equal amounts, with each having corresponding cytotoxicity [65].

The studies described here clearly demonstrate the need for careful chemical manipulation of the surface of the NPs, and with distinctive specificity for the intended medical application. Furthermore, suppositions made upon these *in vitro* approaches can often be regarded as superficial and fall short of what is needed. Many studies have promising outcomes, for example, responses such as effective cell death and uptake can be found to be greater in response to AuNP–drug conjugates compared to drug alone. However, when the effect upon normal, non-cancerous cells is often overlooked and not investigated, it is difficult to be confident that these NP modifications would reduce toxicity to healthy non-cancerous tissue. Therefore, identification of suitable surface moieties (e.g., functionalization, polymer matrices) for adequate targeting, while retaining the biologically inert properties of NPs, is essential for metal-based NPs to progress further toward medical applications.

18.3.2
Carbon-Based Nanoparticles

NP constructs formed of carbon possibly offer the most diverse group applicable to nanomedicine. A few examples include carbon nanotubes (CNTs) implemented as drug or gene delivery systems [66–69], as targeting and photosensitizing agents [70], as tissue scaffolding [71], or used in the treatment of arthritis [69], or to aid imaging techniques [72–74]. Graphene nanostructures also show promise for improved drug delivery systems [75], effective photodynamic therapies and imaging techniques [76–79], as well as biosensors [80]. Fullerenes have been adapted for use as gene delivery vectors [81] in cancer treatments [12,82,83] or as theranostic devices [84]. Nanodiamonds have also been studied based upon their potential to be an advantageous cancer treatment [85,86]. Of all these materials, CNTs have been associated with particularly rampant, non-medical associated toxicity [87], and are therefore the focus of this section.

It has been discussed in previous sections of this chapter, that surface functionalization has proven to be vitally important to avoid unwanted toxicity of medically-oriented metal NPs. In terms of CNTs, this concept can be considered even more critical. When dealing with materials such as CNTs, it can be perceived as extremely questionable to intentionally introduce CNTs into the human body for therapeutic motives. With the potential for CNTs to elicit a negative biological response, the potential risk associated with exposure is significant. *In vitro* studies have reported CNT-induced cell death, oxidative stress, and (pro-)inflammatory conditions to occur following CNT exposure across a variety of exposure methods, concentrations, and in numerous cell phenotypes [88–90]. The driving force of these responses has been the CNT structure and morphology (particularly lengths of greater than 20 μm, which has been associated with frustrated phagocytosis (Figure 18.1), compared to other physical

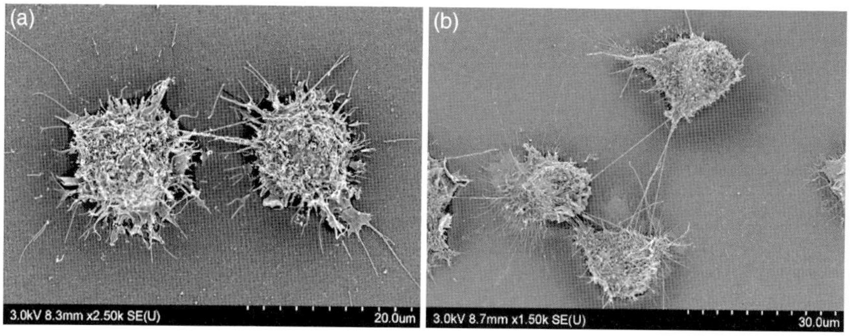

Figure 18.1 Scanning electron microscope images of (a) short MWCNT (<20 μm) (as indicated by the white arrow) and (b) long MWCNT (>50 μm) treated J774A.1 mouse macrophage cells *in vitro*. Cells are shown to effectively phagocytose short CNTs, while long CNTs induce length-dependent frustrated phagocytosis, which is implicit in CNT-induced toxicity. A Hitachi S-4800 FEG SEM scanning electron microscope was used; the scale bars are shown at the bottom right corner of each image.

and chemical factors such as trace elemental (e.g., iron) content [91–98]. However, there are conflicting reports *in vitro*, where CNTs, particularly single-walled (SW) CNTs have elicited low cytotoxicity, and low levels of oxidant or (pro-)inflammatory mediators [99–102]. While *in vivo* toxicity patterns generated by CNTs have been likened to the pathogenicity of asbestos, with strong (pro-)inflammatory responses, mutagenesis, the formation of fibrous lesions and granulomas [100,103–108]. Chronic one-year inhalation studies of SWCNT in mice, indicate retention within the lung and a small level of translocation to the lymphatic system, with a pattern of disease progression throughout this exposure time, although no lung cancers were identified [109]. Interestingly, the toxicity pattern of SWCNT differed from that of asbestos and carbon nanofibers (CNF), with asbestos and CNF inducing greater inflammation, and SWCNT eliciting more fibrosis [109].

In light of the reservations towards the use of CNT in a medical setting, the first hurdle is to address if CNTs are potential advantageous, therapeutic agents, is to determine their biopersistence. Second, to determine and then effectively control their degradation. The pathogenicity described by many, akin to that of asbestos, is reliant on bioaccumulation and biopersistence; therefore, if CNTs were to be degraded it would be an initial step towards their possible removal, but more importantly toward reducing their "asbestos-like" potential pathogenicity. The degradation of CNTs is considered to be highly, but not solely, dependent on the role of alveolar macrophages and recruited neutrophils, specifically by the action of myeloperoxidase derived from neutrophils [110,111], which forms hypochlorite as a result of myeloperoxidase activity [112]. Studies into these reactions, have confirmed degradation of CNTs by these processes, have a lower (pro-)inflammatory response [110,111]. Nonetheless, as in all cases, the biodistribution and ultimate site of deposition of CNTs within the body will often dictate how safe their use would be, and where secondary exposure may occur. Therefore, such degradation processes may not be relevant to all organs in which CNTs locate, highlighting the necessity to deduce the biodurability of CNTs throughout the human body.

Functionalization can be used for avoidance and targeting, firmly assigning the necessity for degradation. When taurine-functionalized CNTs of 10–600 nm were administered directly into the lungs of mice, the lungs retained approximately 20% CNT material one-month postexposure, with no observed CNTs present in secondary organs. Whilst, with intravenous administration, the CNTs rapidly accumulated within the heart, lungs, but predominately within the liver, with 80% remaining in the liver one-month post-exposure. With oral gavage, CNTs were only evident within the GI tract and fecal excretions [113]. Moreover, also using hydrophobic CNTs, intravenous injection of SWCNTs resulted in substantial deposition and lengthy retention in many organs, but particularly the RES of the liver and spleen, with most deposits observed in the lung tissue [114]. However, other studies have shown, regardless of administration route, easy translocation of CNTs throughout organs and body tissues when CNTs were hydrophilic, with ultimate and rapid excretion in feces and urine [115]. Likewise, DTPA-functionalized, iodine-labeled CNTs did not accumulate in the expected organs, such as the liver or spleen with intravenous administration, but were again excreted in urine [116]. Further evidence of effective clearance was demonstrated by Liu *et al.* [117] using PEGylated CNTs administered intravenously, where low level CNT accumulation was observed in the liver or spleen; instead CNTs were well retained in the blood, and eventually cleared. This distribution data indicates that with careful and suitable functionalization the exposure of NPs to secondary organs, and their concomitant toxicity can be adequately reduced, mainly through altering CNTs surface chemistry from hydrophobic to hydrophilic.

For effective functionalization, covalent bonding is often preferred; practically, this is done through oxidation of CNT surfaces, increasing hydrophilicity, and removing unwanted impurities, as well as providing sites for further functionalization [118]. Carboxylated CNTs, when administered intravenously in mice, are rapidly cleared from the body, with less retention and lower, or no, toxicity observed in the RES when compared to pristine CNTs, which has been attributed to greater hydrophilicity [119]. With enhanced excretion and lower RES retention confirmed with oxidized, DTPA-functionalized CNTs [120]. As previously emphasized throughout the chapter, PEG coating of NPs can aid applications in numerous ways, including altering the pattern of blood protein adsorption, and avoidance of circulating and RES oriented macrophages, ultimately increasing their retention in the circulatory system [121]. Alterations in CNT PEGylation would further allow control over the length of blood retention time and renal excretion [117,122]. However, non-covalent attachment does have benefits for reducing the toxicity of CNTs applied in medicine, albeit these methods may not produce stable bonding, as there is easy replacement or removal of bound molecules. Attached surface proteins would be noncovalently bound, and for example, the binding of lung surfactant proteins, such as the short palate, lung, and nasal epithelium clone-1 protein, to SWCNT surfaces can not only modify (pro-)inflammatory responses of macrophages to SWCNT *in vitro*, but also reduce progressive respiratory fibrosis *in vivo* [123]. While other studies have highlighted the less effective clearance based on non-covalent bonding, as functionalization of SWCNTs with Pluronic F108 leads to substantial deposition in the liver due to replacement of Pluronic F108 by blood plasma proteins and subsequent agglomeration [124], with Tween 80-coated SWCNT also depositing within the liver, spleen, and lungs at relatively high numbers [114].

With these modifications in place, it is easy to see how applicable and even safe CNTs may be in medicine. The great promise CNTs have in nanomedicine is rightly given, illuminated by proposed multifunctional treatments, such as the targeting and destruction of B-lymphoma cells *in vivo*, through monoclonal antibodies for tumor specific surface markers, such as CD20 or CD22, attached to CNT exteriors, and destruction of targeted cancer cells through intracellular delivery of cancer drugs, or by thermal ablation [125,126]. While PEGylated CNTs with the additional conjugation to paclitaxel (PTX) have been shown, *in vivo*, to supress tumor growth in mice, which the authors attribute to the PEG-aided retention in circulation leading to the increased uptake of PTX through CNT enhanced permeation [127]. Furthermore, with particular physical attributes of CNTs there is also promise for improving imaging techniques, including molecular sensing based on CNT near infrared fluorescence emissions [128], and thermoacoustic imaging for detection of targeted lesions with a greater spatial resolution than traditional imaging methods [72]. With therapeutic delivery enhanced by loading of CNTs with drugs such as anti-inflammatory dexamethasone [129], or delivery of erythropoietin (EPO) via the small intestine, where, among other NPs, CNTs were shown to provide the highest serum EPO levels after administration [130]. It is clear the structure and chemistry of CNTs allow multiple, simultaneous functionalization, where treatments, diagnostics, and targeting moieties can be added to the same material [131], yet due to their associated toxicity, extreme caution should be taken in their use within medical applications.

18.3.3
Polymer-Based Nanoparticles

With unique characteristics and a certain level of freedom in the design process, polymer-based NPs (PNPs) are an attractive candidate for use in drug delivery, diagnostics, or theranostics, with research thus far focused on diseases such as arthritis and cancer [132]. PNPs can be based on synthetic synthesis methods, or isolated from natural sources. In terms of intrinsic toxicity, poly (lactic-co-glycolic acid) (PLGA), for example, is one of the most prevalent PNPs found in pre-clinical trials due to their associated FDA (US Food and Drug Administration) approval and an assumption that it is nontoxic and therefore proposed for use in the treatment of a wide range of diseases from cancer to diabetes [133].

However, PLGA NPs that can be broken down in the body by hydrolytic enzymes to produce 'assumed' safe by-products, such as lactic acid and glycolic acid, which have previously been reported as cytotoxic *in vitro* [134,135]. Moreover, PLGA has demonstrated limited loading capacity [133], which can consequently lead to a higher administered dose of NPs to maintain comparable drug levels. This, again, may contribute to an increased cytotoxicity that is not observed for other NPs, such as the well-established Doxil liposomal NP constructs [136].

However, increasing interest in PNPs has stemmed from the advanced biocompatibility potential that can be attributed to PNPs compared to other NP constructs used in this field, such as liposomal or metallic NPs [137]. Specifically, PNP functionalities useful for medical applications include biodegradability, high storage stability, sustained cargo release, increased circulation time, and protection of sensitive cargos; all of these attributes can improve the safety of nanomedicines in general [138]. PNPs are, themselves, very stable in solution [139], but as highlighted in section 18.3.1.1 polymer coating of NPs can be used to enhance NP biodurability, and therefore retention time in circulation [55], and moreover, to enable functionalization with cell targeting agents [33]. This, again, is an important consideration for polymer-based nanomedicines, to avoid secondary exposure and potential accumulation in secondary organs; as demonstrated in Figure 18.2, primary hepatocytes can effectively internalize 20 nm polystyrene NPs. One of the most commonly used polymers is PEG, which is often used to coat NPs composed of other materials. Due to the neutral charge of PEG, a high density PEG coating of magnetic Fe_3O_4 NPs provided a diagnostic tool to improve MRI imaging [121,140]. Furthermore, the addition of PEG shields against opsonization,

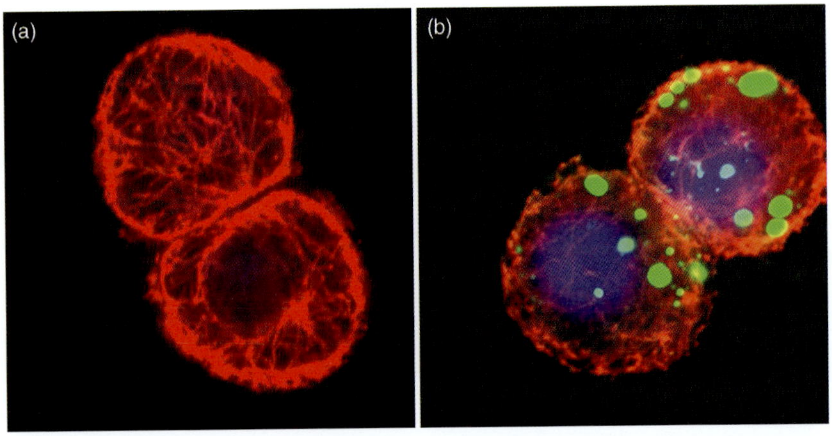

Figure 18.2 Confocal laser scanning microscopy images of (a) primary rat hepatocyte couplets (RHC) and (b) RHC treated with 20 nm polystyrene beads *ex vivo*. Tubulin staining appears as red (primary antibody: anti-α-tubulin monoclonal antibody; secondary antibody: Alexa Fluor 633), nucleus as blue (Hoescht), and fluorescent polystyrene NPs (Molecular Probes, OR, USA) as green.

resulting in less proteins binding to the surface, allowed NPs to escape the RES more efficiently than uncoated NPs. Consequently, reducing the occurrence of cellular internalization of these NPs and increasing circulation time, resulted in less frequent treatments and reduced cytotoxicity [141].

Although for some applications it would be beneficial to reduce cell–particle interactions, whereas for others it is not, such as for cancer therapeutics or gene delivery. A major hurdle for any NP used to deliver DNA is cell and nuclear membrane penetration of target cells [135,142]. A polyplex of Poly (N-(2-hydroxypropyl) methacrylamide) (HPMA) and methacrylamide functionalized with varying lengths of L-lysine repeat units actively target the cells' nucleus in human cervical carcinoma (HeLa) cells *in vitro* [143]. However, L-lysine length dictated the aspect ratio of these PNPs, which in turn dictated treatment efficacy, with PNPs of lower aspect ratios having enhanced nuclear accumulation [84]. While HPMA is an alternative to PEG with similar stealth like properties, it has the added benefit of numerous functionalization sites allowing for the conjugation of multiple compounds. HPMA also benefits from a higher storage stability compared to liposomal NPs, and when conjugated with popular anti-cancer drugs such as doxorubicin or paclitaxel, has improved treatment efficacy, but also reduced superfluous toxicity, compared to cargo alone [144,145]. L-lysine functionalization of PNPs may also influence routes of cellular uptake, and therefore intracellular trafficking events. Whereas, L-arginine-functionalized PNPs display an affinity for caveolae-mediated endocytosis in Cos7 cells (monkey kidney cells), resulting in transport to the Golgi apparatus and endoplasmic reticulum [146].

In the intravenous treatment of tumors with leaky vasculature, particles under 200 nm demonstrate passive targeting of cancer cells via the enhanced permeability and retention (EPR) effect. Due to this size effect, the preference of NPs is to accumulate in cancer cells, while remaining unable to penetrate normal vasculature [147]. Although utilization of the ERP effect is not unique to PNPs it has been used consistently in the treatment in cancer with clinically approved PNPs such as intravenously administered Genexol [148]. In addition, this micellar formulation can provide slow sustained release of Pactiltaxel through diffusion and relaxation of polymer chains that could reduce both the frequency of drug administration and the toxic side effects [149]. The chemotherapy agent, Pactiltaxel, contained within Genexol's block copolymer (poly (ethylene glycol) - block-poly (D, L-lactide)) is difficult to formulate due to its poor solubility, and although it is an effective anticancer treatment, there is additional adverse toxicity associated with its current clinical use [150,151]. Genexol, on the other hand, displayed low toxicity to nontargeted healthy cells, and increased the sensitivity of cancer cells to radiation therapy, compared to the traditional Pactiltaxel treatment method, demonstrating how PNPs can be used to deliver clinically adept drugs, while maintaining a relatively good drug-safety profile.

Naturally occurring polymers, such as chitosan [152–156], also have a variety of therapeutic applications such as for arthritis [152], or as drug carriers [153–155] or gene therapy [156], and can be applied in multifunctional particles to aid in administration to particularly complex systems. One such application is found in oral drug exposures. The oral administration for cancer therapy, therefore via the gastrointestinal (GI) tract, has received much interest, as using this method can potentially deliver prolonged circulation of the drug (and drug-carrier) as well as enhanced cancer cell exposure to relatively low levels of cancer treatment, when compared to intravenous injection. However, although most cancer therapeutics are considered for the oral route, most are not used due to their poor solubility and poor stability, which leads to low bioavailability and increased cytotoxicity [157]. To aid in these matters, complex NP formulations may be of use. The complexity of these formulations are needed to successfully navigate this route of exposure, including circumventing the variable pH levels of the GI tract, bypass mucosal membrane barriers to reach the circulatory system, and avoid the action of digestive and metabolizing enzymes [158]. Polymer-based materials are useful for these exposure routes as they can remain stable in the acidic environment, while are disrupted within the small intestines and colon [159]. Due to their biodegradability, polymeric NPs are often chosen for delivery of drugs in cancer therapy, for example, poly(lactide-co ε-caprolactone)-d-α-tocopheryl polyethylene glycol 1000 succinate (PLA-PCL-TPGS) NPs can be used to encapsulate the broad-spectrum anticancer drug paclitaxel [160]. However, for use as an orally administered agent, this simple complex would not be sufficient to overcome the next hurdle of oral administration, translocation to the circulatory system. This can be achieved, however, through further conjugation of chitosan, which due to its positive charge encourages mucoadhesion [161], but also facilitates the disruption of epithelial tight junctions allowing NPs to pass the mucosal barrier via the paracellular pathway [160]. As previously highlighted, chitosan conjugation with AuNPs can elicit considerable cell toxicity, however, with further alterations chitosan toxicity can be placated, such as with thiolation, which modulates the biocompatibility and reduces cell toxicity [160]. Other examples of how complex PNPs can be used to overcome biological barriers of clinical relevance include the delivery of siRNA to cancer cells, where NP constructs are formed of cyclodextrin, siRNA, PEG, and transferrin. However, it should be noted that although these modifications allow targeted, effective treatment, it may be problematic for the pharmaceutical industry to scale up production of certain PNPs, due to the multiple chemical reactions and purifications that are needed. These prohibitory costs of production, but also batch-to-batch variation, may cause a major stumbling block for the translation of PNPs from the bench-top (laboratory) to the bed-side (clinical use) [162].

18.3.4 Biological-Based Nanoparticles

The use of biologically derived components in nanomedicine is an interesting concept. In terms of administering treatments for lung cancer, biologically formed NPs, including liposomes and micelles, display a greater ability for lung retention than inorganic NPs, including silica, PEG, and quantum dots [163]. Although the use of organic biological material provides useful and effective methods in traditional NP "carrier" scenarios for the targeting and delivery of therapeutics, such as lipid carriers [164], here focus is given to relatively novel biologically derived nano structures, which are formed of uniquely cell-based constructions.

It seems feasible that the use of cell-derived, and therefore naturally occurring and organic, NPs may provide better acceptance by the host when compared to exposure of inorganic engineered NPs, and furthermore, cell-derived membrane vesicles would have naturally occurring moieties intrinsically suited to targeting. As these properties eliminate the introduction of exogenous inorganic carriers and surfactants to the host, it is logical to consider that biologically derived NPs could reduce unwanted toxicity during therapy. Exosomes are nanosized membrane vesicles, which are released from numerous cell types; it is believed that these NPs transfer information between cells without cell to cell contact through, for example, antigen presentation, and are involved in T-lymphocyte T-cell responses and tolerance or hypersensitivity reactions [165]. In fact, this exact principle has been associated with the enhanced toxicity of NPs. Long-term and/or systemic inflammation induced by NPs is difficult to interpret if clearance has been effective, and more so when NPs do not harbor the necessary epitopes to induce certain responses. However, it is believed that NPs can elicit adaptive immune responses controlled by NP-induced release of cellular exosomes [166]. For example, the release of exosomes into bronchoalveolar fluid in response to intratracheal instillation of iron oxide NPs was effectively used to stimulate conditions of hypersensitivity, through activation and differentiation of antigen-presenting cells such as dendritic cells and macrophages, leading to T-lymphocyte priming and culminating in a Th1-like hypersensitivity immune responses [167].

The advantage of applying these organic NP constructs to nanomedicine is that given the right stimulus, these exosomes induce antigen-specific T-lymphocyte-driven inflammatory responses, which can be focused on tumors [168,169], as they consist of tumor specific antigens that allow tumor-specific T-lymphocyte responses, and the expansion of T-lymphocyte repertoires for specific tumors [170]. These studies often use exosomes directly secreted from tumor cells; however, recent advancement of these methods has led to multiple steps, and novel refinements. With these refinements it is possible to reduce the unwanted side-effects associated with the previously outlined methods, such as the impedance of NK cell function and suppression of NK cell cytotoxic activity associated with tumor cell-derived exosomes, which can result in increased cancer growth efficiency tumor targeting can also be achieved by using exosomes derived from dendritic cells (DC). This has previously been tested with immature-DC or LPS-matured DC, where the most effective T-lymphocyte responses were shown for mature DC [173,174]. This method has been applied as a technique for self-immunization against tumors, and as such has been practically tested in phase I clinical trials for cancer therapy. Both clinical trials were considered to be effective as the DC-derived exosomes were well tolerated with little toxicity, and occasional therapeutic response to the treatment [175,176]. There has since been further refinement of this methodology, to enable more efficient tumor targeting and to allow the targeting of a broader spectrum of tumors. Specifically, nanosized membrane vesicles were isolated from homogenized DCs that share similarities with DC exosomes in their MHC molecules and expressed antigens [177]. This has been further developed by Tian *et al.* [178], who prepared DC membrane vesicles *in vitro* with the exposure of DCs to exosomes generated in *ex vivo* murine melanoma (B16) and Lewis lung carcinoma (LLC) cells. The resultant B16- and B16/LLC-derived DC membrane vesicles not only initiated strong T-lymphocyte expansion and T-lymphocyte specific responses *in vitro* and *in vivo*, but also generated a cytotoxic T-lymphocyte population *in vivo*. Furthermore, T-lymphocyte-dependent cytotoxicity of melanoma and LLC cells was observed *ex vivo*, with good tumor specificity (i.e., localization of the NPs). Moreover, these treatments were able to significantly delay tumor growth *in vivo* when applied as an immunization strategy, again with good tumor specificity.

18.4 Summary

Currently, despite some clinical promise, the use and translation of nanomedicine from the lab bench to the clinical setting has been relatively slow [1]. There are numerous reasons for this, most notably is the difficulty of efficiently reproducing the synthesis of NPs in sufficient quantity and with identical properties. Coupled with this, there is a current lack of understanding of the relationship between *in vitro* physicochemical properties of NPs and their *in vivo* fates, their potential toxicity *in vivo*, and the scarcity of current methods of screening NPs rapidly in a manner that predicts the *in vivo* behavior of NPs [179]. While this is the overall objective, it must be emphasized that the current research being focused upon in this area has shown essential and important information as to which materials are currently at a stage where toxicity is at a relatively low level *in vitro*, providing a firm platform for developing NP-based therapeutics (e.g., polymeric or biologically-derived NPs) for in vivo use. Whilst some NPs are already in use in the clinic, the use of other materials for use in nanomedicine (e.g., CNTs) may be more distant, owing to their heightened intrinsic toxicity. In both these cases, but particularly the latter, it is essential that during development the properties that make each material toxic are suitably considered. With this consideration, it has been shown that many potentially detrimental events, such as biopersistence and bioaccumulation in non-target cells and tissues, can be circumvented, ensuring that NP-based therapeutics do not elicit negative side-effects over both an acute and chronic period. While nanomedicine will inevitably receive further, heightened attention as nanotechnology advances, it is essential that a direct link and correlation is made between research pertaining to the medical application of NPs and non-medical based research in which fundamental nanosafety considerations are foremost; linking these disciplines will facilitate the safe progression of this rapidly developing field of nanotechnology.

References

1 Oberdörster, G. (2010) Safety assessment for nanotechnology and nanomedicine: concepts of nanotoxicology. *J. Intern. Med.*, **267** (1), 89–105.
2 Kermanizadeh, A. *et al.* (2015) Nanomaterial translocation – the biokinetics, tissue accumulation, toxicity and fate of materials in secondary organs – a review. *Crit. Rev. Toxicol.*, **45** (10), 837–872.
3 Kreyling, W.G. *et al.* (2014) Air–blood barrier translocation of tracheally instilled gold nanoparticles inversely depends on particle size. *ACS Nano.*, **8** (1), 222–233.
4 Kreyling, W.G. *et al.* (2002) Translocation of ultrafine insoluble iridium particles from lung epithelium to extrapulmonary organs is size dependent but very low. *J. Toxicol. Environ. Health A*, **65** (20), 1513–1530.
5 Kreyling, W.G. *et al.* (2009) Size dependence of the translocation of inhaled iridium and carbon nanoparticle aggregates from the lung of rats to the blood and secondary target organs. *Inhal. Toxicol.*, **21** (supl), 55–60.
6 Oberdörster, G. *et al.* (2005) Principles for characterizing the potential human health effects from exposure to nanomaterials: elements of a screening strategy. *Part Fibre Toxicol.*, **2** (1), 1–35.
7 Kreyling, W.G. *et al.* (2013) Differences in the biokinetics of inhaled nano- versus micrometer-sized particles. *Acc. Chem. Res.*, **46** (3), 714–722.
8 Zhao, J. and Castranova, V. (2011) Toxicology of nanomaterials used in nanomedicine. *J. Toxicol. Environ. Health B*, **14** (8), 593–632.
9 Zhang, J. *et al.* (2008) Uptake of oleoyl-chitosan nanoparticles by A549 cells. *Nanomed. Nanotech. Biol. Med.*, **4** (3), 208–214.
10 Bharali, D.J. and Mousa, S.A. (2010) Emerging nanomedicines for early cancer detection and improved treatment: current perspective and future promise. *Pharmacol. Ther.*, **128** (2), 324–335.
11 Lin, P.-C. *et al.* (2006) Ethylene glycol-protected magnetic nanoparticles for a multiplexed immunoassay in human plasma. *Small*, **2** (4), 485–489.
12 Kang, S.-G. *et al.* (2012) Molecular mechanism of pancreatic tumor metastasis inhibition by Gd@C82(OH)22 and its implication for *de novo* design of nanomedicine. *Proc. Natl. Acad. Sci. USA*, **109** (38), 15431–15436.
13 Liang, Y.-X. *et al.* (2011) CNS regeneration after chronic injury using a self-assembled nanomaterial and MEMRI for real-time *in vivo* monitoring. *Nanomed. Nanotech. Biol. Med.*, 7 (3), 351–359.
14 Zhou, W. *et al.* (2005) Drug-loaded, magnetic, hollow silica nanocomposites for nanomedicine. *Nanomed. Nanotech. Biol. Med.*, **1** (3), 233–237.
15 Pouliquen, D. *et al.* (1992) Investigation of the magnetic properties of iron oxide nanoparticles used as contrast agent for MRI. *Magn. Reson. Med.*, **24** (1), 75–84.
16 Byrne, U.T.E. *et al.* (2009) High-throughput quantification of Alzheimer's disease pathological markers in the post-mortem human brain. *J. Neurosci. Methods*, **176** (2), 298–309.
17 Taylor, E.N. *et al.* (2012) Superparamagnetic iron oxide nanoparticles (SPION) for the treatment of antibiotic-resistant biofilms. *Small*, **8** (19), 3016–3027.
18 Nel, A. *et al.* (2013) Nanomaterial toxicity testing in the 21st century: use of a predictive toxicological approach and high-throughput screening. *Acc. Chem. Res.*, **46** (3), 607–621.

19 Zhu, Y., Eaton, J.W., and Li, C. (2012) Titanium dioxide (TiO_2) nanoparticles preferentially induce cell death in transformed cells in a bak/bax-independent fashion. *PLoS One*, **7** (11), e50607.

20 Escamilla-Rivera, V. *et al.* (2016) Protein corona acts as a protective shield against Fe3O4-PEG inflammation and ROS-induced toxicity in human macrophages. *Toxicol. Lett.*, **240** (1), 172–184.

21 Khan, S. *et al.* (2015) Kinetics of protein adsorption on gold nanoparticle with variable protein structure and nanoparticle size. *J. Chem. Phys.*, **143** (16), 164709.

22 Aggarwal, P. *et al.* (2009) Nanoparticle interaction with plasma proteins as it relates to particle biodistribution, biocompatibility and therapeutic efficacy. *Adv. Drug. Deliv. Rev.*, **61** (6), 428–437.

23 Wang, Q., Perez, J.M., and Webster, T.J. (2013) Inhibited growth of *Pseudomonas aeruginosa* by dextran- and polyacrylic acid-coated ceria nanoparticles. *Int. J. Nanomedicine*, **8**, 3395–3399.

24 Zhao, F. *et al.* (2011) Cellular uptake, intracellular trafficking, and cytotoxicity of nanomaterials. *Small*, **7** (10), 1322–1337.

25 Sereemaspun, A., Rojanathanes, R., and Wiwanitkit, V. (2008) Effect of gold nanoparticle on renal cell: an implication for exposure risk. *Ren. Fail.*, **30** (3), 323–325.

26 Chen, Z. *et al.* (2008) Bio-distribution and metabolic paths of silica coated CdSeS quantum dots. *Toxicol. Appl. Pharmacol.*, **230** (3), 364–371.

27 Mercer, R.R. *et al.* (2013) Extrapulmonary transport of MWCNT following inhalation exposure. *Part. Fibre Toxicol.*, **10** (1), 1–14.

28 Valdiglesias, V. *et al.* (2016) Are iron oxide nanoparticles safe? Current knowledge and future perspectives. *J. Trace. Elem. Med. Bio.*, doi: 10.1016/j.jtemb.2016.03.017

29 Daniel, M.-C. and Astruc, D. (2004) Gold nanoparticles: assembly, supramolecular chemistry, quantum-size-related properties, and applications toward biology, catalysis, and nanotechnology. *Chem. Rev.*, **104** (1), 293–346.

30 Niidome, Y. *et al.* (2006) Pulsed-laser induced fragmentation and dissociation of DNA immobilized on gold nanoparticles. *Mol. Cryst. Liq. Cryst.*, **445** (1), 201/[491]–206/[496].

31 Ardao, I. *et al.* (2012) Rational nanoconjugation improves biocatalytic performance of enzymes: aldol addition catalyzed by immobilized rhamnulose-1-phosphate aldolase. *Langmuir*, **28** (15), 6461–6467.

32 Peng, C. *et al.* (2012) PEGylated dendrimer-entrapped gold nanoparticles for *in vivo* blood pool and tumor imaging by computed tomography. *Biomaterials*, **33** (4), 1107–1119.

33 Reuveni, T. *et al.* (2011) Targeted gold nanoparticles enable molecular CT imaging of cancer: an *in vivo* study. *Int. J. Nanomedicine*, **6**, 2859–2864.

34 Brown, S.D. *et al.* (2010) Gold nanoparticles for the improved anticancer drug delivery of the active component of oxaliplatin. *J. Am. Chem. Soc.*, **132** (13), 4678–4684.

35 Cheng, Y. *et al.* (2011) Addressing brain tumors with targeted gold nanoparticles: a new gold standard for hydrophobic drug delivery? *Small*, **7** (16), 2301–2306.

36 Huo, S. *et al.* (2014) Ultrasmall gold nanoparticles as carriers for nucleus-based gene therapy due to size-dependent nuclear entry. *ACS Nano.*, **8** (6), 5852–5862.

37 Malathi, S. *et al.* (2013) Green synthesis of gold nanoparticles for controlled delivery. *Adv. Mat. Lett.*, **4** (12), 933–940.

38 Bhumkar, D. *et al.* (2007) Chitosan reduced gold nanoparticles as novel carriers for transmucosal delivery of insulin. *Pharm. Res.*, **24** (8), 1415–1426.

39 Shukla, R. *et al.* (2005) Biocompatibility of gold nanoparticles and their endocytotic fate inside the cellular compartment: a microscopic overview. *Langmuir*, **21** (23), 10644–10654.

40 Brandenberger, C. *et al.* (2010) Effects and uptake of gold nanoparticles deposited at the air–liquid interface of a human epithelial airway model. *Toxicol. Appl. Pharmacol.*, **242** (1), 56–65.

41 Gu, Y.-J. *et al.* (2009) Nuclear penetration of surface functionalized gold

nanoparticles. *Toxicol. Appl. Pharmacol.*, **237** (2), 196–204.

42 Pan, Y. *et al.* (2007) Size-dependent cytotoxicity of gold nanoparticles. *Small*, **3** (11), 1941–1949.

43 Jiang, W. *et al.* (2008) Nanoparticle-mediated cellular response is size-dependent. *Nat. Nanotechnol.*, **3** (3), 145–150.

44 Schaeublin, N.M. *et al.* (2011) Surface charge of gold nanoparticles mediates mechanism of toxicity. *Nanoscale*, **3** (2), 410–420.

45 Hauck, T.S., Ghazani, A.A., and Chan, W.C.W. (2008) Assessing the effect of surface chemistry on gold nanorod uptake, toxicity, and gene expression in mammalian cells. *Small*, **4** (1), 153–159.

46 Connor, E.E. *et al.* (2005) Gold nanoparticles are taken up by human cells but do not cause acute cytotoxicity. *Small*, **1** (3), 325–327.

47 Boyles, M.S.P. *et al.* (2015) Chitosan functionalisation of gold nanoparticles encourages particle uptake and induces cytotoxicity and pro-inflammatory conditions in phagocytic cells, as well as enhancing particle interactions with serum components. *J. Nanobiotechnol.*, **13** (1), 1–20.

48 Schlinkert, P. *et al.* (2015) The oxidative potential of differently charged silver and gold nanoparticles on three human lung epithelial cell types. *J. Nanobiotechnol.*, **13** (1), 1–18.

49 Regiel-Futyra, A. *et al.* (2015) Development of noncytotoxic chitosan–gold nanocomposites as efficient antibacterial materials. *ACS Appl. Mater. Interfaces*, **7** (2), 1087–1099.

50 Iyer, A.K. *et al.* (2006) Exploiting the enhanced permeability and retention effect for tumor targeting. *Drug Discov. Today*, **11** (17–18), 812–818.

51 Chanda, N. *et al.* (2010) Bombesin functionalized gold nanoparticles show *in vitro* and *in vivo* cancer receptor specificity. *Proc. Natl. Acad. Sci. USA*, **107** (19), 8760–8765.

52 Goodman, C.M. *et al.* (2004) Toxicity of gold nanoparticles functionalized with cationic and anionic side chains. *Bioconjugate Chem.*, **15** (4), 897–900.

53 Bartneck, M. *et al.* (2012) Effects of nanoparticle surface-coupled peptides, functional endgroups, and charge on intracellular distribution and functionality of human primary reticuloendothelial cells. *Nanomed. Nanotech. Biol. Med.*, **8** (8), 1282–1292.

54 Cai, Q.-Y. *et al.* (2007) Colloidal gold nanoparticles as a blood-pool contrast agent for X-ray computed tomography in mice. *Invest. Radiol.*, **42** (12), 797–806.

55 Kim, D. *et al.* (2011) Amphiphilic polymer-coated hybrid nanoparticles as CT/MRI dual contrast agents. *Nanotechnology*, **22** (15), 155101.

56 Popovtzer, R. *et al.* (2008) Targeted gold nanoparticles enable molecular CT imaging of cancer. *Nano. Lett.*, **8** (12), 4593–4596.

57 Hainfeld, J.F. *et al.* (2011) Micro-CT enables microlocalisation and quantification of Her2-targeted gold nanoparticles within tumour regions. *Brit. J. Radiol.*, **84** (1002), 526–533.

58 Perrault, S.D. *et al.* (2009) Mediating tumor targeting efficiency of nanoparticles through design. *Nano. Lett.*, **9** (5), 1909–1915.

59 Zhang, G. *et al.* (2009) Influence of anchoring ligands and particle size on the colloidal stability and *in vivo* biodistribution of polyethylene glycol-coated gold nanoparticles in tumor-xenografted mice. *Biomaterials*, **30** (10), 1928–1936.

60 Rosell, R. *et al.* (2009) Screening for epidermal growth factor receptor mutations in lung cancer. *N. Engl. J. Med.*, **361** (10), 958–967.

61 Lee, K.J. *et al.* (2014) Novel peptides functionally targeting *in vivo* human lung cancer discovered by *in vivo* peptide displayed phage screening. *Amino Acids*, **47** (2), 281–289.

62 Lee, T.-Y. *et al.* (2007) Peptide-mediated targeting to tumor blood vessels of lung cancer for drug delivery. *Cancer Res.*, **67** (22), 10958–10965.

63 McGuire, M.J. *et al.* (2014) Identification and characterization of a suite of tumor targeting peptides for non-small cell lung cancer. *Sci. Rep.*, **4**, 4480.

64 Sadauskas, E. *et al.* (2007) Kupffer cells are central in the removal of nanoparticles from the organism. *Part Fibre Toxicol.*, **4** (1), 1–7.

65 Su, S. *et al.* (2013) iRGD-coupled responsive fluorescent nanogel for targeted drug delivery. *Biomaterials*, **34** (13), 3523–3533.

66 Bhirde, A.A. *et al.* (2009) Targeted killing of cancer cells *in vivo* and *in vitro* with EGF-directed carbon nanotube-based drug delivery. *ACS Nano*, **3** (2), 307–316.

67 Kostarelos, K. *et al.* (2007) Cellular uptake of functionalized carbon nanotubes is independent of functional group and cell type. *Nat Nano*, **2** (2), 108–113.

68 Al-Jamal, K.T. *et al.* (2011) Functional motor recovery from brain ischemic insult by carbon nanotube-mediated siRNA silencing. *Proc. Natl. Acad. Sci. USA*, **108** (27), 10952–10957.

69 Sacchetti, C. *et al.* (2014) Polyethylene-glycol-modified single-walled carbon nanotubes for intra-articular delivery to chondrocytes. *ACS Nano.*, **8** (12), 12280–12291.

70 Kam, N.W.S. *et al.* (2005) Carbon nanotubes as multifunctional biological transporters and near-infrared agents for selective cancer cell destruction. *Proc. Natl. Acad. Sci. USA*, **102** (33), 11600–11605.

71 Bosi, S. *et al.* (2015) From 2D to 3D: novel nanostructured scaffolds to investigate signalling in reconstructed neuronal networks. *Sci. Rep.*, **5**, 9562.

72 De La Zerda, A. *et al.* (2008) Carbon nanotubes as photoacoustic molecular imaging agents in living mice. *Nat Nano*, **3** (9), 557–562.

73 Ghosh, D. *et al.* (2014) Deep, noninvasive imaging and surgical guidance of submillimeter tumors using targeted M13-stabilized single-walled carbon nanotubes. *Proc. Natl. Acad. Sci. USA*, **111** (38), 13948–13953.

74 Delogu, L.G. *et al.* (2012) Functionalized multiwalled carbon nanotubes as ultrasound contrast agents. *Proc. Natl. Acad. Sci. USA*, **109** (41), 16612–16617.

75 Ma, X. *et al.* (2012) A functionalized graphene oxide-iron oxide nanocomposite for magnetically targeted drug delivery, photothermal therapy, and magnetic resonance imaging. *Nano Res.*, **5** (3), 199–212.

76 Ge, J. *et al.* (2014) A graphene quantum dot photodynamic therapy agent with high singlet oxygen generation. *Nat. Commun.*, **5**, 4596.

77 Shi, X. *et al.* (2013) Graphene-based magnetic plasmonic nanocomposite for dual bioimaging and photothermal therapy. *Biomaterials*, **34** (20), 4786–4793.

78 Yang, K. *et al.* (2012) Multimodal imaging guided photothermal therapy using functionalized graphene nanosheets anchored with magnetic nanoparticles. *Adv. Mater.*, **24** (14), 1868–1872.

79 Yang, K. *et al.* (2010) Graphene in mice: ultrahigh *in vivo* tumor uptake and efficient photothermal therapy. *Nano. Lett.*, **10** (9), 3318–3323.

80 Liu, Y. *et al.* (2010) Biocompatible graphene oxide-based glucose biosensors. *Langmuir*, **26** (9), 6158–6160.

81 Maeda-Mamiya, R. *et al.* (2010) *In vivo* gene delivery by cationic tetraamino fullerene. *Proc. Natl. Acad. Sci. USA*, **107** (12), 5339–5344.

82 Pan, Y. *et al.* (2015) Gd–metallofullerenol nanomaterial suppresses pancreatic cancer metastasis by inhibiting the interaction of histone deacetylase 1 and metastasis-associated protein 1. *ACS Nano.*, **9** (7), 6826–6836.

83 Liu, Y. *et al.* (2015) Gd-metallofullerenol nanomaterial as non-toxic breast cancer stem cell-specific inhibitor. *Nat. Commun.*, **6**, 5988.

84 Yameen, B. *et al.* (2014) Insight into nanoparticle cellular uptake and intracellular targeting. *J. Control. Release*, **190**, 485–499.

85 Wang, X. *et al.* (2014) Epirubicin-adsorbed nanodiamonds kill chemoresistant hepatic cancer stem cells. *ACS Nano.*, **8** (12), 12151–12166.

86 Chow, E.K. *et al.* (2011) Nanodiamond therapeutic delivery agents mediate enhanced chemoresistant tumor treatment. *Sci. Transl. Med.*, **3** (73), 73ra21–73ra21.

87 Donaldson, K. *et al.* (2006) Carbon nanotubes: a review of their properties in

relation to pulmonary toxicology and workplace safety. *Toxicol. Sci.*, **92** (1), 5–22.

88 Kalbacova, M. *et al.* (2006) The study of the interaction of human mesenchymal stem cells and monocytes/macrophages with single-walled carbon nanotube films. *Phys. Status Solidi B*, **243** (13), 3514–3518.

89 Hirano, S., Kanno, S., and Furuyama, A. (2008) Multi-walled carbon nanotubes injure the plasma membrane of macrophages. *Toxicol. Appl. Pharmacol.*, **232** (2), 244–251.

90 Murr, L.E. *et al.* (2005) Cytotoxicity assessment of some carbon nanotubes and related carbon nanoparticle aggregates and the implications for anthropogenic carbon nanotube aggregates in the environment. *Int. J. Environ. Res. Publ. Health*, **2** (1), 31–42.

91 Boyles, M.S.P. *et al.* (2015) Multi-walled carbon nanotube induced frustrated phagocytosis, cytotoxicity and pro-inflammatory conditions in macrophages are length dependent and greater than that of asbestos. *Toxicol. In Vitro*, **29** (7), 1513–1528.

92 Cheng, C. *et al.* (2009) Toxicity and imaging of multi-walled carbon nanotubes in human macrophage cells. *Biomaterials*, **30** (25), 4152–4160.

93 Rothen-Rutishauser, B. *et al.* (2010) Relating the physicochemical characteristics and dispersion of multiwalled carbon nanotubes in different suspension media to their oxidative reactivity *in vitro* and inflammation *in vivo*. *Nanotoxicology*, **4** (3), 331–342.

94 Karlsson, H.L. *et al.* (2008) Copper oxide nanoparticles are highly toxic: a comparison between metal oxide nanoparticles and carbon nanotubes. *Chem. Res. Toxicol.*, **21** (9), 1726–1732.

95 Kim, J.S. *et al.* (2010) Determination of cytotoxicity attributed to multiwall carbon nanotubes (MWCNT) in normal human embryonic lung cell (WI-38) line. *J. Toxicol. Environ. Health A*, **73** (21–22), 1521–1529.

96 Pulskamp, K. *et al.* (2007) Human lung epithelial cells show biphasic oxidative burst after single-walled carbon nanotube contact. *Carbon*, **45** (11), 2241–2249.

97 Brown, D.M. *et al.* (2007) An *in vitro* study of the potential of carbon nanotubes and nanofibres to induce inflammatory mediators and frustrated phagocytosis. *Carbon*, **45** (9), 1743–1756.

98 Clift, M. *et al.* (2013) Assessing the impact of the physical properties of industrially produced carbon nanotubes on their interaction with human primary macrophages *in vitro*. *BioNanoMaterials*, **14**, 239–248.

99 Kagan, V.E. *et al.* (2006) Direct and indirect effects of single walled carbon nanotubes on RAW 264.7 macrophages: role of iron. *Toxicol. Lett.*, **165** (1), 88–100.

100 Shvedova, A.A. *et al.* (2005) Unusual inflammatory and fibrogenic pulmonary responses to single-walled carbon nanotubes in mice. *Am. J. Physiol. – Lung Cell Mol. Physiol.*, **289** (5), L698–L708.

101 Davoren, M. *et al.* (2007) *In vitro* toxicity evaluation of single walled carbon nanotubes on human A549 lung cells. *Toxicol. In Vitro*, **21** (3), 438–448.

102 Yacobi, N.R. *et al.* (2007) Nanoparticle effects on rat alveolar epithelial cell monolayer barrier properties. *Toxicol. In Vitro*, **21** (8), 1373–1381.

103 Murphy, F.A. *et al.* (2012) The mechanism of pleural inflammation by long carbon nanotubes: interaction of long fibres with macrophages stimulates them to amplify pro-inflammatory responses in mesothelial cells. *Part. Fibre Toxicol.*, **9** (1), 1–15.

104 Poland, C.A. *et al.* (2008) Carbon nanotubes introduced into the abdominal cavity of mice show asbestos-like pathogenicity in a pilot study. *Nat. Nano.*, **3** (7), 423–428.

105 Murphy, F.A. *et al.* (2011) Length-dependent retention of carbon nanotubes in the pleural space of mice initiates sustained inflammation and progressive fibrosis on the parietal pleura. *Am. J. Pathol.*, **178** (6), 2587–2600.

106 Muller, J. *et al.* (2005) Respiratory toxicity of multi-wall carbon nanotubes. *Toxicol. Appl. Pharmacol.*, **207** (3), 221–231.

107 Mercer, R.R. *et al.* (2008) Alteration of deposition pattern and pulmonary response as a result of improved dispersion of aspirated single-walled carbon nanotubes in a mouse model. *Am. J. Physiol. – Lung Cell Mol. Physiol.*, **294** (1), L87–L97.

108 Shvedova, A.A. *et al.* (2008) Inhalation vs. aspiration of single-walled carbon nanotubes in C57BL/6 mice: inflammation, fibrosis, oxidative stress, and mutagenesis. *Am. J. Physiol. – Lung Cell Mol. Physiol.*, **295** (4), L552–L565.

109 Shvedova, A.A. *et al.* (2014) Long-term effects of carbon containing engineered nanomaterials and asbestos in the lung: one year postexposure comparisons. *Am. J. Physiol. – Lung Cell Mol. Physiol.*, **306** (2), L170–L182.

110 Shvedova, A.A. *et al.* (2012) Impaired clearance and enhanced pulmonary inflammatory/fibrotic response to carbon nanotubes in myeloperoxidase-deficient mice. *PLoS One*, **7** (3), e30923.

111 Kagan, V.E. *et al.* (2010) Carbon nanotubes degraded by neutrophil myeloperoxidase induce less pulmonary inflammation. *Nat. Nano.*, **5** (5), 354–359.

112 Vlasova, I.I. *et al.* (2011) Myeloperoxidase-induced biodegradation of single-walled carbon nanotubes is mediated by hypochlorite. *Russ. J. Bioorg. Chem.*, **37** (4), 453–463.

113 Deng, X. *et al.* (2007) Translocation and fate of multi-walled carbon nanotubes *in vivo*. *Carbon*, **45** (7), 1419–1424.

114 Yang, S.-t. *et al.* (2007) Biodistribution of pristine single-walled carbon nanotubes *in vivo*. *J. Phys. Chem. C*, **111** (48), 17761–17764.

115 Wang, H. *et al.* (2004) Biodistribution of carbon single-wall carbon nanotubes in mice. *J. Nanosci. Nanotech.*, **4** (8), 1019–1024.

116 Singh, R. *et al.* (2006) Tissue biodistribution and blood clearance rates of intravenously administered carbon nanotube radiotracers. *Proc. Natl. Acad. Sci. USA*, **103** (9), 3357–3362.

117 Liu, Z. *et al.* (2008) Circulation and long-term fate of functionalized, biocompatible single-walled carbon nanotubes in mice probed by Raman spectroscopy. *Proc. Natl. Acad. Sci. USA*, **105** (5), 1410–1415.

118 Wepasnick, K.A. *et al.* (2011) Surface and structural characterization of multi-walled carbon nanotubes following different oxidative treatments. *Carbon*, **49** (1), 24–36.

119 Jain, S. *et al.* (2011) Toxicity of multiwalled carbon nanotubes with end defects critically depends on their functionalization density. *Chem. Res. Toxicol.*, **24** (11), 2028–2039.

120 Al-Jamal, K.T. *et al.* (2012) Degree of chemical functionalization of carbon nanotubes determines tissue distribution and excretion profile. *Angew. Chem. Int. Ed.*, **51** (26), 6389–6393.

121 Jokerst, J.V. *et al.* (2011) Nanoparticle PEGylation for imaging and therapy. *Nanomedicine*, **6** (4), 715–728.

122 Sacchetti, C. *et al.* (2013) Surface polyethylene glycol conformation influences the protein corona of polyethylene glycol-modified single-walled carbon nanotubes: potential implications on biological performance. *ACS Nano.*, **7** (3), 1974–1989.

123 Di, Y.P. *et al.* (2013) Dual acute proinflammatory and antifibrotic pulmonary effects of short palate, lung, and nasal epithelium clone–1 after exposure to carbon nanotubes. *Am. J. Respir. Cell Mol. Biol.*, **49** (5), 759–767.

124 Cherukuri, P. *et al.* (2006) Mammalian pharmacokinetics of carbon nanotubes using intrinsic near-infrared fluorescence. *Proc. Natl. Acad. Sci. USA*, **103** (50), 18882–18886.

125 McDevitt, M.R. *et al.* (2007) Tumor targeting with antibody-functionalized, radiolabeled carbon nanotubes. *J. Nucl. Med.*, **48** (7), 1180–1189.

126 Chakravarty, P. *et al.* (2008) Thermal ablation of tumor cells with antibody-functionalized single-walled carbon nanotubes. *Proc. Natl. Acad. Sci. USA*, **105** (25), 8697–8702.

127 Liu, Z. *et al.* (2008) Drug delivery with carbon nanotubes for *in vivo* cancer treatment. *Cancer Res.*, **68** (16), 6652–6660.

128 Barone, P.W. *et al.* (2005) Near-infrared optical sensors based on single-walled carbon nanotubes. *Nat. Mater.*, **4** (1), 86–92.

129 Murakami, T. *et al.* (2004) Drug-loaded carbon nanohorns: adsorption and release of dexamethasone *in vitro*. *Mol. Pharm.*, **1** (6), 399–405.

130 Venkatesan, N. *et al.* (2005) Liquid filled nanoparticles as a drug delivery tool for protein therapeutics. *Biomaterials*, **26** (34), 7154–7163.

131 Prato, M., Kostarelos, K., and Bianco, A. (2008) Functionalized carbon nanotubes in drug design and discovery. *Acc. Chem. Res.*, **41** (1), 60–68.

132 Muthu, M. *et al.* (2014) Nanotheranostics – application and further development of nanomedicine strategies for advanced theranostics. *Theranostics*, **4** (6), 660–677.

133 Danhier, F. *et al.* (2012) PLGA-based nanoparticles: an overview of biomedical applications. *J. Control. Release*, **161** (2), 505–522.

134 Singh, R.P. and Ramarao, P. (2013) Accumulated polymer degradation products as effector molecules in cytotoxicity of polymeric nanoparticles. *Toxicol. Sci.*, **136** (1), 131–143.

135 Nie, Y. *et al.* (2012) Investigation of PEG-PLGA-PEG nanoparticles-based multipolyplexes for IL-18 gene delivery. *J. Biomater. Appl.*, **26** (8), 893–916.

136 Mendes, L.P. *et al.* (2015) Biodegradable nanoparticles designed for drug delivery: The number of nanoparticles impacts on cytotoxicity. *Toxicol. In Vitro*, **29** (6), 1268–1274.

137 Acharya, S. and Sahoo, S.K. (2011) PLGA nanoparticles containing various anticancer agents and tumour delivery by EPR effect. *Adv. Drug. Deliv. Rev.*, **63** (3), 170–183.

138 Conde, J. *et al.* (2014) Revisiting 30 years of biofunctionalization and surface chemistry of inorganic nanoparticles for nanomedicine. *Front Chem.*, **2**, 48.

139 Grillo, R. *et al.* (2012) Poly (ε-caprolactone)nanocapsules as carrier systems for herbicides: Physico-chemical characterization and genotoxicity evaluation. *J. Hazard. Mater.*, **231–232**, 1–9.

140 Xie, J. *et al.* (2007) Controlled PEGylation of monodisperse Fe3O4 nanoparticles for reduced non-specific uptake by macrophage cells. *Adv. Mater.*, **19** (20), 3163–3166.

141 Li, S.-D. and Huang, L. (2010) Stealth nanoparticles: high density but sheddable PEG is a key for tumor targeting. *J. Control. Release*, **145** (3), 178–181.

142 Witzigmann, D. *et al.* (2015) Biocompatible polymer–peptide hybrid-based DNA nanoparticles for gene delivery. *ACS Appl. Mater. Interfaces*, **7** (19), 10446–10456.

143 Shi, J. *et al.* (2013) Effect of polyplex morphology on cellular uptake, intracellular trafficking, and transgene expression. *ACS Nano.*, **7** (12), 10612–10620.

144 Hu, C.-M.J. *et al.* (2014) Polymeric nanotherapeutics: clinical development and advances in stealth functionalization strategies. *Nanoscale*, **6** (1), 65–75.

145 Lammers, T. and Ulbrich, K. (2010) HPMA copolymers: 30 years of advances. *Adv. Drug. Deliv. Rev.*, **62** (2), 119–121.

146 Li, H. *et al.* (2013) Endoplasmic reticulum localization of poly (ω-aminohexyl methacrylamide)s conjugated with (L-)-arginines in plasmid DNA delivery. *Biomaterials*, **34** (32), 7923–7938.

147 Sun, L. *et al.* (2015) Strategies of polymeric nanoparticles for enhanced internalization in cancer therapy. *Colloid Surf. B.*, **135**, 56–72.

148 Werner, M.E. *et al.* (2013) Preclinical evaluation of genexol-PM, a nanoparticle formulation of paclitaxel, as a novel radiosensitizer for the treatment of non-small cell lung cancer. *Int. J. Radiat. Oncol. Biol. Phys.*, **86** (3), 463–468.

149 Zhang, K. *et al.* (2014) PEG–PLGA copolymers: their structure and structure-influenced drug delivery applications. *J. Control. Release*, **183**, 77–86.

150 Wang, R., Billone, P.S., and Mullett, W.M. (2013) Nanomedicine in action: an overview of cancer nanomedicine on the market and in clinical trials. *J. Nanomaterials*, **2013**, 1–1.

151 Chen, D.-B. *et al.* (2001) *In vitro* and *in vivo* study of two types of long-circulating solid lipid nanoparticles containing paclitaxel. *Chem. Pharm. Bull.*, **49** (11), 1444–1447.
152 Howard, K.A. *et al.* (2008) Chitosan/siRNA Nanoparticle-mediated TNF-[alpha] knockdown in peritoneal macrophages for anti-inflammatory treatment in a murine arthritis model. *Mol. Ther.*, **17** (1), 162–168.
153 Li, F. *et al.* (2009) Anti-tumor activity of paclitaxel-loaded chitosan nanoparticles: an *in vitro* study. *Mater. Sci. Eng. C*, **29** (8), 2392–2397.
154 Kim, J.-H. *et al.* (2008) Self-assembled glycol chitosan nanoparticles for the sustained and prolonged delivery of antiangiogenic small peptide drugs in cancer therapy. *Biomaterials*, **29** (12), 1920–1930.
155 Zhang, N. *et al.* (2010) Effective protection and controlled release of insulin by cationic β-cyclodextrin polymers from alginate/chitosan nanoparticles. *Int. J. Pharm.*, **393** (1–2), 213–219.
156 Katas, H. and Alpar, H.O. (2006) Development and characterisation of chitosan nanoparticles for siRNA delivery. *J. Control. Release*, **115** (2), 216–225.
157 Thanki, K. *et al.* (2013) Oral delivery of anticancer drugs: challenges and opportunities. *J. Control. Release*, **170** (1), 15–40.
158 Luo, C. *et al.* (2014) Emerging integrated nanohybrid drug delivery systems to facilitate the intravenous-to-oral switch in cancer chemotherapy. *J. Control. Release*, **176**, 94–103.
159 Ibekwe, V.C. *et al.* (2006) An investigation into the *in vivo* performance variability of pH responsive polymers for ileo-colonic drug delivery using gamma scintigraphy in humans. *J. Pharm. Sci.*, **95** (12), 2760–2766.
160 Jiang, L. *et al.* (2013) Thiolated chitosan-modified PLA-PCL-TPGS nanoparticles for oral chemotherapy of lung cancer. *Nanoscale Res. Lett.*, **8** (1), 1–11.
161 Bernkop-Schnürch, A., Hornof, M., and Zoidl, T. (2003) Thiolated polymers—thiomers: synthesis and *in vitro* evaluation of chitosan–2-iminothiolane conjugates. *Int. J. Pharm.*, **260** (2), 229–237.
162 Lammers, T. *et al.* (2012) Drug targeting to tumors: principles, pitfalls and (pre-) clinical progress. *J. Control. Release*, **161** (2), 175–187.
163 Garbuzenko, O.B. *et al.* (2014) Inhalation treatment of lung cancer: the influence of composition, size and shape of nanocarriers on their lung accumulation and retention. *Cancer Biol. Med.*, **11** (1), 44–55.
164 Taratula, O. *et al.* (2013) Nanostructured lipid carriers as multifunctional nanomedicine platform for pulmonary co-delivery of anticancer drugs and siRNA. *J. Control. Release*, **171** (3), 349–357.
165 Valadi, H. *et al.* (2007) Exosome-mediated transfer of mRNAs and microRNAs is a novel mechanism of genetic exchange between cells. *Nat. Cell Biol.*, **9** (6), 654–659.
166 Zhu, M. *et al.* (2012) Exosomes as extrapulmonary signaling conveyors for nanoparticle-induced systemic immune activation. *Small*, **8** (3), 404–412.
167 Zhu, M. *et al.* (2012) Nanoparticle-induced exosomes target antigen-presenting cells to initiate Th1-type immune activation. *Small*, **8** (18), 2841–2848.
168 Raposo, G. *et al.* (1996) B lymphocytes secrete antigen-presenting vesicles. *J. Exp. Med.*, **183** (3), 1161–1172.
169 Zitvogel, L. *et al.* (1998) Eradication of established murine tumors using a novel cell-free vaccine: dendritic cell derived exosomes. *Nat. Med.*, **4** (5), 594–600.
170 Andre, F. *et al.* (2002) Malignant effusions and immunogenic tumour-derived exosomes. *Lancet*, **360** (9329), 295–305.
171 Liu, C. *et al.* (2006) Murine mammary carcinoma exosomes promote tumor growth by suppression of NK cell function. *J. Immunol.*, **176** (3), 1375–1385.
172 Clayton, A. *et al.* (2008) Human tumor-derived exosomes down-modulate NKG2D expression. *J. Immunol.*, **180** (11), 7249–7258.

173 Admyre, C. *et al.* (2006) Direct exosome stimulation of peripheral humanT cells detected by ELISPOT. *Eur. J. Immunol.*, **36** (7), 1772–1781.

174 Thery, C. *et al.* (2002) Indirect activation of naive CD4+ T cells by dendritic cell-derived exosomes. *Nat. Immunol.*, **3** (12), 1156–1162.

175 Escudier, B. *et al.* (2005) Vaccination of metastatic melanoma patients with autologous dendritic cell (DC) derived-exosomes: results of thefirst phase I clinical trial. *J. Transl. Med.*, **3** (1), 1–13.

176 Morse, M.A. *et al.* (2005) A phase I study of dexosome immunotherapy in patients with advanced non-small cell lung cancer. *J. Transl. Med.*, **3** (1), 1–8.

177 Kovar, M. *et al.* (2006) Direct stimulation of T cells by membrane vesicles from antigen-presenting cells. *Proc. Natl. Acad. Sci. USA*, **103** (31), 11671–11676.

178 Tian, X. *et al.* (2012) A membrane vesicle-based dual vaccine against melanoma and Lewis lung carcinoma. *Biomaterials*, **33** (26), 6147–6154.

179 Linkov, I., Satterstrom, F.K., and Corey, L.M. (2008) Nanotoxicology and nanomedicine: making hard decisions. *Nanomed. Nanotech. Biol. Med.*, **4** (2), 167–171.

19
Translation to the Clinic: Preclinical and Clinical Pharmacology Studies of Nanoparticles – The Translational Challenge

Rachel Tyson,[1,2,3,4,5] *Leah Osae,*[1,2,3,4,5] *Andrew J. Madden,*[1] *Andrew T. Lucas,*[1,2,3,4,5] *and William C. Zamboni*[1,2,3,4,5]

[1]*University of North Carolina at Chapel Hill (UNC), Eshelman School of Pharmacy, Division of Pharmacotherapy and Experimental Therapeutics, 120 Mason Farm, Genetics Medicine Building, Chapel Hill, NC 27599-7360, USA*
[2]*University of North Carolina at Chapel Hill, Eshelman School of Pharmacy, Center for Pharmacogenomics and Individualized Therapy, 301 Pharmacy Lane, Chapel Hill, NC 27599, USA*
[3]*UNC Lineberger Comprehensive Cancer Center (LCCC), 450 West Drive, Chapel Hill, NC 27514, USA*
[4]*UNC Lineberger Comprehensive Cancer Center (LCCC), Carolina Center of Cancer Nanotechnology Excellence, 450 West Drive, Chapel Hill, NC 27514, USA*
[5]*The North Carolina Center of Innovation Network (NC COIN), North Carolina Medical Innovation Network, 2901 East Lee Street, Greensboro, NC 27401, USA*

19.1
Introduction

Major advances in carrier-mediated agents (CMAs), which include nanoparticles (NPs), nanosomes, and conjugates, have revolutionized drug delivery capabilities over the past decade. Although providing numerous advantages, such as greater solubility, duration of exposure, and delivery to the site of action over their small-molecule (SM) counterparts, there is substantial variability in systemic clearance and distribution, tumor delivery, and pharmacological effects (efficacy and toxicity) of these agents. This chapter provides an overview of factors that affect the pharmacokinetics and pharmacodynamics of CMAs in preclinical models and patients, especially in the treatment of cancer, and the translational challenges associated with these pharmacological factors.

19.2
Nanoparticle Formulations

The number of available nanoparticle-based drug systems has seen exponential growth in the past decade. In 2006 alone, nearly 130 nanotechnology-based

Pharmaceutical Nanotechnology: Innovation and Production, First Edition. Edited by Jean Cornier, Arno Kwade, Andrew Owen, and Marcel Van de Voorde.

products were estimated to be undergoing the drug development process worldwide [1]. While the number of agents used clinically is still limited, the plethora of emerging potential therapeutic agents warrant the need for detailed studies of their unique pharmacology and mechanism of actions in humans. Caron *et al.* summarize the currently available and late-stage development of chemotherapeutic CMAs in supplementary Table S1 [2]. In this chapter, we focus on factors that affect the pharmacokinetics (PK) and pharmacodynamics (PD) of anticancer CMAs in patients, and we hypothesize that many concepts presented in this chapter will be applicable to the vast field of agents to soon enter the clinic.

19.3 Pharmacokinetic Characterization

The disposition of CMAs depends upon the carrier and not on the therapeutic entity until the drug gets released [3]. The nomenclature used to describe CMA pharmacokinetics includes encapsulated (the drug within or bound to the carrier), released (active drug that gets released from the carrier), and sum total (encapsulated drug plus released drug) [4,5]. After the drug is released from its carrier, it is pharmacologically active and subject to the same routes of metabolism and clearance as the noncarrier form of the drug [5]. In theory, the PK disposition of the drug after release from the carrier should be the same as after administration of the small-molecule or standard formulations. Thus, the pharmacology and PK of CMAs are complex and comprehensive. Analytical methods must be performed in order to assess the disposition of encapsulated or released forms of the drug in plasma and tumor [6]. Considerable interpatient variability exists in the PK/PD of CMAs, and while the exact factors are unclear, it is hypothesized that the mononuclear phagocyte system (MPS) (or reticuloendothelial system) plays a key role [7].

The PK of liposomal encapsulated drug and released drug is very different, and compared with conventional small-molecule anticancer agents, the PK variability in liposomal formulations is often much greater [5,8]. Interindividual variability in drug exposure, represented by area under the concentration versus time curve (AUC), of encapsulated drug can be 20- to 100-fold. Factors with the potential to affect CMA PK include CMA-associated physical characteristics and host-associated characteristics [9]. Perhaps the greatest influence on the PK variability of CMA, however, is the MPS. Figure 19.1 illustrates the unique clearance mechanisms associated with CMA as compared with conventional small molecules [2,10].

19.4 Mononuclear Phagocyte System

Once a nanoparticle enters the bloodstream, it encounters plasma proteins and immune cells [11]. The interaction and subsequent effects of nanoparticle therapeutics on the immune system have not been fully elucidated, but at present are

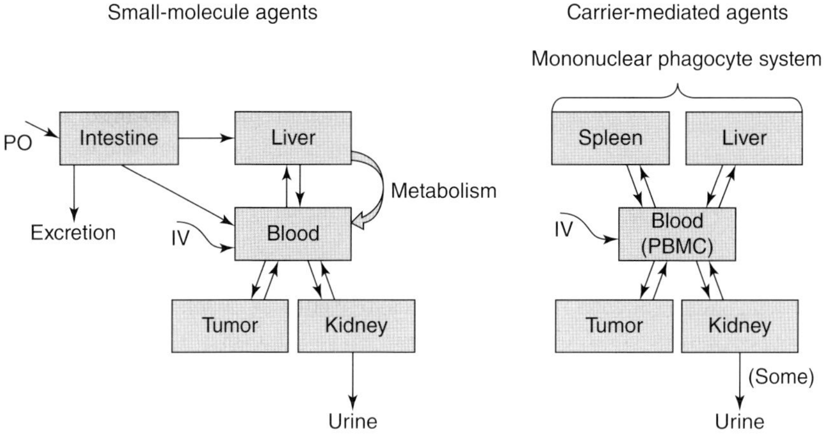

Figure 19.1 Small-molecule anticancer agents undergo a standard route of metabolism and elimination, including enterohepatic recycling and removal through the kidney. Carrier-mediated agents, which are engulfed by phagocytes, are however contained primarily in compartments such as the spleen, liver, and peripheral blood mononuclear cells. (Adapted with permission from Ref. [2]. Copyright 2012, John Wiley & Sons, Inc.)

generally placed into one of two categories: (i) responses to nanoparticles that are specifically modified to stimulate the immune system (e.g., vaccine carriers), and (ii) undesirable interactions and/or side effects [12]. In this chapter, we will focus on the latter, which may have profound clinical implications. Here we describe the MPS and the mechanisms of CMA uptake. In the latter section, we will describe how MPS function affects CMA PK/PD.

Nanoparticle uptake by immune cells can occur in circulating monocytes, platelets, leukocytes, and dendritic cells (DC) of the bloodstream [11,12]. In addition, nanoparticles can be taken up in tissues by phagocytes, such as Kupffer cells in the liver, DC in the lymph nodes, macrophages, and B cells in the spleen [11]. Figure 19.2 illustrates the interaction and clearance of CMA with these immune cells, collectively termed the MPS. Uptake mechanisms may occur through different pathways and are often facilitated by the adsorption of opsonins to the nanoparticle surface and subsequent phagocytosis [2].

Many nanoparticles have been developed for the purpose of evading rapid clearance from the bloodstream and thereby extending systemic circulation time [11]. While this allows for a greater probability of nanoparticle delivery to a target site, an increase in circulation time results in a proportional increase of duration of contact with components of the immune system [11]. CMA PK/PD varies between human patients and can be attributed to many variables, including duration of contact and overall activity of MPS components. In addition, we continue to explore the interspecies relationship of MPS function and CMA PK. We have seen a positive association between murine models and humans, which will be touched upon later in the chapter [13].

Nanoparticles can be modified to evade the MPS system that is theoretically essential for longer circulation and effective delivery to the target site. Historically,

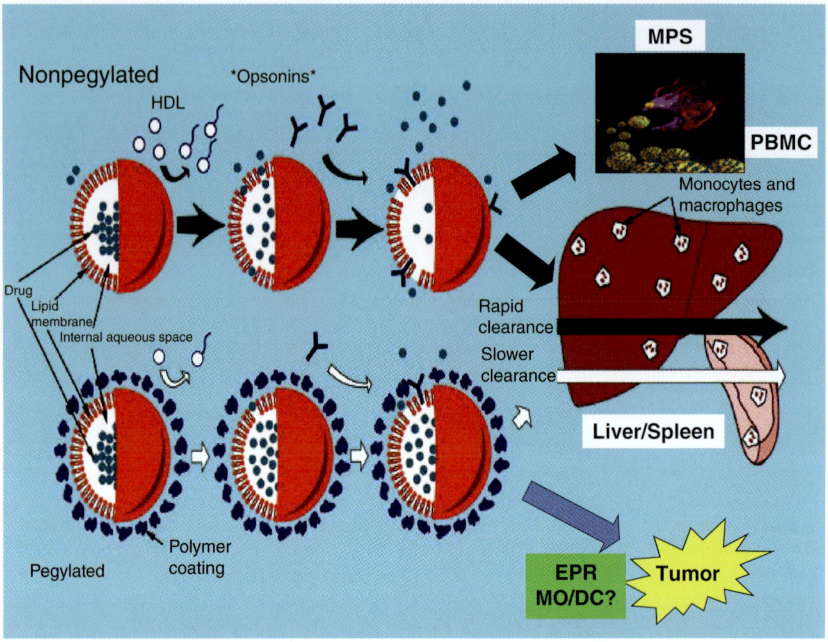

Figure 19.2 Clearance of nanoparticles and CMAs via the mononuclear phagocyte system (MPS). When nonstabilized liposomal agents were first tested, they were found to only minimally increase the circulation time of the small-molecule agent encapsulated within the carrier (rapid clearance). However, stabilization with polyethylene glycol (PEG) has helped to reduce and uptake CL of CMA by MPS (slower clearance). While the clearance of pegylated liposomes are slower than non-PEGylated liposomes, both are phagocytized by peripheral blood mononuclear cells (PBMCs), phagocytes of the liver, and spleen. Greater tumor exposure is seen after administration of PEGylated liposomes, in part due to the enhanced permeability and retention (EPR) effect and possibly the MPS in tumors. (Adapted with permission from Ref. [2]. Copyright 2012, John Wiley & Sons, Inc.)

PEG on the surfaces of CMAs has been used to evade the MPS. DPAs or discoidal polymeric nanoconstructs (a mix of lipid chains and hydrophobic and hydrophilic polymers inside a silicon template) is another method to modify nanoparticles [14]. These were injected into mice with nonorthotopic brain tumors, with promising results. The nanoconstructs were shown to have a half-life of 24 h and 20% of the dose (per gram tumor) accumulated in small malignant masses. Elements of the geometry, surface properties, and the stiffness help these particles escape the mononuclear phagocyte system.

19.5 Delivery of CMA in Tumor

While conventional drugs encounter numerous obstacles *en route* to their target, CMAs can take advantage of leaky vasculature of tumor to extravasate into tissue via the enhanced permeability and retention effect (EPR) [15,16]. Furthermore, the poor lymphatic drainage in tumors leads to accumulation of the CMA for prolonged duration, allowing them to release the drug in tumor cells over time. Passive targeting exploits the classical features of tumor biology in order to increase exposure of CMA in the tumor.

In theory, EPR has been the primary route of CMA delivery to tumors, but heterogenicity of EPR between tumor types and the inability to ensure uniform delivery to all regions of the tumor are forcing researchers to dive deeper into EPR fundamentals and the effects of tumor vasculature [17–19]. Unevenly distributed blood flow, dense microenvironment, and variations in vessel permeability play an important role in the distribution and penetration of CMAs to tumor [20]. Better and more effective CMAs that exploit EPR are needed, while also employing methods to address structural hindrances in tumor microenvironment. Jain and coworkers, well known for their efforts in the field of tumor vasculature, attribute the EPR effect to physiological contributions such as vascular pore dimensions, vascular structure, surrounding stroma, and MPS function [17]. From a preclinical perspective, there is a need for tumor models that accurately represent the types of tumors seen in patients in order to conduct informative profiling and developmental studies of CMAs [17]. It is thought that metastatic, orthotopic, and genetically engineered mouse models (GEMMs) are better options for CMA studies than flank tumor xenografts [17]. However, systematic studies of several types of CMAs in each tumor model have not been reported and are desperately needed to advance the field of CMA in the treatment of cancer. Clinically, there is a need for diagnostic aids to determine EPR activity in patients and predict responders to individual CMAs [17].

Active targeting of CMAs may further improve tumor delivery and activity by allowing the CMA to bind to specific cells in tumor using surface-attached ligands capable of recognizing and binding to cells of interest [21]. Relative to normal cells, tumor cells have certain overexpressed surface receptors or antigens that maximize the specificity of binding of targeted agents. One such strategy for the tumor-targeted drug delivery is the development of immunoliposomes. For example, anti-HER2-targeted liposomal doxorubicin was associated with higher efficacy compared to its nontargeted counterpart in a breast cancer model [22]. While antibody-mediated targeting has been the method of choice, other targeting strategies using nucleic acids, carbohydrates, peptides, aptamers, and vitamins are also being evaluated [18].

MM-302, currently in early-phase clinical studies, incorporates anti-HER2 scFv-PEG-DSPE conjugates into the outer surface of PEGylated liposomal doxorubicin (PLD). In preclinical models, MM-302 has shown superior antitumor activity to free doxorubicin and PLD in HER2 over expressing tumors with a pharmacokinetic profile similar to that of PLD. In addition, MM-302 expressed a favorable cardiosafety profile compared to free doxorubicin [23].

Several preclinical studies support extensive tumor delivery and prolonged exposure of PEGylated liposomes in tumors [5]. The development of PEGylated liposomes, which contain lipid conjugated to polyethylene glycol (PEG), was based on a theory that their incorporation into nanosomes would evade the immune system and help prolong duration of exposure [9]. This is consistent with higher antitumor activity of Doxil in preclinical models compared with doxorubicin and with clinical activity in patients with refractory ovarian cancer and Kaposi sarcoma [24]. In studies comparing the disposition of PEGylated liposomal CKD-602 (S-CKD602) and nonliposomal CKD-602 in mice bearing A375 human melanoma xenografts, S-CKD602 provided pharmacokinetic advantages in plasma, tumor, and tumor ECF at 1/30th of the dose [25].

Tumor exposure and antitumor activity of liposomal anticancer agents were found to be related to the presence of the MPS in tumors [25]. This was demonstrated in mice bearing SKOV-3 human ovarian and A375 human melanoma xenografts [25]. The ratio of S-CKD602 in tumor to plasma was 1.7-fold higher in mice bearing SKOV-3 compared with A375 [25]. The ratio of released CKD-602 to S-CKD602 in tumor was twofold higher in mice bearing SKOV-3 compared with A375 [25]. The staining of MPS cells was 4.5-fold higher in SKOV-3 compared with A375 ($p < 0.0001$) [25]. In addition, SKOV-3 was fourfold more sensitive to S-CKD602 compared with A375 [25]. The increased tumor delivery and release of CKD-602 from S-CKD602 in SKOV-3 ovarian compared with A375 melanoma xenografts was consistent with the increased staining of MPS cells in SKOV-3 suggesting that variability in the MPS in different tumors may affect the tumor disposition and activity of nanosomal anticancer agents [25].

In another study using murine colon tumor xenografts, the sum total tumor platinum exposure was fourfold higher with PEGylated liposomal cisplatin (SPI-077) compared with nonliposomal cisplatin [26]. In spite of fourfold higher exposure associated with SPI-77 compared with cisplatin, this did not translate into antitumor activity in clinical trials. Consistent with the lack of antitumor effects in patients, a subsequent study showed that SPI-077 entered tumors but did not release platinum into tumor extracellular fluid and formed significantly less Pt-DNA adducts than cisplatin [6]. Therefore, as with all drugs, it is important that the disposition of both encapsulated and released versions of liposomes be evaluated in tumors of patients for successful development of CMA. To address this, microdialysis has been used to study the relationship between unbound Pt in tumor ECF and total Pt in tumor homogenates, as well as formation of Pt–DNA adducts (a measure of the cytotoxic exposure within cancer cells) in a group of female C57BL/6 bearing B15 melanoma flank tumors [6]. Overall, CMAs have great utility for targeting many different tumor types and degree of efficacy is influenced by many variables, including MPS activity that may influence the release of drug from liposomes and other CMAs.

To tackle the issue of low tumor delivery of both CMAs and SM agents, a number of different methods have been evaluated. Jain and colleagues attempted to increase the penetration of antibodies and viral nanoparticles into tumor by pretreating tumors with collagenase [27–29]. Collagenase resulted in a two- to threefold increase in the penetration of these agents into tumor over noncollagenase-treated tumors. Similarly, pretreatment with the hormone relaxin, which induces the degradation and structural changes to collagen, has increased the delivery of antibodies and macromolecules to tumors by two- to threefold [27–30]. Pretreatment with losartan, which reduces stromal collagen and hyaluronan production and leads to increased vascular perfusion, produced only a 74% increase in 5-FU delivery to tumors compared with 5-FU alone [31]. The priming of tumors with low-dose IV administration of traditional chemotherapy drugs prior to the administration of liposomal formulations has also been evaluated to increase liposomal tumor delivery, but it only increased the delivery of these agents by approximately twofold [32]. Moreover, potential changes in MPS function and the clearance of CMAs after priming chemotherapy need to be evaluated to fully determine if these effects are related to tumor changes or inhibiting the systemic clearance of CMAs. In addition, conventional radiation therapy (RT) has been reported to only moderately (0.2- to 3-fold) enhance drug delivery to tumors and is associated with toxicities [29]. In summary, the current methods only increased the tumor delivery of CMAs from 0.5 to threefold.

Microbeam radiation therapy (MRT) is a novel radiation therapy treatment that has been shown to eradicate tumor without damaging the function of normal tissues exposed to the same high-dose radiation in animal studies [33]. MRT utilizes an array of parallel microplaner beams delivering periodically oscillating high- and low-dose regions in the treatment volume. It has been hypothesized that the changes in microvasculature induced by MRT can be used to enhance drug delivery to tumors. Thus, the effects of MRT on the tumor PK of PEGylated liposomal doxorubicin (PLD) in preclinical tumor models were evaluated [33]. Studies were performed in mice bearing T11, a syngeneic orthotopic tumor transplant model of triple-negative breast cancer. Prior to administration of PLD, mice received a single treatment of 28 Gy or 34 Gy (peak dose at skin entrance) MRT at the tumor site (treatment area is ~1 cm × 1 cm), or no radiation treatment. All groups were then administered PLD at 6 mg/kg IV × 1 at 16 h after MRT. The PK of PLD in plasma and tumor was evaluated. MRT treatment prior to PLD administration significantly improves the delivery of PLD to tumors (4–22-fold) without altering the plasma PK. In addition, higher doses of MRT resulted in a greater increase in the delivery of PLD to tumors. The improved delivery of PLD to tumors may be due to MRT's acute effects on tumor microvasculature; however, the exact mechanism needs to be further evaluated.

19.6 Methods to Target Brain Tumors

Treating primary or metastatic tumors within the central nervous system (CNS) remains extremely challenging. Numerous approaches are being explored to enhance drug delivery and anticancer efficacy, and the use of nanoparticles and CMAs provides a promising approach to enhance delivery to the brain and brain tumors. The mechanism of CMA delivery to the brain is not fully understood, but hypotheses such as nanoparticle altered distribution and longer blood circulation time may allow enhanced permeation of drugs that have the ability to cross the blood–brain barrier (BBB). In addition, brain tumors may also employ similar EPR effect as solid tumors in other parts of the body, which may be the foundation of enhanced delivery to the CNS compared to small-molecule drug [34–36]. However, the magnitude of the EPR effect in intracranial tumors is relatively weak compared to that of peripheral tumors. Explanations for this finding claim smaller pore size for solute passage in these tumor types compared with peripheral tumors [37,38]. Systematic studies evaluating these mechanisms are needed.

Anders *et al.* utilized an intracranial model of aggressive triple negative breast cancer in athymic mice to evaluate the pharmacological disposition and activity of PLD compared with small-molecule doxorubicin. Treatment with PLD resulted in approximately 1500-fold higher plasma and 20-fold higher intracranial tumor sum total doxorubicin AUC compared with small-molecule doxorubicin [39]. PLD, measured as sum total doxorubicin, was detected at 96 h in plasma and tumor, while small-molecule doxorubicin was undetectable after 24 h in plasma and tumor. Median survival of PLD-treated animals was 32 days (CI 31–38), which was significantly longer than tumor grafts exposed to phosphate-buffered saline alone (26 days [CI 25–28]; $p = 0.0012$) or mice treated with small-molecule doxorubicin (23.5 days [CI 18–28], $p = 0.0002$) [39]. Survival curves are shown in Figure 19.3. These data suggest that PLD is a treatment option for patients with intracranial metastatic breast cancer.

Researchers are taking advantage of PLD with its inherent longer half-life and better brain penetration compared to small-molecule doxorubicin by adding other structural moieties that may enhance brain tumor delivery and efficacy. Preclinical studies of PLD with a glutathione coating (2B3-101) have also shown promising results in brain cancer models. Glutathione, an endogenous tripeptide,

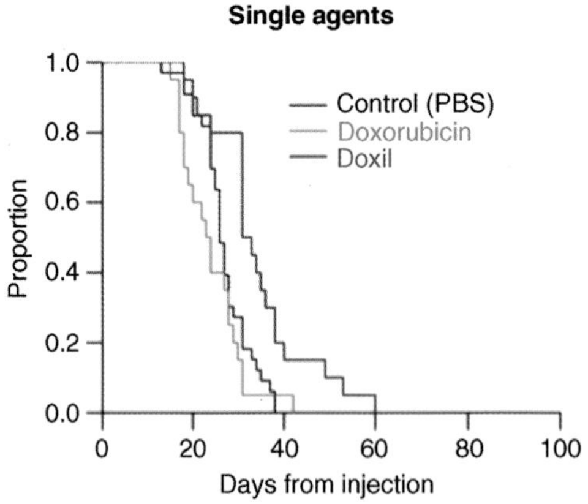

Figure 19.3 Efficacy studies in an intracranial model of breast cancer. Median survival (from times of intracranial cell line injection) of animals treated with control (PBS, black), nonliposomal doxorubicin (NonL-doxo, green) 6 mg/kg IV weekly, and PEGylated liposomal doxorubicin (PLD, blue) 6 mg/kg IV weekly in a murine model of intracranial breast cancer [39]. (Copyright 2013, Anders *et al.*).

is actively transported across the BBB. This inherent property is thought to facilitate 2B3-101 in gaining access into the brain. Mouse models treated with 2B3-101 have shown greater inhibition of brain tumor growth with significant increase in median survival time compared to PLD [40].

An alternative targeting strategy utilizing spherical nucleic acids (SNAs) nanoparticle conjugates has shown promise in targeting oncogenes within glioma tumor cells [41]. The ensuing dismantling of cancer-promoting signals is believed to cause tumor cell apoptosis. These SNAs consist of small interfering RNA (siRNA) coating a gold core. Researchers have created a prototypical SNA that has the ability to cross the BBB, where it can enter the tumor and exert its effect on a known oncogene (Bcl2L12) (56). In murine models, systemic delivery of a particular siRNA-loaded SNA (siL12-2-SNA) rapidly accumulated in xenograft brain tumor tissue, where impaired tumor growth and increased survival were noted. Ultimately, CMAs are of high therapeutic interest for targeting difficult-to-treat organs such as the brain due to its characteristic targeted approach of delivering active drug.

Another method for targeting drugs across the blood–brain barrier involves harnessing a natural process called receptor-mediated transcytosis (RMT). RMT is used by proteins in the body to cross the blood–brain barrier. The protein transferrin (Tf) uses this mechanism and can be incorporated into nanoparticles to improve brain delivery. The ability of 80 nm gold nanoparticles containing Tf to cross the blood–brain barrier was examined in a study by Clark and Davis [42]. These nanoparticles also included an acid-cleavable linkage between the Tf and nanoparticle core. After the particle crosses the barrier, acidification allows release of the nanoparticle to the brain. These modified nanoparticles were found to enter the brain of mice in larger amounts compared with a similar nanoparticle without a cleavable Tf.

Due to the fact that nanoparticles can come in all shapes and sizes, it is pertinent to study which types might be the most effective at facilitating drug delivery. In one study, two polymer nanoparticles were compared to determine their ability to cross the blood–brain barrier. While both of the preparations were able to cross, PLA-HPG-Ad (a block copolymer of polylactic acid and hyperbranched polyglycerol with adenosine on the surface) was found to have a higher brain uptake [43]. In the case of this NP, 0.8% of the injected dose found its way into the brain, compared to less than 0.5% of the other nanoparticle form.

19.7 Physical Characteristics

19.7.1 Particle Size

Many groups have demonstrated that tumor uptake of nanoparticles can depend on particle size. In one study of liposomes, particles that had a hydrodynamic diameter between 100 and 200 nm had a fourfold higher rate of uptake in tumors compared to particles less than 50 nm or greater than 300 nm [44]. These findings were replicated by Charrois and Allen, who found that liposomes ranging between 8 and 160 nm resulted in a significantly greater accumulation in tumor compared with liposomes greater than 240 nm [45]. It has been shown that particles with a hydrodynamic diameter smaller than 50 nm or greater than 300 nm have much shorter blood circulation times compared to particles with a hydrodynamic diameter between 100 and 200 nm, due to increased uptake by the MPS [44]. It is hypothesized that the shorter circulation times of particles smaller than 50 nm or greater than 300 nm do not allow the particles enough tumor exposure to take advantage of the EPR effect, leading to lower tumor accumulation [44]. However, the optimal size of nanoparticles needed to increase blood circulation time and delivery to tumors remains unknown and may be influenced by the type of carrier and tumor. As particle size can affect what accumulates in tumor, it can also influence the concentrations that can be measured in plasma as well as eventual efficacy and toxicity measures.

19.7.2 Particle Shape

Particle shape has also been studied to determine the effect on MPS particle recognition. Particle replication in nonwetting templates (PRINT) technology is a soft lithography process used to fabricate monodisperse populations of PLGA particles with high loadings of anticancer drugs [46]. The PRINT® particle fabrication technique was used to fabricate two different monodisperse shape-specific PLGA particles loaded with the chemotherapeutic docetaxel [47]. The pharmacokinetics of two cylindrical-shaped particles – one with a diameter of 80 nm and a height of 320 nm (PRINT-Doc-80 × 320), and one with a diameter of 200 nm and a height of 200 nm (PRINT-Doc-200 × 200) – were compared with small-molecule (SM) docetaxel in mice bearing SKOV-3 flank xenografts. The concentration versus time profiles for plasma, tumor, and tissues are shown in Figure 19.4. The docetaxel plasma exposure exceeded the increase by 20-fold for both particles compared to SM docetaxel. Additionally, the volume of distribution of docetaxel in PRINT formulations was ∼18-fold (PRINT-Doc-80 × 320) and ∼33-fold (PRINT- Doc-200 × 200) lower than SM docetaxel. The prolonged duration of docetaxel in plasma when dosed with PRINT formulations subsequently led to increased tumor exposure of docetaxel from 0 to 168 h. Thus, particles shaped to have a large aspect ratio may be preferred to decrease clearance by organs of the MPS.

19.7.3 Surface Modification

In an attempt to minimize opsonization and the subsequent rate of MPS uptake, the most commonly used strategy is to conjugate PEG onto the surface [48]. Sadzuka *et al.* conducted a PK study using CPT-11 loaded into bare liposomes

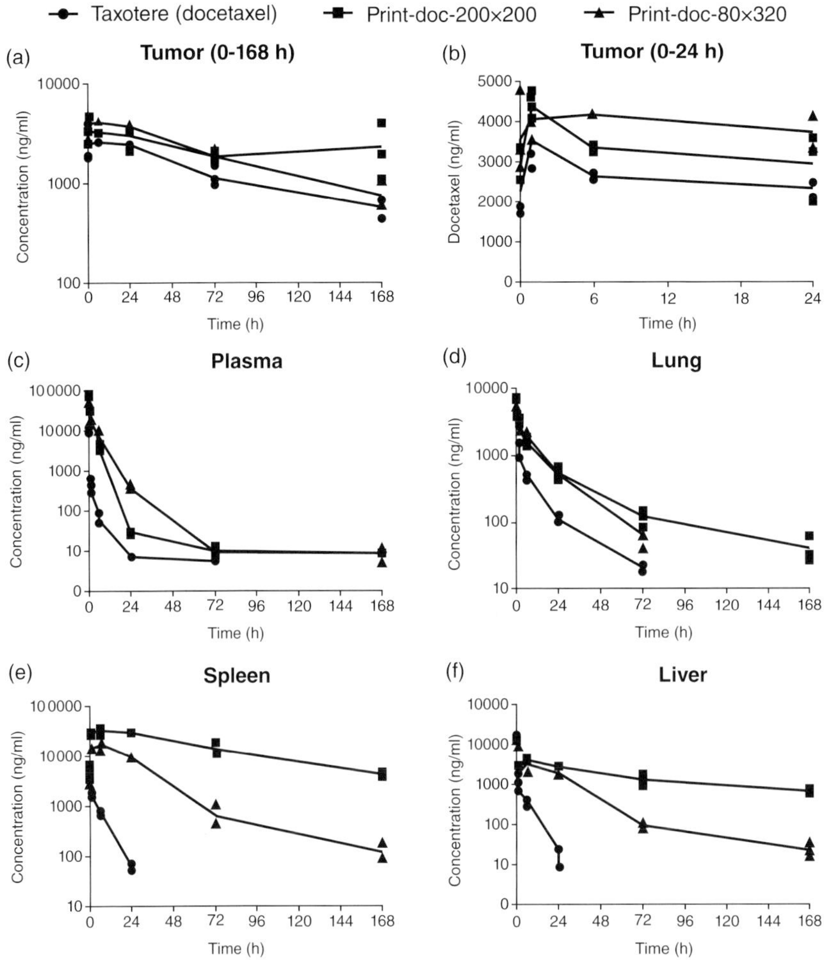

Figure 19.4 Doc concentration versus time curve for (a) tumor (0–168 h), (b) tumor (0–24 h), (c) plasma, (d) lung, (e) spleen, and (f) liver. Doc concentration values for each mouse are represented by (●) for Taxotere, (■) for PRINT-Doc-200 × 200 particles, and (▲) for PRINT-Doc-80 × 320 particles. The lines are connected by the mean value for each time point. (Adapted with permission from Ref. [47]. Copyright 2013, Elsevier Ltd.)

or PEGylated liposomes [49]. They found that the overall exposure in plasma of CPT-11 contained within a PEGylated liposome was sixfold higher than that of non-PEGylated liposomes.

19.7.4 Surface Charge

Drummond *et al.* have studied the effects of surface charge on particle clearance and found that uncharged liposomes have a lower clearance than either positively or negatively charged liposomes [50]. This is believed to be due to reduced opsonization on the uncharged liposomal surface, which leads to less MPS uptake [51]. Levchenko *et al.* conducted a study in which they prepared liposomes of 200 nm in size with different charges and studied tissue distribution over time [52]. They found that the rate of clearance from blood was significantly higher for negatively charged particles versus uncharged particles [52]. Additionally, the negative particles had a higher rate of MPS uptake in the liver compared to the uncharged particles, indicating that phagocytic cells resident to the liver preferentially take up negatively charged particles and increase the rate of clearance of particles from blood [52]. The most common surface modification, PEGylation, comes into play here, as Levchenko has shown that PEGylation can shield the negative charge on liposomes, leading to a significantly reduced rate of liver uptake and prolonged blood circulation [52].

19.7.5
Particle Dose

Chu *et al.* studied the effects of particle dose on particle clearance [53]. Docetaxel-loaded PRINT nanoparticles with identical size, shape, and surface chemistry, but with variable docetaxel loading, were created [53]. The two different formulations of nanoparticles had 9% (9%-NP) and 20% (20%- NP) docetaxel drug loading [53]. Both formulations were administered at identical docetaxel doses of 10 mg/kg that resulted in a total NP dose of 109 mg/kg in the 9%-NP group compared to only 50 mg/kg in the 20%-NP group [53]. The 9%-NP formulation that is associated with administration of a higher number of NPs was found to have a superior pharmacokinetic profile and enhanced efficacy compared to that of the 20%-NP [52]. Figure 19.5 shows the pharmacokinetic profiles of the two formulations in various tissues [53]. The 9%-NP docetaxel increased tumor docetaxel exposure and reduced liver, spleen, and lung exposure compared to that of 20%-NP docetaxel [53]. Chu *et al.* theorizes that the higher particle dose associated with the 9%-NP formulation may have saturated the MPS of the liver and spleen resulting in reduced docetaxel accumulation at those sites accounting for the increased tumor docetaxel exposure relative to the 20%-NP group [53]. While Chu *et al.* did not present any data on the MPS function or activity, there are ongoing studies to investigate the effect of particle dose on the MPS.

19.8
The Effect of MPS on CMA PK and PD

A phase I study looked at the relationship between the disposition of the CMA S-CKD602 (PEGylated liposomal CKD-602, a camptothecin analog) and changes in monocytes and absolute neutrophil count (ANC) [54]. The control of this study was changes in monocytes and ANC after patients with refractory solid tumors received nonliposomal CKD-602 [54]. The percent decrease in ANC and

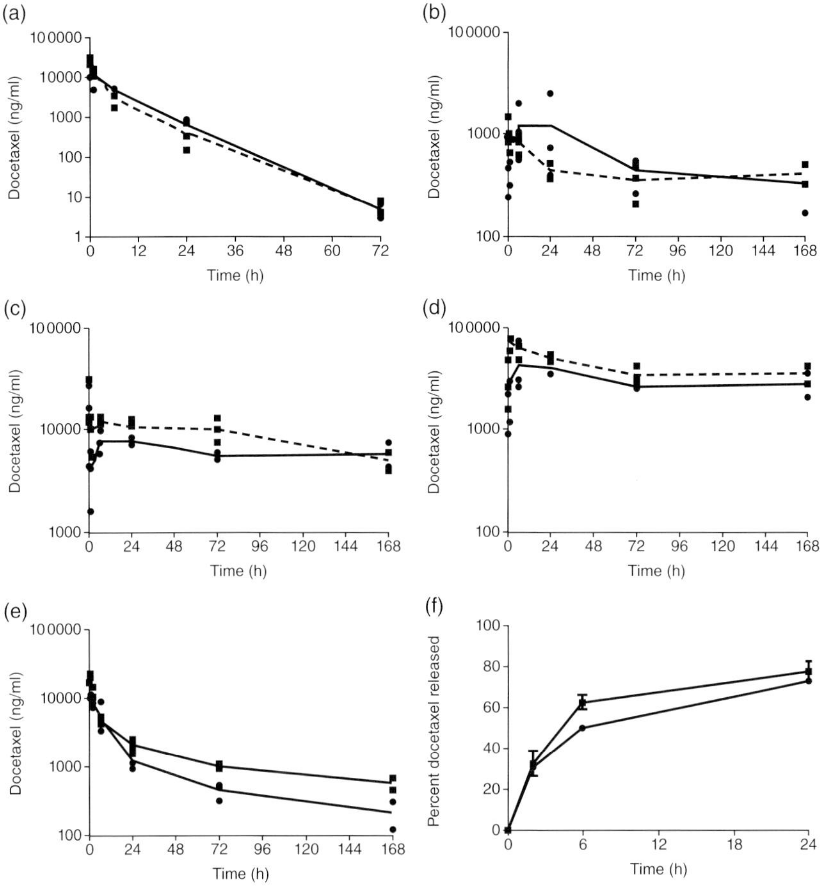

Figure 19.5 Pharmacokinetics of docetaxel with different loadings in PRINT PLGA nanoparticles. Pharmacokinetic profiles of (a) plasma, (b) tumor, (c) liver, (d) spleen, and (e) lung. (f) *In vitro* release kinetics of 9%-NP (●) and 20%-NP (■). Each replicate is shown and the lines are connected by the mean of three replicates. (Adapted with permission from Ref. [53]. Copyright 2013, Elsevier Ltd.)

monocytes from baseline to nadir from the blood of all patients administered S-CKD602 on cycle 1 was measured. The mean ± SD percent decrease in ANC and monocytes at nadir was 42 ± 30 and 58 ± 34%, respectively ($p = 0.001$). The ratio of percent decrease in monocytes to ANC at the nadir was 2.1 ± 2.0. The percent decrease in ANC and monocytes at nadir in the blood of patients was also assessed after administration of nonliposomal CKD-602. After administration, the percent decrease in ANC and monocytes were 86 ± 11 and 87 ± 12%, respectively ($p > 0.05$). The ratio of percent decrease in monocytes to ANC was 1.0 ± 0.2. The results suggest that monocytes are more sensitive to S-CKD602 compared with neutrophils. The increased sensitivity also appears to be related to the liposomal formulation and not the released drug from the liposome or the small-molecule formulation.

PEG-modified liposomal doxorubicin, or PEGL-DOX, is used to treat recurrent ovarian cancer [55]. This treatment is effective and does not cause many side effects, but can result in hand-foot syndrome (HFS), also referred to as palmar-plantar erythrodysesthesia (PPE). When severe, this skin-specific reaction can make it difficult to continue optimal treatment. In a comparison study between DOX and PEGL-DOX, it was found that only PEGL-DOX caused HFS. An explanation for this difference is due to extravasation following long-term circulation of the PEGL-DOX in the body. The study also noted the presence of reactive oxygen species (ROS) that resulted from DOX/copper ions interacting in the skin. ROS causes a cascade of events that stimulate chemokines, leading to an inflammatory state. Thus, the occurrence of PPE may be associated with MPS-related factors.

As already stated, the mechanism for the PPE toxicity associated with PLD is unknown. In a study analyzing blood monocyte subpopulations (classical, nonclassical, and intermediate), it was hypothesized that monocytes involved in eliminating PLD are related to PLD's toxicity. Classical (CD 14++ CD16-), nonclassical (CD14+ CD16++), and intermediate (CD14++ CD16+) monocyte subpopulations were compared between PPE patients and healthy patients (Figure 19.6) [56]. No direct relation between total monocyte count and the occurrence of PPE was found [57]. However, the monocyte populations changed from classical to nonclassical suggesting that PLD does change the phenotype of monocytes, which is consistent with studies presented earlier.

Some of the significant variability in the pharmacokinetic dispositions of CMA versus small molecules were found to be related to linear and nonlinear clearance of S-CKD602 in patients [58]. In the previously mentioned study, despite being treated with the same dose of 1.7 mg/m^2, some patients were found to have linear clearance, while the majority portrayed nonlinear clearance [58]. Those with linear clearance had a plasma concentration versus time profile of CKD-602 with a distribution phase and an elimination phase [58]. For patients with nonlinear clearance, the plasma concentration versus time profile of CKD-602 yielded little change from 0 to 24 h [58]. The incidence of linear or nonlinear clearance was found to be associated with the dose of S-CKD602 administered [58]. At doses from 0.1 to 1.1 mg/m^2, the S-CKD602 sum total and encapsulated CKD-602 plasma concentrations were best described using a model with linear clearance in all the patients ($n = 33$) [58]. At doses of 1.7–2.5 mg/m^2, the S-CKD602 sum total and encapsulated CKD-602 plasma concentrations were best described using a model with linear ($n = 2$) and nonlinear ($n = 10$) clearances [58]. The observation of nonlinear PK at higher doses of CMA coincides with the hypothesis of MPS uptake in particle clearance and its subsequent saturation. However, there was significant interpatient variability in clearance with patients exhibiting linear and nonlinear clearance at the same dose.

The PhenoGLO–high-throughput screening platform (HTSP) is an *ex vivo* flow cytometry-based system used to measure the clearance of nanoparticles by

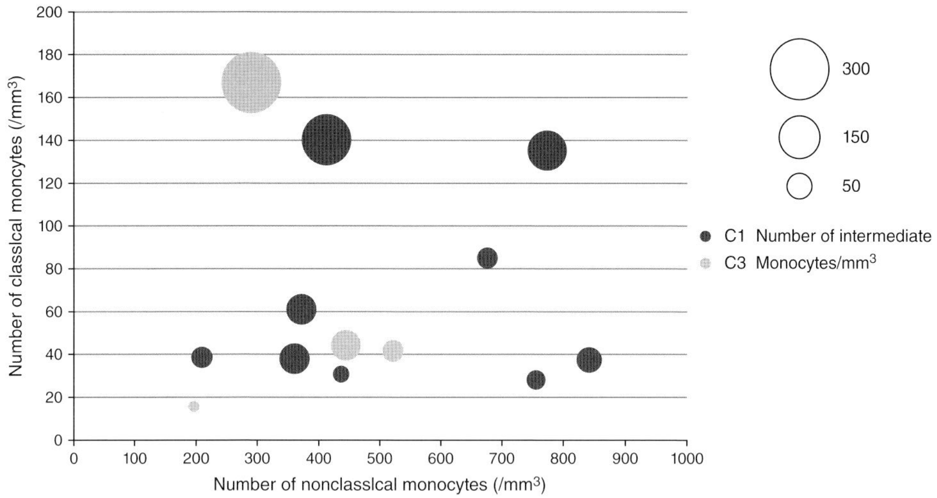

Figure 19.6 Distribution of monocyte subpopulations in nine patients receiving PLD on cycle 1 (C1) and cycle 3 (C3). Nine patients had the analysis at C1 and four patients at C3. (Adapted with permission from Ref. [56]. Copyright 2015, Springer, Berlin.)

the MPS and bidirectional interaction between the MPS and nanoparticles and conjugates [17]. Monocyte and dendritic cell (DC) function, as assessed by phagocytosis and oxidative burst, can predict the PK of PEGylated liposomal NPs in several species as well as in patients [13]. Caron *et al.* measured MO/DC phagocytosis and reactive oxygen species production in mice, rats, dogs, and patients with refractory solid tumors that had been administered a PEGylated liposomal drug formulations [13]. Preclinical pharmacokinetic studies of PLD, CKD-602 (S-CKD602), and cisplatin (SPI-077) were performed at the maximum tolerated dose [13]. Monocyte/DC function was also evaluated in patients with recurrent epithelial ovarian cancer (EOC) administered PLD [13]. Figure 19.7 shows that across species, a positive association was observed between monocyte/DC function and clearance of all three PEGylated liposomes. In patients with EOC, associations also were observed between PLD clearance and phagocytosis ($R^2 = 0.43$, $p = 0.04$) and ROS production ($R^2 = 0.61$, $p = 0.008$) in blood monocytes/DC (Figure 19.8) [13]. These findings suggest that probes of MPS function may help predict PEGylated liposome clearance across species, PLD clearance in patients with EOC, and perhaps utilized to find the correct dose of PLD and other CMAs in the future [13].

19.9 Age

PK studies of Doxil administered in three phase I and II studies in patients with solid tumors and in patients with AIDS-related Kaposi's sarcoma were performed.

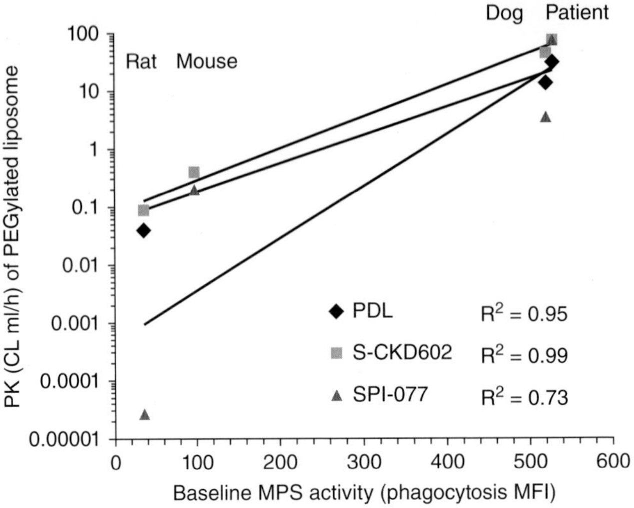

Figure 19.7 Relationship between phagocytosis in MO/DC from blood and CL of PEGylated liposomal agents in mice, rats, dogs, and patients. The mean values for three species are represented by individual symbols, with (◆) as PLD, (■) as S-CKD602, and (▲) as SPI-077. The species data are in vertical columns from left to right: rats, mice, dogs, and patients. The best fit line for each group is represented by the solid lines. Across species, a positive association was observed between cell function and CL of PEGylated liposomes. (Adapted with permission from Ref. [13]. Copyright 2013, The American Society for Pharmacology and Experimental Therapeutics.)

The mean ± SD clearance of sum total Doxil in patients <60 and ≥60 years old were 54.6 ± 28.5 and 23.3 ± 10.8 ml/(h · m^2), respectively ($p < 0.0001$) [59]. A more recent study focusing on the effect of age on doxorubicin PK and toxicity after administration of PLD was published earlier this year [60]. A total of 35 patients (≥70 years old) were enrolled in the study. The mean $t_{1/2}$ of the first three cycles of PLD in patients >77 versus ≤77 years old was 99 h versus 72 h ($p = 0.02$). A more profound 42% increase in mean $t_{1/2}$ was seen when comparing octogenarians with patients in their 70s, ($p = 0.005$) [60].

Age-related effects on PD of CMAs have also been reported. The relationship between neutropenia and monocytopenia after administration of S-CKD602 was tested by evaluating the percent decrease and rate of decrease of ANC and monocytes in patients <60 and ≥60 years of age [58]. Based on overall exposure to encapsulated S-CKD602, it appears that there is a greater reduction in monocytes at the nadir in patients <60 years of age versus patients ≥60 years of age [58]. This study concluded that monocytes are more sensitive than neutrophils to S-CKD602, increased sensitivity is related to the encapsulated liposomal formulation of CKD-602, and that age impacts this interaction [58]. This is consistent with the age-related effects on the CL of PEGylated liposomes.

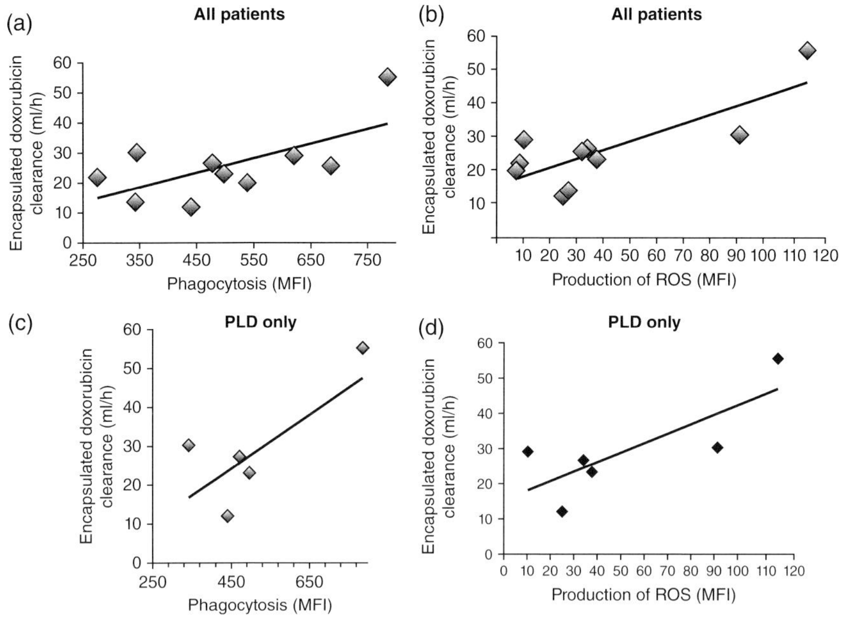

Figure 19.8 Relationship between MO/DC function and encapsulated doxorubicin CL in patients presented in a linear regression model. Measuring phagocytosis and production of ROS of MO/DC from patient blood samples at baseline (prior to the start of chemotherapy) was used as a phenotypic probe of MPS function and encapsulated doxorubicin CL. Each (♦) represents an individual patient, and the solid line is the regression line. (a) Phagocytic activity (MFI) is significantly correlated with CL of encapsulated doxorubicin in 10 patients receiving PLD alone or PLD + carboplatin ($R^2 = 0.43$, $p = 0.04$). (b) Production of reactive oxygen species: MFI is significantly correlated with CL of encapsulated doxorubicin in 10 patients receiving PLD alone or PLD + carboplatin ($R^2 = 0.61$, $p = 0.008$). (c) Phagocytic activity: MFI is significantly correlated with CL of encapsulated doxorubicin in six patients receiving PLD alone ($R^2 = 0.57$, $p = 0.03$). (d) Production of reactive oxygen species: MFI is significantly correlated with CL of encapsulated doxorubicin in six patients receiving PLD alone ($R^2 = 0.61$, $p = 0.001$). (Adapted with permission from Ref. [13]. Copyright 2013, The American Society for Pharmacology and Experimental Therapeutics.)

Age has also been reported to be associated with the toxicity and efficacy of CMA. Figure 19.9 from Gusella *et al.* shows the relationship between age, PLD half-life, and palmar-plantar erythrodysesthesia, a hallmark side effect of PLD. Both increasing age and PLD plasma half-life correlated with PPE severity [60]. In a multicenter phase II trial of elderly patients ($n = 60$) with metastatic breast cancer who were treated with Doxil, severe nonhematological toxicities were correlated to patient age >80 years old [61]. In terms of efficacy, an increase in age was found to be inversely proportional to progression free survival; however, no correlation between age and overall survival was found [61]. Alterations in

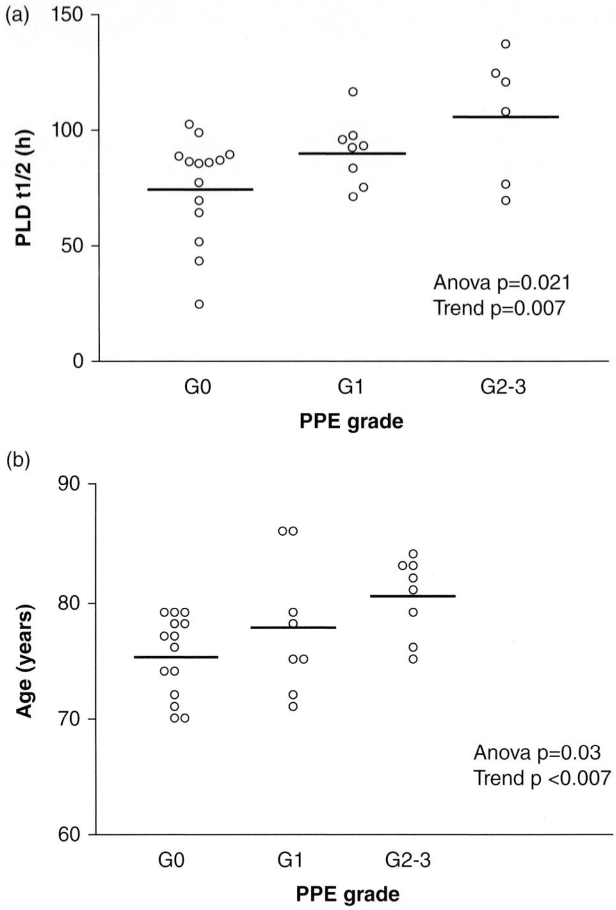

Figure 19.9 HFS (also called PPE) in association with PLD $t_{1/2}$ (a) and age (b). Longer PLD $t_{1/2}$ and advanced age were associated with an overall greater severity PPE grade. (Adapted with permission from Ref. [60]. Copyright 2014, Springer, Berlin.)

the PK and PD of CMA may involve age-related decline in immune system functioning, specifically the association of aging with the function of monocytes [62]. In theory, there is a loss of MPS activity or function in elderly patients that decreases the clearance of CMA by MPS and leads to increased drug exposures and toxicity in elderly patients.

19.10 Gender

Gender was also found to be one of the many factors contributing to the PK/PD variability of CMAs. The effect of gender on clearance of Doxil ($n = 70$), IHL-305

($n = 39$), and S-CKD602 ($n = 45$) was evaluated in PK studies conducted as part of phase I and II studies [63]. Female patients had a 2.4-fold lower overall clearance of Doxil ($p < 0.001$), a 1.4-fold lower overall clearance of IHL-305, and a 1.3-fold lower overall clearance of S-CKD602 compared with male patients [63]. In addition, an evaluation of the plasma PK disposition of TLI (liposomal topotecan) and S-CKD602 in male and female rats found the clearance of TLI and S-CKD602 to be 1.2- and 1.4-fold ($p = 0.009$) lower in female rats compared with male rats, respectively [64]. The basis for the differences in the PK and PD of CMA associated with gender is unclear with some ideas suggesting differences attributed to sex hormones on immune cell function [63,64].

19.11
Tissue and Organ Effects

19.11.1
Body Habitus

Defined as the physical characteristics of an individual leading to a body type of underweight, normal weight, or overweight, body habitus has been suggested to play an important role in PK of drugs cleared by the MPS [58,59]. Common terms used to describe an individual's body habitus include body mass index (BMI) and body surface area (BSA).

PK studies of Doxil were conducted as part of three phase I and II studies in patients with solid tumors (34 patients) and in patients with AIDS-related Kaposi's sarcoma (36 patients) [58]. BSA and BMI were evaluated as potential factors that affect the clearance of Doxil [59]. The linear regression coefficient between BSA and Doxil clearance on cycle 1 was $R^2 = 0.25$. BSA contributed to a relative reduction in variability of clearance by 8.6% [59]. There was no significant relationship found between Doxil clearance on cycle 1 and body composition as measured by actual body weight/ideal body weight (ABW/IBW) or BMI ($R^2 = 0.22$ and 0.13, respectively) [59]. However, it was reported that patients with a lean body composition (ABW/IBW <1.35) had a higher plasma exposure of S-CKD602 compared with patients with an ABW/IBW $\geq$1.35 ($p = 0.02$), perhaps due to a smaller volume of distribution [58]. While there was no relationship found between body composition and Doxil clearance in this study, this could be due to a lower number of patients enrolled [59]. Additional data collection through CMA clinical pharmacology studies is warranted in order to further explore the potential relationship between body composition and nanoparticle clearance.

19.11.2
Presence of Liver Tumors

In a phase I pharmacokinetic study evaluating encapsulated and released CKD-602, 45 patients were enrolled, of which 26 individuals had tumor(s) of all types in their liver [65]. Linear and nonlinear pharmacokinetic models were constructed for encapsulated CKD-602, and it was determined that liver tumor was a significant covariate for maximum velocity. Including liver tumor as a covariate in the model decreased the variation in V_{max} by 29%, meaning that liver tumors (primary or metastases) were outliers from the general population and influenced CMA PK [65]. The interpatient variability in S-CKD602 pharmacokinetic disposition could possibly be explained by the presence of metastatic liver tumors, as the V_{max} of patients with these tumors is 1.5-fold higher than those patients without liver tumors [65]. These data suggest that patients with liver tumor may have 35% lower plasma exposure of encapsulated CKD-602, leaving them at risk for having a lower response potential. This finding is interesting as, historically, most studies show a decrease in clearance of small-molecule drugs when patients have tumors in the liver [66,67].

19.12 Drug–Drug Interactions

Drug–drug interactions have been reported to influence the PK and PD of CMAs. In a drug interaction study, the PK of Doxil when given as a single agent and in combination with a taxane, either paclitaxel ($n = 10$) or docetaxel ($n = 9$), was evaluated. Both paclitaxel and docetaxel increased the Doxil AUC ($p = 0.002$ and 0.039, respectively) and decreased the clearance of Doxil ($p = 0.013$ and 0.16, respectively). Administering paclitaxel produced a more significant increase in systemic exposure of Doxil than coadministration with docetaxel. These findings may explain a high incidence of toxicity observed at relatively low doses of Doxil when coadministered with paclitaxel compared with docetaxel [68]. In addition, a phase I study of patients with solid tumors ($n = 26$) showed that treatment with cisplatin followed by Doxil increased the clearance of Doxil compared to patients receiving single-agent Doxil. A possible mechanism for this accelerated clearance of Doxil is transient macrophage activation induced by cisplatin [69].

In a phase I study of factors influencing the interpatient variability in the pharmacokinetic disposition of S-CKD602, the effect of prior chemotherapy on the pharmacokinetic disposition of S-CKD602 was evaluated [58]. Patients with advanced malignancies received S-CKD602 IV every 3 weeks. Patients who received prior therapy with Doxil ($n = 5$) had a 2.2-fold higher exposure of sum total AUC/dose S-CKD602 compared with patients who did not receive prior Doxil ($n = 39$) ($p = 0.045$) [58]. In addition, the encapsulated AUC/dose of S-CKD602 in patients previously treated with Doxil ($n = 5$) was 1.8-fold higher compared with patients who did not receive Doxil ($n = 34$) ($p = 0.11$). However, prior Doxil therapy did not alter the disposition of released CKD-602 [58]. There was no relationship found between the disposition of S-CKD602 and the number of PLD cycles or the time interval between stopping PLD and starting S-CKD602 [58]. It is unclear if changes in S-CKD602 PK were related to Doxil or patient-related factors as all patients who received Doxil were patients with refractory ovarian cancer already exposed to chemotherapy.

Bevacizumab is a recombinant humanized monoclonal VEGF-A antibody that inhibits the binding of human VEGF-A to its receptors. Combination treatment of locally recurrent or metastatic breast cancer patients ($n = 39$) with bevacizumab at 10 mg/kg IV and Doxil at 20 mg/m^2 IV every 2 weeks resulted in the premature discontinuation of a single-arm phase II trial due to higher than anticipated toxicity [70]. The most significant toxicity noted was grade 3 PPE that occurred in an unusually high proportion of patients (41%), suggesting an additive toxic effect of combined bevacizumab and Doxil treatment [70]. Possible suggested mechanisms of this synergistic toxicity include (i) direct pharmacological interaction between Doxil and bevacizumab;(ii) effects of bevacizumab on the vasculature of soles, palms, and possibly the oral mucosa, resulting in increased accumulation of Doxil in these areas; and (iii) bevacizumab impairing wound healing of dermal and mucosal injuries [70].

Drug efflux pumps are capable of transporting foreign substances and drugs out of cells. Drug efflux proteins in the cellular membrane remove drugs at the site of action upon drug delivery to tumors. The most commonly studied drug efflux pump is Pgp (P-glycoprotein), a cell membrane ATP-binding cassette (ABC) transporter protein encoded by the *MDR1* gene [71]. High expression of drug efflux pumps within cells or tissues may confer drug resistance to many diseases and cancers treated with drugs that are susceptible to efflux [72]. Pgp inhibitors can be coupled with drugs in order to enhance drug efficacy in patients. For example, preclinical and clinical trials show that the taxane chemotherapeutic docetaxel can be used concurrently with Pgp inhibitors such as cyclosporine A, valspodar, and elacridar in order to enhance drug delivery to tumors [73]. Cancer stem cells tend to overexpress drug efflux proteins, which can lead to drug resistance. Nanomedicines have been used to evade efflux transporters via several approaches, such as delivering therapeutic agents that affect self-renewing embryonic signaling pathways in cancer stem cells, by administering drug efflux protein inhibitors, or by using combinations of chemotherapies with amphiphilic Pluronic block copolymers [74]. In addition, the constituents of the nanoparticle carrier may have direct effects on blocking Pgp efflux [74].

19.13 Prior Treatment

In addition to the high interpatient variability in the PK of NPs, there may also be high intrapatient variability in PK of NPs. Gabizon *et al.* reported that the clearance of sum total PLD decreased by approximately 25–50% from

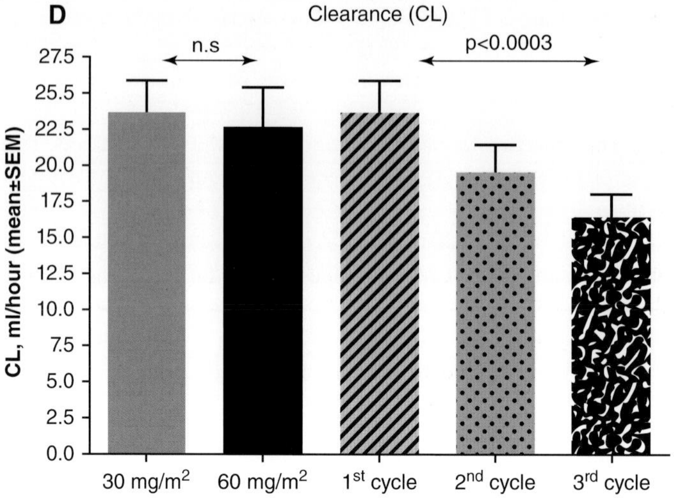

Figure 19.10 Clearance of PLD post-chemotherapy cycle in human subjects. Bars represent mean values and SEM (standard error of the mean) of clearance of PLD by dose and cycle. *P* values shown were calculated by repeated measures of ANOVA. (Adapted with permission from Ref. [75]. Copyright 2008, Springer, Berlin.)

cycle 1 to 3 in patients with ovarian cancer (Figure 19.10) [75]. La-Beck *et al.* reported that this reduction in clearance of Doxil from cycle 1 to cycle 3 was associated with a reduction in precycle monocyte count [59]. These studies suggest that there is a reduction in the clearance of liposomes over time that is associated with a reduction in MPS function. Thus, dose reductions may be needed in subsequent cycles to minimize the risk of toxicity [75]. However, how the reductions in the dose of PLD should be performed in each patient is unclear due to high inter- and intrapatient variability in changes in MPS function. By phenotypically probing patient MPS function prior to administering each cycle of PLD is of interest to guide patient-specific dosing [13]. Studies are ongoing to evaluate the use of phenotypic probes of MPS as a method to individualize the dose of PLD.

19.14 Translational Challenges

A breadth of studies have begun to emphasize the importance of preclinical animal models in understanding and evaluating the interaction between CMAs and the immune system, including the MPS, which ultimately influences CMA PK (clearance and distribution) and PD (efficacy and toxicity). It is fundamental to study representative preclinical tumor models that recapitulate patients with tumors (xenografts versus GEMM) and evaluate the interplay between CMAs and the immune system, including the MPS, chemokines, hormones, and other immune modulators. It will be essential to take into account the tumor types and the tumor microenvironment, including phenotyping of the MPS and mediators (e.g., chemokines), when evaluating CMAs for cancer therapy and translating into humans from preclinical models.

Most current data on PK and PD of CMAs were related to liposome/PEGylated liposomes due to the historical use of liposomes; thus, there is a need for additional data on factors and other CMA subtypes and/or formulations. Future studies also need to be performed to determine if similar relationships between chemokines and other immune modulators exist for these other CMA formulations. However, future studies could be complicated by the fact that certain GEMM models may not yet exist, underlying the importance of beginning to characterize and understand the unique signaling occurring within individual xenograft models and its potential effects on PK disposition. Finally, further study is required to evaluate whether the clearance of CMAs can be scaled across species using other measurements of the MPS or other factors to better predict efficacy and toxicity.

19.15 Future Perspectives on PK and PD

Due to the unique and variable clearance mechanisms of CMAs, it is important to create, validate, and utilize assays and models that represent EPR effect and MPS function and use them to evaluate factors that alter PK and PD of CMAs during all phases of development. There are many properties that make CMAs unique from the active small-molecule drug that is contained within the nanocarrier. These differences lead to significant variability in the PK and PD of CMAs. It has been shown that physical properties, the MPS, presence of tumors in the liver, EPR effect, drug–drug interactions, age, gender, body habitus, and prior treatment all contribute in varying degrees to the PK disposition and PD endpoints of CMAs in preclinical models and in patients. However, these factors do not fully explain all of the PK/PD variability of NPs/CMAs and thus the development of phenotypic probes of the MPS that account for all encompassing factors may be a more appropriate approach to predicting the PK/PD of NP in animal models and patients (Figure 19.11). These probes could also be used to individualize the dose of NPs throughout therapy, as there is high inter- and intrapatient variability in MPS function and NP PK. Studies in animal models and patients using phenotypic probes of MPS function to predict the clearance of PEGylated liposomal agents support this plan [13]. Additional areas of research that can aid in our understanding of how these agents are handled and how we may predict their actions in patients include more sensitive and accurate analytical PK methods, pharmacogenomics, and identification of the optimal preclinical models.

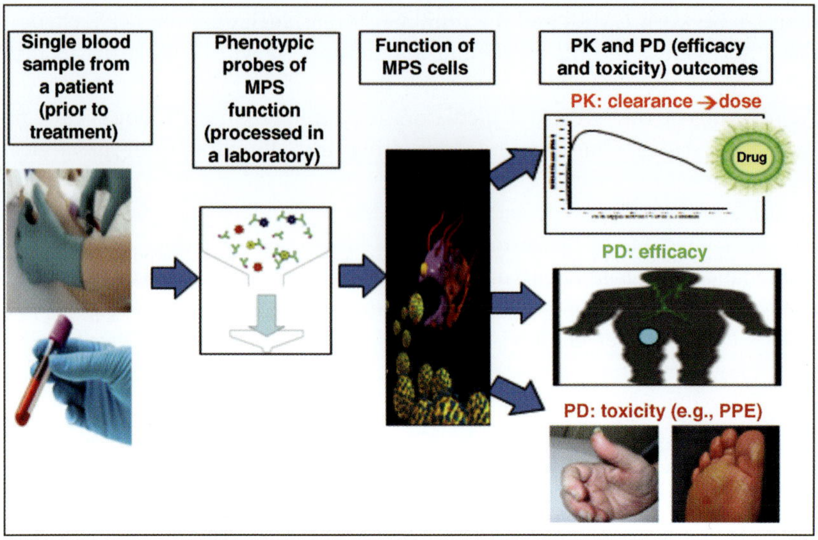

Figure 19.11 Summary of the process to use a phenotypic probe of MPS function in blood to measure MPS function in patients who would predict NP PK, efficacy and, toxicity. This type of probe could be used as a test that could retrospectively be used to explain patients with highly variable PK and PD. This type of probe could also be used as a method to individualize the dose of NPs as needed [13].

References

1 Ge, Y., Tiwari, A., and Li, S. (2011) Nanomedicine: bridging the gap between nanotechnology and medicine. *Adv. Mater. Lett.*, **2** (1), 1–2.

2 Caron, W.P., Song, G., Kumar, P., Rawal, S., and Zamboni, W.C. (2012) Interpatient pharmacokinetic and pharmacodynamic variability of carrier-mediated anticancer agents. *Clin. Pharmacol. Ther.*, **91** (5), 802–812.

3 Laginha, K., Mumbengegwi, D., and Allen, T. (2005) Liposomes targeted via two different antibodies: assay, B-cell binding and cytotoxicity. *Biochim. Biophys. Acta*, **1711** (1), 25–32.

4 Yurkovetskiy, A.V., Hiller, A., Syed, S. *et al.* (2004) Synthesis of a macromolecular camptothecin conjugate with dual phase drug release. *Mol. Pharm.*, **1** (5), 375–382.

5 Zamboni, W.C. (2005) Liposomal, nanoparticle, and conjugated formulations of anticancer agents. *Clin. Cancer Res.*, **11** (23), 8230–8234.

6 Zamboni, W.C., Gervais, A.C., Egorin, M.J. *et al.* (2004) Systemic and tumor disposition of platinum after administration of cisplatin or STEALTH liposomal–cisplatin formulations (SPI-077 and SPI-077 B103) in a preclinical tumor model of melanoma. *Cancer Chemother. Pharmacol.*, **53** (4), 329–336.

7 Laverman, P., Boerman, O.C., Oyen, W.J.G., Corstens, F.H.M., and Storm, G. (2001) *In vivo* applications of PEG liposomes: unexpected observations. *Crit. Rev. Ther. Drug Carrier Syst.*, **18** (6), 551–566.

8 Schell, R.F., Sidone, B.J., Caron, W.P. *et al.* (2014) Meta-analysis of inter-patient pharmacokinetic variability of liposomal and non-liposomal anticancer agents. *Nanomedicine*, **10** (1), 109–117.

9 Zamboni, W.C. (2008) Concept and clinical evaluation of carrier-mediated anticancer agents. *Oncologist*, **13** (3), 248–260.

10 Hume, D.A., Ross, I.L., Himes, S.R., Sasmono, R.T., Wells, C.A., and Ravasi, T. (2002) The mononuclear phagocyte system revisited. *J. Leukoc. Biol.*, **72** (4), 621–627.

11 Dobrovolskaia, M.A., Aggarwal, P., Hall, J.B., and McNeil, S.E. (2008) Preclinical studies to understand nanoparticle interaction with the immune system and its potential effects on nanoparticle biodistribution. *Mol. Pharm.*, **5** (4), 487–495.

12 Dobrovolskaia, M.A. and McNeil, S.E. (2007) Immunological properties of engineered nanomaterials. *Nat. Nanotechnol.*, **2** (8), 469–478.

13 Caron, W.P., Lay, J.C., Fong, A.M. *et al.* (2013) Translational studies of phenotypic probes for the mononuclear phagocyte system and liposomal pharmacology. *J. Pharmacol. Exp. Ther.*, **347** (3), 599–606.

14 Key, J., Palange, A.L., Gentile, F., Ayral, S., Stigliano, C., Di Mascolo, D., De Rosa, E., Cho, M., Lee, Y., Singh, J., and Decuzzi, P. (2015) Soft discoidal polymeric nanoconstructs resist macrophage uptake and enhance vascular targeting in tumors. *ACS Nano*, **9** (12), 11628–11641.

15 Alonso, M.J. (2004) Nanomedicines for overcoming biological barriers. *Biomed. Pharmacother.*, **58** (3), 168–172.

16 Matsumura, Y. and Maeda, H. (1986) A new concept for macromolecular therapeutics in cancer chemotherapy: mechanism of tumoritropic accumulation of proteins and the antitumor agent smancs. *Cancer Res.*, **46** (12 Pt 1), 6387–6392.

17 Prabhakar, U., Maeda, H., Jain, R.K. *et al.* (2013) Challenges and key considerations of the enhanced permeability and retention effect for nanomedicine drug delivery in oncology. *Cancer Res.*, **73** (8), 2412–2417.

18 Peer, D., Karp, J.M., Hong, S., Farokhzad, O.C., Margalit, R., and Langer, R. (2007) Nanocarriers as an emerging platform for cancer therapy. *Nat. Nanotechnol.*, **2** (12), 751–760.

19 Stylianopoulos, T. and Jain, R.K. (2013) Combining two strategies to improve perfusion and drug delivery in solid tumors. *Proc. Natl. Acad. Sci. USA*, **110** (46), 18632–18637.

20 Chauhan, V.P. and Jain, R.K. (2013) Strategies for advancing cancer nanomedicine. *Nat. Mater.*, **12** (11), 958–962.

21 Torchilin, V.P. (2005) Recent advances with liposomes as pharmaceutical carriers. *Nat. Rev. Drug Discov.*, **4** (2), 145–160.

22 Park, J.W., Hong, K., Kirpotin, D.B. *et al.* (2002) Anti-HER2 immunoliposomes: enhanced efficacy attributable to targeted delivery. *Clin. Cancer Res.*, **8** (4), 1172–1181.

23 Wickham, T., Reynolds, J., Drummond, D. *et al.* (2010) Preclinical safety and activity of MM-302, a HER2-targeted liposomal doxorubicin designed to have an improved safety and efficacy profile over approved anthracyclines. *Merrimack Pharm.* doi: 10.1158/0008-5472.SABCS10-P3-14-09.

24 Vaage, J., Barbera-Guillem, E., Abra, R., Huang, A., and Working, P. (1994) Tissue distribution and therapeutic effect of intravenous free or encapsulated liposomal doxorubicin on human prostate carcinoma xenografts. *Cancer*, **73** (5), 1478–1484.

25 Zamboni, W.C., Strychor, S., Joseph, E. *et al.* (2007) Plasma, tumor, and tissue disposition of STEALTH liposomal CKD-602 (S-CKD602) and nonliposomal CKD-602 in mice bearing A375 human melanoma xenografts. *Clin. Cancer Res.*, **13** (23), 7217–7223.

26 Newman, M.S., Colbern, G.T., Working, P.K., Engbers, C., and Amantea, M.A. (1999) Comparative pharmacokinetics, tissue distribution, and therapeutic effectiveness of cisplatin encapsulated in long-circulating, pegylated liposomes (SPI-077) in tumor-bearing mice. *Cancer Chemother. Pharmacol.*, **43** (1), 1–7.

27 Brown, E., McKee, T., di Tomaso, E. *et al.* (2003) Dynamic imaging of collagen and its modulation in tumors *in vivo* using second-harmonic generation. *Nat. Med.*, **9** (6), 796–800.

28 Choi, J., Credit, K., Henderson, K. *et al.* (2006) Intraperitoneal immunotherapy for metastatic ovarian carcinoma: resistance of intratumoral collagen to antibody penetration. *Clin. Cancer Res.*, **12**, 1906–1912.

29 McKee, T.D., Grandi, P., Mok, W. *et al.* (2006) Degradation of fibrillar collagen in a human melanoma xenograft improves the efficacy of an oncolytic herpes simplex virus vector. *Cancer Res.*, **6**, 2509–2513.

30 Perentes, J.Y., McKee, T.D., Ley, C.D. *et al.* (2009) *In vivo* imaging of extracellular matrix remodeling by tumor-associated fibroblasts. *Nat. Methods*, **6** (2), 143–145.

31 Chauhan, V.P., Martin, J.D., Liu, H., Lacorre, D.A., Jain, S.R., Kozin, S.V. *et al.* (2013) Angiotensin inhibition enhances drug delivery and potentiates chemotherapy by decompressing tumour blood vessels. *Nat Commun.*, **4**, 2516.

32 Lu, D., Wientjes, M.G., Lu, Z., and Au, J.L.S. (2007) Tumor priming enhances delivery and efficacy of nanomedicines. *J. Pharmacol. Exp. Ther.*, **322**, 80–88

33 Xiao, S.C., Madden, A.J., Rivera, J., Santos, C., Darr, D., Hunter, L., and Zamboni, W.C. The effects of microbeam radiation therapy on the pharmacokinetics of PEGylated liposomal doxorubicin in a triple negative breast cancer GEM model. doi: 10.1158/1538-7445.AM2015-4516.

34 Siegal, T., Horowitz, A., and Gabizon, A. (1995) Doxorubicin encapsulated in sterically stabilized liposomes for the treatment of a brain tumor model: biodistribution and therapeutic efficacy. *J. Neurosurg.*, **83** (6), 1029–1037.

35 Koukourakis, M.I., Koukouraki, S., Giatromanolaki, A. *et al.* (1999) Liposomal doxorubicin and conventionally fractionated radiotherapy in the treatment of locally advanced non-small-cell lung cancer and head and neck cancer. *J. Clin. Oncol.*, **17** (11), 3512–3521.

36 Sharma, U.S., Sharma, A., Chau, R.I., and Straubinger, R.M. (1997) Liposome-mediated therapy of intracranial brain tumors in a rat model. *Pharm. Res.*, **14** (8), 992–998.

37 Hobbs, S.K., Monsky, W.L., Yuan, F. *et al.* (1998) Regulation of transport pathways in tumor vessels: role of tumor type and microenvironment. *Proc. Natl. Acad. Sci. USA*, **95** (8), 4607–4612.

38 Liu, Y. and Lu, W. (2012) Recent advances in brain tumor-targeted nano-drug delivery systems. *Expert Opin. Drug Deliv.*, **9** (6), 671–686.

39 Anders, C.K., Adamo, B., Karginova, O. *et al.* (2013) Pharmacokinetics and efficacy of PEGylated liposomal doxorubicin in an intracranial model of breast cancer. *PLoS One*, **8** (5), e61359.

40 Gaillard, P.J., Appeldoorn, C.C., Dorland, R. *et al.* (2014) Pharmacokinetics, brain delivery, and efficacy in brain tumor-bearing mice of glutathione pegylated liposomal doxorubicin (2B3-101). *PLoS One*, **9** (1), e82331.

41 Jensen, S.A., Day, E.S., Ko, C.H. *et al.* (2013) Spherical nucleic acid nanoparticle conjugates as an RNAi-based therapy for glioblastoma. *Sci. Transl. Med.*, **5** (209), 209ra152.

42 Clark, A.J. and Davis, M.E. (2015) Increased brain uptake of targeted nanoparticles by adding an acid-cleavable linkage between transferrin and the nanoparticle core. *Proc. Natl. Acad. Sci. USA*, **112** (40), 12486–12491.

43 Saucier-Sawyer, J.K., Deng, Y., Seo, Y.-E., Cheng, C.J., Zhang, J., Quijano, E., and Saltzman, W.M. (2015) Systemic delivery of blood–brain barrier-targeted polymeric nanoparticles enhances delivery to brain tissue. *J. Drug Target.*, **23**, 7–8.

44 Liu, D., Mori, A., and Huang, L. (1992) Role of liposome size and RES blockade in controlling biodistribution and tumor uptake of GM1-containing liposomes. *Biochim. Biophys. Acta*, **1104** (1), 95–101.

45 Charrois, G.J. and Allen, T.M. (2003) Rate of biodistribution of STEALTH liposomes to tumor and skin: influence of liposome diameter and implications for toxicity and therapeutic activity. *Biochim. Biophys. Acta*, **1609** (1), 102–108.

46 Rolland, J.P., Maynor, B.W., Euliss, L.E., Exner, A.E., Denison, G.M., and DeSimone, J.M. (2005) Direct fabrication and harvesting of monodisperse, shape-specific nanobiomaterials. *J. Am. Chem. Soc.*, **127**, 10096–10100.

47 Chu, K.S., Hasan, W., Rawal, S. *et al.* (2013) Plasma, tumor and tissue pharmacokinetics of Docetaxel delivered via nanoparticles of different sizes and shapes in mice bearing SKOV-3 human

ovarian carcinoma xenograft. *Nanomedicine*, **9** (5), 686–693.
48 Li, S.D. and Huang, L. (2008) Pharmacokinetics and biodistribution of nanoparticles. *Mol. Pharm.*, **5** (4), 496–504.
49 Sadzuka, Y., Hirotsu, S., and Hirota, S. (1998) Effect of liposomalization on the antitumor activity, side-effects and tissue distribution of CPT-11. *Cancer Lett.*, **127** (1–2), 99–106.
50 Drummond, D.C., Noble, C.O., Hayes, M.E., Park, J.W., and Kirpotin, D.B. (2008) Pharmacokinetics and *in vivo* drug release rates in liposomal nanocarrier development. *J. Pharm. Sci.*, **97** (11), 4696–4740.
51 Drummond, D.C., Meyer, O., Hong, K., Kirpotin, D.B., and Papahadjopoulos, D. (1999) Optimizing liposomes for delivery of chemotherapeutic agents to solid tumors. *Pharmacol. Rev.*, **51** (4), 691–743.
52 Levchenko, T.S., Rammohan, R., Lukyanov, A.N., Whiteman, K.R., and Torchilin, V.P. (2002) Liposome clearance in mice: the effect of a separate and combined presence of surface charge and polymer coating. *Int. J. Pharm.*, **240** (1–2), 95–102.
53 Chu, K.S., Schorzman, A.N., Finniss, M.C. *et al.* (2013) Nanoparticle drug loading as a design parameter to improve docetaxel pharmacokinetics and efficacy. *Biomaterials*, **34** (33), 8424–8429.
54 Zamboni, W.C., Maruca, L.J., Strychor, S. *et al.* (2011) Bidirectional pharmacodynamic interaction between pegylated liposomal CKD-602 (S-CKD602) and monocytes in patients with refractory solid tumors. *J. Liposome Res.*, **21** (2), 158–165.
55 Yokomichi, N., Nagasawa, T., Coler-Reilly, A., Suzuki, H., Kubota, Y., Yoshioka, R., Tozawa, A., Suzuki, N., and Yamaguchi, Y. (2013) Pathogenesis of hand-foot syndrome induced by PEG-modified liposomal doxorubicin. *Hum. Cell*, **26** (1), 8–18.
56 Ajgal, Z., Chapuis, N., Emile, G., Cessot, A., Tigaud, J.M., Huillard, O., Boudou-Rouquette, P., Fontenay, M., Goldwasser, F., and Alexandre, J. (2015) Risk factors for pegylated liposomal doxorubicin-induced palmar-plantar erythrodysesthesia over time, assessment of monocyte count and baseline clinical parameters. *Cancer Chemother. Pharmacol.*, **76** (5), 1033–1039.
57 Ajgal, Z., Chapuis, N., Emile, G., Cessot, A., Tigaud, J.M., Huillard, O., Boudou-Rouquette, P., Fontenay, M., Goldwasser, F., and Alexandre, J. (2015) Risk factors for the pegylated liposomal doxorubicin-induced palmar-plantar erythrodysesthesia over time: assessment of monocyte count and baseline clinical parameters. *Cancer Chemother. Pharmacol.*, **76** (5), 1033–1039.
58 Zamboni, W.C., Strychor, S., Maruca, L. *et al.* (2009) Pharmacokinetic study of pegylated liposomal CKD-602 (S-CKD602) in patients with advanced malignancies. *Clin. Pharmacol. Ther.*, **86** (5), 519–526.
59 La-Beck, N.M., Zamboni, B.A., Gabizon, A. *et al.* (2012) Factors affecting the pharmacokinetics of pegylated liposomal doxorubicin in patients. *Cancer Chemother. Pharmacol.*, **69** (1), 43–50.
60 Gusella, M., Bononi, A., Modena, Y. *et al.* (2014) Age affects pegylated liposomal doxorubicin elimination and tolerability in patients over 70 years old. *Cancer Chemother. Pharmacol*, **73** (3), 517–524.
61 Falandry, C., Brain, E., Bonnefoy, M. *et al.* (2011) Impact of geriatric vulnerability parameters on pegylated liposomal doxorubicin (PLD) tolerance and outcome in elderly patients with metastatic breast cancer: results of the DOGMES multicenter phase II GINECO trial. *J. Clin. Oncol.*, **29**, 9122.
62 Lloberas, J. and Celada, A. (2002) Effect of aging on macrophage function. *Exp. Gerontol.*, **37** (12), 1325–1331.
63 La-Beck, N., Wu, H., Infante, J. *et al.* (2010) The evaluation of gender on the pharmacokinetics (PK) of pegylated liposomal anticancer agents. *J. Clin. Oncol.*, **28**, e13003.
64 Song, G., Wu, H., La-Beck, N. *et al.* (2010) Effect of gender on pharmacokinetic disposition of pegylated liposomal CKD-602 (S-CKD602) and optisomal topotecan (TLI) in rats. *AACR*. doi: 10.1158/1538-7445.am10-3700.

65 Wu, H., Ramanathan, R.K., Zamboni, B.A. *et al.* (2011) Population pharmacokinetics of pegylated liposomal CKD-602 (S-CKD602) in patients with advanced malignancies. *J. Clin. Pharmacol*, **52** (2), 180–194.

66 Robieux, I., Sorio, R., Borsatti, E. *et al.* (1996) Pharmacokinetics of vinorelbine in patients with liver metastases. *Clin. Pharmacol. Ther.*, **59** (1), 32–40.

67 Twelves, C.J., O'Reilly, S.M., Coleman, R.E., Richards, M.A., and Rubens, R.D. (1989) Weekly epirubicin for breast cancer with liver metastases and abnormal liver biochemistry. *Br. J. Cancer*, **60** (6), 938–941.

68 Lyass, O., Hubert, A., and Gabizon, A.A. (2001) Phase I study of doxil-cisplatin combination chemotherapy in patients with advanced malignancies. *Clin. Cancer Res.*, 7 (10), 3040–3046.

69 Volk, L.D., Flister, M.J., Chihade, D., Desai, N., Trieu, V., and Ran, S. (2011) Synergy of nab-paclitaxel and bevacizumab in eradicating large orthotopic breast tumors and preexisting metastases. *Neoplasia*, **13** (4), 327–338.

70 Rochlitz, C., Ruhstaller, T., Lerch, S. *et al.* (2011) Combination of bevacizumab and 2-weekly pegylated liposomal doxorubicin as first-line therapy for locally recurrent or metastatic breast cancer: a multicenter, single-arm phase II trial (SAKK 24/06). *Ann. Oncol.*, **22** (1), 80–85.

71 Murray, S., Briasoulis, E., Linardou, H., Bafaloukos, D., and Papadimitriou, C. (2012) Taxane resistance in breast cancer: mechanisms, predictive biomarkers and circumvention strategies. *Cancer Treat. Rev.*, **38** (7), 890–903.

72 Urano, N., Fujiwara, Y., Doki, Y., Kim, S.J., Miyoshi, Y., Noguchi, S., Miyata, H., Takiguchi, S., Yasuda, T., Yano, M., and Monden, M. (2006) Clinical significance of class III β-tubulin expression and its predictive value for resistance to docetaxel-based chemotherapy in gastric cancer. *Int. J. Oncol.*, **28** (2), 375–381.

73 Breedveld, P., Beijnen, J.H., and Schellens, J.H. (2006) Use of P-glycoprotein and BCRP inhibitors to improve oral bioavailability and CNS penetration of anticancer drugs. *Trends Pharmacol. Sci.*, **27** (1), 17–24.

74 Zhao, Y., Alakhova, D.Y., and Kabanov, A.V. (2013) Can nanomedicines kill cancer stem cells? *Adv. Drug Deliv. Rev.*, **65**, 1763–1783.

75 Gabizon, A., Isacson, R., Rosengarten, O., Tzemach, D., Shmeeda, H., and Sapir, R. (2008) An open-label study to evaluate dose and cycle dependence of the pharmacokinetics of pegylated liposomal doxorubicin. *Cancer Chemother. Pharmacol.*, **61** (4), 695–702.

20
Regulatory Issues in Nanomedicines

Marisa Papaluca, Falk Ehmann, Ruben Pita, and Dolores Hernan

European Medicines Agency – EMEA, 7 Westferry Circus Canary Wharf, Canary Wharf, London E14 4HB, UK

20.1
Nanomedicines and the Pharmaceuticals Regulatory Framework in Europe

The European regulatory system for medicines is based on a network of all national medicines regulatory authorities for both human and veterinary medicines in the 28 Member States of the European Union and the European Economic Area. The oversight of medicines in the Member States is governed by a single set of legislation[1] and regulatory science requirements implemented either via a centralized coordinated route (centralized procedure, leading to a single marketing authorization binding in all member states, reserved for certain types of medicines as discussed below) or via a decentralized system manned by each member state.

The European Medicines Agency (hereafter "the Agency") is responsible for the coordination of the scientific support and regulatory evaluation of Marketing Authorizations in the centralized procedure, reserved for new and innovative medicines, medicines intended for rare diseases, and other conditions representing a major public health burden such as diabetes, cancer, neurodegenerative disease, HIV-related conditions, viral diseases, and immunological diseases. The Agency also coordinates the pharmacovigilance of other medicines available in the European market. The Agency provides with scientific opinions, based on the evaluation of the evidence available for a medicines benefits/risks balance. The European Commission grants and manages the actual Marketing Authorization of medicines with their legal instruments in consultation with the member states national competent authorities (NCAs). In this way, the overall pharmaceutical framework

1) Directive 2001/83/EC Regulation (EC) No 726/2004. Available at http://ec.europa.eu/health/human-use/legal-framework/index_en.htm.

Pharmaceutical Nanotechnology: Innovation and Production, First Edition. Edited by Jean Cornier, Arno Kwade, Andrew Owen, and Marcel Van de Voorde.

results in a coherent system notwithstanding the differences still in place related to national rules for patients' access pricing and reimbursement.

EMAs responsibilities for medicines regulatory oversight are legally defined in a number of European Regulations and Directives and are implemented with the seven main scientific committees[2)], which are an integral part of the Agency and its scientific secretariat, also providing the logistics, infrastructures, organizational, and managerial support. The work of the committees is focusing on different aspects of medicines lifecycle and include scientific support to innovative medicines and methods[3)], designation of orphan status [1], classification and evaluation of Advanced Therapies Medicinal Products[4)], opinions on binding pediatric investigation plans (PIPs) [2], scientific opinion on the granting of Marketing Authorization [3] and medicines life cycle oversight of benefits and risks, providing independent information, and as mentioned above, the coordination of the EU pharmacovigilance[5)] work on risk management, risks minimization, and safety monitoring of medicines prior and after authorization for use in the clinical setting.

To enable promising new medicines to get to patients at the earliest appropriate time, the Agency is also exploring with the scientific committees and the partners in the regulatory framework, flexible licensing pathways, and a life-span approach with clinical development, licensing, reimbursement, medicines use in clinical practice, and monitoring, which is viewed as a continuum.

The resources and expertise available to regulate medicines to the highest scientific standards consist of thousands of experts across Member States, which contribute in a dynamic and flexible way to the work of the EMA scientific committees composed of regulators appointed by the NCAs for their expertise in pharmaceuticals evaluation and regulatory decision-making. The EMA Scientific Committees act in consultation, as appropriate, with clinical specialists, patients

2) The European Medicines Agency (EMA) has seven scientific committees that carry out its scientific assessments. This page provides a general overview of how the committees operate. Available at http://www.ema.europa.eu/ema/index.jsp?curl=pages/about_us/general/general_content_000217.jsp&mid=.

3) The EMA can give scientific advice and protocol assistance to companies involved in developing medicines. For human medicines, scientific advice and protocol assistance are given by the Committee for Medicinal Products for Human Use (CHMP) on the recommendation of the Scientific Advice Working Party (SAWP). Available at http://www.ema.europa.eu/ema/index.jsp?curl=pages/regulation/general/general_content_000049.jsp&mid=WC0b01ac05800229b9.

4) The Committee for Advanced Therapies (CAT) is the committee at the EMA that is responsible for assessing the quality, safety and efficacy of advanced-therapy medicinal products (ATMPs) and following scientific developments in the field. It is a multidisciplinary committee, gathering together some of the best available experts in Europe. It was established in accordance with Regulation (EC) No 1394/2007 on ATMPs. Available at http://www.ema.europa.eu/ema/index.jsp?curl=pages/about_us/general/general_content_000266.jsp&mid=WC0b01ac05800292a4.

5) The Pharmacovigilance Risk Assessment Committee (PRAC) is the committee at the European Medicines Agency that is responsible for assessing and monitoring safety issues for human medicines. Available at http://www.ema.europa.eu/ema/index.jsp?curl=pages/about_us/general/general_content_000537.jsp&mid=WC0b01ac058058cb18.

representatives, Health Technology Assessment experts, specialists and other stakeholders, both as a gatekeeper and an enabler [4] to pharmaceutical innovation for the benefit of patients. The dialog and collaborative approach not only amid scientific disciplines but also with civil society[6] involved in the development, patients' access, and use of medicines is characteristic of the networking functioning of the Agency. The EMA medicines evaluation and regulatory science standards setting also avails itself of international scientific collaboration via bilateral and multiregional agreements, particularly for innovative and high technology medicines, technologies, methods, and biomarkers that have the potential to address unmet medical needs.

The EU medicines regulatory framework is in constant evolution to address public health needs as they emerge, taking into account the progress in molecular understanding of the diseases (targeted therapies), changing clinical patterns, and epidemiology of diseases as related to aging (frailty and polymedications), globalization (infectious diseases outbreaks and pandemics), life-style (obesity and diabetes epidemic), and impact that authorized medicines themselves have on diseases (e.g., emergence of antimicrobial resistance, viral strains mutation, disease modifiers in arthritis and chronic conditions such as certain types of cancers).

To fulfill its tasks, it is therefore essential that the Agency maintains and fosters the links of the European Medicines Regulatory Network with the civil society, collaboration with Institutions (e.g., European Commission and WHO), and international partners (e.g., U.S. Food and Drug Administration and Japanese Medical Products Agency) from one side and with the advances in academic, translational, and applied science on the other side to ensure that novel products addressing the health needs of the citizens of Europe and beyond, can be optimally developed and made accessible.

20.2 The European Medicines Agency and Nanomedicines

In the context of fostering development of innovative medicines to address patient and public health needs, the Agency, taking into account the experience in this emerging science by its Innovation Task Force[7], identified in nanotechnology-based medicinal products (in this chapter referred to as

6) The EMA is at the core of the European Union's (EU's) medicine and health system, and aims to protect human and animal health. To ensure that the system works effectively, the Agency works closely with its partners and stakeholders, and is a proactive member of important networks in Europe and beyond. Available at http://www.ema.europa.eu/ema/index.jsp?curl=pages/partners_and_networks/general/general_content_000212.jsp&mid=.

7) The Innovation Task Force (ITF) is a multidisciplinary group that includes scientific, regulatory and legal competences. It was set up to ensure coordination across the European Medicines Agency and to provide a forum for early dialogue with applicants. Available at http://www.ema.europa.eu/ema/index.jsp?curl=pages/regulation/general/general_content_000334.jsp&mid=WC0b01ac05800ba1d9.

nanomedicines) the potential in a wide range of applications. Enabling new modes of action, as well combining mechanical, chemical, metabolic, pharmacological, and immunological properties, nanomedicines may provide benefit to patients in a number of ways. But equally, nanomedicines can present a range of technological, scientific, regulatory, and legal uncertainties, which require an early awareness, appropriate scientific, and methodological expertise, and consensus on the most appropriate regulatory requirements.

From the Agency viewpoint, the current approach of the Scientific Committees is adequate for the evaluation of nanomedicines as they progress in clinical development and clinical use. As for any medicinal product, nanomedicinal products will have to be characterized, their fate and toxicology will have to be established as part of their quality, safety and efficacy evaluation, and the appropriateness of test methods will have to be demonstrated. Before marketing, toxicology and ecotoxicology for a specific nanomedicinal product, as well as the methodologies used for the evaluation of toxicity, would be assessed in the context of the evaluation of the Marketing Authorization Application, which foresees evaluation of benefits and risks to patients as well as an environmental risk assessment. The current benefit/risk balance evaluation model is flexible enough to conclude on an individual product basis, proportionate evidentiary standards applicable to such novel and innovative medicinal products.

When it comes to nanomedicine properties such as better targeting, novel delivery modes, better bioavailability of existing substances [5], or novel mechanism of action, the Agency has already discussed a number of situations in Scientific Advice, reviewed full marketing authorizations applications and provided positive scientific opinions for the marketing of nanomedicines exhibiting some of these properties (e.g., see stealth liposomes, multilamellar liposomes, nanoparticles, nanocrystal colloidal dispersions such as Caelix, Mepact, Abraxane, and Rapamune)[8]. Nanostructure scaffolds as part of combined engineered tissues for tissue replacement have already been considered by the Committee on Advanced Therapy Medicinal Products[9] and novel versatile polymers, new imaging nanomedicines, and microenvironment-responsive nanomedicines still in development are discussed at the Innovation Task Force level and in the context of Scientific Advice.

8) The EMA publishes an European public assessment reports (EPAR) for every medicine granted a central marketing authorisation by the European Commission following an assessment by the EMA's Committee for Medicinal Products for Human Use (CHMP). Available at http://www.ema.europa.eu/ema/index.jsp?curl=pages/medicines/landing/epar_search.jsp&mid=WC0b01ac058001d124.

9) Companies can consult the EMA to determine whether a medicine they are developing is an advanced-therapy medicinal product (ATMP). The procedure allows them to receive confirmation that a medicine, which is based on genes, cells or tissues, meets the scientific criteria for defining an ATMP. Available at http://www.ema.europa.eu/ema/index.jsp?curl=pages/regulation/general/general_content_000296.jsp&mid=WC0b01ac058007f4bc.

Methodological limitations for the evaluation of certain aspects of nanomedicines, for example, influence of shape and flexibility on the functionalities of the nanosystem, often remain linked to the level of scientific knowledge: it is therefore essential that the sponsors approach the Agency at a very early stage so as to discuss and develop a common understanding of what methods are mature for inclusion in development and which still remain speculative in research. This is especially important to ensure that such imitations do not constitute a bottleneck for the development and approval of a nanomedicines, provided that the overall evidence progressively generated in studies carried out in quality, preclinical, clinical, and clinical domains are coherent, methodologically robust, and convincingly showing that benefits out weight potential and yet undefinable risks.

In view of the accumulated experience in evaluation of nanomedicines, the increasing demand from sponsors of scientific advice for their development and the interest from stakeholders and partners on the topic, the Agency in 2009 established a European expert group[10)] composed of high profile academics and regulatory science specialists, which since its inception interacted and continues to interact with regulatory scientist focusing on the same topic from the U.S. Food and Drug Administration, the Japan PMDA, and other regulatory agencies. In 2011, the scientific Committee for Medicines for Human use (CHMP) reinforced the nanomedicines expert group with the addition of further specialists (particularly in the manufacturing, quality, nonclinical safety, and pharmacokinetics regulatory science domains) to expand the expertise available for addressing a number of hot issues in the evaluation of nanomedicines, including limitations for the full characterization, definition of critical parameters related to the scale-up of manufacturing, relevance of certain nonclinical models, specific issues in pharmacokinetic studies, concern for long-term safety, and environmental risks.

20.3
Is It Important to Define Nanomedicines?

To date there is no universally accepted definition of nanomedicines. The definition as provided by the Agency on the Website reads: "Nanotechnology is defined as the use of tiny structures – less than 1000 nanometers across – that are designed to have specific properties". In this simple statement, there are

10) The EMA follows the latest developments in nanotechnology that are relevant to the development of medicines. Recommendations from the Agency's Committee for Medicinal Products for Human Use (CHMP) have already led to the approval of a number of medicines based on nanotechnology. Available at http://www.ema.europa.eu/ema/index.jsp?curl=pages/special_topics/general/general_content_000345.jsp&mid=WC0b01ac05800baed9.

embedded three concepts that represent the basis for the Agency's reflection on the description of nanomedicines:

- There is mention of structures and not just of substances.
- The structures are designed on purpose and not just happen to be at nanoscale.
- The structures have specific properties not obtainable with the isolated individual components of the nanostructure.

The European Commission in 2011 issued a Commission Recommendation [6] on a definition for nanomaterial as follows: "'*Nanomaterial' means a natural, incidental or manufactured material containing particles, in an unbound state or as an aggregate or as an agglomerate and where, for 50% or more of the particles in the number size distribution, one or more external dimensions is in the size range 1–100 nm.*" In the "Whereas" (17) to the Recommendation, the Commission states that there are "*special circumstances* [. . .] *in the pharmaceutical sector*", and that the definition "*should not prejudice the use of the term 'nano' when defining certain pharmaceuticals*".

Nanotechnology presents itself as a technology holding the promise of accelerating innovation in the medical field, as one of the key enabling technologies both for pharmaceuticals and devices. For medicines, nanotechnology has only partially been exploited in manufacturing and in other pharmaceuticals domains but there is growing evidence to indicate its usefulness as the knowledge and ability grows of controlling molecular and biological behaviors of molecular systems at the nanoscale level. Biocompatible nanopolymers have shown the ability to optimize manufacturing yields being used in three-dimensional cell culture, separation/purification of cells and proteins, for the manufacturing of a biological pharmaceutical [7]; liposomal formulation have proven effective in modifying biodistribution and tolerability of highly active but toxic molecules useful for the treatment of life-threatening diseases and has the ability to determine time-controlled delivery of multiple complementary active substances, to modify responsiveness of tissues and cellular micro-environments [8].

Novel applications of nanotechnology currently in translation from discovery to development of clinical applications include nanostructures that allow finely controlled transport across biological barriers and manipulation of cell functions, such as the immunocompetent dendritic cells [9], integrated implantable sensory systems with multifunctional chemical structures targeting disease pathways and monitoring their pharmacological action [10]. In the gray area of borderline products between pharmaceuticals and medical devices, some innovative products combining diagnostic and therapeutic functions are already available to patients in some of the EU member states, on the market or in clinical trials such as NanoTherm™ [11] and Nanobiotix [12].

From the research arena, data are emerging on the possibility to introduce novel therapeutic approaches combining the benefits of pharmaceutical properties with the ones of engineered properties of surfaces, shapes, and charge, manipulated at the nanoscale level (e.g., conjugated molecules on the surface of responsive magnetic nanoparticles, virus-like nanoparticles [13]). Nanotechnology allows the production of intentionally functionalized structures that are very diverse and with properties that until recently, being those nanosystems almost exclusively in the domain of fundamental research, were not subject to any particular regulatory framework.

Now, that from the research emerging as nanomedicines are moving into clinical applications, it is becoming clear that functionalized nanosystems can blur the borders between devices and pharmaceuticals as the nanoscale properties activates, in a fully interdependent way, mechanisms of action that are metabolic, immunological, pharmacological, as well as chemical and physical. Therefore, it is anticipated that the key criterion for differentiating medicines from medical device that is, the Mechanism of Action may require additional considerations to define the most appropriate regulatory requirements.

The field of nanotechnology is expanding very rapidly and new nanosystems continue to emerge, and it is therefore most likely too premature to come to a stringent definition to separate out nanosystems from other pharmaceuticals. The differences in characteristics and functionalities among different types of nanomedicines may be greater than the differences in characteristics compared to established chemicals or biological substances. It is therefore sensible at this point in time not to pursue the quest of an all-inclusive definition of nanomedicines, but rather approach the specificities of each on-purpose built nanosystem for medical purpose and identify the appropriate regulatory requirements.

It is important however to develop at least a common working description of what a nanomedicine is, as the regulatory frameworks for the development and authorization of devices and pharmaceuticals in Europe are very different, and regulatory uncertainty is one of the major obstacles for the translation from scientific concept to health products.

20.4 Communicating About Nanomedicines

The Agency's regulatory science work on nanomedicines has been made transparent to the community via a range of different tools: in addition to the launch of a dedicated web page, the Agency has consulted the scientific community with reflection papers, statements, and debates in public conferences as well as publications in peer-reviewed scientific journals.

In order to share the experience accrued in the Regulatory framework with the scientific evaluation of nanomedicines and to open the dialog on the scientific and methodology challenges of innovative nanotechnology-based medicinal products [14], in 2006 the Agency published the first regulatory reflection paper on nanotechnology-based medicinal products for human use [15] and launched a web page dedicated to nanotechnology. In 2011, the Agency's Scientific Committee for medicinal products for human use (CHMP) assigned the task of drafting reflection papers addressing the current regulatory experience on nanomedicines at EU level to the nanomedicines expert group, to make the information available to the sponsors and the research community. Based on the experience developed in the context of Scientific Advice and evaluation of Marketing Authorization Applications successfully, general regulatory principles have been addressed for liposomal formulations developed with reference to an innovator product [16], iron oxide nanoparticles for the treatment of iron deficient anemia [17], and surface coating of nanomedicines [18], of particular interest as the first generation of nanomedicines, including liposomal formulations, iron-based preparations, and nanocrystal-based medicines started to come off patent. In addition to the reflection papers mentioned above, a technical paper coauthored in 2013 by F. Ehmann *et al.* [19] presented considerations on the regulatory requirements for the marketing authorization of what have been nicknamed "nanosimilar" medicinal products. The fact that the level of complexity of the nanomedicines concerned (e.g., different types and molecular arrangements of liposomal formulations and iron nanoparticles) clearly indicates that such products cannot be characterized by physicochemical means only [20] and calls for additional data to be generated by the sponsors to prove that the generic has the same or similar characteristics of the innovator product. Conceptually, therefore the approach is similar to the one successfully implemented for biosimilars with stepwise quality, nonclinical and clinical comparative tests necessary to obtain market authorization.

Collaborations with European Institutions, such as the European Commission Directorates and its scientific bodies (e.g., the Scientific Committee on Emerging and Newly Identified Health Risks (SCENIHR), the Joint Research Center (JRC), and the European Food Safety Authority (EFSA), have been very productive in developing a coherent approach to nanomedicines, supporting policies that took into account progress and experience accumulated in neighboring frameworks.

Open discussions at conferences have also provided useful opportunities to communicate with the scientific community on regulatory requirements and issues specific to nanomedicines. Independent fora including conferences organized by the European Technology Platform on Nanomedicine (ETPN), the Products Quality Research Institute (IPQRI) and the FDA in 2014 [21] and the CLINAM annual conferences [22] – provided dedicated open regulatory sessions for discussion with the scientific community every year, and discussed benefits and challenges arising from the application of nanotechnologies in medicines.

20.5
Liposomal Formulations: State of Play at the EMA

Liposomes are classically described as artificially prepared vesicles composed of one or more concentric lipid bilayers enclosing one or more aqueous compartments. They include, but are not limited to, mono- and multilamellar liposomes, multivesicular liposomes, and polymer-coated liposomes. Liposomes have traditionally been used as a delivery system for one or more active pharmaceutical ingredients, showing their clinical added value by modifying the disposition or release of the active substance(s) administrated to the patient by comparison to their traditional equivalents (free active substance) or by enabling new delivery routes, such as inhalation, of existing active substances. As we will consider later in this chapter, developments in liposomal technology can extend clinical use beyond traditional use of a passive delivery system of an active substance.

Liposomal medicinal products have been approved in the EU since the 1990s, the variety and number of approved products is however still to reach its full potential if one considers how prolific the technology is in scientific articles, patents, and products undergoing clinical development. The currently approved products are mainly, but not exclusively, targeted for use in oncology. The table below provides a nonexhaustive list of approved liposomal medicinal products in the EU; references to the *in vivo* benefits stemming from the use of liposomes, for example, when compared to their traditional free active equivalents, are included in the Table 20.1 when publically available.

Also very relevant to public health is the repurposing of known active substances by the use of liposomal technology to improve their clinical profile and hence achieve a significant benefit in the context of the Orphan Legislation (Table 20.2).

In February 2013, the EMA released its first reflection paper on liposomes: Reflection paper on the data requirements for intravenous liposomal products developed with reference to an innovator liposomal product,[11] to address an identified need to increase the certainty with regards the quality, nonclinical, and clinical data expected to be submitted in support of a marketing authorization of intravenous liposomal products developed with reference to an innovator liposomal product. The reflection paper is intended to facilitate a decision on the

- pharmaceutical data needed as evidence of product comparability between test and reference or after changes to a liposomal product, to support comparative safety and efficacy;
- necessity of preclinical and clinical studies and circumstances that may allow to waive certain studies;
- consideration of the design of relevant *in vivo* nonclinical studies and the potential role for *in vitro* models.

It is further explained that the principles outlined in the reflection paper should also be considered to be applicable to novel "liposome-like" and vesicular products which may be under development including those to be administered by routes other than intravenous administration, that is, the views expressed may be used beyond comparability exercises between test and reference liposomal product and can be extrapolated to other delivery systems similar to liposomes.

11) http://www.ema.europa.eu/docs/en_GB/document_library/Scientific_guideline/2013/03/WC500140351.pdf.

Table 20.1 Nonexhaustive list of liposomal medicinal products granted a marketing authorization in the EU.

Trade name (active substance)	Platform/technology	Indication	MAH	Approval
Caelyx® (doxorubicin)	API in sterically stabilized pegylated liposomes, to increase blood circulation (long-acting) and reduce cardiotoxicity	Multiple myeloma, ovarian neoplasms, breast neoplasms, Kaposi sarcoma	Janssen-Cilag International NV	06/1996
	SmPC reference: "(. . .) Of the 418 patients treated with Caelyx 50 mg/m²/cycle, and having a baseline measurement of left ventricular ejection fraction (LVEF) and at least one follow depodur-up measurement assessed by MUGA scan, 88 patients had a cumulative anthracycline dose of >400 mg/m² an exposure level associated with an increased risk of cardiovascular toxicity with conventional doxorubicin (. . .)"[a)]			
Myocet® (doxorubicin)	Liposome-encapsulated doxorubicin–citrate complex to reduce cardiac toxicity and to increase tumor tissue distribution	Breast neoplasms	Cephalon Europe	07/2000
	SmPC reference: "(. . .) Analyses of cardiotoxicity in clinical trials have shown a statistically significant reduction in cardiac events in patients treated with Myocet compared to patients treated with conventional doxorubicin at the same dose in mg. A meta-analysis showed a statistically significant lower rate of both clinical heart failure ($RR = 0.20$, $p = 0.02$) and clinical and subclinical heart failure combined ($RR = 0.38$, $p < 0.0001$) in patients treated with Myocet versus conventional doxorubicin (. . .)"[b)]			
Visudyne® (verteporfin)	Liposomal formulation of semisynthetic mixture of porphyrins	Degenerative myopia, age-related macular degeneration	Novartis Europharm Ltd.	07/2000
DepoCyte® (cytarabine)	Multivesicular liposomes with unique structure of multiple nonconcentric aqueous chambers (DepoFoam®)	Meningeal neoplasms	Pacira Limited	07/2001
	SmPC reference: *"Median progression-free survival (defined as time to neurological progression or death) for all treated patients was 77 versus 48 d for DepoCyte versus unencapsulated cytarabine, respectively. The proportion of patients alive at 12 mo was 24% for DepoCyte versus 19% for unencapsulated cytarabine".*[c)]			
Mepact® (mifamurtide)	fully synthetic analog of a component of *Mycobacterium sp.* cell wall encapsulated in multilamellar liposomes to facilitate activation of macrophages	high-grade resectable nonmetastatic osteosarcoma	IDM PHARMA SAS	03/2009

	EPAR reference: "(. . .) *MEPACT is a liposomal formulation specifically designed for in vivo targeting to macrophages by intravenous infusion*; SmPC: *(. . .) Liposomal MTP-PE is [muramyl tripeptide phosphatidyl ethanolamine] selectively taken up by macrophages and monocytes and slowly broken down within the cell. Cellular released L-MTP-PE may signal through the NOD2 receptor, an intracellular protein that induces NF-κB activation (. . .)*"[d)]			
AmBisome® (amphoteracin B)	Non PEGylated formulation of liposomal Amphoteracin B	Severe systemic and/or deep mycoses, and visceral leishmaniasis in immuno-competent patients	Gilead Sciences International Limited	09/1998 (UK)
	SmPC reference: "*Due to the size of the liposomes, there is no glomerular filtration and renal elimination of AmBisome, thus avoiding interaction of amphotericin B with the cells of the distal tubuli and reducing the potential for nephrotoxicity seen with conventional amphotericin B presentations*"[e)]			
Depodur® (morphine)	Multivesicular liposomes with unique structure of multiple nonconcentric aqueous chambers (DepoFoam®)	Relief of postoperative pain following major orthopedic, abdominal, or pelvic surgery	Flynn Pharma Limited PLC[f)]	04/2006 (UK)
	SmPC reference: "*(. . .) sustained-release formulation of the active ingredient morphine sulfate designed for epidural administration. (. . .) The analgesic action of Depodur persists for up to 48 h*"[g)]			
Epaxal® (hepatitis A vaccine)	Immunopotentiating reconstituted influenza virosome	Active immunization against hepatitis A	Crucell Italy	12/1999

a) Caelyx® product information. Available at http://www.ema.europa.eu/ema/index.jsp?curl=pages/medicines/human/medicines/000089/human_med_000683.jsp&mid=WC0b01ac058001d124.
b) European Medicines Agency Myocet® product information. Available at http://www.ema.europa.eu/ema/index.jsp?curl=pages/medicines/human/medicines/000297/human_med_000916.jsp&mid=WC0b01ac058001d124.
c) http://www.ema.europa.eu/docs/en_GB/document_library/EPAR_-_Product_Information/human/000317/WC500035649.pdf.
d) European Medicines Agency Mepact® product information and assessment history publically. Available at http://www.ema.europa.eu/ema/index.jsp?curl=pages/medicines/human/medicines/000802/human_med_000899.jsp&mid=WC0b01ac058001d124.
e) http://www.mhra.gov.uk/home/groups/spcpil/documents/spcpil/con1439527267991.pdf.
f) http://www.flynnpharma.com/about-us/news/depodur-marketing-ceased.
g) http://www.mhra.gov.uk/home/groups/par/documents/websiteresources/con2023837.pdf.

Table 20.2 Liposomal medicinal products with Orphan Designation.[a)]

Product and designated orphan indication	Designation date	Grounds for significant benefit as claimed by sponsor
Amikacin sulfate (liposomal) Treatment of *Pseudomonas aeruginosa* lung infection in cystic fibrosis	25/07/2006	Amikacin sulfate (liposomal) might be of potential significant benefit for the treatment of cystic fibrosis mainly because it may provide a major contribution to patient care.
Doxorubicin hydrochloride (liposomal) Treatment of soft tissue sarcoma	27/10/2006	Doxorubicin hydrochloride (liposomal) might be of potential significant benefit for the treatment of soft tissue sarcoma mainly because it might improve the long-term outcome of the patients.
Paclitaxel (liposomal) Treatment of pancreatic cancer	31/10/2006	Paclitaxel (liposomal) might be of potential significant benefit for the treatment of pancreatic cancer, because it may improve the long-term outcome of the patients. According to the sponsor, paclitaxel (liposomal) will, by binding specifically to the cells that line blood vessels, inhibit the growth of newly formed blood vessels, contribute to the destruction of the tumor.
Cisplatin (liposomal) Treatment of pancreatic cancer	08/06/2007	The inclusion of cisplatin in liposomes is expected to increase the concentration of the drug in the cancer cells, compared to normal cells, and decrease the adverse effects of the active substance.
Vincristine sulfate liposomes Treatment of acute lymphoblastic leukemia	08/07/2008	In this medicine, vincristine is contained in liposomes. This is expected to improve the way the medicine works compared with the conventional form of the medicine, by slowing down the clearance of the medicine from the body.
Topotecan hydrochloride (liposomal) Treatment of glioma	05/09/2008	The liposomal delivery system improves the way the medicine works compared with the conventional form of the medicine, since it can be injected directly into the brain, concentrating the medicine at the site of the tumor and reducing side effects by reducing the amount of free active substance in the blood.
Gadodiamide (liposomal) Treatment of glioma	03/12/2008	Gadodiamide (liposomal) is expected to show how much of the tumor the medicine has reached and to indicate where more treatment may be needed. It is also expected to help to see that any catheters (small tubes inserted into the veins) are correctly placed.
Daunorubicin (liposomal) Treatment of acute myeloid leukemia	03/12/2008	When it is contained within liposomes, it is expected to remain in the patient's body for longer than "free" daunorubicin, which might lead to the improved treatment of patients with this condition.

Ciprofloxacin (liposomal) Treatment of cystic fibrosis	24/07/2009	The liposomal formulation for inhalation may allow delivery of higher amounts of ciprofloxacin directly into the lungs compared with existing formulations of ciprofloxacin. Also, the liposomal formulation is expected to reduce the bitterness of the medicine, allowing it to be given by inhalation, and it is expected to remain in the patient's lungs for longer than free ciprofloxacin.
Doxorubicin hydrochloride (in heat-sensitive liposomes) Treatment of hepatocellular carcinoma	23/02/2011	The doxorubicin is contained within liposomes, which allow the active substance to accumulate mainly in the liver. The liposomes used in this medicine are heat-sensitive particles that release the doxorubicin when their temperature reaches 39.5 °C. When this medicine is used together with radiofrequency ablation, the heat from the probe provokes the release of doxorubicin within the tumor, which is expected to improve the antitumor effects of this treatment.
Nanoliposomal irinotecan Treatment of pancreatic cancer	09/12/2011	The nanoliposomes are expected to accumulate within the tumor and release the medicine slowly over time, thereby decreasing the rate at which the irinotecan is removed from the body and allowing it to act for longer; this is expected to improve the treatment of patients with this condition.
Liposomal combination of cytarabine and daunorubicin Treatment of acute myeloid leukemia	11/01/2012	The liposomes are expected to remain in the patient's body for longer than free cytarabine and daunorubicin and accumulate in the patient's bone marrow. The liposomes protect the anticancer medicines from being metabolized early, the extended residence time at the site of action is expected to enhance their effect on cancer cells.

a) Information extracted from the Register of designated Orphan Medicinal Products: http://ec.europa.eu/health/documents/community-register/html/orphreg.htm.

The document is divided into three main parts, quality, nonclinical, and clinical requirements. The first part details general parameters applicable to the majority of liposomes, such as the quality, purity, and stability of lipids and other critical excipients; liposome morphology, mean size and size distribution, aggregates; fraction of encapsulated active substance (amount of free/entrapped); stability of the active substance, lipids, and functional excipients in the finished product; *in vitro* drug substance release rate from the liposome in physiologically/clinically relevant media. The first list is followed by an additional list of parameters that may be applicable to some types of liposomes according to their design and intended *in vivo* performance: maintenance of liposomal formulation integrity in plasma; determination of liposomal "surface" charge; pH of internal compartment for pH-gradient loaded liposomes; characterization of physical state of the active substance inside the liposome; distribution of drug substance within liposome; quality and purity of the PEG starting material is essential for the later quality of the medicinal product; details of linkage chemistry (such as PEG-lipid or similar constructs with or without PEG); and stability of PEG-lipid conjugation. The importance of determining the impact of any change to the manufacturing process of the liposomes, or its constituents, is emphasized due to the potential impact on the clinical performance of the medicinal product; it goes further to state that *in vivo* studies may be necessary to demonstrate that any changes do not affect the safety and efficacy profile of the product when results from physicochemical testing indicate a change in the *in vitro* properties of the product.

The nonclinical section starts with an important statement with regards the battery of *in vivo* studies recommended to demonstrate bioequivalence: "(. . .) the complexity of the particular liposomal formulation will determine whether comparative nonclinical studies could be reduced and if appropriate, it may be decided on a case-by-case basis which studies could be waived". Later in the same section, the expectations about which elements to quantify (encapsulated and unencapsulated drug in blood/plasma and unencapsulated drug in tissue, in addition to traditional methods for total drug and metabolite in blood/plasma and tissues) are stated while it is recognized that there is insufficient regulatory experience to support specific decision criteria for comparability of tissue distribution. Replicate study designs are recommended and all estimates and data displays should include quantification of uncertainty. Advice is also provided with regards which doses to study and which modeling methods to use.

The last section of the paper on clinical requirements starts with dose considerations and highlights that when bioequivalence studies cannot be performed in certain doses due to, for example, ethical reasons, assessment of therapeutic equivalence in each indication will require individual consideration. Pharmacokinetic characteristics of total, encapsulated, and unencapsulated drug are expected to be measured, but recognizing that conventional pharmacokinetic metrics such as AUC and C_{max} might not give sufficient indication of the rate of release at the target sites. The reflection paper invites the applicant to submit an evaluation of additional pharmacokinetic parameters such as distribution and elimination. More recently in silico modeling has been considered as a promising exploratory tool to refine PK characterization of medicines, but not specific recommendations are made at present for liposomal systems, new or follow-on. With regards to safety, the document states that full-scale clinical trial data is not expected at the time of authorization; however, the clinical safety of similar liposomal products should be closely monitored in accordance with current EU legislation and pharmacovigilance guidelines.

The paper concludes with the reflection that experience with liposomal formulations developed with reference to an innovator is still limited, consequently only general recommendations can be given and developers are advised to seek product-specific scientific advice.

As mentioned above, there is still an unharnessed potential for new medicinal products using liposomal technology to provide new therapeutic alternatives to the existing armamentarium. The next-generation liposomes may focus on further specialization of the traditional use of liposomes as a delivery system by manipulation of the bilayer properties so the active substance(s) are released in tissues at specific temperatures and thus enabling an improved tissue targeting; by the versatility of its structure to simultaneously incorporate substances with different chemical properties in the inner environment or at its surface thus allowing itself to be a promising vaccine delivery system carrying different types of antigens and adjuvants; or for peritoneal dialysis with transmembrane pH gradient liposomes.

20.6 Nanosimilar Colloidal Intravenous Iron-Based Preparations

The European Medicines Agency regulatory requirements and considerations on nanosized colloidal iron-based preparations developed with reference to an innovator product (reference medicinal product) are described in the CHMP Reflection Paper (RP), published in March 2015 [23]. Nanosized colloidal intravenous iron-based preparations were first used in humans in the 1930s, and since then they have been widely used to treat iron-deficiency anemia. These products have a complex structure comprising a polynuclear iron(III) hydroxide core surrounded by modified carbohydrate polymer coatings. Examples include high- or low-molecular-weight dextran, gluconate, sucrose, and carboxymaltose.

Differences in the production process or composition with reference to an innovator product may lead to diverse product characteristics that will impact on safety and therapeutic performance. The Reflection Paper discusses the principles for developing and evaluating nanosimilar colloidal intravenous iron-based preparations designed as a treatment for iron-deficiency anemia, developed with reference to a nanosized colloidal innovator product.

The overarching principle is that development of a specific product should take into account the critical product attributes of the innovator (reference medicinal product), and the evidence that supports its use when designing the

Table 20.3 Nonexhaustive list of Iron nanoparticles for the treatment of anemia granted a marketing authorization in the EU.

Product	MAH
CosmoFer	Pharmacosmos UK Limited
Diafer 50 mg/ml solution for injection	Pharmacosmos UK Limited
Monofer 100 mg/ml solution for injection/infusion	Pharmacosmos UK Limited
Venofer (iron sucrose)	Vifor Pharma UK Limited

quality, nonclinical, and clinical development program. Early contact of the sponsors with the Agency is recommended. Challenges for these products are the manufacturing scale-up and the scale of the clinical data required, which will depend on how accurately the physicochemical and nonclinical characterization can be used to predict differences that could influence the efficacy and safety of the product. Discussion between the regulators and the scientific community is ongoing (Table 20.3).

When administered by the parenteral route the nanosized iron complexes are internalized by cells and localization to liver macrophages or hepatocytes has been noted after intravenous administration. This trafficking and/or accumulation of iron-based products in any cell type could be a safety concern.

As described in the RP, the difficulty to fully characterize and define iron complex-based particles using quality methods alone together with uncertainties on how quality attributes relate to *in vivo* performance, requires further investigations. As a result, quality comparability and demonstration of similar plasma concentrations of iron alone, that is, conventional bioequivalence studies in humans, would not be sufficient for the assurance of comparability of the *in vivo* fate and the resulting toxicological and pharmacological effects of these products. Therefore, nonclinical data are required in addition to human clinical PK data. The extent of supplementary nonclinical and clinical data required is discussed the RP and, as for biosimilars, it depends on how accurately the physicochemical and nonclinical characterization can be used to predict differences that could influence the safety and efficacy of the product.

Therefore, the RP is intended to assist in the generation of relevant quality, nonclinical, and PK clinical comparative data to support a marketing authorization for this type of products and is intended to facilitate a decision on

- the pharmaceutical data needed as evidence of product similarity between test and reference products to support comparative safety and efficacy and
- consideration to the types of nonclinical and clinical studies that are required to support the quality data in order to demonstrate similarity.

It is also mentioned that the principles outlined in the RP should also be used when considering the data requirements to support changes to the manufacture and control of existing iron-based nanosized colloidal products.

The discussion is divided in three main sections: quality, nonclinical, and clinical.

The first section focuses on the quality attributes of nanosized iron-based products that may have a major impact on efficacy and safety, namely, the stability of the iron–carbohydrate complex (in other words, the fraction of labile iron released at the time of administration and the short-term stability in plasma, as labile iron has well known direct toxic effects and may influence pharmacokinetics and body distribution, the physicochemical properties of the carbohydrate matrix, and the physicochemical properties of the iron and iron–carbohydrate complex, including size and of the iron core and size and size distribution of the iron–carbohydrate complex.

Correctly identifying the parameters that define relevant physicochemical properties of a nanosized iron-based colloidal product is critical to ensure its quality. The paper also outlines the general parameters to be considered for these products: quality standard for carbohydrates used in the manufacture of the active substance and finished product (description, source and characterization, manufacture, assay, impurity profile, and stability characteristics); structure and composition of carbohydrate matrix; spectroscopic properties; identification and control of key intermediates in the manufacturing process; size of the iron core; amount of labile iron released from the product when administered; polymorphic form of the iron comprising the core; impurities (e.g., ratio of divalent and trivalent iron); morphology; ratio of bound carbohydrate to iron; particle size, size distribution, charge, and surface properties of the iron–carbohydrate complexes; degradation path for the iron–carbohydrate complex; where justified, a reliable and discriminating method for determining degradation kinetics; stability on storage of the product and in-use stability. It is also stressed the importance of adequately characterize and set the specification of the carbohydrate starting materials. It also describes two methods to determine labile iron *in vitro* as a means to demonstrate similarity and assure safety.

This section continues with general recommendations on establishing pharmaceutical comparability between test and reference products.

The nonclinical part starts with a general statement on the need to validate the methods of analysis and continues with a discussion on the importance to perform distribution studies in a relevant animal model to evaluate distribution, metabolism and excretion of these nanoparticles and of their *in vivo* degradation or solubilization products. Particular emphasis should focus on the distribution, accumulation, and retention in at least three compartments: plasma, reticular endothelial system (RES), and target tissues/organs. These studies should provide pivotal evidence of the comparability of the *in vivo* disposition of nanoparticular iron products, as it is not possible to fully explore distribution in humans from blood/plasma data alone.

Since the coated nanoparticles will be gradually degraded, total iron measurements will not reflect the physiological level of iron or the oxidation status. Therefore, the RP recommends the time-dependent measurement of overall iron content in different tissues to reflect the degradation profile of the nanoparticle.

Although there is insufficient regulatory experience with comparative nonclinical biodistribution studies to demonstrate similarity of iron-based nanocolloidal products at present, it is proposed to strive for the use of quantitative statistical approaches to show equivalence, and sponsors are encouraged to seek scientific advice. Furthermore, it is strongly recommended that criteria for comparability in distribution and clearance in comparison to the reference product are clearly defined and justified by the sponsor in advance of the study. Applicants are advised to seek scientific advice in this context. The clinical implications of any noted differences in tissue distribution between test and reference product should be carefully discussed. It is remarked that in this case, toxicity studies are not sensitive enough to demonstrate differences.

The clinical section mainly describes the pharmacokinetics studies and safety and efficacy studies to be performed. The importance to validate the analytical methods to confirm absence of impact from sample processing procedures in the bioanalytical results is also stressed in this section.

In general terms, if the quality comparability, nonclinical data, and the human PK study demonstrate similarity, a further therapeutics equivalence study to demonstrate comparable safety and efficacy would not be needed. However, if minor differences with the reference medicinal product are identified, this study might be necessary to address their impact on safety and efficacy, as the pharmacokinetics and intracellular fate *in vivo* of these products are not fully understood, and demonstration of similar plasma concentrations of iron might not necessarily correlate with therapeutic performance. End points to be considered include ferritin, transferrin saturation, hemoglobin, total iron dose administered over study, and total EPO dose administered over study. Safety end points could include anaphylactoid reaction rate, nontransferring-bound iron (NTBI), overall adverse event rate, markers of oxidative stress, and free radical activity.

Iron products can cause hypersensitivity or other reactions that can, in rare cases, be severe. In addition, the potential release of free, unbound iron may produce both short-term and chronic toxic effects due to oxidative stress. Therefore, product characterization is required with respect to the labile iron present at the time of administration and the stability of the formulation in plasma.

20.7 International Landscape and Convergence on Nanomedicines

Since early 2000 the potential of nanotechnology in the field of medical sciences has been evident, and various regions [24] of the world invested significant [25] effort in fostering the fundamental sciences that converge in nanotechnology both individually and via common endeavors such as the International Organization for Standardization (ISO) and the Organization for Economic Co-operation and Development (OECD) work for standardization and harmonization of methods. A number of studies have been published showing a variable landscape of the main actors in nanotechnology, ranging from Academic centers to startups, spin-offs, and small- and medium-size enterprises and of the funding [26] made available to this multidisciplinary, versatile, and fully evolving science, with China on the research and development lead, followed closely by the United States, and then by Japan, Germany, and the European Union. Until recently in Europe, the main body of R&D advances of nanotechnology in life sciences was happening at the level of research Institutes and Academic centers, while in the United States, the balance was toward health technology enterprises.

The impact of nanotechnology on the public health sector has been gradually growing over the years, but with a clear gap between discovery and translation in health products, thus with a limited number of nanomedicines having been approved in the European Union and globally [27]. However, in view of the increasing numbers of clinical trials ongoing in areas of high public health burden (cancer, diabetes, disorders of the immune system, viral diseases, and rare diseases) and of the convergence between nanotechnology and other main advances in science and technology such as discoveries in molecular pathways, immunology, omics sequencing, and manipulation techniques, it is expected that the rate of translation of products (both nanomedicines and medical devices) will increase significantly in terms of numbers and variety. Late in 2007, the Agency joined international reflection hosted by the FDA on how to define the characteristics of medicines based on nanotechnology, in conjunction with experts of other Regulatory Agencies from the United States, Japan, Canada, and Australia. The group discussed and shared information on relevant on-going guidelines [28] and scientific and legislative initiatives in the various Regions. An exchange of information and experiences also started bringing fruitful learning from neighboring frameworks such as cosmetics, medical devices, and consumers' products at large. The groups, chaired by the Agency, also developed a working descriptor of nanomedicines for "internal use" so that the different authorities across the world could share experience and discuss each other's approach to the regulation of the field and ensure that development of the regulatory science would be complementary and open to input from other actors in the field (e.g., the work of the ISO Technical Committee 299 dedicated to Nanotechnologies). Building on the collective effort of the international expert group, the Agency organized on 2–3 September 2010 the First International scientific workshop on nanomedicines [29]. Some 200 European and international participants from 27 countries, including Australia, Canada, India, Japan, and the United States, discussed benefits and challenges arising from the application of nanotechnologies to medicines. Participants also included representatives from patients' organizations, health care professionals' organizations, academia, regulatory authorities, and the pharmaceutical industry.

In the context of the international collaboration, a reflection paper of block copolymer micelles, jointly developed by experts from Japanese regulatory authority (Pharmaceuticals and Medical Devices Agency (PMDA) and the Ministry of Health, Labour, and Welfare (MHLW) and EMA: this is the first reflection paper in the field addressing a next-generation type of system nanomedicine not yet authorized in any Region, but that entered exploratory

Table 20.4 Nonexhaustive list of block copolymer micelles in clinical trials.

Trade name	Incorporated drug	Polymer	Phase in clinical trials	Indication
SP1049C-202-UK	Doxorubicin	PEO-b-PPO-b-PEO	Phase II	Adenocarcinoma of the easophagus
Paxceed™	Palclitaxel	PLA-b-mPEG	Phase II	Rheumatoid arthritis
Genexol™-PM	Paclitaxel	PLA-b-PEG	Phase III	Metastatic breast or advanced pancreatic cancer

clinical trials in Europe and other Regions for the treatment of solid cancers (Table 20.4)[12].

In 2015, the International Pharmaceuticals Regulatory Forum (IPRF) took on board the establishment and governance of the International nanomedicines expert group enriched with the support of many Regional authorities, including FDA, Health Canada, Japan, Swiss medic, the Association of Southeast Asian Nations (ASEAN), and the Brazilian regulatory Agency (National Health Surveillance Agency or ANVISA (Agência Nacional de Vigilância Sanitária), among others. The newly established IPRF Nanomedicines Working Group[13] got the mandate of sharing nonconfidential information, promoting consensus findings on regulatory standards and convergence focused on nanomedicines/nanomaterial in drug products and borderline and combination products. Regulatory cooperation includes work sharing, in specific areas with other related international bodies and collaboration of training organization. Of note is that in 2016, for the first time information and mapping [30] of the activity on nanomedicines in the participating regions has been made available, providing a precious starting point for understanding current regulations and points of potential convergence on most critical issues. Deliverables for the 2015/2016 work plan include

- information sharing and mapping (annual regulatory updates);
- compilation, mapping, and discussion on terminology and definitions with focus on the classification of nanomedicines/nanotechnology in drug products;
- compilation of information for understanding synergies between the nanomedicine safety and nanomedicine toxicology fields;
- compilation of investigations required for "generic" nanomedicines/nanotechnology in drug products used in regulatory procedures;

12) List of the European Medicines Agency's scientific guidelines on nanomedicines. Available at http://www.ema.europa.eu/ema/index.jsp?curl=pages/regulation/general/general_content_000564.jsp&mid=WC0b01ac05806403e0.
13) IPRF Nanomedicines Working Group Mandate. Available at https://www.i-p-r-f.org/en/working-groups/nanomedicines-working-group/.

- mapping and exchange of requirements for nanomedicine/nanotechnology in drug product class specific guidance (e.g., liposomal formulations); and
- exchange and mapping of general Critical Quality Attributes (CQA) principles for nanomedicines/nanotechnology in drug products.

20.8 Conclusions and Way Forward

The current European regulatory framework is adequate to ensure the oversight of current nanomedicines. Regulatory science shall address the challenges of next-generation nanomedicines answering the fundamental question of how the established principles of benefit/risk analysis, can be enriched by the advances in the understanding of nanotechnology properties, especially considering the high potential of nanomedicines to address with a wide range of different, efficient, and innovative approaches the many unmet medical needs [31].

However, because of the multidisciplinary nature of nanotechnology [32] and the anticipated complexity of next-generation nanomedicines [33,34], it is recommended that emerging and specific issues [35] related to manufacturing, quality, safety and efficacy, and clinical use of novel nanomedicines are addressed from the regulatory science perspective, via the platforms available to ensure smooth transition from research to development and to patients' access.

While a single global technical definition applicable to all nanomedicines may not feasible or useful at this time, it is important to emphasize that in the European Union there exists the commitment and a single strategy to support innovation. The Agency shall work together with the innovators to ensure that clarity is given about the applicable regulatory framework to the new nanosystems, whether pharmaceutical or medical device, in view of the fact that requirements and support available varies significantly in the two domains, and integration of experiences and knowledge will often be necessary for successful development and patients' benefits. Under the current legislation, the mechanism of action is key to the decision on whether a product should be regulated as a medicinal product or a medical device (Directive 2001/83/EC, Article 1.2 (b)); for example, a nanoproduct with a primary physical action would fall under the medical devices regulation. The emerging complexity of nanomedicines may lead to borderline cases where the boundary between medical device and medicinal product may be more difficult to determine, for example, devices for administering medicinal products where the device and the medicinal product form a single integral product designed to be used exclusively in the given combination and which are not reusable or refillable [36], or where there is a combination of multiple modes of action with which neither mode is secondary to the other [37]. The differences in regulation between the medicinal products and medical devices are extensive[14] [38,39]. Developers of novel medical

14) European Commission Medical Devices Regulatory framework webpage. Available at http://ec.europa.eu/health/medical-devices/regulatory-framework/index_en.htm.

products moving from research to development should understand which requirements would be applicable to their technologies.

Sponsors of novel nanomedicines are therefore urged to seek the support available via the Innovation Task Force[15] at an early stage, and the newly established EU Innovation Offices Network (European Union Medicines Agencies Network Strategy to 2020 – Working together to improve health) to discuss and plan for Regulatory and Scientific advice at individual national or EU level on the strategy for development and follow up advices on the acceptability of methodologies.

The Agency's tools for opinion making are proven to be the main avenues to development success and patients' access [40]. Early dialog is crucial to support innovation not only in Europe but also in the context of global medicines development [41] for the benefit of global health and to inform international convergence in policies and regulatory requirements.

References

1 European Medicines Agency (2015) The Committee for Orphan Medicinal Products (COMP) is the committee at the European Medicines Agency that is responsible for reviewing applications from people or companies seeking'orphan-medicinal-product designation'. This designation is for medicines to be developed for the diagnosis, prevention or treatment of rare diseases that are life-threatening or very serious. Available at http://www.ema.europa.eu/ema/index.jsp?curl=pages/about_us/general/general_content_000263.jsp&mid=WC0b01ac0580028e30.

2 European Medicines Agency (2006) The Pediatric Committee (PDCO) is the committee at the European Medicines Agency that is responsible for assessing the content of pediatric investigation plans and adopting opinions on them. This includes assessing applications for full or partial waivers and assessing applications for deferrals. The PDCO was established in accordance with the Pediatric Regulation (Regulation (EC) 1901/2006. Available at http://www.ema.europa.eu/ema/index.jsp?curl=pages/about_us/general/general_content_000265.jsp&mid=WC0b01ac0580028e9d.

3 European Medicines Agency (2004) The Committee for Medicinal Products for Human Use (CHMP) is responsible for preparing the Agency's opinions on all questions concerning medicines for human use, in accordance with Regulation (EC) No 726/2004. Available at http://www.ema.europa.eu/ema/index.jsp?curl=pages/about_us/general/general_content_000094.jsp&mid=WC0b01ac0580028c79.

4 Ehmann, F. *et al.* (2013) Gatekeepers and enablers: how drug regulators respond to a challenging and changing environment by moving toward a proactive attitude. *Clin. Pharmacol. Ther.* **93**(5), 425–432.

5 Butcher, Neville J. *et al.* (2016) Drug delivery: unravelling the stealth effect. *Nat. Nanotechnol.*, **11** (4), 310–331.

6 EU (2011) Commission recommendation of 18 October 2011 on the definition of nanomaterial (2011/696/EU). *OJ.*, **275**, 38–40.

7 Ogawa, K. *et al.* (2014) Recent patent applications in three-dimensional cell culture. *Nat. Biotechnol.*, **32**, 1004.

15) ITF webpage. Available at http://www.ema.europa.eu/ema/index.jsp?curl=pages/regulation/general/general_content_000334.jsp&mid=WC0b01ac05800ba1d9.

8 Chou, H.Y. *et al.* (2010) Hydrogel-delivered GM-CSF overcomes nonresponsiveness to hepatitis B vaccine through the recruitment and activation of dendritic cells. *J. Immunol.*, **185**, 5468–5475.

9 Buonaguro, L. *et al.* (2011) Developments in virus-like particle-based vaccines for infectious diseases and cancer. *Expert Rev. Vaccines*, **10**, 1569–1583.

10 Veiseh, O. *et al.* (2015) Managing diabetes with nanomedicine: challenges and opportunities. *Nat. Rev. Drug Discov.*, **14**, 45–57.

11 MagForce (2016) Mag Force a nanomedicine company. Available at http://www.magforce.de/en/home.html (accessed Jan. 2016).

12 Nanobiotix (2016) Nanobiotix a nanomedicine company. http://www.nanobiotix.com/news/ (accessed Jan. 2016).

13 Jennings, G.T. and Bachmann, M.F. (2009) Immunodrugs: therapeutic VLP-based vaccines for chronic diseases. *Annu. Rev. Pharmacol. Toxicol.*, **49**, 303–326.

14 Global survey of companies pursuing 'nanomedicine' indicating that nanotechnology is taking root in the drug and medical device industry. Wagner, V., Dullaart, A., Bock, A.K., and Zweck, A. (2006) The emerging nanomedicine landscape. *Nat. Biotechnol.*, **24** (10), 1211–1217.

15 European Medicines Agency (2006) Reflection paper on nanotechnology-based medicinal products for Human Use. Available at http://www.ema.europa.eu/docs/en_GB/document_library/Regulatory_and_procedural_guideline/2010/01/WC500069728.pdf.

16 European Medicines Agency (2013) Reflection paper on the data requirements for intravenous liposomal products developed with reference to an innovator liposomal product. Available at http://www.ema.europa.eu/docs/en_GB/document_library/Scientific_guideline/2013/03/WC500140351.pdf.

17 European Medicines Agency (2015) Reflection paper on the data requirements for intravenous iron-based nano-colloidal products developed with reference to an innovator medicinal product. Available at http://www.ema.europa.eu/docs/en_GB/document_library/Scientific_guideline/2015/03/WC500184922.pdf.

18 European Medicines Agency (2013) Reflection paper on surface coatings: general issues for consideration regarding parenteral administration of coated nanomedicine products. Available at http://www.ema.europa.eu/docs/en_GB/document_library/Scientific_guideline/2013/08/WC500147874.pdf.

19 Ehmann, F. *et al.* (2013) Next-generation nano-medicines and nanosimilars: EU regulators' initiatives relating to the development and evaluation of nanomedicines. *Nanomedicine (Lond.)*, **8** (5), 849–856.

20 Mühlebach, Stefan *et al.* (2015) Regulatory challenges and approaches to characterize nanomedicines and their follow-on similars. *Nanomedicine*, **10** (4), 659–674.

21 Bartlett, J.A. *et al.* (2015) Summary report of PQRI workshop on nanomaterial in drug products: current experience and management of potential risks. *AAPS J.*, **17** (1), 44–64.

22 Clinical Nanomedicine and Targeted Medicine (2016) Enabling technologies for personalized medicine. Available at https://www.clinam.org/images/stories/pdf/conference.pdf.

23 European Medicines Agency (2015) Data requirements for intravenous iron-based nano-colloidal products developed with reference to an innovator medicinal product. Available at http://www.ema.europa.eu/ema/index.jsp?curl=pages/regulation/general/general_content_000564.jsp&mid=WC0b01ac05806403e0.

24 DeFrancesco, L. (2003) Little science, big bucks. *Nat. Biotechnol.*, **21**, 1127–1129.

25 Hullmann, A. (2006) Who is winning the global nanorace? *Nat. Nanotechnol.*, **1**, 81–83.

26 Shapira, P. and Wang, J. (2010) Follow the money. *Nature*, **468**, 627–628.

27 Betty, Y.S. and Kim, M.D. (2010) Nanomedicine. *N. Engl. J. Med.*, **363**, 2434–2443.

28 FDA (2014) Guidance for industry considering whether an FDA-regulated

product involves the application of nanotechnology. Available at http://www.fda.gov/RegulatoryInformation/Guidances/ucm257698.htm.

29 European Medicines Agency's workshop on nanomedicines (2009) http://www.ema.europa.eu/ema/index.jsp?curl=pages/news_and_events/events/2009/12/event_detail_000095.jsp&mid=WC0b01ac058004d5c3.

30 IPRF Nanomedicines Working group (2016) Information sharing and mapping. Available at https://www.i-p-r-f.org/files/7414/5387/7778/IPRF_Nanomedicines_WG_-_info_mapping_Jan2016.pdf.

31 Papaluca, M. *et al.* (2015) White spots in pharmaceutical pipelines–EMA identifies potential areas of unmet medical needs. *Expert Rev. Clin. Pharmacol.*, **8** (3), 353–360.

32 Porter, A.L. and Youtie, J. (2009) Where does nanotechnology belong in the map of science? *Nat. Nanotechnol.*, **4** (9), 534–536. doi: 10.1038/nnano.2009.207

33 Jhaveri, A.M. *et al.* (2014) Multifunctional polymeric micelles for delivery of drugs and siRNA. *Pharmacol.*, **5**, 77.

34 Rizzo, L.Y. *et al.* (2013) Recent progress in nanomedicine: therapeutic, diagnostic and theranostic applications. *Curr. Opin. Biotechnol.*, **24** (6), 1159–1166.

35 Bowman, D.M. and Gatof, J. (2015) Reviewing the regulatory barriers for nanomedicine: global questions and challenges. *Nanomedicine*, **10** (21), 3275–3286.

36 MHRA (2013) Guidance on legislation – borderlines between medical devices and medicinal products. Available at http://www.mhra.gov.uk/home/groups/dts-bs/documents/publication/con286964.pdf.

37 Lebourgeois, C. (2008) Device and drug combination products: a new regulatory, reimbursement and marketing challenge. Lifescience Online.

38 Parvizi, N. and Woods, K. (2014) Regulation of medicines and medical devices: contrasts and similarities. *Clin. Med.*, **14** (1), 6–12.

39 Chowdhury, N. (2010) Regulation of nanomedicines in the EU: distilling lessons from the pediatric and the advanced therapy medicinal products approaches. *Nanomedicine (Lond)*, **5** (1), 135–142.

40 Hofer, M.P., Jakobsson, C., Zafiropoulos, N., Vamvakas, S., Vetter, T., Regnstrom, J., and Hemmings, R.J. (2015) Regulatory watch: impact of scientific advice from the European Medicines Agency. *Nat. Rev. Drug Discov.*, **14** (5), 302–303.

41 Noorlander, C.W. *et al.* (2015) Horizon scan of nanomedicinal products. *Nanomedicine*, **10**, 1599–1608.

21
Social Studies of Nanopharmaceutical Research

Michael Schillmeier

University of Exeter, Department of Sociology & Philosophy, Amory Building, Rennes Drive, Exeter, EX4 4RJ, UK

21.1
Engaging with Ethical, Legal, and Social Implications of Nanoresearch

Since the Human Genome Project in the 1990s, ELSI accounts (i.e., the discussions of ethical, legal, and social implications of science and technology) have gained substantial importance and have drawn attention to the "coproduction" [1] of science, technology, and society [2]. ELSI accounts echo a long tradition of engaging with social, historical, political, and philosophical issues regarding the development of science and technology. Moreover, since the late 1970s, "science and technology studies" (STS) have been involved in understanding the concrete problems, questions, and issues of research practices [3]. Clearly, STS and ELSI accounts play an important role in understanding the different and changing ways of how science and technology both shape and are shaped by societal organization, cultural production, and related interests and values [4].

With the emergence of nanoscience and nanotechnology, STS and ELSI accounts have discussed in detail the ethical and social issues of "nano" as well as the importance of public understanding and engagement with science and technology [5]. It is argued that "ethical considerations are the foundations of healthy progress, and must be openly participatory in their undertaking." [6] However, due to the specificities of nano and nanopharmacy, current ethical studies do not share a common perception of what the exact ethical issues are [7]. Moreover, it remains undecided if nanopharmacy challenges the canon of bioethical issues as they can be found in other emerging fields within the life sciences [8]. General ethical issues like patient's rights, autonomy and responsibility, responsible innovation, risk/benefit analysis in clinical trials, issues of missing definitions, standardization and characterization, global challenges of regulation [9], human enhancement, misuse of medical technologies and bioterrorism, environmental safety, and so on dominate current ethical debates and

Pharmaceutical Nanotechnology: Innovation and Production, First Edition. Edited by Jean Cornier, Arno Kwade, Andrew Owen, and Marcel Van de Voorde.

are hardly novel concerns. Still, it is important not to act as if ethical issues of nanopharmacy can be deferred to more general debates about bioethics. Ethical issues are part of the specificity of every research agenda, the more so if it is governed by a myriad of uncertainties and possible risks as is the case with nanotechnological research [10].

A crucial set of ethical issues, next to the ones briefly mentioned above, concerns the questions of higher costs, affordability, equal accessibility, and distribution of clinically available nanomedicines. Hall *et al.* [11] have argued that "the higher costs of the clinically available nanodrugs may be attributed more to the fact that they are "newer" and more effective than their pharmaceutical principles alone, with the added manufacturing costs playing a minor role." Although an ethical problem in itself, it poses a more general ethical question concerning the affordability, accessibility, and distribution of nanopharmaceuticals. I suggest that a general *ethos* should foster the idea of "good" nanopharmacy. The ethos I propose could read as follows: *What appears as good nanopharmacy for the poor is equally good for those who are better off, or consider themselves more privileged.* Moreover, nanopharmacy also needs to engage with the limits of the ethics of Big Pharma as well as the problem of "institutional corruption and the pharmaceutical industry" [12].

21.2
Nanopharmacy and the "Culture of Promise"

The French philosopher of science and mathematician Michel Serres has argued that the object of science is not a given, but it is science that creates its objects and, if necessary, desists from them. The objects of science generate the "horizon of knowledge" and related research processes and practices that define what kind of objects become part of science and which are excluded. Moreover, as we know from the history of pharmaceutical research, even a well-functioning medicine is never a finished "best" product, but is always open for improvement. Thus, in many ways the scientific "object is project" as Serres has put it bluntly [13].

Undoubtedly, the objects of nanopharmacy (as well as the question of ethics) are very much projects. In the case of chemotherapeutics, for instance, such projects span a horizon of innovative pharmacological thoughts from the late nineteenth century up to now. This can be seen in Paul Ehrlich's idea of targeted drug delivery via a "magic bullet," [14] which was advocated in 1906 and still plays a vital role in imagining current project-objects in nanopharmacy [15].

With the "project-objects" in pharmacy comes a "culture of promise" to provide medical and pharmaceutical improvements and benefits for the treatment of diseases [16]. The "culture of promise" gained temporary climax by highlighting the revolutionary prospect of delivering drugs and nanomedicines measurable in a nanometer size range. It was meant to lead to improved pharmacokinetics and pharmacodynamics, which in turn ought to enable more specific, efficient, less toxic, and lower cost medicines for the majority of diseases and their multiple side effects. Although improvements in pharmacological research and related visions contribute to effective healthcare practices, the excessive culture of promise in nanotechnology research have set unrealistic targets and even have been counterproductive for nanopharmaceutical research itself if the promised results and goals could not be met.

This asymmetry between promise and actuality creates a problem that risks becoming a source of distrust in nanopharmaceutical research. The more so if it promotes an unconsidered and iterative slogan of "fast science" and its science policies that make absent concrete problems and issues of specific research investigations on a nanoscale [16]. Hence, the "culture of promise" is not just an innocent attribution of the "goodwill" of science, but also deeply affects how research is carried out as a matter of fast science. The latter comprises the shortening of research projects, the pressure of the "publish or perish" ideology, the dominant interest of publishing merely positive results and obscuring negative ones or "dead ends," the increasing power of economic reasoning that governs scientific research practices, and so on.

All these requirements of fast science may be at odds with the demands of what I like to call "good translation" in nanopharmacological research. Good translation includes, for instance, precise characterization of a new drug formulation as well as the reproducibility of an experimental design to meet the standards of a stable and consistent medicine, but also the full recognition that nanopharmacy is not an independent research activity but assembles a wide range of scientific and nonscientific actors. All these actors need to gain an equal stake in nanopharmacy. In addition, all procedures and interactions with heterogeneous actors and their interest and expertise require a *slowing down* rather than a *speeding up of* scientific practices. Unfortunately, however, the agenda of fast science and the related "culture of promise" have nothing creative to contribute. On the contrary, this prevailing policy reinforces the fierce rules of accelerating and intensifying global competition rather than aiming at good translation. To be sure, competition is good as long as it allows us to respond to and address, in a *responsible* way, the requirements of novel fields of research such as nanopharmaceutical agendas, in which the application of good pharmaceutical solutions to a medical issue is an ongoing project rather an accomplished goal.

21.3
From "Science Meets Society" to Translation as a Social Process

Responsible research has to focus on *improving* the translational processes of nanopharmaceutical medicines for all actors involved – from bench to bedside. This also means that the notion of "translation," which focuses on applied research in healthcare and gained widespread recognition in fast science accounts, needs reconsideration. First, and most importantly, the notion of translation should not be conflated with a smooth process of linear progression or "best way" of research development. Rather, we find at every step of nanopharmaceutical research different processes of translation that can be better understood as complications that arise from their application. Complications start with the prospect of immature and often unrealistic ideas that turn into a concrete research question, which may develop into preclinical *in vitro* experimentation that, if the researcher is lucky, may translate into *in vivo* experimentation. This may further translate into a cascade of clinical trials and, if successful, into an approved nanomedicine, which then translates into a prescription of a drug that translates into different effects while interacting with different and changing physiology as well as (possibly) with other prescribed drugs. This long and interlaced sentence portrays awkwardly but adequately the high probability that ideas may not translate into applicable end products. However, it also tells us that there is no way of cutting this process short if we wish to improve given medicines.

Moreover, the nanopharmaceutical process of translation relates cognitive objects (ideas) with material experimentation, molecular processes with cells and organisms, animal models with human bodies, the laboratory with other laboratories, assets with computers, pharmacology and toxicology [17], the laboratory with the clinic, laboratory experimentation with highly specific patient needs, the characterization of nano-objects with regulatory challenges and requirements, nanomaterials with ethical challenges and philosophical reflection, pharmaceutical efficacy with economic reasoning and political interests, and so forth. It assembles what I like to call the *social complexity of nanopharmacy*, which relates and composes heterogeneous processes and actors, requirements, and obligations [18]. Moreover, each process of translation may feed back on earlier stages of translation and alter their understanding and composition. Untranslatability or failures of translation may provoke novel forms of experimental practices that suggest new forms of translation that may entail unexpected results or undesirable side effects.

Hence, each process of translation links as well as creates different processes and materialities, different requirements, different obligations, and different trials that decide upon the quality of the research project-object and its future. Thus, translation refers to a set of practices that constantly alters the processes and objects involved. Each phase of translation presents a *complication* and thus adds complexity to the overall process of nanopharmaceutical research and usage. It assembles a process of multiple translations, which although not comparable, aim to compose compatible relations across and with different scales of action (nano/micro/macro).

It is of the utmost importance that social studies of nanopharmacy engage with and analyze the myriad of translations as they become apparent in current research activities. Accordingly, social studies of nanopharmacy are not restricted to the rather abstract and misleading idea of "science meets society" as put forward by the rhetoric of fast science, as if "science" and "society" refer to two different spaces of reality. It doesn't help "science" much when merely informing the nonscientific audience about work in order to gain trust and recognition. As Weitze and Heckl [19] have argued, the corresponding idea of "public understanding of science," which suggests that society lacks understanding and thus "proper information and explanation could bring together science and society," has been "proven to be empirically wrong." It appears similarly abstract and misconceived to argue that it is the society that needs to critically assess the effects of science from the outside.

The idea of "public engagement with science" advocates a different route, which is not *about* science, but a way to collaborate, practice, and experiment *with* science, although the experimental practices differ from the laboratory experimentation. As I have argued elsewhere, the concept of "publics," as envisaged by authors like John Dewey, Walter Lippman, and others, offers an innovative way of engaging with scientific practice and emerging technologies, linking lab experimentation with all the relevant actors (e.g., patients, clinicians, researchers, regulators, concerned citizens, NGOs, policy makers, industry, and so forth) who are concerned with a specific nanomedical or nanopharmaceutical issue:

> Nanomedical publics bring together people (and their practices and objects) who share a concern for an issue for which no immediate answers and fixed solutions are given (or can be expected). Publics, then, engage with the ambiguities and uncertainties of scientific research practices, their relevant objects of concern and their possible effects inside and outside the scientific laboratory [20].

Generally speaking, social studies of nanopharmacy are obliged to care about all the different processes of translation as they may occur in the development and usage of nanomedicines. In that sense, social studies of nanopharmacy involve the analysis and collaboration with all the diverse actors – ideas and materials, human and nonhuman, scientific and social scientific, scientific and nonscientific, bodies and technologies, the clinic and patients – as necessary mediators, who/which affect and are affected by nanopharmaceutical research.

21.4 Metaphors and Nanopharmacy

Social studies of nanopharmacy also suggest that the way we imagine and talk about research issues and objects has a significant impact on how nanomedicines are produced as well as how health and illness is understood. Current studies of nanopharmacy underline that the prevailing idea of the "magic bullet" and the related "culture of promise" of nanopharmacy and nanomedicine mirror "the engineering values of control, precision, efficiency, and surveillance" which are "dominantly framed in terms of *military metaphors*" [21–23]. STS scholar Sacha Loeve states that

> in the current context of crisis of pharmaceutical innovation, military metaphors do provide a persuasive means to sustain a climate of 'general mobilisation' similar to wartime. In using them, researchers, start-ups, clinicians and patients may feel that despite their diverse stakes and interests, they take part in a crusade in which they are all united – both the crusaders and the crusaded (i.e. patients) – against a common enemy [24].

For Loeve, military or ballistic metaphors are poorly chosen to account for the different processes of how nanoparticles interact with changing environments. They underestimate the body being an active, dynamic, and heterogeneous system. The military metaphor not only transports a rather under-complex understanding of disease and the body, it also configures the patient as a "fighter" and thus plays a powerful, but also ambivalent description both of experiencing illnesses (like cancer) and its modes of medical engagement [24]. However, Loeve also notes that current nanopharmaceutical and nanomedical research agendas are informed by a change from military metaphors toward "ecological" metaphors as well as a wide range of nonmilitary metaphors used by patient experiences of their illness ("journey," "dance," "drama"). Hence, the multiplication of metaphors refers (1) to more complex, diverse, and individually experienced understandings of disease and the body, (2) to the social and cultural dimensions of illness, (3) to the changing medical ways of dealing with and caring about disease, and (4) to an understanding of nanopharmaceutical objects as milieu-dependent medicines [24].

In such a reading, metaphors in nanopharmacy are historically changing tools of understanding, shaping, and engaging with health and illness in research and clinical practices. Thus, the employment of different metaphors mirrors and evokes different developments and cultures of nanomedicines [25,26]. They may contribute to a more complex and thus more realistic understanding of illness, related processes of interacting human bodies, and the relevance of changing and diverse (inner and outer) environments. Clearly, the ideas of "being at war with" or the "magic bullet" offer rather under-complex and limited imaginaries to do so. Vincent and Loeve [27] rightly stress that "addressing drugs to a specific site and releasing the right dose in the right place at the right moment in the complex environment of a living body requires more than a magic bullet."

21.5
Nanopharmacy and "Personalized Medicine"

The nanopharmaceutical promise entails the prospect of moving from the development of highly standardized "block buster" and "one size fits all" pharmaceutics toward targeting the precise nanomedical formulas and doses that reflect the *individual situation of illness(es)*, its differences in disease emergence and its idiosyncratic responses to treatments.

This promised relationship between nanopharmaceutical development and personalized medicine is thought to promote and further unfold a new "episteme" [28] in medicine, that is, a way of locating and understanding diseases and patients as well a the fundamental reorganization of healthcare in general [29,30]. However, as the STS scholar and philosopher Xavier Guchet and others have shown recently, the relationship between nanomedicine, nanopharmacy, and personalized medicine is not straightforward. Rather, it assembles *polysemic* understandings and conflicting expectations of/from personalized medicine and articulates controversies over the concrete meaning of "person" and "personalization" *within* biomedical research agendas [31]. Moreover, personalized nanopharmacy needs to pay attention to the increasing importance given to research findings in epigenetics, which highlight the significance of different and shifting human/environment relationships in understanding individual disease formation and their effects [32]. Up to now, it remains unresolved whether the progress in personalized nanopharmacy will compliment and improve novel developments of "patient-centered" forms of care or if it merely extends the current trend of the technomolecular gaze in medicine and, thus strengthens the biomedicalization and individualization of disease at the expense of social and patient centered models of healthcare.

The future of personalized nanopharmacy is imagined to "enhance[s] the autonomy of the patient and user by giving them more control, but at the same time shifts responsibility and liability to the service providers and product developers as the medical professionals slowly move out of the picture" [33,34]. Such a technologically mediated individualism unfolds the neoliberal figure of the competent and self-responsible individual. In effect, medical power becomes partly disentangled from the medical profession and is instead distributed among technological and market-driven networks, as well as clever and autonomous individuals [34]. Clearly, such a technocratic perspective through which the patient becomes a rational "user" of technologies and the "client" of service providers not only creates the neoliberal myth of the autonomous patient, but also presupposes the autonomous, rational, capable, and well-connected individual.

By installing the "healthy," able, and autonomous person, the image of technologically mediated pharmacy and medicine makes absent the everyday life of experiencing illness and the associated requirements and obligations. The prevailing argument that nanotechnological advances in medicine and pharmacy shift the responsibility from the medical system to the individual who is thereby thought to gain autonomy, is a rather problematic assumption of facets of a neoliberal discourse that requires the "autonomous subject" for its reasoning and economy driven strategies. It also assumes a rather simplistic, one-sided, and normative understanding of technology as a fixed tool of improvement and enhancement. By making this point clear I do not wish to downplay the importance of patients gaining their own voice or the possibilities of technological advance in pharmacy and healthcare settings. Quite the contrary, the future of personalized nanopharmacy cannot do without a shift toward an in-depth view of the situated and specific requirements of patients' needs as well as the perspectives and experiences of the different patients. We need to empower patients and patient groups to engage with medical and pharmacological research in the prevention, diagnosis, and treatment of diseases. Cleary, the engagement of patients with nanopharmacological research and application is not well established and needs novel spaces of interaction between patients, interested citizens, research agendas, medical practice, the pharmacy, and the clinic. It needs to be observed with vigilant eyes if and how strategies of propagating biomolecular understandings of health and illness will create empowering experiences of the individual or if it just names the shift from medical to more technocratic forms of power.

Although the patients play an important role in the current nanomedical rhetoric, they rarely play an active part in the nanopharmaceutical research processes. Rather, they remain merely vulnerable individuals in the course of clinical trials and clinical practices. They may also become victims of disillusion suffering from a "culture of promise" that promises unrealistic results that cannot be achieved in a short period of time. The constructive role of patients and patient advocacy groups is vital, precisely when (object and technologically mediated) risks and uncertainties dominate the diagnosis and the treatment of diseases with nanopharmaceuticals that not only treat diseases, but also unfold a wide range of uncertainties and risks [35]. Emerging risks and uncertainties that cannot be adequately dealt with by the prevailing rationalist model of risk/benefit analysis of science *troubles* the relationship between patient, nanopharmaceutical treatment, and the classical idea of informed consent. As Timmermanns *et al.* [36] have pointed out: "As long as nanopharmaceuticals are associated with risks, but also with significant uncertainty and ignorance ('unknown unknowns'), it may prove as an impossible task to inform affected persons adequately."

In such a situation where middle- and long-term effects and possible acute individual side-effects may be unknowingly produced by pharmaceuticals, for which nanopharmacy can not offer a reliable risk/benefit analysis and established treatments, the individual (or a subgroup) becomes the bearer of "second order risks" that escape the scientific reasoning of calculable probabilities [37]. Second order risks are those uncertainties and risks that are produced by the progress of our current institutions, for which at the same time no institutionalized remedies are available if they produce adverse effects.

21.6 Concluding Remarks

Although there is a long-standing and growing body of fine empirical and conceptual studies on science and technologies including the social studies of nanoscience, nanotechnology, and nanomedicine, it should be critically noted that scientists have little awareness of these literatures. Cooperations between the different fields of nanoresearch and STS or ELSI projects are primarily motivated by current requests for grant applications and directives of science policymakers and rarely born directly from research issues and problems. It should also be noted that the idea of converging technologies and the demand for transdisciplinary work, necessary for an adequate understanding of nanoscaled processes in medicine and pharmacy, does not include social sciences and STS. However, it seems to me that the time is more than ripe for transdisciplinary research agendas to include from the very beginning the cooperation with social sciences, and invest in diverse forms of public engagement [38]. The engagement of and with a plurality of actors – scientific and nonscientific – should not be seen as an obstacle but, rather, should be internalized as the ultimate basis for a collectively responsible process of scientific experimentation. Nanopharmacy can play a pioneering role in rethinking scientific practices understood as a social accomplishment that engages in the inclusion of *all* relevant and interested actors involved in emerging healthcare technologies and novel research practices.

References

1 Jasanoff, Sh. (ed.) (2004) *States of Knowledge: The Co-Production of Science and the Social Order*, Routledge, London.

2 Schillmeier, M. (2015) What ELSI/A makes big and small in nanotechnology research, in *Absence in Science, Security and Policy: From Research Agendas to Global Strategies* (eds B. Rappert and B. Palmer), Palgrave Macmillan, Houndmills, UK, pp. 55–77.

3 (a) Knorr-Cetina, K. (1995) Laboratory studies: the cultural approach to the study of science, in *Handbook of Science and Technology Studies* (eds Sh. Jasanoff *et al.*), Sage, London, pp. 140–166. (b) Latour, B. (1987) *Science in Action: How to Follow Scientists and Engineers through Society*, Harvard University Press, Cambridge, MA. (c) Latour, B. (1988) *The Pasteurization of France*, Harvard University Press, Cambridge, MA. (d) Latour, B. and Woolgar, St. (1986) *Laboratory Life: The Construction of Scientific Facts*, Princeton University Press, Princeton (originally published in 1979).

4 (a) The literature is vast, but for an introduction, see, for example, Gibbons, M., Limoges, C., Nowotny, H., Schwartzmann, S., Scott, P., and Trow, M. (1994) *The New Production of Knowledge: The Dynamics of Science and Research in Contemporary Societies*, Sage, Los Angeles. (b) Nowotny, H., Scott, P., and Gibbons, M. (2001) *Rethinking Science, Knowledge and the Public in the Age of Uncertainty*, Polity, London. (c) Keller, E.F. (2002) *The Century of the Gene*, Harvard University Press, Harvard. (d) Rheinberger, H.J. (2010) *An Epistemology of the Concrete: Twentieth-Century Histories of Life*, Duke University Press, Durham.

5 (a) For a brief but critical summative discussion, see Schillmeier, M. (2015) What ELSI/A makes big and small in nanotechnology research, in *Absence in Science, Security and Policy: From Research Agendas to Global Strategies* (eds B. Rappert and B. Palmer), Palgrave Macmillan, Houndmills, UK, pp. 55–77. (b) For a specific focus on nanomedicine, see Schillmeier, M., Barz, M., and Luxenhofer, R. (2015) Quo vadis nanomedicine? *Nanomedicine*, **10** (20/21), 3089–3091.

6 Hall, R.M., Sun, T., and Ferrari, M. (2012) A portrait of nanomedicine and its bioethical implications. *J. Law Med. Ethics*, **14** (4), 763–779.

7 (a) Timmermans, J., Zhao, Y., van den Hoven, J. (2011) Ethics and nanopharmacy: value sensitive of new drugs. *Nanoethics*, **5**, 269–283. (b) See also Costa, H.S., Sethe, S., Pego, A.P., and Olsson, A.S. (2011) Scientists' perception of ethical issues in nanomedicine. *Nanomedicine*, **6** (4), 681–691. (c) Kazemi, A., Majidinia, M., and Jamali, A.A. (2014) The question of ethics in nanomedicine. *J. Clin. Res. Bioeth.*, **5** (4), 193. (d) Resnik, D.B. and Tinkle, S.S. (2007) Ethics in nanomedicine. *Nanomedicine*, **2** (3), 345–350.
8 Kuiken, T. (2011) Nanomedicine and ethics: is there anything new or unique? *Nanobiotechnology*, **3**, 111–118.
9 Bowman, D.M. and Gatof, J. (2015) Reviewing the regulatory barriers for nanomedicine: global questions and challenges. *Nanomedicine*, **10** (21), 3275–3286.
10 See, for example, the symposium: Wolf, S.M., McCullough, J., Kahn, J.P., Jones, C. (2012) (eds) Nanodiagnostics and nanotherapeutics: building research ethics and oversight. *J. Law Med. Ethics*, **40** (4), 841–847.
11 Hall, R.M., Sun, T., and Ferrari, M. (2012) Nanomedicine and its bioethical implications. *J. Law Med. Ethics*, **40** (4), 776.
12 See, for example, the special issue Institutional corruption and the pharmaceutical industry. *J. Law Med. Ethics*, **41** (3), 544–746.
13 Serres, M. (1992) *Hermes II: Interferenz*, Merve, Berlin, p. 81 (originally published in 1972).
14 Ehrlich, P. (1960) Address delivered at the dedication of the Georg-Speyer-Haus, in *The Collected Papers of Paul Ehrlich* (ed. F. Himmelweit), Pergamon Press, London, pp. 53–63 (originally published in 1906).
15 Schillmeier, M., Barz, M., and Luxenhofer, R. (eds) (2015) Quo vadis nanomedicine? *Nanomedicine*, **10** (20/21), 3089–3091.
16 Schillmeier, M. (2015) Caring about social complexity in nanomedicine. *Nanomedicine*, **10** (20), 3181–3193.
17 See, for example, PourGashtasbi, G. (2015) Nanotoxicology and challenges of translation. *Nanomedicine*, **10** (20), 3121–3129.
18 Schillmeier, M. (2015) Caring about social complexity in nanomedicine. *Nanomedicine*, **10** (20), 3181–3193.
19 Weitze, M.-D. and Heckl, W.M. (2015) Communicating science in the making – challenges and opportunities. *Nanomedicine*, **10** (20), 3099.
20 Schillmeier, M. (2015) 3189.
21 Loeve, S. (2015) Of drug administration, war and oïkos. Mediating cancer with nanomedicines. *Nanomedicine*, **10** (21), 3261–3274.
22 Loeve, S., Vincent, B.B., and Gazeau, F. (2013) Nanomedicine metaphors: from war to care. Emergence of an ecological approach. *Nano Today*, **8** (6), 560–565.
23 See, for example, Franzen, S. and Lommel, S.A. (2009) Targeting cancer with 'smart bombs': equipping plant virus nanoparticles for a 'seek and destroy' mission. *Nanomedicine*, **4** (5), 575–588.
24 Vincent, B.B. and Loeve, S. (2014) Metaphors in nanomedicine: the case of targeted drug delivery. *Nanoethics*, **8** (1), 1–17.
25 Annas, G.J. (1995) Reframing the debate on health care reform by replacing our metaphors. *N. Engl. J. Med.*, **332** (11), 744–747.
26 Camus, J.T.W. (2009) Metaphors of cancer in scientific popularization articles in the British press. *Discourse Stud.*, **11** (4), 465–495.
27 Vincent, B.B. and Loeve, S. (2014) Metaphors in nanomedicine: the case of targeted drug delivery. *Nanoethics*, **8** (1), 1–17.
28 Foucault, M. (1973) *The Birth of the Clinic. An Archaeology of Medical Perception*, Tavistock Publications Limited, London.
29 Weston, A.D. and Hood, L. (2004) Systems biology, proteomics, and the future of health care: towards predictive, preventive, and personalized medicine introduction: paradigm changes in health care. *J. Proteome Res.*, **3**, 179–196.
30 Guchet, X. (2015) 'What's in a word? The person of personalized (Nano) medicine. *Nanomedicine*, **10** (20), 3167–3179.
31 (a) Guchet, X. (2015) 'What's in a word? The person of personalized (Nano) medicine. *Nanomedicine*, **10** (20), 3167–3179. (b) See also Pokorska-Bocci, A., Alison, St., Sagoo, G.S., Hall, A., Kroese, M.,

and Hillary, B. (2014) Personalized medicine: what's in a name? *Personal. Med.*, **11** (2), 197–210. (c) Tutton, R. (2012) Personalizing medicine: futures present and past. *Soc. Sci. Med.*, **74**, 1721–1728.

32 Chadwick, R. and O'Connor, A. (2013) Epigenetics and personalized medicine: prospects and ethical issues. *Personal. Med.*, **10** (5), 463–471.

33 Timmermans, J., Zhao, Y., and Hoven, J.v. d. (2011) Ethics and nanopharmacy: value sensitive of new drugs. *Nanoethics*, **5**, 279.

34 Kuiken, T. (2011) Nanomedicine and ethics: is there anything new or unique? *Nanobiotechnology*, **3**, 111–118.

35 See in the case of HIV and other diseases Callon, M., Lascoumes, P., and Barthe, Y. (2001) *Acting in an Uncertain World: An Essay on Technical Democracy*, The MIT Press, Cambridge/ MA./London, England.

36 Timmermans, J., Zhao, Y., and van dan Hoven, J. (2011) Ethics and nanopharmacy: value sensitive of new drugs. *Nanoethics*, **5**, 274.

37 On second order risks' that unfold beyond the modernist framework of calculative probabilities, see Beck, U. (1992) *Risk Society: Towards a New Modernity*, Sage, London.

38 See, for example, Schillmeier, M. (2015) Caring about social complexity in nanomedicine. *Nanomedicine*, **10** (20), 3181–3193.

Part Four
Pharmaceutical Applications of Nanomaterials

22
Nanoparticles for Imaging and Imaging Nanoparticles: State of the Art and Current Prospects

Thomas Maldiney[1–4] *and Nathalie Mignet*[5]

[1]*PSL Research University, Chimie ParisTech, Unité de Technologies Chimiques et Biologiques pour la Santé (UTCBS), 11 Rue Pierre et Marie Curie, 75005 Paris, France*
[2]*CNRS, UTCBS UMR 8258, 75006 Paris, France*
[3]*Université Paris Descartes, Sorbonne-Paris-Cité, UTCBS, 75006 Paris, France*
[4]*INSERM, UTCBS U 1022, 75006 Paris, France*
[5]*University Paris Descartes, Faculty of Pharmacy, 4 avenue de l' Observatoire, 75006 Paris, France*

22.1
Introduction

Nanomedicines are defined as objects of nanometric size designed for human health, either for drug delivery or imaging. Initially designed to improve drug delivery, they showed great interest in terms of drug solubility, improved pharmacokinetic, and reduced toxicity, thus improving their pharmaceutical index. These advantages have been mostly evidenced using liposomes, which were the first nanoparticles on the market. Since the evidence of these structures by Alex Bangham in 1963, numerous studies have been reported on these self-assembled nanosystems that are the most advanced materials for drug delivery in terms of clinical applications [1]. In 2015, it was not only the liposomes that reached the market. Novel nanoparticles also got approval for drug delivery as well as for diagnosis purposes, and a number of nanoparticles entered clinical trials, noticeably as active therapeutic objects.

As discussed by Weissleder and Pittet a few years ago, nanotechnologies offer a precious tool to explore the molecular pathway and singularity of cancer [2]. Indeed, they provide an experimental key to probe the complexity of biological systems and understand the physiopathological mechanisms associated with various diseases. Ever since, numerous technological advances are being investigated in order to exploit the unique optical, physical, and chemical properties of these materials within the nanometer scale [3]. As a result, nanoparticles are now largely suggested as diagnostic and contrast agents in liver, spleen, or lymphatics, the main constituents of the reticuloendothelial system [4]. Moreover,

Pharmaceutical Nanotechnology: Innovation and Production, First Edition. Edited by Jean Cornier, Arno Kwade, Andrew Owen, and Marcel Van de Voorde.

they can also enable the localization and migration studies of cells with therapeutic interests [5]. Although some doubts have been expressed about the future and clinical perspectives of nanoparticles [6], their translational potential has already been demonstrated, notably in patients with acute myocardial infarction [7]. Today, nano-objects have become part of the imaging modality, capable of bringing more information to the physician for diagnosis, treatment follow-up, and/or personalized medicine, also called companion diagnostic.

In this chapter, we were interested in both describing the nanoparticles useful for imaging and highlighting the interest of imaging to make advances in the field of nanomedicine. Initially, one of the main reasons to image nanoparticles was to understand the fate of nano-objects and obtain a rapid idea about blood resilience of nanoparticles *in vivo*. The main idea underlying these studies was the conception of nanomaterials with improved properties, such as stealthiness or targeting abilities [8,9]. These advances in nanoparticles were also made possible by the concomitant innovations in imaging techniques. Easy-to-handle systems now available in academia helped to bridge the gap between *in vitro* studies in flask or cells and *in vivo* animal studies. Until now, nanoparticles have been approved by the FDA for liver metastases diagnosis using magnetic resonance imaging (MRI) or ultrasound imaging [10]. One can expect that more nanomedicines will be approved in the near future [11], notably regarding the actual clinical trials described in the last part of this chapter.

22.2 Conception of Nanotechnologies for Imaging

Technical issues such as lack of resolution will not be improved using nanoparticles, however, sensitivity is one of the limits for which nanoparticles can bring some improvements. We recently prepared a thorough review on this topic "Nanomedicines developed to improve nonradiative imaging techniques: fluorescence, magnetic resonance imaging and ultrasound." The questions to be addressed for improving the signal are dependent on each imaging modality. Understanding the fundamentals for each modality allowed designing nanoparticles capable of increasing the signal and thus leading to a better signal-to-noise ratio [10].

22.2.1 Nanoparticles Designed for Optical Imaging

This is particularly true for fluorescence imaging due to the background obtained from endogenous proteins after applying an excitation wavelength. Distinction between excited and emitted photons, from background and labeled molecules, remains a challenge. Therefore, the molecular or nanoparticular imaging agent should present a large stokes shift (separation between excitation and emission wavelengths), be bright, emit in the near-infrared regions to limit tissue absorbance, and preferentially exhibit a lifetime longer than endogenous excited molecules. Indeed, such challenge regarding the necessity to significantly improve the signal-to-noise ratio can be met by having recourse to two main strategies, largely exploited among the scientific community.

The first strategy relies on the idea that a strong increase in the emission signal would be sufficient to gain a higher sensitive detection for *in vivo* imaging (Scheme 22.1). In this case, the autofluorescence from endogenous chromophores in the living organism is left unchanged, and efforts concentrate on improving the global optical properties of the probe, that is to say the total amount of light emerging from the nanoparticulate system. This is notably the case for quantum dots, among the most popular inorganic optical probes of the later decade, that certainly displays one of the highest quantum yields [12]. Other optical imaging agents have proven highly interesting properties and targeting efficacy, but contrary to the other nanoparticles intended for optical imaging, the emission wavelength of quantum dots can be adjusted by varying the size of the crystal core [13]. Such singular effect, also known as the quantum confinement effect, was first described in the 1980s and largely studied by physicists who investigated several applications for quantum dots in transistors, solar cells, and LEDs. Most of the commercialized quantum dots are composed of an inorganic core based on a hybrid structure comprising cadmium, selenium, tellurium, or indium. The diameter of quantum dots generally ranges from 2 to 10 nm. As an example, a 2 nm wide cadmium–selenium nanoparticle emits a luminescence signal around 475 nm when its 8 nm wide counterpart shines at 650 nm. However, the degradation products of these first semiconductors during biological applications, mainly due to the significant release of cadmium ions or other heavy metals, were shown to be responsible for irreversible cell toxicity and immune response with blood components [14]. Therefore, recent studies dealt with different cores that could present comparable properties and advantages toward degradation and biocompatibility. To this end, the cytotoxicity of quantum dots was then reduced by introducing indium-based materials or working on encapsulation of the core in order to provide a more biocompatible core–shell structure and prevent reticuloendothelial system accumulation. Despite all these efforts, the detailed biochemical and pharmacological mechanism associated with the degradation and metabolism of quantum dots *in vivo* remains unclear, hindering further clinical applications of quantum dots [15].

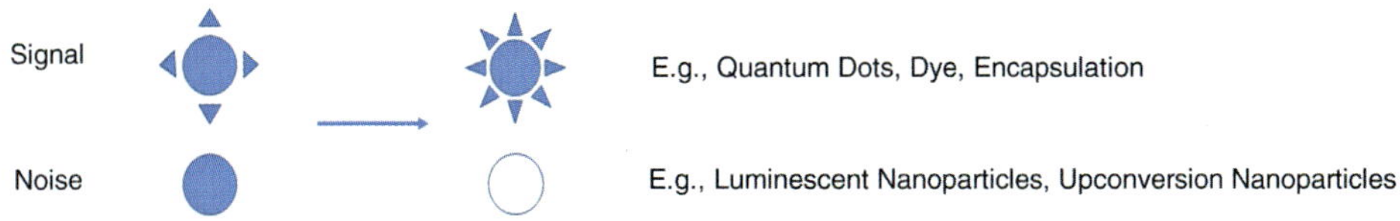

Scheme 22.1 Strategies for contrast-enhanced imaging in optical imaging. Increasing the signal-to-noise ratio either requires increasing the signal or limiting the background signal. Examples of nanoparticles regarding the first approach are quantum dots, liposomes, or emulsion filled with dyes [12,16]. The second approach is possible, thanks to luminescent nanoparticles [17] and upconversion nanoparticles [18].

Considered as noncytotoxic as regard to inorganic nanoparticles, self-assembled nanosystems composed of organic lipids or polymer scaffolds have also been proposed for the grafting or encapsulation of fluorescent dyes. One of the main probes used is indocyanin green (ICG) since it has already been approved by the FDA. Moreover, compared to other cyanins, ICG exhibit the longest wavelength in the near-infrared region, with a wide emission spectra ranging from 750 to 900 nm, which is well positioned in the so-called transparency window. However, ICG suffers from the fact that its emission is highly dependent on its environment, which makes it difficult to quantify. Moreover, it is rapidly eliminated from the bloodstream. Therefore, encapsulation was proposed as a means to increase its stability and reduce the effect of the environment on the emission wavelength. ICG was encapsulated into micelles, emulsions, or liposomes and showed enhanced fluorescent signal and stability. The interest of these systems would be to specifically detect and highlight a target, as demonstrated with silicates targeting transferrin [19], mixed ethyloxazoline–caprolactone micelles targeting the folate receptor [20], or mannose or RGD liposomes containing ICG [16,21].

The second strategy to improve detection sensitivity *in vivo* focuses on the background signal (Scheme 22.1). Pursuing the idea that a significant decrease of the background signal during optical acquisition would largely increase the signal-to-noise ratio and contribute to improve the global optical detection *in vivo*, several research groups have developed original alternatives dedicated to optical imaging in living animal. Among these nanotechnologies, europium-based liposomes have been proposed as a means to follow the biodistribution of liposomes post *in vivo* injection. *Ex vivo* quantification was still required but considerably simplified, thanks to the longer lifetime of the europium complexes [22]. More recently, upconversion nanoparticles (UCNPs) have been proposed. Made of lanthanide-doped fluorides or oxides, these materials are excited in the near-infrared region at low-energy radiation with photons that do not trigger any autofluorescence signal, and consequently emit photons of higher energy (in the tissue transparency window). Upconversion results from a non-linear effect that requires at least two metastable energy states to store the energy of absorbed pump photons. The combined energy of these pump photons is responsible for the emission of a higher energy photon. In addition to these singular optical properties, UCNPs possess many advantages that make them highly interesting candidates for *in vivo* imaging. As an example, the optical properties can be adjusted at will by varying the synthesis method – the composition of core, the size, or the dopant nature and concentration. Besides, these materials were shown to be easily accessible to surface engineering (inert coating, silanization, organic ligand adsorption, etc.) [18].

Along with the description of the first class of nanoparticles, we have seen that efficient solutions and alternatives to molecular probes could be envisioned for optical imaging in living animals. However, no matter how bright is the signal from these optical probes – quantum dots, molecular-based luminophores, or even the most recent upconversion nanoparticles, the common link between all these technologies lies in the absolute dependency on constant excitation light. In other words, the emission signal from these compounds strictly requires the concomitant use of an excitation source. As an example, due to the intrinsic physical properties of the photoluminescence phenomenon – that rarely exceeds the millisecond, the emission from quantum dots or any other fluorescent probe vanishes when the excitation source is switched off.

Sticking to the hypothesis that a complete extinction of the autofluorescence signal from living tissues would increase the detection sensitivity *in vivo*, le Masne de Chermont *et al.* lately introduced a new approach to optical imaging, based on the use of nanomaterials with a longer emission lifetime, called persistent luminescence nanoparticles [17]. Derived from thermoluminescence, persistent luminescence relates to a particular optical phenomenon in which the excitation energy can be stored by the material and then slowly released upon ambient thermal energy under the form of a photonic emission that can last from several hours to a few days following the end of the excitation. Thus, acting as optical capacitors, these nanoparticles can be activated before the injection to living animals. However, as the excitation source is completely suppressed during the acquisition, the use of persistent luminescence nanoparticles allows circumventing the autofluorescence signal from endogenous chromophores as well as highly sensitive and real-time *in vivo* optical imaging [23]. The first generation of persistent luminescence nanoparticles was initially composed of a semiconductor silicate-based structure doped with rare-earth cations, but the past 5 years have witnessed several advances and developments, ranging from crystal composition [24] to the optimization of surface functionalization [25], in order to improve the global optical and biological properties of these probes. Notably, recent work reported the ability to regain persistent luminescence signal *in vivo* at any time (Figure 22.1), up to several months following the initial injection to living mice [26]. As of now, the related imaging systems are not currently used in clinic, but developments are ongoing to improve biocompatibility of these materials and provide adequate materials for preclinical [27] and clinical evaluation.

Obviously, the present list of nanoparticles mentioned above should not be taken as an exhaustive panel of all the available techniques and ongoing developments intended for optical imaging. To cite some of the other important technologies, carbon nanodots [28], carbon nanotubes [29], gold nanoparticles [30], or nitrogen-vacancy centers in diamond-based nanoscale sensors [31] represent valuable alternatives to the optical nano-tools described above. The reader can also refer to several reviews on the topic [32,33].

No matter how hard people keep working on the improvement of signal sensitivity, optical imaging remains widely known to provide both a rather poor spatial resolution due to significant scattering from living matter in the traditional near-infrared window (NIR-I, 700–950 nm) [34] and a limited tissue penetration depth [35]. More recently, optical imaging in the second near-infrared window (NIR-II, 1000–1400 nm) has attracted increasing attention of the scientific community due to its very low autofluorescence signal and negligible tissue scattering [36]. Interestingly, this technique was shown to provide high-resolution

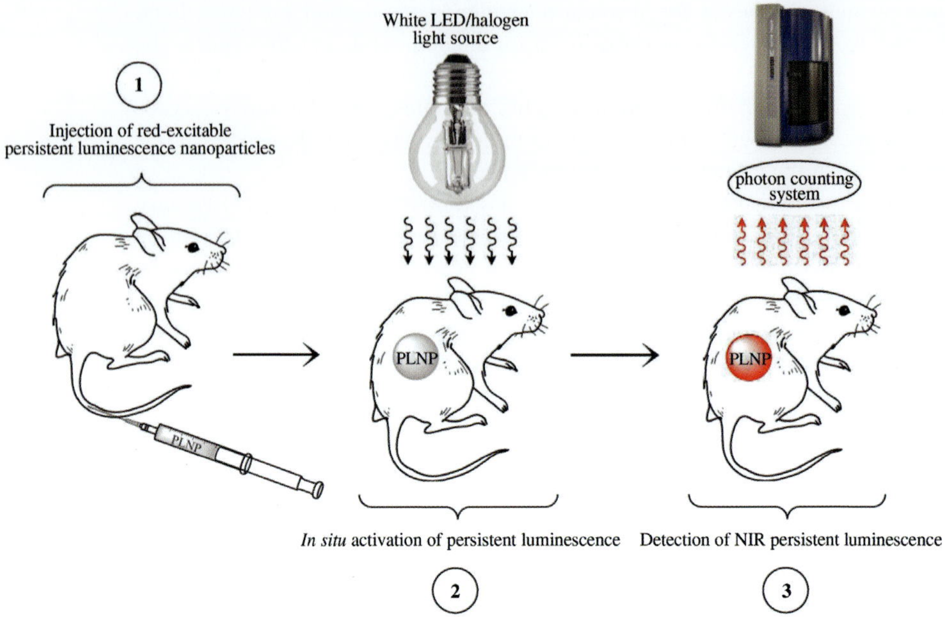

Figure 22.1 Schematic representation of *in vivo* optical imaging with persistent luminescence nanoparticles. (Adapted with permission from Ref. [26]. Copyright 2014, Nature Publishing Group.)

optical images affording a maximal penetration depth (Figure 22.2), usually >5 mm [37]. Thus, great efforts have been made toward the discovery of novel NIR-II emitting optical probes devoted to *in vivo* imaging in small animals [38,39].

Unfortunately, the preclinical and clinical exploitation of the NIR-II optical probes are not yet achieved due to the lack of sensitive and low-cost cameras in this infrared region. Indeed, contrary to the common silicon-based detectors used within the traditional NIR-I, NIR-II cameras require semiconductor alloys with narrower bandgaps such as InGaAs and HgCdTe (Figure 22.2a). However, as Figure 22.2b–g clearly highlights the ability of these new probes emitting in the NIR-II to allow a dynamic visualization of the vascular system or lymphatic drainage with impressive spatial resolution, we can expect a clinical evaluation of such systems in the near future. Altogether, such major improvements should play an important role in diagnosis and hold great promises for future preclinical or even clinical applications.

22.2.2
Particles Designed for Ultrasound Imaging

Microbubbles were developed for ultrasound imaging. These spheres, composed of a gas core surrounded by a protein, lipid, or polymeric shell, exhibit different

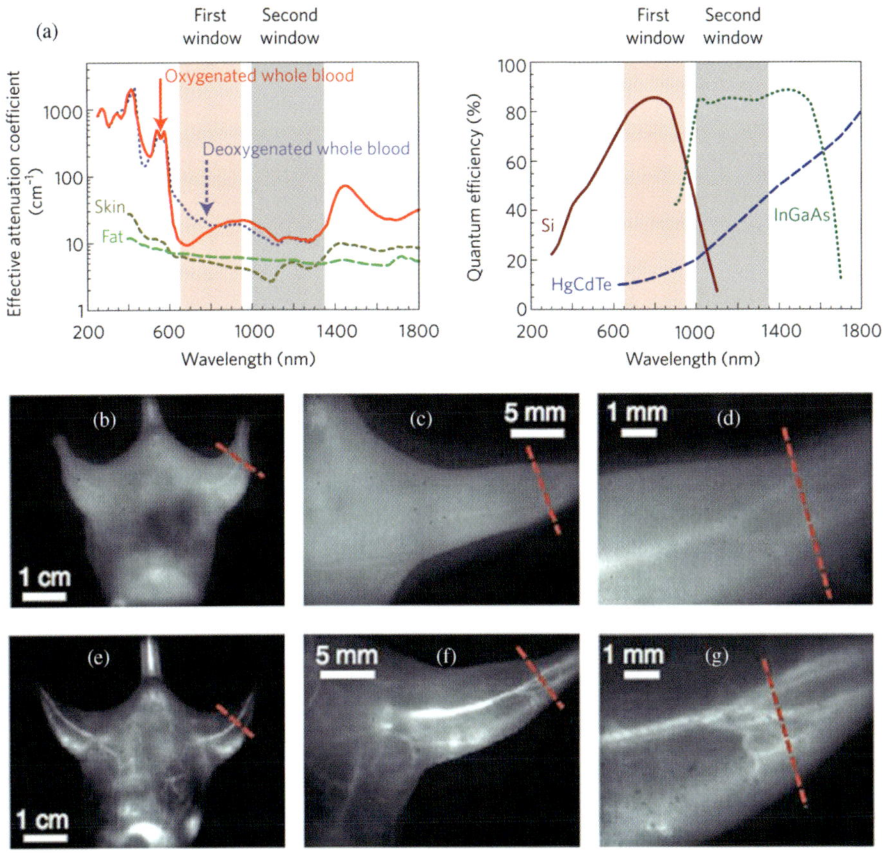

Figure 22.2 Second window for *in vivo* imaging, (a) Optical windows and sensitivity curves for different cameras. (Adapted with permission from Ref. [36]. Copyright 2009, Rights Managed by Nature Publishing Group.) Optical imaging in the NIR-I (b–d) and NIR-II (e–g) using carbon nanotubes. (Adapted with permission from Ref. [39]. Copyright 2012, Nature Publishing Group.)

refractive indices as regard to the tissue; moreover, they are able to oscillate under ultrasound leading to a nonlinear response responsible for the signal enhancement (Scheme 22.2) [40].

This finding led to commercialized microbubbles to perform enhanced ultrasound imaging. As regard to gas expansion, these objects are not in the nanometer range, unless the fluorinated gas is encapsulated as a liquid [42]. However, the liquid-to-gas transition requires a higher frequency than what is usually used for ultrasound imaging. These nano-objects responsive to ultrasound stimuli are mostly developed for drug delivery, in particular to reach deep tissues [43]. Gas-filled microbubbles developed for ultrasound imaging are in the 1–4 μm range, contain air, perfluorobutane, or sulfur hexafluoride gas, and are surrounded by albumin or lipidic shells. They exhibit a lifetime of approximately 10 min, such

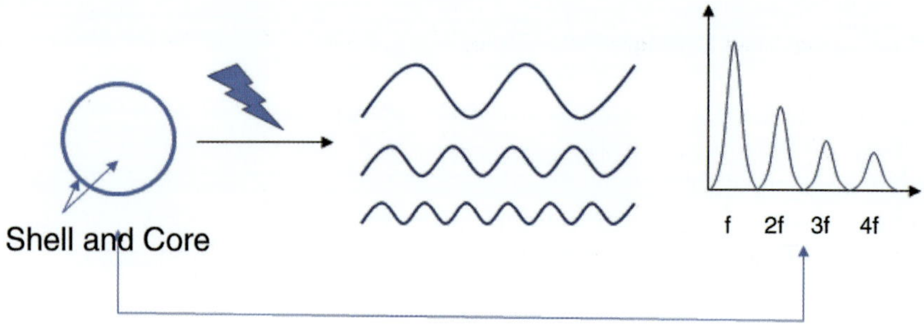

Scheme 22.2 Contrast-enhanced ultrasound imaging, thanks to the nonlinear response of microbubbles to ultrasound. Shell and core design will impact the nonlinear response, as shown by Dayton's *et al.* [41].

as the commercially available microbubbles developed by Schering AG (Levovist), Bracco Int. (Sonovue), GE Healthcare (Optison, Sonazoid), Alliance Pharma (Imagent), and Bristol Meyers (Definity) [44]. Liver applications (Figure 22.3) and hypervascular metastases can be detected with these agents, thanks to enhanced ultrasound contrast. Tumor vascular architecture can also be observed using contrast-enhanced ultrasound, allowing a better grading of tumor stage [45]. Contrast-enhanced ultrasound was also proposed to accurately diagnose incomplete radio frequency treatment for liver and renal carcinoma. Residual tumor vasculature was shown using contrast-enhanced ultrasound, in particular for highly vascular foci [46]. The limit of the technique is that using harmonics and frequencies at low mechanical index reduces the spatial resolution and the overall image quality. However, targeting microbubbles are currently being evaluated as the next microbubbles generation to discriminate between molecular and functional imaging [47,48].

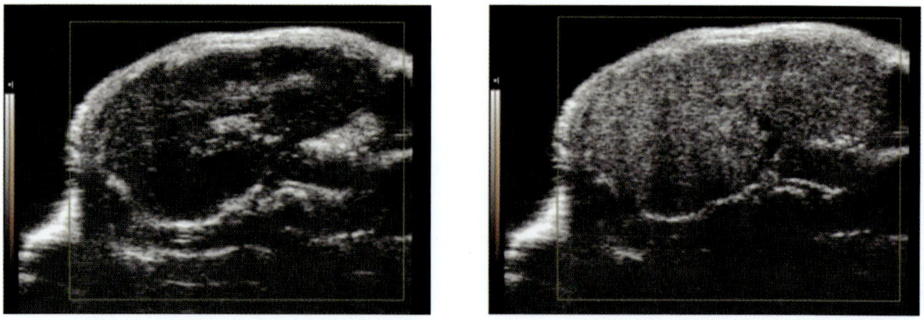

Figure 22.3 Enhanced ultrasound imaging of a liver prior and post injection of microbubbles developed for gene delivery triggered by ultrasound [49]. (Courtesy of G. Renault, from the ultrasound imaging platform Cochin, Paris Descartes University.)

22.2.3
Particles Designed for Magnetic Resonance Imaging

MRI signal issued from water proton relaxation provides anatomic and functional information. Contrast-enhanced imaging is very interesting for MRI to increase its sensitivity that, associated with 3D resolution, returns a perfectly localized signal. Two classes of contrast agents have been reported affecting either the T_1 or T_2 relaxation times and leading to hyper- or hyposignals. Clinical contrast agents are composed of gadolinium that primarily affects the T_1 relaxation time leading to brighter signals (Scheme 22.3). This is the case of DOTAREM, for instance, that increases the MRI signal and is rapidly eliminated from the bloodstream. As for all molecular agents, its half-life is relatively short (less than 5 min), which would be a limitation for specific contrast agents. For this reason, a number of nanoparticles have been proposed for MRI signal enhancement. Iron oxide is the most reported with more than 3500 citations in 25 years and the most evaluated in current clinical trial. Iron oxides are superparamagnetic agents that can be functionalized for surface property modification. Usually covered with citrate ions or dextran polymers, they have been transferred to clinic. A large number of studies have dealt with the coverage of various copolymers to render these nanoparticles stealth; this is the case for polyions [50], polyglycerol [51], or polyphosphonate [52] polymers grafted onto the iron oxide surface. As of now, they are mainly used precisely because they are taken up by the reticuloendothelial system [53]. Specific agents obtained by grafting ligands onto the surface of iron oxide nanoparticle have been scarcely proposed, but usually give attractive results such as VCAM-1 targeting [54], P-selectin with fucoidan [55], glypican-3 [56], EGF receptor [57], or beta-1 [58] targeting.

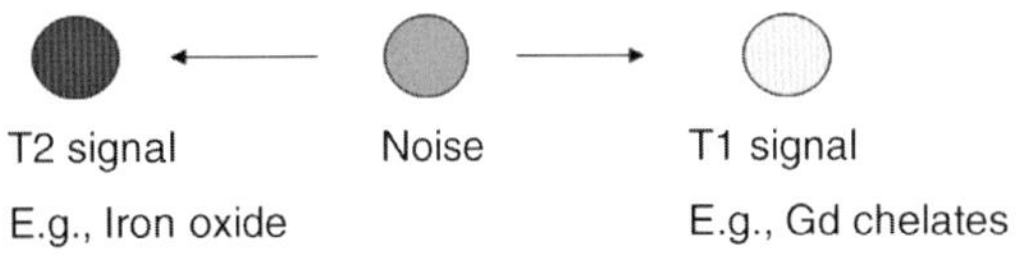

Scheme 22.3 Increasing the signal-to-noise ratio for contrast-enhanced MRI. Representative conventional hyposignal obtained from iron oxide and hypersignal obtained from gadolinium chelates.

In terms of positive contrast imaging agent, mostly gadolinium-based chelates have been proposed and incorporated into self-assembled systems such as liposomes [59] or onion-like vesicles [60], or grafted onto the surface of nanoparticles such as dendrimers [61] or ultrasmall nanoparticles [62].

None of them have reached the clinic as yet; however, from these studies, we learnt that a certain number of properties were key elements to obtaining positive contrast agents. Macromolecular complex is stumbling lower than molecular complexes, which then has to be recovered from a fast rotational correlation

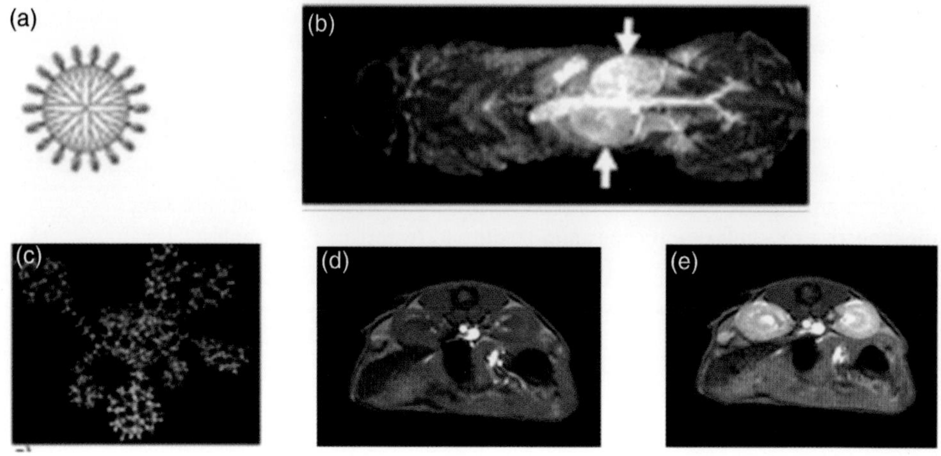

Figure 22.4 Examples of ultrasmall nanoparticles capable of providing a positive signal enhancement in the kidney using magnetic resonance imaging. (a and b) Dendrimers of the fourth generation. (Adapted with permission from Ref. [63]. Copyright 2011, Elsevier Inc.) (c–e) Axial images of kidney prior and postinjection of Aguix nanoparticles [64]. (Courtesy of G. Ramniceanu and B.T. Doan, Platform Imaging Facility, Paris Descartes University (piv.parisdescartes.fr/spip.php?article1839).)

time or a fast proton exchange rate. Although the former can be tuned by the flexibility of the linker between the chelate and the nanoparticle, a faster proton exchange rate can be obtained by increasing the number of protons to be exchanged. The number of gadolinium chelates on the surface of dendrimers [63] or ultrasmall silicate nanoparticles [62] makes them until now the most attractive positive MRI agents for the future (Figure 22.4). The large surface-to-size ratio, associated with the very small size of these nanoparticles, plays a major role in their tumbling motion, without mentioning the importance of their pharmacokinetic. Dendrimer biodistribution can be simply altered by changing the core [63]. All these criteria have to be taken into account to obtain a relevant positive contrast agent for MRI.

22.3 *In Vivo* Nanoparticle Imaging to Gain Insight into Nanomedicine Biodistribution and Stability

22.3.1 Nanoparticle Biodistribution

The initial studies on liposomes paved the way for *in vivo* imaging of nanoparticles. As sensitivity was required to evaluate the percentage of liposomes per organ, radioactivity was mainly used. Therefore, the first studies on liposome biodistribution have been performed with ^{14}C- or ^{3}H-labeled liposomes [8]. Since then, other probes have been used, such as fluorescence or delayed fluorescence showing that it was also possible to obtain similar results post lipid extraction [22][1]. Until now, radioactive probes are used to provide a quantified amount of nanoparticles in various organs, in particular for nanoparticles that could potentially be transferred to the clinic, as pharmacokinetic is an element that will have to be well documented for the agencies. Some nonexhaustive examples of these can be found with lactosylated albumin [65], for the hybrid gadolinium oxide nanoparticles [66], gold nanoparticles [67], or polyamidoamine dendrimer [68].

22.3.2
Imaging Nanoparticles to Optimize Surface and Size with Reference to Their Biodistribution and Clearance

The half-life of liposomes revealed that the liposomes were eliminated very fast. Covering their surface with hydrophilic polymer such as poly(ethylene glycol) led to the notion of stealthiness where liposomes could escape the recognition by opsonins and subsequent elimination by the macrophages [69,70]. Since then, a better understanding of the interaction of the nanoparticles with the blood constituents led to a better description of the protein corona at the surface of nanoparticles plunged into a biological environment [71,72], varying according to the nanoparticle size and surface [73,74].

To prevent the adsorption of proteins, pegylation was applied to any type of nanoparticles. It allowed a more precise understanding of the physiological issues associated with the fate of nanoparticles *in vivo*. As an example, quantum dots were initially described as powerful imaging agents and a potential alternative to molecular-based imaging system due to their outstanding optical properties *in vitro*, but rapidly turned out to be of precious help *in vivo*. Indeed, their photostability and physical steadiness gave access to an unpreceded *in vivo* follow-up and to an extensive study of the influence of numerous surface properties on their global distribution following systemic injection in living animals. Notably, several groups reported not only the stealth effect of PEG-covered quantum dots [75], describing both the influence of PEG chain length and its global conformation to the biodistribution of the inorganic nanoparticles, but also several other ways to prevent major accumulation within the reticuloendothelial system [76,77]. However, the later work of Hammond and coworkers employs 50 nm wide quantum dots to demonstrate the unique character of layer-by-layer assembly of polyelectrolytes to increase *in vivo* stability and long blood elimination half-life [78]. We can also quote the important and recent efforts toward zwitterionic coatings [79]. They were shown to greatly reduce nonspecific adsorption of proteins and lipids on the surface of nanoparticles and

1) Mignet and Scherman revue MMB Ch 30, 2010.pdf.

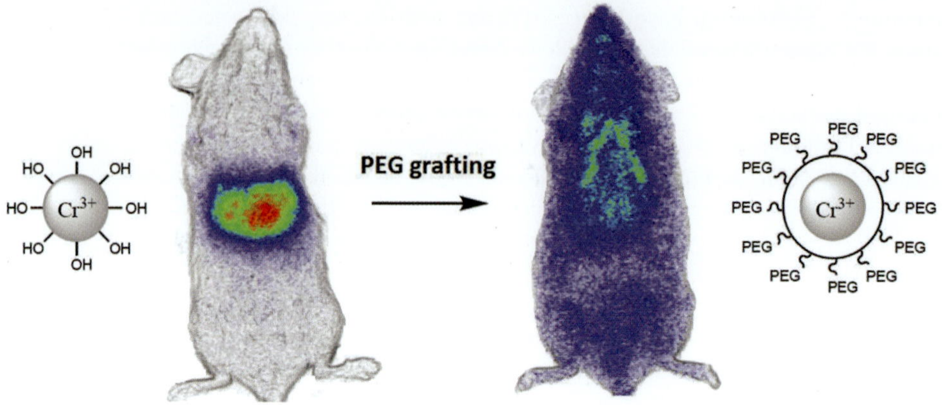

Figure 22.5 Biodistribution of chromium-doped persistent luminescence nanoparticles (PLNPs) following systemic administration in living mice. The left image corresponds to the biodistribution of negatively charged PLNPs that largely accumulate within liver. The right image shows the biodistribution of the same nanoparticles after PEG grafting that manage to evade the global reticuloendothelial retention. (Adapted with permission from Ref. [23]. Copyright 2011, American Chemical Society.)

to counter opsonization and scavenging by the mononuclear phagocyte system, thereby preventing the formation of the protein corona [80].

Similar studies exploring the influence of surface state on the biodistribution of nanoparticles were also accessible through the use of persistent luminescence nanoparticles (Figure 22.5). The initial proof of concept *in vivo* confirmed the importance of surface charge in the global clearance of these objects after systemic injection [17]. Nanoparticles with a global positive surface charge were shown to largely accumulate within lung capillaries due to probable aggregation of the nanoparticles. On the contrary, negatively charged nanoparticles were rapidly cleared from the blood circulation within the two major organs composing the reticuloendothelial system, mainly liver and spleen. Such accumulation could be successfully delayed after a proper functionalization of the surface with PEG moieties [25] and by increasing aminosilane layer thickness of stealth persistent luminescence nanoparticles [81]. Similarly, gadolinium-labeled dendrimers of the fourth or fifth generation circulated more than 1 h with minimal liver and kidney uptake postpegylation [82].

In addition to these surface effects, controlling the size of the nanoparticles was also shown to be of particular interest in order to delay or prevent the somehow inevitable confinement within the reticuloendothelial organs. It is now largely assumed that decreasing the size of the nanoparticles from several tens of nanometers to about 10 nm, sometimes less when possible, can significantly increase their blood half-life *in vivo* and hinder subsequent liver or spleen accumulation. Such result was demonstrated for a large panel of different nanoparticles, including liposomes [83], dendrimers [82], upconversion nanoparticles [84], quantum dots [85], persistent luminescence nanoparticles [17], and many others. Nanoparticles of smaller size such as ultrasmall cationic superparamagnetic iron oxide nanoparticles exhibiting a 7 nm diameter was shown to distribute between kidney and liver (Scheme 22.4) [86]. Fast renal accumulation was obtained for ultrasmall silicate nanoparticles by both MRI and PET imaging [62]. This critical size effect provided a solid base for the development and rational design of targeted nanoparticles dedicated to biological applications. As an example, we can quote the use of quantum dots as a model system to define the adequate hydrodynamic diameter and global surface charge that allowed rapid body elimination of nanometer-sized objects by renal filtration. In this study, the authors suggest a direct link and correspondence between their result, mainly a size criterion, and the putative clinical utility of the studied nanoparticles [87].

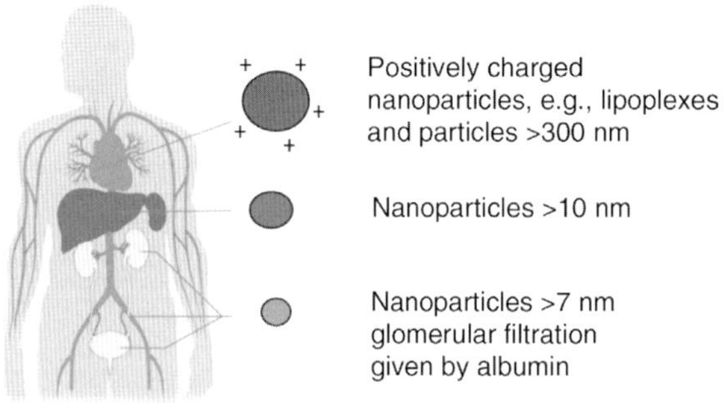

Scheme 22.4 General distribution of nanoparticles as regard to their size and charge. This schematic view does not take into account nanoparticle density.

22.3.3
Imaging Nanoparticle to Optimize Their Intrinsic Stability

The question that can be addressed is the integrity of the nanoparticle post *in vivo* injection. To answer this question, several dyes have in general been used to label several components of the nanoparticle and the pharmacokinetic of each labels were compared. This way, the stability of the nanoparticle in its totality can be addressed and optimized. This has been earlier addressed for drug delivery systems to provide evidence that the drug was associated with the nanoparticle postinjection. This was particularly described for encapsulated doxorubicin as the drug emit is fluorescent, which obviously simplified the studies. Indeed, it reduces the risk of modifying the nanoparticle behavior by the encapsulation of another dye, which would not have similar physicochemical properties as the encapsulated drug. As an example, the intrinsic fluorescence of doxorubicin allowed following its accumulation into murine BFS-1 sarcoma using thermosensitive liposomes, showing that doxorubicin was mostly released when heat above 42 °C was applied [88].

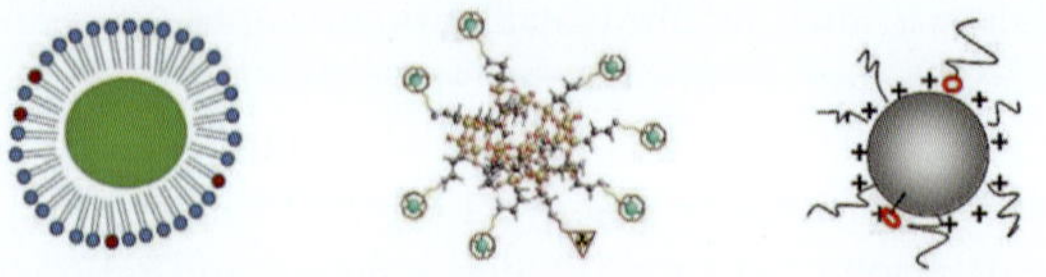

(a) (b) (c)

Figure 22.6 Examples of multimodal nanoparticles to assess stability of oil filled nanovesicles (a) (adapted from Ref [60]), ultrasmall nanoparticles as a bimodal PET/MRI preclinical study (b) adapted from Ref. [94]), and double labeling of gas-filled microbubbles to be able to follow the devenir of the lipid microbubbles that become invisible to ultrasound (c) (adapted from Ref [49]).

This question of particle integrity is particularly relevant for self-assembled nanosystems such as micelles, liposomes, emulsions, or amphiphilic polymers whose formation is reversible. Förster resonance energy transfer that occurs only when two complementary fluorophores are in proximity has been proposed to follow micelle stability [89], to follow emulsion integrity postincubation in serum [90], to evidence the effect of the PEG on nanoemulsion stability *in vivo* [91], or to follow polymeric nanoparticle integrity *in vivo* [92]. Mostly, lipidic probes have been used within these studies. Such information is fundamental to improving the stability of the nanoparticles or selecting the more appropriate applications in full knowledge (Figure 22.6).

Apart from nanoparticle stability, bimodal imaging can also be a mean to gain information from preclinical imaging [93] or to complement information obtained from a single imaging modality. As an example, longer term imaging of microbubbles when they are not visible to ultrasound imaging (Figure 22.6).

22.4 Translational Interest of Nanoparticles for Medical Imaging

22.4.1 Macrophage Imaging by Nanoparticle Uptake

What has been established from the first studies on liposomes [94] to the more recent studies is that nanoparticles of a usual size of 20–200 nm, which are not decorated by an inert coating, are recognized by soluble blood constituents called opsonins, which will induce the phagocytosis of nanoparticles by macrophages. This drawback has proved to be an advantage for inflammation processes observation, and it is anticipated that nanoparticles specific to immune cell subtypes will have an emerging role in diagnostic and therapy. A thorough review on the interest of macrophages imaging by nanoparticle has been recently published [95].

Iron oxides have been the most studied in this field. However, due to strong competition or reduced number of applied clinical act, few iron oxides that were approved were later on withdrawn from the market. This is the case for Feridex (endorem, AMAG Pharma), Resovist (Cliavist), and Sinerem (Combidex, Guerbet).

Few clinical trials are ongoing in order to take advantage of macrophage imaging in various pathologies. Due to its iron content, ferumoxytol, a medication used for anemia, has been turned to an imaging agent that is currently in clinical trial in various diseases. It is tested to observe macrophage infiltration in kidney transplant, as a means to indicate if the transplant will be rejected (GE Healthcare, 2015). It has also been proposed for cardiovascular inflammation and can be found in phase II clinical trial for myocardial inflammation for acute myocardial infarction [7]. In the field of cancer, lymph node imaging represents a preoperative staging of pancreatic cancer. Lymph node imaging is based on abnormal accumulation of iron oxide nanoparticles in malignant nodes [96]. Iron oxide nanoparticles coated with dextran, ferumoxtran-10, is tested in clinic for lymph node imaging in prostate and bladder cancer [97]. It was also tested as means to detect lymphocytic infiltration of pancreatic islets in type 1 mellitus diabetes (Jostin Diabetes Center [98]), and in multiple sclerosis (Stanford University [98]). These few examples of clinical trials in the last 5 years indicate the potential of this approach that is applicable to a large range of diseases. A number of research studies are conducted in various imaging modalities to provide the next generation of nanoparticles, promising for medical applications, as a help for surgery, for disease gradation, or for new applications such as acute inflammation or transplant rejection.

22.4.2
Blood Pool Agent

Blood pool agents (BPAs) are intravascular contrast agents. Due to their size, they remain longer in the intravascular space and diffuse less than small molecules in the interstitial space. As a consequence, longer acquisition time can be performed to provide better images. Moreover, additional information can be obtained if combined with first-pass arterial agents. Vasculature permeability measurement, blood volume, perfusion, and endovascular leaks could benefit from these agents.

The first FDA-approved blood pool agent is Gadofosveset (Vasovist® or Ablavar, Bayer Schering Pharma AG, Berlin/Germany), which is a gadolinium derivative capable of binding albumin, thanks to its diphenylcyclohexyl group. This agent provides a better diagnostic for the detection of vascular stenosis and aneurysms using enhanced magnetic resonance angiography (MRA) [99]. Other molecules such as gadocoletic acid (Bracco SpA) or gadomelitol (Guerbet) are currently being investigated for coronary MRI and pulmonary embolism, respectively [98,100]. There are, however, a few disadvantages of using reversible protein binding agents. The reversibility rate will depend on the affinity of the agent toward albumin, exchange with other proteins can occur, and unbound chelates can also be present that complicates the interpretation of the images, as well as the quantification, as albumin-bound chelates will exhibit a higher relaxivity. For these reasons, nanoparticles have been proposed as blood pool agents. Indeed, as the size is a crucial parameter for the agent to be maintained longer in the blood than molecular complexes, small-size macromolecules or nanoparticles could give a more reliable signal, even though we know now that the protein corona model proposed rapid exchange of protein to the surface of nanoparticles as well. Dendrimer such as Gadomer-17 (Schering) was evaluated to visualize small vessels formed in response to ischemia in a rabbit model of ischemia and indicated that the absence of leakage of this agent led to higher signal-to-noise ratio and a better visualization compared to small contrast agent such as DTPA.Gd [101]. Alternative macromolecules and nanoparticles contrast agents have been reviewed earlier [102], as well as emerging lymphatic agents [103], and more information can be found on a dedicated Web site to blood pool agents [104]. X-ray blood pool agents such as iodinated liposomal or polymeric nanoparticles have also been reviewed before [105].

22.4.3
Targeted Nanoparticles

Targeting ligands binding to receptors expressed in vascular diseases and preferably available from the lumen can be conjugated to nanoparticles, to enable the selective accumulation of the nanoparticle complexes to the diseased tissues. Although considered as a hard-to-reach approach 10 years ago, targeted nanoparticles have now entered clinical trial whether it is for drug delivery or for imaging.

Lymph node imaging with silica nanoparticles functionalized with RGD ligands and cyanin 5,5 is currently being investigated in clinic. The objective being not only to detect lymph node but also to provide direct evidence of pathological lymph nodes. The ultimate goal is to allow the surgeon to distinguish between diseased and nondiseased lymph nodes and draw a lymph node mapping of the diseased ones prior surgery [106].

As another example, de Jong and coworkers indicated in 2000 that targeted contrast-enhanced ultrasound can potentially have many applications in both medical diagnostics and medical therapeutics [107]. Today, the first clinical trials using targeting microbubbles have been performed. Comparison of nontargeted versus VEGFR2-targeted lipid-filled microbubbles showed that the nontargeted microbubbles are quickly washed out, while the targeting microbubbles specifically adhere to their receptors [48].

The use of targeted nanoparticles could expand the diagnostic capabilities of current vascular imaging by detecting specific molecular processes that play a role in the pathophysiology of vascular disease. Obviously, inflamed tissues, tumors, and thrombus appear attractive targets for functionalized nanoparticles.

Table 22.1 Summary of the current nanoparticles, mainly used in the various imaging modalities.

Modality	Type of nanoparticles	Size	Pros	Cons	Transfer to clinic	References
MRI	**Iron oxide**	3–100 nm	Already commercialized Degradation pathway well known High signal T1 imaging for the future	Commercialization suspended by a number of firms	Commercially available Number of clinical trials going on based on metastases uptake	[7,50–57,86,97]
	Dendrimers	3–10 nm	Small-size ^{19}F MRI proposed for the future	Most of them are nondegradable	Phase I clinical trial for drug delivery	[61,63,68,82]
	AGUIX	3–5 nm	Small-size MRI and X-rays for cancer Renal excretion Degradable	Rapid excretion	Phase I clinical trial for image-guided therapy against glioblastoma	[62,66,93]
MRI and/or optical	**Liposomes**	80–500 nm	Imaging and drug delivery Ferromagnetic liposomes Well tolerated	Size Polydispersity	Commercially available as drug delivery systems Clinical trial as surgery help	[1,8,16,21,22,59,60,69,83,88] (see footnote 1)
	Polymer/ polymersomes	15–200 nm	Imaging and drug delivery Polymer-coated NP	Size Polydispersity Stability Degradability and toxicity depend on the polymers	Commercially available as drug delivery systems. Not evaluated as contrast agent	[20,70,71,74,89,92]

(continued)

Table 22.1 (*Continued*)

Modality	Type of nanoparticles	Size	Pros	Cons	Transfer to clinic	References
	Carbon nanotubes	20 nm to 5 μm	Optical, MRI and opto-acoustics possibilities Possibility of second transparency window (NIR II)	Degradability and toxicity evaluated	Clinical trial with carbon nanotube X-ray, not as injected materials	[10,31,35]
Optical	**QD**	2–50 nm	Small size High quantum yield Possibility of NIR II	Not degradable	Not yet	[12–15,29,32,75–77,85,87]
	Persistent luminescence	20–200 nm	High signal-to-noise ratio Can evolve toward NIR II	No glomerular filtration Degradability Poor quantum yield	Not yet	[17,23–27,81]
	Gold	3–40 nm	Interest for optoacoustics, optical imaging, and heat Small size	Degradability	Not yet	[4,36,67]
	UPCNPs	5–50	NIR II agents envisioned	Degradability	Not yet	[18,84]
US	**MB**	0.1–10 μm	Ultrasound imaging and sonoporation targeted MB	Low half-life Size	Commercially available	[10,43–49,107]

The disadvantages and advantages of nanoparticles, with reference to their future role as contrast agents.

22.5
Conclusion

Nanoparticles in the field of imaging is a fast developing field with exciting opportunities for the future. A tremendous amount of work is performed in research to find innovative nanomaterials with improved properties in particular for optical imaging, but for magnetic resonance and ultrasound imaging as well. Nanoparticles have found their way to the clinic in CT, MRI, and ultrasound imaging for diagnostic and surgery help. Their size and surface properties are the main criteria that may change their pharmacokinetic, elimination, and recognition by macrophages. These physicochemical properties are precisely what led them to few applications, in the field of cancer, cardiovascular diseases, and other inflammatory diseases. As the role of macrophages is getting more deciphered, their specific recognition will undoubtedly be implemented in the future generation of nanoparticles that already have the capacity to improve the sensitivity of imaging modalities. Overall, the understanding of the physicochemical properties of the nanoparticles combined with the protein corona effect on the distribution of targeted and untargeted nanoparticles will ultimately expand the area of applications of the nanomedicine together with the advances in the knowledge of biomarkers that will also provide additional possibility to implement targeting features for future applications.

We summarized the main interest of nanoparticles for various imaging modalities in the future in Table 22.1. In terms of optical imaging, upconversion nanoparticles, luminescent nanoparticles, and NIR II contrast agents should expand in the near future the applications of optical imaging agents. For all imaging modalities, biodistribution is obviously a key factor that primarily depends on the size of the nanoparticles, but also on their surface charge, their density, and their shape. The rare examples of nanoparticles under 7 nm, meaning a size under the glomerular filtration, fundamentally displaced the knowledge on the field of nanoparticle with the need for new characterization methods and techniques. It also gave highly interesting examples of ultrasmall iron oxide nanoparticles, dendrimers, or ultrasmall Aguix nanoparticles. Finally, the use of imaging to assess drug delivery protocols is excellent example of theranostics and will ultimately expand the transfer of nanoparticles to the clinic.

References

1 Immordino, M.L., Dosio, F., and Cattel, L. (2006) Stealth liposomes: review of the basic science, rationale, and clinical applications, existing and potential. *Int. J. Nanomedicine*, **1**, 297–315.

2 Weissleder, R. and Pittet, M.J. (2008) Imaging in the era of molecular oncology. *Nature*, **452**, 580–589.

3 Chapman, S., Dobrovolskaia, M., Farahani, K., Goodwin, A., Joshi, A., Lee, H., Meade, T., Pomper, M., Ptak, K., Rao, J. *et al.* (2013) Nanoparticles for cancer imaging: the good, the bad, and the promise. *Nano Today*, **8**, 454–460.

4 Ocampo-García, B., Fde, M.R., Ferro-Flores, G., De León-Rodríguez, L.,

Santos-Cuevas, C., Morales-Avila, E., de Murphy, C., Pedraza-López, M., Medina, L., and Camacho-López, M. (2011) 99mTc-labelled gold nanoparticles capped with HYNIC-peptide/mannose for sentinel lymph node detection. *Nucl. Med. Biol.*, **38**, 1–11.

5 Grimm, J. and Scheinberg, D. (2011) Will nanotechnology influence targeted cancer therapy? *Semin. Radiat. Oncol.*, **21**, 80–87.

6 Kiessling, F., Marianne, E., Grimm, J., and Lammers, T. (2014) Nanoparticles for imaging: top or flop? *Radiology*, **273**, 10–28.

7 Alam, S., Shah, A., Richards, J., Lang, N., Barnes, G., Joshi, N., MacGillivray, T., McKillop, G., Mirsadraee, S., Payne, J. *et al.* (2012) Ultrasmall superparamagnetic particles of iron oxide in patients with acute myocardial infarction: early clinical experience. *Circ. Cardiovasc. Imaging*, **5**, 559–565.

8 Parr, M., Ansell, S., Choi, L., and Cullis, P. (1994) Factors influencing the retention and chemical stability of poly (ethylene glycol)–lipid conjugates incorporated into large unilamellar vesicles. *Biochim. Biophys. Acta*, **1195**, 21–30.

9 Kunjachan, S., Ehling, J., Storm, G., Kiessling, F., and Lammers, T. (2015) Noninvasive imaging of nanomedicines and nanotheranostics: principles, progress, and prospects. *Chem. Rev.*, **115**, 10907–10937.

10 Richard, C., Doan, B.-T., and Mignet, N. (2016) Increased sensitivity for medical imaging using non-ionizing nanomedicine as contrast agents, in *Nanotheranostic for Personalised Medicine* (eds P. Couvreur and S. Mura), Oxford Press.

11 Weissleder, R. and Nahrendorf, M. (2015) Advancing biomedical imaging. *Proc. Natl. Acad. Sci. USA*, **112**, 14424–14428.

12 Liab, J. and Zhu, J.-J. (2013) Quantum dots for fluorescent biosensing and bio-imaging applications. *Analyst*, **138**, 2506–2515.

13 Michalet, X., Pinaud, F., Bentolila, L., Tsay, J., Doose, S., Li, J.J., Sundaresan, G., Wu, A., Gambhir, S., and Weiss, S. (2005) Quantum dots for live cells, *in vivo* imaging, and diagnostics. *Science*, **307**, 538–544.

14 Lovrić, J., Cho, S.J., Winnik, F.M., and Maysinger, D. (2005) Unmodified cadmium telluride quantum dots induce reactive oxygen species formation leading to multiple organelle damage and cell death. *Chem. Biol.*, **12**, 1227–1234.

15 Tsoi, K.M., Dai, Q., Alman, B.A., and Chan, W.C. (2013) Are quantum dots toxic? Exploring the discrepancy between cell culture and animal studies. *Acc. Chem. Res.*, **46**, 662–671.

16 Jeong, J., Lee, C., Cheong, S., Kim, E., Hwang, H., Na, K., Lim, S., Sohn, M., and Jeong, H. (2013) The effect of mannosylation of liposome-encapsulated indocyanine green on imaging of sentinel lymph node. *J. Liposome Res.*, **23**, 291–297.

17 le Masne de Chermont, Q., Chaneac, C., Seguin, J., Pelle, F., Maîtrejean, S., Jolivet, J.-P., Gourier, D., Bessodes, M., and Scherman, D. (2007) Nanoprobes with near-infrared persistent luminescence for *in vivo* imaging. *Proc. Natl. Acad. Sci. USA*, **104**, 9266–9271.

18 Chatterjee, D., Rufalhah, A., and Zhang, Y. (2008) Upconversion fluorescence imaging of cells and small animals using lanthanide doped nanocrystals. *Biomaterials*, **29**, 937.

19 Barth, B.M., Sharma, R., Altino, E.İ., Morgan, T.T., Sriram, S., Kaiser, J.M., Mcgovern, C., Matters, G.L., Jill, P., Kester, M. *et al.* (2010) Bioconjugation of calcium phosphosilicate composite nanoparticles for selective targeting of human breast and pancreatic cancers *in vivo*. *ACS Nano*, **4**, 1279–1287.

20 Yan, L. and Qiu, L. (2015) Indocyanine green targeted micelles with improved stability for near-infrared image-guided photothermal tumor therapy. *Nanomedicine (Lond.)*, **10**, 361–373.

21 Ding, J., Feng, M., Wang, F., Wang, H., and Guan, W. (2015) Targeting effect of PEGylated liposomes modified with the Arg–Gly–Asp sequence on gastric cancer. *Oncol. Rep.*, **34**, 1825–1834.

22 Mignet, N., Le Masne de Chermont, Q., Randrianarivelo, T., Seguin, J., Richard,

C., Bessodes, M., and Scherman, D. (2006) Liposome biodistribution by time resolved fluorimetry of lipophilic europium complexes. *Eur. Biophys. J.*, **35**, 155–161.

23 Richard, C., Maldiney, T., le Masne de Chermont, Q., Seguin, J., Wattier, N., Courties, G., Apparailly, F., Bessodes, M., Scherman, D., Loménie, N. *et al.* (2012) Persistent luminescence nanoparticles for bioimaging. *Adv. Intell. Soft Comput.*, **120**, 37–53.

24 Maldiney, T., Lecointre, A., Viana, B., Bessière, A., Bessodes, M., Gourier, D., Richard, C., and Scherman, D. (2011) Controlling electron trap depth to enhance optical properties of persistent luminescence nanoparticles for *in vivo* imaging. *J. Am. Chem. Soc.*, **133**, 11810–11815.

25 Maldiney, T., Richard, C., Seguin, J., Wattier, N., Bessodes, M., and Scherman, D. (2011) Effect of core diameter, surface coating, and PEG chain length on the biodistribution of persistent luminescence nanoparticles in mice. *ACS Nano*, **5**, 854–862.

26 Maldiney, T., Bessière, A., Seguin, J., Teston, E., Sharma, S.K., Viana, B., Bos, A.J., Dorenbos, P., Bessodes, M., Gourier, D. *et al.* (2014) The *in vivo* activation of persistent nanophosphors for optical imaging of vascularization, tumours and grafted cells. *Nat. Mater.*, **13**, 418–426.

27 Maldiney, T., Ballet, B., Bessodes, M., Scherman, D., and Richard, C. (2014) Mesoporous persistent nanophosphors for *in vivo* optical bioimaging and drug-delivery. *Nanoscale*, **6**, 13970–13976.

28 Wang, J., Liu, G., Leung, K., Loffroy, R., Lu, P., and Wang, Y. (2015) Opportunities and challenges of fluorescent carbon dots in translational optical imaging. *Curr. Pharm. Des.*, **21**, 5401–5416.

29 Akizuki, N., Aota, S., Mouri, S., Matsuda, K., and Miyauchi, Y. (2015) Efficient near-infrared up-conversion photoluminescence in carbon nanotubes. *Nat. Commun.*, **16**, 8920.

30 Huang, X. and El-Sayed, M. (2010) Gold nanoparticle: optical properties and implementations in cancer diagnosis and photothermal therapy. *J. Adv. Res.*, **1**, 13–28.

31 Schirhagl, C., Chang, K., Loretz, M., and Degen, C.L. (2014) Nitrogen-vacancy centers in diamond: nanoscale sensors for physics and biology. *Annu. Rev. Phys. Chem.*, **65**, 83–105.

32 Choi, H. and Frangioni, J. (2010) Nanoparticles for biomedical imaging: fundamentals of clinical translation. *Mol. Imaging*, **9**, 291–310.

33 Wolfbeis, O. (2015) An overview of nanoparticles commonly used in fluorescent bioimaging. *Chem. Soc. Rev.*, **44**, 4743–4768.

34 Lim, Y., Kim, S., Nakayama, A., Scott, N., Bawendi, M., and Frangioni, J. (2003) Selection of quantum dot wavelengths for biomedical assays and imaging. *Mol. Imaging*, **2**, 50–64.

35 Gao, X.H., Cui, Y.Y., Levenson, R.M., Chung, L.W., and Nie, S. (2004) *In vivo* cancer targeting and imaging with semiconductor quantum dots. *Nat. Biotechnol.*, **22**, 969–976.

36 Smith, A., Mancini, M., and Nie, S. (2009) Second window for *in vivo* imaging. *Nat. Nanotechnol.*, **4**, 710–711.

37 Welsher, K., Sherlock, S., and Dai, H. (2011) Deep-tissue anatomical imaging of mice using carbon nanotube fluorophores in the second near-infrared window. *Proc. Natl. Acad. Sci. USA*, **108**, 8943–8948.

38 Li, C., Zhang, Y., Wang, M., Zhang, Y., Chen, G., Li, L., Wu, D., and Wang, Q. (2014) *In vivo* real-time visualization of tissue blood flow and angiogenesis using Ag2S quantum dots in the NIR-II window. *Biomaterials*, **35**, 393–400.

39 Hong, G., Lee, J., Robinson, J., Raaz, U., Xie, L., Huang, N., Cooke, J., and Dai, H. (2012) Multifunctional *in vivo* vascular imaging using near-infrared II fluorescence. *Nat. Med.*, **18**, 1841–1846.

40 Faez, T., Emmer, M., Kooiman, K., Versluis, M., van der Steen, A., and de Jong, N. (2013) 20 years of ultrasound contrast agent modeling. *IEEE Trans. Ultrason. Ferroelectr. Freq. Control*, **60**, 7–20.

41 Dayton, P.A., Zhao, S., Bloch, S.H., Schumann, P., Penrose, K., Matsunaga,

T.O., Zutshi, R., Doinikov, A., and Ferrara, K.W. (2006) Application of ultrasound to selectively localize nanodroplets for targeted imaging and therapy. *Mol. Imaging*, **5**, 160–174.

42 Sheeran, P.S., Luois, S., Dayton, P.A., and Matsunaga, T.O. (2011) Formulation and acoustic studies of a new phase-shift agent for diagnostic and therapeutic ultrasound. *Langmuir*, **27**, 10412–10420.

43 Delalande, A., Postema, M., Mignet, N., Midoux, P., and Pichon, C. (2012) Ultrasound and microbubble-assisted gene delivery: recent advances and ongoing challenges. *Ther. Deliv.*, **3**, 1199.

44 Correas, J., Bridal, L., Lesavre, A., Méjean, A., Claudon, M., and Hélénon, O. (2001) Ultrasound contrast agents: properties, principles of action, tolerance, and artifacts. *Eur. Radiol.*, **11**, 1316–1328.

45 Maheo, K., Chevalier, S., Vibet, S., Bougnoux, P., Richard, S., Serriere, S., Bleuzen, A., Tranquart, F., and Goupille, C. (2012) Non-invasive quantification of tumor vascular architecture during docetaxel chemotherapy. *Breast Cancer Res.*, **134**, 1013–1025.

46 Hoeffel, C., Pousset, M., Timsit, M.O., Elie, C., Mejean, A., Merran, S., Tranquart, F., Khairoune, A., Joly, D., Richard, S., Helenon, O., and Correas, J.M. (2010) Radiofrequency ablation of renal tumours: diagnostic accuracy of contrast-enhanced ultrasound for early detection of residual tumour. *Eur. Radiol.*, **20**, 1812.

47 Payen, T., Dizeux, A., Baldini, C., Le Guillou-Buffello, D., Lamuraglia, M., Comperat, E., Lucidarme, O., and Bridal, S. (2015) VEGFR2-targeted contrast-enhanced ultrasound to distinguish between two anti-angiogenic treatments. *Ultrasound Med. Biol.*, **41**, 2202–2211.

48 Bzyl, J., Lederle, W., Rix, A., Grouls, C., Tardy, I., Pochon, S., Siepmann, M., Penzkofer, T., Schneider, M., Kiessling, F. *et al.* (2011) Molecular and functional ultrasound imaging in differently aggressive breast cancer xenografts using two novel ultrasound contrast agents (BR55 and BR38). *Eur. Radiol.*, **21**, 1988–1995.

49 Manta, S., Delalande, A., Bessodes, M., Bureau, M.-F., Scherman, D., Pichon, C., and Mignet, N. (2016) Characterization of positively charged lipid shell microbubbles with tunable resistive pulse sensing (TRPS) method: a technical note. *Ultraound. Med. Biol.*, **42**, 624–630.

50 Kokuryo, D., Anraku, Y., Kishimura, A., Tanaka, S., Kano, M., Kershaw, J., Nishiyama, N., Saga, T., Aoki, I., and Kataoka, K. (2013) SPIO-PICsome: development of a highly sensitive and stealth-capable MRI nano-agent for tumor detection using SPIO-loaded unilamellar polyion complex vesicles (PICsomes). *J. Control Release*, **169**, 220–227.

51 Arsalani, N., Fattahi, H., Laurent, S., Burtea, C., Vander Elst, L., and Muller, R. (2012) Polyglycerol-grafted superparamagnetic iron oxide nanoparticles: highly efficient MRI contrast agent for liver and kidney imaging and potential scaffold for cellular and molecular imaging. *Contrast Media Mol. Imaging*, **7**, 185–194.

52 Torrisi, V., Graillot, A., Vitorazi, L., Crouzet, Q., Marletta, G., Loubat, C., and Berret, J.-F. (2014) Preventing corona effects: multiphosphonic acid poly (ethylene glycol) copolymers for stable stealth iron oxide nanoparticles. *Biomacromolecules*, **15**, 3171–3179.

53 Jokerst, J.V., Lobovkina, T., Zare, R.N., and Gambhir, S.S. (2011) Nanoparticle PEGylation for imaging and therapy. *Nanomedicine (Lond.)*, **6**, 715–728.

54 Fréchou, M., Beray-Berthat, V., Raynaud, J., Mériaux, S., Gombert, F., Lancelot, E., Plotkine, M., Marchand-Leroux, C., Ballet, S., Robert, P. *et al.* (2013) Detection of vascular cell adhesion molecule-1 expression with USPIO-enhanced molecular MRI in a mouse model of cerebral ischemia. *Contrast Media Mol. Imaging*, **8**, 157–164.

55 Suzuki, M., Bachelet-Violette, L., Rouzet, F., Beilvert, A., Autret, G., Maire, M., Menager, C., Louedec, L., Choqueux, C., Saboural, P. *et al.* (2015) Ultrasmall superparamagnetic iron oxide nanoparticles coated with fucoidan for

molecular MRI of intraluminal thrombus. *Nanomedicine (Lond.)*, **10**, 73–87.
56 Park, J., Stephen, Z., Sun, C., Veiseh, O., Kievit, F., Fang, C., Leung, M., Mok, H., and Zhang, M. (2011) Glypican-3 targeting of liver cancer cells using multifunctional nanoparticles. *Mol. Imaging*, **10**, 69–77.
57 Hsieh, W., Liang, C., Chieh, J., Wang, S., Lai, I., Chen, J., Chang, F., Tseng, W., Yang, S., Wu, C. *et al.* (2012) *In vivo* tumor targeting and imaging with anti-vascular endothelial growth factor antibody-conjugated dextran-coated iron oxide nanoparticles. *Int. J. Nanomedicine*, 7, 2833–2842.
58 Wang, D., Fei, B., Halig, L.V., Qin, X., Hu, Z., Xu, H., Wang, Y.A., Chen, Z., Kim, S., Shin, D.M. *et al.* (2014) Targeted iron-oxide nanoparticle for photodynamic therapy and imaging of head and neck cancer. *ACS Nano*, **8**, 6620–6632.
59 Strijkers, G.J., Kluza, E., van Tilborg, G.A.F., van der Schaft, D.W.J., Griffioen, A.W., Mulder, W.J.M., and Nicolay, K. (2010) Paramagnetic and fluorescent liposomes for target-specific imaging and therapy of tumor angiogenesis. *Angiogenesis*, **13**, 161–173.
60 Doan, B.-T., Crauste-Manciet, S., Bourgaux, C., Dhotel, H., Jugé, L., Brossard, D., Scherman, D., Bessodes, M., Cuenod, C.-A., and Mignet, N. (2014) Lipidic spherulites as magnetic resonance imaging contrast agents. *New J. Chem.*, **38**, 5190–5197.
61 Kojima, C., Ph, D., Turkbey, B., Ogawa, M., Ph, D., Bernardo, M., Ph, D., Kobayashi, H., and Ph, D. (2012) Dendrimer-based MRI contrast agents: the effects of PEGylation on relaxivity and pharmacokinetics. *Nanomedicine*, **7**, 1001–1008.
62 Truillet, C., Bouziotis, P., Tsoukalas, C., Brugière, J., Martini, M., Sancey, L., Brichart, T., Denat, F., Boschetti, F., Darbost, U. *et al.* (2015) Ultrasmall particles for Gd-MRI and (68) Ga-PET dual imaging. *Contrast Media Mol. Imaging*, **10**, 309–319.
63 Longmire, M., Ogawa, M., Choyke, P., and Kobayashi, H. (2014) Dendrimers as high relaxivity MR contrast agents. *WIREs Nanomed. Nanobiotechnol.*, **6**, 155–162.
64 Lux, F., Mignot, A., Mowat, P., Louis, C., Dufort, S., Bernhard, C., Denat, F., Boschetti, F., Brunet, C., Antoine, R. *et al.* (2011) Ultrasmall rigid particles as multimodal probes for medical applications. *Angew Chem. Int. Ed.*, **50**, 12299–12303.
65 Chaumet-Riffaud, P., Martinez-Duncker, I., Marty, A., Richard, C., Prigent, A., Moati, F., Sarda-mantel, L., Scherman, D., Bessodes, M., and Mignet, N. (2010) Synthesis and application of lactosylated, 99m Tc chelating albumin for measurement of liver function. *Bioconj. Chem.*, **21**, 589–596.
66 Kryza, D., Taleb, J., Janier, M., Marmuse, L., Miladi, I., Bonazza, P., Louis, C., Perriat, P., Roux, S., Tillement, O. *et al.* (2011) Biodistribution study of nanometric hybrid gadolinium oxide particles as a multimodal SPECT/MR/optical imaging and theragnostic agent. *Bioconjug. Chem.*, **22**, 1145–1152.
67 Alric, C., Miladi, I., Kryza, D., Taleb, J., Lux, F., Bazzi, R., Billotey, C., Janier, M., Perriat, P., Roux, S. *et al.* (2013) The biodistribution of gold nanoparticles designed for renal clearance. *Nanoscale*, **5**, 5930–5939.
68 Ghai, A., Singh, B., Panwar, H., Schultz, M., Parmar, A., Kumar, P., Sharma, S., Dhawan, D., and Kumar, M. (2015) Radiolabeling optimization and characterization of (68)Ga labeled DOTA-polyamido-amine dendrimer conjugate – animal biodistribution and PET imaging results. *Appl. Radiat. Isot.*, **105**, 40–46.
69 Mayhew, E., Lasic, D., Babbar, S., and Martin, F. (1992) Pharmacokinetics and antitumor activity of epirubicin encapsulated in long-circulating liposomes incorporating a polyethylene glycol-derivatized phospholipid. *Int. J. Cancer*, **51**, 302–309.
70 Needham, D., McIntosh, T., and Lasic, D. (1992) Repulsive interactions and mechanical stability of polymer-grafted lipid membranes. *Biochim. Biophys. Acta*, **1108**, 40–48.

71 Gref, R., Lück, M., Quellec, P., Marchand, M., Dellacherie, E., Harnisch, S., Blunk, T., and Müller, R. (2000) "Stealth" corona-core nanoparticles surface modified by polyethylene glycol (PEG): influences of the corona (PEG chain length and surface density) and of the core composition on phagocytic uptake and plasma protein adsorption. *Colloids Surf. B Biointerfaces*, **18**, 301–313.

72 Tenzer, S., Docter, D., Rosfa, S., Wlodarski, A., Kuharev, J., Rekik, A., Knauer, S., Bantz, C., Nawrot, T., Bier, C. *et al.* (2011) Nanoparticle size is a critical physicochemical determinant of the human blood plasma corona: a comprehensive quantitative proteomic analysis. *ACS Nano*, **5**, 7155–7167.

73 Lundqvist, M., Stigler, J., Elia, G., Lynch, I., Cedervall, T., and Dawson, K. (2008) Nanoparticle size and surface properties determine the protein corona with possible implications for biological impacts. *Proc. Natl. Acad. Sci. USA*, **105**, 14265–14270.

74 Natte, K., Friedrich, J., Wohlrab, S., Lutzki, J., von Klitzing, R., Österle, W., and Orts-Gil, G. (2013) Impact of polymer shell on the formation and time evolution of nanoparticle–protein corona. *Colloids Surf. B Biointerfaces*, **1**, 213–220.

75 Walling, M., Novak, J.A., and Shepard, J. (2009) Quantum dots for live cell and *in vivo* imaging. *Int. J. Mol. Sci.*, **10**, 441–491.

76 Ballou, B., Lagerholm, B.C., Ernst, L.A., Bruchez, M.P., and Waggoner, A.S. (2004) Noninvasive imaging of quantum dots in mice. *Bioconjug. Chem.*, **15**, 79–86.

77 Fischer, H.C., Liu, L., Pang, K.S., and Chan, W.C.W. (2006) Pharmacokinetics of nanoscale quantum dots: *in vivo* distribution, sequestration, and clearance in the rat. *Adv. Funct. Mater.*, **16**, 1299–1305.

78 Poon, Z., Lee, J.B., Morton, S.W., and Hammond, P.T. (2011) Controlling *in vivo* stability and biodistribution in electrostatically assembled nanoparticles for systemic delivery. *Nano Lett.*, **11**, 2096–2103.

79 Shrake, R., Demillo, V., Ahmadiantehrani, M., Zhu, X., Publicover, N., and Hunter, K. (2015) Facilitated preparation of bioconjugatable zwitterionic quantum dots using dual-lipid encapsulation. *J. Colloid Interface Sci.*, **437**, 140.

80 Pombo García, K., Zarschler, K., Barbaro, L., Barreto, J., O'Malley, W., Spiccia, L., Stephan, H., and Graham, B. (2014) Zwitterionic-coated "Stealth" nanoparticles for biomedical applications: recent advances in countering biomolecular corona formation and uptake by the mononuclear phagocyte system. *Small*, **10**, 2516–2529.

81 Maldiney, T., Rémond, M., Bessodes, B., Scherman, D., and Richard, C. (2015) Controlling aminosilane layer thickness to extend the plasma half-life of stealth persistent luminescence nanoparticles *in vivo*. *J. Mater. Chem. B*, **3**, 4009–4016.

82 Kojima, C., Turkbey, B., Ogawa, M., Bernardo, M., Regino, C., Bryant, L.H., Jr., Choyke, P., Kono, K., and Kobayashi, H. (2011) Dendrimer-based MRI contrast agents: the effects of PEGylation on relaxivity and pharmacokinetics. *Nanomedicine*, **7**, 1001–1008.

83 Fanciullino, R., Mollard, S., Correard, F., Giacometti, S., Serdjebi, C., Iliadis, A., and Ciccolini, J. (2014) Biodistribution, tumor uptake and efficacy of 5-FU-loaded liposomes: why size matters. *Pharm. Res.*, **31**, 2677–2684.

84 Chen, F., Bu, W., Cai, W., and Shi, J. (2013) Functionalized upconversion nanoparticles: versatile nanoplatforms for translational research. *Curr. Mol. Med.*, **13**, 1613–1632.

85 Schipper, M., Iyer, G., Koh, A., Cheng, Z., Ebenstein, Y., Aharoni, A., Keren, S., Bentolila, L., Li, J., Rao, J. *et al.* (2009) Particle size, surface coating, and PEGylation influence the biodistribution of quantum dots in living mice. *Small*, **5** (1), 126–134.

86 Uchiyama, M., Toma, S., Rodrigues, S., Shimada, A., Loiola, R., Cervantes Rodríguez, H., Oliveira, P., Luz, M., Rabbani, S., Toma, H. *et al.* (2015) Ultrasmall cationic superparamagnetic iron oxide nanoparticles as nontoxic and efficient MRI contrast agent and

magnetic-targeting tool. *Int. J. Nanomedicine*, **10**, 4731–4746.

87 Choi, H., Liu, W., Misra, P., Tanaka, E., Zimmer, J., Itty Ipe, B., Bawendi, M., and Frangioni, J. (2007) Renal clearance of quantum dots. *Nat. Biotechnol.*, **25**, 1165–1170.

88 Li, L., ten Hagen, T., Hossann, M., Süss, R., van Rhoon, G., Eggermont, A., Haemmerich, D., and Koning, G. (2013) Mild hyperthermia triggered doxorubicin release from optimized stealth thermosensitive liposomes improves intratumoral drug delivery and efficacy. *J. Control Release*, **168**, 142–150.

89 Chen, H., Kim, S., He, W., Wang, H., Low, P., Park, K., and Cheng, J. (2008) Fast release of lipophilic agents from circulating PEG-PDLLA micelles revealed by *in vivo* Förster resonance energy transfer imaging. *Langmuir*, **24**, 5213–5217.

90 Gravier, J., Sancey, L., Hirsjärvi, S., Rustique, E., Passirani, C., Benoît, J., Coll, J., and Texier, I. (2014) FRET imaging approaches for *in vitro* and *in vivo* characterization of synthetic lipid nanoparticles. *Mol. Pharm.*, **11**, 3133–3144.

91 Lainé, A., Gravier, J., Henry, M., Sancey, L., Béjaud, J., Pancani, E., Wiber, M., Texier, I., Coll, J., Benoit, J. *et al.* (2014) Conventional versus stealth lipid nanoparticles: formulation and *in vivo* fate prediction through FRET monitoring. *J. Control Release*, **188**, 1–8.

92 Garcia-Amorós, J., Tang, S., Zhang, Y., Thapaliya, E., and Raymo, F. (2016) Self-assembling nanoparticles of amphiphilic polymers for *in vitro* and *in vivo* FRET imaging. *Top. Curr. Chem.*, **370**, 29–59.

93 Truillet, C., Bouziotis, P., Tsoukalas, C., Sancey, L., Denat, F., Boschetti, F., Stellas, D., Anagnostopoulos, C., Koutoulidis, V., Moulopoulos, L., Lux, F., Perriat, P., and Tillement, O. (2014) Innovative multimodal DOTA/NODA nanoparticles for MRI and PET imaging for tumor detection. *EJNMMI Phys.*, **1**, A80.

94 Tahover, E., Patil, Y., and Gabizon, A. (2015) Emerging delivery systems to reduce doxorubicin cardiotoxicity and improve therapeutic index: focus on liposomes. *Anticancer Drugs*, **26**, 241–258.

95 Weissleder, R., Nahrendorf, M., and Pittet, M. (2014) Imaging macrophages with nanoparticles. *Nat. Mater.*, **13**, 125–138.

96 McDermott, S., Thayer, S., Fernandez-Del Castillo, C., Mino-Kenudson, M., Weissleder, R., and Harisinghani, M. (2013) Accurate prediction of nodal status in preoperative patients with pancreatic ductal adenocarcinoma using next-gen nanoparticle. *Transl. Oncol.*, **6**, 670–675.

97 Birkhäuser, F., Studer, U., Froehlich, J., Triantafyllou, M., Bains, L., Petralia, G., Vermathen, P., Fleischmann, A., and Thoeny, H. (2013) Combined ultrasmall superparamagnetic particles of iron oxide-enhanced and diffusion-weighted magnetic resonance imaging facilitates detection of metastases in normal-sized pelvic lymph nodes of patients with bladder and prostate cancer. *Eur. Urol.*, **64**, 953–960.

98 Data from the websites 2016. www.clinicaltrials.gov.

99 Goyen, M. (2008) Gadofosveset-enhanced magnetic resonance angiography. *Vasc. Heal. Risk Manag.*, **4**, 1–9.

100 Keilholz, S., Bozla, R., Fujiwara, N., Mata, J., Berr, S., Corot, C., and Hagspiel, K. (2009) MR diagnosis of a pulmonary embolism: comparison of P792 and Gd-DOTA for first-pass perfusion MRI and contrast-enhanced 3D MRA in a rabbit model. *Korean J. Radiol.*, **10**, 447–454.

101 Jaspers, K., Versluis, B., Leiner, T., Dijkstra, P., Oostendorp, M., van Golde, J., Post, M., and Backes, W. (2011) MR angiography of collateral arteries in a hind limb ischemia model: comparison between blood pool agent Gadomer and small contrast agent Gd-DTPA. *PLoS One*, **26**, e16159.

102 Bumb, A., Brechbiel, M., and Choyke, P. (2010) Macromolecular and dendrimer based magnetic resonance contrast agents. *Acta Radiol.*, **51**, 751–767.

103 Sevick-Muraca, E., Sunkuk Kwon, S., and Rasmussen, J. (2014) Emerging lymphatic imaging technologies for mouse and man. *J. Clin. Invest.*, **124**, 905–914.

104 Data from the websites 2016. www.bloodpoolagents.us.

105 Hallouard, F., Anton, N., Choquet, P., Constantinesco, A., and Vandamme, T. (2010) Iodinated blood pool contrast media for preclinical X-ray imaging applications: a review. *Biomaterials*, **31**, 6249–6268.

106 Benezra, M., Penate-medina, O., Zanzonico, P.B., Schaer, D., Ow, H., Burns, A., Destanchina, E., Longo, V., Herz, E., Iyer, S. *et al.* (2011) Multimodal silica nanoparticles are effective cancer-targeted probes in a model of human melanoma, *Oncolog*, **121**, 2768–2780.

107 De Jong, N., Frinking, P., Bouakaz, A., and Ten Cate, F. (2000) Detection procedures of ultrasound contrast agents. *Ultrasonics*, **38**, 87.

23
Nanoparticle-Based Physical Methods for Medical Treatments

Christine Ménager

Sorbonne Universités, UPMC Univ Paris 06, CNRS, UMR 8234, laboratoire PHENIX, 4 place Jussieu, F-75005, Paris, France.

23.1
Photothermal Therapy

The use of light to cause damage to diseased cells through localized heat generation is referred to as photothermal therapy (PTT).

Many photothermal methodologies rely on the use of metallic nanostructures because of their unique plasmonic properties, which have been reviewed thoroughly in the literature [1,2]. For metallic nanostructures, the absorption of light results from the surface plasmon resonance (SPR). In metals, the conduction electrons at the surface of the nanoparticle collectively oscillate with a corresponding excitation of a resonant wavelength of light (Figure 23.1a). Upon absorption of a photon, the metallic nanoparticle surface can dissipate the absorbed energy into the surrounding solution via intrinsic-to-external phonon–phonon coupling, with subsequent local heating.

23.1.1
Gold Nanoparticles

Gold nanoparticles have the advantages of greater absorption cross section, greater solubility, efficient absorption at longer wavelengths, and facile conjugation with targeting molecules and drugs. These properties make gold nanoparticles promising candidates for PTT of cancer. Examples of the use of gold nanoparticles in PTT are abundant in the literature, and we focus here on gold nanoparticles that absorb in the near-infrared (NIR) region of the spectrum, such as nanorods and gold–silica nanoshells.

Most colloidal synthetic methods for obtaining gold nanoparticles follow a similar strategy, whereby solvated gold salt is reduced in the presence of surface-capping ligands, which prevent aggregation of the particles by electrostatic and/or physical repulsion. Particle size is adjusted by varying the ratio of gold ion to

Pharmaceutical Nanotechnology: Innovation and Production, First Edition. Edited by Jean Cornier, Arno Kwade, Andrew Owen, and Marcel Van de Voorde.

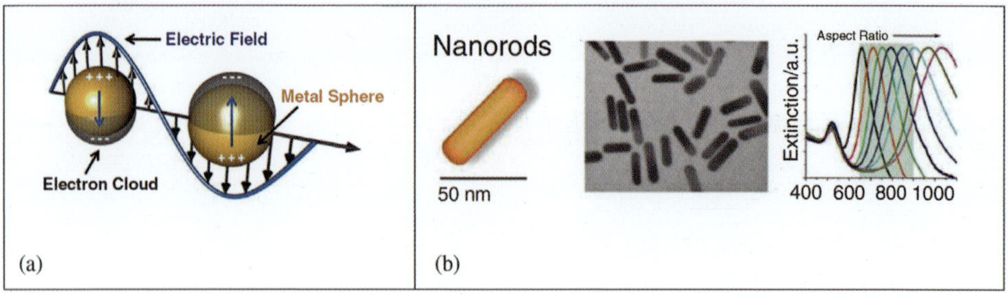

Figure 23.1 (a) Scheme illustrating surface plasmon resonance, which arises when incident light couples to the conduction band electrons of a metal nanoparticle and drives their collective oscillation. (With permission from Ref. [3]. Copyright 2013, Wiley-VCH Verlag GmbH.). (b) Graphical illustration, transmission electron micrograph, and synthetically tunable extinction spectra for gold nanorods. Spectral redshifts are indicated for the increasing aspect ratio. The NIR tissue transmission window is depicted as a green box in each spectrum. (Adapted with permission from Ref. [4]. Copyright 2011, Royal Society of Chemistry.)

reducing agent or gold ion to stabilizer; larger (and typically less monodisperse) sizes are obtained from larger ratios. Variations in shape (nanorods, nanocubes, nanocages, nanoplates, etc.) can also lead to unique scattering properties.

One of the more frequently used PTT agents is the gold nanorod, which is readily synthesized since the pioneering work of Murphy *et al.* [5]. The main advantage of gold nanorods in comparison to spherical nanoparticles is the existence of a second SPR band, which absorbs in the NIR spectral range. The resulting nanorod solutions exhibit plasmon resonance modes for their short (transverse) and long (longitudinal) axes polarization (Figure 23.1b).

A number of preclinical laser-based strategies have coupled different gold nanoparticle platforms (including nanospheres, nanoshells, nanorods, and nanocages) with phototherapy to produce antitumor effects. Much of the preclinical literature highlighting nanoparticle gold as an anticancer therapy has been reviewed [4].

El-Sayed *et al.* [6] first demonstrated the use of gold nanorods for *in vivo* cancer PTT. They showed that the method was capable of inhibiting tumor growth and, in many cases, inducing complete tumor resorption following a single 10 min laser exposure (Figure 23.2).

The first use of anisotropic gold nanoparticles in targeted photothermal therapy was conducted by the Halas research group using silica@Au nanoshells functionalized with antibodies such as anti-HER2. Nanoshells are nanostructures with a silica core and a thin gold shell with tunable optical extinction in the vis-NIR spectrum, depending on the diameter of both the core and the shell. Upon NIR irradiation, nanoshells are used to ablate various cancerous cell lines *in vitro* and have been used successfully in the *in vivo* treatment of cancer in animal models. The antibodies direct the gold nanoparticles toward the cancer cells because they conjugate with the surface cell markers that are overexpressed by

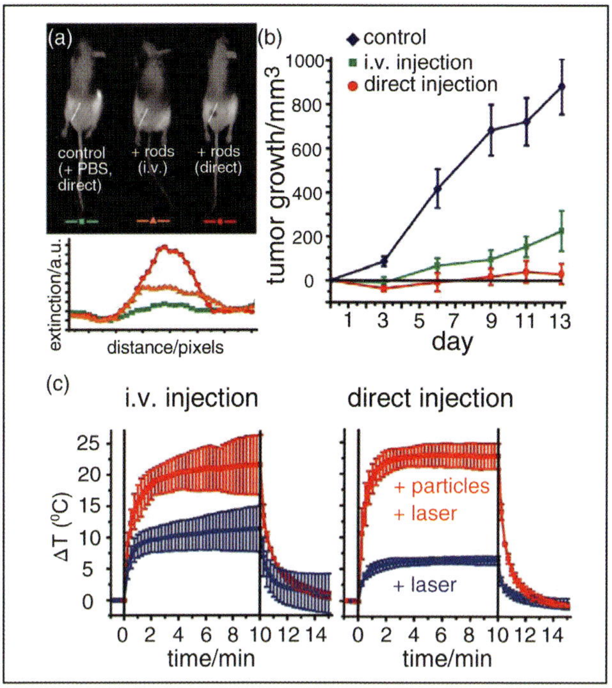

Figure 23.2 *In vivo* near-infrared (NIR) laser photothermal therapy using gold nanorod contrast agents. PEGylated gold nanorods were injected intravenously (i.v.) and locally in carcinoma-bearing nude mice. NIR imaging (a) indicated significantly increased NIR laser absorption and scattering by nanorods accumulated at the rear flank tumor sites. Changes in tumor volume (b) were recorded over 2 weeks following a single laser exposure, indicating significant tumor growth remission for both direct and i.v.-administered nanorods, as well as resorption of >57% of the directly injected tumors and 25% of the i.v.-treated tumors. Real-time intratumoral temperature probe measurements (c) correlated with heating (>20 °C) of the nanorod-treated tumors at the time of tumor resorption or remission. (Adapted with permission from Ref. [7]. Copyright 2008, Elsevier Science B.V.)

cancer cells. These antibodies are linked to orthopyridyl disulfide–PEG–*n*-hydrosuccinimide (OPSS-PEG-NHS) bound to the Au surface through strong Au—S bonds. The advantage of the PEG linker is that it provides enhanced permeability and retention (EPR) effect involving the new blood vessels formed at the tumor site. This type of PTT was first demonstrated in mice with subcutaneous tumors measuring 1 cm. Analysis showed that the PTT produced tissue damage over a similarly sized area as that exposed to laser irradiation. Magnetic resonance thermal imaging shows an average temperature increase of 37 °C after 5 min of irradiation, which is sufficient to induce irreversible tissue damage. Nanoshell-free samples showed an average increase of 9 °C, which is considered to be safe for cell viability [8]. Further experiments showed animal survival times of >90 days [9].

Despite the seemingly ease of nanoshell synthesis and the desirable plasmonic properties, these particles are relatively large in size (130 nm) compared with other NIR-absorbing gold nanoparticles. This size may decrease their accumulation in some cancerous tissues or impede their elimination from the body. Nonetheless, AuraLase, a product based on gold nanoshells, is being commercialized by Nanospectra Biosciences, Inc. and is currently in the process of US Food and Drug Administration (FDA)-sanctioned human pilot studies.

23.1.2 Carbon Nanomaterials

Carbon nanomaterials or nanocarbons have been studied for theranostic purposes because of their unique physical and chemical properties. Nanocarbons are classified into sp^2 carbon nanomaterials such as zero-dimensional fullerenes, one-dimensional carbon nanotubes (CNTs), and two-dimensional grapheme.

23.1.2.1 Carbon Nanotubes

Single-wall carbon nanotubes (SWCNTs) have attracted significant attention because of their outstanding physical properties such as fluorescence, hyperthermia by NIR absorption, hydrophobic drug loading, and photoacoustic imaging [10]. CNTs are commonly synthesized by the discharge method, laser method, ball milling method, or chemical vapor deposition method. However, to be applicable in biomedical purposes, SWCNTs need to be a few hundred nanometers in length at most and be readily dispersible in water. Therefore, a number of techniques have been developed to cut SWCNTs to appropriate lengths and to sort them. Surface modification methods to endow water solubility to SWCNTs have also been developed.

SWCNTs hold a particular interest because of their extraordinary photon-to-thermal energy conversion efficiency with a high absorption cross section of NIR light. Choi and coworkers reported the *in vivo* obliteration of solid malignant tumors by the combined treatment of SWCNTs and NIR irradiation [11]. The photothermally treated mice displayed complete destruction of the tumors without harmful side effects or recurrence of tumors over 6 months, whereas the untreated tumors in control mice grew continuously until the death of the mice. Most of the injected SWCNTs were excreted almost completely from the mice in about 2 months through the biliary or urinary pathway. These results suggest that SWCNTs may act as an effective photothermal agent and may point the way to future cancer therapeutics. Dai and coworkers demonstrated a high tumor uptake of SWCNTs through passive nontargeted accumulation following intravenous injection and elimination of tumor masses by the photothermal pathway induced by very low-NIR laser power of only 0.6 W/cm^2 [12]. The SWCNTs exhibited an optical absorbance at 808 nm, which was about 328% greater than that of Au NRs at the same mass concentration of 0.35 mg/ml. This finding indicated a good performance of SWCNTs for *in vivo* tumor imaging and PTT. Although SWCNTs at an injected dose of 3.6 mg/kg afforded ablation of tumors with NIR irradiation at a power of 0.6 W/cm^2, Au NRs at an injected dose of 35 mg/kg required a power of 2 W/cm^2 for tumor elimination. In addition, no toxicity of the SWCNTs was observed *in vivo* throughout the treatment process.

23.1.2.2 Nanographene

Liu *et al.* studied the *in vivo* behaviors of PEGylated nanographene sheets (NGS) using a fluorescent labeling method. *In vivo* fluorescence imaging revealed high tumor uptake levels of NGS in several xenograft tumor mouse models. They also demonstrated the usefulness of NGS for photothermal therapy by using strong optical absorbance in the NIR region [13].

Moreover, no obvious signs of toxicity were observed in histology examination, blood chemistry, and whole-blood analysis of NGS-injected mice. NGS with a biocompatible coating may thus be a novel type of 2D nanomaterial with great potential in cancer therapy.

23.2 Photodynamic Therapy

PDT is known as a promising addition to the conventional armory against cancer. PDT, in general, is considered to be minimal invasive and nondamaging to healthy tissue. It involves the administration of a tumor-localizing photosensitizer (PS) followed by local illumination of the tumor with light of a specific wavelength to activate the PS. The excited PS then transfers its energy to molecular oxygen, thus generating cytotoxic reactive oxygen species (ROS), such as singlet oxygen ($^1O_2$) that can oxidize key cellular macromolecules leading to tumor cell ablation.

In principle, two classes of photosensitizers are discussed for PDT: molecular photosensitizers (most often porphyrin-based) and inorganic nanoparticles. Despite the widespread and rapidly growing applications, PDT has yet to gain clinical acceptance as a first-line oncological intervention due to certain limitations: lack of an ideal PS, challenges in formulating PS, choosing the right light dosimetry for a complete and effective treatment, difficulties in planning the treatment, and monitoring the treatment response. Nanoparticles represent an emerging technology in the field of PDT that can overcome most of the limitations of classical PS [14]. In the following section, two examples of such nanomaterials are presented.

23.2.1 TiO_2 Nanoparticles

In recent years, TiO_2 has been regarded as potential photosensitizing agent for PDT due to its low toxicity, physiological inertness, excellent biocompatibility, and unique photocatalytic activity. Certain nanoscale materials such as TiO_2 NPs have the ability to generate ROS, due to their unique optical absorption properties, thus allowing them to behave as PSs by itself. The greatest problem

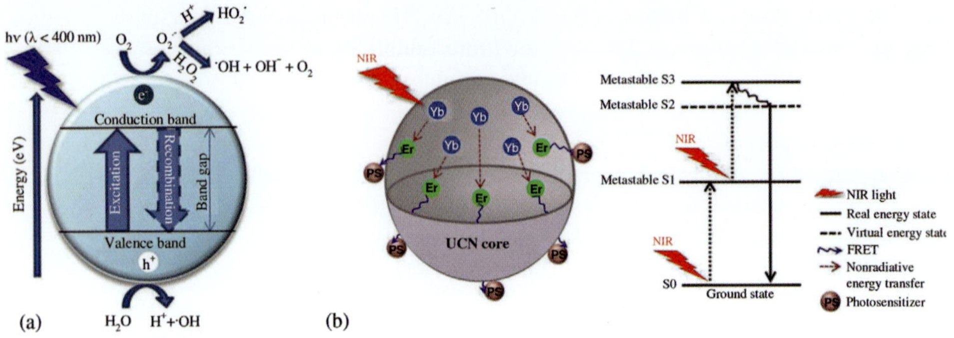

Figure 23.3 (a) Schematic illustration of photodynamic reaction upon light irradiation on TiO_2 nanoparticle. ($^{\bullet}OH$, hydroxyl radical, $O_2^{\bullet -}$, superoxide anion, $HO_2^{\bullet -}$, hydroperoxyl radical, and H_2O_2). (b) Schematic of energy transfer from UCN core to the attached PS and corresponding energy diagram. (Adapted with permission from Ref. [14]. Copyright 2016, American Chemical Society.)

for photodynamic use of TiO_2, however, remains absorption of light in the UV part of the spectrum that constitutes only 5% of the white light spectrum. In order to make TiO_2 nanoparticles amenable for practical applications, the nanoparticles must be modified to respond to the visible light in this optical window. Different methods have been developed to extend the optical absorption of TiO_2 in the visible region. Interaction of TiO_2 nanoparticles with enediol molecules (including catechols and squaric or ascorbic acid containing compounds) was the first approach that held promise for extending the optical absorption to the visible region for biological or medical applications.

Under irradiation with UV light with energy greater than the bandgap energy of TiO_2 (i.e., shorter than 400 nm), the electrons in the valence band of TiO_2 are excited to the conduction band, thus resulting in the formation of photoinduced hole–electron pairs (Figure 23.3a). These photoinduced electrons and holes possess strong reduction and oxidation properties that can interact with surrounding O_2 and H_2O molecules to generate various ROS, such as hydroxyl radical ($OH^{\bullet}$), superoxide anion radical ($O_2^{\bullet -}$), and hydrogen peroxide (H_2O_2), which react with biological molecules, such as lipids, proteins, and DNA, and eventually kill cancer cells.

The detailed mechanism of UV-induced phototoxic effect of TiO_2 nanoparticles was reported on a series of human cancer cells. However, only a few studies have reported the *in vivo* application of TiO_2 nanoparticles for PDT in animal models. Generally, the TiO_2 particles were either administered intratumorally or subcutaneously over the tumor tissue, rather than intravenous delivery due to its insolubility and aggregation issues in physiological environment.

Following administration of TiO_2 nanoparticles, the tumors were irradiated with UV light after the skin was surgically removed to expose the tumor. This is because the penetration depth of UV light (300–400 nm) into the tissue is limited to a few fractions of a millimeter. Cai *et al.* reported significant suppression of HeLa cells implanted in nude mice for up to 30 days, compared with those receiving TiO_2 alone or UV irradiation alone [15].

23.2.2 Upconversion Nanoparticles (UCN)

Recently, it has become increasingly necessary to develop new PSs that could be excited at NIR range to augment the scope and applicability of PDT especially for the treatment of solid and large tumors. This is where the UCN technology becomes very useful, because UCNs could act as delivery agents of the PS and also convert the NIR light to visible light required for the activation of associated PS at much deeper levels in the tissues.

UCNs are nanometer-sized materials that convert low-energy light to high-energy light through sequential excitation with multiple photons, via an anti-Stokes emission process. Materials exhibiting such photon upconversion are usually comprised of host lattices of ceramic materials, embedded with transition metal, actinide, or lanthanide ions such as Yb^{3+}, Er^{3+}, and Tm^{3+}. Such materials possess multiple "real" metastable electronic states that can principally be used to generate upconversion luminescence (Figure 23.3b) [14].

While two-photon excitation requires simultaneous absorption of two photons using a virtual state with a lifetime scale of femtosecond, upconversion process requires sequential absorption using a real metastable state with a lifetime on the order of microseconds.

The biggest challenge in the application of UCNs for PDT *in vivo* has been the delivery of the particles such that they selectively accumulate in the tumor, preventing systemic toxicity. Most of the studies reported delivery of UCNs via intratumoral injections. This route of administration was chosen as the particles synthesized initially were large and aggregated in the physiological media.

The first study to demonstrate systemic administration of a 42 nm UCN carrying Chlorin e6 (Ce6) was by Park *et al.* [16]. Ce6 was attached via both physical adsorption to phospholipid layer and covalent conjugation to the amino group on UCN, achieving stable and highest PS payload (>1000 Ce6 molecules/UCN). Due to the presence of the biocompatible polymer PEG, these UCNs carrying Ce6 had better circulation half-life than free-Ce6. Particles mainly accumulated in the liver and spleen; however, the amount dropped considerably 7 days post-injection, reducing long-term toxic effects. Following *in vivo* PDT at 980 nm, there was a sixfold decrease in tumor size among the treated group, thus clearly demonstrating its potential as PDT agent.

23.3 Magnetic Hyperthermia

Among various nanoparticles that are currently being developed, magnetic nanoparticles show great promise as hyperthermia-inducing agents. Magnetic nanoparticles produce heat through various energy loss pathways under an external alternating magnetic field.

23.3.1 Magnetic Iron Oxide Nanoparticles

The choice of magnetic materials for *in vivo* use of nanoparticles is restricted by the requirement of biocompatibility. Iron oxide nanoparticles have been used in most studies to date. The FDA and the European Medicines Agency have already approved the medical use of magnetic iron oxides that include magnetite (Fe_3O_4-mixed Fe^{2+} and Fe^{3+} ions) and maghemite γ-Fe_2O_3, which retains the same spinel structure as magnetite but is fully oxidized to Fe^{3+}. In contrast to other inorganic materials, adequately coated iron oxide nanoparticles are generally considered to be biocompatible. After endocytosis, iron oxide nanoparticles are degraded in endosomes and released as iron ions. Possible toxic effects of the released free iron ions can be avoided by maintaining iron homeostasis. The excess iron ions are incorporated into ferritin proteins for iron detoxification and storage.

Iron oxide nanoparticles exemplify the unique properties that can result from formulating materials on a nanoscale. Iron oxide nanoparticles possess a superparamagnetic property. In the presence of an external magnetic field, superparamagnetic iron oxide nanoparticles (SPIONs) can provide strong paramagnetic signals at very low doses, which makes them excellent contrast agents in magnetic resonance imaging (MRI). These agents can also be used as an energy transfer mediator by transforming an external magnetic field to heat.

High-quality magnetic nanoparticles can be synthesized by chemical methods such as coprecipitation [17], thermal decomposition [18], sol–gel process [19], and hydrothermal reaction [20]. Compared with top-down approaches, these bottom-up methods enable the synthesis of uniformly sized nanoparticles. Typical magnetic nanoparticles obtained by bottom-up synthesis comprise a magnetic core and organic (e.g., polysaccharides, polymers, and small molecules) or inorganic shells (e.g., silica and other nanoparticles). Although the physical properties of nanoparticles are determined by their inorganic core, their surface properties also play an important role, especially in effective interfacing (e.g., ensuring biocompatibility and specific localization) with biological systems such as proteins, cells, and tissues.

When magnetic nanoparticles are exposed to an oscillating magnetic field, magnetic energy is dissipated as thermal energy through two distinct mechanisms as the particle returns to its equilibrium state. Brownian relaxation describes the dissipation associated with friction losses caused by the rotation of a nanoparticle in the surrounding medium, and Néel relaxation is related to the rotation of the magnetic moments within the nanoparticle magnetic core (Figure 23.4a). When nanoparticles are inside biological tissue, the contribution of Brownian relaxation to heat generation can be hindered by the relatively high viscosity of the medium surrounding the particle. For hyperthermia applications,

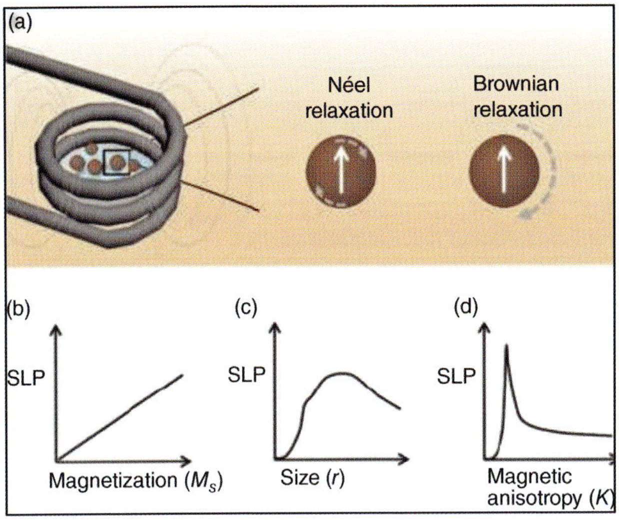

Figure 23.4 (a) Thermal dissipation process from magnetic nanoparticles under AMF showing Néel and Brownian relaxation processes. Panels (b–d) show the relationship between specific loss power and saturation magnetization value (M_s), particle size (r), and magnetic anisotropy constant (K), respectively. (Adapted with permission from Ref. [21]. Copyright 2015, American Chemical Society.)

nanoparticle designs that maximize the heat released through the Néel mechanism are therefore favored. Aside from increasing the strength and frequency of the applied magnetic field, the heat generated may be increased by optimizing parameters such as nanoparticle size, shape, and material, as well as grain structure, which can affect the hysteresis properties such as remanence and coercivity. Furthermore, monodisperse nanoparticle samples have the highest associated energy transfer.

In the case of Néel relaxation, the characteristic relaxation time of a magnetic nanoparticle (MNP) system is given by $\tau_N = \tau_0 \exp[KV/kT]$, where k is the Boltzmann constant, T is the temperature, V is the particle volume, and K is the anisotropy constant. By contrast, Brownian relaxation time is described as $\tau_B = 4\pi\eta r^3/(kT)$ and depends on the viscosity of the medium (η) in addition to temperature. In each situation, the faster relaxation mechanisms will dominate, and the effective relaxation time may be defined as $\tau_{eff} = \tau_N\tau_B/(\tau_N + \tau_B)$. As a consequence of the magnetization rotation under AMF, an increase in temperature with time ($\Delta T/\Delta t$) at a given MNP mass concentration (m) can be measured and used to determine the specific absorption rate (SAR), which is defined in the equation $SAR = C(\Delta T/\Delta t)(1/m)$, where C is the sample specific heat capacity, also called specific loss power (SLP). This value is widely used to compare the heating capacity of different MNPs [22]. SLP values depend on the magnetization, size, and anisotropy of the magnetic material (Figure 23.4b–d).

The hyperthermia procedure, which is based on heat generation within cancer cells, takes advantage of the greater sensitivity of tumor cells to temperature compared with normal tissues. Whereas thermoablation (46–56 °C) causes tumor destruction by direct cell necrosis, hyperthermia (42–45 °C) induces changes in cellular functions by damaging intracellular proteins (i.e., release of heat shock proteins, induction, and regulation of apoptosis) related to cell survival and proliferation. Hyperthermia treatment causes minimal damage to normal tissues. Although the use of magnetic nanoparticles for tumor hyperthermia was first reported 30 years ago, it took until 2003 for magnetic nanoparticle-based hyperthermia therapy to enter clinical trials (at Charité–University Medicine Berlin). In the trials, superparamagnetic iron oxide–aminosilane-type core–shell nanoparticles were injected into the tumor area and subjected to a 100 kHz oscillating magnetic field. Under the magnetic field, the coated nanoparticles spread in the tumor tissue (thermal bystander effect), which improved the cellular uptake and avoided rapid removal by macrophages [23]. This phenomenon allows a single injection of nanoparticles to be sufficient for 10 consecutive treatment sessions, which minimizes the invasiveness of the therapy.

Different products, including NanoTherm™, are on the market for the local treatment of solid tumors (glioblastoma multiforme, prostate cancer, and pancreatic cancer). Although the SLP values of superparamagnetic iron oxide nanoparticles increase as the frequency (f) and/or the amplitude (H) of the magnetic field increases, it is recommended that the product of the frequency and the amplitude (Hf) should be smaller than 5×10^9 A/(m s) for the safety of patients.

Many magnetic nanoparticles, including Fe_2O_3 coated with stabilizers and Fe_3O_4 encapsulated in cationic liposomes, have been tested for magnetic hyperthermia, and this form of hyperthermia is clinically approved in Europe for the treatment of glioblastoma [24].

NanoTherm therapy is currently applied for the treatment of prostate cancer in the United States. The purpose of this study, which will enroll up to 120 men, is to demonstrate that NanoTherm therapy can focally ablate cancer lesions for patients who have Gleason Score 7 prostate cancer and are under active surveillance. The Gleason Score is internationally recognized to classify the extent and growth of a prostate tumor. Today, patients receive standard therapy such as surgery, radiation, or chemotherapy when reaching this diagnostic value. By ablating the lesions, patients are expected to maintain active surveillance and avoid all the well-known side effects of standard therapy, such as impairment of urinary and sexual functions.

However, apoptotic hyperthermia is basically ineffective and has been shown to be insufficient for cancer treatment because cells typically acquire resistance to induced thermal stress, which is called thermotolerance. Cells can resist thermal stress when exposed to a mild temperature. Therefore, repeated higher temperature treatment is generally required to induce sufficient cancer cell death, although this treatment causes undesired necrosis and damage to normal tissue. The use of a low temperature while still retaining high therapeutic efficacy is one of the critical and challenging issues facing the application of apoptotic hyperthermia research in the clinical setting. Recent reports show promising ways to improve MH efficacy, and the first approach is targeted intracellular

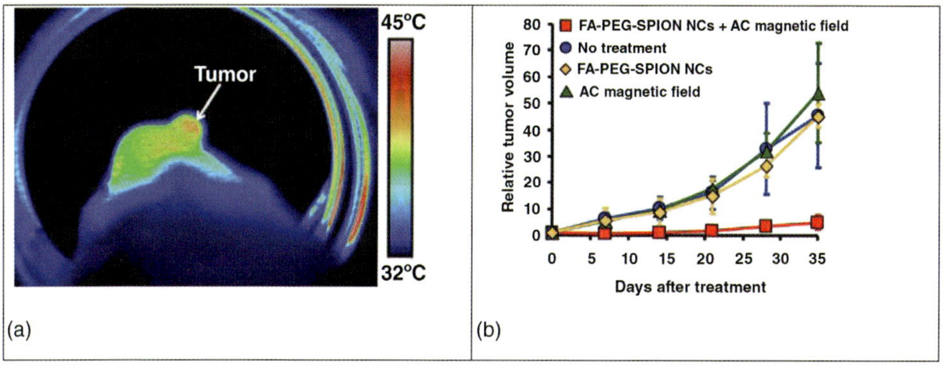

Figure 23.5 (a) Thermal image of a mouse 24 h after intravenous injection of folic acid (FA) and PEG-functionalized superparamagnetic nanoparticle clusters (FA-PEG-SPION NCs) under an AC magnetic field with $H = 8$ kA/m and $f = 230$ kHz. (b) Tumor growth behavior, FA-PEG-SPION NCs, application of an AC magnetic field, and application of an AC magnetic field 24 h after intravenous injection of the functionalized magnetic clusters ($n = 5$). (Taken from Ref. [25]. Copyright 2013, Ivyspring International Publisher.)

hyperthermia. One interesting system comprises folic acid (FA) and PEG-functionalized superparamagnetic nanoparticle clusters. These clusters are injected i.v., and AFM (8 kA/m, 230 kHz) has been applied to significantly inhibit tumor growth in tumor-bearing mice (Figure 23.5) [25].

23.4 Radiotherapy

23.4.1 Hafnium Oxide Nanoparticles

Hafnium oxide (HfO_2) is another example of an inorganic metallic compound that is emerging as a unique nanoformulation. Nanoparticles of hafnium oxide possess unique properties, which are used to enhance the therapeutic effectiveness of radiotherapy. Hafnium has a high atomic number ($Z = 72$), which makes it an attractive candidate as a radiosensitizing agent. Hafnium oxide nanoparticles are radioenhancers and are used in combination with radiotherapy as a physical mode of action to destroy cancer cells in solid tumors. Activation of nanoparticles increases the energy deposited where they are injected, which increases cancer cell death and the efficacy of radiotherapy. As the tumor is irradiated, high-energy photons from external beam radiotherapy are absorbed by tissues and generate electrons, which then activate hafnium oxide nanoparticles. Once activated, hafnium oxide nanoparticles also emit high-energy electrons, which increase the production of free radicals and other reactive oxygen species (ROS), and thus increase the ability of radiation to target and destroy cancer cells through double-stranded DNA damage. This technology is based on physics and may be applied across all radiotherapy indications. All preclinical models have shown a systematic superiority of hafnium oxide with radiotherapy for cell killing compared with radiotherapy alone. Clinical development programs are running with these kinds of particles for six indications across Europe, the United States, and the Asia-Pacific region: a registration trial of soft tissue sarcoma, and phase I and II trials of liver cancers, prostate cancer, head and neck cancer, and rectal cancer [26].

23.5 Sonodynamic Therapy

Sonodynamic therapy (SDT) is a recently developed anticancer treatment in which ultrasound is used to activate the cytotoxic effects of chemical compounds, known as sonosensitizers. SDT diverges from photodynamic therapy (PDT) in that drug activation is achieved through ultrasound rather than light. SDT can overcome the main drawback of PDT related to the limited depth penetration of light. Whether pulsed or continuous, ultrasound is considered to be safer and more readily accepted by the patient than either radiotherapy or chemotherapy. In addition, ultrasound may be used as an external control of the time, dose, and location of drug release, providing tailor-made and localized cancer therapy [27]. The ability of US to activate some sensitizers such as porphyrin and 5-aminolevulinic acid has led researchers to consider sonodynamic therapy as an alternative to light-based PDT. As we have mentioned in the chapter concerning the PDT, it is well known that upon exposure to ultraviolet light, TiO_2 particles can produce electrons, which lead to the formation of ROS [28]. Owing to the nonradiative nature of US, SDT seems to be a more viable option for activating TiO_2 NPs to generate ROS. Nonetheless, *in vivo* cancer therapy using TiO_2 NPs and SDT has not been investigated, rather primarily ascribed to their poor tumor targetability and instability in biological fluids. Park and coworkers reported on hydrophilized $HTiO_2$ NPs that produce ROS *in vivo* when activated by US to eradicate tumors. They demonstrated that TiO_2 NP-based SDT generate a high level of ROS both *in vitro* and *in vivo*. To evaluate $^1O_2$ generation *in vivo*, fluorescence images of the tumor tissue were obtained 12 h after systemic administration of Cy5.5-labeled $HTiO_2$ NPs. The red fluorescence in the tumor image shows that the $HTiO_2$ NPs were distributed evenly in US-treated and nontreated animal groups. Without US treatment, the $^1O_2$ signal (green) was rarely detected in the tumor tissue. Interestingly, in the US-treated mouse, strong fluorescence was observed mostly around blood vessels in tumor tissue (Figure 23.6). In addition, the upregulation of proinflammatory cytokines and interleukins (ILs) in tumor tissue after SDT was verified [29].

Quantitative analysis indicated that US-treated tumor tissue contained 29.7-fold more $^1O_2$ molecules than nontreated tissue. On the other hand, a significant reduction in tumor size ($p < 0.005$) was observed in mice treated with $HTiO_2$

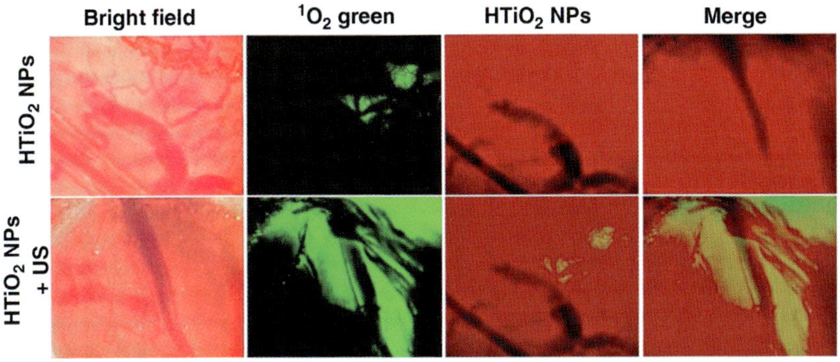

Figure 23.6 *In vivo* fluorescent imaging of the tumor site to observe $^1O_2$ (green) and $HTiO_2$ NP (red) 12 h after SDT. Scale bar: 1000 μm. (Taken from Ref. [29]. Copyright 2016, Macmillan Publishers Limited.)

NPs and US compared with controls. $HTiO_2$ NPs (5 mg/kg) plus US treatment suppressed tumor volume to below 700 mm^3 over 24 days. It implies that there is a correlation between tumor regression and ROS generation by US-activated $HTiO_2$ NPs. In addition, a substantial amount of vascular damage was observed in tumors treated with $HTiO_2$ NPs (5 mg/kg) and US from day 17. The extent of damage was increased with the treatment progress.

Although the mechanism of ROS generation during US treatment is not fully understood, sonoluminescence is believed to be a key phenomenon to generate ROS.

23.6 Cryosurgery

Cryosurgery (CS) is the application of extreme cold to destroy abnormal or diseased tissue. It is appropriate for treating localized diseases and solid tumors larger than 1 cm, but tiny or diffuse metastases are usually not affected by cryosurgery. Generally, all tumors that can be reached by cryoprobes during an operation are treatable. However, in many clinical cases, freezing alone does not completely destroy the targeted tumor, possibly because the freezing rate does not produce massive ice nucleation in tumor cells, especially at the edge of the tumor. Consequently, a major concern of conventional CS is maximizing the freezing efficiency, and thus avoiding insufficient freezing between multiple cryoprobes.

A new conceptual modality for nanocryosurgical ablation of tumors has been proposed recently. The main strategy is to apply MgO nanoparticles, which are nontoxic, biodegradable, and have few side effects in the human body, to mediate the freezing procedure effectively. Detailed investigation through animal experiments and nucleation analysis has demonstrated that delivery of MgO nanoparticles into the target tissues can significantly improve the cryosurgical outcome. The formation of an iceball during the freezing process is accelerated and the iceball is enlarged because of the excellent thermal properties of MgO nanoparticles. In addition, this method promotes the generation of ice nuclei and thus increases cryoinjury to the target cells. Therefore, combining the biodegradability and nontoxicity of MgO nanoparticles with their relatively lightweight properties and excellent thermal properties should help in the development of high-performance cryosurgery [30].

23.7 Future Perspectives

Undoubtedly, future applications will benefit from both the improved performance of the physical methods presented in this chapter (e.g., PTT, PDT, MH, and SDT) resulting from technical progress and the discovery of new particles that exhibit useful properties. For example, the use of light for the excitation of the surface plasmon of metallic nanoparticles to produce heat is a promising physical treatment for cancer, although its disadvantage is the limited penetration depth of only a few centimeters. Therefore, it has been suggested that techniques to deliver NIR light into deeper tissues should exploit fiber-optic probes; meeting this challenge remains a crucial task. The problem with the use of an alternative magnetic field to produce heat is very different. There is no absorption of the magnetic field by tissues, but it remains technologically difficult to generate a focalized alternative magnetic field in deep tissues. As already discussed, the heat dissipation is very sensitive to the magnetic properties of nanoparticles (e.g., saturation magnetization and magnetic anisotropy) and to the surrounding environments (e.g., solvent viscosity, magnetic field frequency, and amplitude). Therefore, extensive research has focused on the control of magnetism to optimize the applicability of heat generation and, independently, on the development of an external magnetic field setup that generates a focused AMF.

On the other hand, combination therapy, which uses more than one therapeutic approach, has shown great potential for the treatment of cancer and some other serious diseases. They often combine chemotherapeutic with a physical treatment like PDT; however, the combination of physical treatments such as those discussed in this chapter can lead to very interesting synergistic effect. One recent study illustrates the combination of different physical treatments with the combined use of PDT and magnetic hyperthermia in the same treatment [31]. The authors designed an optimized smart nanoplatform based on dually loaded hybrid liposomes to achieve enhanced tumor therapy. The aqueous core was highly loaded with iron oxide nanoparticles, while the lipid bilayer was supplied with a photosensitizer payload. The double cargo translated into double functionality: generation of singlet oxygen under laser excitation and heat production under alternating magnetic field stimulation, coupling photodynamic therapy (PDT) to magnetic hyperthermia (MHT). These liposomes address both therapeutic agents within tumor cells, and the combined PDT/MHT therapy resulted in complete cancer cell death *in vitro* while total solid tumor ablation was achieved in an *in vivo* rodent model.

Wang and coworkers prepared a multifunctional nanoplatform by covalently grafting graphene oxide with UCNPs, obtaining GO–UCNP composite, which was demonstrated to be effective for the loading of photosensitizer to realize a synergistic treatment effect of cancer cells *in vitro* by combining PTT with PDT [32].

In the past decades, much effort has been channeled in the development of multifunctional theranostic agents where a number of diverse diagnostic and therapeutic functionalities have been incorporated in a single nanoplatform for a "see and treat" approach. In addition to that, standardized physicochemical characterization, validation, and safety protocols must be established to achieve pure and homogeneous nanoparticles that can yield precise and reproducible results. The major bottleneck for the translation of these theranostic agents into clinical practice is the absence of standardized procedures to assess its *in vivo* biodistribution, detailed pharmacokinetic pharmacodynamic (PK–PD) analysis, short- and long-term effects of the nanomaterials *in vivo*, and its clearance from the system. This was exactly the reason behind the development of standardized evaluation protocols for rigorous characterization of nanoparticle's physicochemical properties, *in vitro* immunological and cytotoxic characteristics, as well as administration, distribution, metabolism, and elimination (ADME)/toxicity profiles in animal models; to facilitate the regulatory review of nanotechnology-based cancer therapeutics; and fast track the clinical trial process.

References

1 Dreaden, E.C., Alkilany, A.M., Huang, X., Murphy, C.J., and El-Sayed, M.A. (2012) The golden age: gold nanoparticles for biomedicine. *Chem. Soc. Rev.*, **41** (7), 2740–2779.

2 Doane, T.L. and Burda, C. (2012) The unique role of nanoparticles in nanomedicine: imaging, drug delivery and therapy. *Chem. Soc. Rev.*, **41** (7), 2885.

3 Langville, M.R., Personick, M.L., and Mirkin, C.A. (2013) Plasmon-mediated syntheses of metallic nanostructures. *Angew. Chem., Int. Ed.*, **52**, 13910–13940.

4 Dreaden, E.C., Mackey, M.A., Huang, X., Kang, B., and El-Sayed, M.A. (2011) Beating cancer in multiple ways using nanogold. *Chem. Soc. Rev.*, **40** (7), 3391.

5 Murphy, C.J., Sau, T.K., Gole, A.M., Orendorff, C.J., Gao, J., Gou, L., Hunyadi, S.E., and Li, T. (2005) Anisotropic metal nanoparticles: synthesis, assembly, and optical applications. *J. Phys. Chem. B*, **109** (29), 13857–13870.

6 El-Sayed, I., Huang, X., and Elsayed, M. (2006) Selective laser photo-thermal therapy of epithelial carcinoma using anti-EGFR antibody conjugated gold nanoparticles. *Cancer Lett.*, **239** (1), 129–135.

7 Dickerson, E., Dreaden, E., Huang, X., Elsayed, I., Chu, H., Pushpanketh, S., Mcdonald, J., and Elsayed, M. (2008) Gold nanorod assisted near-infrared plasmonic photothermal therapy (PPTT) of squamous cell carcinoma in mice. *Cancer Lett.*, **269** (1), 57–66.

8 Hirsch, L., Stafford, R.J., Bankson, J.A., Sershen, S.R., Rivera, B., Price, R.E., Hazle,

J.D., Halas, N.J., and West, J.L. (2003) Nanoshell-mediated near-infrared thermal therapy of tumors under magnetic resonance guidance. *Proc. Natl. Acad. Sci. USA*, **100** (23), 13549–13554.

9 Lal, S., Clare, S.E., and Halas, N.J. (2008) Nanoshell-enabled photothermal cancer therapy: impending clinical impact. *Acc. Chem. Res.*, **41** (12), 1842–1851.

10 Muthu, M.S., Leong, D.T., Mei, L., and Feng, S.-S. (2014) Nanotheranostics: application and further development of nanomedicine strategies for advanced theranostics. *Theranostics*, **4** (6), 660–677.

11 Moon, H.K., Lee, S.H., and Choi, H.C. (2009) *In vivo* near-infrared mediated tumor destruction by photothermal effect of carbon nanotubes. *ACS Nano*, **3** (11), 3707–3713.

12 Robinson, J.T., Welsher, K., Tabakman, S.M., Sherlock, S.P., Wang, H., Luong, R., and Dai, H. (2010) High performance *in vivo* near-IR imaging and photothermal cancer therapy with carbon nanotubes. *Nano Res.*, **3** (11), 779–793.

13 Yang, K., Zhang, S., Zhang, G., Sun, X., Lee, S.-T., and Liu, Z. (2010) Graphene in mice: ultrahigh *in vivo* tumor uptake and efficient photothermal therapy. *Nano Lett.*, **10** (9), 3318–3323.

14 Lucky, S.S., Soo, K.C., and Zhang, Y. (2015) Nanoparticles in photodynamic therapy. *Chem. Rev.*, **115** (4), 1990–2042.

15 Cai., R., Kubota, Y., Shuin, H., Hashimoto, K., and Fujishima, A. (1992) Induction of cytotoxicity by photoexcited TiO_2 particles. *Cancer Res.*, **52**, 2346.

16 Park, Y.I., Kim, H.M., Kim, J.H., Moon, K.C., Yoo, B., Lee, K.T., Lee, N., Choi, Y., Park, W., Ling, D., Na, K., Moon, W.K., Choi, S.H., Park, H.S., Yoon, S.Y., Suh, Y.D., Lee, S.H., and Hyeon, T. (2012) Theranostic probe based on lanthanide-doped nanoparticles for simultaneous *in vivo* dual-modal imaging and photodynamic therapy. *Adv. Mater.*, **24**, 5755–5761.

17 Bacri, J.-C., Perzynski, R., Salin, D., Cabuil, V., and Massart, R. (1990) Ionic ferrofluids: a crossing of chemistry and physics. *J. Magn. Magn. Mater.*, **85**, 27–32.

18 Hyeon, T., Lee, S.S., Park, J., Chung, Y., and Na, H.B. (2001) Synthesis of highly crystalline and monodisperse maghemite nanocrystallites without a size-selection process. *J. Am. Chem. Soc.*, **123** (51), 12798–12801.

19 Itoh, H. and Sugimoto, T. (2003) Systematic control of size, shape, structure, and magnetic properties of uniform magnetite and maghemite particles. *J. Colloid Interface Sci.*, **265** (2), 283–295.

20 Xuan, S., Hao, L., Jiang, W., Gong, X., Hu, Y., and Chen, Z. (2007) Preparation of water-soluble magnetite nanocrystals through hydrothermal approach. *J. Magn. Magn. Mater.*, **308** (2), 210–213.

21 Lee, N., Yoo, D., Ling, D., Cho, M.H., Hyeon, T., and Cheon, J. (2015) Iron oxide based nanoparticles for multimodal imaging and magnetoresponsive therapy. *Chem. Rev.*, **115** (19), 10637–10689.

22 Colombo, M., Carregal-Romero, S., Casula, M.F., Gutiérrez, L., Morales, M.P., Böhm, I.B., Heverhagen, J.T., Prosperi, D., and Parak, W.J. (2012) Biological applications of magnetic nanoparticles. *Chem. Soc. Rev.*, **41** (11), 4306.

23 Jordan, A., Scholz, R., Wust, P., Fähling, H., Krause, J., Wlodarczyk, W., Sander, B., Vogl, T., and Felix, R. (1997) Effects of magnetic fluid hyperthermia (MFH) on C3H mammary carcinoma *in vivo*. *Int. J. Hyperthermia*, **13** (6), 587–605.

24 Thiesen, B. and Jordan, A. (2008) Clinical applications of magnetic nanoparticles for hyperthermia. *Int. J. Hyperthermia*, **24** (6), 467–474.

25 Hayashi, K., Nakamura, M., Sakamoto, W., Yogo, T., Miki, H., Ozaki, S., Abe, M., Matsumoto, T., and Ishimura, K. (2013) Superparamagnetic nanoparticle clusters for cancer theranostics combining magnetic resonance imaging and hyperthermia treatment. *Theranostics*, **3** (6), 366–376.

26 Marill, J., Anesary, N.M., Zhang, P., Vivet, S., Borghi, E., Levy, L., and Pottier, A. (2014) Hafnium oxide nanoparticles: toward an *in vitro* predictive biological effect? *Radiat. Oncol.*, **9** (1), 150.

27 Serpe, L., Foglietta, F., and Canaparo, R. (2012) Nanosonotechnology: the next challenge in cancer sonodynamic therapy. *Nanotechnol. Rev.*, **1** (2), 173–182.

28 Wang, J., Guo, Y., Liu, B., Jin, X., Liu, L., Xu, R., Kong, Y., and Wang, B. (2011) Detection and analysis of reactive oxygen species (ROS) generated by nano-sized TiO_2 powder under ultrasonic irradiation and application in sonocatalytic degradation of organic dyes. *Ultrason. Sonochem.*, **18** (1), 177–183.

29 You, D.G., Deepagan, V.G., Um, W., Jeon, S., Son, S., Chang, H., Yoon, H.I., Cho, Y.W., Swierczewska, M., Lee, S., Pomper, M.G., Kwon, I.C., Kim, K., and Park, J.-H. (2016) ROS-generating TiO_2 nanoparticles for non-invasive sonodynamic therapy of cancer. *Sci. Rep.*, **6**, 23200.

30 Di, D.-R., He, Z.-Z., Sun, Z.-Q., and Liu, J. (2012) A new nano-cryosurgical modality for tumor treatment using biodegradable MgO nanoparticles. *Nanomedicine*, **8** (8), 1233–1241.

31 Di Corato, R., Béalle, G., Kolosnjaj-Tabi, J., Espinosa, A., Clément, O., Silva, A.K.A., Ménager, C., and Wilhelm, C. (2015) Combining magnetic hyperthermia and photodynamic therapy for tumor ablation with photoresponsive magnetic liposomes. *ACS Nano*, **9** (3), 2904–2916.

32 Wang, Y., Wang, H., Liu, D., Song, S., Wang, X., and Zhang, H. (2013) Graphene oxide covalently grafted upconversion nanoparticles for combined NIR mediated imaging and photothermal/photodynamic cancer therapy. *Biomaterials*, **34**, 7715–7724.

24
Nanodrugs in Medicine and Healthcare: Oral Delivery

Alejandro Sosnik[1,2]

[1]*Technion-Israel Institute of Technology, Department of Materials Science and Engineering, Laboratory of Pharmaceutical Nanomaterials Science, Technion City, Haifa 3200003, Israel*
[2]*Technion-Israel Institute of Technology, Russell Berrie Nanotechnology Institute (RBNI), Technion City, Haifa 3200003, Israel*

24.1
General Aspects and Challenges of Oral Drug Delivery

Oral administration is the most patient compliant route owing to minimal invasiveness, painfulness, ease-of-use (and no need of trained personnel), cost-effectiveness, reproducibility of the administration, and feasibility in the whole range of patient ages [1]. These advantageous features rely on the availability of a broad spectrum of so-called conventional solid, semisolid, and liquid dosage forms adjustable to the patient needs [2]. These formulations are scalable and relatively cheap. Accordingly, it comprised 38% of the total drug delivery in 2012 and it is forecasted to grow from a \$49 billion in 2010 to a \$97 billion market in 2017 [3]. At the same time, drugs delivered by the oral route are exposed to an aggressive biological environment that jeopardize their chemical integrity and their pharmacological or biological activity before they reach the systemic circulation [4]. Peptides and proteins represent the paradigm of instability by the oral route [5–7] and significant efforts are being devoted to enable the oral administration of proteins of chronic use (e.g., insulin) [8]. Another challenge pertains to the complex structure and the properties of the gastrointestinal tract (especially of the intestine where most of the drugs undergo absorption) that change in its different portions. The gastrointestinal tract reaches complete anatomical and functional maturity over the first years of life; for example, children present very substantial changes in the gastric pH over the first few days and weeks. The complexity of the structure of the gastrointestinal tract is exemplified for the intestinal wall in Figure 24.1 [9].

A crucial component of the digestive system is the mucus that covers the gastrointestinal wall and represents the first barrier for absorption from the lumen. In addition, the gastrointestinal absorption of poorly water-soluble molecules is

Pharmaceutical Nanotechnology: Innovation and Production, First Edition. Edited by Jean Cornier, Arno Kwade, Andrew Owen, and Marcel Van de Voorde.

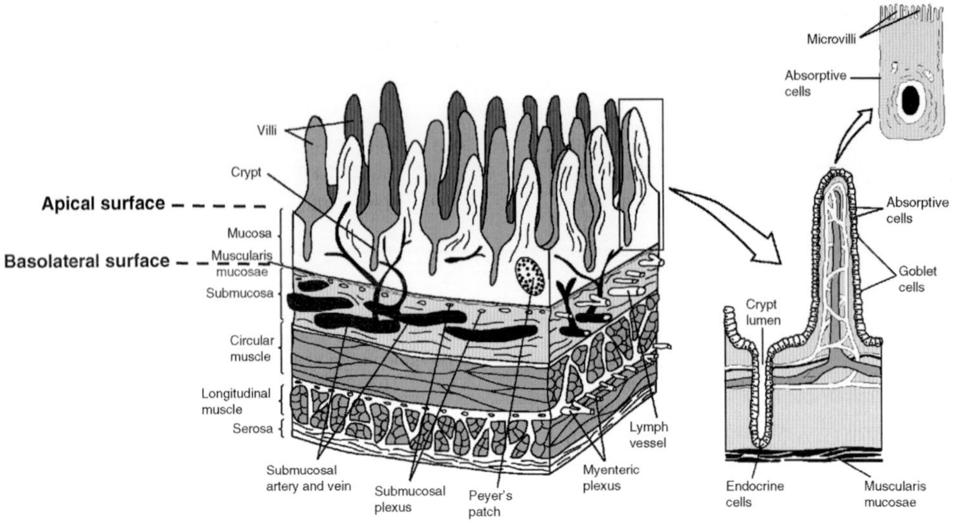

Figure 24.1 Structure of the intestinal wall. (Reproduced with modifications from Ref. [9] with permission of Elsevier.)

usually limited due to incomplete or late dissolution, resulting in low oral bioavailability. This biopharmaceutical drawback has also contributed to increased attrition rates in the drug development process, a more noteworthy phenomenon since the widening implementation of combinatorial chemistry and high-throughput screening [10]. Another hurdle to ensure drug absorption in the intestine is low permeability through membranes [11,12] and the presence of pumps that actively remove them in the basolateral-to-apical direction during absorption [13,14].

Finally, many drugs undergo first-pass metabolism (to a greater extent in the liver and to a lower one in the intestinal wall), thus limiting bioavailability [15]. Conventional pharmaceutical products usually fail to provide a comprehensive solution to all these drawbacks. In this framework, a broad spectrum of innovative technologies, from the early drug micronization to the more recent nanonization of pure drugs, to the design of more complex polymeric and lipid nanocarriers have been explored to maximize the oral bioavailability of drugs. This chapter provides an overview of the nanotechnology approaches emphasizing their clinical potential and status and the limitations posed for bench-to-bedside translation.

24.2
Pure Drug Micronization as a Conceptual Preamble to More Complex Drug Delivery

The reduction of the pure drug particle size to the micrometer scale, namely, micronization, was incorporated in the early 1960s to increase surface area and drug dissolution rates and since then it has become one of the most extensively used technological strategies to improve oral bioavailability of drugs in the clinical practice [16–18]. In this scenario, it represented the conceptual basis to the more recently implemented nanonization processes that will be discussed subsequently [19,20].

24.3 Nanotechnology Platforms for Improved Oral Drug Delivery

With the advent of the ability to control, mass produce, and fully characterize structures at the nanosize level, nanotechnologies have gained a great deal of attention in pharmaceutical design and development giving place to the budding of new research areas such as nanopharmaceuticals and nanodrug delivery currently investigated for the diagnosis, prophylaxis, and treatment of disease [21]. Most research is being oriented toward treating cancer by the intravenous route [22,23]. For instance, the first FDA-approved nanomedicine was Doxil®, a liposomal intravenous formulation of doxorubicin [24]. At the same time, the gap between academic research and clinical translation is very profound [25], highlighting a number of unsolved issues, including insufficient improvement of drug performance, difficult production of sophisticated systems under industrial setups, and expensive or cost-inviable scalability [26,27]. Regardless of the inherent potential of nanomedicines to improve oral therapies, investigation of nanotechnologies for oral administration has been much more constrained [28]. Regardless of the complexity of the nanotechnology approach, the pharmacokinetics expected for an innovative oral nanopharmaceutical of even of an approved drug demands comprehensive bioequivalence studies [29]. This stage is crucial to ensure safety and efficacy and it is not deprived of ethical concerns [30].

24.3.1 Pure Drug Nanoparticles

Pure drug nanoparticles are produced by top-down (e.g., high-pressure homogenization or nanomilling) and bottom-up (e.g., nanoprecipitation) techniques and nanoparticles are usually stabilized with surfactants [19,20,31]. Since it is a carrier-less approach, it constitutes the simplest and most easily scalable nanotechnology to improve the oral bioavailability of poorly water-soluble drugs and amorphous, semicrystalline or crystalline pharmaceutical products can be formulated in solid [32] and liquid formats [33,34]. Additional features of pure drug nanoparticles are increase of saturation solubility and of mucoadhesiveness to the intestinal mucosa [35] and eventually sustained release and prolongation of the half-life [36–38]. It is still intriguing that regardless of the feasibility of the approach and the commercial availability of industrial equipment, the number of pure drug nanoparticle products for oral administration on the market and preclinical and clinical trials is relatively small (Table 24.1).

Table 24.1 Pure drug nanocrystals for oral administration on the market or under preclinical and clinical trial.

Drug	Commercial name/ Company	Pharmacological activity	Production method	Status	Reference
Sirolimus	Rapamune®/Wyeth	Immunosuppressant	Top-down, media milling	Commercially available	[38]
Aprepitant	Emend®/Merck	Antiemetic	Top-down, media milling	Commercially available	[39]
Fenofibrate	Tricor®/Abbott	Hypercholesterolemia	Top-down, media milling	Commercially available	[39]
Fenofibrate	Triglide™/First Horizon Pharmaceutical	Hypercholesterolemia	Top-down, high-pressure homogenization	Commercially available	[39]
Megestrol acetate	Megace® ES/Par Pharmaceutical	Appetite stimulant	Top-down, media milling	Commercially available	[39]
Griseofulvin	Gris-PEG®/Novartis	Antifungal	Bottom-up, coprecipitation	Commercially available	[40]
Nabilone	Cesamet®/Lilly	Antiemetic	Bottom-up, coprecipitation	Commercially available	[40]
Morphine sulfate	Avinza/King Pharmaceuticals	Psychostimulant	Top-down, ball milling	Commercially available	[38]
Dexmethylphenidate HCl	Focalin® XR/Novartis	Psychostimulant in attention-deficit hyper-activity disorder (ADHD) and narcolepsy	Top-down, ball milling	Commercially available	[38]
Methylphenidate HCl	Ritalin® LA/Novartis	Psychostimulant in attention-deficit hyper-activity disorder and narcolepsy	Top-down, ball milling	Commercially available	[38]
Tizanidine HCl	Zanaflex Capsules™/ Accorda	Muscle relaxant	Top-down, ball milling	Commercially available	[38]

Insulin	BioSante	Diabetes	—	Phase I	[38]
Fenofibrate	SkyePharma	Hypercholesterolemia	—	Phase I	[38]
Calcium phosphate	BioVant®/BioSante	Vaccine adjuvant	—	Phase I	[38]
Testosterone	—	Male hypogonadism	Top-down, nanomilling	Phase I	[41]
Investigational guanylhydrazone	Semapimod®/Cytokine PharmaSciences	TNF-inhibitor, anti-inflammatory and anti-immune diseases	—	Phase II	[39]
Megestrol acetate	Par Pharmaceuticals, Inc.	Weight loss associated with AIDS	Top-down, ball milling	Phase II	[38]
2-Methoxy estradiol	Panzem® NCD/ EntreMed	Ovarian cancer Recurrent glioblastoma multiforme Prostate cancer	Top-down, ball milling	Phase II	[38]
2-Methoxy estradiol/ temozolomide	Panzem® NCD with temozolomide/ EntreMed	Antitumoral	Top-down, ball milling	Phase II	[38]
2-Methoxy estradiol/ bevacizumab[a)]	Panzem® NCD with Avastin/EntreMed	Antitumoral	Top-down, ball milling	Phase II	[38]
2-Methoxy estradiol/ sunitinib maleate	Panzem® NCD with sunitinib/EntreMed	Antitumoral	Top-down, ball milling	Phase II	[38]
Fenofibrate	Solvay Pharmaceuticals	Sleep apnea syndrome	Top-down, ball milling	Phase II	[38]
Cytokine inhibitor	Cytokine inhibitor/ PharmaSciences	Crohn's disease	Top-down, ball milling	Phase II	[38]
Undisclosed antibiotic[b)]	Baxter NANOEDGE	Anti-infective	—	Phase II	[38]
Danazol	—	Estrogen antagonist	Top-down, media milling	*In vivo* (dog)	[42]
Naproxen	—	Anti-inflammatory	Top-down, media milling	*In vivo* (rat)	[43]
Cilostazol	—	Antiplatelet agent	Top-down, media milling	*In vivo* (dog)	[44]

(*continued*)

Table 24.1 (*Continued*)

Drug	Commercial name/ Company	Pharmacological activity	Production method	Status	Reference
Ketoprofen	—	Anti-inflammatory	Top-down, media milling	*In vivo* (dog)	[45]
Cyclosporine	—	Immunosuppressant	Top-down, high-pressure homogenization	*In vivo* (pig)	[46]
Spironolactone	—	Diuretic	Top-down, high-pressure homogenization	*In vivo* (rat)	[47]
Itraconazole	—	Antifungal	Bottom-up, precipitation	*In vivo* (rat)	[48]
Efavirenz	-/Tandem Nano Ltd.	Antiretroviral	Bottom-up, spray drying	*In vivo (rats)*	[49]
Indinavir free base	—	Antiretroviral	Bottom-up, nanoprecipitation and supercritical fluids	*In vivo (dogs)*	[36,37,50]
Efavirenz	-/Tandem Nano Ltd.	Antiretroviral	Bottom-up, emulsion-templated freeze-drying technique	*In vivo (rats)*	[51]

a) Bevacizumab in the combination is administered i.v.
b) Oral and i.v. administration.

This is in opposition to several long-acting nanosuspensions undergoing preclinical and clinical evaluation (e.g., rilpivirine, cabotegravir, paliperidone) or already on the market (e.g., olanzapine, medroxyprogesterone) by the intramuscular route.

24.3.2 Dendrimers and Other Branched Nanocarriers

Dendrimers are highly branched macromolecules that display a well-defined three-dimensional nanometer-scale architecture with very narrow molecular weight distribution (usually ~1) and extremely high functionality that enables both the encapsulation and complexation of drugs [52,53]. By tuning the number of synthetic cycles, the size, the surface functionality and charge, and the accessibility of drug molecules to the macromolecular core can be modified and accordingly the encapsulation capacity and the release kinetics. Poly(amidoamine) (PAMAM) dendrimers were the first family to be produced and commercialized [54], although due to high toxicity, especially of the amine-terminated derivatives, they have not been approved [55]. At the same time, they have inspired the design of more biocompatible molecules based on biocompatible polymeric precursors and led to the development of the active poly(lysine)-based dendrimer SPL7013 formulated in a gel (VivaGel®, Starpharma) that has been clinically trialed for prophylaxis of sexually transmitted infections, including HIV [56,57].

Aiming to better control the synthesis and the scalability under pilot and industrial setups, simplified versions of nanocarriers such as dendrons and dendritic polymers have been also developed [58]. Most of the drug delivery studies have been mainly oriented to parenteral and topical release [59]. However, since hyperbranched polymers can facilitate permeation across membranes [60], absorption by the Peyer's patches in the intestine [61], and adhesion to mucosal tissues, their investigation for oral drug delivery has gained interest. The inhibition of efflux pumps of the ATP-bindings cassette superfamily in the gastrointestinal tract is a complementary mechanism that boosts the systemic concentration of orally administered drugs [62]. Most of the attempts to deliver drug-loaded dendrimers by the oral route employed pristine or surface-coated PAMAMs that displayed better compatibility and loaded the cargo by capitalizing on electrostatic interactions or simple encapsulation [63–70]. Due to the fact that PAMAMs are not approved, these works represent a modest step toward clinical translation. The same could be claimed for some studies that did not assess the encapsulation of any specific cargo [62,64,65]. These findings point out the preliminary nature of the research niche at the crossroad of dendrimers and oral route.

24.3.3 Polymeric Micelles

Polymeric micelles are nanostructures (usually <100 nm) formed by the self-assembly of amphiphilic copolymers above the critical micellar concentration

(CMC) [71]. The most popular amphiphiles are A–B diblocks and A–B–A triblocks where A and B represent the hydrophilic and the hydrophobic blocks, respectively. To overcome the physical instability of these nanocarriers under extreme dilution to final concentrations close or below the CMC, unimolecular micelles have also been investigated [72]. The hydrophobic blocks form an inner domain known as core that is capable of hosting hydrophobic molecules and the hydrophilic ones and the outer corona that is in direct contact with the dispersant (e.g., water). As previously described for other nanotechnologies, polymeric micelles were employed mainly for the intravenous administration of anticancer drugs [71,73]. At the same time, their potential as oral drug nanocarriers has been increasingly highlighted [74–76], although only a few works reported preclinical data [77,78], stressing the immature state of this unique research avenue. For example, Lee *et al.* encapsulated paclitaxel in micelles produced with block copolymers of poly(ethylene glycol) (PEG) and poly(2-(4-vinylbenzyloxy)-*N,N*-diethylnicotinamide) [79]. The oral bioavailability of the drug was 12.4% of the i.v. dose. Satturwar *et al.* used PEG-*b*-poly(alkyl(meth)acrylate-*co*-methacrylic acid) micelles for the encapsulation and pH-responsive release of candesartan cilexetil [80]. Even though the proof of concept was demonstrated, no *in vivo* results were reported. Other studies investigated the encapsulation of cyclosporine A [81,82], paclitaxel [83], vorinostat [84], nifedipine [85], dexibuprofen [86], docetaxel [87], and camptothecin [88]. Our research group has comprehensively investigated pristine and chemically modified commercially available (and in some cases approved) poly(ethylene oxide)-*b*-poly(propylene oxide) (PEO-PPO) block copolymers to improve the aqueous solubility and oral bioavailability of the antiretroviral efavirenz in the treatment of pediatric HIV and conducted a comprehensive preclinical evaluation [89,90] that enabled the preliminary clinical trial of the micellar formulation in one adult healthy volunteer [91]. In another work, the antituberculosis drug rifampicin was encapsulated into "flower-like" polymeric micelles made of poly(epsilon-caprolactone)-*b*-poly(ethylene glycol)-*b*-poly(epsilon-caprolactone) copolymers and its acid degradation in the stomach partially prevented, resulting in a significant increase of the oral bioavailability with respect to the free drug [92]. This performance was observed even in the presence of the water-soluble isoniazid, another antituberculosis drug that is coadministered with rifampicin and that catalyzes its degradation. In a recent study, Dian *et al.* encapsulated quercetin in polymeric micelles of a polyvinyl caprolactam-polyvinyl acetate polyethylene glycol graft copolymer (Soluplus®) and increased the oral bioavailability by 286% and prolonged the half-life by 2.19-fold [93].

The oral bioavailability of the micelles themselves has been a matter of discussion. The very low absorption in the intestine and systemic bioavailability of polymeric micelles has been suggested [76], although Mathot *et al.* showed that some of them can cross the intestinal epithelium by a saturable mechanism and reach an oral bioavailability of up to 40% [94,95]. This behavior could be probably attributed to the circulation of nonassembled unimers rather than of assembled structures in the bloodstream. It is reasonable to expect that this outcome will depend on the size and the chemical nature of the micellar surface. The main drawbacks that remain unsolved are the relatively low physical stability of polymeric micelles under extreme dilution, the weak interaction with mucosa, and the inability to sustain the release of the cargo. In this context, development of more sophisticated polymeric micelles is called for to enhance their overall oral performance [96].

24.3.4 Nanoemulsions

Nanoemulsions are systems formed by two immiscible liquid phases where one liquid (usually the oily phase) is dispersed in the form of nanosized droplets (20–200 nm) in the other (usually the aqueous phase) and stabilized with nonionic or amphoteric surfactants adsorbed at the interface [77,97,98]. The oil droplets serve as reservoir of poorly water-soluble drugs. The emulsification energy of some systems is low and thus they undergo self-emulsification once the oily phase is added to water and gently stirred. These systems are known as self-emulsifying drug delivery systems (SEDDSs) [99]. As previously discussed for other platforms, nanoemulsions have been more extensively explored for routes other than the oral one (e.g., topical and transdermal) [99]. However, some attempts include the oral delivery of simvastatin [100], coenzyme Q_{10} [101], heparin [102], breviscapine [103], proteins [104], and anticancer drugs [105]. Only a few oral SEDDSs products have reached the market [106]. For example, Neoral® and Sandimmune®, self-emulsifying systems of cyclosporine A, are a gold-standard therapy to prevent organ rejection following transplantation [107,108] – the former displaying a more predictable and efficient intestinal absorption than the latter. In addition, liquid formulations of the protease inhibitors ritonavir (Norvir®) and saquinavir (Fortovase®) have also been developed using this approach [106]. However, the low control of the droplet size and size distribution represents a disadvantage to ensure low pharmacokinetic variability [108].

24.3.5 Solid Lipid Nanoparticles

Solid lipid nanoparticles (SLNs) are colloidal systems where the lipid phase is a solid at room temperature, as opposed to nanoemulsions where it is a liquid [109–111]. SLNs have been conceived to overcome biopharmaceutical disadvantages such as physicochemical stability and complex production processes displayed by the more popular liposomes; liposomes are difficult for implementation by the oral route due to very low stability in the aggressive conditions of the gastrointestinal tract. In general, the higher the aqueous solubility of the cargo, the lower the encapsulation capacity of SLNs. Thus, methods at room temperature and 0 °C have been developed. Otherwise, highly hydrophobic drugs can be encapsulated by hot homogenization [109–111]. The use of SLNs as oral drug delivery systems was introduced in the mid-1990s. To improve their stability in the stomach, SLNs were encapsulated within gastro-resistant capsules or incorporated into pellets and tablets [110]. One intrinsic limitation of SLNs is the crystallization of the lipid components that might result in the expulsion of the payload under storage conditions [112]. This phenomenon motivated the development of nanostructured lipid carriers (NLCs), a lipid nanocarrier where the crystallization is more controlled and prevented to some extent, and concomitantly the encapsulation capacity and the physical stability enhanced. It is worth stressing that most studies initially focused on SLNs, probably due to an easier developmental process [113]. However, NLCs represent a technology that enables a better control of the encapsulation and release and thus they have been the matter of more recent studies [113]. In both cases, a longer residence time in the gastrointestinal tract with respect to other lipid nanocarriers (e.g., SEDDSs) would be of great appeal. The most relevant examples of SLNs and NLCs for oral administration are presented in Table 24.2 [111,113].

Table 24.2 SLNs and NLCs for the improvement of the oral pharmacokinetics of drugs.

Drug	Type of carrier	Main goal/outcome	Reference
All-*trans* retinoic acid	SLN	Improvement of oral bioavailability	[114]
Apomorphine	SLN	Improvement of oral bioavailability and brain regional distribution	[115]
α-Asarone	SLN	Improvement of oral bioavailability and tissue biodistribution	[116]
Buspirone hydrochloride	SLN	Improvement of oral bioavailability	[117]
Camptothecin	SLN	Improvement of biodistribution and sustained release and targeting	[118]
Carvedilol	SLN	Improvement of oral bioavailability, lymphatic uptake and reduction of hepatic first-pass	[119]
Clozapine	SLN	Improvement of oral bioavailability and tissue distribution	[120]
Cryptotanshinone	SLN	Improvement of oral bioavailability and change in metabolism	[121]
Cyclosporine A	SLN	Reduction of bioavailability variability and avoidance of the huge initial plasma concentration	[122]
Curcumin	SLN	Improvement of oral bioavailability and sustained release	[123]
Digoxin	SLN	Improvement of oral bioavailability	[124]
Etoposide	NCL	Improvement of oral bioavailability	[125]
Fenofibrate	SLN	Improvement of oral bioavailability	[126]

Fenofibrate	NCL	Improvement of oral bioavailability	[127]
Iloperidone	NCL	Improvement of oral bioavailability	[128]
Insulin	Lectin-modified SLN	Reduction of enzymatic degradation and improvement of oral bioavailability	[129]
Insulin	SLN	Improvement of oral bioavailability	[130–132]
Lovastatin	NLC	Improvement of encapsulation capacity, stability in the gastrointestinal tract and oral bioavailability	[133]
Luteolin	NCL	Improvement of oral bioavailability	[134]
Melatonin	SLN	Sustained release	[135]
Methotrexate	SLN	Improvement of oral bioavailability and lymphatic absorption	[136]
Miconazole	NCL	Similar oral pharmacokinetics of oral gel	[137]
Montelukast	NCL	Improvement of oral bioavailability	[138]
N_3-*O*-toluyl-fluorouracil	Cationic and anionic SLN	Improvement of oral bioavailability	[139,140]
Nitrendipine	SLN	Reduction of hepatic first-pass and improvement of oral bioavailability	[141]
Octadecylamine	SLN	Improvement of oral bioavailability and lymphatic absorption and prolonged release	[142]
Pentoxifylline	SLN	Reduction of hepatic first-pass and improvement of oral bioavailability	[143]
Praziquantel	SLN	Improved oral bioavailability and prolonged systemic circulation	[144,145]
Quercetin	SLN	Improved oral bioavailability	[146]
Quercetin	NCL	Improved oral bioavailability	[147]
Resveratrol	NCL	Higher physical stability of the drug and minimal expulsion compared to SLN	[148]
Rifampicin, isoniazid, and pyrazinamide	SLN	Prolonged systemic circulation and improved antituberculosis efficacy	[149]
Salmon calcitonin	SLN without and with coating	Prolonged systemic effect	[150,151]
Saquinavir mesylate	NCL	Improvement of transport across Caco2 cell monolayers	[152]
Silymarin	NCL	Improvement of oral bioavailability with respect to commercially available Legalon®	[153]
Simvastatin	SLN, NLC	Improvement of oral bioavailability	[154]
Spironolactone	SLN	Improvement of oral bioavailability	[155]
Spironolactone	NCL	Change of metabolic profile	[156]
Tamoxifen	NCL	Improvement of oral bioavailability and prolongation of half-life	[157,158]

(continued)

Table 24.2 (*Continued*)

Drug	Type of carrier	Main goal/outcome	Reference
Tripterin	Cell-penetrating peptide-coated NCL	Improvement of oral bioavailability	[159]
Vinpocetine	SLN	Improvement of oral bioavailability	[160]
Vinpocetine	NLC	Improvement of oral bioavailability	[161]

Source: Reproduced with modifications from Refs [110,112] with permission from Springer and Elsevier, respectively.

24.3.6 Polymeric Nanoparticles

Due to the ability to stabilize sensitive active agents, sustain their release, and increase permeability through membranes and bioavailability and biodistribution, polymeric nanoparticles are the most popular polymeric drug nanocarriers [162–164]. Together with liposomes, they attracted most of the investigational efforts over the last decades and were most successfully translated into clinics, mainly supported by the previous experience with polymeric microparticles. Based on the preparation technique, two structures can be produced: (i) solid matrix particles where the drug is homogeneously dispersed as a solid or at the molecular level and (ii) hollow capsules where a drug core is surrounded by a polymeric membrane [162]. A long list of natural, synthetic, and semisynthetic experimental and approved polymers and copolymers have been investigated for the production of nanoparticles and their administration mainly by parenteral routes [164]. Conversely, only a few products for the intravenous treatment of cancer have been marketed [25,165]. By the oral route, polymeric nanoparticles can improve the pharmacokinetics of the cargo, enabling localized delivery in the gastrointestinal tract (e.g., colonic release) or increase the systemic delivery. The number of scientific papers in this area is immense and discussing all of them is beyond the scope of this chapter. For this, readers are referred to a comprehensive review recently published by Kumari *et al.* [163]. One of the works that deserves special attention due to the ability to dramatically prolong the half-life of a cargo formed by several drugs in the systemic circulation is the one conducted by Khuller and coworkers that investigated the coencapsulation of several antituberculosis drugs within poly(lactic-*co*-glycolic) acid (PLGA) nanoparticles [166–169]. In this pioneering work, the authors demonstrated the ability of different orally administered nanoparticles to maintain constant drug levels in plasma for several weeks and thus replace a daily administration regimen and obtain similar preclinical results in a murine model of the disease. It was clear that to display such performance, the nanoparticles had to undergo absorption in the gastrointestinal tract. However, this piece of work did not address this aspect. In a later study, Semete *et al.* studied the biodistribution of PLGA nanoparticles following oral administration and they confirmed that these nanoparticles indeed reach the systemic circulation and redistribute to different organs [170]. Owing to the ability to isolate the cargo, polymeric nanoparticles have also become very appealing for the oral delivery of peptides, proteins, vaccines, genes, and other sensitive molecules [171–173] and nanoencapsulation of insulin emerging as one of the most intensively investigated areas [174]. Regretfully, as previously discussed for other platforms, no clinical trials have been reported employing these innovative products, and approved products that exploit this nanotechnology for the oral route are not yet commercially available.

24.4
Conclusive Remarks

The limited success rate of the translational process in nanomedicine is exceptional, as recently stressed for the therapy of cancer [25]. One of the major challenges is the reproducible, traceable, and cost-viable scale-up of nanopharmaceuticals that demands the simplification of the production processes to reduce costs and the minimization of the use of toxic solvents to prevent environmental concerns. In this framework, production technologies such as spray-drying and electrohydrodynamic atomization that are currently available at the laboratory and pilot scales are being intensively investigated at the academic and industrial levels. These techniques together with the implementation of computational approaches [175] and more rational and simplistic designs might become key (and unavoidable) players to make innovative pharmaceuticals a reality [176,177].

Acknowledgments

The author thanks the financial support of Technion, the Phyllis and Joseph Gurwin Fund for Scientific Advancement, and the European Union's Seventh Framework Programme under grant agreement #612675-MC-NANOTAR.

References

1 MarketsandMarkets (2015) North American Drug Delivery Technologies Market 2017. Available at www.beforeitsnews.com (accessed October 22).

2 Strickley, R.G., Iwata, Q., Wu, S., and Dahl, T.C. (2008) Pediatric drugs: a review of commercially available oral formulations. *J. Pharm. Sci.*, **97** (5), 1731–1774.

3 GBI Research (2012) Oral Drug Delivery Market Report. Contract Pharma. Available at http://www.contractpharma.com/issues/2012-06/view_features/oral-drug-delivery-market-report (accessed October 22, 2015).

4 Gavhane, N. and Yadav, A.V. (2012) Loss of orally administered drugs in GI tract. *Saudi Pharm. J.*, **20** (4), 331–334.

5 Park, K., Kwon, I.C., and Park, K. (2011) Oral protein delivery: current status and future prospect. *React. Funct. Polym.*, **71** (3), 280–287.

6 Singh, R., Singh, S., and Lillard, J.W. (2008) Past, present, and future technologies for oral delivery of therapeutic proteins. *J. Pharm. Sci.*, **97** (7), 2497–2523.

7 Renukuntla, J., Vadlapudi, A.D., Patel, A., Boddu, S.H.S., and Mitra, A.K. (2013) Approaches for enhancing oral bioavailability of peptides and proteins. *Int. J. Pharm.*, **447** (1–2), 75–93.

8 Fonte, P., Araújo, F., Reis, S., and Sarmento, B. (2013) Oral insulin delivery: how far are we? *J. Diabetes Sci. Technol.*, **7** (2), 520–531.

9 Rumsey, R.D.E. (1998) Structure and function of the small intestine, in *Encyclopedia of Human Nutrition*, 2nd edn, Academic Press, pp. 929–938.

10 Stegemann, S., Leveiller, F., Franchi, D., de Jong, H., and Lindén, H. (2007) When poor solubility becomes an issue: from early stage to proof of concept. *Eur. J. Pharm. Sci.*, **31** (5), 249–261.

11 Amidon, G.L., Lennernas, H., Shah, V.P., and Crison, J.R. (1995) A theoretical basis for a biopharmaceutic drug classification: the correlation of *in vitro* drug product dissolution and *in vivo* bioavailability. *Pharm. Res.*, **12** (3), 413–420.

12 Martinez, M.N. and Amidon, G.L. (2002) A mechanistic approach to understanding the factors affecting drug absorption: a review of fundamentals. *J. Clin. Pharmacol.*, **42** (6), 620–643.

13 Kwon, H., Lionberger, R.A., and Yu, L.X. (2004) Impact of P-glycoprotein-mediated intestinal efflux kinetics on oral bioavailability of P-glycoprotein substrates. *Mol. Pharm.*, **1** (6), 455–465.

14 Sosnik, A. (2013) Reversal of multidrug resistance by the inhibition of ATP-binding cassette pumps with generally regarded as safe (GRAS) nanopharmaceuticals: a review. *Adv. Drug Deliv. Rev.*, **65** (13–14), 1828–1851.

15 Pond, S.M. and Tozer, T.N. (1984) First-pass elimination: basic concepts and clinical consequences. *Clin. Pharmacokinet.*, **9** (1), 1–25.

16 Atkinson, R.M., Bedford, C., Child, K.J., and Tomich, E.G. (1962) Effect of particle size on blood griseofulvin-levels in man. *Nature*, **193**, 588–589.

17 Rasenack, N. and Müller, B.W. (2004) Micron-size drug particles: common and novel micronization techniques. *Pharm. Dev. Technol.*, **9** (1), 1–13.

18 Kawabata, Y., Wada, K., Nakatani, M., Yamada, S., and Onoue, S. (2011) Formulation design for poorly water-soluble drugs based on biopharmaceutics classification system: basic approaches and practical applications. *Int. J. Pharm.*, **420** (1), 1–10.

19 Müller, R.H. and Peters, K. (1998) Nanosuspensions for the formulation of poorly soluble drugs: I. Preparation by a size-reduction technique. *Int. J. Pharm.*, **160** (2), 229–237.

20 Junghanns, J.-U.A.H. and Müller, R.H. (2008) Nanocrystal technology, drug delivery and clinical applications. *Int. J. Nanomedicine*, **3** (3), 295–310.

21 Bawarski, W.E., Chidlowsky, E., Bharali, D.J., and Mousa, S.A. (2008) Emerging nanopharmaceuticals. *Nanomedicine*, **4** (4), 273–282.

22 Chauhan, V.P. and Jain, R.K. (2013) Strategies for advancing cancer nanomedicine. *Nat. Mater.*, **12**, 958–962.

23 Xu, X., Ho, W., Zhang, X., Bertrand, N., and Farokhzad, O. (2015) Cancer nanomedicine: from targeted delivery to combination therapy. *Trends Mol. Med.*, **21** (4), 223–232.

24 Barenholz, Y. (2012) Doxil® – the first FDA-approved nano-drug: lessons learned. *J. Control. Release*, **160** (2), 117–134.

25 Venditto, V.J. and Szoka, F.C., Jr. (2013) Cancer nanomedicines: so many papers and so few drugs!. *Adv. Drug Deliv. Rev.*, **65** (1), 80–88.

26 Muthu, M.S. and Wilson, B. (2012) Challenges posed by the scale-up of nanomedicines. *Nanomedicine (Lond.)*, **7** (3), 307–309.

27 Paliwal, R., Babu, R.J., and Palakurthi, S. (2014) Nanomedicine scale-up technologies: feasibilities and challenges. *AAPS PharmSciTech*, **15** (6), 1527–1534.
28 Feng, S.S., Zhao, L., and Tang, J. (2011) Nanomedicine for oral chemotherapy. *Nanomedicine (Lond.)*, **6** (3), 407–410.
29 Duncan, R. and Gaspar, R. (2011) Nanomedicine(s) under the microscope. *Mol. Pharm.*, **8** (6), 2101–2141.
30 Resnik, D.B. and Tinkle, S.S. (2007) Ethical issues in clinical trials involving nanomedicine. *Contemp. Clin. Trials*, **28** (4), 433–441.
31 Merisko-Liversidge, E.M. and Liversidge, G.G. (2008) Drug nanoparticles: formulating poorly water-soluble compounds. *Toxicol. Pathol.*, **36** (1), 43–48.
32 Heng, D., Ogawa, K., Cutler, D.J., Chan, H.-K., Raper, J.A., Ye, L., and Yun, J. (2010) Pure drug nanoparticles in tablets: what are the dissolution limitations. *J. Nanopart. Res.*, **12** (5), 1743–1754.
33 Rabinow, B.E. (2004) Nanosuspensions in drug delivery. *Nat. Rev. Drug Discov.*, **3**, 785–796.
34 Chavhan, S.S., Petkar, K.C., and Sawant, K.K. (2011) Nanosuspensions in drug delivery: recent advances, patent scenarios, and commercialization aspects. *Crit. Rev. Ther. Drug Carrier Syst.*, **28** (5), 447–488.
35 Junyaprasert, V.B. and Morakul, B. (2015) Nanocrystals for enhancement of oral bioavailability of poorly water-soluble drugs. *Asian J. Pharm. Sci.*, **10** (1), 13–23.
36 Imperiale, J.C., Nejamkin, P., Del Sole, M.J., Lanusse, C., and Sosnik, A. (2015) Novel protease inhibitor nanoparticle-in-microparticle delivery system leads to a dramatic improvement of the oral pharmacokinetics in dogs. *Biomaterials*, **37**, 383–394.
37 Imperiale, J.C. and Sosnik, A. (2015) Pure nanocrystals of a poorly water-soluble protease inhibitor sustain the release by the oral route: a new generation of nanocarrier-less nano-delivery systems? Annual Meeting of the Controlled Release Society, Edinburgh, Scotland.
38 Shegokar, R. and Müller, R.H. (2010) Nanocrystals: industrially feasible multifunctional formulation technology for poorly soluble actives. *Int. J. Pharm.*, **399** (1–2), 129–139.
39 Center for Drug Evaluation and Research (2015) *Orange Book: Approved Drug Products with Therapeutics Equivalence Evaluations*. 29th edn, Food and Drug Administration, Rockville, MD. Available at http://www.accessdata.fda.gov/scripts/cder/ob/default.cfm (October 10, 2015).
40 de Waard, H., Frijlink, H.W., and Hinrichs, W.L. (2011) Bottom up preparation techniques for nanocrystals of lipophilic drugs. *Pharm. Res.*, **28** (5), 1220–1223.
41 Page, S.T., Bremmer, W.J., Clark, R.V., Bush, M.A., Zhi, H., Caricofe, R.B., Smith, P.M., and Amory, J.K. (2008) Nanomilled oral testosterone plus dutasteride effectively normalizes serum testosterone in normal men with induced hypogonadism. *J. Androl.*, **29** (2), 222–227.
42 Liversidge, G.G. and Cundy, K.C. (1995) Particle size reduction for improvement of oral bioavailability of hydrophobic drugs: I. Absolute oral bioavailability of nanocrystalline danazol in Beagle dogs. *Int. J. Pharm.*, **125** (1), 91–97.
43 Liversidge, G.G. and Conzentino, P. (1995) Drug particle size reduction for decreasing gastric irritancy and enhancing absorption of naproxen in rats. *Int. J. Pharm.*, **125** (2), 309–313.
44 Jinno, J., Kamada, N., Miyake, M., Yamada, K., Mukai, T., Odomi, M., Toguchi, H., Liversidge, G.G., Higaki, K., and Kimura, T. (2006) Effect of particle size reduction on dissolution and oral absorption of a poorly water-soluble drug, cilostazol, in Beagle dogs. *J. Control. Release*, **111** (1–2), 56–64.
45 Vergote, G.J., Vervaet, C., Van Driessche, I., Hoste, S., De Smedt, S., Demeester, J., Jain, R.A., Ruddy, S., and Remon, J.P. (2002) *In vivo* evaluation of matrix pellets containing nanocrystalline ketoprofen. *Int. J. Pharm.*, **240** (1–2), 79–84.
46 Müller, R.H., Runge, S., Revelli, V., Mehnert, W., Thünemann, A.F., and Souto, E.B. (2006) Oral bioavailability of cyclosporine: solid lipid nanoparticles

(SLN) versus drug nanocrystals. *Int. J. Pharm.*, **317** (1), 82–89.

47 Lungguth, P., Hanafy, A., Frenzel, D., Grenier, P., Nhamias, A., Ohlig, T., Vergnault, G., and Spahn-Langguth, H. (2005) Nanosuspension formulations for low-soluble drugs: pharmacokinetic evaluation using spironolactone as model compound. *Drug Dev. Ind. Pharm.*, **31** (3), 319–329.

48 Mou, D., Chen, H., Wan, J., Xu, H., and Yang, X. (2011) Potent dried drug nanosuspensions for oral bioavailability enhancement of poorly soluble drugs with pH-dependent solubility. *Int. J. Pharm.*, **413** (1–2), 237–244.

49 Tshweu, L., Katata, L., Kalombo, L., Chiappetta, D.A., Hocht, C., Sosnik, A., and Swai, H. (2014) Enhanced oral bioavailability of the antiretroviral efavirenz nano-encapsulated in poly(epsilon-caprolactone) nanoparticles by a spray-drying method. *Nanomedicine (Lond.)*, **9** (12), 1821–1833.

50 Imperiale, J.C., Bevilacqua, G., Rosa, P.T.V., and Sosnik., A. (2014) Production of pure indinavir free-base nanoparticles by a supercritical anti-solvent (SAS) method. *Drug Dev. Ind. Pharm.*, **40** (12), 1607–1615.

51 McDonald, T.O., Giardiello, M., Martin, P., Siccardi, M., Liptrott, N.J., Smith, D., Roberts, P., Curley, P., Schipani, A., Khoo, S.H., Long, J., Foster, A.J., Rannard, S.P., and Owen, A. (2014) Antiretroviral solid drug nanoparticles with enhanced oral bioavailability: production, characterization, and *in vitro–in vivo* correlation. *Adv. Healthc. Mater.*, **3** (3), 400–411.

52 Tomalia, D.A. (2005) Birth of new molecular architecture: dendrimers as quantized building blocks for nanoscale synthetic polymer chemistry. *Prog. Polym. Sci.*, **30** (3–4), 294–324.

53 Mignani, S., El Kazzouli, S., Bousmina, M., and Majoral, J.-P. (2013) Expand classical drug administration ways by emerging routes using dendrimer drug delivery systems: a concise overview. *Adv. Drug Deliv. Rev.*, **65** (10), 1316–1330.

54 Esfand, R. and Tomalia, D.A. (2001) Poly(amidoamine) (PAMAM) dendrimers: from biomimicry to drug delivery and biomedical applications. *Drug Discov. Today*, **6** (8), 427–436.

55 Labieniec-Watala, M. and Watala, C. (2015) PAMAM dendrimers: destined for success or doomed to fail? Plain and modified PAMAM dendrimers in the context of biomedical applications. *J. Pharm. Sci.*, **104** (1), 2–14.

56 Rupp, R., Rosenthal, S.L., and Stanberry, L.R. (2007) VivaGel™ (SPL7013 Gel): a candidate dendrimer – microbicide for the prevention of HIV and HSV infection. *Int. J. Nanomedicine*, **2** (4), 561–566.

57 Price, C.F., Tyssen, D., Sonza, S., Davie, A., Evans, S., Lewis, G.R., Xia, S., Spelman, T., Hodsman, P., Moench, T.R., Humberstone, A., Paull, J.R.A., and Tachedjian, G. (2011) SPL7013 gel (VivaGel®) retains potent HIV-1 and HSV-2 inhibitory activity following vaginal administration in humans. *PLoS One*, **6** (9), e24095.

58 Gillies, E.R. and Fréchet, J.M.J. (2005) Dendrimers and dendritic polymers in drug delivery. *Drug Discov. Today*, **10** (1), 35–43.

59 Cheng, Y., Xu, Z., Ma, M., and Xu, T. (2008) Dendrimers as drug carriers: applications in different routes of drug administration. *J. Pharm. Sci.*, **97** (1), 123–143.

60 Kitchens, K.M., El-Sayed, M.E., and Ghandehari, H. (2005) Transepithelial and endothelial transport of poly(amidoamine) dendrimers. *Adv. Drug Deliv. Rev.*, **57** (15), 2163–2176.

61 Sakthivel, T., Toth, I., and Florence, A.T. (1999) Distribution of a lipidic 2.5nm diameter dendrimer carrier after oral administration. *Int. J. Pharm.*, **183** (1), 51–55.

62 Liu, Y., Tee, J.K., and Chiu, G.N. (2015) Dendrimers in oral drug delivery application: current explorations, toxicity issues and strategies for improvement. *Curr. Pharm. Des.*, **21** (19), 2629–2642.

63 D'Emanuele, A. and Attwood, D. (2005) Dendrimer–drug interactions. *Adv. Drug Deliv. Rev.*, **57** (15), 2147–2162.

64 Wiwattanapatapee, R., Carreno-Gomez, B., Malik, N., and Duncan, R. (2000)

Anionic PAMAM dendrimers rapidly cross adult rat intestine *in vitro*: a potential oral delivery system? *Pharm. Res.*, **17** (8), 991–998.
65 Florence, A.T., Sakthivel, T., and Toth, I. (2000) Oral uptake and translocation of a polylysine dendrimer with a lipid surface. *J. Control. Release*, **65** (1–2), 253–259.
66 D'Emanuele, A., Jevprasesphant, R., Penny, J., and Attwood, D. (2004) The use of a dendrimer-propranolol prodrug to bypass efflux transporters and enhance oral bioavailability. *J. Control. Release*, **95** (3), 447–453.
67 Tripathi, P.K., Khopade, A.J., Nagaich, S., Shrivastava, S., Jain, S., and Jain, N.K. (2002) Dendrimer grafts for delivery of 5-fluorouracil. *Pharmazie*, **57** (4), 261–264.
68 Man, N., Cheng, Y.Y., Xu, T.W., Ding, Y., Wang, X.M., Li, Z.W., Chen, Z.C., Huang, G.Y., Shi, Y.Y., and Wen, L.P. (2006) Dendrimers as potential drug carriers. Part II: Prolonged delivery of ketoprofen by *in vitro* and *in vivo* studies. *Eur. J. Med. Chem.*, **41** (5), 670–674.
69 Huang, X., Wu, Z., Gao, W., Chen, Q., and Yu, B. (2011) Polyamidoamine dendrimers as potential drug carriers for enhanced aqueous solubility and oral bioavailability of silybin. *Drug Dev. Ind. Pharm.*, **37** (4), 419–427.
70 Hayes, P.Y., Ross, B.P., Thomas, B.G., and Toth, I. (2006) Polycationic lipophilic-core dendrons as penetration enhancers for the oral administration of low molecular weight heparin. *Bioorg. Med. Chem.*, **14** (1), 143–152.
71 Sosnik, A. (2013) Temperature- and pH-sensitive polymeric micelles for drug encapsulation, release and targeting, in *Smart Materials for Drug Delivery* (eds C. Alvarez-Lorenzo and A. Concheiro) Royal Society of Chemistry, London, pp. 115–147.
72 Newkome, G.R., Moorefield, C.N., Baker, G.R., Saunders, M.J., and Grossman, S.H. (1991) Unimolecular micelles. *Angew. Chem., Int. Ed. Engl.*, **30** (9), 1178–1180.
73 Cabral, H. and Kataoka, K. (2014) Progress of drug-loaded polymeric micelles into clinical studies. *J. Control. Release*, **190**, 465–476.
74 Francis, M.F., Cristea, M., and Winnik, F.M. (2004) Polymeric micelles for oral drug delivery: why and how. *Pure Appl. Chem.*, **76** (7–8), 1321–1335.
75 Bromberg, L. (2008) Polymeric micelles in oral chemotherapy. *J. Control. Release*, **128** (2), 99–112.
76 Gaucher, G., Satturwar, P., Jones, M.-C., Furtos, A., and Leroux, J.-C. (2010) Polymeric micelles for oral drug delivery. *Eur. J. Pharm. Biopharm.*, **76** (2), 147–158.
77 Sant, V.P., Smith, D., and Leroux, J.-C. (2005) Enhancement of oral bioavailability of poorly water-soluble drugs by poly(ethylene glycol)-*block*-poly(alkyl acrylate-*co*-methacrylic acid) self-assemblies. *J. Control. Release*, **104** (2), 289–300.
78 Lu, Y. and Park, K. (2013) Polymeric micelles and alternative nanonized delivery vehicles for poorly soluble drugs. *Int. J. Pharm.*, **453** (1), 198–214.
79 Lee, S.C., Huh, K.M., Lee, J., Cho, Y.W., Galinsky, R.E., and Park, K. (2007) Hydrotropic polymeric micelles for enhanced paclitaxel solubility: *in vitro* and *in vivo* characterization. *Biomacromolecules*, **8** (1), 202–208.
80 Satturwar, P., Eddine, M.N., Ravenelle, F., and Leroux, J.C. (2007) pH-responsive polymeric micelles of poly(ethylene glycol)-*b*-poly(alkyl(meth)acrylate-*co*-methacrylic acid): influence of the copolymer composition on self-assembling properties and release of candesartan cilexetil. *Eur. J. Pharm. Biopharm.*, **65** (3), 379–387.
81 Zhang, Y., Li, X., Zhou, Y., Fan, Y., Wang, X., Huang, Y., and Liu, Y. (2010) Cyclosporin A-loaded poly(ethylene glycol)-*b*-poly(D,L-lactic acid) micelles: preparation, *in vitro* and *in vivo* characterization and transport mechanism across the intestinal barrier. *Mol. Pharm.*, **7** (4), 1169–1182.
82 Yu, H., Xia, D., Zhu, Q., Zhu, C., Chen, D., and Gan, Y. (2013) Supersaturated polymeric micelles for oral cyclosporine A delivery. *Eur. J. Pharm. Biopharm.*, **85** (3), 1325–1336.
83 Dahmani, F.Z., Yang, H., Zhou, J., Yao, J., Zhang, T., and Zhang, Q. (2012)

Enhanced oral bioavailability of paclitaxel in pluronic/LHR mixed polymeric micelles: preparation, *in vitro* and *in vivo* evaluation. *Eur. J. Pharm. Sci.*, **47** (1), 179–189.

84 Mohamed, E.A., Zhao, Y., Meshali, M.M., Remsberg, C., Borg, T.M., Foda, A.M.M., Takemoto, J.K., Sayre, C.L., Martinez, S.E., Davies, N.M., and Forrest, M.L. (2012) Vorinostat with sustained exposure and high solubility in poly(ethylene glycol)-*b*-poly(DL-lactic acid) micelle nanocarriers: characterization and effects on pharmacokinetics in rat serum and urine. *J. Pharm. Sci.*, **101** (10), 3787–3798.

85 Yang, Y.-H. and Ding, P.-T. (2015) Study on the preparation of nifedipine-loaded oral copolymer micelles and its pharmacokinetics in rats. *Cell Biochem. Biophys.*, **71** (1), 155–160.

86 Abdelbary, G. and Amal Makhlouf, A. (2014) Adoption of polymeric micelles to enhance the oral bioavailability of dexibuprofen: formulation, *in-vitro* evaluation and *in-vivo* pharmacokinetic study in healthy human volunteers. *Pharm. Dev. Technol.*, **19** (6), 717–727.

87 Dou, J., Zhang, H., Liu, X., Zhang, M., and Zhai, G. (2014) Preparation and evaluation *in vitro* and *in vivo* of docetaxel loaded mixed micelles for oral administration. *Colloids Surf. B Biointerfaces*, **114**, 20–27.

88 Tian, Y., Shi, C., Zhang, X., Sun, Y., Wang, J., Zhang, Y., Yang, J., Wang, L., Wang, L., and Mao, S. (2015) Nanomicelle based peroral delivery system for enhanced absorption and sustained release of 10-hydrocamptothecin. *J. Biomed. Nanotechnol.*, **11** (2), 262–273.

89 Chiappetta, D.A., Hocht, C., Taira, C., and Sosnik, A. (2010) Efavirenz-loaded polymeric micelles for pediatric anti-HIV pharmacotherapy with significantly higher oral bioavailability. *Nanomedicine (Lond.)*, **5** (1), 11–23.

90 Chiappetta, D.A., Hocht, C., Taira, C., and Sosnik, A. (2011) Oral pharmacokinetics of the anti-HIV efavirenz encapsulated within polymeric micelles. *Biomaterials*, **32** (9), 2379–2387.

91 Sosnik, A. and Carcaboso, A. (2014) Nanomedicines in the future of pediatric therapy. *Adv. Drug Deliv. Rev.*, **73**, 140–161.

92 Moretton, M.A., Hotch, C., Taira, C., and Sosnik, A. (2014) Encapsulation of rifampicin within flower-like polymeric micelles enhances the oral bioavailability in a pediatric fixed dose combination with isoniazid. *Nanomedicine (Lond.)*, **9** (11), 1635–1650.

93 Dian, L., Yu, E., Chen, X., Wen, X., Zhang, Z., Qin, L., Wang, Q., Li, G., and Wu, C. (2014) Enhancing oral bioavailability of quercetin using novel soluplus polymeric micelles. *Nanoscale Res. Lett.*, **9**, 684.

94 Mathot, F., van Beijsterveldt, L., Préat, V., Brewster, M., and Ariën, A. (2006) Intestinal uptake and biodistribution of novel polymeric micelles after oral administration. *J. Control. Release*, **111** (1–2), 47–55.

95 Mathot, F., des Rieux, A., Ariën, A., Schneider, Y.J., Brewster, M., and Préat, V. (2007) Transport mechanisms of mmePEG750P(CL-*co*-TMC) polymeric micelles across the intestinal barrier. *J. Control. Release*, **124** (3), 134–143.

96 Sosnik, A. and Menaker Raskin, M. (2015) Polymeric micelles in mucosal drug delivery: challenges towards clinical translation. *Biotechnol. Adv.*, **33** (6), 1380–1392.

97 Chen, H.B., Khemtong, C., Yang, X.L., Chang, X.L., and Gao, J.M. (2011) Nanonization strategies for poorly water-soluble drugs. *Drug Discov. Today*, **16** (7–8), 354–360.

98 Fryd, M.M. and Mason, T.G. (2012) Advanced nanoemulsions. *Annu. Rev. Phys. Chem.*, **63**, 493–518.

99 Spernath, A. and Aserin, A. (2006) Microemulsions as carriers for drugs and nutraceuticals. *Adv. Colloid Interface Sci.*, **128–130**, 47–64.

100 Bok Ki Kang, B.K., Lee, J.S., Chon, S.K., Jeong, S.Y., Yuk, S.H., Khang, G., Lee, H.B., and Cho, S.H. (2004) Development of self-microemulsifying drug delivery systems (SMEDDS) for oral

bioavailability enhancement of simvastatin in Beagle dogs. *Int. J. Pharm.*, **274** (1–2), 65–73.

101 Kommuru, T.R., Gurley, B., Khan, M.A., and Reddy, I.K. (2001) Self-emulsifying drug delivery systems (SEDDS) of coenzyme Q10: formulation development and bioavailability assessment. *Int. J. Pharm.*, **212** (2), 233–246.

102 Kim, S.K., Lee, E.H., Vaishali, B., Lee, S., Lee, Y.-K., Kim, C.-Y., Moon, H.T., and Byun, Y. (2005) Tricaprylin microemulsion for oral delivery of low molecular weight heparin conjugates. *J. Control. Release*, **105** (1–2), 32–42.

103 Ma, Y., Li, H., and Guan, S. (2015) Enhancement of the oral bioavailability of breviscapine by nanoemulsions drug delivery system. *Drug Dev. Ind. Pharm.*, **41** (2), 177–182.

104 Sun, H., Liu, K., Liu, W., Wang, W., Guo, C., Tang, B., Gu, J., Zhang, J., Li, H., Mao, X., Zou, Q., and Zeng, H. (2012) Development and characterization of a novel nanoemulsion drug-delivery system for potential application in oral delivery of protein drugs. *Int. J. Nanomedicine*, **7**, 5529–5543.

105 Mei, L., Zhang, Z., Zhao, L., Huang, L., Yang, X.-L., Tang, J., and Feng, S.-S. (2013) Pharmaceutical nanotechnology for oral delivery of anticancer drugs. *Adv. Drug Deliv. Rev.*, **65** (6), 880–890.

106 Gursoy, R.N. and Benita, S. (2004) Self-emulsifying drug delivery systems (SEDDS) for improved oral delivery of lipophilic drugs. *Biomed. Pharmacother.*, **58** (3), 173–182.

107 Coukell, A.J. and Plosker, G.L. (1998) Cyclosporin microemulsion (Neoral): a pharmacoeconomic review of its use compared with standard cyclosporin in renal and hepatic transplantation. *Pharmacoeconomics*, **14** (6), 691–708.

108 Keown, P. and Niese, D. (1998) Cyclosporine microemulsion increases drug exposure and reduces acute rejection without incremental toxicity in *de novo* renal transplantation. *Kidney Int.*, **54** (3), 938–944.

109 Müller, R.H., Mäder, K., and Gohla, S. (2000) Solid lipid nanoparticles (SLN) for controlled drug delivery: a review of the state of the art. *Eur. J. Pharm. Biopharm.*, **50** (1), 161–177.

110 Üner, M. and Yener, G. (2007) Importance of solid lipid nanoparticles (SLN) in various administration routes and future perspectives. *Int. J. Nanomedicine*, **2** (3), 289–300.

111 Das, S. and Chaudhury, A. (2011) Recent advances in lipid nanoparticle formulations with solid matrix for oral drug delivery. *AAPS PharmSciTech*, **12** (1), 62–76.

112 Westesen, K., Bunjes, H., and Koch, M.H.J. (1997) Physicochemical characterization of lipid nanoparticles and evaluation of their drug loading capacity and sustained release potential. *J. Control. Release*, **48** (2–3), 223–236.

113 Beloqui, A., Solinis, M.A., Rodriguez-Gascon, A., Almeida, A.J., and Preat, V. (2015) Nanostructured lipid carriers: promising drug delivery systems for future clinics. *Nanomedicine*, **12** (1), 143–161.

114 Hu, L., Tang, X., and Cui, F. (2004) Solid lipid nanoparticles (SLNs) to improve oral bioavailability of poorly soluble drugs. *J. Pharm. Pharmacol.*, **56** (12), 1527–1535.

115 Tsai, M.J., Huang, Y.B., Wu, P.C., Fu, Y.S., Kao, Y.R., Fang, J.Y., and Tsai, Y.H. (2011) Oral apomorphine delivery from solid lipid nanoparticles with different monostearate emulsifiers: pharmacokinetic and behavioral evaluations. *J. Pharm. Sci.*, **100** (2), 547–557.

116 Wang, D., Wang, X., Li, X., and Ye, L. (2008) Preparation and characterization of solid lipid nanoparticles loaded with α-asarone. *PDA J. Pharm. Sci. Technol.*, **62** (1), 56–65.

117 Varshosaz, J., Tabbakhian, M., and Mohammadi, M.Y. (2010) Formulation and optimization of solid lipid nanoparticles of buspirone HCl for enhancement of its oral bioavailability. *J. Liposome Res.*, **20** (4), 286–296.

118 Yang, S., Zhu, J., Lu, Y., Liang, B., and Yang, C. (1999) Body distribution of camptothecin solid lipid nanoparticles after oral administration. *Pharm. Res.*, **16** (5), 751–757.

119 Sanjula, B., Shah, F.M., Javed, A., and Alka, A. (2009) Effect of poloxamer 188 on lymphatic uptake of carvedilol-loaded solid lipid nanoparticles for bioavailability enhancement. *J. Drug Target.*, **17** (3), 249–256.

120 Manjunath, K. and Venkateswarlu, V. (2005) Pharmacokinetics, tissue distribution and bioavailability of clozapine solid lipid nanoparticles after intravenous and intraduodenal administration. *J. Control. Release*, **107** (2), 215–228.

121 Hu, L., Xing, Q., Meng, J., and Shang, C. (2010) Preparation and enhanced oral bioavailability of cryptotanshinone-loaded solid lipid nanoparticles. *AAPS PharmSciTech*, **11** (2), 582–587.

122 Muller, R.H., Runge, S., Ravelli, V., Mehnert, W., Thunemann, A.F., and Souto, E.B. (2006) Oral bioavailability of cyclosporine: solid lipid nanoparticles (SLN®) versus drug nanocrystals. *Int. J. Pharm.*, **317** (1), 82–89.

123 Kakkar, V., Singh, S., Singla, D., and Kaur, I.P. (2011) Exploring solid lipid nanoparticles to enhance the oral bioavailability of curcumin. *Mol. Nutr. Food Res.*, **55** (3), 495–503.

124 Hu, L., Jia, H., Luo, Z., Liu, C., and Xing, Q. (2010) Improvement of digoxin oral absorption in rabbits by incorporation into solid lipid nanoparticles. *Pharmazie*, **65** (2), 110–113.

125 Zhang, T., Chen, J., Zhang, Y., Shen, Q., and Pan, W. (2011) Characterization and evaluation of nanostructured lipid carrier as a vehicle for oral delivery of etoposide. *Eur. J. Pharm. Sci.*, **43** (3), 174–179.

126 Hanafy, A., Spahn-Langguth, H., Vergnault, G., Grenier, P., Tubic Grozdanis, M., Lenhardt, T., and Langguth, P. (2007) Pharmacokinetic evaluation of oral fenofibrate nanosuspensions and SLN in comparison to conventional suspensions of micronized drug. *Adv. Drug Deliv. Rev.*, **59** (6), 419–426.

127 Tran, T.H., Ramasamy, T., Truong, D.H., Choi, H.G., Yong, C.S., and Kim, J.O. (2014) Preparation and characterization of fenofibrate-loaded nanostructured lipid carriers for oral bioavailability enhancement. *AAPS PharmSciTech*, **15** (6), 1509–1515.

128 Mandpe, L. and Pokharkar, V. (2013) Quality by design approach to understand the process of optimization of iloperidone nanostructured lipid carriers for oral bioavailability enhancement. *Pharm. Dev. Technol.*, **20** (3), 320–329.

129 Zhang, N., Ping, Q., Huang, G., Xu, W., Cheng, Y., and Han, X. (2006) Lectin-modified solid lipid nanoparticles as carriers for oral administration of insulin. *Int. J. Pharm.*, **327** (1–2), 153–159.

130 Zhang, Z., Lv, H., and Zhou, J. (2009) Novel solid lipid nanoparticles as carriers for oral administration of insulin. *Pharmazie*, **64** (9), 574–578.

131 Sarmento, B., Martins, S., Ferreira, D., and Souto, E.B. (2007) Oral insulin delivery by means of solid lipid nanoparticles. *Int. J. Nanomedicine*, **2** (4), 743–749.

132 Zhang, N., Ring, Q., Huang, G., Han, X., Cheng, Y., and Xu, W. (2006) Transport characteristics of wheat germ agglutinin-modified insulin-liposomes and solid lipid nanoparticles in a perfused rat intestinal model. *J. Nanosci. Nanotechnol.*, **6** (9–10), 2959–2966.

133 Chen, C.C., Tsai, T.H., Huang, Z.R., and Fang, J.Y. (2010) Effects of lipophilic emulsifiers on the oral administration of lovastatin from nanostructured lipid carriers: physicochemical characterization and pharmacokinetics. *Eur. J. Pharm. Biopharm.*, **74** (3), 474–482.

134 Liu, Y., Wang, L., Zhao, Y., He, M., Zhang, X., Niu, M., and Feng, N. (2014) Nanostructured lipid carriers versus microemulsions for delivery of the poorly water-soluble drug luteolin. *Int. J. Pharm.*, **476** (1–2), 169–177.

135 Priano, L., Esposti, D., Esposti, R., Castagna, G., De Medici, C., Fraschini, F., Gasco, M.R., and Mauro, A. (2007) Solid lipid nanoparticles incorporating melatonin as new model for sustained oral and transdermal delivery systems. *J. Nanosci. Nanotechnol.*, **7** (10), 3596–3601.

136 Paliwal, R., Rai, S., Vaidya, B., Khatri, K., Goyal, A.K., Mishra, N., Mehta, A., and

Vyas, S.P. (2009) Effect of lipid core material on characteristics of solid lipid nanoparticles designed for oral lymphatic delivery. *Nanomedicine*, **5** (2), 184–191.
137 Mendes, A.I., Silva, A.C., Catita, J.A., Cerqueira, F., Gabriel, C., and Lopes, C.M. (2013) Miconazole-loaded nanostructured lipid carriers (NLC) for local delivery to the oral mucosa: improving antifungal activity. *Colloids Surf. B Biointerfaces*, **111** (1), 755–763.
138 Patil-Gadhe, A. and Pokharkar, V. (2014) Montelukast-loaded nanostructured lipid carriers: Part I. Oral bioavailability improvement. *Eur. J. Pharm. Biopharm.*, **88** (1), 160–168.
139 Liu, D.H., Liu, C.X., Zou, W.W., and Zhang, N. (2010) Enhanced gastrointestinal absorption of N_3-*O*-toluylfluorouracil by cationic solid lipid nanoparticles. *J. Nanopart. Res.*, **12** (3), 975–984.
140 Liu, C., Liu, D., Bai, F., Zhang, J., and Zhang, N. (2010) *In vitro* and *in vivo* studies of lipid-based nanocarriers for oral N_3-*o*-toluyl-fluorouracil delivery. *Drug Deliv.*, **17** (5), 352–363.
141 Kumar, V.V., Chandrasekar, D., Ramakrishna, S., Kishan, V., Rao, Y.M., and Diwan, P.V. (2007) Development and evaluation of nitrendipine loaded solid lipid nanoparticles: influence of wax and glyceride lipids on plasma pharmacokinetics. *Int. J. Pharm.*, **335** (1–2), 167–175.
142 Yuan, H., Chen, J., Du, Y.Z., Hu, F.Q., Zeng, S., and Zhao, H.L. (2007) Studies on oral absorption of stearic acid SLN by a novel fluorometric method. *Colloids Surf. B Biointerfaces*, **58** (2), 157–164.
143 Varshosaz, J., Minayian, M., and Moazen, E. (2010) Enhancement of oral bioavailability of pentoxifylline by solid lipid nanoparticles. *J. Liposome Res.*, **20** (2), 115–123.
144 Yang, L., Geng, Y., Li, H., Zhang, Y., You, J., and Chang, Y. (2009) Enhancement of the oral bioavailability of praziquantel by incorporation into solid lipid nanoparticles. *Pharmazie*, **64** (2), 86–89.
145 Xie, S., Pan, B., Wang, M., Zhu, L., Wang, F., Dong, Z., Wang, X., and Zhou, W. (2010) Formulation, characterization and pharmacokinetics of praziquantel-loaded hydrogenated castor oil solid lipid nanoparticles. *Nanomedicine (Lond.)*, **5** (5), 693–701.
146 Li, H., Zhao, X., Ma, Y., Zhai, G., Li, L., and Lou, H. (2009) Enhancement of gastrointestinal absorption of quercetin by solid lipid nanoparticles. *J. Control. Release*, **133** (3), 238–244.
147 Sun, M., Nie, S., Pan, X., Zhang, R., Fan, Z., and Wang, S. (2014) Quercetin-nanostructured lipid carriers: characteristics and anti-breast cancer activities *in vitro*. *Colloids Surf. B Biointerfaces*, **113** (1), 15–24.
148 Neves, A.R., Lúcio, M., Martins, S., Lima, J.L., and Reis, S. (2013) Novel resveratrol nanodelivery systems based on lipid nanoparticles to enhance its oral bioavailability. *Int. J. Nanomedicine*, **8** (1), 177–187.
149 Pandey, R., Sharma, S., and Khuller, G.K. (2005) Oral solid lipid nanoparticle-based antitubercular chemotherapy. *Tuberculosis*, **85** (5–6), 415–420.
150 Garcia-Fuentes, M., Prego, C., Torres, D., and Alonso, M.J. (2005) A comparative study of the potential of solid triglyceride nanostructures coated with chitosan or poly(ethylene glycol) as carriers for oral calcitonin delivery. *Eur. J. Pharm. Sci.*, **25** (1), 133–143.
151 Martins, S., Silva, A.C., Ferreira, D.C., and Souto, E.B. (2009) Improving oral absorption of salmon calcitonin by trimyristin lipid nanoparticles. *J. Biomed. Nanotechnol.*, **5** (1), 76–83.
152 Beloqui, A., Solinís, M.A., Rodríguez-Gascón, A., del Pozo-Rodríguez, A., des Rieux, A., and Préat, V. (2013) Mechanism of transport of saquinavir-loaded nanostructured lipid carriers across the intestinal barrier. *J Control. Release*, **166** (2), 115–123.
153 Shangguan, M., Lu, Y., Qi, J., Han, J., Tian, Z., Xie, Y., Hu, F., Yuan, H., and Wu, W. (2014) Binary lipids-based nanostructured lipid carriers for improved oral bioavailability of silymarin. *J. Biomater. Appl.*, **28** (6), 887–896.
154 Tiwari, R. and Pathak, K. (2011) Nanostructured lipid carrier versus solid lipid nanoparticles of simvastatin:

comparative analysis of characteristics, pharmacokinetics and tissue uptake. *Int. J. Pharm.*, **415** (1–2), 232–243.

155 Langguth, P., Hanafy, A., Frenzel, D., Grenier, P., Nhamias, A., Ohlig, T., Vergnault, G., and Spahn-Langguth, H. (2005) Nanosuspension formulations for low-soluble drugs: pharmacokinetic evaluation using spironolactone as model compound. *Drug Dev. Ind. Pharm.*, **31** (3), 319–329.

156 Beloqui, A., Solinís, M.A., Delgado, A., Évora, C., Isla, A., and Rodríguez-Gascón, A. (2014) Fate of nanostructured lipid carriers (NLCs) following the oral route: design, pharmacokinetics and biodistribution. *J. Microencapsul.*, **31**, 1–8.

157 Shete, H., Chatterjee, S., De, A., and Patravale, V. (2013) Long chain lipid based tamoxifen NLC. Part II: Pharmacokinetic, biodistribution and *in vitro* anticancer efficacy studies. *Int. J. Pharm.*, **454** (1), 584–592.

158 Shete, H.K., Selkar, N., Vanage, G.R., and Patravale, V.B. (2014) Tamoxifen nanostructured lipid carriers: enhanced *in vivo* antitumor efficacy with reduced adverse drug effects. *Int. J. Pharm.*, **468** (1–2), 1–14.

159 Chen, Y., Yuan, L., Zhou, L., Zhang, Z.H., Cao, W., and Wu, Q. (2012) Effect of cell-penetrating peptide-coated nanostructured lipid carriers on the oral absorption of tripterine. *Int. J. Nanomedicine*, **7**, 4581–4591.

160 Luo, Y., Chen, D., Ren, L., Zhao, X., and Qin, J. (2006) Solid lipid nanoparticles for enhancing vinpocetine's oral bioavailability. *J. Control. Release*, **114** (1), 53–59.

161 Zhuang, C.Y., Li, N., Wang, M., Zhang, X.N., Pan, W.S., Peng, J.J., Pan, Y.-S., and Tang, X. (2010) Preparation and characterization of vinpocetine-loaded nanostructured lipid carriers (NLC) for improved oral bioavailability. *Int. J. Pharm.*, **394** (1–2), 179–185.

162 Sosnik, A., Carcaboso, A., and Chiappetta, D.A. (2008) Polymeric nanocarriers: new endeavors for the optimization of the technological aspects of drugs. *Recent Pat. Biomed. Eng.*, **1** (1), 43–59.

163 Kumari, A., Yadav, S.K., and Yadav, S.C. (2010) Biodegradable polymeric nanoparticles based drug delivery systems. *Colloids Surf. B Biointerfaces*, **75** (1), 1–18.

164 Rao, J.P. and Geckeler, K.E. (2011) Polymer nanoparticles: preparation techniques and size-control parameters. *Prog. Polym. Sci.*, **36** (7), 887–913.

165 Hafner, A., Lovrić, J., Lakoš, G.P., and Pepić, I. (2014) Nanotherapeutics in the EU: an overview on current state and future directions. *Int. J. Nanomedicine*, **9**, 1005–1023.

166 Pandey, R., Zahoor, A., Sharma, S., and Khuller, G.K. (2003) Nanoparticle encapsulated antitubercular drugs as a potential oral drug delivery system against murine tuberculosis. *Tuberculosis*, **83** (6), 373–378.

167 Pandey, R. and Khuller, G.K. (2006) Oral nanoparticle-based antituberculosis drug delivery to the brain in an experimental model. *J. Antimicrob. Chemother.*, **57** (6), 1146–1152.

168 Zahoor, A., Pandey, R., Sharma, S., and Khuller, G.K. (2006) Pharmacokinetic and pharmacodynamic behavior of antitubercular drugs encapsulated in alginate nanoparticles at two doses. *Int. J. Antimicrob. Agents*, **27** (5), 409–416.

169 Sharma, A., Sharma, S., and Khuller, G. PK. (2004) Lectin-functionalized poly(lactide-*co*-glycolide) nanoparticles as oral/aerosolized antitubercular drug carriers for treatment of tuberculosis. *J. Antimicrob. Chemother.*, **54**, 761–766.

170 Semete, B., Booysen, L., Lemmer, Y., Kalombo, L., Katata, L., Verschoor, J., and Swai, H.S. (2010) *In vivo* evaluation of the biodistribution and safety of PLGA nanoparticles as drug delivery systems. *Nanomedicine*, **6** (5), 662–671.

171 Damgé, C., Pinto Reis, C., and Maincent, P. (2008) Nanoparticle strategies for the oral delivery of insulin. *Expert Opin. Drug Deliv.*, **5** (1), 45–68.

172 des Rieux, A., Fievez, V., Garinot, M., Schneider, Y.-J., and Préat, V. (2006) Nanoparticles as potential oral delivery systems of proteins and vaccines: a

mechanistic approach. *J. Control. Release*, **116** (1), 1–27.

173 Jung, T., Kamm, W., Breitenbach, A., Kaiserling, E., Xiao, J.X., and Kissel, T. (2000) Biodegradable nanoparticles for oral delivery of peptides: is there a role for polymers to affect mucosal uptake? *Eur. J. Pharm. Biopharm.*, **50** (1), 147–160.

174 Fonte, P., Araújo, F., Silva, C., Pereira, C., Reis, S., Santos, H.A., and Sarmento, B. (2015) Polymer-based nanoparticles for oral insulin delivery: revisited approaches. *Biotechnol. Adv.*, **33**, 1342–1354.

175 Mackenzie, R., Booth, J., Alexander, C., Garnett, M.C., and Laughton, C.A. (2015) Multiscale modeling of drug–polymer nanoparticle assembly identifies parameters influencing drug encapsulation efficiency. *J. Chem. Theory Comput.*, **11**, 2705–2713.

176 Sosnik, A. and Seremeta, K.P. (2015) Advantages and challenges of the spray-drying technology for the production of pure drug particles and drug-loaded polymeric carriers. *Adv. Colloids Interface Sci.*, **223**, 40–54.

177 Sosnik, A. (2014) Production of drug-loaded polymeric nanoparticles by electrospraying technology. *J. Biomed. Nanotechnol.*, **10** (9), 2200–2217.

25
Steroidal Nanodrugs Based on Pegylated Nanoliposomes Remote Loaded with Amphipathic Weak Acids Steroid Prodrugs as Anti-Inflammatory Agents

Keren Turjeman and Yechezkel Barenholz

The Hebrew University-Hadassah Medical School, Institute for Medical Research Israel-Canada (IMRIC), Department of Biochemistry and Molecular Biology, Laboratory of Membrane and Liposome Research, Ein Karem, 91120 Jerusalem, Israel

25.1
A Short Relevant Background on Inflammatory and Autoimmune Diseases

Inflammation is a vital physiological response for the survival of the organism. It is involved in many pathological states: autoimmune disease, cystic fibrosis, cancer, lupus, diabetes type-1, asthma, allergic diseases, atherosclerosis, acute cardiovascular events, postsurgery healing, and sepsis [1,2]. Such pathological states can be collectively referred to as diseases that have an inflammatory component. The high prevalence of such diseases and their very heavy burden on an individual and on the society has made the scientific community consider diseases with an inflammatory component to be one of the major target for twenty-first century medicine. The inflammatory process [2–4] is composed of three phases: acute inflammation, immune response, and chronic inflammation. Chronic inflammation has several characteristics that differentiate it from acute inflammation:

1) Change in local leukocyte population, mainly from neutrophils to macrophages and lymphocyte T and B cells.
2) Change in profile of inflammatory mediators, from autacoids to more potent inflammatory mediators secreted by the activated macrophages, lymphocytes, and fibroblasts, which include interleukins, tumor necrosis factor-α, interferons, and platelet-derived growth factor.
3) The persistent attack of immunoactive cells leads to massive tissue damage mediated by activated granulocytes and other leukocytes, which release toxic agents such as granular proteins (e.g., cathepsin, serine proteases, eosinophil collagenase, eosinophil cationic protein, and lactoferrin) and free radicals (e.g., hydrogen peroxide, nitric oxide, and hydroxyl radicals).
4) The inability of tissue regeneration leads to constant formation of granulation tissue characterized by angiogenesis and fibrosis processes.

Pharmaceutical Nanotechnology: Innovation and Production, First Edition. Edited by Jean Cornier, Arno Kwade, Andrew Owen, and Marcel Van de Voorde.

Therefore, it is clear that if chronic inflammation is left uncontrolled, severe damage will occur, which can lead to morbidity, as in rheumatoid arthritis, and even death, as in multiple sclerosis. However, in autoimmune diseases and other chronic inflammatory pathologies, clearing the noxious agent is not possible. The current therapeutic strategies are either immunosuppression or suppressing the inflammatory response. Glucocorticosteroids (GCs) are widely used, highly efficacious anti-inflammatory drugs; however, their use is limited due to their severe side effects. In Table 25.1, some therapeutic strategies [5–10] are shown.

Table 25.1 Common therapeutic strategies for treating inflammation [5–10].

Therapeutic agent	Therapeutic effect
Anti-inflammatory	
Non-steroidal anti-inflammatory drugs (NSAIDs) (aspirin, ibuprofen, diclofenac)	• Inhibiting cyclooxygenase enzyme (COX-1 and 2), which is responsible for the production of prostaglandins (important inflammatory mediators).
Glucocorticoids	• Reduce inflammation or swelling by binding toglucocorticoid receptors . The activated GR complex, in turn, upregulates the expression of anti-inflammatory proteins in the nucleus and represses the expression of proinflammatory proteins in the cytosol. • Inhibiting phospholipase A_2, diminishing eicosanoid production. • Inhibiting various leukocyte inflammatory events (epithelial adhesion, emigration, chemotaxis, phagocytosis, respiratory burst, etc.). • Suppress cyclooxygenase expression.
Immunosuppressive	
Interferons	• IFN-β, represses the production of Th1 cytokines as well as the activation of monocytes. • IFN-γ, triggers apoptosis of lymphocytes.
TNF-α binding proteins (monoclonal antibodies, circulating TNF-α receptors)	• Binding to TNF-α. • Inhibiting the synthesis of IL-1 and IL-6 and the adhesion of lymphocyte-activating protein.
Small biological agents	• Fingolimod increases the expression or changes the function of certain adhesion molecules in lymphocytes, so they accumulate in the lymphatic tissue and their number in the circulation is diminished. • Myriocin, a very potent inhibitor of serine palmitoyltransferase, 10–100 times more potent than Cyclosporine.
Antibodies (T-cell receptor-directed antibodies, IL-2- receptor-directed antibodies)	• Inhibiting T cells and causing cell lysis • They are used as a quick and potent immunosuppression method to prevent the acute rejection reaction.

Drugs acting on immunophilins (cyclosporine, tacrolimus, sirolimus)	• Inhibiting the growth and differentiation of T cells. • Binding to immunophilins leading to inhibition of the activity of calcineurine, a trans-activator of IL-2 transcription.
Mycophenolate	• Acts as a noncompetitive, selective, and reversible inhibitor of inosine-5′-monophosphate dehydrogenase (IMPDH), which is a key enzyme in the *de novo* synthesis of guanosine nucleotide. • In contrast to other human cell types, lymphocytes B and T are very dependent on this process.
Glucocorticoids	• Suppressing the cell-mediated immunity. • Inhibiting genes that code for the cytokines (IL-1, IL-2, IL-3, IL-4, IL-5, IL-6, IL-8, and TNF-γ). • Reducing the T-cell proliferation. • Suppressing the humoral immunity, diminishing both B cell clone expansion and antibody synthesis.

25.2 Drug Delivery Systems (DDS) Based on Nanoparticles (NP) for the Treatment of Diseases That Involve Inflammation

An important and long-term goal of the pharmaceutical industry is to develop therapeutic agents that can be selectively delivered to specific areas in the body to maximize the therapeutic index. Drugs given systemically provide therapeutic efficacy, but can also exhibit adverse reactions. The "magic bullet" concept, first theorized by Paul Ehrlich in 1891, represents the first early description of the drug-targeting paradigm [11]. The aim of drug targeting is to deliver drugs to the right place, at the right concentration, for the right period of time. The challenge of increasing a drug's therapeutic effect, with a concurrent minimization of side effects, can be optimized through proper design and DDS engineering [12–14]. Nanoparticles are stable, solid colloidal particles consisting of biodegradable polymer or lipid materials and range in size from 10 to 1000 nm. Drugs can be absorbed onto the particle surface, entrapped inside the polymer/lipid, or dissolved within the particle matrix [15]. Examples of common DDS are given in Table 25.2. Many of the advantages of a drug delivered via a nanocarrier are related to the unique pharmacokinetic properties of the carrier. When a drug is associated with a carrier, its clearance (Cl) decreases (the half-life ($t_{1/2}$) increases), the volume of distribution decreases, which means that the carrier with the drug remains longer in the blood compartment, and the area under the time versus concentration curve (AUC) increases, which means prolonged drug plasma distribution [16–18]. The majority of pharmaceutical research into the utility of nanoparticle DDS has been in the area of oncology where the enhanced permeability and retention (EPR) effect has significantly contributed to cancer-targeting drug design [19–21]. This effect is based on the fact that cancer tissue vasculature, unlike vasculature of normal healthy tissues, is "leaky," that is, penetrable by large molecules and even for small particles, allowing them to

Table 25.2 Common nanoparticle-based drug delivery systems (DDS).

Name	Description
Polymeric micelles	Self-assembled block co-polymers, that in aqueous solution arrange to form an outer hydrophilic layer and an inner hydrophobic core. The miceller core can be loaded with a water-insoluble therapeutic agent.
Liposomes	Lipid structures that can be made "stealth" by PEGylation and further conjugated to antibodies for targeting.
Dendrimers	Monodispered symmetric macromolecules built around a small molecule with an internal cavity surrounded by a large number of reactive end groups.
Biodegradable polymeric nanoparticles (PNPs)	Prepared from biocompatible and biodegradable polymers. The drug is dissolved, entrapped, encapsulated or attached to a nanoparticles matrix.
Inorganic (ceramic) particles	Fabricated using inorganic compounds including silica, alumina, titania, and so on. Their surfaces can be easily modified with different functional groups.
SLN	Spherical solid lipid nanoparticles dispersed in water or in aqueous surfactant solution.

extravasate and accumulate in the interstitial space of the diseased tissue. In tumors, such accumulation is additionally facilitated by the lack of a lymphatic system, which is responsible for the drainage of macromolecules from normal tissues. It has been found that the effective pore size in the endothelial lining of the blood vessels in most peripheral human tumors ranges from 200 to 600 nm in diameter, and the EPR effect allows for passive targeting to tumors based on this cut-off size of the leaky vasculature [22]. This is an efficient strategy for anticancer drug design, allowing high selectivity, improved therapeutic efficacy, and decreased toxicity [19–21,23,24]. Evidence suggests that the EPR phenomenon is not exclusive to solid neoplasms and is evident where vascular permeability is increased, for example, inflammation [23,25]. Therefore, both in cancer and in inflammatory diseases, drug efficacy is improved and toxicity may be reduced as a consequence of preferential accumulation at disease sites through the EPR effect, which is a passive targeting to the diseased tissue, combined with a lower concentration of the drug in healthy tissues [26]. Additional strategies for the treatment of inflammation using nanotechnology include the following:

1) *Targeting macrophages* – The potential of macrophages for rapid recognition and clearance of foreign particles has provided a rational approach to macrophage-specific targeting with nanoparticles.
2) *Targeting pro-inflammatory molecules* – A major effort is underway to fine-tune the migration of neutrophils into inflamed organs. Recent advancements of the understanding of the cell adhesion molecules have impacted the design and development of drugs (i.e., peptides, proteins) for the

potential treatment of cancer, cardiovascular diseases, and autoimmune diseases [27–29]. However, more detailed information on the mechanism(s) of internalization and intracellular trafficking of cell adhesion molecules is required for delivering drug molecules to a specific cell type or for diagnosis of cancer and other diseases.

25.3 Glucocorticosteroid as Anti-Inflammatory Agents

From the early days of the discoveries of cortisone and cortisol, numerous biochemical studies have focused on the mechanisms by which these GCs exert their anti-inflammatory immunosuppressive effects. A brief summary of the physiological mechanisms is presented here [1,30–35]. Cortisol and synthetic GCs passively traverse the cell membrane due to their semilipophilicity. In the cell, the GC binds with high affinity to the glucocorticoid receptor (GR), which causes dissociation of GR-bound proteins such as HSP90, HSP70, Src, and p23, and then in this form the GC/GR complex exerts its physiological effect in three different ways: (1) binding to GR DNA-responsive elements, (2) interaction with inflammatory transcription factors, and (3) nongenomic pathways. Collectively, these molecular mechanisms result in potent immunosuppressive and anti-inflammatory effects that lead to decrease in vascular permeability, inhibition of leukocyte migration, inhibition of T cell and B cell proliferation, reduction of the number of circulating granulocytes, reduction in the production of inflammatory mediators (i.e., cytokines, prostaglandins, and leukotrienes), and reduction in free radical production. Short-term treatment with GCs in life-threatening inflammatory states such as severe asthmatic conditions (even at high doses) is considered to be safe and, so far, irreplaceable in spite its toxic effects. However, when exposure to GCs is long term, such as in autoimmune diseases, then severe toxic adverse effects emerge. These are the result of two main factors: the free passage of the semilipophilic GC into cells and the fact that GCs have broad pharmacodynamics; namely, GC-responsive elements are found in almost any cell type [32,35]. Therefore, on long-term treatment, the prolonged systemic presence of GCs results in vast uncontrolled genomic effects in all responsive tissues. These effects are similar to the pathological state of hypercortisolism, and are also known as exogenous Cushing's syndrome (Table 25.3). Chemical modifications partially solve problems of unfavorable biodistribution mostly when intralesional administration is enabled. For example, the GC acetate prodrugs are much more hydrophobic than the GC drugs (e.g., methylprednisolone acetate compared to methylprednisolone). Hence, upon intralesional injection this is translated to much slower dispersion into the systemic circulation from site of injection, since it has to be first dissolved in the fluids of the intralesional site, and only then it can disperse into the vascular space and into the systemic circulation [36]. Other examples that utilize this approach include intralesional administration of GC prodrugs by the use of inhalers in asthma, enemas in inflammatory bowel diseases, and intra-articular injection of GCs in

Table 25.3 The physiological effects of long-term exposure to GCs.

Physiological system	Effect
Cardiovascular system	Hypertension
Kidneys	Water and salt retention for GCs that have mineralocorticoid activity such as cortisol and prednisolone. Renal calculi.
Central nervous system	Depression, psychosis, euphoria, apathy, lethargy pseudotumor cerebri.
Endocrine system	Decreased gonadotrophin release, decreased GH release, decreased TSH release. Suppression of the hypothalamic–pituitary–adrenal axis. Adrenal gland atrophy.
Gastrointestinal system	Peptic ulcer disease, pancreatitis with fat necrosis, fatty infiltration of the liver.
Carbohydrate, protein, lipid metabolism	Insulin resistance increase in gluconeogenesis, hepatic glycogen deposition, free-fatty-acid production (increased lipolysis), deposition of visceral and central adipose tissue, cholesterol, and triglycerides. Protein catabolism. Decreased HDL.
Skin, muscle, connective tissue	Skin thinning, muscular atrophy, collagen breakdown, protein catabolism.
Bone, calcium metabolism	Inhibition of osteoblast function, osteoporosis, decreased linear growth (children), decreased intestinal calcium absorption, hypercalciuria.
Blood, immune system	Neutrocytophilia, lymphocytopenia. Immunosuppression.
Eye	Glaucoma, posterior subcapsular cataracts.

monoarthritis. Although this form of administration improved significantly the therapeutic index of GCs, it is important to note that success in this form of therapy is quite limited as it is suitable for cases where the inflammation is limited to a small number of inflamed sites and short-term therapy is sufficient. For example, when there is a case of monoarthritis such as inflammation of the elbow joint due to sport injury, then such therapy is beneficial. However, when there are sporadic sites of inflammations, such as polyarthritis or when the site of inflammation is not accessible for intralesional injection, as in the cases of multiple sclerosis and Sjögren's syndrome, then another delivery approach is needed. Furthermore, the local administration results only in a short-term limited effect, as GCs intralesionally injected eventually diffuse from the inflamed site leading again to problems of unfavorable biodistribution, which may end up in exogenous Cushing's syndrome [37,38]. In order to solve issues of unfavorable pharmacokinetics and improve therapeutic index of GCs in a way suitable for most diseases with an inflammatory component, a totally different approach should be applied. Such an approach should combine targeting ability to the inflamed site (regardless of the location of the inflammation) with superior pharmacokinetics. Namely, the optimal GC treatment will be a drug delivery approach that will bring the GC to the inflamed site, while avoiding unspecific biodistribution to other GC-responsive organs such as the liver. In addition, in the inflamed site, in order for the GC to be bioavailable to the wide spectrum of immunoactive cells, the drug delivery system should either be phagocytosed, or the encapsulated GC should slowly diffuse out of the drug delivery system into the inflamed site influencing both nonphagocytotic and phagocytotic immunoactive cells. These requirements can be met through the delivery of the GC by the use of nano sterically stabilized liposomes (NSSLs).

25.4
Steroidal Nanodrugs Based on Pegylated Nanoliposomes Remote Loaded with Amphipathic Weak Acids Steroid Prodrugs as Anti-Inflammatory Agents

There are ~15 liposome-based DDS formulations, mostly of anticancer and antifungal drugs, now approved for clinical use [39]. A good example of such approved anticancer sterically stabilized nanoliposome formulation is the first FDA approved nanodrug, Doxil®, and the antifungal, AmBisome® [40,41]. One of the key features of liposomes' attractiveness as a drug delivery system is the large versatility in their composition and method of preparation [42–45]. This combination results in liposomes that are versatile in morphology, size distribution, lamellarity, and trapped aqueous volume. All of this, with the ability to match the method of preparation to the different stability of the agent, are to be encapsulated [44]. In the past two decades, we have witnessed the development of long-circulating drug carriers within the nanoscale size range. Numerous interesting approaches for design and engineering of such long-circulating vehicles have been described [46–48]. Among them, surface stabilization of nanoparticles and liposomes with a range of nonionic surfactants or polymeric or lipopolymeric macromolecules has proved to be one of the most successful approaches for keeping the particles in the blood for prolonged periods of time [49]. This chapter will discuss our two decade-long experience with NSSLs for the treatment of diseases with an inflammatory component. These ~80-nm-long circulating liposomes are specifically designed to utilize the vascular abnormalities (and leakiness) of the blood vessels that are present in inflamed or tumorous tissues. They are able to extravasate through gaps within the endothelial lining that are smaller than 100 nm in the case of inflamed tissue. When designing a liposome for medical application, another important physical feature, besides the packing parameter (PP), that needs to be considered is the membrane phase behavior [50]. This parameter is important, as it can predict what will be the partition coefficient and relative permeability of the liposome bilayer membrane. Three main phases are recognized: the solid ordered = SO, the liquid disordered = LD, and the liquid ordered = LO [50]. The phase in which a membrane will be depends on lipid composition, medium composition, pH, and its T_m (the temperature at which transition from the SO-to-LD phase occurs). It can be followed by various methods, of which the most common is differential scanning calorimetry (DSC). The SO phase is characterized by a high conformational trans/gauche ratio, leading to densely packed hydrocarbon chains, and a slow translational/lateral diffusion coefficient (10^{-11} cm^2/s), as well as small free volume. The LD phase is characterized by a high conformational gauche/trans ratio, disordered hydrocarbon chains, and faster translational diffusion coefficients (10^{-8} cm^2/s) [51]. These differences in dynamics and structure of the lipid bilayer explain the low permeability of the SO phase (below the T_m) and higher permeability of the LD phase (above the T_m). In terms of medical application, if a liposome bilayer is composed of a phospholipid with a T_m below 37 °C, when these liposomes are used *in vivo* the membrane will be in the LD phase. This will cause encapsulated agents to be released faster than from liposomes with membranes composed of lipid with T_m above 37 °C, thus in the body it will be in the SO phase. The LO phase is unique because it requires the presence of membrane-active sterols such as cholesterol. The LO phase was first proposed by Ipsen *et al.*, in 1987 [52], as being in between the SO and LD phases; thus membrane-active sterols are defined as sterols that enable a transformation of a phospholipid bilayer from either LD or SO phase into the LO phase [50,53]. In addition, it was found that membrane-active sterols stabilize the LO phase over a wide range of compositions and temperatures, and the incorporation of the membrane-active sterol in the lipid bilayer is characterized by a large increase in membrane thickness, which results in reduction of the membrane permeability [50]. Recent studies have shown that the presence of membrane-active sterols have the ability to decrease the number of water molecules at the membrane surface [54], leading to stronger association between phospholipid hydrocarbon chains through van der Waals interactions and thus further reducing the membrane free volume [55–57]. All of these unique features of the LO phase make it relatively impermeable, and highly stable on the shelf and in biological fluids *in vivo*. Therefore, the LO phase and liposome-forming lipids with high $T_m \geq 37$ °C are used extensively for *in vivo* applications, as exemplified by the FDA-approved liposomal drug Doxil [58].

25.5 Methods for Loading Drugs into Liposomes

In order for the liposome to serve as drug carrier, it has to encapsulate the desired drug or agent. Liposomes are unique drug carriers due to their two environments available for loading: the membrane and the intraliposome aqueous phase [58]. Two main approaches exist for encapsulating drugs into liposomes: passive and remote loading (also referred to as active loading) [58].

25.5.1 Passive Drug Loading

Passive loading is defined as a loading of drug/agent during liposome preparation. For a stable encapsulation of drugs by the passive loading method [58], only highly hydrophobic or highly hydrophilic drugs (both defined by octanol/

buffer partition coefficient [59]) can be used. Hydrophobic drugs are either added to the lipids used to form the liposomes prior to their hydration (and thus they become part of the liposome lipid bilayer during the hydration step) or, alternatively, they are added to preformed liposomes (the first approach is preferable). However, encapsulation of highly hydrophobic molecules in the lipid bilayer is limited due to the high packing parameter (>0.1) and, based on the additive packing parameter principles, excess of drug will increase the additive packing parameter (>1.0), where micro- and macroscopical phase separation will occur between the drug and the liposome bilayer [58]. Hydrophilic drugs/agents are passively encapsulated by adding them to the hydration medium during the hydration step. Thus, as liposomes are formed they enclose the aqueous medium that contains the agents, thereby encapsulating the drugs in the intraliposome aqueous phase. Although this method is simple and widely used, it suffers from several limitations related to drug solubility and, when combined with the nano volume of the intraliposome aqueous phase, it results in a low drug-to-lipid/liposome ratio and low encapsulation efficiency.

25.5.2 Remote (Active) Drug Loading

Remote loading [58,60,61] uses a different approach. The term remote come from the two stages required. First, the desired liposomes (based on composition, structure, and size distribution) are prepared in a way that will allow molecules that are amphipathic weak acids or bases to be loaded at the desired time into the intraliposome aqueous phase of these preformed liposomes. Remote loading is based on the unique property of the drug agent to be loaded against a concentration gradient. This explains why it is also referred to as an active loading. The remote loading is driven thermodynamically by transmembrane pH or ion gradients, which allow amphipathic weak acids or bases to diffuse across the membrane in their uncharged form followed by their ionization in the intraliposome aqueous phases, which results in their accumulation there. The agent's level of ionization determines the level of its uncharged species, and is dependent on the pK_a of the agent and local pH at inraliposome aqueous phase [62]. The basic assumption is that this approach requires the encapsulated agent to have a reasonable aqueous solubility. In a way, the active (remote) loading imitates bioenergetic principles in which ion or pH forms a transmembrane gradient in cells and subcellular organelles. In addition, it requires that the liposomes used for the loading will have the driving force caused by the transmembrane gradient, which will "pump" the amphipathic weak acid or base to be loaded and concentrate in the intraliposome aqueous phase of the liposome. This unique methodology was utilized by biochemists and liposomologists, as evident in the early studies of Ramos *et al.* [63], who used radiolabeled amphipathic acetic acid to measure the electrochemical gradient of protons in *Escherichia coli* membrane vesicles, and by the work of Nichols and Deamer [64], which showed that amphipathic amines (weak bases) such as catecholamines could be encapsulated in liposomes that exhibit a pH gradient where intraliposome pH was lower than that of the extraliposome bulk medium. Later this approach was applied by Cullis and coworkers [65] for loading amphipathic weak base drugs into liposomes, driven by a pH gradient. In our laboratory, these methods were further developed by using preformed liposomes in which pH and ion gradients were created by the use of salts of either the amphipathic bases [61] or the weak acids [60], where both can be presented as uncharged and charged species, that is, ammonia/ammonium or acetic acid/acetate, while the counterion is originally of either a strong acid or base such as SO_4^{2-} or Ca^{2+}, respectively. Thus, we are using an ammonium sulfate gradient [61,66] for entrapping amphipathic weak bases and a calcium acetate gradient [60,66] for entrapping amphipathic weak acids. These types of ion gradients create a pH gradient that is advantageous over a simple pH gradient, where a large reservoir of the amphipathic ion is much larger than the buffer capacity of a simple pH gradient, thus enabling a more efficient and stable encapsulation. In addition, the counterion can be selected so that it will induce (or not induce) a precipitation of the entrapped agent in the intraliposome aqueous phase as a drug–counterion salt, which further stabilizes the loading procedure [66]. This concept is exemplified by Doxil, the first nanoliposome drug approved by the FDA, in 1995, and since then in clinical use worldwide. In Doxil, the amphipathic weak base doxorubicin [58] is remotely loaded into NSSL by means of an ammonium sulfate transmembrane gradient to form doxorubicin sulfate crystals in the intraliposome aqueous phase [40].

25.6 Comparing Various Approaches Used for Formulating Liposomal GCs

From a historical perspective, in the early stage of research related to liposomal GCs, the dominant approach was to utilize the lipophilic nature of GCs and to encapsulate them in the liposome lipidic bilayer. However, this approach when applied to the conventional available GCs was based on the misconception that the GCs could be maintained in the lipid bilayer. But, as it turned out, such encapsulation has encountered a major limitation of stability, as GCs are not lipophilic enough, but rather semilipophilic, as is apparent from their relatively high mass aqueous solubility and log*D* values. For instance, cholesterol, one of the liposome membrane components, has a log*D* of 9.85 (at pH 7.0) [67] and mass solubility of 6e−9 g/l, while hydrocortisone has a much lower log*D* of 1.43 (at pH 7.0) and mass solubility of 0.16 g/l. These physicochemical features suggest that, in fact, GCs such as hydrocortisone are not suitable for "encapsulation" in the liposome bilayer, since upon dilution they will desorb to the aqueous medium, leaving the liposomes behind, without the drug. This is similar to what was described before for liposome membrane–associated doxorubicin [68,69]. A good example of such behavior for a GC was described in the study by Mishina *et al.* [70], where the authors report that >50% of encapsulated methylprednisolone leaks to the bulk medium during

10 days storage even without dilution. Two approaches are currently used. The first is to make chemical modifications to the GC, so it will be highly hydrophobic (log$D$ >9.0). This was demonstrated in 1976 by Shaw *et al.* [71], who used the cortisol–palmitate ester as a prodrug, which is transformed into cortisol (the active drug) by ubiquitous esterases. In 2006, this approach was revisited by Teshima *et al.* [72], who used the more potent prednisolone–palmitate ester. However, this approach suffers from a major drawback imposed by the fact that the mol % of GC–palmitate in the lipid bilayer is limited, as this molecule is not a "liposome-forming lipid" [73]. In addition, due to its large packing parameter, there is a rather low limit to its membrane level, above which formation of liposomes is prevented [73] as the liposome lipid bilayer cannot accommodate a high level of the GC–palmitate without losing its integrity and/or being transformed into a nonlamellar phase. This explains why the drug in the liposome bilayer is limited to a drug-to-lipid ratio of 0.1.

The second approach is best presented by Storm and coworkers [74–77]. These authors used highly hydrophilic nonamphipathic acidic GC prodrugs such as prednisolone phosphate, which was encapsulated passively in the intraliposome aqueous phase. However, the second approach also suffers from the same drawback as the first, that is, low drug-to-lipid ratio. In this case, the reason is different from that in the first approach and is related to limitations of the passive loading process, mainly the very small volume of the NSSL [42,58]. Also, this approach suffers from the additional disadvantage of a very poor loading efficiency (≤5%) [74,75]. Not less important, the two approaches lack a controlled release of the encapsulated GC during systemic circulation and at the inflammation sites, as the palmitate–GC incorporation is found to be highly stable during incubation in plasma [72], and release of the encapsulated prednisolone phosphate is possible only upon physical disruption of the liposome bilayer [76]. Furthermore, the use of NSSL presents a special paradox: on the one hand, the absolute need for nanoliposomes, as only they have reach efficiently the inflammation sites and, on the other hand, the NSSL exhibits extremely small trapped aqueous volumes and therefore the amount of drug is very low, even for drugs which are highly soluble. Namely, for such a formulation to reach a therapeutically sufficient drug level at the inflammation site, a large amount of NSSL has to be administrated. This may cause various types of toxicities [78,79]. However, when applying the remote loading approach, the very small trapped aqueous volume of nanoliposomes actually supports faster and higher drug accumulation and intraliposome precipitation. The steroid prodrugs are amphipathic weak acids, and a highly efficient (>90%) and stable GC encapsulation was obtained based on a transmembrane calcium acetate gradient (Figure 25.1) [80]. The intraliposomal CaAc concentration is high and the concentration in the external medium is low. Acetate anion reacts with water to form acetic acid and hydroxyl ion. Acetic acid is able to cross the lipid membrane, where in the bulk medium it is diluted and dissociates again to acetate ion. Alkaline conditions are formed to the extent that the equilibrium of acetate shifts the reaction to the unprotonated state of the acetate anion. Weak amphipathic acid (D) is able to cross the lipid

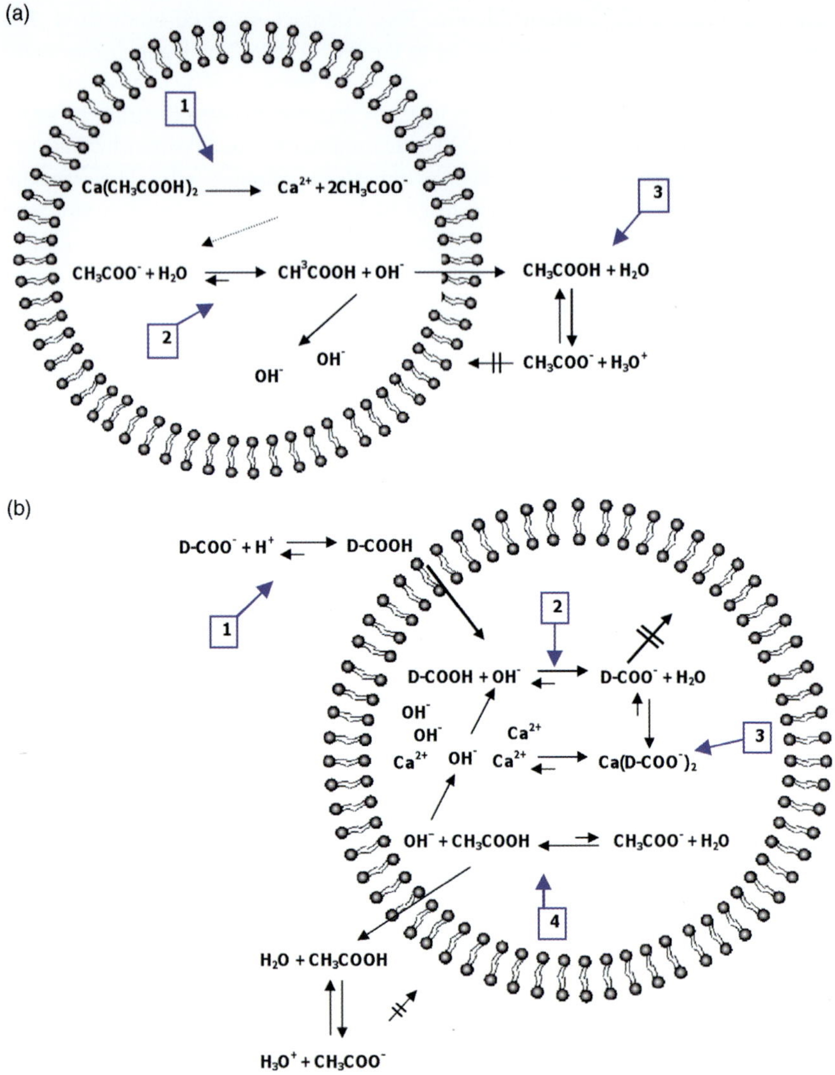

Figure 25.1 Principles and mechanism of NSSL transmembrane calcium acetate gradient-driven remote loading and release mechanisms of amphipathic weak acids such as MPS. (a) Fabrication stage of NSSL having transmembrane calcium acetate gradient. Calcium acetate at the desired concentration is passively loaded into intraliposome aqueous phase during lipid hydration to form multilamellar liposomes. Calcium acetate is removed from the extraliposome medium resulting in intraliposome high/extraliposome-low calcium acetate gradient. The nonprotonated charged acetate is in pH-dependent equilibrium with the uncharged protonated acetic acid ($pKa = 4.75$). Acetic acid (but neither acetate nor calcium ions) can diffuse across the liposome membrane to the external medium. The release of acetic acid induces pH increase in the intraliposome aqueous phase to the extent that the equilibrium of acetate shifts the reaction to the direction of the nonprotonated, charged acetate anion, and therefore release of acetic acid is slowed down or

membrane in its protonated form. Inside the aqueous phase, the drug encounters alkaline conditions; this causes deprotonation. The unprotonated drug forms a precipitate with the calcium ions. The deprotonation and the formation of precipitate cause the protonation of acetate, which in turn, leaves the aqueous phase that further propels the process of loading and helps to maintain conditions in which equilibrium is favorable for deprotonation of drug.

Some examples of the different strategies that were used over the years for formulating liposomal GCs are presented in Table 25.4.

25.7 The Use of Liposomes Loaded with Steroids as Anti-Inflammatory Agents: A Brief Historical Perspective

The attractiveness of liposomes as a drug delivery system for GC has led researchers to try to use liposomes for treating diseases that involve inflammation. Presented below is a brief historical description of the advances that were made.

1978 – Dingle *et al.* [98] used MLV that encapsulates the hydrophobic cortisol–palmitate prodrug to treat rats induced with arthritis. It was observed that intra-articular injections of these liposomes resulted in a long localization of the liposome in inflamed joints (site of the injection) concomitantly with controlled release of cortisol by ester hydrolysis of cortisol palmitate. This development was a major breakthrough as the therapeutic effect of cortisol was improved at least 10-fold compared with intra-articular injection of free cortisol. However, these liposomes are limited to local application and not suitable for systemic use.

1981 – The next achievement in this field came with the understanding of the unique physiology of inflammation, where dramatic changes occur in the microanatomy of blood capillaries, that is, at the inflammation site, including increased vascular permeability (vascular gaps >100 nm). Liposomologists sought to use these inflammation-related features as the Achilles' heel of the disease, as it enables one to achieve passive targeting and accumulation of liposomes at the inflammation site, carrying with them imaging reagents and

practically stops. (b) These preformed liposomes are "eager" to "pump in" the amphipathic weak acid GC (drug-D) from the extraliposome medium. When an amphipathic weak acid GC prodrug (i.e., MPS) is added to the extraliposome aqueous medium, it diffuses across the membrane into the intraliposome aqueous phase in its protonated (unionized) form. In the alkaline intraliposome aqueous phase (see b1) it undergoes deprotonation (ionization). The deprotonated (ionized DCOO-) of the weak acid drug will form a salt with Ca^{2+} [$Ca(MPS)_2$], which precipitates in the nanoaqueous volume of the nanoliposome due to its high concentration and low solubility product. These two processes, the deprotonation of the amphipathic weak acid GC and the concomitant formation of a calcium salt, lead to lowering of the intraliposomal pH, thereby reducing the intraliposome pH. This translates into favorable conditions for the protonation of more acetic acid, which induces is the repeating and recycling the conditions described above. *Source:* Avnir 2011 [80].

Table 25.4 Examples for different strategies used so far for formulating liposomal GCs.

Loading approach	Drug	Liposomal category	Route of administration	References
Remote loading	Methylprednisolone hemisuccinate (MPS)	PEGylated nano liposomes	Systemic: intravenous, subcutaneous	[80–82]
	Betamethasone hemisuccinate	PEGylated nano liposomes	Systemic: intravenous	[82,83]
Passive loading	Hydrocortisone	Multilamellar liposomes	Local: intra-articular	[84] [77,85]
	Dexamethasone	PEGylated liposomes	Systemic: intravenous	[77]
	Prednisolone			
	Budesonide	PEGylated liposomes	Systemic: intravenous	[86]
		Non-PEGylated liposomes	Local: aerosols	[87–89]
	Prednisolone phosphate	Non-PEGylated liposomes	Systemic: intravenous	[90,91]
		PEGylated liposomes		
	Dexamethasone phosphate	Oligolamellar and multilamellar	Local: intra-articular	[92] [92]
		RGD–PEG liposomes	Systemic: intravenous	[93]
		Non-PEGylated liposomes	Systemic: intravenous	[94,95]
		PEGylated liposomes	Systemic: intravenous	
	Budesonide phosphate	PEGylated liposomes	Systemic: intravenous	[84]
	Beclomethasone Dipropionate	PEGylated liposomes	Local: aerosols	[77,85]
		Non-PEGylated liposomes		
Loading in the lipid bilayer	Cortisol palmitate, cortisol octanoate	Different liposomal formulations (DPPC/EPC, DMPC, DPPC, or DSPC)	Local: intra-articular	[96,97]

anti-inflammatory drugs. In 1981 Morgan *et al.* [99] were one of the first groups to demonstrate this unique effect. In their study, they report that injection of 99 mTc radiolabeled MLV localizes in the abscess of rats induced by intramuscular injection of *Staphylococcus aureus* into rat thigh.

1982 – Detailed and extensive pharmacokinetics and biodistribution studies have shown that, in general, after iv injections, liposomes are quickly accumulated by the reticuloendothelial system (RES) and localized mainly in organs such as the spleen and liver. The pioneering studies by senior and Gregoriadis' group [100,101] demonstrate the decreased RES uptake of liposomes by using nanoscale liposomes composed of zwitterionic sphingomyelin and other neutral liposome-forming lipids, either in the SO or in the LO phase.

1991 – Another major advance was made by introduction of "stealth" liposomes, also known as sterically stabilized liposomes (SSL) [18,30,102,103]. The first generation of SSL was based on a lipid composition of sphingomyelin, cholesterol, and GM ganglioside or included hydrogenated phosphatidylinositol (PI). However, in these liposomes, steric stabilization was dependent on the animal species [104].

The second generation of SSL was based on achieving steric stabilization using the lipopolymer PEG-DSPE in which a polyethylene glycol (PEG) moiety is attached to the primary amino group of distearoyl phosphatidylethanolamine (1,2-distearoyl-*sn*-glycero-3-phosphoethanolamine = DSPE) (Figure 25.2).

For steric stabilization, it is required that the PEG moiety will be of molecular mass > 750 Da, and most often 2000 Da (referred to as 2000-PEG-DSPE) is used. The reason that DSPE lipid is used for the attachment of PEG is that its desorption from the liposome is slower than the clearance rate of the NSSL containing this type of lipopolymer. The incorporation of 2000-PEG-DSPE into a lipid bilayer under conditions that bilayer stability is maintained is limited to the range of up to 9 mol % for small and large unilamellar vesicles (SUV and LUV,

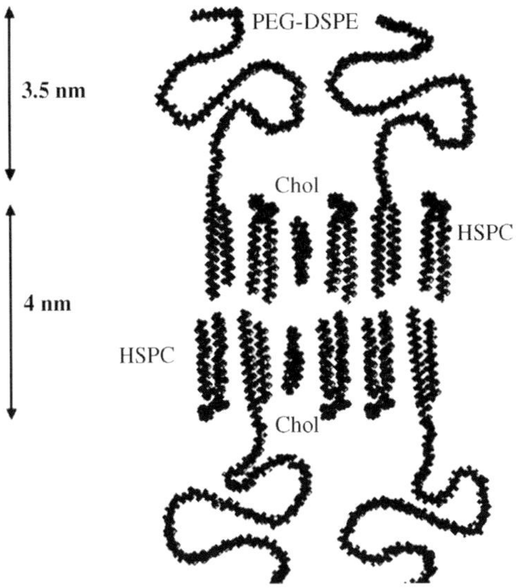

Figure 25.2 Schematic presentation 2000-PEG-DSPE incorporated in a phospholipidic bilayer.

respectively). This limit is due to the very large highly hydrated head group and therefore it has a small packing parameter (PP) [54,105,106], which reduces the additive packing parameter (APP) of the system, and below APP of 0.74, micelles will start forming [54]. It is reported that the presence of such lipopolymer in the liposome bilayer results in the effect of physical steric stabilization that is explained by the high hydration of the PEG moiety, in which every ethylene oxide group binds 3–4 water molecules by hydrogen bonding [105]. Thus, a hydration shell is formed around the liposome while reducing the amount of water in the membrane/water interface. The formation of such a hydration shell increases the stability of SSL as it prevents the passive and active binding of immunoactive biological agents such as immunoglobulins, opsonins, and proteins of complement from biological fluids, as well as better retaining the encapsulated drug [107–109]. Therefore, this leads to reduction of uptake by phagocytotic cells such as macrophages of the RES system *in vivo*, which translates to a prolonged circulation half-life, concomitantly enhancing accumulation of liposomes in inflammation and tumor sites [18,75,102,110]. In inflammatory-related diseases, SSL and especially nano SSL (NSSL) have been extensively used since 1992 for imaging purposes [110,111] and as a drug delivery system, encapsulating anti-inflammatory drugs such as glucocorticoids [74,75], methotrexate [112], the antibiotics (ciprofloxacin) [113], and the enzyme superoxide dismutase [114] (antioxidant therapy). In all of these examples, a superior therapeutic effect of the drug encapsulated in NSSL over the nonencapsulated free drug was demonstrated, as explained by the much longer circulation time and passive targeting to the inflammation site.

25.8
Lessons Learned from Experimental Animal Models of Diseases That Involve Inflammation

This section will discuss our almost two-decade-long experience with NSSL for the treatment of diseases with an inflammatory component [115]. Preclinical studies using six different animal models for diseases that involve inflammation (different EAE mice models for MS, AIA rat model for RA, MRL-lpr/Ipr mice model for lupus, carrageenan or zymosan induced Inflammation in mice, Mdx mice model for DMD, and *Plasmodium berghei* Anka model for CM) demonstrate that the liposomal nanodrug therapeutic efficacy is superior to that of the free drug and to many drugs currently used to treat these diseases [80–82,116–118]. These nanodrugs accumulate selectively at sites of enhanced vascular permeability, such as inflamed tissues. Accumulation of drug-loaded NSSL at these sites, followed by drug release there, explains their superior therapeutic efficacy *in vivo*. Due to their high potency, the liposomal drugs can be administered less frequently, and can improve therapeutic efficacy as well as patient safety and compliance, thereby improving steroid therapeutic index.

25.8.1
Pharmacokinetics (PK) and Biodistribution (BD) Advantages of Steroidal Nanodrugs

We have previously demonstrated pharmacokinetics (PK) and biodistribution (BD) advantages of NSSL–MPS in different mammalian species [80,116].

In the acute EAE mice model, while nonencapsulated MPS is rapidly cleared in minutes ($t_{1/2}$ of ~9 min), encapsulated MPS is cleared in hours ($t_{1/2}$ of ~12 h) (Figure 25.3a). At 1 h postinjection, the MPS ratio of brain-to-liver

(a)
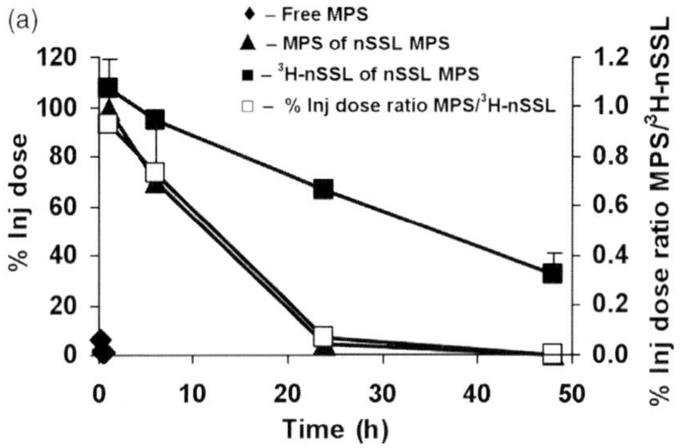

Figure 25.3 Representative results of treatment with steroidal liposomes in EAE mice model. (a) *In vivo* pharmacokinetic study in mice of ^{3}H-nSSL-MPS and of free MPS [80]. Pharmacokinetics of free MPS (◆), MPS of nSSL–MPS (▲), ^{3}H-nSSL of nSSL–MPS (■), and the ratio between encapsulated MPS and its carrier ^{3}H-nSSL (□). The change in this ratio with time is used as a method to calculate *in vivo* MPS release rate from ^{3}H-nSSL-MPS. (b) Comparison of the therapeutic efficacy of NSSL–MPS and nonliposomal (free) MPS in acute EAE mice model. SJL/J mice ($n = 10$) were treated by IV injections on days 10, 12, 14 with: NSSL–MPS 50 mg/kg BW (▲), free MPS 50 mg/kg BW (◆), and dextrose 5% (control) (■) [80]. (c) Comparison of therapeutic efficacy of NSSL–MPS with clinically available drugs, copaxone and betaferon on acute EAE mouse model. SJL/J mice ($n = 10$) were treated by IV injections on days 8, 11, and 14 with: NSSL–MPS 50 mg/kg BW (▲); copaxone 250 μg (▼); betaferon 2000 units (●); dextrose 5% (control) (■) [80]. (d) Treatment with NSSL–MPS reduced inflammation and demyelination in brains and spinal cords of mice with AT–EAE compared with free-MPS-treated mice and control mice. Brains and spinal cords were obtained on day 13 post T-cell transfer. Black arrows indicate infiltrating inflammatory cells; white arrow indicates demyelination. Representative viii & v-stained brains (i,ii,iii,v,vii) and spinal cord (c,f,h) sections from control (1–iii), as well as NSSL–MPS (iii–v) and free-MPS-treated EAE mice (vi,viii) show extensive inflammation involving perivascular infiltrates of mononuclear leukocytes (arrows) within the cerebral parenchyma and spinal cords of CTRL mice and free-MPS-treated mice (arrows). In the NSSL–MPS treated group, much fewer infiltrating cells were observed. LFB staining demonstrates extensive demyelination in the control spinal cord (x) and a decrease in myelin density in the free MPS treated group (ix, xii) around blood vessels compared with NSSL–MPS treated mice (xi), demonstrating densely organized myelin sheaths. Original magnification of x 40 [101]. (e) Brain tissue characteristics of acute EAE mice using magnetic resonance imaging. Ventricles volume measurement normalized to total brain volume. The ventricles volume in the EAE group (G1) was bigger than the volume in the naïve and NSSL–MPS (10 mg/kg) treated groups (G0 and G2) [100]. (f) T2 images of representative mice brains. (i) G0 – naïve group, (ii) G1 –EAE group, (iii) G2 – EAE treated with NSSL–MPS (10 mg/kg) group [100].

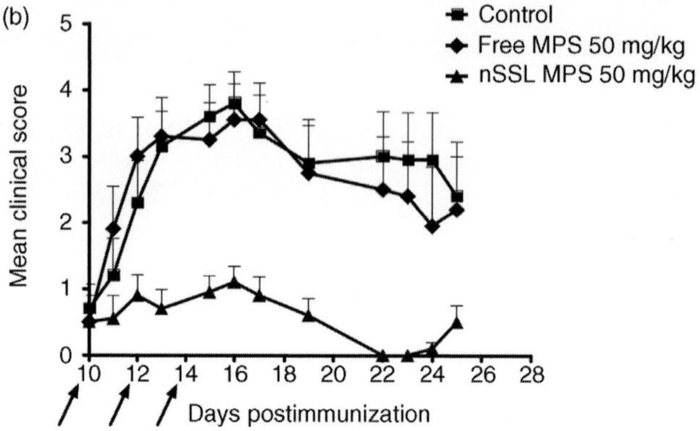

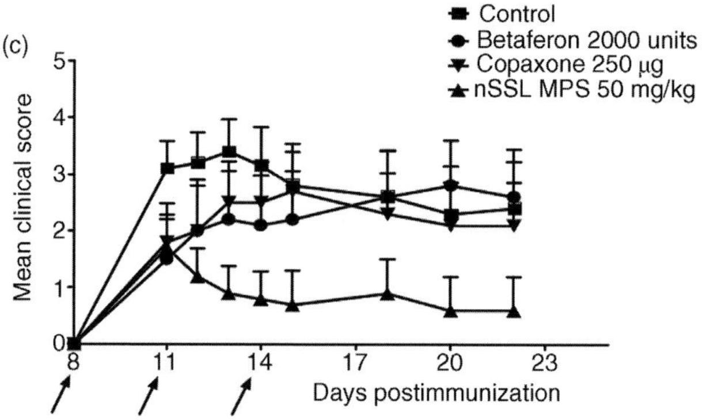

Figure 25.3 (*Continued*)

distribution is 12 times higher for liposomal MPS than for free MPS, and at 24 h postinjection only MPS derived from NSSL is found in the brain (Table 25.5). This enhanced permeability to the brain may be explained by changes in the vascular system that occur due to the inflammation typical of the EAE brain [119,120]. Interestingly, during the first hour post-IV injection, the liver gets much higher levels of nonencapsulated (free) MPS than of MPS derived from NSSL–MPS. This suggests much less GC first-pass metabolism, which is relevant to GC side effects [121]. Similar results were also obtained with other liposome-encapsulated water-soluble glucocorticoid prodrugs, for example, beta-methasone hemisuccinate (BMS), for treatment of experimental cerebral malaria (ECM) [118]. Our results show selective accumulation of BMS in the brains of diseased mice, which can be explained by blood–brain barrier (BBB) damage that is prominent in ECM. Results in the adjuvant-induced arthritis (AIA) rat model also show the PK superiority of the liposomal MPS over the free drug ($t_{1/2}$ of 11 h compared to $t_{1/2}$ <10 min for the free

(d)

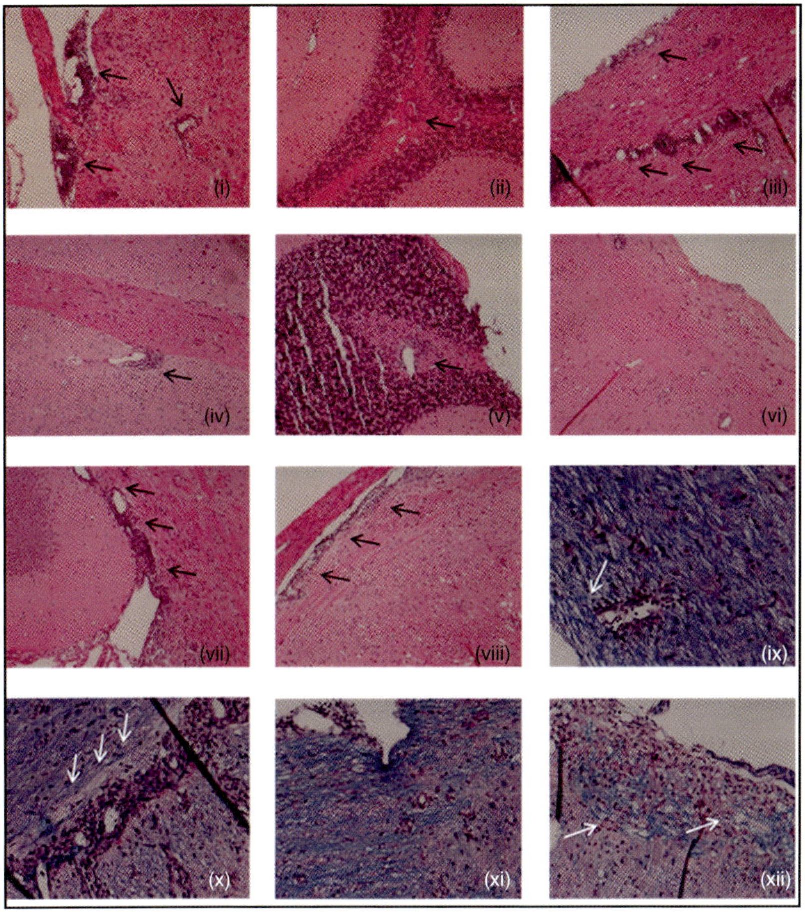

Figure 25.3 (*Continued*)

drug), as well as drug accumulation and a slow release rate at the inflamed paw. In humans and in large animals having large blood volume, drug release may be much faster than in small animals [122]. Therefore, we also studied the pharmacokinetics of NSSLs–MPS in a 15-kg Beagle dog, demonstrating again a much longer circulation time of the liposomal MPS, with a mean residence time (MRT) of ~9 h compared to less than 15 min for the free MPS. The PK similarity between the species and the superiority of the liposomal drug over the free drug in various PK parameters are prerequisite for therapeutic efficacy and suggest that the observed pharmacokinetic advantages will also be retained in humans, similar to what was demonstrated for doxorubicin [123].

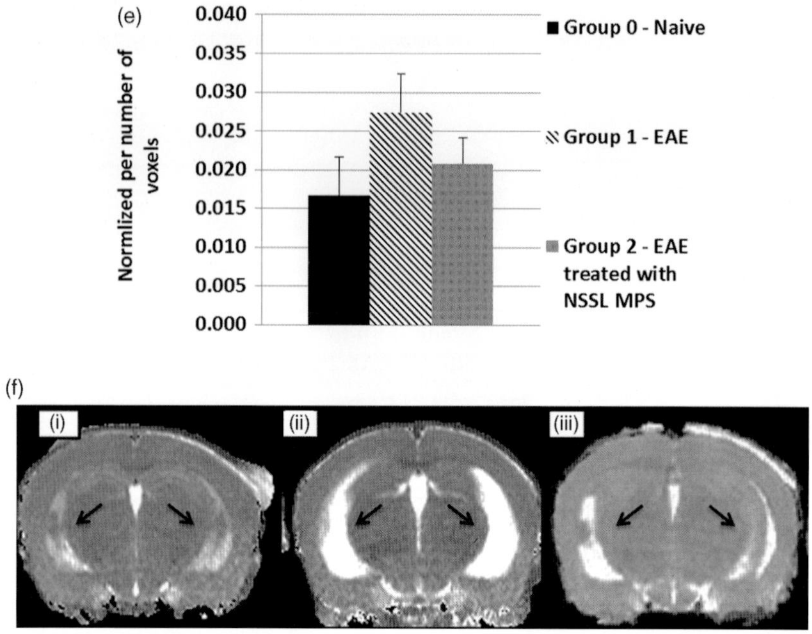

Figure 25.3 (*Continued*)

25.8.2 NSSL-Based Steroidal Nanodrugs Improve Significantly the Anti-Inflammatory Therapeutic Efficacy over the Same Steroids Given "As Is"

We have investigated the GC nanodrug's therapeutic efficacy in several murine models for disease with an inflammatory component. Our results using animal models of rheumatic arthritis, multiple sclerosis, cerebral malaria, lupus, Duchenne muscular dystrophy, carrageenan, or zymosan-induced inflammation showed that these nanodrugs have therapeutic efficacies superior to the same steroid administered "as is" and to other drugs and/or biologicals currently used to treat these diseases [80–82,116–118,124]. Representative results in the acute EAE model are presented in Figure 25.3b and c.

Table 25.5 Accumulation of MPS originating from NSSL–MPS and of free MPS in the liver and brain of acute EAE-induced mouse [80].

Formulation	Time (h)	Liver[a)]	Brain[a)]	Brain/liver ratio
Free MPS	0.3	112.30	0.36	0.003
Free MPS	24	1.10	0.00	0.000
NSSL–MPS	1	48.82	3.65	0.075
NSSL–MPS	24	3.01	0.54	0.180

a) μg MPS/gr organ.

25.8.3
Treatment with Liposomal Steroids Affects Cytokines Secretion and Tissue Pathology

In addition to the effect on the disease, NSSL–GC also suppressed the secretion of proinflammatory cytokines, but did not change the levels of TGF-β in AIA rats [82]. These results suggest that part of the beneficial therapeutic effect of NSSL–MPS on arthritis may be induced by suppression of the secretion of the proinflammatory cytokines TNF-α, IL-6, and IFN-β by activated lymphocytes.

In EAE mice, H&E and LFB staining clearly showed that the differences in therapeutic efficacy correspond to differences in neuropathology (Figure 25.3d) [81]. Treatment with NSSL–MPS reduced inflammation and demyelination in brains and spinal cords of mice with AT-EAE compared with free-MPS-treated mice and control mice. The reduction in T-cell infiltration of the nervous system could lead to clinical benefits by reducing ongoing demyelination, as was demonstrated by LFB staining, thus allowing the remyelination that normally occurs during recovery from EAE to restore neurological functions. These differences observed by histological staining were accompanied with changes in the brain tissue characteristics compared to the control group observed by MRI [81]. For example, the ventricles measurements showed significantly larger ventricles in the EAE group compared to the naïve and treated mice (Figure 25.3f and g). This pathology was previously indicated in the EAE model [125]. The MoA in EAE is likely related to the ability of steroids to act as immunosuppressors, to reduce edema, inhibit demyelination, and restore BBB abnormalities, which together ameliorate tissue damage. Indeed, in a model for cerebral malaria [83], treatment with NSSL–BMS suppressed cerebral inflammation affecting the levels of different cytokines, chemokines, and cell markers, as well as diminishing hemorrhage and edema, correlating with reduced clinical score. Also in MRL-lpr/lpr mice, a mice model for lupus, the therapeutic superiority of NSSL–MPS administered weekly compared with daily injections of free MPS had a beneficial effect on disease pathology by reducing proliferation of lymphoid tissue and renal damage [117].

25.8.4
Replacing Steroids with Nanosteroidal Drugs Results in Reduced Toxicity

Our results in the various animal models mentioned above suggest strongly that treatment with steroidal nanodrug (NSSL–GC) is improving steroid therapeutic index over the same steroid uses as-is. This effect is a combination of improvement of the therapeutic efficacy concomitantly with reducing significantly toxicities and side effects. Furthermore, one of the main advantages of administrating steroidal nanodrugs over the same GCs prodrugs as-is, is that it is efficacious to the same or better level at 5–10-fold lower concentration than the same steroid given as-is. For example, in mdx mice treated twice a week with either NSSL–MPS (5 mg/kg or 2 mg/kg), or free MPS (5 mg/kg) or placebo for 14 months, treatment with the free MPS had a clear bone catabolic effect in comparison with the control group, while treatment with liposomal MPS at 2 and 5 mg/kg mitigated this effect.

The advantage of this steroidal nanodrug demonstrating reduced toxicity was also exemplified in our previously published work [116–118]. Treatment of ECM, using the murine *P. berghei* ANKA model mice with free BMS at a dose of 5–20 mg/kg resulted in significant acute toxicity, including mice death. The use of NSSL–BMS completely abolished BMS toxicity and dramatically improved the therapeutic efficacy of the treatment [118]. We also tested the effect of treatment with 10 mg/kg NSSL–MPS on liver and kidney functions of the AIA rats [116]. Liver function, renal function, and blood glucose levels were in the normal range. There was no evidence of any histopathologic changes in liver specimens from any of the liposome-treated rats. Furthermore, NSSL–MPS injected at the "peak" of the disease either subcutaneously or intravenously suppressed AIA significantly, even when compared with higher doses of the free drugs or to TNF-α antagonists. Free MPS, at 2–25-fold higher concentrations was ineffective [82].

We have shown [117] that long-term treatment of MRL-lpr/lpr mice (model for systemic lupus erythematosus) with a weekly injection of 25 mg/kg of NSSL–MPS is superior to a daily injection of 5 mg/kg of free MPS. Mice treated with NSSL–MPS for 4.5 months had reduced spleen size and lymphadenopathy, followed by a decrease in body weight gain; less severe glomerular disease and less renal damage as evaluated by lower urea levels and increased survival, compared with the free-MPS treated mice.

NSSL–GCs are passively targeted to the inflamed tissue due to the enhanced permeability of the inflamed tissue vasculature, reducing steroid level in unwanted tissues. Therefore, more of the drug is reaching the inflamed site where it is slowly released at zero-order kinetics without changing the corticosteroid MoA. Thus, treatment with NSSL–GC enables to achieve the desired therapeutic efficacy, while reducing significantly the amount of drug that is administrated and prolonging the time between injections.

The highly efficacious anti-inflammatory therapeutic feature of these liposomal-GC formulations supports further development of NSSL as potential therapeutic agents for diseases with an inflammatory component.

References

1 Rhen, T. and Cidlowski, J.A. (2005) Antiinflammatory action of glucocorticoids – new mechanisms for old drugs. *N. Engl. J. Med.*, **353**, 1711–1723.

2 Rock, K.L., Latz, E., Ontiveros, F., and Kono, H. (2009) The sterile inflammatory response. *Annu. Rev. Immunol.*, **28**, 321–342.

3 Murphy, K.M., Travers, P., and Walport, M. (2012) *Janeway's Immunobiology*, Garland Science, New York, NY.

4 Playfair, J.H.L. and Chain, B.M. (2012) *Immunology at a Glance*, Wiley-Blackwell.

5 Gillett, N. and Chan, C. (2000) Applications of immunohistochemistry in

the evaluation of immunosuppressive agents. *Hum. Exp. Toxicol.*, **19**, 251–254.
6 de Lima Souza, T.R.C., Marques, G.S., de Medeiros Vieira, A.C.Q., and de Freitas, J.C.R. (2012) *State of the Art of Anti-Inflammatory Drugs*, (ed. F. Badria), p. 115.
7 Østensen, M., Khamashta, M., Lockshin, M., Parke, A., Brucato, A. *et al.* (2006) Anti-inflammatory and immunosuppressive drugs and reproduction. *Arthritis Res. Ther.*, **8**, 209.
8 Barnes, P.J. (2006) Corticosteroids: the drugs to beat. *Eur. J. Pharmacol.*, **533**, 2.
9 Pisetsky, D.S. and Ward, M.M. (2012) Advances in the treatment of inflammatory arthritis. *Best Pract. Res. Clin. Rheumatol.*, **26**, 251–261.
10 Wood, A.J. and O'Dell, J.R. (2004) Therapeutic strategies for rheumatoid arthritis. *N. Engl. J. Med.*, **350**, 2591–2602.
11 Gensini, G.F., Conti, A.A., and Lippi, D. (2007) The contributions of Paul Ehrlich to infectious disease. *J. Infect.*, **54**, 221–224.
12 Singh, R. and Lillard, J.W., Jr. (2009) Nanoparticle-based targeted drug delivery. *Exp. Mol. Pathol.*, **86**, 215–223.
13 LaVan, D.A., McGuire, T., and Langer, R. (2003) Small-scale systems for *in vivo* drug delivery. *Nat. Biotechnol.*, **21**, 1184–1191.
14 Kipp, J. (2004) The role of solid nanoparticle technology in the parenteral delivery of poorly water-soluble drugs. *Int. J. Pharm.*, **284**, 109–122.
15 Kreuter, J. (1983) Evaluation of nanoparticles as drug-delivery systems. II: Comparison of the body distribution of nanoparticles with the body distribution of microspheres (diameter greater than 1 micron), liposomes, and emulsions. *Pharm. Acta Helv.*, **58**, 217–226.
16 Barenholz, Y. and Lasic, D.L. (eds) (1996) Liposomes: models for bilogical phenomena, in *Handbook of Nonmedical Aplications of Liposomes* (eds Y. Barenholz and D. Lasic), CRC Press, Boca Raton, FL.
17 Gabizon, A., Catane, R., Uziely, B., Kaufman, B., Safra, T. *et al.* (1994) Prolonged circulation time and enhanced accumulation in malignant exudates of doxorubicin encapsulated in polyethylene-glycol coated liposomes. *Cancer Res.*, **54**, 987–992.
18 Gabizon, A., Shmeeda, H., and Barenholz, Y. (2003) Pharmacokinetics of pegylated liposomal doxorubicin: review of animal and human studies. *Clin. Pharmacokinet.*, **42**, 419–436.
19 Maeda, H., Fang, J., Inutsuka, T., and Kitamoto, Y. (2003) Vascular permeability enhancement in solid tumor: various factors, mechanisms involved and its implications. *Int. Immunopharmacol.*, **3**, 319–328.
20 Maeda, H., Wu, J., Sawa, T., Matsumura, Y., and Hori, K. (2000) Tumor vascular permeability and the EPR effect in macromolecular therapeutics: a review. *J. Control. Release*, **65**, 271–284.
21 Greish, K. (2007) Enhanced permeability and retention of macromolecular drugs in solid tumors: a royal gate for targeted anticancer nanomedicines. *J. Drug Target.*, **15**, 457–464.
22 Torchilin, V.P. (2007) Targeted pharmaceutical nanocarriers for cancer therapy and imaging. *AAPS J.*, **9**, E128–147.
23 Duncan, R. (2003) The dawning era of polymer therapeutics. *Nat. Rev. Drug Discov.*, **2**, 347–360.
24 Maeda, H., Bharate, G., and Daruwalla, J. (2009) Polymeric drugs for efficient tumor-targeted drug delivery based on EPR-effect. *Eur. J. Pharm. Biopharm.*, **71**, 409–419.
25 Shenoy, V., Vijay, I., and Murthy, R. (2005) Tumour targeting: biological factors and formulation advances in injectable lipid nanoparticles. *J. Pharm. Pharmacol.*, **57**, 411–421.
26 Koo, O.M., Rubinstein, I., and Onyuksel, H. (2005) Role of nanotechnology in targeted drug delivery and imaging: a concise review. *Nanomedicine*, **1**, 193–212.
27 Schiffelers, R.M., Koning, G.A., ten Hagen, T.L., Fens, M.H., Schraa, A.J. *et al.* (2003) Anti-tumor efficacy of tumor vasculature-targeted liposomal doxorubicin. *J. Control. Release*, **91**, 115–122.

28 Gupta, A.S., Huang, G., Lestini, B.J., Sagnella, S., Kottke-Marchant, K. *et al.* (2005) RGD-modified liposomes targeted to activated platelets as a potential vascular drug delivery system. *Thromb. Haemost.*, **93**, 106–114.
29 Chen, X., Plasencia, C., Hou, Y., and Neamati, N. (2005) Synthesis and biological evaluation of dimeric RGD peptide-paclitaxel conjugate as a model for integrin-targeted drug delivery. *J. Med. Chem.*, **48**, 1098–1106.
30 Czock, D., Keller, F., Rasche, FM., and Haussler, U. (2005) Pharmacokinetics and pharmacodynamics of systemically administered glucocorticoids. *Clin. Pharmacokinet.*, **44**, 61–98.
31 Buttgereit, F., Straub, R.H., Wehling, M., and Burmester, G.R. (2004) Glucocorticoids in the treatment of rheumatic diseases: an update on the mechanisms of action. *Arthritis Rheum.*, **50**, 3408–3417.
32 Yanovski, J.A. and Cutler, G.B., Jr. (1994) Glucocorticoid action and the clinical features of Cushing's syndrome. *Endocrinol. Metab. Clin. North Am.*, **23**, 487–509.
33 Dubois, E.F.L. (2005) Clinical potencies of glucocorticoids: what do we really measure? *Curr. Respir. Med. Rev.*, **1**, 103–108.
34 Franklin Adkinson, N. Jr., Yunginger, J.W., Busse, W.W., Bochner, B.S., Simons, F.E.R., and Holgate, S.T. (2003) *Glucocorticoids Middleton's Allergy: Principles and Practice*, Mosby, Inc., pp. 870–913.
35 Krakoff, L.R. (1988) Glucocorticoid excess syndromes causing hypertension. *Cardiol. Clin.*, **6**, 537–545.
36 Samtani, M.N., Lohle, M., Grant, A., Nathanielsz, P.W., and Jusko, W.J. (2005) Betamethasone pharmacokinetics after two prodrug formulations in sheep: implications for antenatal corticosteroid use. *Drug Metab. Dispos.*, **33**, 1124–1130.
37 Abma, E.M., Blanken, R., and De Heide, L.J. (2002) Cushing's syndrome caused by topical steroid therapy for psoriasis. *Neth. J. Med.*, **60**, 148–150.
38 Wicki, J., Droz, M., Cirafici, L., and Vallotton, M.B. (2000) Acute adrenal crisis in a patient treated with intraarticular steroid therapy. *J. Rheumatol.*, **27**, 510–511.
39 Allen, T.M. and Cullis, P.R. (2004) Drug delivery systems: entering the mainstream. *Supramol. Sci.*, **303**, 1818–1822.
40 Barenholz, Y.C. (2012) Doxil® – the first FDA-approved nano-drug: lessons learned. *J. Control. Release*, **160**, 117–134.
41 Boswell, G., Buell, D., and Bekersky, I. (1998) AmBisome (liposomal amphotericin B): a comparative review. *J. Clin. Pharmacol.*, **38**, 583–592.
42 Lichtenberg, D. and Barenholz, Y. (1988) Liposomes: preparation, characterization, and preservation. *Methods Biochem. Anal.*, **33**, 337–462.
43 Mozafari, M.R. (2005) Liposomes: an overview of manufacturing techniques. *Cell. Mol. Biol. Lett.*, **10**, 711–719.
44 Crommelin, D.J. and Storm, G. (2003) Liposomes: from the bench to the bed. *J. Liposome Res.*, **13**, 33–36.
45 Barenholz, Y. and Crommelin, D.J. (1994) Liposomes as pharmaceutical dosage forms, in *Encyclopedia of Pharmaceutical Technology* (ed. J. Swarbick and J.C. Boylan), Marcel Dekker Inc., New York, pp. 1–39.
46 Moghimi, S.M., Hunter, A.C., and Murray, J.C. (2001) Long-circulating and target-specific nanoparticles: theory to practice. *Pharmacol. Rev.*, **53**, 283–318.
47 Kwon, G.S. and Kataoka, K. (2012) Block copolymer micelles as long-circulating drug vehicles. *Adv. Drug Deliv. Rev.*, **64**, 237–245.
48 Müllner, M., Dodds, S.J., Nguyen, T.-H., Senyschyn, D., Porter, C.J. *et al.* (2015) Size and rigidity of cylindrical polymer brushes dictate long circulating properties *in vivo*. *ACS Nano*, **9**, 1294–1304.
49 Moghimi, S.M. and Hunter, A.C. (2000) Poloxamers and poloxamines in nanoparticle engineering and experimental medicine. *Trends Biotechnol.*, **18**, 412–420.
50 Barenholz, Y. (2004) Sphingomyelin and cholesterol: from membrane biophysics and rafts to potential medical

applications. *Subcell. Biochem.*, **37**, 167–215.
51 Simons, K. and Vaz, W.L. (2004) Model systems, lipid rafts, and cell membranes. *Annu. Rev. Biophys. Biomol. Struct.*, **33**, 269–295.
52 Ipsen, J.H., Karlstrom, G., Mouritsen, O.G., Wennerstrom, H., and Zuckermann, M.J. (1987) Phase equilibria in the phosphatidylcholine-cholesterol system. *Biochim. Biophys. Acta*, **905**, 162–172.
53 Ben-Yashar, V. and Barenholz, Y. (1989) The interaction of cholesterol and cholest-4-en-3-one with dipalmitoylphosphatidylcholine. Comparison based on the use of three fluorophores. *Biochim. Biophys. Acta*, **985**, 271–278.
54 Garbuzenko, O., Barenholz, Y., and Priev, A. (2005) Effect of grafted PEG on liposome size and on compressibility and packing of lipid bilayer. *Chem. Phys. Lipids*, **135**, 117–129.
55 Mouritsen, O.G. and Jorgensen, K. (1994) Dynamical order and disorder in lipid bilayers. *Chem. Phys. Lipids*, **73**, 3–25.
56 Samuni, A.M., Lipman, A., and Barenholz, Y. (2000) Damage to liposomal lipids: protection by antioxidants and cholesterol-mediated dehydration. *Chem. Phys. Lipids*, **105**, 121–134.
57 Hirsch-Lerner, D., Zuidam, D., and Barenholz, Y. (1998) Physiochemical characterization of DOTAP-containing lipoplexes by fluorescent probes: relevance to lipofection, in *Targetting of Drugs Strategies for Stealth Therapeutic Systems* (eds G. Gregoriadis and B. McCormack), Plenum, New York, pp. 169–183.
58 Barenholz, Y. (2003) Relevancy of drug loading to liposomal formulation therapeutic efficacy. *J. Lipos. Res.*, **13**, 1–8.
59 Stein, W.D. (1986) *Transport and Diffusion Across Cell Membranes*, Academic Press.
60 Clerc, S. and Barenholz, Y. (1995) Loading of amphipathic weak acids into liposomes in response to transmembrane calcium acetate gradients. *Biochim. Biophys. Acta*, **1240**, 257–265.
61 Haran, G., Cohen, R., Bar, L.K., and Barenholz, Y. (1993) Transmembrane ammonium sulfate gradients in liposomes produce efficient and stable entrapment of amphipathic weak bases. *Biochim. Biophys. Acta*, **1151**, 201–215.
62 Clerc, S. and Barenholz, Y. (1998) A quantitative model for using acridine orange as a transmembrane pH gradient probe. *Anal. Biochem.*, **259**, 104–111.
63 Ramos, S., Schuldiner, S., and Kaback, H.R. (1976) The electrochemical gradient of protons and its relationship to active transport in *Escherichia coli* membrane vesicles. *Proc. Natl. Acad. Sci. USA*, **73**, 1892–1896.
64 Nichols, J.W. and Deamer, D.W. (1976) Catecholamine uptake and concentration by liposomes maintaining p/gradients. *Biochim. Biophys. Acta*, **455**, 269–271.
65 Madden, T.D., Harrigan, P.R., Tai, L.C., Bally, M.B., Mayer, L.D., Cullis, P.R. *et al.* (1990) The accumulation of drugs within large unilamellar vesicles exhibiting a proton gradient: a survey. *Chem. Phys. Lipids*, **53**, 37–46.
66 Zucker, D., Marcus, D., Barenholz, Y., and Goldblum, A. (2009) Liposome drugs' loading efficiency: a working model based on loading conditions and drug's physicochemical properties. *J. Control. Release*, **139**, 73–80.
67 American Chemical Society (2006) *Scifinder Scholar*, Washington, DC.
68 Gabizon, A., Chisin, R., Amselem, S., Druckmann, S., Cohen, R. *et al.* (1991) Pharmacokinetic and imaging studies in patients receiving a formulation of liposome-associated adriamycin. *Br. J. Cancer*, **64**, 1125–1132.
69 Amselem, S., Cohen, R., and Barenholz, Y. (1993) *In vitro* tests to predict *in vivo* performance of liposomal dosage forms. *Chem. Phys. Lipids*, **64**, 219–237.
70 Mishina, E.V., Straubinger, R.M., Pyszczynski, N.A., and Jusko, W.J. (1993) Enhancement of tissue delivery and receptor occupancy of methylprednisolone in rats by a liposomal formulation. *Pharm. Res.*, **10**, 1402–1410.
71 Shaw, I.H., Knight, C.G., and Dingle, J.T. (1976) Liposomal retention of a modified

anti-inflammatory steroid. *Biochem. J.*, **158**, 473–476.

72 Teshima, M., Kawakami, S., Fumoto, S., Nishida, K., Nakamura, J. *et al.* (2006) PEGylated liposomes loading palmitoyl prednisolone for prolonged blood concentration of prednisolone. *Biol. Pharm. Bull.*, **29**, 1436–1440.

73 Kumar, V.V. (1991) Complementary molecular shapes and additivity of the packing parameter of lipids. *Proc. Natl. Acad. Sci. USA*, **88**, 444–448.

74 Metselaar, J.M., Wauben, M.H., Wagenaar-Hilbers, J.P., Boerman, O.C., and Storm, G. (2003) Complete remission of experimental arthritis by joint targeting of glucocorticoids with long-circulating liposomes. *Arthritis Rheum.*, **48**, 2059–2066.

75 Schmidt, J., Metselaar, J.M., Wauben, M.H., Toyka, K.V., Storm, G. *et al.* (2003) Drug targeting by long-circulating liposomal glucocorticosteroids increases therapeutic efficacy in a model of multiple sclerosis. *Brain*, **126**, 1895–1904.

76 Metselaar, J.M., van den Berg, W.B., Holthuysen, A.E., Wauben, M.H., Storm, G. *et al.* (2004) Liposomal targeting of glucocorticoids to synovial lining cells strongly increases therapeutic benefit in collagen type II arthritis. *Ann. Rheum. Dis.*, **63**, 348–353.

77 van den Hoven, J.M., Hofkens, W., Wauben, M.H., Wagenaar-Hilbers, J.P., Beijnen, J.H. *et al.* (2011) Optimizing the therapeutic index of liposomal glucocorticoids in experimental arthritis. *Int. J. Pharm.*, **416**, 471–477.

78 Szebeni, J., Baranyi, L., Savay, S., Milosevits, J., Bunger, R. *et al.* (2002) Role of complement activation in hypersensitivity reactions to Doxil and hynic PEG liposomes: experimental and clinical studies. *J. Liposome Res.*, **12**, 165–172.

79 Storm, G., Oussoren, C., Peeters, P.A.M., and Barenholz, Y. (1993) *Tolerability of Liposomes In Vivo, Liposome Technology*, 2nd edn (ed. G. Gregoriadis), CRC Press, Boca Raton, FL, pp. 345–383.

80 Avnir, Y., Turjeman, K., Tulchinsky, D., Sigal, A., Kizelsztein, P. *et al.* (2011) Fabrication principles and their contribution to the superior *in vivo* therapeutic efficacy of nano-liposomes remote loaded with glucocorticoids. *PloS One*, **6**, e25721.

81 Turjeman, K., Bavli, Y., Kizelsztein, P., Schilt, Y., Allon, N. *et al.* (2015) Nano-drugs based on nano sterically stabilized liposomes for the treatment of inflammatory neurodegenerative diseases. *PloS One*, **10**, e0130442.

82 Ulmansky, R., Turjeman, K., Baru, M., Katzavian, G., Harel, M. *et al.* (2012) Glucocorticoids in nano-liposomes administered intravenously and subcutaneously to adjuvant arthritis rats are superior to the free drugs in suppressing arthritis and inflammatory cytokines. *J. Control. Release*, **160**, 299–305.

83 Waknine-Grinberg, J.H., Even-Chen, S., Avichzer, J., Turjeman, K., Bentura-Marciano, A. *et al.* (2013) Glucocorticosteroids in nano-sterically stabilized liposomes are efficacious for elimination of the acute symptoms of experimental cerebral malaria. *PloS One*, **8**, e72722.

84 Davidenkova, E., Ternova, N., Rozenberg, O., Noskin, L., Loshakova, L. *et al.* (1984) Relationship between prolongation of antiinflammatory activity of hydrocortisone incorporated into liposomes and their lipid composition in experimental arthritis. *Bull. Exp. Biol. Med.*, **97**, 716–718.

85 Schmidt, J., Metselaar, J.M., and Gold, R. (2003) Intravenous liposomal prednisolone downregulates *in situ* TNF-α production by T-cells in experimental autoimmune encephalomyelitis. *J. Histochem. Cytochem.*, **51**, 1241–1244.

86 Parmar, J., Singh, D., Hegde, D.D., Lohade, A., Soni, P. *et al.* (2010) Development and evaluation of inhalational liposomal system of budesonide for better management of asthma. *Indian J. Pharm. Sci.*, **72**, 442.

87 Hofkens, W., Storm, G., Van Den Berg, W., and Van Lent, P. (2011) Liposomal targeting of glucocorticoids to the inflamed synovium inhibits cartilage matrix destruction during murine

antigen-induced arthritis. *Int. J. Pharm.*, **416**, 486–492.
88 Hofkens, W., Grevers, L.C., Walgreen, B., De Vries, T.J., Leenen, P.J. *et al.* (2011) Intravenously delivered glucocorticoid liposomes inhibit osteoclast activity and bone erosion in murine antigen-induced arthritis. *J. Control. Release*, **152**, 363–369.
89 Metselaar, J., Van den Berg, W., Holthuysen, A., Wauben, M., Storm, G. *et al.* (2004) Liposomal targeting of glucocorticoids to synovial lining cells strongly increases therapeutic benefit in collagen type II arthritis. *Ann. Rheum. Dis.*, **63**, 348–353.
90 Bonanomi, M., Velvart, M., Stimpel, M., Roos, K., Fehr, K. *et al.* (1987) Studies of pharmacokinetics and therapeutic effects of glucocorticoids entrapped in liposomes after intraarticular application in healthy rabbits and in rabbits with antigen-induced arthritis. *Rheumatol. Int.*, **7**, 203–212.
91 Koning, G.A., Schiffelers, R.M., Wauben, M.H., Kok, R.J., Mastrobattista, E. *et al.* (2006) Targeting of angiogenic endothelial cells at sites of inflammation by dexamethasone phosphate-containing RGD peptide liposomes inhibits experimental arthritis. *Arthritis Rheum.*, **54**, 1198–1208.
92 Rauchhaus, U., Schwaiger, F.-W., and Panzner, S. (2009) Separating therapeutic efficacy from glucocorticoid side-effects in rodent arthritis using novel, liposomal delivery of dexamethasone phosphate: long term suppression of arthritis facilitates interval treatment. *Arthritis Res. Ther.*, **11**, 1–9.
93 Hofkens, W., van den Hoven, J.M., Pesman, G.J., Nabbe, K.C., Sweep, F.C. *et al.* (2011) Safety of glucocorticoids can be improved by lower yet still effective dosages of liposomal steroid formulations in murine antigen-induced arthritis: comparison of prednisolone with budesonide. *Int. J. Pharm.*, **416**, 493–498.
94 Konduri, K.S., Nandedkar, S., Düzgünes, N., Suzara, V., Artwohl, J. *et al.* (2003) Efficacy of liposomal budesonide in experimental asthma. *J. Allergy Clin. Immunol.*, **111**, 321–327.
95 Waldrep, J.C., Keyhani, K., Black, M., and Knight, V. (1994) Operating characteristics of 18 different continuous-flow jet nebulizers with beclomethasone dipropionate liposome aerosol. *Chest J.*, **105**, 106–110.
96 Shaw, I., Knight, C., and Dingle, J. (1976) Liposomal retention of a modified anti-inflammatory steroid. *Biochem. J.*, **158**, 473–476.
97 Phillips, N.C., Thomas, D., Knight, C.G., and Dingle, J.T. (1979) Liposome-incorporated corticosteroids. II. Therapeutic activity in experimental arthritis. *Ann. Rheum. Dis.*, **38**, 553–557.
98 Dingle, J.T. (1978) Articular damage in arthritis and its control. *Ann. Intern. Med.*, **88**, 821–826.
99 Morgan, J.R., Williams, K.E., Davies, R.L., Leach, K., Thomson, M. *et al.* (1981) Localisation of experimental staphylococcal abscesses by 99MTC-technetium-labelled liposomes. *J. Med. Microbiol.*, **14**, 213–217.
100 Senior, J. and Gregoriadis, G. (1982) Stability of small unilamellar liposomes in serum and clearance from the circulation: the effect of the phospholipid and cholesterol components. *Life Sci.*, **30**, 2123–2136.
101 Senior, J., Crawley, J.C., and Gregoriadis, G. (1985) Tissue distribution of liposomes exhibiting long half-lives in the circulation after intravenous injection. *Biochim. Biophys. Acta*, **839**, 1–8.
102 Gabizon, A. and Martin, F. (1997) Polyethylene glycol-coated (pegylated) liposomal doxorubicin. Rationale for use in solid tumours. *Drugs*, **54** (4), 15–21.
103 Gabizon, A.A. (2001) Stealth liposomes and tumor targeting: one step further in the quest for the magic bullet. *Clin. Cancer Res.*, **7**, 223–225.
104 Allen, T.M., Hansen, C., and Rutledge, J. (1989) Liposomes with prolonged circulation times: factors affecting uptake by reticuloendothelial and other tissues. *Biochim. Biophys. Acta*, **981**, 27–35.
105 Tirosh, O., Barenholz, Y., Katzhendler, J., and Priev, A. (1998) Hydration of polyethylene glycol-grafted liposomes. *Biophys. J.*, **74**, 1371–1379.

106 Allen, T.M., Hansen, C., Martin, F., Redemann, C., and Yau-Young, A. (1991) Liposomes containing synthetic lipid derivatives of poly(ethylene glycol) show prolonged circulation half-lives *in vivo*. *Biochim. Biophys. Acta*, **1066**, 29–36.

107 Senior, J., Delgado, C., Fisher, D., Tilcock, C., and Gregoriadis, G. (1991) Influence of surface hydrophilicity of liposomes on their interaction with plasma protein and clearance from the circulation: studies with poly(ethylene glycol)-coated vesicles. *Biochim. Biophys. Acta*, **1062**, 77–82.

108 Lasic, D.D., Martin, F.J., Gabizon, A., Huang, S.K., and Papahadjopoulos, D. (1991) Sterically stabilized liposomes: a hypothesis on the molecular origin of the extended circulation times. *Biochim. Biophys. Acta*, **1070**, 187–192.

109 Torchilin, V.P., Omelyanenko, V.G., Papisov, M.I., Bogdanov, A.A., Jr., Trubetskoy, V.S. *et al.* (1994) Poly (ethylene glycol) on the liposome surface: on the mechanism of polymer-coated liposome longevity. *Biochim. Biophys. Acta*, **1195**, 11–20.

110 Boerman, O.C., Oyen, W.J., van Bloois, L., Koenders, E.B., van der Meer, J.W. *et al.* (1997) Optimization of technetium-99m-labeled PEG liposomes to image focal infection: effects of particle size and circulation time. *J. Nucl. Med.*, **38**, 489–493.

111 Boerman, O.C., Storm, G., Oyen, W.J., and van Bloois, L., van der Meer, J.W. *et al.* (1995) Sterically stabilized liposomes labeled with indium-111 to image focal infection. *J. Nucl. Med.*, **36**, 1639–1644.

112 Williams, A.S., Jones, S.G., Goodfellow, R.M., Amos, N., and Williams, B.D. (1999) Interleukin-1beta (IL-1beta) inhibition: a possible mechanism for the anti-inflammatory potency of liposomally conjugated methotrexate formulations in arthritis. *Br. J. Pharmacol.*, **128**, 234–240.

113 Bakker-Woudenberg, I.A., ten Kate, M.T., Guo, L., Working, P., and Mouton, J.W. (2002) Ciprofloxacin in polyethylene glycol-coated liposomes: efficacy in rat models of acute or chronic *Pseudomonas aeruginosa* infection. *Antimicrob. Agents Chemother.*, **46**, 2575–2581.

114 Cruz, M.E., Manuela Gaspar, M., Barbara, M., Martins, F., and Luisa Corvo, M. (2005) Liposomal superoxide dismutases and their use in the treatment of experimental arthritis. *Methods Enzymol.*, **391**, 395–413.

115 Turjeman, K. and Barenholz, Y. (2016) Liposomal nano-drugs based on amphipathic weak acid steroid prodrugs for treatment of inflammatory diseases. *J. Drug Target.*, 1–41.

116 Avnir, Y., Ulmansky, R., Wasserman, V., Even-Chen, S., Broyer, M. *et al.* (2008) Amphipathic weak acid glucocorticoid prodrugs remote-loaded into sterically stabilized nanoliposomes evaluated in arthritic rats and in a Beagle dog: a novel approach to treating autoimmune arthritis. *Arthritis Rheum.*, **58**, 119–129.

117 Moallem, E., Koren, E., Ulmansky, R., Pizov, G., Barlev, M. *et al.* (2016) A liposomal steroid nano-drug for treating systemic lupus erythematosus. *Lupus*, **25** (11), 1209–1216.

118 Waknine-Grinberg, J.H., Even-Chen, S., Avichzer, J., Turjeman, K., Bentura-Marciano, A. *et al.* (2013) Glucocorticosteroids in nano-sterically stabilized liposomes are efficacious for elimination of the acute symptoms of experimental cerebral malaria. *PLoS One*, **8** (8), e72722.

119 Gold, R., Linington, C., and Lassmann, H. (2006) Understanding pathogenesis and therapy of multiple sclerosis via animal models: 70 years of merits and culprits in experimental autoimmune encephalomyelitis research. *Brain*, **129**, 1953–1971.

120 Floris, S., Blezer, E., Schreibelt, G., Döpp, E., Van der Pol, S. *et al.* (2004) Blood–brain barrier permeability and monocyte infiltration in experimental allergic encephalomyelitis. *Brain*, **127**, 616–627.

121 Schleimer, R., Spahn, J., Covar, R., and Szefler, S. (2003) Chapter 52. Glucocorticoids. *Middleton's Allergy Principles and Practices*, 6th edn, Mosby, Inc, Philadelphia, pp. 870–913.

122 Gabizon, A.A., Barenholz, Y., and Bialer, M. (1993) Prolongation of the circulation time of doxorubicin encapsulated in liposomes containing a polyethylene

glycol-derivatized phospholipid: pharmacokinetic studies in rodents and dogs. *Pharm. Res.*, **10**, 703–708.

123 Gabizon, A., Shmeeda, H., and Barenholz, Y. (2003) Pharmacokinetics of pegylated liposomal doxorubicin. *Clin. Pharmacokinet.*, **42**, 419–436.

124 Guo, J., Waknine-Grinberg, J.H., Mitchell, A.J., Barenholz, Y., and Golenser, J. (2014) Reduction of experimental cerebral malaria and its related proinflammatory responses by the novel liposome-based β-methasone nanodrug. *Biomed. Res. Intern.*, **2014**, 292471.

125 Karlik, S., Munoz, D., Louis, J.S., and Strejan, G. (1999) Correlation between MRI and clinico-pathological manifestations in Lewis rats protected from experimental allergic encephalomyelitis by acylated synthetic peptide of myelin basic protein. *Magn. Reson. Imaging*, **17**, 731–737.

26
Nanodrugs in Medicine and Healthcare: Pulmonary, Nasal and Ophthalmic Routes, and Vaccination

Christel C. Müller-Goymann and Mukta Paranjpe

Technische Universität Braunschweig, Institut für Pharmazeutische Technologie, Mendelssohnstr. 1, 38106 Braunschweig, Germany

26.1
Introduction

Colloidal drug delivery systems have been studied extensively for many decades. These systems act as a platform or as carriers for different drugs for different routes of administration [1–4]. Systems such as solid lipid nanoparticles (SLN), polymeric nanoparticles, and liposomes are of particular interest in this chapter. Routes of administration such as pulmonary, nasal, or ocular ones are non-invasive routes of administration and offer numerous advantages over conventional peroral route of administration whereas, vaccination usually requires parenteral administration, that is, intramuscular or subcutaneous injection. The nasal route for vaccination is of particular interest with regard to avoiding injections and increasing immune responses. All these routes can be utilized for local or systemic delivery of an active pharmaceutical ingredient (API) depending on the disease and nature of the API. Nanoparticle-based systems offer numerous functionalities such as improved bioavailability, improved drug encapsulation and protection of the API, and higher encapsulation efficiency of lipophilic drugs, to name a few. In the case of lipid-based nanoparticles, the use of physiological lipids in the formulation improves the bioavailability, as well as biodegradability. In addition, these lipids have high stability and low toxicity profiles. Owing to these advantages, nanoparticle-based systems are particularly attractive formulations in comparison with the traditional drug delivery systems.

Several lipid-based formulations have been successful in phase 3 studies, for example, for the treatment of cystic fibrosis patients with chronic *Pseudomonas aeroginosa* lung infection as Arikace® (Amikacin dry liposomal formulation) [5], Pulmaquin® (Ciprofloxacin liposomal formulation) [6], as well as for respiratory distress syndrome Alveofact®, a bovine pulmonary surfactant liposomal formulation [7]. Liposomal formulations encapsulating a variety of different APIs have been approved for nasal and ophthalmic administration as well as for

Pharmaceutical Nanotechnology: Innovation and Production, First Edition. Edited by Jean Cornier, Arno Kwade, Andrew Owen, and Marcel Van de Voorde.

vaccination. LipoNasal® hay fever nasal spray is a medical product supporting and promoting the natural healing process in irritation and inflammation of the nasal mucosa by forming a thin protecting layer onto the nasal mucosa [8]. Liposomal dispersions to be sprayed onto the closed eyelid such as TEARS AGAIN® or LipoNit® treat the dry eye syndrome (keratoconjunctivitis sicca). The liposomes spread well over the eyelid edge into the tear film where they reestablish the natural composition of the tear fluid and protect the latter against evaporation [9,10]. Saponin incorporation into liposomes causes a transformation to soccer-ball-like hollow structures [11]. Antigens can be attached to these 40–50 nm sized particles, which are used as strong adjuvants in veterinary vaccines due to their immunostimulating effects, for example, Equip® F ad us. vet., Equilis® Prequenza, CattleMaster Gold® [12–14]. Many other lipid and polymer-based nanoparticles are under investigation for pulmonary, nasal, ocular routes, and for vaccination. Apart from the treatment of diseases and for vaccination, different nanoparticles are also studied for diagnostic purposes, for example, Endorem®, which is an aqueous suspension of dextrane-stabilized iron oxide nanoparticles as superparamagnetic contrast agent in magnetic resonance imaging MRI [15].

This chapter will focus on different types of nanoparticles, manufacturing processes, challenges faced in manufacturing, advantages over conventional systems, different kinds of nanoparticles for different routes of administration, and future therapies based on nanoparticles.

26.2 Different Routes of Administration

26.2.1 Pulmonary Route

The lungs are responsible for the gas exchange and supply of oxygen to all the cells. The structure and function of the lungs make them ideal for gas exchange. Pulmonary route offers various advantages over traditional peroral route of drug administration. The availability of large surface area, rapid absorption, and increased bioavailability owing to high vascularization makes the lungs especially attractive candidates for pulmonary drug delivery [16]. Apart from these advantages, the lungs ubiquitously contain phospholipids and phospholipid-based surface proteins in the mucosal secretions [17]. These surface proteins enhance the efficacy of phospholipid-based formulations by increasing acceptability and tolerance in the lung tissue [18].

Currently, numerous drugs originally used via traditional peroral route, have been formulated as nanoparticle-based systems for pulmonary application [19]. Anti-infective drugs such as amphotericin B, rifampicin, isoniazid, and so on are currently developed as either polymer-based or lipid-based nanoparticles and thorough physicochemical characterization along with animal studies have

Table 26.1 Combined selective references for pulmonary, ophthalmic, nasal, and vaccination routes.

API category/disease	Type of particle	Reference
Lung disorders Anti-inflammatory, antiasthma, pulmonary hypertension, antioxidants, anticancer	Solid lipid nanoparticles, lipid microparticles, liposomes	[22–28]
Lung infections Tuberculosis, cystic fibrosis	Solid lipid nanoparticles, lipid microparticles, liposomes	[29–31]
Nasal infections/allergies/systemic effects Acute rhinitis, pollen sensitivity, hypertension, brain targeting of viral infections, brain tumors, stroke	Solid lipid nanoparticles, chitosan microparticles, liposomes, nanoemulsions	[8,32–37]
Ophthalmic infections/allergies/ocular diseases of the anterior and posterior segment of the eye Allergic conjunctivitis, dry eye syndrome, glaucoma, diabetic retinopathy, wet age-related macular degeneration (AMD)	Solid lipid nanoparticles (SLN), lipid microparticles, polymer nanoparticles, nanoemulsions, liposomes	[9,10,38–49]
Vaccination Influenza	Solid lipid nanoparticles, lipid microparticles, virosomes, ISCOM	[50–54]
Proteins, peptides Insulin		[55–57]
Surfactant, gene, antibody		[58]

shown promising results for possible human administration [20,21]. In addition to the anti-infectives, other API categories such as antioxidants, anti-inflammatory, anticancer, vascular drug therapy, surfactants, and protein-based systems are also under development for possible pulmonary drug delivery system (see Table 26.1). The most challenging aspect in the development of nanoparticle-based drug delivery systems for various routes is the maintenance of the colloidal state properties after administration. In spite of development in the design and manufacturing of nanoparticle-based systems, only a few formulations are available on commercial scale.

26.2.2 Nasal Route

Apart from local effects of commercial nasal spray formulations of corticosteroid suspensions and of solutions of α_1 and α_2 sympathomimetic APIs such as xylometazoline or oxymetazoline [59,60], the systemic availability of a multitude of APIs from nasal administration is comparably fast as that from parenteral administration due to excellent blood circulation and a mucosal area of about 170 cm^2 with less tight junctions compared to the gastroendothelium and the blood brain barrier [61]. Nasal administration avoids injection and is thus more acceptable for the patient. Compared to peroral administration the API enters the blood circulation faster from the nasal route than from the gastrointestinal tract together with the advantage of avoiding a first pass effect in the liver [32].

The physicochemical characteristics of an API such as molecular weight, partition coefficient, sufficient to high solubility in mucus, and compatibility with tissue are of major importance for the systemic availability. Due to the olfactory mucosa in the upper region of the nasal cavity, the API should preferably be odorless. It has been shown that microbial, viral, and parasite infections may find their way directly to the brain, most probably by the olfactory nerve as the first cranial nerve [62–64]. Such nano- and micron-sized infectious particles drew a lot of interest during the last decade with regard to targeting the brain with nano-sized carriers for the treatment of CNS deseases. A superior drug targeting of the brain of animal models has been demonstrated when nanoparticles were given via the nasal route in comparison to drug solutions [65]. However, the experiments did not undoubtedly demonstrate whether the nanoparticles themselves were absorbed and the drug released afterwards or vice versa.

Based on viral infections via the nasal route such as influenza A, nasal influenza vaccination was widely studied and proved to be an excellent alternative to parenteral immunization because of the additional mucosal immune response [66]. Furthermore, avoiding injection is of special interest for the vaccination of children. Fluenz® Tetra was approved in 2013 by the European Medicines Agency (EMA) as the first nasally administered influenza vaccine in Europe. It is a suspension of four strains of live attenuated influenza A viruses for the immunization of children and adolescents from 24 months up to 18 years of age whereas, parenteral vaccination is normally done with three strains of inactivated viruses. The US Food and Drug Administration (FDA) has already granted marketing authorization to nasal suspensions of three strains of live attenuated influenza viruses under the name of FluMist® in 2003 and switched to FluMist Quadrivalent in 2012 with four strains [67]. In recent years, the research focus is on the development of different types of nanoparticles as adjuvants for the nasal delivery of vaccines against a variety of further mucosa-related infections such as hepatitis B [68].

26.2.3
Ophthalmic Route

The therapy of eye diseases is mainly done topically via ophthalmic administration of preferably aqueous formulations, that is, eye drops, because the ocular bioavailability of the majority of APIs is insufficient from the systemic circulation after peroral administration due to a strong blood retina barrier. Toward the environment, the cornea of the eye represents the main barrier and is one of the tightest tissues of the body [69]. Furthermore, eye drops remain in contact with the eye only for a short period of time before being diluted by tear fluid and drained. In addition, the area of absorption is small as to about 123 mm^2 [70]. Therefore, only sufficiently lipophilic small molecules penetrate into the corneal epithelium and permeate further into the anterior chamber whereas, hydrophilic and high molecular weight molecules such as antibodies or aptamers need to be directly injected into the vitreous humor of the eye.

Pegaptanib was the first aptamer for the treatment of wet age-related macular degeneration (AMD) and was approved by the FDA in 2004 under the name Macugen®. This pegylated single strand nucleic acid binds to the vascular endothelial growth factor (VEGF) as an antagonist and thus suppresses neovascularization. In 2011, the monoclonal antibody fragment ranibizumab was granted approval for the same treatment under the name Lucentis®. Again the mechanism of action is an antagonism of VEGF and thus a suppression of neoangiogenesis [58]. Apart from large hydrophilic molecules, corticosteroids such as the small lipophilic molecule triamcinolone acetonide are intravitreally injected as crystalline suspension for the treatment of AMD and other eye diseases [71]. The suspension represents a depot for prolonged effect. In order to obtain a long lasting effect of topical ophthalmic administration, dispersions of drug-loaded solid lipid nanoparticles are of particular interest [72].

26.2.4
Vaccination

Parenteral vaccination with live attenuated viruses or microorganisms generally results in a strong immune response of the vaccinated organism – either human or animal – whereas inactivated vaccines, split vaccines, or toxoid vaccines such as tetanus vaccine require the addition of an adjuvant to give high amounts of antibodies and a long-lasting protection. Aluminum hydroxide precipitates are widely used as particulate inorganic adjuvants, while the approval of oil in water emulsions or modified liposomes are less frequent in marketed vaccines [73,74]. Since liposomes consist of cholesterol and phospholipids as natural membrane constituents, their immunogenicity is insufficient unless modified by the incorporation of immunogenic additives. The solubilization of surface proteins from influenza A virus, that is, hemagglutinin and neuraminidase, by liposomes and the presentation of these proteins on the surface of the liposomes transforms the latter to virosomes that enable sufficient immunogenicity for a hepatitis A vaccine and a high antibody concentration within a short period of time (10 days) along with higher tolerability compared to aluminum hydroxide-adjuvanted hepatitis A vaccines [75]. The first marketing authorization was granted to virosome-adjuvanted hepatitis A vaccines in 2003 under the brand names HAVpur® and Epaxal®.

Another modification of liposomes with regard to saponin incorporation also provides high adjuvant effects. Purified extracts of triterpene saponins from *Quillaja saponaria Molina* (Quillajaceae) or *Quillaja brasiliensis* interact with liposomes forming 40–50 nm spherical cage-like particles as carriers for correspondent antigens, especially subunit antigens to enhance the immune response [11–13]. Such immunostimulating complexes are named ISCOMs and have proven their adjuvant efficiency in marketed veterinary vaccines in the case of Quil A or highly purified QS 21 from *Q. saponaria Molina* (Equip, Equilis). Since the hemolytic property of QB 90 from *Q. brasiliensis* is weaker than that of Quil A and QS 21 but it also stimulates both the cellular and humoral immune response as was tested in a bovine viral diarrhea virus vaccine in mice [76,77], ISCOMs with QB 90 are therefore considered a promising vaccine adjuvant even for vaccination of humans.

26.3 Different Types of Nanoparticles for Different Routes of Administration

Colloidal drug delivery systems have been of special interest in pharmaceutical as well as food industry. Colloidal drug carriers such as solid lipid nanoparticles, polymeric nanoparticles as well as liposomes and lipid nanocarriers are of special interest for administration of different active pharmaceutical ingredient (API) molecules via different routes of administration. Polymeric nanoparticles with different polymers are advantageous due to high drug solubility and sustained release properties [78,79]. Nevertheless, it is important for polymeric nanoparticles to have toxicological and degradation profiles as not all polymers are completely biodegradable [80]. Lipid-based nanoparticles are more acceptable as they are physiological part of membranes of, for example, the lung tissue along with low toxicity and biodegradable properties [81].

Lipid emulsions have been used since a long time as parenteral nutrition therapy for infants as well as adults. Parenteral nutrition therapy comprises mainly emulsions of long chain triglycerides (LCT) as well as middle chain triglycerides (MCT) [82]. Currently, studies have shown that along with LCT and MCT, fish oil also has an anti-inflammatory effect for parenteral therapy for patients with acute respiratory distress syndrome (ARDS) [83]. For pulmonary application, in order to obtain maximum drug loading and sustained release of the API, matrix-based systems consisting of solid lipid are believed to be more suitable as the API is incorporated in the lipid core or deposited at the lipid core surface.

26.4 Manufacturing Processes of Nanoparticles

A large number of methods for the preparation of nanoparticle dispersions have been described in great detail in the literature. The manufacturing processes can be distinguished into two categories such as bottom-up processes and top-down processes. Bottom-up processes include solvent injection [84] and solvent evaporation methods [85]. These methods are generally limited to lab scale only and also have major disadvantages like use of organic solvents that can prove toxic for various noninvasive routes of application.

Top-down processes comprise sonication by using ultrasonic treatment, high shear processes utilizing rotor–stator mechanism and the most commonly used high-pressure homogenization. All the mentioned methods are based on the principle of breaking of the droplets using shear forces. Sonication requires high energy and is limited to small volumes. In addition, hazard of metal contamination is a major disadvantage. Particles produced using sonication are large with large polydispersity indices indicating multimodal particle size distribution. Although rotor–stator machines utilize high energy, the forces are not sufficient to break down the droplets into nanometer range. Rotor–stator devices have limited application and are mostly used in food industry and in manufacturing of cosmetic preparations [86]. In order to enable production on large scale with sufficiently high forces to break up the droplets into nanometer range, high-pressure homogenizers are the devices of choice. Homogenization can be hot or cold [87]. For dispersed phase above 40%, hot or melt homogenization is a suitable method. For hot melt homogenization, the device may be used at elevated temperature to produce nanoemulsions at temperature 10 K higher than the melting temperature of the lipid matrix [2]. High-pressure homogenizers also have disadvantages such as large volume requirements and extensive cleaning procedures [88,89]. Recently, a novel method has been introduced by Finke *et al.* utilizing microchannel homogenization for the manufacturing of solid lipid nanoparticles. This method requires a small sample volume, with low dead volume and offers easy cleaning procedures. Besides, the microchannel homogenization device may be utilized for preparing samples at elevated temperatures by maintaining the entire set-up in a temperature-controlled water bath [88,90]. Multiple microchannel geometries and their influence on particle size distribution as well as variations in process parameters such as number of cycles and pressure drop have been described in detail by Finke *et al.*

For the preparation of liposomes, the lipid film method is a frequently used method [91]. The lipid film method is used for preparing liposomes consisting of phospholipids and cholesterol in specific molar ratios. The lipid components are dissolved in a suitable organic solvent, followed by the addition of API in the solvent mixture and subsequent removal of solvent under vacuum. Lipid film formed as a result of solvent evaporation is then rehydrated using an aqueous buffer solution, followed by either sonication or extrusion to obtain liposomes with small particle size. The major disadvantage of the lipid film method is the residual solvent. Traces of residual solvent play a major role in maintenance of particle size distribution after manufacturing. Solvent residues often tend to increase the particle size of the liposomes along with multimodal particle size distribution. As liposomal formulations are intended for internal administration, this residual solvent may be toxic. Solvent-free small- and large-scale extrusion methods for preparation of solid lipid nanoparticles as well as liposomes have been described in literature [22,92–94].

26.5 Different Diseases Targeted Via Nanoparticle-Based Drug Delivery Systems

26.5.1 Pulmonary Diseases

Currently, numerous drugs originally used via traditional peroral route, have been formulated as nanoparticle-based systems for pulmonary application. Anti-infective drugs such as amphotericin B, rifampicin, isoniazid, and so on, are currently developed as polymer-based or lipid-based nanoparticles and thorough physicochemical characterization along with animal studies have shown promising results for possible human administration. In addition to the anti-infectives, other API categories such as antioxidants, anti-inflammatory, anticancer, vascular drug therapy, surfactants, and protein-based systems are also under development for possible pulmonary drug delivery system [95]. The most challenging aspect in the development of nanoparticle-based drug delivery systems for pulmonary application is the maintenance of the colloidal state properties after nebulization. In spite of development in the design and manufacturing of nanoparticle-based systems, only a few formulations are available on commercial scale. This indicates there is still need to investigate these systems effectively in order to manufacture them on industrial scale as well as acceptable for patients for pulmonary application [23]. Selected references of nanoparticle-based systems for pulmonary application are provided in Table 26.1.

26.5.2 Nasal Diseases

Apart from local therapeutics against acute rhinitis and hay fever rhinitis, systemic effects of nasal administration of drug-loaded liposomal sprays and solid lipid nanoparticle dispersions have been reported and are appropriate to treat diseases such as hypertension [32,33]. A direct nose-to-brain targeting via the olfactory nerve has also been proposed for a variety of diseases such as viral infections, brain tumors, and stroke [34–37]. Cyclosporine A acts as a neuroprotective agent against stroke. Its intranasal administration as an oil-in-water nanoemulsion (CsA-NE) exhibited superior uptake in brain regions such as olfactory bulbs, mid brain, and hind brain, compared with both nasal and intravenous administration of a CsA solution and intravenous administration of the nanoemulsion [37]. Selected references of nanoparticle-based systems for nasal application are provided in Table 26.1.

26.5.3 Ophthalmic Diseases

In contrast to local colloidal therapeutics against infections [38–40], allergic conjunctivitis [41], and dry eye syndrome [9,10,42,43], intraocular diseases require penetration across the cornea into the anterior segment of the eye or even further into the posterior segment of the eye. For glaucoma treatment [44–46], a variety of nanotechnology-based systems have been studied, ranging from drug nanocrystals to colloidal carriers such as liposomes, polymeric and lipid nanoparticles, and chitosan nanoparticles. Diabetic retinopathy and wet AMD needs intraocular administration of the respective API-loaded nanotechnology-based systems [47–49]. Selected references of nanoparticle-based systems for ophthalmic application are provided in Table 26.1.

26.5.4 Vaccination

Recent progress in the design of nanoparticulate vaccine delivery includes modified liposomes such as virosomes and immune-stimulating complexes (ISCOMs), lipid-based particles, nanostructures composed of natural and synthetic polymers, and lipid-polymer hybrid nanoparticles [50,51]. Despite parenteral administration as the main route for vaccination, special focus is on adjuvant effects of the nasal route for vaccination [52–54]. Selected references of nanoparticle-based systems for vaccination are provided in Table 26.1.

26.6 Challenges Faced in Formulation Development of Nanoparticle-Based Systems

Although colloidal systems such as lipid- and polymer-based nanoparticles have shown promising results on lab scale in various *in vitro* and *ex vivo* studies involving various disease models, their application on commercial scale has not yet achieved success. The most important challenge in colloidal systems is the maintenance of the colloidal state post administration. The increasing variety of suggested applications, and encouraging results from different stages of clinical trials, need to be augmented by simple production processes and a variety of quality control assays. In addition, many studies have been performed in *in vitro* and *ex vivo* models. The greater challenge here is the *in vitro–in vivo* correlation and also consideration of physiological factors and diseased state. In the past, products such as Exubera® (inhaled insulin) was introduced in the market, but had to be withdrawn as a result of failure to gain acceptance among the patients and physicians due to its expense and putative side effects despite its effectiveness [55–57]. Attempts of other pharmaceutical companies to use intrapulmonary insulin delivery have recently also failed (e.g., Afrezza®) but are presently being made as well as some minor attempts to use intranasal delivery systems. Intranasal insulin delivery faces a smaller surface area (about 170 cm^2) with quite different absorption characteristics in nasal epithelium and its associated vasculature. Many factors including composition and character of the nasal mucus affect absorption.

For a colloidal formulation intended for pulmonary or nasal application, along with the right choice of matrix and API, correct device type plays an important part in effective pulmonary and intranasal drug delivery. Unsuccessful device was a major reason for the failure of Exubera [55]. Both, the development of the nebulization device along with the formulation development should be performed in parallel. Device parameters such as flow rate, type of mechanism used to nebulize the droplets, and device attachments such as spacers, T-attachment, masks play a vital role. Apart from device parameters, patient's age, and breathing frequency, appropriate use of the nebulization device should also be considered. The formulation should maintain the colloidal properties post nebulization and should be stable over longer shelf life. Optimization of all these parameters will certainly enable development of an appropriate device along with a suitable matrix and API for a successful drug delivery.

Challenges faced in ocular and intravitreal delivery need to consider the outstanding anatomy and functionalities of the eye in the context of pharmaceutical manufacturing (sterile formulations). Government regulations require highest quality issues with regard to the manufacturing process and the stability of the nanotechnology-based formulation. Issues comprise the scalability of the manufacturing process, reliability and reproducibility of the final product and its long-term stability in the context of chemical, physical, physicochemical, and microbiological issues. Increasing the number of parameters in a nanotechnology-based system such as the introduction of surface modifications or ligands also increases the challenge to assess the pharmacokinetics, pharmacodynamics, and toxicology of the formulation subsequent to administration. In addition, clinical trials are usually more complex and thus more costly than those for conventional formulations. The cost-benefit analysis may be a limitation to the clinical translation in comparison to existing therapies [96,97].

For vaccination purposes, liposome-derived virosomes hold promise as adjuvant for influenza A vaccine (Inflexal®) and hepatitis A vaccine (Epaxal, HAVpur). However, industrial scale-up of sophisticated manufacturing processes is still a challenge to be addressed [98].

In conclusion, nasal, pulmonary, and ocular drug delivery systems, as well as nanoparticulate delivery systems as adjuvant in vaccination are certainly promising systems and do have lot of potential for the treatment of and protection against various diseases.

References

1 Mueller, R. (2000) Solid lipid nanoparticles (SLN) for controlled drug delivery – a review of the state of the art. *Eur. J. Pharm. Biopharm.*, **50**, 161–177.

2 Mueller, R. (2007) Lipid nanoparticles: recent advances. *Adv. Drug Deliv. Rev.*, **59**, 375–376.

3 Couvreur, P., Tulkens, P., Roland, M., Trouet, A., and Speiser, P. (1977) Nanocapsules: a new type of lysosomotropic carrier. *FEBS Lett.*, **84**, 323–326.

4 Gregoriadis, G., Leathwood, P.D., and Ryman, B.E. (1971) Enzyme entrapment in liposomes. *FEBS Lett.*, **14**, 95–99.

5 Clancy, J.P., Dupont, L., Konstan, M.W., Billings, J., Fustik, S., Goss, C.H., Lymp, J., Minic, P., Quittner, A.L., Rubenstein, R.C.

et al. (2013) Phase II studies of nebulised Arikace in CF patients with Pseudomonas aeruginosa infection. *Thorax*, **68**, 818–825.

6 Ong, H., Traini, D., Cipolla, D., Gonda, I., Bebawy, M., Agus, H., and Young, P. (2012) Liposomal nanoparticles control the uptake of ciprofloxacin across respiratory epithelia. *Pharm. Res.*, **29**, 3335–3346.

7 Zhang, L., Cao, H.-Y., Zhao, S., Yuan, L.-J., Han, D., Jiang, H., Wu, S., and Wu, H.-M. (2015) Effect of exogenous pulmonary surfactants on mortality rate in neonatal respiratory distress. *Pharmacol. Ther.*, **34**, 46–54.

8 Weston, L.A. and Mösges, R. (2010) Treating seasonal allergic rhinoconjunctivitis with a liposomal nasal spray. *Allergologie*, **33**, 196–204.

9 Dausch, D., Lee, S., Dausch, S., Kim, J.C., Schwert, G., and Michelson, W. (2006) Comparative study of treatment of the dry eye syndrome due to disturbances of the tear film lipid layer with lipid-containing tear substitutes: Efficacy of lipid-containing tear substitutes. *Klin. Monatsbl. Augenheilkd.*, **223**, 974–983.

10 Pult, H., Gill, .F., and Riede-Pult, B.H. (2012) Effect of three different liposomal eye sprays on ocular comfort and tear film. *Cont. Lens Anterior Eye*, **35**, 203–207.

11 Pedersen, J.S., Oliveira, C.L., Hübschmann, H.B., Arleth, L., Manniche, S., Kirkby, N., and Nielsen, H.M. (2012) Structure of immune stimulating complex matrices and immune stimulating complexes in suspension determined by small-angle X-ray scattering. *Biophys. J .*, **102**, 2372–2380.

12 Paillot, R., Fraser, S., Prowse-Davis, L., Rash, N., Montesso, F., Slootmans, N., Thomas, A., Besognet, B., Meinert, T., Ons, E., and Salt, J. (2015) ISCOM-based equine influenza vaccine: Duration of immunity and randomised clinical trials to assess an accelerated schedule of immunisation and efficacy. *Trials Vaccinol.*, **4**, 61–70.

13 Paillot, R. and Prowse, L. (2012) ISCOM-matrix-based equine influenza (EIV) vaccine stimulates cell-mediated immunity in the horse. *Vet. Immunol. Immunopathol.*, **145**, 516–521.

14 Van Donkersgoed, J., van den Hurk, J.V., McCartney, D., and Harland, R.J. (1991) Comparative serological response in calves to eight commercial vaccines against infectious bovine rhinotracheitis, parainfluenza-3, bovine respiratory syncytial, and bovine viral diarrhea viruses. *Can. Vet. J.*, **32** (12), 727–733.

15 Laniado, M. and Chachuat, A. (1995) The endorem tolerance profile. *Der Radiologe*, **35**, S266–270.

16 Kelly, L.J. (2004) The respiratory system, in *Essentials of Human Physiology for Pharmacy*, CRC Press, Boca Raton, FL, pp. 239–277.

17 Rang, H.P., Dale, M.M., Ritter, J.M., and Flower, R.J. (2012) Respiratory system, in *Rang and Dale's Pharmacology*, 7th edn, Elsevier Churchill Livingstone, Edinburgh, p. 345.

18 Beck-Broichsitter, M., Ruppert, C., Schmehl, T., Günther, A., and Seeger, W. (2014) Biophysical inhibition of synthetic vs. naturally-derived pulmonary surfactant preparations by polymeric nanoparticles. *BBA-Biomembranes*, **1838**, 474–481.

19 Patton, J.S., Brain, J.D., Davies, L.A., Fiegel, J., Gumbleton, M., Kim, K.-J., Sakagami, M., Vanbever, R., and Ehrhardt, C. (2010) The particle has landed – characterizing the fate of inhaled pharmaceuticals. *J. Aerosol Med. Pulm. D*, **23**, S71–S87.

20 Lim, Y.H., Tiemann, K.M., Hunstad, D.A., Elsabahy, M., and Wooley, K.L. (2016) Polymeric nanosparticles in development for treatment of pulmonary infectious diseases. *WIREs Nanomed. Nanobiotechnol.*. doi: 10.1002/wnan.1401

21 Kalhapure, R.S., Suleman, N., Mocktar, C., Seedat, N., and Govender, T. (2015) Nanoengineered drug delivery systems for enhancing antibiotic therapy. *J. Pharm. Sci.*, **104**, 872–905.

22 Paranjpe, M., Neuhaus, V., Finke, J.H., Richter, C., Gothsch, T., Kwade, A., Büttgenbach, S., Braun, A., and Müller-Goymann, C.C. (2013) *In vitro* and *ex vivo* toxicological testing of sildenafil-loaded solid lipid nanoparticles. *Inhal. Toxicol.*, **25**, 536–543.

23 Cipolla, D., Gonda, I., and Chan, H.-K. (2013) Liposomal formulations for inhalation. *Ther. Deliv.*, **4**, 1047–1072.

24 Chiraz, J.-M., Andrieu, V., Elaissari, A., and Fessi, H. (2011) Beclomethasone-loaded lipidic nanocarriers for pulmonary drug delivery: preparation, characterization and *in vitro* drug release. *J. Nanosci. Nanotech.*, **11**, 1841–1851.

25 Elhissi, A., Islam, M.A., Arafat, B., Taylor, M., and Ahmed, W. (2010) Development and characterisation of freeze-dried liposomes containing two anti-asthma drugs. *Micro Nano Lett.*, **5**, 184.

26 Wang, P., Zhang, L., Peng, H., Li, Y., Xiong, J., and Xu, Z. (2013) The formulation and delivery of curcumin with solid lipid nanoparticles for the treatment of on non-small cell lung cancer both *in vitro* and *in vivo*. *Mater. Sci. Eng. C*, **33**, 4802–4808.

27 Lee, W.-H., Loo, C.-Y., Traini, D., and Young, P.M. (2015) Inhalation of nanoparticle-based drug for lung cancer treatment: advantages and challenges. *Asian J. Pharm. Sci.*, **10**, 481–489.

28 Hajos, F., Stark, B., Hensler, S., Prassl, R., and Mosgoeller, W. (2008) Inhalable liposomal formulation for vasoactive intestinal peptide. *Int. J. Pharm.*, **357**, 286–294.

29 Liu, C., Shi, J., Dai, Q., Yin, X., Zhang, X., and Zheng, A. (2013) *In vitro* and *in vivo* evaluation of ciprofloxacin liposome for pulmonary administration. *Drug Dev. Ind. Pharm.*, **41**, 272–278.

30 Manca, M., Sinico, C., Maccioni, A., Diez, O., Fadda, A., and Manconi, M. (2012) Composition influence on pulmonary delivery of rifampicin liposomes. *Pharmaceutics*, **4**, 590–606.

31 Varshosaz, J., Ghaffari, S., Mirshojaei, S.F., Jafarian, A., Atyabi, F., Kobarfard, F., and Azarmi, S. (2013) Biodistribution of amikacin solid lipid nanoparticles after pulmonary delivery. *BioMed Res. Int.*, **2013**, 1–8.

32 Aboud, H.M., El Komy, M.H., Ali, A.A., El Menshawe, S.F., and Abd Elbary, A. (2016) Development, optimization and evaluation of carvedilol-loaded solid lipid nanoparticles for intranasal drug delivery. *AAPS PharmSciTech*. doi: 10.1208/s12249-015-0440-8.

33 Saindane, N.S., Pagar, K.P., and Vavia, P.R. (2013) Nanosuspension based *in situ* gelling nasal spray of carvedilol: development, *in vitro* and *in vivo* characterization. *AAPS PharmSciTech*, **14**, 189–199.

34 Dalpiaz, A., Fogagnolo, M., Ferraro, L., Capuzzo, A., Pavan, B., Rassu, G., Salis, A., Giunchedi, P., and Gavini, E. (2015) Nasal chitosan microparticles target a zidovudine prodrug to brain HIV sanctuaries. *Antiviral Res.*, **123**, 146–157.

35 Md, S., Mustafa, G., Baboota, S., and Ali, J. (2015) Nanoneurotherapeutics approach intended for direct nose to brain delivery. *Drug Dev. Ind. Pharm.*, **41**, 1922–1934.

36 Zhuang, X., Teng, Y., Samykutty, A., Mu, J., Deng, Z., Zhang, L., Cao, P., Rong, Y., Yan, J., Miller, D., and Zhang, H.G. (2016) Grapefruit-derived nanovectors delivering therapeutic miR17 through an intranasal route inhibit brain tumor progression. *Mol. Ther.*, **24**, 96–105.

37 Yadav, S., Gattacceca, F., Panicucci, R., and Amiji, M.M. (2015) Comparative biodistribution and pharmacokinetic analysis of cyclosporine-A in the brain upon intranasal or intravenous administration in an oil-in-water nanoemulsion formulation. *Mol. Pharm.*, **12**, 1523–1533.

38 Law, S.L., Huang, K.J., and Chiang, C.H. (2000) Acyclovir-containing liposomes for potential ocular delivery: corneal penetration and absorption. *J. Control. Release*, **63**, 135–140.

39 Bozdag, S., Dillen, K., Vandervoort, J., and Ludwig, A. (2005) The effect of freeze-drying with different cryoprotectants and gamma-irradiation sterilization on the charateristics of ciprofloxacin HCl-loaded poly(D,L-lactide-glycolide)nanoparticles. *J. Pharm. Pharmacol.*, **57**, 699–707.

40 Dillen, K., Bozdag, S., Vandervoort, J., and Ludwig, A. (2007) Evaluation of the physicochemical characteristics and activity of various kinds of ciprofloxacin HCl-loaded cationic nanoparticles. *J. Drug Del. Sci. Technol.*, **17**, 49–56.

41 Souto, E.B., Doktorovova, S., Gonzales-Mira, E., Egea, M.A., and Garcia, M.L. (2010) Feasibility of lipid nanoparticles for ocular delivery of anti-inflammatory drugs. *Curr. Eye Res.*, **35**, 537–552.

42 Sall, K., Stevenson, O.D., Mundorf, T.K., and Reis, B.L. (2000) Two multicenter randomized studies of the efficacy and safety of cyclosporine ophthalmic emulsion in moderate to severe dry eye disease. *Ophthalmology*, **107**, 631–639.

43 De Campos, A.M., Sanchez, A., and Alonso, M.J. (2001) Chitosan nanoparticles: a new vehicle for the improvement of the delivery of drugs to the ocular surface. Application to cyclosporine A. *Int. J. Pharm.*, **224**, 159–168.

44 Ammar, H.O., Salama, H.A., Ghorab, M., and Mahmoud, A.A. (2009) Nanoemulsion as a potential ophthalmic delivery system for dorzolamide hydrochloride. *AAPS PharmSciTech*, **10**, 808–819.

45 Kim, N.J., Harris, A., Gerber, A., Tobe, L.A., Amireskandari, A., Huck, A., and Siesky, B. (2014) Nanotechnology and glaucoma: a review of the potential implications of glaucoma medicine. *Br. J. Ophthalmol.*, **98**, 427–431.

46 Fangueiro, J.F., Veiga, F., Silva, A.M., and Souto, E.B. (2016) Ocular drug delivery – new strategies for targeting anterior and posterior segments of the eye. *Curr. Pharm. Des.*, **22**, 1135–1146.

47 Pescina, S., Sonvico, F., Santi, P., and Nicoli, S. (2015) Therapeutics and carriers: the dual role of proteins in nanoparticles for ocular delivery. *Curr. Top. Med. Chem.*, **15**, 369–385.

48 Fangueiro, J.F., Silva, A.M., Garcia, M.L., and Souto, E.B. (2015) Current nanotechnology approaches for the treatment and management of diabetic retinopathy. *Eur. J. Pharm. Biopharm.*, **95**, 307–322.

49 Bochot, A. and Fattal, E. (2012) Liposomes for intravitreal drug delivery: a state of the art. *J. Control. Release*, **161**, 628–634.

50 Sahdev, P., Ochyl, L.J., and Moon, J.J. (2014) Biomaterials for nanoparticle vaccine delivery systems. *Pharm. Res.*, **31**, 2563–2582.

51 Brito, L.A. and O'Hagan, D.T. (2014) Designing and building the next generation of improved vaccine adjuvants. *J. Control. Release*, **190**, 563–579.

52 Sharma, R., Agrawal, U., Mody, N., and Vyas, S.P. (2015) Polymer nanotechnology based approaches in mucosal vaccine delivery: challenges and opportunities. *Biotechnol. Adv.*, **33**, 64–79.

53 Cevher, E., Salomon, S.K., Somavarapu, S., Brocchini, S., and Alpar, H.O. (2015) Development of chitosan-pullulan composite nanoparticles for nasal delivery of vaccines: *in vivo* studies. *J. Microencapsul*, **32**, 769–783.

54 Illum, L., Jabbal-Gill, I., Hinchcliffe, M., Fisher, A.N., and Davis, S.S. (2001) Chitosan as a novel nasal delivery system for vaccines. *Adv. Drug Deliv. Rev.*, **51**, 81–96.

55 Mack, G.S. (2007) Pfizer dumps Exubera. *Nat. Biotechnol.*, **25**, 1331–1332.

56 Hollander, P.A., Blonde, L., Rowe, R., Mehta, A.E., Milburn, J.L., Hershon, K.S., Chiasson, J.-L., and Levin, S.R. (2004) Efficacy and safety of inhaled insulin (Exubera) compared with subcutaneous insulin therapy in patients with type 2 diabetes results of a 6-month, randomized, comparative trial. *Diabetes Care*, **27**, 2356–2362.

57 Henkin, R.I. (2010) Inhaled insulin-intrapulmonary, intranasal, and other routes of administration: mechanisms of action. *Nutrition*, **26**, 33–39.

58 Klettner, A. and Roider, J. (2008) Comparison of bevacizumab, ranibizumab, and pegaptanib *in vitro*: efficiency and possible additional pathways. *Invest. Ophthalmol. Vis. Sci.*, **49**, 4523–4527.

59 Newman, S.P., Moren, F., and Clarke, S.W. (1987) Deposition pattern of nasal sprays in man. *Rhinology*, **26**, 111–120.

60 Newman, S.P., Moren, F., and Clarke, S.W. (1987) The nasal distribution of metered dose inhalers. *J. Laryngol. Otol.*, **101**, 127–132.

61 Bagger, M. and Bechgaard, E. (2004) A microdialysis model to examine nasal drug delivery and olfactory absorption in rats using lidocaine hydrochloride as a model drug. *Int. J. Pharm.*, **269**, 311–322.

62 Becker, Y. (1995) HSV-1 brain infection by the olfactory nerve route and virus latency and reactivation may cause learning and behavioral deficiencies and violence in children and adults: a point of view. *Virus Genes*, **10**, 217–226.

63 St. John, J.A., Ekberg, J.A.K., Dando, S.J., Meedeniya, A.C.B., Horton, R.E., Batzloff,

M., Owen, S.J., Holt, S., Peak, I.R., Ulett, G.C., Mackay-Sim, A., and Beacham, I.R. (2014) Burkholderia pseudomallei penetrates the brain via destruction of the olfactory and trigeminal nerves: implications for the pathogenesis of neurological melioidosis. *mBio*, **5** (2), e00025–14. doi: 10.1128/mBio.00025-14.

64 Cervantes-Sandoval, I., Serrano-Luna, J.J., Garcia-Latorre, E., Tsutsumi, V., and Shibayama, M. (2008) Characterization of brain inflammation during primary amoebic meningoencephalitis. *Parasitol. Int.*, **57**, 307–315.

65 Mistry, A., Stolnik, S., and Illum, L. (2009) Nanoparticles for direct nose-to-brain delivery of drugs. *Int. J. Pharm.*, **379**, 146–157.

66 Read, R.C., Naylor, S.C., Potter, C.W., Bond, J., Jabbal, GillI., Fisher, A., Illum, L., and Jennings, R. (2005) Effective nasal influenza vaccine delivery using chitosan. *Vaccine*, **23**, 4367–4374.

67 Belshe, R.B., Edwards, K.M., Vesikari, T., Black, S.V., Walker, R.E., Hultquist, M., Kemble, G., and Connor, E.M. (2007) Live attenuated versus inactivated influenza vaccine in infants and young children. *N. Engl. J. Med.*, **356**, 685–696.

68 Slütter, B., Bal, S., Keijzer, C., Mallants, R., Hagenaars, N., Que, I., Kaijzel, E., van Eden, W., Augustijns, P., Löwik, C., Bouwstra, J., Broere, F., and Jiskoot, W. (2010) Nasal vaccination with N-trimethyl chitosan and PLGA based nanoparticles: nanoparticle characteristics determine quality and strength of the antibody response in mice against the encapsulated antigen. *Vaccine*, **28**, 6282–6291.

69 Sosnova-Netukova, M., Kuchynka, P., and Forrester, J.V. (2007) The suprabasal layer of corneal epithelial cells represents the major barrier site to the passive movement of small molecules and trafficking leukocytes. *Br. J. Ophthalmol.*, **91**, 372–378.

70 Dua, H.S., Gomes, J.A.P., and Singh, A. (1994) Corneal epithelial wound healing. *Br. J. Ophthalmol.*, **78**, 401–408.

71 Jonas, J.B., Söfker, A., Hayler, J., and Degenring, R.F. (2003) Intravitreal crystalline triamcinolone acetonide as an additional tool in pars plana vitrectomy for complicated proliferative vitreoretinopathy? *Acta Ophthalmol. Scand.*, **81**, 663–665.

72 Almeida, H., Amaral, M.H., Lobao, P., Frigerio, C., and Lobo, J.M.S. (2015) Nanoparticles in ocular delivery systems for topical administration: promises and challenges. *Curr. Pharm. Des.*, **21**, 5212–5224.

73 Baylor, N.W., Egan, W., and Richman, P. (2002) Aluminum salts in vaccines – US perspective. *Vaccine*, **20**, S18–S23.

74 O'Hagan, D.T., Ott, G.S., Nest, G.V., Rappuoli, R., and Giudice, G.D. (2013) The history of MF59$^{(®)}$ adjuvant: a phoenix that arose from the ashes. *Expert Rev. Vaccines*, **12**, 13–30.

75 Gluck, R., Mischler, R., Brantschen, S., Just, M., Althaus, B., and Cryz, S.J. Jr. (1992) Immunopotentiating reconstituted influenza virus virosome vaccine deliverysystem for immunization against hepatitis A. *J. Clin. Invest.*, **90**, 2491–2495.

76 Cibulski, S.P., Mourglia-Ettlin, G., Teixeira, T.F., Quirici, L., Roehe, P.M., Ferreira, F., and Silveira, F. (2016) Novel ISCOMs from Quillaja brasiliensis saponins induce mucosal and systemic antibody production, T-cell responses and improved antigen uptake. *Vaccine*, **34**, 1162–1171.

77 Cibulski, S.P., Silveira, F., Mourglia-Ettlin, G., Teixeira, T.F., Dos Santos, H.F., Yendo, A.C., de Costa, F., Fett-Neto, A.G., Gosmann, G., and Roehe, P.M. (2016) Quillaja brasiliensis saponins induce robust humoral and cellular responses in a bovine viral diarrhea virus vaccine in mice. *Comp. Immunol. Microbiol. Infect. Dis.*, **45**, 1–8.

78 Beck-Broichsitter, M., Merkel, O.M., and Kissel, T. (2012) Controlled pulmonary drug and gene delivery using polymeric nano-carriers. *J. Control. Release*, **161**, 214–224.

79 Beck-Broichsitter, M., Schmehl, T., Gessler, T., Seeger, W., and Kissel, T. (2012) Development of a biodegradable nanoparticle platform for sildenafil: formulation optimization by factorial design analysis combined with application of charge-modified branched polyesters. *J. Control. Release*, **157**, 469–477.

80 Park, S., Jeong, E.J., Lee, J., Rhim, T., Lee, S.K., and Lee, K.Y. (2013) Preparation and characterization of nonaarginine-modified chitosan nanoparticles for siRNA delivery. *Carbohydr. Polym.*, **92**, 57–62.

81 Nassimi, M., Schleh, C., Lauenstein, H.-D., Hussein, R., Lübbers, K., Pohlmann, G., Switalla, S., Sewald, K., Müller, M., Krug, N. *et al.* (2009) Low cytotoxicity of solid lipid nanoparticles in *in vitro* and *ex vivo* lung models. *Inhal. Toxicol.*, **21**, 104–109.

82 Calder, P.C. (2009) Hot topics in parenteral nutrition. Rationale for using new lipid emulsions in parenteral nutrition and a review of the trials performed in adults. *Proc. Nutr. Soc.*, **68**, 252–260.

83 Hecker, M., Ott, J., Sondermann, C., Schaefer, M.B., Obert, M., Hecker, A., Morty, R., Vadasz, I., Herold, S., Rosengarten, B. *et al.* (2014) Immunomodulation by fish-oil containing lipid emulsions in murine acute respiratory distress syndrome. *Crit. Care*, **18**, R85.

84 Schubert, M. (2003) Solvent injection as a new approach for manufacturing lipid nanoparticles – evaluation of the method and process parameters. *Eur. J. Pharm. Biopharm.*, **55**, 125–131.

85 Soppimath, KumareshS., Aminabhavi, TejrajM., Kulkarni, AnandraoR., and Rudzinski, Walter E. (2001) Biodegradable polymeric nanoparticles as drug delivery devices. *J. Control. Release*, **70**, 1–20.

86 Rodgers, T.L. and Cooke, M. (2012) Rotor–stator devices: the role of shear and the stator. *Chem. Eng. Res. Des.*, **90**, 323–327.

87 Friedrich, I. and Müller-Goymann, C. (2003) Characterization of solidified reverse micellar solutions (SRMS) and production development of SRMS-based nanosuspensions. *Eur. J. Pharm. Biopharm.*, **56**, 111–119.

88 Finke, J., Schur, J., Richter, C., Gothsch, T., Kwade, A., Büttgenbach, S., and Müller-Goymann, C. (2012) The influence of customized geometries and process parameters on nanoemulsion and solid lipid nanoparticle production in microsystems. *Chem. Eng. J.*, **209**, 126–137.

89 Finke, J.H. (2014) Manufacturing colloidal drug delivery systems in customized microsystems: characterization of process efficiency and interactions. Cumulative thesis. Braunschweig.

90 Gothsch, T., Finke, J.H., Beinert, S., Lesche, C., Schur, J., Büttgenbach, S., Müller-Goymann, C., and Kwade, A. (2011) Effect of microchannel geometry on high-pressure dispersion and emulsification. *Chem. Eng. Technol.*, **34**, 335–343.

91 Torchilin, V. P. and Weissig, V. (2003) *Liposomes – A Practical Approach*, Oxford University Press, New York.

92 Joseph, S. and Bunjes, H. (2012) Preparation of nanoemulsions and solid lipid nanoparticles by premix membrane emulsification. *J. Pharm. Sci.*, **101**, 2479–2489.

93 Joseph, S. and Bunjes, H. (2013) Influence of membrane structure on the preparation of colloidal lipid dispersions by premix membrane emulsification. *Int. J. Pharm.*, **446**, 59–62.

94 Zheng, S., Alkan-Onyuksel, H., Beissinger, R.L., and Wasan, D.T. (1999) Liposome microencapsulations without using any organic solvent. *J. Dispers. Sci. Technol.*, **20**, 1189–1203.

95 Paranjpe, M. and Müller-Goymann, C.C. (2014) Nanoparticle-mediated pulmonary drug delivery: a review. *Int. J. Mol. Sci.*, **15**, 5852–5873.

96 Narang, A.S., Chang, R.K., and Hussain, M.A. (2013) Pharmaceutical development and regulatory considerations for nanoparticles and nanoparticulate drug delivery systems. *J. Pharm. Sci.*, **102**, 3867–3882.

97 Zylberberg, C. and Matosevic, S. (2016) Pharmaceutical liposomal drug delivery: a review of new delivery systems and a look at the regulatory landscape. *Drug Deliv.*. doi: 10.1080/10717544.2016.1177136.

98 Madni, A., Sarfraz, M., Rehman, M., Ahmad, M., Akhtar, N., Ahmad, S., Tahir, N., Ijaz, S., Al-Kassas, R., and Löbenberg, R. (2014) Liposomal drug delivery: a versatile platform for challenging clinical applications. *J. Pharm. Pharm. Sci.*, **17**, 401–426.

27
Neurodegenerative Diseases – Alzheimer's Disease

Maria Gregori and Francesca Re

University of Milano-Bicocca, School of Medicine and Surgery, via Cadore 48, Monza 20900, Italy

27.1
Introduction

Alzheimer's disease (AD) is a progressive neurodegenerative brain disease that slowly destroys memory and cognitive skills, currently affecting 24 million people worldwide, with 4.6 million new cases each year [1]. A major pathological hallmark of AD is the formation of neuritic plaques within the brains of patients, composed primarily of filamentous aggregates (fibrils) of the amyloid beta peptide (Aβ), a small peptide of 39–42 amino acids formed in abnormal amounts by an aberrant cleavage of amyloid precursor protein (APP) [2]. According to the amyloid hypothesis [3], accumulation of Aβ aggregates in the brain is the primary driving force in AD pathogenesis, contributing directly to oxidative stress, mitochondrial dysfunction, impaired synaptic transmission, disruption of membrane integrity, and impaired axonal transport, which lead to neurodegeneration [4]. Current treatments are based on enhancement of remaining cognitive function, thus providing only short-term benefits; therefore, given the pivotal role played by Aβ in AD, novel treatments under development aim to interfere with Aβ production or with the formation of Aβ aggregates. Moreover, at the time of diagnosis, AD is usually already at a mild to moderate stage. To make early intervention possible, more sensitive diagnostic techniques are needed. Another tricky issue to be considered in the search of new therapeuthic and diagnostic agents for AD is that the blood–brain barrier (BBB), a layer of specialized brain microvascular endothelial cells that protects the brain from potential hazardous substances in the blood flow, makes the brain impermeable to the majority of potential good candidates [5]. In this scenario, nanoparticles (NPs) have been proposed as interesting tool potentially able to solve the unmet problem of enhancing drug transport across the BBB, thanks to the possibility of functionalizing their surface with proper BBB ligands, thus exploiting

Pharmaceutical Nanotechnology: Innovation and Production, First Edition. Edited by Jean Cornier, Arno Kwade, Andrew Owen, and Marcel Van de Voorde.

physiological mechanisms of transport to the brain [6]. In this chapter, possible strategies for the development of novel AD therapies and diagnosis involving the use of NP will be discussed.

27.2
Diagnosis

27.2.1
Detection of Amyloid Plaques

Current imaging of amyloid plaques in the brain is based on positron emission tomography (PET) [7]. The more popular tracer is Pittsburgh Compound-B (PiB) [8], but the short half-life of carbon-11 limits its clinical viability. In 2012, the FDA approved florbetapir F18 that may have more general clinical use due to its longer half-life (~110 min) [9]. However, PET has serious drawbacks such as low spatial resolution, high cost, and patient exposure to radiation. In contrast, magnetic resonance imaging (MRI) does not involve ionizing radiation, has higher spatial resolution, and is generally available in the clinical setting. However, MRI without amyloid specific probes was reported to detect plaques only with a high magnetic field (9.4 T) and very long scanning time [10–12]. In the search of probes that could both specifically bind to Aβ plaques and be visualized by MRI, superparamagnetic iron oxide (SPIO) NPs functionalized with Aβ ligands are greatly investigated. SPIO NP are composed by a core of magnetite (Fe_3O_4) or maghemite (Fe_2O_3) surrounded by an hydrophilic layer and have the ability to efficiently enhance the T_2 relaxation rate of water protons, providing darker color compared to unlabeled tissues [13]. Cheng *et al.* proposed SPIO NP stabilized by amphiphilic block copolymer (polyethylene glycol–polylactic acid (PEG–PLA)) and conjugated with curcumin (Cur-MNPs) as Aβ ligand [14]. Amyloid plaques were visualized as dark spots by *ex vivo* MRI after intravenous injection of Cur-MNPs in Tg2576 mice taken as AD model; moreover, immunohistochemical staining confirmed that amyloid plaques and iron oxide NP colocalized. Another Aβ ligand used for SPIO NP functionalization is 1,1-dicyano-2-[6-(dimethylamino)naphthalene-2-yl] propene [15]. A significant T_2* signal loss was detected in the hippocampal area of AD rats after intravenous injection of these NPs, but not in non-AD rats. However, in this case, mannitol was used to artificially open the BBB. On the contrary, ultrasmall SPIO NPs coupled with a cyclic heptapeptide derived from a phage display library (C-IPLPFYN-C) and have high affinity to $A\beta_{1-42}$ are able to cross the BBB without any facilitating strategy and accumulate in the brain 90 min after their injection in NMRI mice, as assessed by MRI in healthy mice. Tests with these NPs on transgenic mice, aimed at confirming the potential of early AD diagnosis, are still lacking [16]. A more complete work describes the preparation of USPIO NP functionalized with $A\beta_{1-42}$ peptide for the staining of the AD plaques, and with PEG to facilitate

BBB passage, called USPIO-PEG- Aβ_{1-42} [17]. After femoral injection of USPIO-PEG-Aβ_{1-42} in APP/PS1 mice, *in vivo* μMRI showed many dark spots that correlated with the amyloid plaque distribution found histologically. As control, few spots were seen after injection of USPIO alone in the same mice or USPIO-PEG-Aβ_{1-42} in control wild-type mice.

Despite the large clinical use of monoclonal antibodies (mAb) to the diagnosis and therapy of an array of human disorders [18], only one example in literature describes the use of immune SPION as contrast agents for AD diagnosis. SPIO linked to an anti-APP mAb showed to penetrate the BBB and to act as contrast agent for the imaging of plaques in double transgenic AD mice. In fact, the number of MRI-visible plaques per brain increased from 347 ± 45 in the control AD mice to 668 ± 86 in the mice treated with anti-APP-SPION [19].

To accelerate the application of SPION in the clinics, a better understanding of the consequences that SPION administration would have in the brain, such as interactions with amyloid beta and neurotoxicity, is essential. Mirsadeghi *et al.* investigated the roles of size and charge of the PEG-coated SPION on Aβ fibrillation, finding that positively charged SPION promote fibrillation at significantly lower particle concentrations than negatively charged or uncharged SPIONs. Moreover, a significant increase in the lag time of Aβ fibrillation was found by decreasing the size of the negatively charged SPION from 65.1 to 49.5 nm [20]. About the possible neurotoxicity of such systems, it is reported that exposure to SPION for 6 h caused a strong generation of reactive oxygen species (ROS) and cell toxicity in the microglia, due to lysosomal iron liberation [21].

A different approach involves the use of quantum dot (QDs) for *in vivo* plaques imaging in AD mice. QDs are nanocrystals made of a crystalline core of CdSe surrounded by a ZnS shell, with unique photophysical properties, including broad excitation spectra and narrow emission spectra, size-tunable fluorescence, high resistance to chemical and metabolic degradation, and long fluorescence lifetime [22]. In this case, for Aβ detection, QDs were conjugated with an anti-Aβ_{1-42} antibody. The results demonstrated that this probe after intracerebroventricular injection could effectively track Aβ_{1-42} in the brain of APP transgenic mice [23].

Further studies are needed to better understand which are the best candidates suitable for AD diagnosis, with a better balance between effectiveness and cellular toxicity, without promoting Aβ fibrillation.

27.2.2
Detection of AD Biomarkers

New research in AD biomarkers, such as the development of methods to indirectly estimate levels of brain amyloid plaques from Aβ levels in plasma or cerebrospinal fluid (CSF), have increased the ability to detect evidence of early AD pathology *in vivo* [24,25]. Among all, electrochemical biosensors seem promising because of their simplicity, rapid response, potential real-time and onsite analysis, and compatibility with miniaturization [26]. Various nanomaterials, in particular gold NP (AuNP), have been proposed for signal amplification. Since a single AuNP is loaded with hundreds of labels for a proper AD marker, a significant amplification for the detection of the marker itself is possible. Decreased levels of $A\beta_{1-42}$ and enhanced levels of total and phosphorylated tau in CSF have been used for diagnosis of AD [27]. Thus, different groups investigated new techniques to allow a rapid, sensitive, and inexpensive quantification of Aβ or tau in CSF.

Yu *et al.* prepared a multiwalled carbon nanotubes platform densely packed with AuNP-bearing gelsolin for the detection of Aβ and horseradish peroxidase (HRP) to produce a visible reduction of current in the presence of H_2O_2 and HRP substrate. This methodology was able to detect Aβ down to 28 pM, which is a remarkable result considering that no Aβ antibodies were employed [28]. Liu *et al.* developed a different electrochemical biosensors using AuNP, modified with an Aβ mAb able to capture $A\beta_{(1-16)}$, which in turn is able to capture heme. The complex $A\beta_{(1-16)}$-heme-AuNPs captured by the mAb-covered electrode catalyzed the reduction of O_2 to H_2O_2, allowing Aβ detection with a limit of 10 pM [29].

Gold NP functionalized with an Aβ mAb were also used to construct a dot blot immunoassay. In this case, the detection limit was 11 pM [30]. In all these examples, CSF samples were used to validate the ability of the assays.

Interestingly, Kim *et al.* utilized saliva as a biomarker medium instead of CSF, and correlated the salivary Aβ levels to AD pathological aspects. They developed a magnetoimmunoassay system, based on magnetic silica NPs functionalized with an Aβ mAb able to capture salivary Aβ and to generate a fluorescent signal, thanks to the subsequent binding to QD for Aβ concentration as low as ∼4 pM. Their study indicated that salivary Aβ levels were elevated in AD patients compared with control group. Even if future studies are needed to understand the mechanism of how Aβ peptide accumulates in saliva, this methodology appear to be an easy approach to simply detect pathological alteration that lead to severe AD onset [31].

AuNP-based assays were used for the quantification of tau protein. Stegurová *et al.* exploited a polymerase chain reaction (PCR) combined with sandwich ELISA, with tau protein immobilized by using anti-tau mAbs to PCR plate wells and subsequently detected by immuno-PCR using AuNPs functionalized with both anti-tau mAbs and PCR oligonucleotide template. The limit of detection of this assay was found to be 5 pg/ml [32]. Zengin *et al.* proposed the rapid detection of tau by using a surface-enhanced Raman scattering (SERS)-based sandwich assay that utilizes anti-tau mAb-functionalized silica-coated Fe_2O_3 NP and polyclonal anti-tau immobilized AuNP [33].

Other AD biomarkers, such as volatile organic compounds from the breath, analyzed using carbon nanotubes and AuNP-based sensors [34], and acetylcholinesterase (AChE), detected in the CSF by using a AuNP-based assay [35], have been investigated, but a number of challenges remain for the biomarkers to become widely applied in clinical practice.

27.3
Therapy of Alzheimer's Disease

AD has proven challenging to treat and many unsuccessful therapeutic trials have been made. Current therapies for AD do not modify the course of disease, but they only control the symptoms of the disease. Failed therapies include anti-inflammatory, statins, hormonal therapies, chelators, drugs targeting Aβ and tau. Since clinical trials in advanced AD have been unsuccessful, the scientific research has moved to the prodromal and presymptomatic phases of the disease. Then, it turns out to be a great challenge to identify effective therapies.

27.3.1
Current Therapies

Since cholinergic neurotransmitter activity is low in AD, cholinesterase inhibitors, that is, donepezil, galantamine, and rivastigmine, are currently approved for use in mild and moderate AD. These cholinesterase inhibitors may temporarily improve cognition by reducing the breakdown of the neurotransmitter acetylcholine, but measurable benefit is not seen in most patients treated.

To reduce NMDA receptor-mediated neurotoxicity present in AD, memantine, an NMDA receptor antagonist, is currently used in moderate and severe AD. Memantine has a statistically significant effect on cognition and behavior of patients, but it has no effect on the progression of the disease.

Also antioxidant, anti-inflammatory, antiamyloidogenic, neuroprotective, and cognition-enhancing effects of a variety of nutraceuticals, including curcumin, apigenin, docosahexaenoic acid, epigallocatechin gallate, α-lipoic acid, and resveratrol, have been proposed and used for the potential prevention and treatment of AD.

Antioxidant therapy has been suggested for the prevention and treatment of AD, since many studies demonstrated that oxidative stress plays a central role in a common pathophysiology of neurodegenerative diseases such as AD and Parkinson's disease [36]. However, the results with regard to their efficacy of treating neurodegenerative diseases have been inconsistent.

In this context, nitric oxide (NO) contributes to the maintenance of normal neuronal activity and survival, thus serving as an important regulatory mechanism in the central nervous system. By contrast, accumulating evidence suggests that the normal aging process can trigger excessive production of reactive oxygen/nitrogen species (such as NO), contributing to the etiology of several neurodegenerative diseases, that is, AD. Targeting of protein *S*-nitrosylation, resulting from covalent attachment of an NO group to a cysteine thiol of the target protein, can lead to novel therapeutics [37].

Both oxidative stress and inflammation have been implicated in AD pathogenesis and so consequently antioxidants as well as anti-inflammatory agents have been investigated for AD pharmacotherapy.

Clinical studies evaluating the effects of diclofenac, naproxen, and rofecoxib, however, failed to produce any therapeutic benefit supposedly due to treatment timing, dosing, and agent selection.

Natural products, mostly with potent antioxidant and anti-inflammatory properties, have been a subject of serious investigation for AD treatment. Besides vitamins and other dietary antioxidants, a range of nutraceuticals have been evaluated. Dietary polyphenols, such as resveratrol, curcumin, and tea catechins, have shown therapeutic promise in preclinical AD models. Phytoestrogens have also shown considerable promise in improving cognitive decline in AD patients. Souvenaid is a nutritional supplement of vitamins and lipids that have shown statistically significant benefits on a delayed verbal recall task but no benefit on cognitive and behavioral deficits has been detected. No evidence for cognitive or functional benefit was found using Souvenaid in combination with cholinesterase inhibitors and/or memantine. Ginkgo biloba, acetyl-L-carnitine, curcumin, and coconut oil have also been used for AD, but randomized trial data have not confirmed their benefit obtained instead from basic research. A meta-analyses of clinical trials show that Ginkgo may possibly slow the cognitive decline in AD patients; however, the overall results remain inconclusive [38,39].

27.3.2 Latest Therapeutic Directions

Currently, the use of stem cell therapy is under investigation as therapeutic options for AD. However, treatment with stem cells comes with a number of drawbacks, for instance, the source of these cells, their quantity, and ethical issues. Over recent years, the potential of induced pluripotent stem cells (iPSCs) has been widely investigated and these cells seem promising for production of numerous different tissues both *in vitro* and *in vivo*. One of the major advantages of iPSCs is that they can be made autologous and can provide a sufficient quantity of cells by culturing, making the use of other stem cell sources unnecessary. However, improvement of this therapeutic strategy for AD is necessary to increase the efficiency of reprogramming, the quality of pluripotency, and the safety of these cells before use in human trials [40].

Most of AD therapies are based on the assumption that Aβ accumulation is the primary pathogenic trigger of AD (Aβ-centric therapies). Antiamyloid drugs aim to decrease Aβ production, increase its clearance, or reduce aggregation of the protein. Aβ production can be inhibited by modifying the activity of the β- and γ-secretase enzymes that cleave the amyloid precursor protein. Despite evidence of efficacy for these drugs *in vitro* and *in vivo* in animal models of AD, drugs that inhibit secretases have failed to show any benefit in established disease in clinical trials.

Immunotherapy has been used to increase clearance of Aβ through active (vaccination) or passive (monoclonal antibodies, gamma globulin) immunization. Initial vaccination trials were ceased due to meningoencephalitis, with no cognitive benefit found.

Passive immunotherapy is based on the administration of monoclonal or polyclonal Abs against Aβ. Recently published phase III trials of two mAbs have failed to show any benefit, with vasogenic edema and microhemorrhages identified as a potentially serious adverse event. Of the limited trials of drugs that inhibit the aggregation of Aβ, none have been positive to date. Active immunization has been used to treat AD, by targeting Aβ. The trial was halted by the development of aseptic meningoencephalitis, which occurred in 6% of patients and was caused by a T-cell-mediated autoimmune response.

The amyloid hypothesis has dominated much of the research for AD therapy. However, recent failures for amyloid-based therapies have led some to question whether Aβ is the consequence rather than the cause of AD. Then, the focus has shifted to tau protein. Tau is a protein that stabilizes microtubules. It is abundant in neurons but in AD it is hyperphosphorylated and presents intracellularly in the form of tangles (aggregates). Anti-tau therapies have focused on inhibition of tau aggregation and phosphorylation. Trials of anti-tau therapies in established AD have not yet been successful.

There are numerous other drugs currently available for AD, including intranasal insulin and resveratrol. Resveratrol stimulates the sirtuin pathway. Sirtuin proteins are thought to have an antiaging effect and have been found to promote the activity of alpha secretase. In contrast to beta and gamma secretases, alpha secretase cleaves the amyloid precursor protein into peptides that do not aggregate. Promoting alpha secretase through the sirtuin pathway may potentially reduce the formation of amyloid plaques. A phase II trial of a gene therapy, which is thought to stimulate nerve growth factor, is currently in progress.

Although tremendous efforts have been made to delay AD progression as well as ameliorate and cure AD symptoms, only four cholinesterase inhibitors (donepezil, galantamine, rivastigmine, and tacrine, which is rarely prescribed because of its associated side effects, especially liver damage) and an NMDAR antagonist (memantine) have been approved by the US Food and Drug Administration for AD treatment. However, these drugs are not designed to halt or reverse the underlying process of AD, but rather to compensate for declining brain function. The disease is now recognized as multifactorial and consequently strongly demands more effective treatments. Recently, mounting evidence has shown that successful treatment of neurodegenerative diseases, including AD, Parkinson's disease, and amyotrophic lateral sclerosis, can be achieved through the use of stem cells. Cell therapy may offer an opportunity to treat AD or delay its progression by being able to tackle several factors involved in its pathogenesis at once [41].

27.3.3 Future Directions: Nanomedicine

Many potential drugs for AD treatment could be available, but barriers such as BBB, blood–cerebrospinal fluid barrier, and *p*-glycoproteins restrict the effective and safe drug delivery to the brain in patients with AD. Advancement in nanotechnology-based drug delivery systems and easily multifunctionalizable devices with size on the order of billionth of meter over the last decade exemplifies the effective drug delivery and targeting to the brain with controlled rate in various diseases, including AD. Nanocarriers, as polymeric nanoparticles, liposomes, nanoassembly, and dendrimers, have been studied and investigated as therapeutic options in AD.

Recently, one of the most promising nanotechnology-based approaches for AD therapy is multifunctional liposomes targeting the brain and promoting the disaggregation of Aβ assemblies able to reduce Aβ burden in AD mouse models. These nanoparticles are liposomes bifunctionalized with a peptide derived from the apolipoprotein-E receptor-binding domain for BBB targeting and with phosphatidic acid for Aβ binding.

Treatment of animal models of AD with these liposomes decreased total brain Aβ burden, brain Aβ oligomers, and the treatment ameliorated mouse impaired memory, reaching the brain in an intact form [42].

Aptamers represent the novel class of oligonucleotides holding multiple applications in the area of biomedicine. In the recent times, aptamers were identified to have the potential for penetrating into the deep human crevices and thus can be utilized in addressing the issues of complex neurological disorders. Considering the specificity and stability enhancement by chemical modifications, aptamer-based nanotechnologies may have great potential for future therapeutics and diagnostics (theranostics) [43].

Overall, the development and design of nanosized delivery systems for curcumin and other potential drugs for AD, including liposomes, polymeric nanoparticles and micelles, conjugates, peptide carriers, cyclodextrins, solid dispersions, lipid nanoparticles, and emulsions are under investigation [44,45].

References

1 Ferri, C.P., Prince, M., Brayne, C., Brodaty, H., Fratiglioni, L., Ganguli, M., Hall, K., Hasegawa, K., Hendrie, H., Huang, Y., Jorm, A., Mathers, C., Menezes, P.R., Rimmer, E., Scazufca, M., and Alzheimer's Disease International (2005) Global prevalence of dementia: a Delphi consensus study. *Lancet*, **366** (9503), 2112–2117.

2 Masters, C.L., Simms, G., Weinman, N.A., Multhaup, G., McDonald, B.L., and Beyreuther, K. (1985) Amyloid plaque core protein in Alzheimer disease and Down syndrome. *Proc. Natl. Acad. Sci. USA*, **82**, 4245–4249.

3 Hardy, J. and Selkoe, D.J. (2002) The amyloid hypothesis of Alzheimer's disease: progress and problems on the road to therapeutics. *Science*, **297** (5580), 353–356.

4 Crouch, P.J., Harding, S.M., White, A.R., Camakaris, J., Bush, A.I., and Masters, C.L. (2008) Mechanisms of Abeta mediated neurodegeneration in Alzheimer's disease. *Int. J. Biochem. Cell. Biol.*, **40** (2), 181–198.

5 Wolburg, H., Noell, S., Mack, A., Wolburg-Buchholz, K., and Fallier-Becker, P. (2009) Brain endothelial cells and the glio-vascular complex. *Cell Tissue Res.*, **335** (1), 75–96.

6 Gregori, M., Masserini, M., and Mancini, S. (2015) Nanomedicine for the treatment of Alzheimer's disease. *Nanomedicine (Lond.)*, **10** (7), 1203–1218.

7 Zhang, L., Chang, R.C., Chu, L.W., and Mak, H.K. (2012) Current neuroimaging techniques in Alzheimer's disease and applications in animal models. *Am. J. Nucl. Med. Mol. Imaging*, **2** (3), 386–404.
8 Klunk, W.E., Engler, H., Nordberg, A., Wang, Y., Blomqvist, G., Holt, D.P., Bergstrom, M., Savitcheva, I., Huang, G.F., Estrada, S., Ausen, B., Debnath, M.L., Barletta, J., Price, J.C., Sandell, J., Lopresti, B.J., Wall, A., Koivisto, P., Antoni, G., Mathis, C.A., and Langstrom, B. (2004) Imaging brain amyloid in Alzheimer's disease with Pittsburgh compound-B. *Ann. Neurol.*, **55**, 306–319.
9 Gandhi, H., Hewing, D., Botkin, C., Hubble, W., Turner, J., and Osman, M. (2013) Amyvid: a review and assessment of clinical implementation. *J. Nucl. Med.*, **54**, 2709.
10 Amatsubo, T., Yanagisawa, D., Morikawa, S., Taguchi, H., and Tooyama, I. (2010) Amyloid imaging using high-field magnetic resonance. *Magn. Reson. Med. Sci.*, **9** (3), 95–99.
11 Vanhoutte, G., Dewachter, I., Borghgraef, P., Van Leuven, F., and van der Linden, A. (2005) Noninvasive *in vivo* MRI detection of neuritic plaques associated with iron in APP[V717I] transgenic mice, a model for Alzheimer's disease. *Magn. Reson. Med.*, **53**, 607–613.
12 Jack, C.R.Jr., Wengenack, T.M., Reyes, D.A., Garwood, M., Curran, G.L., Borowski, B.J., Lin, J., Preboske, G.M., Holasek, S.S., Adriany, G., and Poduslo, J.F. (2005) *In vivo* magnetic resonance microimaging of individual amyloid plaques in Alzheimer's transgenic mice. *J. Neurosci.*, **25**, 10041–10048.
13 Laurent, S., Forge, D., Port, M., Roch, A., Robic, C., Vander Elst, L., and Muller, R.N. (2008) Magnetic iron oxide nanoparticles: synthesis, stabilization, vectorization, physicochemical characterizations, and biological applications. *Chem. Rev.*, **108**, 2064–2110.
14 Cheng, K.K., Chan, P.S., Fan, S., Kwan, S.M., Yeung, K.L., Wáng, Y.X., Chow, A.H., Wu, E.X., and Baum, L. (2015) Curcumin-conjugated magnetic nanoparticles for detecting amyloid plaques in Alzheimer's disease mice using magnetic resonance imaging (MRI). *Biomaterials*, **44**, 155–172.
15 Zhang, D., Fa, H.B., Zhou, J.T., Li, S., Diao, X.W., and Yin, W. (2015) The detection of β-amyloid plaques in an Alzheimer's disease rat model with DDNP-SPIO. *Clin. Radiol.*, **70** (1), 74–80.
16 Ansciaux, E., Burtea, C., Laurent, S., Crombez, D., Nonclercq, D., Vander Elst, L., and Muller, R.N. (2015) *In vitro* and *in vivo* characterization of several functionalized ultrasmall particles of iron oxide, vectorized against amyloid plaques and potentially able to cross the blood–brain barrier: toward earlier diagnosis of Alzheimer's disease by molecular imaging. *Contrast Media Mol. Imaging*, **10** (3), 211–224.
17 Wadghiri, Y.Z., Li, J., Wang, J., Hoang, D.M., Sun, Y., Xu, H., Tsui, W., Li, Y., Boutajangout, A., Wang, A., de Leon, M., and Wisniewski, T. (2013) Detection of amyloid plaques targeted by bifunctional USPIO in Alzheimer's disease transgenic mice using magnetic resonance microimaging. *PLoS One*, **8** (2), e57097.
18 Waldmann, T.A. (1991) Monoclonal antibodies in diagnosis and therapy. *Science*, **252** (5013), 1657–1662.
19 Sillerud, L.O., Solberg, N.O., Chamberlain, R., Orlando, R.A., Heidrich, J.E., Brown, D.C., Brady, C.I., Vander Jagt, T.A., Garwood, M., and Vander Jagt, D.L. (2013) SPION-enhanced magnetic resonance imaging of Alzheimer's disease plaques in AβPP/PS-1 transgenic mouse brain. *J. Alzheimers Dis.*, **34** (2), 349–365.
20 Mirsadeghi, S., Shanehsazzadeh, S., Atyabi, F., and Dinarvand, R. (2016) Effect of PEGylated superparamagnetic iron oxide nanoparticles (SPIONs) under magnetic field on amyloid beta fibrillation process. *Mater. Sci. Eng. C Mater. Biol. Appl.*, **59**, 390–397.
21 Petters, C., Thiel, K., and Dringen, R. (2015) Lysosomal iron liberation is responsible for the vulnerability of brain microglial cells to iron oxide nanoparticles: comparison with neurons and astrocytes. *Nanotoxicology*, **19**, 1–11.
22 Alivisatos, A.P. (1996) Semiconductor clusters, nanocrystals, and quantum dots. *Science*, **271**, 933–937.

23 Feng, L., Long, H.Y., Liu, R.K., Sun, D.N., Liu, C., Long, L.L., Li, Y., Chen, S., and Xiao, B. (2013) A quantum dot probe conjugated with aβ antibody for molecular imaging of Alzheimer's disease in a mouse model. *Cell. Mol. Neurobiol.*, **33** (6), 759–765.

24 Sperling, R. and Johnson, K. (2013) Biomarkers of Alzheimer disease: current and future applications to diagnostic criteria. *Continuum (Minneap. Minn.)*, **19** (2 Dementia), 325–338.

25 Rodrigue, K.M., Kennedy, K.M., and Park, D.C. (2009) Beta-amyloid deposition and the aging brain. *Neuropsychol. Rev.*, **19** (4), 436–450.

26 Zhang, S., Xia, J., and Li, X. (2008) Electrochemical biosensor for detection of adenosine based on structure-switching aptamer and amplification with reporter probe DNA modified Au nanoparticles. *Anal. Chem.*, **80** (22), 8382–8388.

27 Dubois, B., Feldman, H.H., Jacova, C., Dekosky, S.T., Barberger-Gateau, P., Cummings, J., Delacourte, A., Galasko, D., Gauthier, S., Jicha, G., Meguro, K., O'brien, J., Pasquier, F., Robert, P., Rossor, M., Salloway, S., Stern, Y., Visser, P.J., and Scheltens, P. (2007) Research criteria for the diagnosis of Alzheimer's disease: revising the NINCDS-ADRDA criteria. *Lancet Neurol.*, **6** (8), 734–746.

28 Yu, Y., Sun, X., Tang, D., Li, C., Zhang, L., Nie, D., Yin, X., and Shi, G. (2015) Gelsolin bound β-amyloid peptides(1–40/1–42): electrochemical evaluation of levels of soluble peptide associated with Alzheimer's disease. *Biosens. Bioelectron.*, **68**, 115–121.

29 Liu, L., Zhao, F., Ma, F., Zhang, L., Yang, S., and Xia, N. (2013) Electrochemical detection of β-amyloid peptides on electrode covered with *N*-terminus-specific antibody based on electrocatalytic O_2 reduction by Aβ(1–16)-heme-modified gold nanoparticles. *Biosens. Bioelectron.*, **49**, 231–235.

30 Wang, C., Liu, D., and Wang, Z. (2012) Gold nanoparticle based dot-blot immunoassay for sensitively detecting Alzheimer's disease related β-amyloid peptide. *Chem. Commun. (Camb.)*, **48** (67), 8392–8394.

31 Kim, C.B., Choi, Y.Y., Song, W.K., and Song, K.B. (2014) Antibody-based magnetic nanoparticle immunoassay for quantification of Alzheimer's disease pathogenic factor. *J. Biomed. Opt.*, **19** (5), 051205.

32 Stegurová, L., Dráberová, E., Bartos, A., Dráber, P., Rípová, D., and Dráber, P. (2014) Gold nanoparticle-based immuno-PCR for detection of tau protein in cerebrospinal fluid. *J. Immunol. Methods*, **406**, 137–142.

33 Zengin, A., Tamer, U., and Caykara, T. (2013) A SERS-based sandwich assay for ultrasensitive and selective detection of Alzheimer's tau protein. *Biomacromolecules*, **14** (9), 3001–3009.

34 Tisch, U., Schlesinger, I., Ionescu, R., Nassar, M., Axelrod, N., Robertman, D., Tessler, Y., Azar, F., Marmur, A., Aharon-Peretz, J., and Haick, H. (2013) Detection of Alzheimer's and Parkinson's disease from exhaled breath using nanomaterial-based sensors. *Nanomedicine (Lond.)*, **8** (1), 43–56.

35 Liu, D., Chen, W., Tian, Y., He, S., Zheng, W., Sun, J., Wang, Z., and Jiang, X. (2012) A highly sensitive gold-nanoparticle-based assay for acetylcholinesterase in cerebrospinal fluid of transgenic mice with Alzheimer's disease. *Adv. Healthc. Mater.*, **1** (1), 90–95.

36 Kim, G.H., Kim, J.E., Rhie, S.J., and Yoon, S. (2015) The role of oxidative stress in neurodegenerative diseases. *Exp. Neurobiol.*, **24** (4), 325–340.

37 Nakamura, T. and Lipton, S.A. (2016) Protein *S*-nitrosylation as a therapeutic target for neurodegenerative diseases. *Trends Pharmacol. Sci.*, **37** (1), 73–84.

38 Waite, L.M. (2015) Treatment for Alzheimer's disease: has anything changed? *Aust. Prescr.*, **38** (2), 60–63.

39 Geldenhuys, W.J. and Darvesh, A.S. (2015) Pharmacotherapy of Alzheimer's disease: current and future trends. *Expert Rev. Neurother.*, **15** (1), 3–5.

40 Pen, A.E. and Jensen, U.B. (2016) Current status of treating neurodegenerative disease with induced pluripotent stem cells. *Acta Neurol. Scand.* doi: 10.1111/ane.12545.

41 Amemori, T., Jendelova, P., Ruzicka, J., Urdzikova, L.M., and Sykova, E. (2015) Alzheimer's disease: mechanism and approach to cell therapy. *Int. J. Mol. Sci.*, **16** (11), 26417–26451.

42 Balducci, C., Mancini, S., Minniti, S., La Vitola, P., Zotti, M., Sancini, G., Mauri, M., Cagnotto, A., Colombo, L., Fiordaliso, F., Grigoli, E., Salmona, M., Snellman, A., Haaparanta-Solin, M., Forloni, G., Masserini, M., and Re, F. (2014) Multifunctional liposomes reduce brain β-amyloid burden and ameliorate memory impairment in Alzheimer's disease mouse models. *J. Neurosci.*, **34** (42), 14022–14031.

43 Sriramoju, B., Kanwar, R., Veedu, R.N., and Kanwar, J.R. (2015) Aptamer-targeted oligonucleotide theranostics: a smarter approach for brain delivery and the treatment of neurological diseases. *Curr. Top. Med. Chem.*, **15** (12), 1115–1124.

44 Ahmad, M.Z., Ahmad, J., Amin, S., Rahman, M., Anwar, M., Mallick, N., Ahmad, F.J., Rahman, Z., Kamal, M.A., and Akhter, S. (2014) Role of nanomedicines in delivery of anti-acetylcholinesterase compounds to the brain in Alzheimer's disease. *CNS Neurol. Disord. Drug Targets*, **13** (8), 1315–1324.

45 Ruozi, B., Belletti, D., Pederzoli, F., Veratti, P., Forni, F., Vandelli, M.A., and Tosi, G. (2014) Nanotechnology and Alzheimer's disease: what has been done and what to do. *Curr. Med. Chem.*, **21** (36), 4169–4185.

Part Five
The Nanopharmaceutical Market

28
A Practical Guide to Translating Nanomedical Products

Raj Bawa[1,2]

[1]*Bawa Biotech LLC, Patent Law Department, 21005 Starflower Way, Ashburn, VA 20147, USA*
[2]*Rensselaer Polytechnic Institute, Department of Biological Sciences, 110 8th St, Troy, NY 12180, USA*

Nano has permeated virtually every sector of the global economy though few in the stock market get excited about it anymore. Over the past two decades, nano has become more sectorized, with nanomedicine and nanoelectronics leading the way. Optimists tout nano as an enabling technology, a sort of next industrial revolution that could enhance the wealth and health of nations.

However, many consider nano to be a repackaging of old terms, concepts, and technologies. There is no standard definition for anything nano, including nanomedicine. In fact, nanomedicine does appear to be a relabeling of earlier terminology [1]. I define it as the science and technology of diagnosing, treating, and preventing disease as well as improving human health via nanoscale tools, devices, interventions, and procedures. It is driven by collaborative research, patenting, commercialization, business development, and technology transfer within diverse areas such as biomedical sciences, chemical engineering, biotechnology, physical sciences, and information technology.

In any case, nanomedicine continues to evolve and play a pivotal role in various industry segments. For instance, nanomedicine's influence on the pharmaceutical, device and biotechnology industries is readily apparent. This decade has witnessed relatively more advances and product development. Areas within nanomedicine (nanoscale drug delivery systems, theranostics, nanoimaging, etc.) could eventually turn out to be a healthcare game-changer by offering patients access to personalized or precision medicine. Another distinctive discipline within nanomedicine referred to as nanopharmacy is also making a major impact. Nanopharmacy emphasizes improving drug pharmacokinetics/pharmacodynamics as well as reducing nonspecific toxicity/immunogenicity in order to attain maximum efficacy and minimum undesirable side effects. Most experts agree that R&D is in full swing and novel nanomedical products, especially in the drug delivery sector (Figure 28.1), are consistently inching their way into the marketplace. There are hundreds of nanomedical products on the market and

Pharmaceutical Nanotechnology: Innovation and Production, First Edition. Edited by Jean Cornier, Arno Kwade, Andrew Owen, and Marcel Van de Voorde.

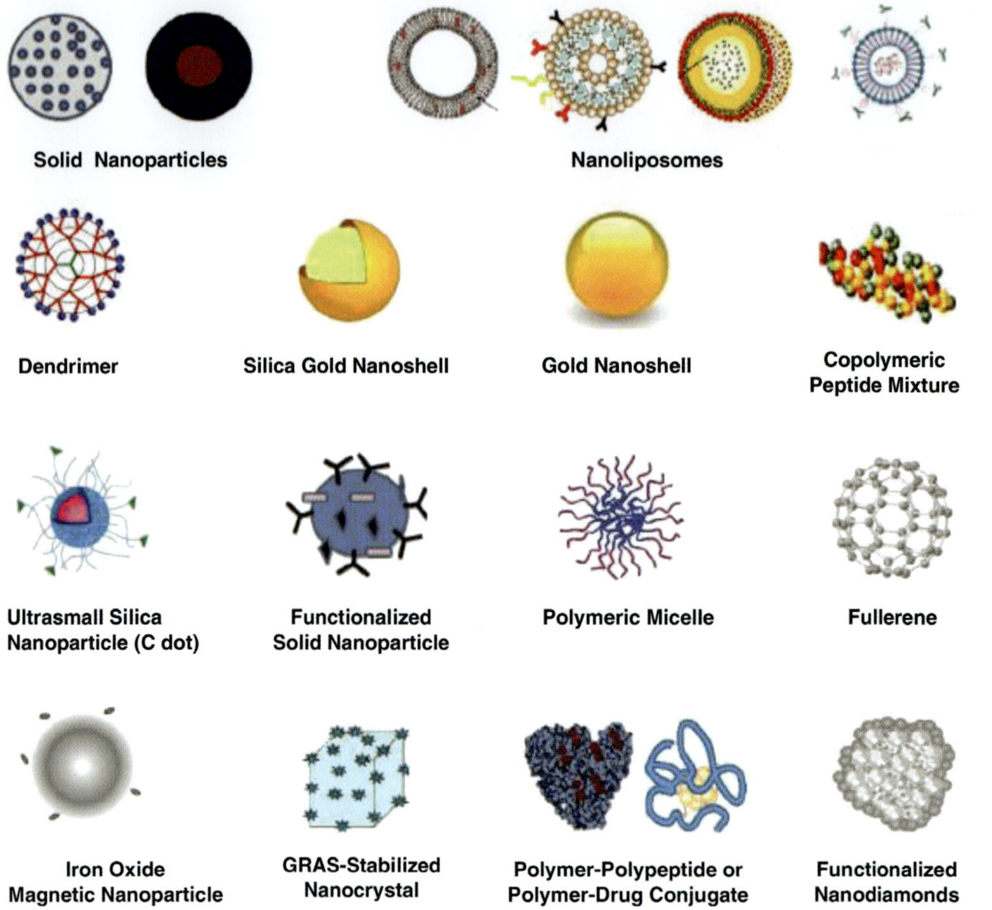

Figure 28.1 Schematic illustrations of nanoscale drug delivery system platforms (nanotherapeutics or nanodrug products). Shown are nanoparticles (NPs) used in drug delivery that are approved, in preclinical development, or in clinical trials. They are generally considered as first- or second-generation multifunctional engineered NPs, generally ranging in diameters from a few nanometers upto a micrometer. Active biotargeting is frequently achieved by conjugating ligands (antibodies, peptides, aptamers, folate, hyaluronic acid, etc.) tagged to the NP surface via spacers or linkers such as PEG or by altering the NP surface characteristics. NPs such as carbon nanotubes and quantum dots, although extensively advertised for drug delivery, are specifically excluded from the figure as this author considers them commercially unfeasible for drug delivery. Nonengineered antibodies and naturally occurring NPs are also excluded. Antibody–drug conjugates are encompassed by the cartoon labeled "polymer–polypeptide or polymer–drug conjugate." This list of NPs is not meant to be exhaustive, the illustrations are not meant to reflect the three-dimensional shape or configuration, and the NPs are not drawn to scale. NPs: nanoparticles; PEG: polyethylene glycol; GRAS: generally recognized as safe; C dot: Cornell dot; ADCs: antibody–drug conjugates. *Copyright © 2017 Raj Bawa. All rights reserved.*

the potential appears vast. Still, revolutionary nanomedical breakthroughs are just promises at this stage.

The positive outlook for nanomedicine continues to be tempered by certain issues and concerns. For example, startups, academia, and companies often exaggerate basic research developments or early-stage preclinical nanomedical discoveries as revolutionary. Potential benefits are frequently overstated or inferred to be very close to application when clear bottlenecks to commercial translation exist. Instead, the focus should be on fabrication of safe and effective nanomedicines that can truly enhance benefit-to-risk ratio [2]. However, what is seen is an overwhelming increase in empirical approaches that tend to find exaggerated *in vivo* biomedical applications for a broad range of emerging and poorly characterized multifunctional, hybrid, or nonbiodegradable nanomaterials (e.g., carbon nanotubes (CNTs), quantum dots, graphene oxide, and certain metallic nanoparticles) that present toxicity and safety concerns [2]. The "nano" prefix is thrown around to suit whatever purpose, whether it is for federal research funding, approval of patents, raising venture capital funds, running for office, or seeking publication of a journal article. All of this is happening while hundreds of over-the-counter products containing silver nanoparticles, nanoscale titanium dioxide, and carbon nanoparticles continue to stream into the marketplace without adequate safety testing, labeling, or regulatory review. For example, nanoscale titanium dioxide, present in powdered Dunkin' Doughnuts and Hostess Donettes, has been classified as a potential carcinogen by the National Institute for Occupational Safety and Health (NIOSH) while the World Health Organization (WHO) has linked it in powder form to various cancers.

Stakeholders, especially investors and consumer-patients, get nervous about the "known unknown" novel applications, uncertain health risks, industry motives, and general lack of governmental transparency. Venture has mostly shied away in recent years, although industry–university alliances have continued to develop. Wall Street's early interest in nano has been somewhat limited over the years, from cautionary involvement to generally shying away. In spite of anemic nanoproduct development, there is no end in sight to publications, press releases, and patent filings. Universities and small businesses have jumped into the fray with industry with the clear intention of patenting as much nano as they can grab. Even governments across the globe, impressed by "nanopotential," continued to stake their claims by doling out billions for research and development (R&D).

Will nanomedicine stocks and venture backed startups deliver on their investment promise by the next decade? Will nanomedicine evolve into a stand-alone industry or will technology behind it enhance and improved many different industries? Whether nanomedicine eventually blossoms into a robust industry, or it continues to incrementally influence medicine and healthcare, one thing is certain: The die is cast and it is here to stay. In the meantime, tempered expectations are in order. Dissecting hope from hype is often difficult. However, like any emerging field, the full picture with respect to nanomedicine is yet to emerge – and we are just getting started!

This chapter aims to increase awareness of broad issues pertaining to nanomedicine translation *per se*; it does not focus on subspecialities like nanodrug delivery or nanopharmacy. The following terms are used interchangeably as they all pertain to a "drug or therapeutic": nanomedicines, nanodrugs, nanotherapeutics, and nanopharmaceuticals. Similarly, the following "technology" terms are used interchangeably: nano, nanotech, and nanotechnology.

28.1
From the Laboratory to the Clinic: Overcoming the Valley of Death

No one can argue that the enormous infusion of public and private investments in biomedical research has yielded drastically less clinical products than expected. The relatively long time for medical products from discovery to ultimate clinical use and the relatively low proportion of discoveries that survived that journey is a problem. There is consensus that the development of (nano) medical products and interventions takes too long, is too expensive, and fraught with failures at every stage of development. There is too wide an innovation gap between basic sciences (preclinical biomedical research) and clinical sciences (development of novel therapeutic options for the patient). This continues to threaten or stall translation of advances in the laboratory to the patient's bedside.

These barriers to translational research are relatively recent. In the 1950s and 1960s, basic (or preclinical) and clinical research were tightly linked in agencies such as the National Institutes of Health (NIH), and clinical research was mainly conducted by physician–scientists who also undertook patient care [3]. In the 1970s, this model changed with the explosion of genetic engineering. Clinical and basic research started to diverge and biomedical research emerged as a unique discipline with its own training. As a result, nowadays most of biomedical research is conducted by highly specialized PhD-scientists while physician-scientists are a minority.

Creating medical products today, including nanomedical, whether they are drugs, devices, or combination products, is a complex process that requires a multiple of scientific disciplines. It is time-consuming, expensive, and enormously challenging. For example, *de novo* drug discovery and development is a 10–17 year process from conception to marketed drug (Figure 28.2). Inherent to this complexity is low solubility and poor bioavailability of the molecules being studied. It may take up to a decade for a drug candidate to just enter clinical trials, with very few tested candidates in trials reaching the clinic. In fact, often, more drugs come off patent each year than are approved by the Food and Drug Administration (FDA). According to a 2014 study by the Tufts Center for the Study of Drug Development, developing a new prescription medicine that gains marketing approval is estimated to cost nearly $2.6 billion [4].

Regardless of the industry or the origin of technology, for a product to become successful it must endure and traverse a most difficult period in its lifetime, the so-called valley of death (Figure 28.3). It is a graveyard for many "good" scientific ideas, technologies, new products, and processes, representing the transition

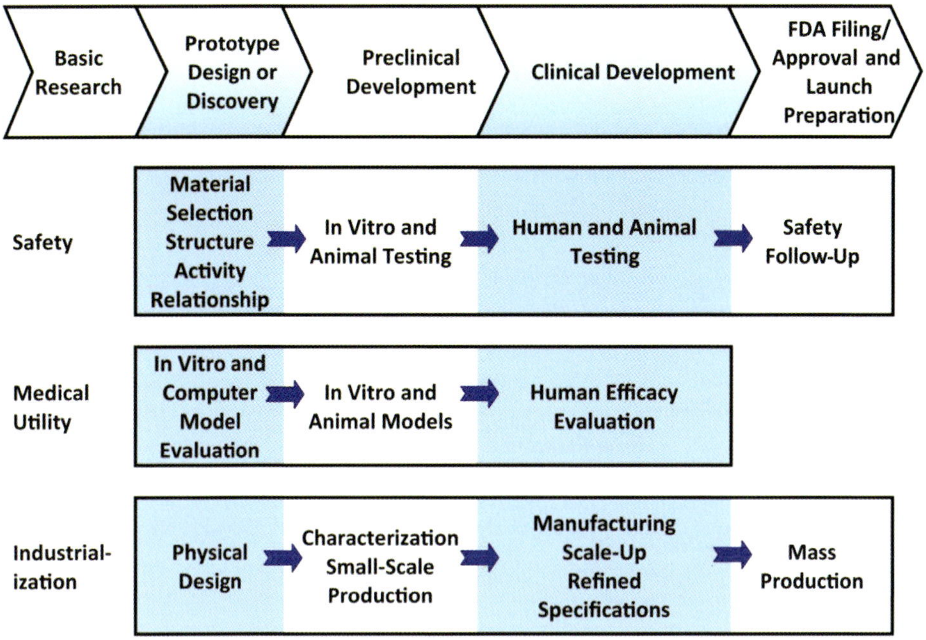

Figure 28.2 An overview of the product development pathway. This figure represents a highly generalized description of activities involving FDA-regulated product development that must be successfully completed at different points. The FDA describes three interdependent subgroups (safety, medical utility, and industrialization) of the general pathway to approval with efficiencies gained in these three subgroups affecting the overall expense and timeline to approval. In summary, development can be conceptualized as a process leading from basic research through a series of developmental steps to a commercial product. Many of the activities involving product development are highly complex and whole industries are devoted to supporting them. Not all are performed for every candidate and many activities are omitted from the figure. If the product being developed is a drug, then first a candidate drug emerges from a drug discovery program. Then, the candidate must successfully complete a series of evaluations of its potential safety and efficacy and must be amenable to mass production. For each candidate finishing the pathway, thousands of candidates are evaluated in the discovery phase. (Figure adapted from the FDA.)

from basic research activities to product development. By extension, the same is true for nanomedicines. All stakeholders – pharma, patients, regulators, patent offices, funders – have suffered and are to blame for the valley of death. Each needs to re-examine its role and become an active, full partner in the biomedical ecosystem so that translational activities are more fruitful. Similarly, although great strides have been made in nanomedicine at the "science" level, especially with respect to drug delivery and nanoimaging, bottlenecks at the "translational" level are impeding commercialization (Table 28.1).

The European Society for Translational Medicine defines translational medicine (TM) as an interdisciplinary branch of the biomedical field supported by

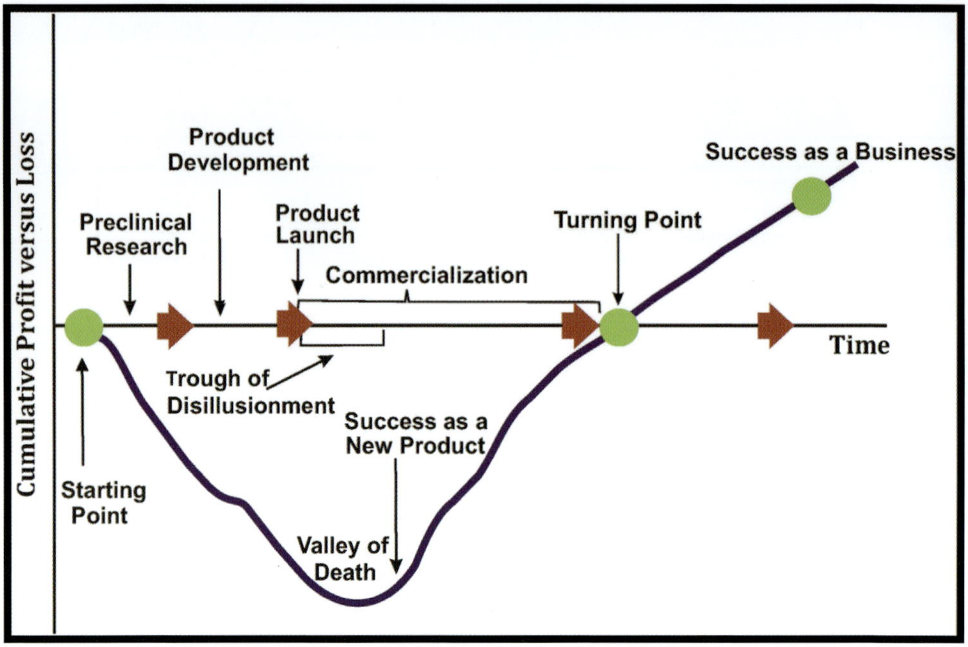

Figure 28.3 The valley of death in commercialization. The valley of death represents the gap that exists between R&D breakthroughs made at the cellular and molecular biology levels on one end and the static levels of new treatments, diagnostics, and preventative tools reaching the market on the other. This is the time when ideas and inventions must undergo technical feasibility review, manufacturing optimization, market demand evaluation, reduction in production costs, and commercialization potential studies. This is when prior to market entry decisions are made whether to proceed or terminate product development. The *upstream* side of the valley of death (the science side) represents basic research inherently fraught with uncertainty, while *downstream* (the business side) represents the more regimented process of product development characterized by manufacturing, marketing, deliverables, deadlines, and budgets. Commercialization is about the translation crossing these two distinct paradigms.

three main pillars (benchside, bedside, and community) with the goal to combine disciplines, resources, expertise, and techniques within these pillars to promote enhancements in prevention, diagnosis, and therapies [5]. Given this, the aim of TM [5] is to facilitate the transition of preclinical or basic research into clinical or medical application, generally via a faster, easier, cheaper, and more efficient route. This allows realizing the social value of science, that is, the production of medical products, applications, and methods that help improve human health. The primary impetus for TM is that there are better ways to move preclinical biomedical research to medical practice more quickly without sacrificing quality or increasing costs. TM invariably involves multidisciplinarity, collaboration, and networking along with novel models, modes of communication, and regulatory systems – all features that are the hallmark of

Table 28.1 Select barriers to nanomedicine translation.

Nomenclature and terminology
Imprecise definition for nano-related terms
Lack of technical specifications, standards, guidelines, best practices, and measurements regarding "nano"
Different terms refer to identical nanomaterials and nanoparticles
Discrepancies and inconsistent definitions in pharma with respect to various terms relevant to drug R&D spills into nanomedicine; FDA, EMA, WHO, etc. cannot agree on definitions central to drug development
Failure of standard-setting organizations (ISO, ASTM, etc.) to produce technical specifications that clarify the issue
Commercial manufacturing and quality control ("the process is the product")
Issues pertaining to separation of undesirables and impurities (by-products, catalysts, starting materials, etc.) during manufacturing; presence of impurities (host cell proteins or protein aggregates formed during processing) may trigger an immune response in patients while protein potency may be impaired via degradation in binding regions
Lack of precise control over nanoparticle/nanomaterial manufacturing parameters and control assays
Many currently used compounds/components for synthesis pose problems for large-scale current Good Manufacturing Practice (cGMP)
Technological challenges experienced during scale-up; scalability complexities regarding enhancing production rate to increase yield
Complexities and high fabrication costs of various nanomaterials, nanoparticles, and nanomedicines; cost of raw materials; expensive and time-consuming separation processes may be required
Reproducibility issues such as control of size distribution and mass
Stability of both the starting materials and the product (aggregation, degradation, etc.)
Batch-to-batch variability; contamination; impurities
Toxicity and immunogenicity
Lack of *in vivo* knowledge regarding the interaction between nanomedical products and complex biosurfaces/tissues
Lack of rational preclinical characterization strategies via multiple techniques
Limited knowledge on biocompatibility and biodistribution of diverse nanomaterials and nanoparticles
Limited prior experience with toxicity assessment of nanoscale therapeutics; small number of approved nanomedicine classes offers limited opportunities for study; lack of standard *in vitro* screening platforms that provide excellent correlation of potential *in vivo* bioperformance and outcome; high-throughput methods for nanomaterial binding, cell internalization and interaction with plasma proteins and immune factors (e.g., complement) not available; biomarker methods for small-molecule analysis not suitable for nanomedicines
Mixed messages emanate from various federal agencies and transnational regulatory bodies regarding safety and toxicity issues on similar/identical nanomaterials and nanoparticles
Immunogenicity of nanotherapeutics, especially protein-based, presents a major challenge to their development; immune responses often directed to these nanotherapeutics, resulting in reduced efficacy of the therapeutic, anaphylaxis in patient, and so on; C activation-related

(*continued*)

Table 28.1 (*Continued*)

adverse effects of liposome-based nanotherapeutics, referred to as C activation-related pseudoallergy (CARPA), is now well accepted
Unpredictable toxicity with respect to the diverse population of nanomaterials and nanoparticles
Limited or lack of advanced tools, technologies, and characterization assays regarding nanomedical products providing potential clarity; critical analysis, and comparison cannot be comprehensive at this stage given the scarcity of clinically approved nanoproducts, heterogeneity of nanomaterials fabricated, lack of appropriate *in silico* modeling tools, and limited guidance from regulatory agencies
Adsorption, distribution, metabolism, and excretion (ADME) studies regarding nanomedicines either lacking altogether or limited in scope; physiochemical properties of engineered nanoparticles directly impact ADME and hence are fundamental determinants of toxicity and efficacy; nanoparticle unpredictability with respect to ADME negatively impacts translational efforts
Consumer confidence
Public's general reluctance to embrace innovative or emerging medical technologies without clearer safety or regulatory guidelines
Perception that many nanoproducts are inherently unsafe
Government and industry suspicion
Media hype and misinformation not effectively countered by academia, government, and industry
Ethical challenges and societal issues not transparently addressed by stakeholders
Funding challenges
Relative scarcity of venture funds due to the perception that most medical nanoproducts lack a good return on investment (ROI)
Prolonged timescale is a detriment to funders and investors
Funders and venture capitalists often not experienced or versed in technological aspects and cannot fully gauge potential for translation
Barriers more steep for nanomedicine with respect to procuring funds to initiate a first-in-human (FIH) clinical trial
Big pharma's continued reluctance to seriously invest in nanomedicine, specially early-stage preclinical research lacking "proof-of-concept" in man
Lack of industry support limits potential to reach FIH clinical trials in any research setting (academic, start-up, small company, etc.)
Due diligence and peer review regarding translational potential of projects or research proposals often lacking during the funding process
Clinical research and trials
Cost, time, and effort required for clinical trials are a deterrent
General lack of knowledge about the FDA/EMA drug or device review process; limited understanding of the various aspects of drug and device laws in various jurisdictions
Challenges in patient recruitment is more acute in nanomedicine due to factors such as strict inclusion/exclusion criterion and delay by ethics committees
Challenges (cost, trial design, selection of participants, data analysis) with respect to international harmonization of bridging studies and the design of global clinical trials

	Lack of consensus on the different procedures, assays, and protocols to be employed during preclinical development and characterization of nanomedicines; this can also impact clinical trial design
Patents and intellectual property	
	Patent review delays, spotty examination, and access to relevant "prior art" at patent offices
	Issuance of invalid patents or patents of unduly broad legal scope by patent offices
	Emerging patent thickets due to a "patent prospector" mentality and issuance of overlapping patent claims
	A general lack of understanding of the patent process by stakeholders
	Patent expiry (the "patent cliff") of blockbuster drugs
	Limited knowledge regarding the basics of intellectual property law in academic circles
Support for small businesses and startups	
	General lack of financial incentives favoring longer term nanomedicine investments
	Limited tax-free bonds for financing, tax credits for capital investments, reduced capital gains tax rates, or investment-specific loan guarantees
	Lack of mentorship and business planning assistance
	Little assistance in attracting private and public funds
	The Small Business Innovation Research (SBIR) process in the United States is more focused on research and less on commercialization
	Lack of centralized audit system from the federal government is costly and slows down work at small businesses
	More nano tools needed in academia and small businesses
Academia and the university professor	
	Overhyped press releases from eminent university laboratories
	Professors behave more like "celebrity-academics" than researchers
	Research often focused on poorly characterized and nonbiodegradable nanomaterial-based platforms
	Fancy animations on laboratory websites exaggerate preclinical data and clinical partnerships with pharma project false hope of translational potential
	Irreproducibility of basic, preclinical research is a major problem at universities
	Awards and research activities that generate publications (*l'art pour l'art*) are more valued than patents
	Focus is often on journal impact factors and attending conferences
	Focus is on research and publications rather than commercialization; some academics even shun commercialization
	Inability or lack of willingness to conform to translational activities; few incentives for translational activities compound the problem
	Lack of coherent technology transfer policy from universities to start-ups
	Lack of communication between clinical researchers and basic scientists
	Evidence of clinical validity and clinical utility of the research being conducted is often lacking
	Lack of interdisciplinary research; lack of a collaborative spirit between industry and academia, or between clinical and basic science researchers
	A deficit in cross-disciplinary or hybrid scientific training at educational institutions
Regulatory uncertainty: baby steps and the bumpy road ahead	
	Confusion and future uncertainty due to "baby steps" undertaken by federal regulatory bodies such as the FDA and EMA

(*continued*)

Table 28.1 (*Continued*)

A lack of clear regulatory or safety guidelines
Governmental regulatory bodies lack technical and scientific knowledge to support risk-based regulation, thereby leaving a significant regulatory void
Issuance of too many nonbinding "draft" guidance documents by the FDA and "position papers" by EMA to make substantive policy changes
Product classification issues blur the regulatory boundaries between various product classes given that many are multimodal hybrid structures
Precautionary stance by regulatory agencies reflects their lack of expertise and experience with nanoscale formulations
National differences in regulatory requirements pose challenges for clinical trials involving international multicenters
Differences between regulatory agencies with regard to the definition of compound characteristics need to be harmonized to clarify the Biopharmaceutical Classification Scheme (BCS)
Bureaucracy and a conservative, insular attitude among government regulators hinders translation
Rise of diverse nano-specific regulatory arrangements and systems contribute to a dense global nanoregulatory landscape, full of gaps and devoid of central coordination; standardization, and harmonization on a global basis is complicated by technical, political, and economic issues
Technology Transfer Offices (TTOs)
TTOs at universities and institutes lack in-depth technical and business expertise
Decisions made in a vacuum or on imperfect analysis; limited experts and informed gatekeepers to do valuation or proper audit of "true" licensing royalties
Issues such as insular nature and high employee turnover indirectly impede translation
Other factors
Key technology benefits not identified early on in product development or research project
Limited infrastructure that becomes outdated quickly due to advances in technology
Relative scarcity of workers trained for nanoproduct development; need for foreign workers poses problems
Crisis of reproducibility in antibody performance due to shortcuts taken by manufacturers and researchers; this has contributed to irreproducibility of preclinical research data in biomedicine which directly impedes nanomedical translation
Absence of outstanding drug researchers in academic settings who are trained to separate "hits" into compounds good, bad, and ugly; academia not as well versed as big pharma when it comes to drug R&D
"True" interdisciplinarity still missing from nanomedicine translation; wide gaps persist between conception of innovative nanomedicine platforms and regulatory clinical approval; traversing the "valley of death" difficult
Misuse of *P*-values are contributing to the irreproducibility of preclinical biomedical research; this indirectly impacts nanomedical translation
Quality assurance (QA) guidelines for basic research lacking or not properly implemented
Lack of ability for tracing data, including which equipment the experiment was conducted on and where the source data are stored

nanomedicine. The growth of TM, in general, has coincided with an ever-changing pharma landscape.

However, in spite of significant investments by the public and private sectors, major issues that led to the emergence of TM in the first place have continued to dog TM and persist along the research–practice continuum (Table 28.1). In the United States, the NIH has made TM a central piece of its so-called NIH Roadmap for Medical Research [6] while the FDA launched a similar "Critical Path Initiative" [7] to address the growing crisis in moving basic discoveries to the market where they can be available to patients. Although both of these governmental initiatives [6,7] were launched over a decade ago, they have proven unsuccessful in dramatically improving the availability of new diagnostic/therapeutic modalities to the American public. This is because both the NIH and FDA have failed to address key blocks in translational research. In fact, experts frequently accuse these federal bureaucracies for neglecting their mandates of translating advances at the preclinical stage in the laboratory to clinical applications in the practice of medicine (i.e., the classical "bench-to-bedside" paradigm).

28.2 Irreproducible Preclinical Research: A Bottleneck for Translation?

We are in the midst of a widening research crisis. The current pervasive culture of science focuses on rewarding flashy, eye-catching, and positive findings. There is an increased emphasis on making provocative statements rather than presenting technical details or reporting basic elements of experimental design. These are some of the factors that have resulted in irreproducible preclinical research in biomedicine, mainly from academia. There are reports that less than one-third of biomedical papers can be reproduced; this is due to sloppy science blamed in part on scientific culture, training, and incentives [8,9]. A survey of nearly 900 members by the American Society for Cell Biology in 2015 found that more than two-thirds of respondents had been on at least one occasion unable to reproduce published results. These results are strikingly similar to another online survey of 1,576 researchers by *Nature* conducted in 2016 [8c] that reported that 70% of researchers have tried and failed to reproduce another scientist's experiments, and more than half have failed to reproduce their own experiments. Irreproducible research delays treatments, wastes time, and squanders research dollars. It is clearly widespread. In fact, it is seen in all disciplines of biomedical research [10–12], with the area most susceptible being research work that employs animal models [10]. Research institution administrators, faculty members, and trainees all share blame here. They must do far more for reproducibility of biomedical research data [13]. Most institutions will, however, not make the necessary moves unless forced by a regulatory or funding body. However, note that there is no evidence to suggest that irreproducibility is caused by scientific misconduct [14]. Various proposals and recommendations, including crowd-sourced analysis of research [15], are being studied as viable options to stem this tide of irreproducible research activities. Obviously, human clinical trials are less at risk from irreproducibility because they are already governed by various regulations that stipulate rigorous design and independent oversight.

Big pharma is particularly concerned about this irreproducibility crisis plaguing biomedical research. Drug companies have reported that one-quarter or fewer of high profile papers are reproducible [13]. In the past, drug screening was mainly performed at pharma and supported internally by outstanding teams of chemists. Over the years, there has been a growing reliance on academia for this upstream drug R&D. In fact, this collaborative innovation between pharma and the academic community is credited with producing key enabling discoveries underlying many marketed blockbusters. Today, preclinical drug discovery research is still primarily conducted and managed by pharma. However, academia now contributes to this effort by conducting basic research into fundamental and mechanistic aspects of human disease biology and discovery of targets whose modulation could have therapeutic potential. The resultant "gold nuggets" that are thus generated by academia are then plucked by pharma to discover and develop drugs that modulate those targets, thereby driving the drug discovery engine. However, this common arrangement is in trouble and the collaborative paradigm is breaking down as much of the research published in academia has proven not to be reproducible by drug companies [16]. Basically, academic target discovery research reproducibility has become suspect [17]. Some of the reasons for this crisis are inherent to the two entities whose mission and focus is distinct (although overlapping in a few areas). For instance, the two have differing expertise and incentives with respect to drug discovery targets, lead discovery programs, hit discovery, lead optimization strategies, interpretation of complex data, and production of high-quality probes.

Another important factor for the imperfect marriage between academia and industry with respect to drug R&D is the absence of outstanding support structure in academic drug research where researchers are typically not trained to separate "hits" into compounds good, bad, and ugly [18]. Many contend that, as a result, naivety about promiscuous, assay-duping molecules is polluting the literature and wasting resources [19].

Shortcuts taken by antibody manufacturers and researchers alike have resulted in a crisis of reproducibility in antibody performance. Obviously, this greatly affects identification of drug targets, thereby contributing to the reproducibility crisis in biomedical research [20]. This discontent has spurred action, with advanced technologies and characterization efforts promising clarity [21]. In the meantime, it may be best that researchers hold back using commercial antibodies rather than further muddy-up preclinical research data with the subsequent negative consequences for TM.

Recently, the American Statistical Association (ASA) issued principles to guide use of the *P*-value and warned that *P*-values cannot be used to determine whether a hypothesis is true or whether the results are important [22]. According to the ASA, misuse of *P*-values is also contributing to this irreproducibility crisis [23].

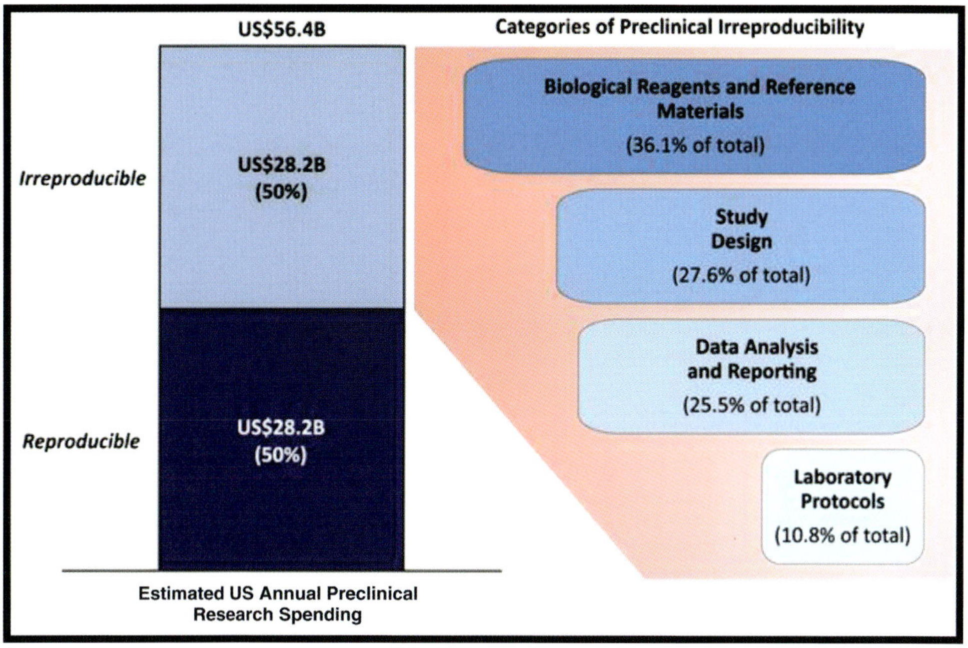

Figure 28.4 Economic costs of irreproducibility. This figure represents the estimated US preclinical research spending and categories of errors that contribute to irreproducibility. Errors in study design and biological reagents and materials contribute to a majority of the approximately US$28 billion annually spent on irreproducible preclinical research in the United States. Note that the percentage value of error for each category is the midpoint of the high and low prevalence estimates for that category divided (weighted) by the sum of all midpoint error rates. Figure reprinted from Ref. [9].

All of this irreproducibility of biomedical research is costly. According to a recent report, about US$28 billion are annually spent on irreproducible preclinical research in the United States (Figure 28.4) [9]. In this regard, because errors in study design and biological reagents and materials contribute to a majority spent, implementing steps to improve preclinical reproducibility should be a priority in these two areas (Table 28.2) [9].

Unfortunately, this reproducibility crisis has coincided with major changes in pharma's productivity as numerous market forces and drivers have continued to dictate a change in its quest for discovering, developing, and delivering novel therapeutics. These include downsizing, mergers and acquisitions (M&As), revenue losses due to patent expirations on blockbusters, enhanced regulatory oversight, high cost of clinical trials, Abbreviated New Drug Application (ANDA) challenges from generic manufacturers, and relative scarcity of new molecular entities (NMEs) due to innovation crisis. In the process, these forces are altering the drug R&D landscape and affecting healthcare delivery. All of this is cause for concern. Clearly, new ground rules, flexible business models, strategic

Table 28.2 Investing in practical solutions to improve preclinical reproducibility rates.

Study design

- Improve training programs at academic institutions to ensure that best practices are reinforced in the areas of core skills, methods, technology, and tools.
- Establish targeted training, coaching, and certification of established principal investigators (PIs) to reinforce application of best practices throughout the research process.
- Establish research funder policies, including funders such as NIH and leading disease foundations, requiring successful completion of training courses at all levels.

Biological reagents and reference materials

- Promote broad adoption by vendors to offer only validated reagents (e.g., antibodies and cell lines) and broad utilization of these reagents by PIs as a documented best practice in the research process.
- Ensure that research funder policies require documented use of validated and monocontaminated reagents, annual reagent authentication throughout the research study, and adequate funding to cover these additional costs.
- Ensure that procedures to document reagent validation and lack of contamination are required by publishers.
- Incentivize the continued development of tools for reagent validation using improved genomics data.
- Define standard operating procedures for biological materials handling throughout the material's life cycle.

Source: Reprinted from Ref. [9].

collaborative partnerships, and competitive business strategies are in order in this post-blockbuster era. In fact, pharma is frequently turning to high-throughput screening and miniaturization technologies such as nanotechnology to enhance or supplement aspects of drug target discovery and drug development. In spite of pharma's strategy of M&A, in-licensing, and an enormous capital investment in R&D, it has been unsuccessful in replacing drugs coming off patent with sufficient NMEs. The number of NMEs reaching the market has not increased in any major way in the past decade (Figure 28.5).

There is a difference between a New Molecular Entity (NME) and New Chemical Entity (NCE) under the US Federal Food, Drug, and Cosmetic Act ("FD&C Act" or "the Act"). They are sometimes used interchangeably; however, they are distinct. In other words, the FDA Center for Drug Evaluation and Research's (CDER's) classification of a drug product as an NME for review purposes is distinct from its determination of whether a drug product is an NCE within the meaning of the Act. An NCE is defined in 21 CFR 314.108(a) as "a drug that contains no active moiety that has been approved by the FDA in any other application submitted under 505(b) of the Act." An active moiety is defined by the FDA as a molecule or ion responsible for the physiological or pharmacological action of the drug substance, excluding those appended portions of the molecule that cause the drug to be an ester, salt (including a salt with hydrogen or

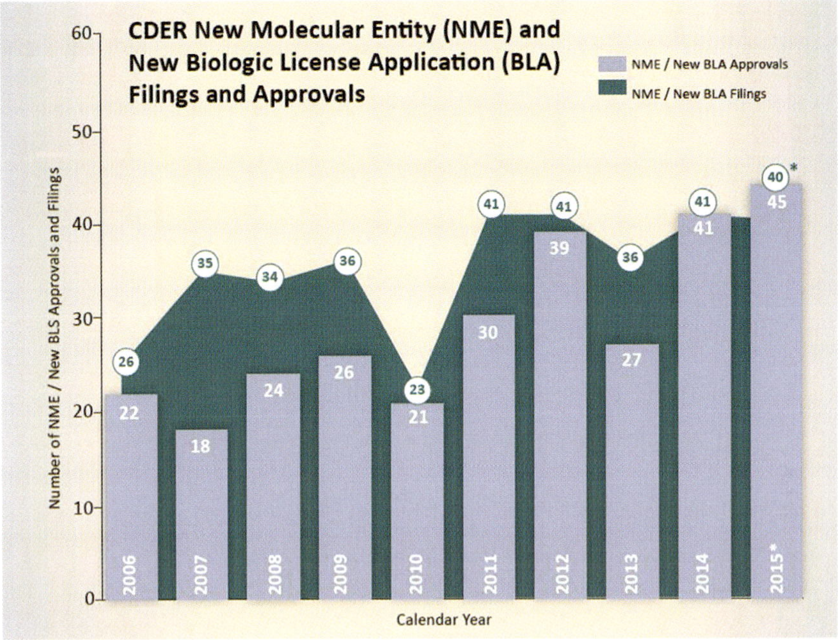

Figure 28.5 Ten-year historic comparison of drug approvals by FDA's Center for Drug Evaluation and Research (CDER). This figure represents New Molecular Entity (NME) and New Biologic License Application (BLA) filings and approvals in each calendar year starting from 2006 until 2015. New drugs approved by the FDA have risen sharply in recent years with the 2015 bounty being the most productive since 1996. However, in 2015, big innovations were in short supply, rejection letters issued by the FDA were surprisingly down, and few drugs stood out as breakthroughs. In fact, many products were more known for their breathtaking price tags and rapidity of FDA approval. The vertical bars indicate the number of New Drug Applications (NDAs) for NMEs approved by CDER from 2006 to 2015. The circled numbers indicate the number of NDAs for NMEs plus BLAs for new therapeutic biologics received by CDER for approval from 2006 until 2015. From 2006 through 2014, CDER has averaged about 28 novel drug approvals per year. CDER approved 45 novel drugs in 2015 (NMEs and new BLAs combined), up from the previous recent record of 41 drugs approved in 2014. Of these, 16 (36%) represented first-in-class designated drugs, 14 (31%) were cancer drugs, about 30% were biologics, 21 (47%) were orphan-designated drugs for rare diseases, and 16 were drugs with a novel mechanism of action.

Notes:

1) *The 2015 filed numbers include those filed in calendar year 2015 plus those currently pending filing (i.e., within their 60-day filing period) in calendar year 2015.
2) NMEs have chemical structures that have never been approved by CDER before. However, in some cases a NME may have actions similar to earlier drugs and may not necessarily offer unique clinical advantages over existing therapies.
3) In rare instances, it may be necessary for FDA to change a drug's NME designation or the status of its application as a novel BLA if new information becomes available.
4) Approvals by the Center for Biologics Evaluation and Research (CBER) are excluded in this drug count.
5) The data in this figure are current as of February 2016.
6) Details on approval requirements for New Drug Applications (NDAs) are found in Section 505(b) of the Food, Drug & Cosmetics Act (FD&C Act) (21 U.S.C. 355(b)). *Figure courtesy of the FDA. Data provided in this legend is courtesy of Drugs@FDA and various drug companies.*

coordination bonds), or other noncovalent derivative (such as a complex, chelate, or clathrate) of the molecule. An NME is a drug that contains an active moiety that has never been approved by the FDA or marketed in the United States. Certain drugs are classified by CDER as NMEs for purposes of regulatory review. Some drugs are characterized as NMEs for administrative purposes, but nonetheless contain active moieties that are closely related to active moieties in products that have been previously been approved by CDER. For example, CDER classifies biological products submitted in an application under Section 351(a) of the Public Health Service Act as NMEs for purposes of regulatory review, regardless of whether it has previously approved a related active moiety in a different product. It is important to note that it is the NCE status, and not NME status, that governs the granting of the 5 years of market exclusivity after approval in the United States, regardless of the patent situation (also known as Hatch–Waxman exclusivity).

28.3
Protecting Inventions via Patents: The Cornerstone of Translation

The protection of intellectual property (IP), within which patents fall, is increasingly important. So far, the process of converting basic research in nanomedicine into commercially viable products has been difficult. IP, obviously, is the lifeblood of any nanoenterprise, both as an enabler of translation and sometimes as a barrier to competition or litigation. Patents can have an impact at all stages in the translation pipeline: preclinical research stage, clinical trial stage, at the point of commercialization, and when the product is in the clinic.

In the context of IP, patents in the nanomedical space are critical. The protection of inventions via patents provides an opportunity for nanomedical companies to recoup the high cost of discovery by preventing competitors from entering the marketplace while the patent is in force. Simply put, securing valid and defensible patent protection from the patent offices is critical to any commercialization effort. Valid patents stimulate market growth and innovation, generate revenue, prevent unnecessary licensing, and reduce infringement lawsuits. Obtaining patents can add value to the bottom line of a company by increasing its intangible assets and, more importantly, enhance the company's power in the marketplace by providing it with the right to stop others from making or using the invention without permission. Understanding the patent process, the patent landscape, and white-space opportunities are essential to translational research and the development of innovations for clinical use. White-space opportunity, a metaphor about opportunity, is defined variously: as a business space where there is little or no competition, or it refers to entirely new markets, or it indicates gaps in existing markets or product lines.

Freedom-to-operate or FTO (also called "product clearance" or "right to use" opinions) is another important patent concept that researchers should become fluent with so that they are aware of the patents in existence when developing novel technologies in the first place. This will help (i) identify technology in development that could potentially infringe valid patents and lead to enforcement action on the part of the patent holder (a time-consuming and expensive process for both parties); and (ii) assist researchers in protecting their own IP by assessing their inventions and the scope of protecting them via patents relative to other art in their field of research. In other words, FTOs are often used to determine whether a particular action, such as testing or commercializing a product, can be done without infringing valid patents belonging to others. Because patents are specific to different jurisdictions, a FTO analysis should relate to particular countries or regions where you want to operate or commercialize your nanoproduct. FTO analysis involves identifying and analyzing patents belonging to others that may subject your company to patent infringement liability. To limit its risk of potential litigation and avoid unnecessary expenses, a FTO should be performed before developing and launching a new product or before acquiring a new company. Preferably, in nanomedicine, it should be done during the preclinical stage so that the company is able to (i) modify the product to work around the patent and avoid future infringement before reaching a point of no return, (ii) identify additional opportunities for patenting or further R&D, or (iii) analyze its business position and have an opportunity to take out a license.

Details on nanopatents, including the legal criteria necessary to obtain a US patent and the prosecution process for obtaining a US patent, can be found elsewhere [24–26].

In spite of scanty product development, nanopatent filings and grants have continued unabated. However, it is no secret that nanopatents of dubious scope and breath, especially on foundational nanomaterials and upstream nanotechnologies, have been routinely granted by patent offices. In fact, "patent prospectors" have been on a global quest for "nanopatent land grabs" since the early to mid-1980s [24–27]. As a result, patent thickets in certain sectors of nanotechnology have arisen that could have a chilling impact on commercialization activities. A patent thicket is a dense web of overlapping patent claims that can potentially impede a company to commercialize new technology. They may also require innovators to reach licensing deals with multiple partners for multiple patents. For example, the US carbon nanotube patent landscape is a tangled mess, mainly due to issuance of multiple US patents in error by the PTO. Also to blame for this is the fact that there is a lack of nanonomenclature whereby inventors and scientists have employed distinct terms to refer to CNTs. As a result, contrary to the foundations of US patent law, various US patents on CNTs have been granted with legally identical claims [28]. The expected negative impact on commercialization and patent litigation has not arrived as of now because CNTs have failed to deliver on the hype. Fabrication of affordable and high-quality CNTs has not materialized and scientists are now pursuing other exciting materials such as graphene instead. Hype and technology often evolve together and, in the case of CNTs, the "peak of inflated expectations" of the 1990s was replaced by the "trough of disillusionment" in the early 2000s [29].

Patent offices continue to be under enormous strain and scrutiny. Issues ranging from poor patent quality, questionable examination practices, inadequate search capabilities, rising attrition, poor examiner morale, and an enormous patent backlog are just a few issues that need reform. The nomenclature issue (next section) is also affecting patent drafting and prosecution at patent offices.

28.4 Terminology and Nomenclature: Lost in Translation

In the heady days of any emerging technology, definitions tend to abound and are only gradually documented in reports, journals, handbooks, and dictionaries. Ultimately, standard-setting organizations such as the International Organization for Standardization (ISO) and American Society for Testing and Materials (ASTM) International produce technical specifications. This evolution is typical and essential, as the development of terminology is a prerequisite for creating a common, valid language needed for effective communication in any field. Clearly, a similar need for an internationally-agreed definition for key nano terms has gained urgency. Nomenclature, technical specifications, standards, guidelines, and best practices are critically needed to advance nano in a safe and responsible manner. Contrary to some commentators, terminology does matter because it prevents misinterpretation and confusion. It is also necessary for research activities, harmonized regulatory governance, accurate patent searching and application drafting, standardization of procedures, manufacturing and quality controls, assay protocols, the grant review process, decisions by policymakers, ethical analysis, public discourse, safety assessment, and more. Also, nomenclature is crucial to any translational and commercialization effort.

Although various "nano" terms, including "nanotechnology," "nanoscience," "nanopharmaceutical," "nanodrug," "nanotherapeutic," "nanomaterial," "nanopharmacy," and "nanomedicine" are widely used, there is confusion, disagreement, and ambiguity regarding their definitions. In fact, there is no precise definition of nanotechnology as applied to pharmaceuticals or in reference to drug delivery. This haunts regulators, patent offices, policymakers, drug formulation scientists, pharma executives, and legal professionals. Clearly, the current definitions for various nano terms are inadequate. All definitions of nanotechnology based on size or dimensions should be dismissed, especially in the context of nanomedicine and nanodrugs, for reasons well articulated elsewhere [30]. There is simply no scientific basis or logic to limiting all nanotechnology to a sub-100 nm limitation [30]. Moreover, nano is not solely a metric of length, and nanoscale researchers do not accept such rigid limitations on dimensionality.

In the absence of any formal definition for a nanotherapeutic formulation (sometimes referred to as Nanoscale Drug Delivery System or NDDS or nanodrug product), I define it as (i) a formulation, often colloidal, containing therapeutic particles (nanoparticles) ranging in size from 1 to 1000 nm; and (ii) either (a) the carrier(s) is/are the therapeutic (i.e., a conventional therapeutic agent is absent) or (b) the therapeutic is coupled (functionalized, solubilized, entrapped, coated, etc.) to a carrier.

Nanoscale therapeutics may have unique properties (nanocharacter) that can be beneficial for drug delivery and other applications but there is no specific size range or dimensional limit where superior properties are found [30–32]. A change in properties of particulate materials in relation to particle size is basically a continuum and there is no clear size cutoff for novel properties as they can happen above 100 nm [30]. Hence, the size limitation below 100 nm cannot be touted as the basis of novel properties of nanotherapeutics. Often, nanotherapeutics (Figure 28.1) are colloidal drug delivery systems having a particle size of 1–1000 nm. Furthermore, there are numerous FDA-approved and/or marketed nanodrug products where the particle size does not fit the sub-100 nanometer profile proposed by the US National Nanotechnology Initiative (NNI) in the early 1990s: Abraxane (~130 nm), Myocet (~190 nm), Amphotec (~130 nm), Epaxal (~150 nm), Inflexal (~150 nm), Lipo-Dox (180 nm), Oncaspar (50–200 nm), Copaxone (1.5–550 nm), and so on. Therefore, the arbitrary sub-nano cutoff proposed by the NNI is irrelevant in the context of nanomedicine. The NNI definition has been correctly criticized over the years [30–32]. It was poorly thought-out and the NNI needs to set the record straight by rescinding it. The FDA, which was involved in the formulation of this inaccurate sub-100 nm NNI definition, has not adopted any "official" regulatory definition for nanotechnology, nanotherapeutic, or nanoscale. However, since 2011, following the publication of a "draft" guidance document, it uses an awkward, loose, and "unofficial" size-based definition. According to the FDA, engineered nanoproducts or products that employ nanotechnology either (i) have at least one dimension in the 1–100 nm range or (ii) are of a size range of up to 1000 nm (i.e., 1 μm), provided the novel/unique properties or phenomenon (including physical/chemical properties or biological effects) exhibited are attributable to these dimensions greater than 100 nm.

Viable *sui generis* definition of nano having a bright-line size range (especially as applied to nanodrugs) blurs with respect to what is truly nanoscale; it is unnecessary, misleading, and in fact, may never be feasible. Given this backdrop, I proposed the following definition of nanotechnology about a decade ago, one that is unconstrained by an arbitrary size limitation or dimension [26]: *The design, characterization, production, and application of structures, devices, and systems by controlled manipulation of size and shape at the nanometer scale (atomic, molecular, and macromolecular scale) that produces structures, devices, and systems with at least one novel/superior characteristic or property.* My definition has four interrelated key features:

- First, it recognizes that the properties and performance of the synthetic, engineered *structures, devices, and systems* are inherently rooted in their nanoscale dimensions. The definition focuses on the unique physiological behavior of these *structures, devices, and systems* that is occurring *at the nanometer scale*; it does not focus on any shape, aspect ratio, specific size, or dimensionality.

- Second, the focus of this flexible definition is on "technology" that has commercial potential from a consumer perspective, not "nanoscience" or basic research conducted in a laboratory setting that may lack commercial implication.
- Third, the *structures, devices, and systems* that result must be *novel/superior* compared to their bulk, conventional counterparts.
- Fourth, the concept of *controlled manipulation* compared to "self-assembly" is critical to the definition.

Apart from creating confusion in the nanomedicine community and among relevant stakeholders, there are concerns that this definitional issue could continue to pose a major bottleneck to translational efforts. It is apparent that it has contributed to the evolving patent thicket in certain sectors along with a lack of specific protocols for preclinical development, slower nanomaterial characterization, and pollution in the scientific literature. If translational nanomedicine is to become robust, it is important that some order, central coordination, and uniformity be introduced at the transnational level to address the rise of diverse nano terms seen in patents, journals, and the press. This is also critical to prevent a significant scientific, legal, and regulatory void from developing, all of which will negatively affect translational efforts.

28.5 Gaps in Regulatory Guidance

Transparent and effective governmental regulatory guidance is critical for nanomedical translation. However, emerging technologies such as nanomedicine are particularly problematic for governmental regulatory agencies to handle, given their independent nature, slow response rate, significant inertia, and a general mistrust of industry. Major global regulatory systems, bodies, and regimes regarding nanomedicines are not fully mature, hampered in part by a lack of specific protocols for preclinical development and characterization. Additionally, in spite of numerous harmonization talks and meetings, there is lack of consensus on procedures, assays, and protocols to be employed during preclinical development and characterization of nanomedicines. On the other hand, there is a rise of diverse nanospecific regulatory arrangements and systems, contributing to a dense global nanotechnology regulatory landscape, full of gaps and devoid of central coordination [33–37]. It is often observed that governmental regulatory bodies lack technical and scientific knowledge to support risk-based regulation, thereby leaving a significant regulatory void. In fact, the "baby steps" the FDA has undertaken over the past decade have led to regulatory uncertainty. The bumpy ride is expected to continue [33].

28.6 Conclusions and Outlook

Efforts are underway to bridge the translational gap between benchtop preclinical research and bedside medial applications with nanoproducts, nanomaterials, nanotherapeutics, and so on. Practical considerations should be at the forefront to streamline and improve translational nanomedicine (Table 28.3). This, in turn, will enable delivering more therapies rapidly, safely, and effectively to patients globally. It is important to optimally integrate healthcare, academia, and industry to achieve changes at various levels along the translational path (Table 28.3). These are critical to transforming nanomedicine and improving the performance of its supply chain for the benefit of all stakeholders.

In a big pharma and biotech setting, enhancing translational nanomedicine will require a corporate cultural change, and senior leadership commitment to advocate and implement the changes. I believe that issues such as effective patent reform, adaptive regulatory guidance, robust governmental efforts, and consumer health are all intertwined and require special attention while addressing nanomedicine translation from the bench to the bedside. In this regard, science-based governance that promotes translation on one hand and balances consumer health on the other is crucial.

A concerted international approach is the only way to overcome the complex barriers confronting translational medicine, and by extension, translational nanomedicine. No one entity, organization, or institution can operate in isolation or undertake the task individually. Serious efforts in the past decade involve streamlining the research approval process and reducing regulatory burdens to push translational medicine. In the United States, the National Center for Advancing Translational Sciences (NCATS) was established in 2012 with its mission to "catalyze the generation of innovative methods and technologies that will enhance the development, testing, and implementation of diagnostics and therapeutics across a wide range of human diseases and conditions" [38]. Similarly, there are other entities dedicated to serving as "adapters" and "deriskers" between basic research entities and commercial organizations (Table 28.4). These key players must come together on a global platform to address issues affecting translational efforts. Despite geographic diversity and organization-specific mandates, they must leverage expertise, share best practices, and pool their experiences. Obviously, integrating and leveraging their cumulative knowledge will lead to improved health outcomes for patients.

It is important that the public's desire for novel nanomedical products, venture community's modest investment, federal infusion of funds, and big pharma's lingering interest in nanomedicine continue. In the end, the long-term prognosis and development of nanomedicine will hinge on effective regulatory policies, issuance of valid patents, clearer safety guidelines, transparency, and full commitment of all stakeholders involved – big pharma, academia, governmental regulatory agencies, policymakers, the venture community, disease advocacy groups, and the consumer-patient. We need everyone on board so that translation

Table 28.3 From the lab to the clinic: improving translational nanomedicine.

- Research scientists in academia should understand the entire supply chain from research to development, including basic concepts relevant to commercialization.
- Granting agencies and peer reviewers that review grants should have expertise in translational medicine, industrial portfolio management, and commercialization of research to properly access feasibility of proposals that have a greater potential for patient application. It is very important that review panels or committees should reflect appropriate balance of technical, business, venture, and commercialization expertise. Proposals and submissions should seek/include criteria to evaluate whether the research is capable of clinical application. Funding projects should be evaluated in terms of realistic potential of making it to the clinic rather than specific disease targets. In other words, the mindset needs to be changed from a "product-" to a "patient"-oriented approach in nanomedical product development.
- There is an urgent need for coordinated education and training programs. Educational institutions and universities should offer more interdisciplinary/hybrid courses and graduate training modules where applied research, business landscaping, intellectual property law, FDA regulatory issues, and the patent process are emphasized. Courses for healthcare personnel, researchers, physicians, pharmacists, and nurses should focus on more in-depth instruction. The public should be educated via more innovative portals of education both directly and through the news media and Internet regarding both the possibilities and limitations of nanomedicine along with its translational potential.
- Academic researchers should be encouraged to develop innovative translatable products. Academic research that is advertised as being applied or translational should have to demonstrate a minimum threshold requirement on realistic chances to help patients prior to funding. Portfolios and projects should be developed and evaluated with an eye on applied research; even basic research should be analyzed to determine such potential. Academia and industry must enhance collaborative efforts to address the nonreproducibility of preclinical research that primarily emanates from academic research laboratories. Universities may consider establishing a "gap fund" to support translation studies in light of diminished grant funding.
- Regional harmonization efforts (rather than global) should be undertaken with respect to bridging studies and the design of clinical trials for nanomedicines.
- Matrices and stringent evaluation criteria should be employed throughout a funded "applied" academic project to see how successful it is with respect to translation and whether it merits continued funding.
- Advanced manufacturing technologies must be explored that enable more control over size and shape that allow surface modifications using covalent and noncovalent approaches to fabricate precisely defined nanoscale drug delivery systems (NDDS). Top-down nanocolloid fabrication techniques such as photolithography, microfluidic synthesis, and molding technology such as particle replication in nonwetting templates are of particular interest to overcome the limitations of conventional bottom-up fabrication methods. Flexible and adaptive manufacturing ("on demand") are important in this context to add to market availability.
- On a case-by-case basis and in conjunction with industry, the FDA (and analogous regulatory agencies) should identify unique safety issues associated with nanoparticles and nanomedical products. The agency should meet its regulatory and statutory obligations by offering technical advice and guidance to industry beyond what its track record currently reflects. With industry input, a comprehensive public databank relating to the biological interactions of engineered nanomaterials (ENMs) should be generated. The FDA should actively seek product safety data from industry where FDA statutory authority exists for premarket review. Furthermore, it should incentivize and encourage voluntary industry submissions of safety data on nanomaterials or products that incorporate nanotechnology

prior to market launch, especially in cases (e.g., cosmetics) where the FDA lacks statutory authority for premarket review. FDA's excessive reliance on publicly available or voluntarily submitted information, adverse event reporting, and on postmarket surveillance activities may not be ideal in the case of engineered nanomaterials (ENMs) for human use.

- Laboratories that focus on clinical applications should implement quality assurance systems such as Good Clinical Practice (GCP), Good Manufacturing Practice (GMP) and Good Laboratory Practice (GLP), especially if submitting data to regulatory agencies.
- Key questions should be asked early on during the development phase of the project: is the idea patentable, will it help patients in a clinical setting, is the clinical hypothesis backed by generated preclinical data, is there freedom-to-operate with respect to the patent estate and commercial landscape, is it likely to be reimbursed by insurance companies, is there a need commercially, is there a significant market size, are major safety issues addressed, is the immunology and pharmacology well studied, are all components (active, carrier, excipient, etc.) well characterized, are there unique safety concerns due to the nanoscale, are there excessive fabrication costs and complexities, and so on.
- Science policymakers should subsidize more risky research strategies, incentivize strategy diversity, and encourage publication of failed experiments/negative data – all of these activities are known to increase the speed of discovery. Medical and basic science journal editors should strengthen the peer-review process, mandate sufficient data and methods to reproduce reported research, seek inclusion of information on data provenance, publish software codes used for data analysis, and seek data manipulation steps done by hand that were not included in the software code.
- University Technology Transfer Offices (TTOs) should be revamped and required to disclose the return-on-investment (ROI) in terms of funds expended on patent prosecution versus licensing royalties generated.
- Quality assurance (QA) guidelines for basic research published by the WHO or RQA should be implemented by laboratories to safeguard data and ensure scientific rigor. Digital manipulation or errors can be minimized or prevented via "read-only files" stored on laboratory instruments. Strengthening data standards and methods transparency in scientific publications should be supported to enable replication of published results. Granting agencies should require proof that instruments have been calibrated and that plans exist for tracing data, including which equipment the experiment was conducted on and where the source data are stored.
- Recognizing genuine requests for scrutiny from harassment in a climate of research transparency is essential to safeguarding the research community and driving translational efforts.
- Consensus-testing protocols to provide benchmarks for the creation of classes of nanoscale materials, both engineered and native, should be developed. In addition, reference classes for ENMs that are synthesized and characterized need to be cataloged prior to translation. This can be accomplished by creating a minimum universal set of characterization techniques via currently available tools and tests. This effort can be supplemented by developing unique tools, imaging modalities, and techniques. Mathematical and computer models for risk/benefit analysis that can monitor quality, safety, and effectiveness *vis-à-vis* standard ENMs are other options. Since minor variations in the physicochemical characteristics of nanotherapeutics (nanomaterial + API) can affect safety, immunogenicity and efficacy, multiple methods based on different principles should be employed during nanomaterial and API assessment. Innovative *in vitro/ex vivo*, *in silico*, and *in vivo* (animal) screening systems, including novel 3D cell systems (3D tumor spheroids), may be required. In this context, it is important to employ methods relevant to the specific route of administration that are standardized, validated, and widely accepted by researchers and regulatory agencies alike. However, it is critical to conduct all these assays and tests under biologically relevant conditions such as the microenvironment of an immunocompromised cancer patient or a patient whose plasma proteins produce "protein coronas."

(*continued*)

Table 28.3 From the lab to the clinic: improving translational nanomedicine.

- Existing methodologies should be adapted, as well as new paradigms should be developed for evaluating *in vivo* animal and clinical data pertaining to safety and efficacy of nanomedical products before and during the product life cycle. Guidance should elaborate specifics as to what kind of data are required at each step of the nanomedical translational process.
- Early sponsor interaction with the FDA in the development process is helpful to identify appropriate pathways to be navigated. File patent applications (regular and provisional) at an early stage to capture upstream aspects of nanomedical products and employ an interdisciplinary team of patent attorneys or patent agents to draft applications. The regulatory review process, patent prosecution at patent offices, and business developments should all be coordinated throughout translation.
- Since there are few protocols to characterize nanomedicines at the physicochemical, biological, and physiological levels, it is essential to develop a research strategy that involves adsorption, distribution, metabolism, and excretion (ADME) studies. An improvement of physiologically based models for the prediction of the impact of formulation changes on drug exposure and its variability is in order. A holistic approach to understanding ADME can be realized through the integration of mechanistic ADME data through the mathematical algorithms that underpin physiologically based pharmacokinetic (PBPK) modeling, routinely utilized to support regulatory submissions for conventional medicines in the United States by the FDA and in Europe by the EMA. Although advances in PBPK reflect significant advances in the predictability of critical pharmacokinetics (PK) parameters from physical chemistry, *in vitro* data and software platforms/databases, challenges persist with respect to making critical decisions in early and clinical drug development and in the selection of individualized dosing regimens.
- Toxicology tests should be developed and physicochemical characterization (PCC) studies for nanomaterials conducted. Although complexity and diversity of nanomedicines pose a problem, biocompatibility and immunotoxicity must be taken into consideration during preclinical assessment. Also, standards that correlate the biodistribution of various nanomaterials with safety/efficacy (by using parameters such as size, surface charge, stability, surface characteristics, solubility, crystallinity, and density) need further assessment.
- Integrating and leveraging cumulative knowledge regarding translational barriers (Table 28.1) will lead to improved health outcomes for patients. International regulatory harmonization efforts and formal treaties with relevant stakeholders should be further explored. The unique entities that have been recently established (Table 28.4) must leverage expertise and pool their experiences despite geographical diversity or organization-specific mandates.
- Allow greater patient input into drug development, regulatory processes and clinical trial design. Manufacturers should seek patient perspective early on in product development. Furthermore, patient information and data should be more readily shared for research, especially with respect to chronic diseases. It is essential to find appropriate balance between safeguarding access to an individual's health information and sharing that data for public health with guaranteed anonymity. However, for these recommendations to become a reality, clearer policies and guidelines may be needed via governmental action so that companies do not risk legal issues, patient privacy is safeguarded and data security is ensured.
- Enhance and streamline institutional review board (IRB) approval process to minimize unnecessary delays and redundancy.
- International harmonization efforts regarding biosimilar versions of biologics need to be undertaken as a large number of nanomedicines are biologics. The EMA guidelines (divided into three sections) versus the FDA issued draft guidance (clearly identifying a stepwise approach) need to be reconciled.

Table 28.4 Major global translational science organizations.

Organization	Mission and objectives	Year Founded	Location
The Center for Drug Research and Development (CDRD) www.cdrd.ca	Headquartered in Vancouver, CDRD is Canada's fully integrated national drug development and commercialization center. Its basic mandate is to successfully bridge the commercialization gap between academia and industry, and translate preclinical research discoveries into new therapies for patients. It works in partnership with academia, industry, government, and foundations to provide expertise and infrastructure to enable researchers from leading health research institutions to advance promising early-stage drug candidates, and transform them into commercially viable investment opportunities for the private sector – and ultimately into innovative new therapies for patients. In doing so, CDRD is actively growing Canada's health sciences industry into a wholly optimized generator of economic prosperity for the country. According to CDRD, it works with excellent organizations to develop funding partnerships aimed at advancing and commercializing selected promising discoveries. Since becoming operational in 2008, it has established four such innovation funds to support projects. CDRD utilizes the expertise of around 100 scientific, commercial, and project management experts located in its facilities covering over 40 000 ft^2 of translational research space with additional sites of specialized expertise in the form of select partnerships across the country. Six related scientific divisions have been created to assist investigators with capabilities and infrastructure supporting the drug development process that mirrors the drug development processes – target validation, screening, medicinal chemistry, drug delivery, pharmacology/toxicology, and biologics. CDRD experts have interacted with about 1700 academic investigators to date, providing commercial education, advice, and input into their technologies. From these discussions, CDRD has taken on approximately 210 drug development (translational) projects, and has collaborated to derisk and advance the technologies toward commercialization. CDRD has already achieved a number of key milestones and	2008	Canada

(continued)

Table 28.4 (*Continued*)

Organization	Mission and objectives	Year Founded	Location
	outcomes, making a significant impact on Canada's drug development environment: 1052 drug development projects evaluated; 828 potential projects/technologies reviewed; 209 projects undertaken (on 134 distinct technologies); 56 projects advanced toward commercialization and/or commercialized (51 ongoing); 12 technologies out-licensed to the private sector or under current development/management; 5 spin-off companies launched; 95 affiliated institutions; 33 new patent families supported with CDRD data; 23 collaborations on scientific publications; $90.7 million in grant funding facilitated for PIs and their CDRD-related projects; over $40 million in international pharmaceutical sector investment attracted; $220 million in incremental commercially focused health research being conducted as a result of CDRD; 157 postdoctoral fellows, co-op students and interns through the CDRD Training Program; and over 98 drug development and commercialization workshops and seminars offered.		
The European Infrastructure for Translational Medicine (EATRIS ERIC) www.eatris.eu	EATRIS provides access to innovative translational research infrastructure and expertise for companies and researchers in need of support for advancing biomedical innovations. It is comprised of over 70 leading academic groups and institutions in 10 European countries. According to EATRIS, this infrastructure provides a single point-of-access to the right expertise and facilities, expedites the development process, and provides access to large and diverse clinical patient cohorts. This is possible since EATRIS is able to leverage its state-of-the-art facilities and knowledge across Europe that reduces translational research risks and bottlenecks. EATRIS institutes offer a pipeline in the areas of advanced therapy medicinal products (ATMP) and biologics; biomarkers; imaging and tracing; small molecules, and vaccines. Since Europe's leading academic hospitals are part of the EATRIS infrastructure, a broad range of patient cohorts, including patients with the burden of rare diseases, are registered in the EATRIS databases. Funders encourage projects that have a high translational potential and that have been shortlisted for funding.	2013	Europe

	The core process involves a four-steps comprising: • *Translational Assessment*: Confirmation of the unmet medical need, clear end product envisaged, innovative character and IP clarity • *Matchmaking*: Identification from the EATRIS database of the innovative infrastructure, facilities and expertise required to support the project, including patient cohorts. • *Exploration:* The client reviews the project content and the EATRIS institutions selected. Definition of the project plan, or optionally the creation of a complete Project Development Plan, including optimal regulatory strategy is undertaken. • *Initiation:* At this final stage, bilateral contracts are executed between the client and EATRIS institution. One or more EATRIS institutions execute the project. Identification of relevant translational tools and facilities for optimal data generation Projects can fall into different categories as follows: • EATRIS helps on addressing scientific and technical challenges to reduce, remove bottlenecks in translational research. • EATRIS works with funders to improve the success chances of their translational projects, through the utilization of innovative academic infrastructure and expertise. • EATRIS aims to create a seamless innovation pipeline for biomedical innovation, and partners with key stakeholders in the science, regulatory, and funding domains to reach these ends. • EATRIS also provides troubleshooting support for certain ongoing projects.		
MRC Technology (MRCT) www.mrctechnology.org	MRCT is an independent life science medical research charity that helps bridge the gap between basic research and commercial application. Its goal is to ensure that promising life science research reaches its full potential in patient treatments and diagnostics, thereby bridging the "valley of death." It is self-funded and works with academic, pharmaceutical, biotechnology, and charity organizations from around the world. It has helped launch 12 drugs and form 18 start-ups, negotiated over 400	2000	UK

(*continued*)

Table 28.4 (*Continued*)

Organization	Mission and objectives	Year Founded	Location
	commercial licenses, and generated over £600+ million in royalty revenues for its academic and charity partners, with global pharma revenues from this research being over £40+ billion. MRCT experts can accelerate research to generate novel small-molecule or biologic drugs. MRCT's Centre for Therapeutics Discovery and Centre for Diagnostics Development can develop new standard assays, adapt older ones, carry out high-throughput screening using in-house compound libraries, or develop structure–activity relationships (SAR) to improve potency, solubility, and physicochemical properties of hit series to turn them into drug-like molecules. MRCT scientists can synthesize antibodies to obtain optimal binding affinity, functional efficacy, and robust biophysical properties to generate a lead candidate. Discoveries are always protected to ensure return on investment if commercialized. intellectual property (IP) and commercialization expertise ensures novel IP and robust supporting data packages suitable for collaborating. According to MRCT, some partners outsource their entire tech transfer operation, from IP management through to commercialization, while others need help run specific projects for their Tech-Transfer Offices (TTOs). According to MRCT, its approach involves the following: • *Identifying and evaluating research:* Expert MRCT teams examine existing research portfolios and look for projects with potential for further development. The teams also offer services to ensure that future research funding is geared toward success. • *Protecting assets with potential:* Specialized IP management expertise on the partner's promising healthcare research is offered. Expert advice on further potential development routes and access to funding is also available. • *Investing in promising projects*: MRCT's specialist drug discovery, diagnostics, and medical device centers are available to both research and industry partners. MRCT		

	also invests their own resources in projects with real potential and have built an excellent record of accomplishment in developing drug targets. • *Partnering with industry:* MRCT develops projects to a stage where they have strong commercial potential, and then work with its industry partners to continue their development to market. Revenue streams are ultimately used to fund further research MRCT has joined the Alliance of Leading Drug Discovery and Development Centres, which aims to improve the rate at which academic research is translated into new medicines. In an effort to identify and develop new treatments for dementia, it has launched a Dementia Consortium with the charity Alzheimer's Research UK, Lilly and Eisai.		
The National Center for Advancing Translational Sciences (NCATS) www.ncats.nih.gov	NCATS at the National Institutes of Health (NIH) was established to transform the translational science process so that new treatments and cures for disease can be delivered to patients faster and more efficiently by identifying system-wide scientific and operational impediments in the translational research. Emphasizing innovation and relying on data and novel technologies, NCATS develops, demonstrates, and disseminates improvements in translational science: the focus is to bring to patients new drugs, diagnostics, and medical devices much faster. NCATS works through an array of funding programs, collaborative research projects, and preclinical and clinical tools designed to catalyze translational medicine. NCATS offers a variety of training and educational opportunities in translational medicine ranging from the Assay Guidance Manual eBook and workshop to research training experiences for scientists, to the Translational Science Training Program for NIH graduate students and postdoctoral researchers. Through its Clinical and Translational Science Awards (CTSA) Program, NCATS supports an innovative national network of more than 50 medical research centers that work together to improve the translational research process via collaboration and innovation in training, research tools, and processes. The NCATS Division of Pre-Clinical Innovation contains multiple programs and research groups that collaborate with academic, nonprofit, and industry researchers to develop promising therapeutic candidates.	2012	US

(continued)

Table 28.4 (*Continued*)

Organization	Mission and objectives	Year Founded	Location
	According to the NCATS, the following are some of the current initiatives and programs: • *Funding Opportunity Announcements (FOAs):* The majority of NCATS awards are for applications sent in response to FOAs. NCATS develops FOAs with an aim to stimulate translational research in areas of greatest need and for identified gaps in diagnostics and therapy development. • *Small Business Grants and Contracts:* NCATS' small business programs, including Small Business Innovation Research (SBIR) and Small Business Technology Transfer (STTR), help entrepreneurs develop and commercialize new translational technologies through grant and contract awards. It supports further development of preclinical and clinical tools, instruments, devices, and related methodologies that may have broad application to translational research. • *Collaboration Opportunities:* NCATS encourages partnerships across all scientific disciplines and research sectors, including with NIH investigators, universities, and medical centers, US federal agencies, small businesses, industry, patient groups, and advocacy organizations • *Expertise and Resources:* NCATS staff offers experts in many different fields relevant to translational research and science policy, from small molecules to human subject protections. It offers a variety of preclinical and clinical tools plus resources for patient/community engagement and health information. • *Scientific Conference Support:* NCATS offers to domestic institutions and organizations, including established scientific or professional societies, scientific conference grants to support high quality, national and internal meetings that are relevant to public health, and the NCATS mission.		

Therapeutic Innovation Australia (TIA) www.therapeuticinnovation.com.au	TIA, a not-for-profit organization funded through Australian Government Department of Education, supports Australian researchers in taking promising medical research from the laboratory and translating it into clinical application. Its mission is to improve the efficiency and effectiveness of translational health research through leveraging investments in research infrastructure. This is accomplished via a national institutional network of 45+ sites located at 11 universities, 12 medical research organizations, 15 hospitals, and clinical networks that enable development of small molecules, biotherapeutics, cell therapies, and biomarkers. TIA forms a central partnering function between researchers, capability managers, and experts in product development from academic and industry sectors. According to TIA, in 2013–2014, TIA supported 67 proof-of-concept products and 80 clinical trials. Its strategy employs the following: • Funding critical research for successful translational outcomes. • Supporting linkage between translational health researchers and closure of infrastructural gaps. • International engagement to maximize translational efficiency. • Provide facilitated pathways for translational researchers in critical areas such as biomarkers, drug development, and cell therapies. TIA is supported through enabling infrastructure that includes a national registry of medical research projects (ATRAX) and an online document repository of 560 open-access generic documents (templates) that can be adapted for use in establishing or extending quality systems (www.iqdocs.org). Seminars that focus on translational science are held to foster collaboration and build understanding between academia and industry.	2011	Australia

becomes more widespread and we can advance innovative nanomedical products to patients, especially in high unmet disease areas. We must endure and traverse the valley of death for the overall benefit of society. Together, we can help drive progress and make the future happen faster. *For the times they are a-changin.*

28.7
Disclosures and Conflict of Interest

The author declares that he has no conflict of interest and has no affiliations or financial involvement with any organization or entity discussed in this chapter. Currently, the author is a Scientific Advisor to Teva Pharmaceutical Industries, Ltd., Israel. No writing assistance was utilized in the production of this chapter and the author has not received any payment for its preparation. Parts of this chapter are adapted, with permission, from the author's recent book chapter [39].

References

1 Weissig, V., Pettinger, T.K., and Murdock, N. (2014) Nanopharmaceuticals (Part 1): products on the market. *Int. J. Nanomed.*, **9**, 4357–4373.

2 Farhangrazi, Z.S. and Moghimi, S.M. (2016) Nanomedicine: shadow and substance, in *Handbook of Clinical Nanomedicine: Law, Business, Regulation, Safety, and Risk* (Eds R. Bawa, G. Audette, and B. Reese), Pan Stanford Publishing, Singapore, pp. 1081–1090.

3 Butler, D. (2008) Crossing the valley of death. *Nature*, **453**, 840–842.

4 Tufts Center for the Study of Drug Development (2016) Available at http://csdd.tufts.edu/news/complete_story/pr_tufts_csdd_2014_cost_study (accessed April 20, 2016).

5 Cohrs, R.J., Martin, T., Ghahramani, P., Bidaut, L., Higgins, P.J., and Shahzad, A. (2015) Translational medicine definition by the European Society for Translational Medicine. *New Horiz. Transl. Med.*, **2**, 86–88.

6 NIH Roadmap for Medical Research (2016) Available at http://pubs.niaaa.nih.gov/publications/arh311/12-13.pdf (accessed March 17, 2016).

7 Woodcock, J. and Woosley, R. (2008) The FDA critical path initiative and its influence on new drug development. *Annu. Rev. Med.*, **59**, 1–12.

8 (a) Baker, M. (2016) Quality time. *Nature*, **529**, 456–458. (b) Baker, M. (2015) Irreproducible biology research costs put at $28 billion per year. *Nature*. doi: 10.1038/nature.2015.1771 (c) Baker, M. (2016) Is there a reproducibility crisis? *Nature*, **533**, 452–454.

9 Freedman, L.P., Cockburn, I.M., and Simcoe, T.S. (2015) The economics of reproducibility in preclinical research. *PLoS Biol.*, **13**, e1002165.

10 Prinz, F., Schlange, T., and Asadullah, K. (2011) Believe it or not: how much can we rely on published data on potential drug targets? *Nat. Rev. Drug Discov.*, **10**, 712–713.

11 Unreliable research: Trouble at the Lab. *The Economist*. Available at go.nature.com/dstij3. (accessed March 14, 2016).

12 Ioannidis, J.P.A. (2005) Why most published research findings are false. *PLoS Med.*, **2** (8), e124.

13 Begley, C.G., Buchan, A.M., and Dirnagl, U. (2015) Institutions must do their part for reproducibility. *Nature*, **525**, 25–27.

14 Collins, F.S. and Tabak, L.A. (2014) Policy: NIH plans to enhance reproducibility. *Nature*, **505**, 612–613.

15 Silberzahn, R. and Uhlmann, E.L. (2015) Many hands make tight work. *Nature*, **526**, 189–191.

16 Fishburn, C.S. (2015) Translational medicine: the changing role of big pharma, in *Principles of Translational Science in Medicine: From Bench to Bedside*, 2nd edn (ed. M. Wehling), Elsevier, pp. 313–325.

17 Errington, T.M. *et al.* (2014) An open investigation of the reproducibility of cancer biology research. *eLife*, **3**. doi: 10.7554/eLife.04333.

18 Dahlin, J.L. and Walters, M.A. (2014) The essential roles of chemistry in high-throughput screening triage. *Future Med. Chem.*, **6** (11), 1265–1290.

19 Baell, J. and Walters, M.A. (2014) Chemical con artists foil drug discovery. *Nature*, **513**, 481–483.

20 Baker, M. (2015) Blame it on the antibodies. *Nature*, **521**, 274–276.

21 Baker, M. (2015) Antibody anarchy: a call to order. *Nature*, **527**, 545–551.

22 Baker, M. (2016) Statisticians issue warning on *P* values. *Nature*, **531**, 151.

23 Wasserstein, R.L. and Lazar, N.A. (2016) The ASA's statement on *p*-values: context, process, and purpose. *AM Static.* doi: 10.1080/00031305.2016.1154108.

24 Bawa, R. (2009) Patenting inventions in bionanotechnology: a primer for scientists and lawyers, in *Bionanotechnology: Global Prospects* (ed. D.E. Reisner), CRC Press, Boca Raton, FL, pp. 309–337.

25 Bawa, R. (2007) Nanotechnology patent proliferation and the crisis at the US Patent Office. *Albany Law J. Sci. Technol.*, **17** (3), 699–735.

26 Bawa, R. (2007) Patents and nanomedicine. *Nanomedicine (Lond.)*, **2** (3), 351–374.

27 Bawa, R. (2017) Emerging issues in nanodrugs and nanomedicine, in *Biotechnology and the Law*, 2nd edn (eds H.B. Wellons and E.S. Ewing), American Bar Association, Chicago, IL.

28 Harris, D. and Bawa, R. (2007) The carbon nanotube patent landscape in nanomedicine: an expert opinion. *Expert Opin. Ther. Patents*, **17** (9), 1165–1174.

29 Davenport, M. (2015) Much ado about small things. *Chem. Eng. News*, **93** (23), 10–15.

30 Bawa, R. (2016) What's in a name? Defining "nano" in the context of drug delivery, in *Handbook of Clinical Nanomedicine: Nanoparticles, Imaging, Therapy, and Clinical Applications* (eds R. Bawa, G. Audette, and I. Rubinstein), Pan Stanford Publishing, Singapore, pp. 127–168.

31 Bawa, R. (2016) Racing ahead: nanomedicine under the microscope, in *Handbook of Clinical Nanomedicine: Law, Business, Regulation, Safety, and Risk* (eds R. Bawa, G. Audette, and B. Reese), Pan Stanford Publishing, Singapore, pp. xxxvii–li.

32 Kreyling, W.G., Semmler-Behnke, M., and Chaudhry, Q. (2010) A complementary definition of nanomaterial. *Nano Today*, **5**, 165–168.

33 Bawa, R. (2016) Baby steps, regulatory uncertainty and the bumpy road ahead, in *Handbook of Clinical Nanomedicine: Law, Business, Regulation, Safety, and Risk*, (eds R. Bawa, G. Audette, and B., Reese), Pan Stanford Publishing, Singapore, pp. 339–383.

34 Tinkle, S., McNeil, S.E., Mühlebach, S., Bawa, R., Borchard, G., Barenholz, Y., Tamarkin, L., and Desai, N. (2014) Nanomedicines: addressing the scientific and regulatory gap. *Ann. N Y Acad. Sci.*, **1313**, 35–56.

35 Owen, A., Rannard, S., Bawa, R., and Feng, S.-S. (2015) Editorial: interdisciplinary nanomedicine publications through interdisciplinary peer-review. *J. Interdiscip. Nanomed.*, **1** (1), 1–5.

36 Hodge, G.A., Bowman, D.M., and Maynard, A.D. (eds) (2010) *International Handbook on Regulating Nanotechnologies*, Edward Elgar Publishing, UK.

37 Bawa, R., Melethil, S., Simmons, W.J., and Harris, D. (2008) Nanopharmaceuticals: patenting issues and FDA regulatory challenges. *SciTech Lawyer*, **5** (2), 10–15.

38 National Center for Advancing Translational Sciences (2016) Available at ncats.nih.gov/ (accessed April 20, 2016).

39 Bawa, R., Bawa, S.R., and Mehra, R. (2016) The translational challenge in medicine at the nanoscale, in *Handbook of Clinical Nanomedicine: Law, Business, Regulation, Safety and Risk* (eds R. Bawa, G.F. Audette, and B.E. Reese), Pan Stanford Publishing, Singapore, pp. 1291–1346.

29
Development and Commercialization of Nanocarrier-Based Drug Products

Marianne Ashford

AstraZeneca, Pharmaceutical Sciences, Innovative Medicines Silk Road Business Park, Charter Way, Macclesfield, Cheshire SK10 2NA, UK

29.1
Drivers for New Medicines

There is still considerable unmet need in many diseases, including infection, cancer, diabetes, and cardiovascular disease, where modern society, increased global mobility, an aging population, and poor lifestyles fuel the need for better medicines. In cancer, particularly, although significant progress has been made and 5-year survival rates in many diseases have increased, there are few cancers where a total cure occurs despite the huge drive for cure over palliative care. In addition, as diagnosis of disease improves with developments in specific biomarkers and imaging, new treatments or even prophylactic therapy should be possible in a number of diseases.

A small-molecule drug still has approximately only 6% chance of reaching the market with the main reasons for failure (~90%) being related to safety or efficacy, thus a lack of robust therapeutic index [1]. To improve efficacy, more drug need to get into the diseased tissue, with less drug in other tissues; thus, greater site specificity is required. Therefore, considerably more work is needed if we are able even to partly realise Nobel Laureate Paul Ehrlich's "magic bullet" concept first envisioned in the 1890s.

The sequencing of the Human Genome completed in 2003 catapulted the understanding of medicine and the function of the genome. It is estimated that only 1–2% of the genome, ~30 000 genes code for disease-modifying proteins, and only ~30% of these proteins can be accessed by traditional small-molecule chemistries, monoclonal antibodies or antibody fragments. This has led to many new modalities being explored for their use as therapeutics such as DNA, mRNA, siRNA, microRNAs, antisense oligonucleotides, and more recently CRISPR-Cas9. These nucleic acid-based drugs interfere with protein production,

Pharmaceutical Nanotechnology: Innovation and Production, First Edition. Edited by Jean Cornier, Arno Kwade, Andrew Owen, and Marcel Van de Voorde.

either via knocking down or by expressing a protein rather than interacting with the expressed protein itself, as is the case with conventional drugs. This opens up "druggable space" and drugs against new targets can be prosecuted as long as the delivery challenges presented by these modalities can be overcome. A nanocarrier that can have a critical functional role in efficient intracellular delivery is likely to be an integral part of the product of these nucleic acid-based drugs.

In cancer, the emergence of resistance [2] and the practice of combination dosing drive the use of nanomedicines for more efficient delivery. By utilizing a nanomedicine approach and an endocytic rather than transmembrane diffusional entry into the cell, the cell surface will have less contact with the drug and multidrug resistance genes are less likely to be upregulated [3,4]. Combination therapy is becoming increasingly common in many diseases, particularly in oncology and infection. The main challenges of combination therapy are achieving synergistic concentrations of the drugs at the cell/tissue of interest at the same time and managing the tolerability of the combination. A nanocarrier can overcome these challenges by co-delivery.

The next generation of nanomedicines is likely to bring many benefits to patients. These include improving the ability to formulate poorly soluble drugs, improving the therapeutic index of drugs in a number of disease settings via a variety of approaches, enabling the delivery of the plethora of new drug modalities that require intracellular delivery, overcoming resistance, and enabling combination dosing. Nanomedicines have the ability to transform not only drug delivery but also drug discovery by enabling new medicinal products for patients with incurable diseases. Figure 29.1 shows the progression of modalities and delivery systems as more specific targeted delivery.

Nanomedicine is an interdisciplinary area, where nanoscience, nanoengineering, nanotechnology, novel biomaterials, novel chemistries, and multifunctional

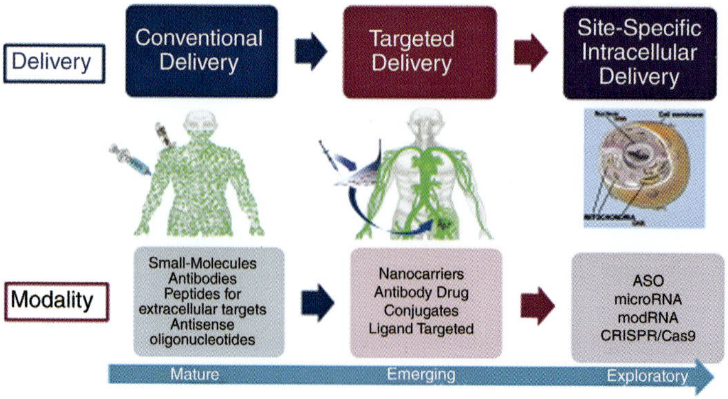

Figure 29.1 Progression of drug delivery.

nanocarriers will interact with life sciences, medicine, and disease understanding to bring new products to patients. Nanopharmacy is becoming an increasingly important discipline to enable their development and commercialization.

29.2 Current Marketed Nanomedicines

The majority of currently marketed nanocarrier formulations are liposomes and pegylated proteins (~40%). Nanomedicines have been shown to improve the therapeutic index of a relatively small number of small-molecule drugs to date (e.g., doxorubicin, amphotericin, paclitaxel, irinotecan). Most of these in the clinic have achieved this therapeutic index benefit, through improved toxicity rather than efficacy. There are many different types of nanomedicines in clinical trials in a range of disease segments (Section 29.4.2, also see Ref. [5]). Many of these are still aimed at improving therapeutic index, although increasingly nanomedicine approaches are being investigated as enabling technologies for intractable targets. The next section considers some of the leading marketed nanomedicine products, rationale for their development, as well as some development/manufacture issues they have encountered.

29.2.1 Amphotericin B Liposomal Products

Amphotericin B is a broad-spectrum antifungal drug; however, it has a number of dose-limiting toxicities, including nephrotoxicity and infusion-related reactions. It is an extremely lipophilic molecule with very low water solubility, so to enable intravenous delivery a number of lipid-based formulations have been developed. These have different lipid compositions and nanoparticle structures resulting in substantially different pharmacokinetic properties and tissue distribution [6].

A liposomal formulation of amphotericin B, AmBisome®, was approved by the EMA in 1990 and the FDA in 1997, for the treatment of severe fungal infections; it was the first marketed liposomal product. In AmBisome, the amphotericin is intercalated within the unilamellar liposomal bilayer and the drug is therefore an integral part of the overall structure of the liposomes. The liposomes consist of hydrogenated soy phosphatidylcholine:cholesterol:distearoyl phosphatidylglycerol (DSPG):amphotericin B in a 2 : 1 : 0.8 : 1 ratio and 9 : 1 lipid to drug ratio. They are 100 nm in diameter and have negative surface charge, which avoids rapid recognition by the MPS resulting in a prolonged circulation time and a large area under the concentration–time curve. Studies with labeled liposomes have shown that they accumulate at sites of fungal infections due to inflammation and an EPR effect. The product is a lyophilized powder that needs to be diluted prior to infusion.

AmBisome is also approved for visceral leishmaniosis, which is a parasitic neglected disease that can be fatal. It is included in the World Health Organization (WHO) Essential Medicines List, although it is difficult to access in many countries due to its high cost. Gilead who is currently the single source supplier and still has some patent exclusivity has partnered with the World Health Organization and other groups to make AmBisome available at discounted prices in developing countries.

A lipid complex of amphoterin B (Abelcet®) is marketed by the Liposome Company and was originally approved in the United States in 1995. It is composed of two lipids l-α-dimyristoyl phosphatidylcholine (DMPC) and l-α-dimyristoyl phosphatidylglycerol (DMPG) in a 7 : 3 molar ratio with an approximate 1 : 3 drug to lipid ratio (by weight). These lipid–amphotericin B complexes appear as large ribbon-like structures with a diameter in the 1.6–11 μm range. Due to this large size, following infusion, the complexes are recognized by macrophages and are taken up rapidly by the tissues of the MPS (e.g., liver and spleen). Consequently, the circulating amphotericin B plasma concentrations are low, the clearance rapid, and volume of distribution large.

Amphotericin B in a 1 : 1 molar ratio with cholesteryl sulfate produces a colloidal dispersion. It was previously marketed as both Amphocil® and Amphotec® and was initially approved in the United Kingdom in 1994 and by the FDA in 1996. Two molecules of amphotericin B bind to two molecules of cholesteryl sulfate, forming a tetramer that has both a hydrophilic and a hydrophobic portion. These tetramers aggregate into spiral arms that form a disk-type structure with a diameter of approximately 122 nm and a thickness of 4 nm. After intravenous infusion, the colloidal dispersion complexes remain largely intact and are rapidly removed from the circulation by cells of the MPS, predominately by Kupfer cells of the liver, and to a lesser extent in the spleen and bone marrow.

29.2.2
Doxil

Doxil® was the first nanomedicine to be approved by the FDA in 1995 for the treatment of Kaposi's sarcoma. This was followed by its European approval in 1997 under the brand name Caelyx. Doxil is currently indicated for ovarian cancer, AIDS-related Kaposi's sarcoma, and multiple myeloma.[1] It is a pegylated liposomal formulation of doxorubicin hydrochloride. The liposomes are ~100 nm in diameter with 10 000–15 000 drug molecules per liposome giving a lipid:drug ratio of 8 : 1. It is composed of fully hydrogenated soy phosphatidylcholine (HSPC), cholesterol, and a lipid with a polyethylene glycol head group (DSPE-PEG2000) in a molar ratio of 56.4 : 38.3 : 5.3. Drug loading is achieved

1) www.doxil.com (March 2016).

using a base exchange mechanism into preformed liposomes. The liposomes contain a high concentration of ammonium sulfate that results in exchange of the doxorubicin, a weak base, for ammonium ions across the lipid bilayer. The concentration of doxorubicin in the liposomes becomes higher than its intrinsic solubility, resulting in precipitation of doxorubicin sulfate crystals inside the liposome.

Reformulation of doxorubicin hydrochloride into this liposomal formulation resulted in reduced cardiotoxicity and alopecia compared to free doxorubicin. Although improving the original dose-limiting toxicities, this formulation resulted in new toxicities, most notably palmar–plantar erythrodysesthesia or "hand-foot syndrome," which is a redness, swelling, blistering and pain on the palms of the hands or soles of feet. This is thought to be due to the long circulation times and "burst" release of doxorubicin as liposomes are compressed as they extravasate through the small peripheral vessels close to the skin.

Doxil due to its PEG coating that inhibits protein adhesion (opsonization) and delays recognition of the liposomes by macrophage phagocytic system has extended circulation times of 3–4 days in humans. This prolonged plasma circulation time together with the enhanced permeability of blood vessels due to the enhanced permeability and retention (EPR) effect results in enhanced tumor accumulation [7]. Doxil is an important clinical drug whose usage continues to grow. It has been well studied and lessons learnt throughout its history have been documented by one of its inventors Barenholz [8].

The supply of Doxil has been plagued by issues since 2011 when the FDA found manufacture and sterility issues at the sterile manufacture facility where it was being manufactured at a CMO. The factory was subsequently closed and supply was interrupted. As commissioning manufacture and supply of a complex product takes time, this made way for a generic alternative. LipoDox was produced by Sun Pharmaceuticals in India to receive accelerated approval by the FDA using its abbreviated new drug application pathway in 2013. This is the first generic nanomedicine and its FDA approval was triggered by the unmet clinical need.

Creating the formulation for Doxil requires 17 different process vessels, specialized equipment, specially trained personnel with dedicated know-how, and takes 5 days. In contrast, a simple intravenous formulation needs only a few process vessels and a couple of steps. The associated process controls and analytical testing of such a complex product and process add to the cost and technical complexity. Sales of Doxil rose steadily until 2010 to $509 M when they took a sharp decline due to the supply issues,[2] which emphasize the importance of a robust manufacturing process and supply chain.

2) www.pharmacircle.com. March 2016.

29.2.3 Other Liposomal Products in Oncology

More recently, in 2015, the FDA approved Merrimack's irinotecan liposome injection, Onivyde®, for metastatic adenocarcinoma of the pancreas cancer in combination with fluorouracil (5-FU) and leucovorin in an expedited review. Irinotecan was originally approved as (Camptosar®) in 1996 for second-line colorectal cancer. It is a prodrug and is converted to the more potent SN38 predominantly in the liver. It was the first topoisomerase drug and appeared a very exciting compound based on preclinical studies in a number of cancer models. This potential, however, has not been realized in the clinic as humans do not produce SN38 as efficiently as mice. A pegylated liposomal formulation with 80 000 irinotecan molecules/liposome (~110 nm diameter) provides a long circulation time that allows greater accumulation in the tumor and local activation and release of SN38 from irinotecan.

Three nonpegylated liposomal formulations have also been approved. Myocet®, a nonpegylated liposomal formulation of the citrate salt of doxorubicin, is on some markets for metastatic breast cancer. It has a POPC:cholesterol molar ratio of 55.8 : 44.2 and the liposomes are about 150–180 nm in diameter. A daunorubicin liposomal formulation was approved in the United States in 1996 for HIV-related Kaposi's sarcoma, this is only 50 nm in diameter and has a DSPC:cholesterol ratio of 2 : 1. More recently, Marqibo®, a ~100 nm liposomal formulation of vincristine with a sphingomyelin:cholesterol mole ratio of 57.4 : 42.6, has been approved by the FDA for the treatment of acute lymphoblastic leukemia. These liposomes are designed so that they are taken up by phagocytic cells of the MPS. They have a shorter circulating half-life compared to Doxil due to the lack of stealth layer. These formulations avoid the high plasma concentrations of free drug but still generate sustained delivery, as the MPS cells act as a reservoir of the free drug that slowly returns into the circulation. A similar approach has been taken in formulations of antimicrobial or antiparasitic drugs.

Depocyt® is a liposomal formulation of cytarabine for intrathecal use and was approved for lymphomatous meningitis by FDA in 2007. Unlike the usual unilamellar or multilamellar liposomes, it is a multivesicular system containing hundreds of water-filled compartments separated by a lipid bilayer and is known as Depofoam®. This structure allows encapsulation of large quantities of drugs and ensures prolonged release.

29.2.4 ABRAXANE®

ABRAXANE or nab-paclitaxel is an albumin-bound paclitaxel injectable suspension that was first approved by the FDA in 2005 and in Europe in 2008 by Abraxis. It is now indicated for the treatment of advanced breast, non-small cell lung and pancreatic cancers and is marketed by Celgene. It makes use of the endogenous plasma protein albumin that is a 67 kDa protein, about 4 nm in diameter and 5 nm long, and reversibly binds to hydrophobic molecules. Albumin is spray-dried with paclitaxel and lyophilized to produce a sterile powder for reconstitution. On reconstitution, a suspension containing ~130 nm paclitaxel albumin-bound particles is formed, which on intravenous injection rapidly dissociate to form smaller particles and unbound paclitaxel [9]. Paclitaxel, which is a poorly soluble taxane, was originally formulated with the polyoxyethylated castor oil Cremophor® EL and dehydrated alcohol as Taxol®. The Cremophor can cause a range of allergic reactions that limit the dose that can be given. Using albumin as a nanocarrier can enable 50% higher doses of paclitaxel (260 versus 175 mg/m^2 per cycle) to be given and therefore better clinical outcomes have been achieved. This reformulation has also enabled the product to be approved in more indications than the original formulation.

Sales of Abraxane were $135 M in its first year and usage continues to grow as new indications are added, with worldwide sales of $848 M in 2014.[2] It is a standard of care in several indications and it is currently going through extensive clinical trials (>20), either as a monotherapy or in several combination regimes.

It is a good example of where a better formulation of a poorly soluble drug, that is, removal of dose-limiting excipients, can enable higher doses to be administered and better efficacy to be achieved. Despite the novelty of the approach, the clinical benefit achieved has enabled a very successful nanomedicine.

29.2.5 Genexol -PM

Genexol -PM is a biodegradable poly(ethylene glycol)poly(D,L lactide) copolymer micellar formulation of paclitaxel. It has a size of 20–50 nm and a drug loading of 16.7% and is presented as a lyophilized powder. It was originally approved in South Korea for advanced breast cancer and non-small cell lung cancer. It subsequently gained in Hungary and Bulgaria but under the trade name Cynviloq™. It is now in a phase III clinical trial in the United States in metastatic or locally recurrent breast cancers designed to show bioequivalence to ABRAXANE. It is again a solubilizing rather than a targeting formulation and on injection, the micelles rapidly dissociate as they are diluted with plasma.

29.2.6 Pegylated Proteins

Pegylation of proteins results in improved solubility, extended circulation times, reduced immunogenicity from the protein, increased stability, and enhanced protection from proteolytic degradation. Pegylation since its conception in the

1970s has been widely used and there are several pegylated proteins as marketed products.

The first of these proteins was ADAGEN®, pegademase bovine where monomethoxypolyethylene glycol (molecular weight 5000) is covalently attached to the adenosine deaminase enzyme. It is an intramuscular injection for enzyme replacement therapy for adenosine deaminase deficiency in patients with severe combined immunodeficiency disease. Two of the most successful pegylated proteins are Pegasys®, Peginterferon alfa-2a, a PEGylated interferon alpha for use in the treatment of chronic hepatitis C and hepatitis B, and Neulasta®, Pegfilgrastim, a PEGylated recombinant methionyl human granulocyte colony-stimulating factor for severe cancer chemotherapy-induced neutropena.

Polyethylene glycol, PEG, is a linear hydrophilic polymer with a long history as a nontoxic polymer and has received "GRAS" status (i.e., generally recognized as safe) by the FDA. PEGylation is currently the most popular method of bioconjugation and has resulted in a number of successful protein products. Molecular weights of PEG up to 40 kDa are employed and a monomethoxy end group (mPEG) tends to be used as these are less immunogenic [10]. From a nanocarrier perspective, however, there are many properties of PEG that are not ideal. PEG is not biodegradable, can accumulate in the body, and be immunogenic; it is polydisperse and some reactions can be nonspecific. Despite this, probably due to its clinical precedence, it is still widely used and many are in clinical trials as pegylated proteins and some companies specialize in PEG technology (e.g., Enzon Pharmaceuticals, Nektar Therapeutics)

29.2.7 Antibody Drug Conjugates

Antibody drug conjugates (ADCs) approved by regulatory authorities include Genentech's KADYCLA® trastuzumab emtansine to treat human epidermal growth factor receptor-2 (HER2) positive metastatic breast cancer and Seattle Genetics ADCETRIS®, brentuximab vedotin, which is approved for relapsed Hodgkin lymphoma and relapsed systemic anaplastic large-cell lymphoma in many countries. KADYCLA contains the cytotoxic DM1 linked to the monoclonal antibody trastuzumab, anything between 0 and 8 DM1 molecules per antibody with average of ~3.5. ADCETRIS contains an antibody against CD30 and monomethyl auristatin E, which is a cytostatic compound with considerable toxicity and therefore cannot be used in its unconjugated form.

Many other ADCs are in clinical trials (~70) and further research toward bi- and multispecific hapten binding antibodies should lead to a next generation of ADCs. Challenges, however, with therapeutic index have been seen as the potency of the cytotoxics has increased and careful linker design is required to prevent premature release and to afford site specificity.

29.3 Developing Nanomedicines

29.3.1 The Development Process

The high-level research and development (R&D) process of a typical medicine includes four main stages: drug discovery – where a new drug candidate is selected, preclinical development – where animal studies to assess efficacy and toxicity are carried out, clinical development –where the concept is tested in man and the safety and efficacy and dose of the drug elucidated, and commercialization. These stages are then subdivided further (Figure 29.2). In the discovery stage, the target is first selected, a hit that will be a particular modality such as a small molecule, antibody, peptide, antisense oligonucleotide, and so on is identified. Following more experimentation a lead compound is generated and then optimized prior to candidate selection. Preclinical development and manufacturing is the first stage of the development process and this is where more significant investment is needed [11]. The clinical stage is generally subdivided into phases: phase I where single and multiple ascending dose safety studies are carried out, phase II where dose setting is determined, and phase III where benefit over existing therapies is established. Depending on the indication, these phases can merge and if extreme benefit is seen, phase II studies can be used as registration studies or the development may leave out phase II and move from phase I to phase III. Registration and launch of the product follows.

Nanomedicines follow a similar path, with a research/concept/idea that will move to a therapeutic project where a preclinical body of evidence will be generated. If successful, the candidate nanomedicine will be moved into development and then into the clinic. In contrast to typical small-molecule drugs and antibodies, it is not just the active pharmaceutical ingredient that will be selected for preclinical development at the time of candidate selection, but, due to the functional nature of the nanocarrier, this should also be selected and the two should be seen as an integrated system. This nanocarrier delivery system also needs to be a good prototype of the final formulation to allow a representative preclinical package to be generated to support the first studies in humans (phase I). For nucleic acid delivery, given that the nanocarrier is liable to enable intracellular delivery and thus drive effect, work will need to begin at research concept phase or target selection phase to enable biological understanding of a new target and

Figure 29.2 Typical research and development process.

its link to disease modification. This phase is significantly earlier in the R&D process than pharmaceutical design and drug delivery groups have typically become involved. It is likely for these new modalities that both the intended delivery system/type of nanocarrier and route of administration may be chosen at this point, so well before candidate nomination. For example, local delivery to a particular tissue, for example, intratumoural, intradermal, or intracardiac, will provide higher concentrations of the nanomedicine in the tissue of interested, which should assist intracellular delivery and the chances of a successful translation into a medicine.

The preclinical development package needs to build a platform of evidence that will derisk the investment and improve chances of success in the clinic. It will also need to contain the necessary toxicity studies to support safe dosing in man. This is normally conducted in two species, rodent and nonrodent, and contains a dose range finding and maximum tolerated dose study plus a repeat dose study, the length of which is determined by the duration of the intended clinical study. Normally, some toxicity studies on the nanocarrier itself, without drug, should be carried out, if not evaluated previously, to support first clinical dosing. If the nanomedicine is a reformulation of an existing approved drug, it may be possible to develop the nanomedicine in the United States under FDA 505(b)(2) regulatory path that utilizes existing safety data and has fewer requirements for clinical studies compared to that of a new chemical entity under the traditional 505(b)(1) application process. This shortened path was introduced to offer cheaper routes to registration for generic alternatives to branded products post patent expiry, but it has also been exploited by alternative delivery technologies, thus expediting commercialization of new formulations that offer therapeutic improvement over existing drugs.

To support both early stages of discovery, preclinical and clinical studies, nanomedicines need to be designed, optimized, produced, and scaled up. Like any manufacture process, the process needs to be robust, reproducible, and resulting materials characterized to ensure the quality of the product produced. The added complexity of many nanocarriers and nanomedicines makes this more challenging and costly than more simple dosage forms.

29.3.2 Improving Translation of Nanomedicines into Clinical Use

29.3.2.1 Lessons Learnt from Traditional Research and Development

Nanomedicines like many drugs have suffered from poor translation into successful clinical medicines [12] and many are critical to the amount of academic research and investments, resulting in limited applications particularly in the medical fields.

It is important that the same lessons are learnt with nanomedicines as those that have been used to reduce the attrition of traditional small-molecule drugs over the last 5 years. A framework based on five important technical determinants of project success and pipeline quality has been recently described [1].

These have become known as the 5 R's: the right target, the right tissue, the right safety, the right patient, and the right commercial potential. In terms of the right target, this means that preclinically the candidate drug must achieve target engagement, a strong linkage between the target and disease must be demonstrated, the candidate drug must show differentiated efficacy, and predictive biomarkers should be available. In addition, the drug must achieve the appropriate level of drug exposure in the target tissue with a full knowledge of the PK–PD properties and drug–drug interactions. Achieving the right safety means that a suitable therapeutic margin is achieved with a detailed understanding of the drug and any metabolites' toxicity profiles. Furthermore, there must be a patient selection hypothesis and appropriate biomarkers in place. Finally, the project must target the correct, commercially attractive, patient population. The 5 R's are some of the key technical determinants of project success and this framework and similar ones used by others have contributed to the rise in number of new medicine approvals over the last couple of years.

This framework should also be rigorously applied to nanomedicine development and commercialization, especially given the added complexity and cost of the development. Applying the principles of the 5 R's framework to developing more effective nanomedicines should be realized by transitioning toward disease-driven nanomedicine design. This involves having an improved understanding of the relationship between disease physiology and nanomedicine behavior as well as building a stronger preclinical data package with a specific line-of-sight to the end clinical application of the nanomedicine in patients. No single nanomedicine will achieve the "right exposure" and the "right efficacy" in all tissues. The diverse range of nanomedicine systems available make it possible to adopt a disease-driven development strategy and transition away from formulation-driven (bottom-up) approaches. From the initiation of a project, it is important to build a clinical line-of-sight and to understand the specific challenges with the standard-of-care, such as excessive normal organ toxicity or unsuitable pharmacokinetic profile. Designing a nanomedicine to overcome a well-defined challenge has a greater chance of success than developing a delivery system and then attempting to align it with an existing clinical challenge. It is essential to consider the relationship between the heterogeneous disease and patient pathophysiology and the physicochemical properties of different nanomedicines to enable the rational selection of the nanomedicine systems that are most appropriate for specific indications. Thus, rational selection criteria are critical in the development of clinically successful and translatable nanomedicines. A disease-driven approach focuses on rationally selecting a drug, the delivery system, and target patient population to balance many different variables to maximize therapeutic activity. In addition, if significant disease heterogeneity exists such as in tumors, using biomarkers or imaging to preselect the most amenable patients/tumor types to participate in clinical trials and receive treatment is likely to improve that outcome of the trial as used in a personalized healthcare approach.

A sixth factor, the right culture, was also identified as a key success factor for projects [1]. This is crucial in encouraging effective decision-making based on these technical determinants, and with nanomedicines that are different to typical small molecule or antibody projects, this sixth factor will play an even more important role.

29.3.2.2 Support from Specialist Groups

A number of groups have been set up to try to catalyze the translation of promising nanomedicines into clinical use. The first of these was the Nanotechnology Characterization Laboratory (NCL), a multidisciplinary laboratory set up in 2004 by the National Cancer Institute, National Institute of Health, and the FDA to support the preclinical characterization of nanotechnology products.[3] The main objectives of the NCL include the establishment and standardization of an analytical cascade for nanomaterial characterization, facilitating the clinical development and regulatory review of nanomaterials for cancer clinical trials, identifying and characterizing the critical parameters related to a nanomaterials' absorption, distribution, metabolism, and excretion (collectively termed ADME) and toxicity, engaging and facilitating academic and industrial-based knowledge sharing, and interfacing with regulatory authorities.

Other groups have been set up in Europe to support the development, translation, and commercialization of nanomedicines such as the European Nanomedicine Technology Platform created in 2006 and more recently a Translational Advisory Board,[4] which is part of the EU ENATRANS project (Enabling NAnomedicine TRANSlation). They will provide free of charge, nonbinding, and strategic advice to promote and guide projects in the nanomedicine area. Unlike the NCL that was set up to support translation of cancer medicines, they will support projects in all disease areas. In addition, a European Nanomedicine Characterization Laboratory (EU-NCL) (www.euncl.eu) was funded and set up in 2015 by the European Commission's Horizon 2020 research and innovation programme and draws on expertise from 8 core members and 14 satellite laboratories including the US NCL. Their aims are very similar to the NCL and include providing a transdisciplinary testing infrastructure covering a comprehensive set of preclinical assays (physical, chemical, *in vitro*, and *in vivo* biological testing) to allow researchers to fully characterize the biodistribution, metabolism, pharmacokinetics, safety profiles, and immunological effects of their medicinal nanoproducts. In addition, they aim to foster the use and deployment of standard operating procedures (SOPs), benchmark materials and quality management for the preclinical characterization of medicinal nanoproducts and promote intersector and interdisciplinary communication.

3) www.ncl.cancer.gov. March 2016.
4) www.enatrans.eu. March 2016.

29.3.3 Preclinical Development

29.3.3.1 *In Vitro* Preclinical Development Testing

The first phase of the testing cascade is a comprehensive test of physicochemical properties of the nanoparticle formulation. Parameters such as the size, size distribution, surface characteristics, composition, presence of stealth layer, and of course the presence of targeting ligands will all affect *in vivo* distribution, efficacy, and tolerability. Particle size and size distribution are such critical measurements for the characterization and quality control (QC) of nanoparticles that now two orthogonal methods of characterization are recommended. Particle size is difficult to determine for nanomaterials, particularly if they are not spherical. Dynamic light scattering (DLS) is widely used for a range of nanoparticle types for both characterization and quality control purposes. It provides average particle size (Z_{ave}), size distribution, and polydispersity, but there are several limitations that need to be understood. Electron microscopy techniques such as transmission electron microscopy and atomic force microscopy are also popular and are used mainly for characterization purposes. They provide morphological information as well as confirmation of size, but are not practical to use as QC tests because sample preparation is challenging and time consuming. Several new techniques are being rapidly developed and increasingly adopted. Tunable resistance pulse sensing, for example, is an impedance-based method relying on a change of resistance as particles pass through a pore over which a voltage is applied, and nanoparticle tracking analysis involves microscopy-based video tracking of particles under Brownian motion utilizing laser light scattering. Both techniques provide greater information than the more traditional techniques, including particle size, distribution, and concentration measurements and are better able to cope with polydispersity and more heterogeneous samples than DLS.

Far more *in vitro* characterization of the formulation is required than for a simple intravenous injection where solubility across the pH range, stability, osmolality, sterility, endotoxins, and some basic blood compatibility tests for hemolysis and platelet aggregation/coagulation tests are carried out. Understanding the immune compatibility of nanocarriers has been identified as one of the most important factors to evaluate in preclinical development. *In vitro* biochemical analyses and cell-based assays can mimic the *in vivo* physiological environment and can therefore address some biological activity, immunological, and toxicity issues. These studies are useful as they should prevent unnecessary costly and labor- and animal-intensive *in vivo* studies, which due to species differences may not be predictive of the human situation. Significant work has now been done to develop a set of predictive immunological *in vitro* tests [13] and these are also described in Chapter 17 “Nanoparticle Toxicity: General Overview and Insights Into Immunological Compatibility.” For more complex nanoformulations that contain an active targeting ligand and/or a nucleic acid drug, a measure of its functionality postmanufacture should also be a key test that is developed and utilized.

The NCL has set out a standardized analytical testing cascade for nanoparticles to support the physicochemical characterization, the preclinical toxicology, pharmacology, and efficacy of nanoparticles, that is, their preclinical development. They have successfully supported the clinical translation over a dozen nanoparticles into the clinic and advise the FDA on CMC regulatory packages. Therefore, it is wise to consult their comprehensive testing cascade and the detailed assay protocols available on their Web site to support the progression of a new nano project. A summary of the recommended preclinical tests is shown in Table 29.1.

Table 29.1 Summary of key *in vitro* tests required during preclinical development.

Type of test	Parameters measured	Assessment	Comment
Physicochemical characterization	Size, size distribution, aggregation	Dynamic light scattering (DLS) measures hydrodynamic radius; transmission electron microscopy, newer methods coming on line	Two orthogonal methods recommended
	Surface charge	Zeta potential to measure net charge of surface of nanoparticle	Care needed regarding solution pH, media
	Surface functionality	Presence of stealth layer, ligand; Cryo-TEM and range of indirect techniques	Important to understand as it affects stability/ biodistribution
	Morphology	Cryo-TEM to allow visualization in solution if possible	Careful sample preparation required
	Topology/ architecture	More complex analytical techniques required such as atomic force microscopy; more techniques are needed	Structural motif of nanoparticle that is spatial relationship of its atoms
	Molecular weight	Gel permeation chromatography	For final material and component characterization
	Purity	Assay	Free drug may need to be controlled
	Chemical composition	Assay	All components of nanoparticle need to be controlled
	Drug loading	Determined via dissolution of nanoparticles or degradation of any chemical bonds	Important to determine amount of free drug

	Stability	Chemical, physical, "in use" stability need to be evaluated	Physical, chemical, and in-use stability. Decision on presentation for clinical trials and product
	Solubility	LC-MS–MS	Also need to have understanding of solubility properties of encapsulated material
Microbiological assessment	Microbial sterility	Tested for microbial contamination via plating and counting techniques	
	Endotoxin testing	Limulus amebocyte lysate (LAL) assays, care needed and appropriate controls.	For detection of Gram-negative bacterial endotoxin
	Mycoplasma testing	Incubation of nanoparticle with a suitable indicator cell line that allows amplification of low-grade mycoplasma growth, a PCR-based method is used for the detection of mycoplasma DNA encoding specific 16S rRNAs	Normally only those formulation derived from animal origin
Drug release	Drug release in buffers/ physiological media	Careful design of release studies required, methods include dual isotope radiolabeled method and *in vitro* blood partitioning assays, detection via LC-MS–MS	Should be carried out in buffers and physiologically relevant media
Hematological assays	Hemolytic properties	Colorimetric determination of effect of nanoformulation on total hemoglobin	Appropriate concentrations need to be considered
	Platelet aggregation	Platelet counting or light transmission methods	Determines potential for anticoagulation or thrombus formation
	Interaction with plasma proteins	2D polyacrylamide gel electrophoresis (PAGE)	Protein adsorption effect MPS uptake/ biodistribution
	Plasma coagulation times	Commercial kits available – Thrombin Clotting Time key test	
In vitro immunological assays	Complement activation assays	PAGE plus Western blot analysis for qualitative assay or Enzyme Immunoassay to determine specific activation pathway	Determines ability to activate innate immune system

(*continued*)

Table 29.1 (*Continued*)

Type of test	Parameters measured	Assessment	Comment
	Measurement cytokine production	Identification and quantification of induced cytokines in fresh whole blood or peripheral blood mononuclear cells (PBMCs) – commercial kits available	Nanoparticles and active may induce cytokines
	Leukocyte proliferation assay	Measurement of a nanoparticles' ability to induce proliferative response of human lymphocytes or to suppress that induced by phytohemagglutinin (PHA-M).	Test the effect of nanoparticle on immunological function of leukocytes
	Effect on cytotoxic activity of NK cells	Cell viability test to determine the capacity of human natural killer (NK) cells to lyse tumorous target cells in the presence of nanoparticle	NK cells are an important part of body's innate defense mechanism
In vitro toxicology tests	Oxidative stress	Measurement glutathione, lipid peroxidation, or ROS as markers of cell oxidative stress in cell lines	
	Cytotoxicity testing	Measurements for necrosis and in cell lines, for example, MTT reduction to check for cell viability/lactate dehydrogenase (LDH) release for membrane integrity	Apoptosis can also be measured via caspase activation assays
	Autophagy	Microscopy and protein modification assays to detect autophagic vacuoles	Nanoparticles may cause adverse lysosomal pathologies/autophagic dysfunction

29.3.3.2 *In Vivo* Preclinical Development

The key *in vivo* studies needed to support first in human studies are pharmacokinetic, toxicological, and efficacy studies.

A thorough understanding of the ADME processes of nanomedicines, ideally of the encapsulated drug, the free drug, and the components of the nanoformulation in blood and tissues is desirable. The key tissues are the target tissue that will determine efficacy and those tissues that are liable to give concern from a toxicological perspective. Given that many nanoformulations are designed for controlled release, determination of tissue residence times is also desirable. Many systems that have moved into clinical development to date, however, have struggled to develop bioanalytical assays to measure both total and free drug concentrations in plasma and tissue. The separation of free drug from a nanoparticle in blood/tissue has caused significant technical challenges and it often means that early clinical studies have been conducted without a knowledge of free drug concentration. This results in the lack of knowledge of pharmacokinetic properties of the nanomedicine in plasma and tissue and no pharmacokinetic–pharmacodynamic (PK–PD) relationship. This lack of understanding increases the risk of failure in later development. Further work and development of better bioanalytical assays are needed to aid future derisked clinical translation. The route of clearance of the drug and nanoparticle components will be required during development, but not necessarily for phase I studies. These are traditionally determined through radiolabeled studies during early clinical development, but this requires radiolabeling of both the free drug and nanocarrier, which depending on the complexity of the formulation and manufacturing process may provide additional technical challenges.

Traditionally, to progress to human studies, GLP toxicity studies are carried out. As mentioned previously, these must be carried out with a representative prototype of the final product. Ideally, the same batch of active and nanocarriers should be used for the GLP toxicity studies and the phase I clinical studies to derisk any differences in batch-to-batch variability at this early stage in the CMC development. For a new chemical entity or where the drug distribution is significantly different from previous formulations, for clinical trials in many countries an acute repeat dose toxicity study in two species (rodent and nonrodent) is required. These studies aim to identify the target organs of acute toxicity for any of the components of the system and to set the human starting dose. Organs rich in macrophages such as the liver and spleen are key targets for intact nanoparticles and vacuolization is common when large numbers of nanoparticles are dosed. In addition to the standard toxicological measurements, careful examination of markers of the immune response should also be carefully studied.

Nanotoxicology is developing as an area of pharmaceutical toxicology in its own right and is an important part of nanopharmacy. Acute toxicity of a nanocarrier usually comprises complement activation, hemolysis, inflammation, oxidative stress, or impaired mitochondrial function. Analyzing chronic toxicity is more demanding, and data are largely missing. Further discussion of nanotoxicology is available in Chapter 15 "Computational Predictive Models for Nanomedicine."

Finally, further efficacy studies to improve understanding in additional disease models and support clinical translation are important studies in this development phase. The unrepresentative nature of many xenograft models in oncology has been criticized for a lack of translation of many cancer nanomedicines. This is particularly the case for differences in the EPR effect between these models and the clinical disease. It is recommended that more sophisticated models such as genetically engineered or patient explant models be adopted more widely and that further understanding of the accumulation, distribution, and retention of nanomedicines within tumors that have similar phenotypes to the disease that the nanomedicine is indicated in are employed [14]. In addition, the unrepresentative nature of the immune systems of many preclinical disease models has been criticized for lack of translation of nanomedicines as the immune system is so important in determining nanocarrier biodistribution [15].

More sophisticated models are required for a range of disease areas. Particularly for intracellular delivery systems, models that encompass human cells and tissues in an appropriate setting preclinically are required to aid understanding and better design. Some of the microphysiological systems that are being developed can help support safety and efficacy understanding, thus aiding more predictable clinical translation [16,17].

29.3.3.3 **Formulation and Process Optimization**

As already discussed, once a nanomedicine candidate is accepted into development, the active pharmaceutical ingredient and nanocarrier should be fixed, with limited changes to the formulation and process following GLP toxicity studies. This is due to the complexity of the formulation and the lack of understanding of the critical quality attributes of the product that may affect its *in vivo* performance. For oral immediate release products, risk to *in vivo* performance differences is determined by the Biopharmaceutics Classification Scheme,[5] and there are known critical quality attributes such as disintegration times, dissolution rates and particle size, and often a good understanding of *in vitro–in vivo* relationships. This is unclear for many nanomedicines and complicated by the fact that plasma pharmacokinetics is unlikely to be a surrogate for activity with nanomedicines. The critical quality attributes of a nanomedicine are liable to be influenced by many factors, including the critical material attributes of the components of the nanocarrier, the critical formulation, and critical process parameters.

In practice, minimizing the risk of changes to *in vivo* performance often means "front loading" of formulation and process optimization prior to GLP toxicity and first in human studies. This means spending significant time and cost at risk prior to knowing if the nanomedicine performs in human testing. Typically, the major cost in pharmaceutical development is spent during phase II and prior to the pivotal phase III studies, once a clinical proof of concept has been generated during phase II. In nanomedicine development, this earlier investment where risk of failure is higher needs to be factored into the business plan for the development and commercialization of the nanomedicine.

The breadth of possible nanocarriers makes it difficult to generalize on formulations and processes to fabricate nanomedicines. All components of the nanocarrier and formulation should be biocompatible and ideally biodegradable, including any linkers or ligands. Any impurities in the components need to be carefully controlled. Often a manufacturer's reported specification is not accurate enough for proper nanoparticle characterization and does not always make

5) www.fda.gov. (March 2016).

it clear how the measurement was made, so proper qualification is required. It is also imperative, early in the R&D process, to consider how the nanocarriers will be scaled up. Currently, little thought to scale-up has been given to many of the highly complex multicomponent systems reported in the academic literature and "developability" and "manufacturability" have not been properly assessed for many materials. Precise control of size, size distribution, and geometry are fundamental to performance and thus controlling these and ensuring batch-to-batch consistency are key. The issues with Doxil manufacture have already been discussed in Section 29.2.2. Achieving well-controlled size and uniformity with a range of innovative biomaterials is paramount for further exploitation of them into functional nanoparticles and their subsequent development into successful nanomedicines in the clinic.

During preclinical development, it is imperative to consider the target product profile and how the product will be administered. This should inform both the minimum drug loading of the nanomedicine, the number of nanoparticles likely to be administered per dose, the dose of the drug and nanocarrier, the product presentation, the route and time of administration (e.g., bolus/infusion), in use stability criteria, and desired shelf life. All of these may pose technical challenges and may inform "developability." If the drug loading is low, like with many of the first-generation nanocarriers such as liposomes and linear polymer conjugates (where drug loading in the nanocarrier is typically less than 5 wt%), excipient concentrations and the number of nanoparticles dosed will be high. Both these may carry a toxicity risk; from the toxicity of the excipients themselves, where unprecedented levels of excipients may need to be dosed in the clinic, or from the large numbers of nanoparticles being dosed, which may saturate the nanoparticle clearance mechanisms within the body. Additionally, from a practical perspective, the injection volume is limited to 5 ml/kg in many preclinical species, which will limit the doses that can be evaluated in efficacy and toxicity studies unless very concentrated nanoparticles can be prepared. Concentration of nanoparticles, in itself, often poses physical stability issues, particularly if they then need to be frozen to ship to the site of preclinical testing. In the clinic, low drug loading will result in a large and undesirable number of vials per dose, which can be unacceptable to patients or clinical staff. To maintain sterility, parenteral formulations are often filled into vials and lyophilized *in situ*; to obtain a reasonable drying process time, the upper limit is ~1 g of solids, thus with 5% drug loading, a 400 mg dose will require eight vials. Increasing the number of vials above this causes challenges to patient, clinical staff, and costs. Consideration of these challenges and processing steps suggest that active agents with reasonably high potency should be chosen for nanoparticle development to help keep doses lower and minimize costs and nanoparticle burden in the body.

Many nanocarriers consist of pharmaceutical excipients not usually used in conventional manufacture, many are composed of macromolecules (either lipids or polymers) that have been specially designed, for example, PLA–PEGs or pegylated lipids. Linear and branched polymers are often polydisperse and if the drug is to be attached via conjugation, this can be random or incomplete, which results in lack of control of the material and resultant nanoparticles. This needs to be addressed with new chemistries or by means to narrow polydispersity easily and at scale. New dendrimer/dendron architectures where there is a more defined structure and architecture and new chemistries for conjugation can remove some of these concerns. Designing novel biomaterials with greater functionality is likely to be an increasing trend, for both securing more functional biomaterials for delivery and securing novel intellectual property (IP) to protect the invention.

Self-assembly of macromolecules is a common method for formation of many types of nanoparticles. These macromolecules generally rely on secondary intermolecular interactions, including hydrophobic–hydrophobic interactions, hydrogen bonding, electrostatic interactions, stereocomplexation, π–π stacking, and host–guest interactions to form their nanostructures. By modifying the chemical building blocks of the macromolecule, the self-assembly processes and the structure and physicochemical properties of the assembled particles can be controlled. A thorough understanding of the physicochemical properties of the components of the nanoparticles, phase transition kinetics, fluid dynamics, and manufacturing processes is required.

Many methods of producing polymeric or lipid nanoparticles or micelles to date have relied on batch mode processing methods such as precipitation, emulsification, and dialysis, which are laborious processes with many steps and often require copious amounts of solvents/water. To ensure reproducibility, a large number of in-process controls are likely to be required. Despite this, these approaches have been scaled up to enable clinical trials and commercial supply of a limited number of nanoparticle types to date. Such process methods mean that the development process is often expensive and scale-up carries a risk of nonreproducible material. In addition, bespoke equipment and/or large spaces and access to large volumes of solvents/water are required for GMP manufacture, which may limit the number of contract manufacturing organizations that are able or willing to take on such a complex and potentially long manufacture. If cytotoxic or highly potent materials that require high containment facilities are also employed, this may further narrow the number of GMP manufacturing options available.

Given the complexity of many nanoparticle production methods, applying the principles of "quality by design" is critical for the success of the product. Investing in process analytical technologies (PAT) will ensure an online/at-line quality assessment approach, which should create longer term savings. Knowing and anticipating the most critical points of the process will facilitate the implementation of automated procedures to resolve problems as they occur in line rather than wasting whole batches later.

Newer preparation methods with better control over particle size and higher degrees of reproducibility and scalability are now being explored, which will enable easier scale-up and development of processes for global manufacture. These are generally flow-based methods that rely on controlling the fluidics and mixing dynamics of solutions of the polymeric or lipidic components or template-assisted systems.

Microfluidic devices enable precise liquid handling within microchannels creating a high surface-to-volume ratio and enabling rapid and controlled micromixing, and thus ensuring efficient and homogeneous mass transfer. These devices can produce a range of nanoparticles such as liposomes, lipid nanoparticles, polymeric nanoparticles, and micelles via a continuous process, thus avoiding issues of batch-to-batch variability. In addition, microfluidic devices give superior control over nanoparticle size and physicochemical properties than many of the more traditional fabrication methods. Nanoparticle size can be manipulated by adjusting the flow rates and therefore mixing times, device/chip geometry, polarity of the solvents, and concentration and composition of the biomaterials used to make the nanoparticles. For example, several microfluidic platforms capable of generating size-tunable polyethylene glycol-*b*-poly(lactic-*co*-glycolic acid) (PEG-*b*-PLGA) nanoparticles with a narrower size distribution, higher drug loading capacity, and an improved batch-to-batch consistency compared with those prepared from a conventional precipitation method have been developed [18,19]. Optimization of microfluidic devices has led to development of microfluidic platforms capable of producing up to 250 g of polymer nanoparticles/day with good control over particle size and size distributions (PDI < 0.1) [20]. However, further work is still required to scale this approach to enable larger batches of nanoparticles for commercial manufacture.

Flash nanoprecipitation is also a simple, continuous, and scalable process that allows the production of block copolymeric nanoparticles. This process uses rapid micromixing to obtain homogeneous supersaturation conditions and controlled precipitation of hydrophobic solutes (organic or inorganic) along with block copolymer self-assembly. The rapid mixing conditions are achieved using confined precipitation geometries with two or more impinging fluid streams, for example, a confined impinging jet mixer or multi-inlet vortex mixer. Nanoparticles with narrow (PDI < 0.15) and controllable size distributions from 30 to 300 nm can be readily obtained by fine-tuning the kinetics of micromixing, mixer geometry, solute nucleation and growth, and block copolymer structure [21]. The versatility offered by flash precipitation means that it can be applied to the production of multifunctional nanoparticles with targeting ligands and composite nanoparticles comprised of inorganic and organic cores with both encapsulated drugs and imaging agents.

The template-assisted systems that have been employed are the layer-by-layer system and particle replication in nonwetting templates (PRINT) technology. The layer-by-layer assembly uses size-controlled core nanoparticles (e.g., gold, silica, calcium phosphate nanocrystals, and PLGA nanoparticles) on which layers of polymers or biological molecules (DNA or RNA) are sequentially deposited. The core nanoparticle can be dissolved and replaced by a drug. Different shapes can be produced by using cores of different geometries. One of the issues with exploiting this processing technique for nanoparticle production has been the challenge of removing the excess materials used in each layering step. A fluidic process incorporating a tangential flow filtration module that is capable of removing excess polymer used during each layering step similar to that used in the formulation of biologicals has been recently developed, which should increase the versatility and scalability of this technique [22].

PRINT technology, is a versatile "top-down" method that has been employed in the preparation of polymeric nanoparticles by Liquidia. PRINT technology uses a highly fluorinated perfluoropolyether elastomer as a mold, which has a very low surface energy that enables it to "harvest" objects easily. It offers excellent control over particle size, shape, and chemical composition. Monodisperse polymeric nanoparticles with sizes ranging 100–500 nm and shapes including spheres, cylinders, disks, cones, and Janus particles have been prepared with high uniformity and in a highly scalable manner. A range of modalities including nucleic acid-based molecules and proteins have been encapsulated [23].

Further work is required to develop these newer processes more fully in order to ensure simpler and more continuous processing in nanopharmacy.

Many nanomedicines are for parenteral delivery, thus sterilization is required. Achieving sterility of nanoparticles is often more challenging than traditional injectables as many of the preferred methods of sterilization such as heat sterilization and radiation sterilization could damage the integrity of the nanoformulation; therefore, filter sterilization methods are often used. This requires the particle size of the nanoformulations to be small enough to pass through a 0.22 μm sterilizing filter, and some development of the process is required to prevent blocking of filters, loss of material, and viscosity issues.

At the end of the fabrication process, a colloidal dispersion is usually produced. This is the way that many liposomal products are currently presented. It is unlikely, however, that such a dispersion will have the chemical or physical stability required to be a final pharmaceutical product with an acceptable shelf life for all nanoparticle formulations. A lyophilization process, therefore, will often be employed to form a lyophile, or a frozen suspension may be provided, at least for early clinical studies. Lyophilization is a long, costly, and complex process, but it should enable the product to be stored under ambient conditions during its shelf life and as a sterile powder for easier transportation. This additional process again adds complexity and cost to the nanoparticle manufacturing process. Alternatively, although not favorable, a frozen product may be acceptable or refrigerated storage may be required. These storage requirements again add cost and complexity to a global supply chain. Often, in practice, such restrictions mean that the product is liable to be wasted due to deviations in storage conditions during global shipments or clinical practice, adding further cost and liability to an already costly and complex development process and supply chain. A shelf life of at least 2 years and ideally 5 years is desirable for a commercial product.

The challenges of the formulation and process development, manufacture, and supply of nanomedicines should not be underestimated. The degree of complexity is higher than many other pharmaceuticals and this is often compounded if cytotoxics or high-potency drugs are incorporated with the additional requirements for product sterility.

29.3.3.4 Analytical Considerations

Analytical requirements required by the Regulatory Authorities are more complex for nanomedicines. The nanomedicine must be capable of being made reproducibly to a very tight analytical standard with a few percent variability and with all impurities known and quantified down to a similar level as defined by ICH guidelines. Often nanocarriers contain polymers, lipids or other macromolecules and components that can be hard to characterize and make reproducibly. These need to be tightly controlled and securely sourced to ensure minimal variability in starting materials. Demonstration of the removal of any toxic excipients used as part of the manufacturing or purification process needs to be performed and controls put on any residual solvents used.

A larger number and broader range of analytical techniques will be required than for traditional dosage form development. The more conventional techniques such as high-performance liquid chromatography (HPLC) and mass spectrometry will need to be adapted for macromolecules and expertise in characterizing larger molecules gained. Additional techniques will need to be developed to understand and fully characterize the nanomedicine from both physical and biophysical perspectives, so as to provide information on the secondary structure, particle size, shape, dynamics, polarity, release kinetics, encapsulation efficiency, ligand density, binding, and functionality. For example, techniques such as high-resolution imaging, *in vitro* assays, surface plasmon resonance (SPR), isothermal titration calorimetry (ITC), differential scanning calorimetry light scattering, circular dichroism, and transmission electron microscopy (TEM) shall all be adopted during the development process and used to characterize materials or set analytical specifications. A range of additional properties will need to be added to the drug specification compared to more traditional dosage forms. A specification will also need to be put on the free drug in the nanocarrier, and this is liable to add to the long-term stability challenges, particularly those intended for infusions where acceptable in-use stability also needs to be factored in.

Nanoparticles should be characterized in biological media relevant to the *in vivo* situation. This is particularly important for drug release, which is likely to be a critical quality attribute in many future nanoparticles, thus adding to the analytical complexity. Various methods for determining drug release from nanoparticles have been reviewed [24], and a novel stable isotope method that provides improvement on existing methods has been recently reported by scientists at the NCL [25]. Further details on analytical characterization are discussed in Chapter 29.

29.3.3.5 Lessons Learnt from NCL

Some of the pitfalls of the many (>300) nanomaterials that have been investigated by the NCL have been summarized [26]. The nanomaterials came from a range of different sources, including government, academia, and industry, and thus different knowledge and experience of the R&D process. The most common issues or challenges encountered were related to nanoparticle synthesis, purification, characterization, and analysis.

Approximately, a third of those nanomaterials submitted to the NCL had endotoxin levels higher than the US FDAs allowable limits. High endotoxin levels are liable to affect interpretation of many safety/immunological assays that may be run as part of the preclinical development package as well as impact *in vivo* studies. Endotoxins are normally assessed in parenteral products using the Limulus Amoebocyte Lysate Test or LAL test, in which a sample containing pyrogens causes gel formation in the lysis product of amoebocyte cells of the giant horseshoe crab *Limulus polyphemus*. Many nanoparticles interfere with the traditional LAL assay and thus careful selection of controls is required to allow appropriate assay interpretation.

Immunological understanding of nanocarriers and their effects on the immune system needs to be improved, particularly for nucleic acid drugs that often stimulate the immune system themselves. This is an area that has previously not received enough attention in the past but is now a growing area of research for those developing novel systems in this area. A list of comprehensive assays and lessons learnt in terms of immunological testing has been recently published by scientists at the NCL [13] and outlined in Chapter 17 "Nanoparticle Toxicity: General Overview and Insights Into Immunological Compatibility."

It is imperative that nanoparticles are characterized under physiological conditions, and that thorough characterization is carried out. Understanding the *in vitro–in vivo* (IVIV) correlation of release rates is important in the design of future clinical studies and defining the critical quality attributes of the product. Investing in a study to determine *in vivo* release rate early on in preclinical models will aid the development process and may well save time and money later. To do this, characterization of free drug separately from total drug in plasma and the associated challenges of developing a robust bioanalytical method need to be overcome. Chemical and physical stability under physiological conditions also need to be assessed.

Like any pharmaceutical development, batch-to-batch consistency is required to deliver a robust formulation and process is required. The complexity of nanoformulations can make this harder to achieve, but this is a key step to determine prior to significant *in vivo* testing and certainly clinical development.

29.3.4
Regulatory Considerations

Despite several nanomedicines being on the market, there is a lack of specific protocols for nanomedicines development. However, recently, the regulatory bodies from the European Medicines Agency from the European Union, Federal Drugs Administration (FDA) from the United States, and the PDMA/MHLW from Japan have been working together to achieve common perspectives in nanomedicine development through the International Committee of Harmonization (ICH) and a number of guidances have been published, as illustrated in Table 29.2. Reviews integrating some of the concepts behind these guidances and some of the key factors and challenges in the regulation of nanomedicines have been recently published [27,28].

Table 29.2 Summary of guidances issued by regulatory authorities on nanomedicine development.

Source	Title	Reference
FDA	FDA. Draft Guidance on Doxorubicin Hydrochloride, February 2010	http://www.fda.gov/downloads/Drugs/ . . . / Guidances/UCM199635.pdf
EMA	Reflection Paper on Non-Clinical Studies for Generic Nanoparticle Iron Medicinal Product Applications	EMA/CHMP/SWP/100 094/2011 http:/ www.ema.europa.eu/docs/eu/docs/en GB document library/Scientific guideline/ 2011/04/WC500 105 048PDF
EMA	Reflection Paper on the Data Requirements for Intravenous Liposomal Products Developed with Reference to an Innovator Liposomal Product	EMA/CHMP/806 058/2009http://www.ema.europa.eu/docs/en_GB/document_library/Scientific_guideline/2011/07/WC500109479.pdf
MHLW/ EMA	Joint MHLW/EMA Reflection Paper on the Development of Block Copolymer Micelle Medicinal Products	EMA/CHMP/13 099/2013http://www.ema.europa.eu/docs/en GB/document library/ Scientific Guideline/2013/02/WC500 138 390PDF
FDA	Liposome Drug Products: Chemistry, Manufacturing, and Controls; Human Pharmacokinetics and Bioavailability; and Labeling Documentation; Draft Guidance for Industry; Availability October 2015	http://www.fda.gov/downloads/drugs/ guidancecomplianceregulatoryinformation/ guidances/ucm070570.pdf

The active component in the nanocarrier, be it a small molecule, nucleic acid, peptide, protein, or antibody will determine whether the nanomedicine will follow the regulations for biological products or new chemical entities. The biologicals have their special regulatory position because they are a family of complex molecules that are difficult if not impossible to fully characterize by physicochemical analytical methods. Many nanomedicines that do not contain biologicals are known as nonbiological complex drugs or NBCDs. These are defined as being a medicinal product, that is not a biological medicine, where the active substance is not a homomolecular structure, but consists of different (closely related and often nanoparticulate) structures that cannot be isolated and fully quantitated, characterized, and/or described by physicochemical analytical means. It is also unknown which structural elements might impact the therapeutic performance. The composition, quality, and *in vivo* performance of NBCDs are highly dependent on the manufacturing processes of both the active ingredient and the formulation. These products raise specific challenges during the development, manufacturing, clinical testing, and quality control processes and also make it challenging for regulators and any follow-on producer. Comparability and interchangeability may need to be established during the entire life cycle due to variations caused by scale-up or process improvements. This explains the "front loading approach" to development described in Section 29.3.3.3 and the earlier recommendation to invest in determining whether an *in vitro–in vivo* correlation is possible/appropriate at least on "drug release." This challenge in proving bioequivalence makes a greater hurdle for follow-up versions or generic nanomedicines and serves to protect the investment of the innovator.

The complexity and diversity of nanomedicines and lack of existing regulations means that a critical role needs to be taken by the various authorities' scientific advice procedures to aid applicants with the development process. It is also imperative that the regional authorities continue to work together globally with key industry and academic stakeholders to provide further guidance and support to the regulatory requirements to ensure the quality of these complex systems can be developed and maintained. The support provided by the NCL and the new EU-NCL aiding the proper standardization and comprehensive characterization of nanomedicines will provide invaluable support in their development.

29.4 Commercialization of Nanomedicines

In order to translate the wealth of academic research (18 143 publications using search term "nanoparticle" in 2015 in PubMed) into viable applications and products, factors such as competitive edge, business plan, and future market size need to be considered. In addition, the adoption of the latest science, technological advances, and understanding in the multidisciplinary areas associated with nanomedicine development and commercialization are required.

This is in an environment where R&D costs continue to rise, regulatory requirements are more stringent, superior efficacy over current treatments needs to be proven, fewer side effects are acceptable, patient populations are shrinking due to increased disease segmentation, and pressures are rising on already limited healthcare budgets. It is essential to perform pharmacoeconomic studies to demonstrate both social and economic added values of any novel products compared with established treatments. Important indicators such as increment in QALYs (quality-adjusted life expectancy years) or costs associated with future consecutive hospitalizations should be considered in the development of any business case plan for nanomedicines.

Due to their high development costs, achieving success of nanomedicines commercially could be further challenged if their proposed application is in a niche indication. However, help is provided from many regulatory authorities around the world, including the FDA and in Europe, which have a harmonized process via the designation of orphan drug status for rare diseases or niche indications. Orphan drug designation is an incentive to encourage pharmaceutical companies to develop drugs for diseases that have a small market and this initiative has been very successful in increasing the number of available medicines in rare diseases [29]. Here, there are clear regulatory paths, support, and help plus financial incentives, including significant tax incentives on R&D costs, increased patent protection, and support with clinical research or creating government-supported R&D. The increased understanding and greater adoption of personalized medicines approaches may mean this route to commercialization can be adopted more frequently and utilized for nanomedicines.

The better the nanomedicine fits within the current healthcare system and medical practice, the more rapidly and likely its adoption by clinicians and acceptance by payers.

29.4.1 Nanotechnology Investment

The continued investment in nanotechnology research in many countries plus the potential applications of nanomedicines in a range of diseases with unmet need will continue to drive their commercialization. The United States was one of the first to make a significant investment in nanotechnology in 2000 with the National Nanotechnology Initiative and has spent US$22 billion with a further US$1.5 billion requested for 2016. The aims of this initiative are advancing world-class R&D programs, fostering the transfer of new technologies into products for commercial and public benefit, developing and sustaining educational resources, a skilled workforce, a dynamic infrastructure and a toolset to advance nanotechnology as well as supporting the responsible development of nanotechnology. Observation suggests a typical 20-year gestation period from scientific discovery to exploitation in the market in a number of other technology areas such as plastics, the internet, biotech and broader nanotechnology [30]. Nanocarriers and their use in drug delivery literature commenced in the 1960s with liposomes, the first dendrimer was described in 1978 and long-circulating PLGA particles in 1994 [21]. Of these, only the liposomes have successfully been commercialized as products to date (Section 29.1.2). However, the latter two are in clinical trials, a dendrimer in phase I with Starpharma's DEP™ docetaxel and a PLA nanoparticle with a PEG stealth layer with BIND Therapeutics ACCURIN® nanoparticles encapsulating different drugs. The application in healthcare of the nanotechnology investment has been accelerated by the formation of a number of alliances such as the National Institute of Health incorporating nanomedicine into its roadmap for medical research and the formation of the National Cancer Institute (NCI) Alliance for Nanotechnology in Cancer, both in 2004. The latter has the aim of advancing a number of promising nanotechnologies for the diagnosis, treatment, and the prevention of cancer. The NCI Alliance for Nanotechnology in Cancer is a comprehensive initiative encompassing the public and private sectors, designed to accelerate the application of the best capabilities of nanotechnology to cancer. The NCI support was further extended in 2015, following the success of the first 10 years of the program demonstrated by over 18 clinical trials being approved for new technologies, over 220 patents filed, 85 companies formed and over 2750 peer-review journal articles (nano.cancer.gov/action).

At a similar time, in Europe, the EU Commission adopted a communication "Towards a European Strategy for Nanotechnology" COM (2004) 338, which proposed institutionalizing European nanoscience and nanotechnology R&D efforts within an integrated and responsible strategy, and which spurred European action plans and ongoing funding for nanotechnology R&D. The application in medicine was initiated in 2004 when the European Science Foundation launched a Scientific Forward Look on Nanomedicine that involved a series of five workshops and a Consensus Conference (November 2004). Subsequently, the European Society for Nanomedicine (ESNAM)[6] and the European Foundation for Clinical Nanomedicine (CLINAM) were established.[7] CLINAM has hosted a yearly conference since 2008 for the many disciplines involved in translation of nanomedicines, and many national platforms have also been established in Europe such as the British Society for Nanomedicine in the UK[8] and Société Française de Nanomédecine in France.[9]

29.4.2 The Nanomedicine Market

The global nanomedicine market is projected to be US$97–129 billion in 2016 with projections of US$136 billion by 2021. This has grown approximately 14% since 2011. This encompasses diagnostics, therapeutics, and regenerative medicine and is dominated by oncology applications. It is estimated that the drug delivery market could represent US$44.6 billion about 46% of the market [31].

Slightly larger figures were reported by Transparency Market Research in their report titled "Nanomedicine Market: Global Industry Analysis, Size, Share, Growth, Trends and Forecast, 2013–2019" where they estimated the global nanomedicine market to be worth US$177.60 by 2019 and US$78.54 billion in 2012, this again being dominated (38%) by oncology indications. They projected a CAGR of ~12% between 2013 and 2019 [32], which is fueled by the rising government support for R&D of nanomedicines around the world, an increase in investment and healthcare collaborations, and high unmet medical needs. According to the report, cardiovascular indications are expected to display the fastest growth owing to the growing geriatric population and increasing demand for nanomedicine-based devices and drugs for the treatment of cardiovascular diseases. The report also analyzed the global nanomedicine market on the basis of geographical regions, including North America, Europe, Asia-Pacific, and rest of the world. The United States is currently leading, but the Asia-Pacific growth is significantly faster than other areas, reflected by its increased investment in nanotechnology.

In 2010, the delivery system market, a subset of the therapeutics market, was estimated as $US 1.3 billion and was split according to the different delivery

6) www.esnam.org (March 2016).
7) www.clinam.org (March 2016).
8) www.britishsocietynanomedicine.org (March 2016).
9) www.sfnano.fr (March 2016).

systems [31]. This analysis contained nanocrystals, as the major part of the market, so only ~50% of these data are relevant to nanocarriers. Within nanocarriers, liposomes and injectable nanoemulsions were the leading marketed nanoparticle technologies. The delivery systems market was projected to be US $136 billion by 2021.

Similarly, analysis of the pharmaceutical database Pharmacircle[2)] shows that liposomes are the main nanoparticle drug delivery technology currently marketed, followed by injectable nanoemulsions (Figure 29.3). Analysis of these nanoparticle technologies in development shows greater diversification of the types of systems with viral and nonviral systems for intracellular delivery being the leading delivery systems (Figure 29.4). This is primarily due to the wealth of early work on vaccines and nucleic acid-based drugs that are aimed at disease targets not easily prosecutable by medicinal chemistry or antibody approaches. The majority of these programs are in the preclinical phase or phase 1. Within the nonviral delivery category, there are a range of delivery systems including cationic/ionizable lipid or polymer nanoparticle based systems and a number using electroporation or other physical means to aid delivery. Liposomes, polymeric, and micellar nanoparticles are the main systems for more small molecules. The main drugs in the nanoparticle technology programs are doxorubicin/doxorubicin hydrochloride (40) and the taxols, paclitaxel (30), and docetaxel (18). The numbers in development are large numbers, particularly in the early phases (890 preclinical development, 339 phase 1, 196 phase 2, 68 in phase 3, 20 in registration phase, data snapshot in March 2016). Nearly 40% of these are in cancer therapeutic area with 80% of these being injectables.

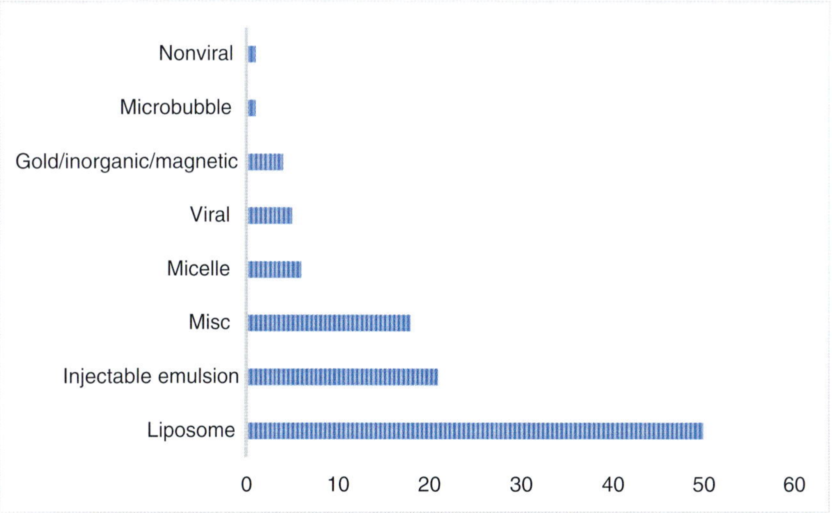

Figure 29.3 Comparison of nanocarrier delivery technologies for marketed nanoparticle products (data collated from Pharmacircle).

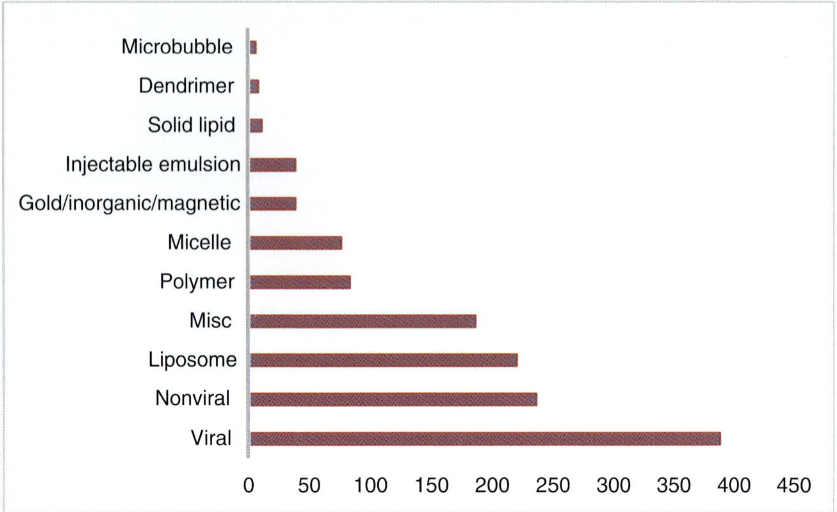

Figure 29.4 Comparison of nanocarrier delivery technologies for nanoparticles in development (data collated from Pharmacircle).

29.4.3 Challenges and Initial Solutions for Nanomedicine Commercialization

Commercialization of nanomedicines includes the nanomedicine design, preclinical development that requires an understanding of ADME properties and toxicology, chemistry and manufacturing controls, clinical studies as well as the instigation of a global supply chain, the securing of IP, and funding for such activities. The challenges for nanomedicine commercialization are partly due to the breadth and diversity of the research, complexity of many of the systems, and the variety of nanomaterials available as well as the complexity of biology and medicine. Some of the challenges encountered in nanomedicine development were discussed in March 2013 at a conference "Nanomedicines: Charting a Roadmap to Commercialization" held by the Nanomedicine Alliance [33].

There are clear regulatory processes involved for the approval of medicinal products and devices for both clinical and commercial use, including many guidelines where significant effort has been made to standardize this internationally (www.ICH.org). It must be remembered, however, that most medicinal products have the active ingredient, to date mainly a small molecule with molecular weight around 500 or a monoclonal antibody with a small number of normally nonfunctional excipients in the product. For nanomedicines, the active ingredient may well be more complex, for instance, antisense oligonucleotide, siRNA, mRNA, and gene, and this is compounded by the composition, structure, and architecture of the nanocarrier itself.

Much of nanomedicine research is done in academic laboratories with ever more complex systems, mixtures of materials, so-called nanohybrids, or nanodevices, combination of inorganic and organic nanoparticles, and novel materials perhaps with little line-of-sight thinking to the possibilities of characterization, scale-up, achieving regulatory approval, or global supply chains. In addition, in-depth knowledge of the disease the nanomedicine is intended to treat is often missing and thus the research seems to be technology or drug delivery driven rather than disease understanding led. The focus or endpoint for much of this academic research is often a preclinical proof of concept of the technology in a relatively narrow area. A more comprehensive preclinical package with work to build confidence in clinical translation is often required to help attract investment from those in a position to rapidly develop and commercialize the products.

Traditionally, small- to medium-size enterprises (SMEs) or drug delivery companies have taken many of these technologies through preclinical development and early clinical studies and then sought out "big Pharma" to further invest or license and develop these into marketed products. Some, however, have tried to develop nanomedicines themselves and run into funding difficulties, which have resulted in long stepwise developments with technologies being transferred between many companies and few reaching the market. This loss of continuity, "piecemeal" development, and often poor design of trials/processes with little line-of-sight thinking have led to high attrition rates and solvency issues for some small companies. The pharmaceutical industry, although sharing the ultimate common goal of bringing innovative medicines to patients in areas of unmet need, has a different focus to academia and many SMEs. The focus is more on return on investment, running a lean business, and reducing attrition rates. Although the pharmaceutical industry has been through a lean period in terms of successful new drug approvals over recent years, it is still profitable in doing business in the traditional way. Finding new targets that can be prosecuted via traditional medicinal chemistry approaches and simple dosage forms via well-trodden regulatory pathways is considerably easier than taking greater risk on new technologies and more complex developments.

In some disease areas such as cancer, where new biology areas (e.g., DNA damage repair, epigenetics, and metabolism) and disease understanding allow targets that can be prosecuted in traditional ways with small molecules; there is perhaps less of a driver/need for nanomedicines in a company's portfolio. However, there still remains a need to prosecute key targets that are considered "intractable" by traditional medicinal chemistry approaches in these diseases and therapeutic index stills remains a big challenge. Conversely, in other disease areas such as cardiovascular, these "easy" targets are fewer and opening up new target space via peptide or nucleic acid approaches will drive the need for novel nanomedicine approaches within the portfolio. Scientific breakthroughs, greater disease understanding, and the need for more site-specific delivery will also drive greater adoption of these technologies in the future.

Some of the key elements that traditionally help commercialization of products such as standardization, clear regulations, and financing are not available for nanomedicines, partly due to their diversity and complexity. At the research stage, it is estimated that only 10% of results are reproducible. Better measurements and standards are desperately needed to further scientific understanding. The existence of the Nanotechnology Characterization Laboratories (the United States and now Europe) and increased communication via several fora should help to address this need. Commercialization has also been hampered by both real and perceived safety concerns related to nanotoxicology, many of which have little or no scientific foundation. Nanotoxicology, however, is growing as a discipline and the importance of dose, route of administration, and biokinetics of nanoengineered materials is being studied and should inform nanomedicine design [34]. Poor communication between disciplines and confusion in the many "nano" terms and volume of literature does not help the commercialization process but considerable effort is now being made to address these issues.

The Alliance for Nanotechnology in Cancer, part of the US' National Cancer Initiative, established the Translation of Nanotechnology in Cancer (TONIC) consortium in 2011 to bring together public, private and academic sectors interested in nanomedicine drug development, with the mission of accelerating the translation and development of nanotechnology solutions for the early detection, diagnosis, and treatment of cancer. The main goals of TONIC include providing Alliance researchers insight into industry needs in technology platforms and drug targets, promoting collaborations between Alliance investigators and industry partners on promising precompetitive and late-stage programs, and serving as a sustained forum for nanotechnology idea exchange. The partnership further provides TONIC members the opportunity to interact with regulatory authorities and the Nanotechnology Characterization Laboratory to promote the qualification, development, and regulatory acceptance of nanotechnologies in cancer. TONIC also encourages the sharing of consortium project results with the scientific community and independent verification opportunities to ensure data reproducibility and robustness. The nanotechnology effort is also being reflected in other disease areas. For example, the emergence of nanotechnology-enabled long-acting antiretroviral medicines has recently resulted in the NIH-funded Long-Acting/Extended Release Antiretroviral Resource Program (LEAP; www.longactinghiv.org) that although in its early stages aims to bring key stakeholders together to foster further development.

In Europe, a new translational hub has also been initiated via the European Nanomedicine Technology Platform to consolidate the many programs and projects and to enhance the innovation capacity of SMEs and academia in order to accelerate the development of nanomedicines toward the market. Three areas have been supported: Enabling NAnomedicine TRANSlation project (ENATRANS) that supports SMEs in the nanobiomedical sector to translate their products from the laboratory phase to clinical applications, NanoFacturing that aims both to scale-up an existing GMP pilot line to a medium-scale sustainable manufacturing process for solid-core nanopharmaceuticals and second to create a large-scale process platform that would serve as the basis for GMP compliant industrial manufacture facility, and the NanoPilot project that will build a GMP pilot line for the production of polymer-based nanopharmaceuticals via a continuous flow microreactors process. The latter two focus on scale-up and fabrication of nanoparticles for the pharmaceutical industry which are major hurdles in translation as discussed above.

In Europe, the support is more visible across a number of different disease areas with applications in cancer, atherosclerosis, diabetes, eye disorders, tissue engineering, combating antibiotic resistance and other infections, Alzheimer's disease, arthritis and inflammatory diseases.

A nanomedicine development and commercialization process will be a more expensive and more complex development than that of a traditional oral or simple parenteral formulation. As a result, the drivers for developing such a product need to be clear and significant clinical benefit will be the key driver for success. A robust business case that includes securing strong IP, an assessment of competition, and projection of return on investment is required. Second to market of a me-too product be it a simple formulation or costly nanomedicine is unlikely to bring return on investment or get approval/adoption in many healthcare systems. Many of the nanomedicines in clinical trials are a reformulation of existing drugs. From a risk perspective, knowing the drug is active clinically will increase probability of success, however the real benefit is likely to come from using nanotechnology to enable novel targets. It is estimated that only one in five of new treatments recuperate the development costs, so it is imperative that if at the outset it is known that costs and complexity will be higher, a robust business case is developed and technical risks are realized and properly mitigated.

A summary of the challenges that need to be addressed to enable successful nanomedicine commercialization is collated in Table 29.3.

Table 29.3 Summary of challenges that need addressing to enable successful nanomedicine commercialization.

Challenge	Area	Comment
Development	Characterization and quality control	Sophisticated/nonstandard analytical equipment with specialized personnel needed
		Quality control process complex
	Scale-up	Laboratory process not amenable to scale-up, few continuous processes, currently low efficiency
		Sterilization processes limited
		Lack of manufacturing facilities willing to take on complex products
	Reproducibility	Small changes may result in changes to product
	Biomaterials	Dedicated/specialized complex excipients required, concerns regarding reproducibility of batches and secure supply
	Dosage form	Acceptable product and shelf life needed for patient/hospitals. In-use stability needs to be considered.

(continued)

Table 29.3 (*Continued*)

Challenge	Area	Comment
	Therapeutic efficacy	Need superiority over existing options and adequate preclinical models
	Bioanalytical methods	Difficulties in measurement of free and encapsulated/conjugated/complexed active
Safety	Biocompatibility	For both nanocarrier and degradation products
	Immune response	Lack of understanding of interaction with immune system
	Bioaccumulation	Impact of long-term retention in body
	Metabolism and excretion	Need to understand for active and nanocarrier, challenges in radiolabeling active/nanocarrier, ADME studies needed for preclinical regulatory package
Regulations		Lack of clear global regulations for many parts of dossier
Intellectual Property (IP)		Lack of freedom to operate, crowded area for many technologies, long development times leading to short patent life
Lack of multidisciplinary platform/team		Lack of appreciation of multidisciplinary nature of nanomedicine development and interplay between various disciplines and link to human disease
Lack of support	Clinician	Apprehension, lack of understanding, challenge with performing clinical trials
	Patient	Lack of awareness, concerns novelty
	Industry	Skepticism regarding different approach, concerns regarding technical challenge, costs, and risk, little precedence

29.4.4
Key Players in Nanomedicines

The number of companies working in the diagnostic and therapeutic nanomedicine fields has grown significantly during the 5-year period 2008–2013, this is illustrated by data collated in the United Kingdom, France, Germany, and the United States (Table 29.4). There is more or less an equal spread and expansion of diagnostic and therapeutic nanomedicine companies. From the therapeutic companies, many offer a technology and are subsequently redeveloping a medicine into a nanoformulation and are small companies or university spin-offs.

Analysis in Pharmacircle[2] indicates that the companies with the largest number of marketed nanoparticle products are the South Korean company Biospectrum with liposomal creams mainly for skin indications, Ltt-Biopharma, a virtual

Table 29.4 Number of companies in nanomedicines – therapy, diagnostics [31].

Country	Number of companies in 2008	Number of companies in 2013	Change %
The United Kingdom	9	28	211
France	12	30	150
Germany	19	101	432
The United States	45	145	222

Japanese company that is focusing on reformulation of drugs for improved therapeutic index and convenience, and the Japanese company Mitsubishi Tanabe Pharma Corporation that has both polymeric and nanoemulsion injectables. These are diverse and often niche products in specific markets.

Interestingly, in development, the companies with the largest number of nanoparticle programs are now primarily biopharmaceutical companies, with Arbutus Biopharma who focus on RNAi and lipid nanoparticle technology, Inovio focusing on cancer and infectious diseases and their DNA immunotherapy-based technology platform and electroporation delivery system, and Alnylam Pharmaceuticals who focus on the translation of RNAi-based therapeutics using a range of delivery techniques leading the way. Celgene is listed as having the most number of nanoparticle programs with small molecule drugs, with its acquisition of Abraxis and its albumin technology.

In the last few years, several large Pharmaceutical Industries have become more involved in nanomedicines and announced collaborations with specialized nanopharmaceutical companies. For example, BIND Therapeutics, who have their ACCURIN™ technology, have collaborations with AstraZeneca, Pfizer, and Merck. Liquidia are collaborating with GSK for inhaled particles made using Liquidia PRINT platform. Starpharma have licensed their dendrimer technology to AstraZeneca for a family of oncology targets. This has allowed the larger Pharma to enable novel candidate drugs in their portfolios with nanotechnology. In addition, Cerulean are collaborating with AstraZeneca in a clinical study using their nanoparticle camptothecin conjugate in combination with AstraZeneca's LYNPARZA™ with the aim of showing synergy in combination with manageable tolerability. These collaborations and bringing industrial expertise and know-how to the development and commercialization of medicines will serve to expedite and increase the exploitation of these exciting and innovative nanotechnologies. In addition, many pharmaceutical companies now have a range of new modalities in their portfolios that need nanoformulations to ensure efficient delivery. Progressing these through the R&D processes should aid the understanding of the nanoparticle development process in all phases and within all disciplines employed and nanopharmacy as a whole. Further information on the commercialization of nanomedicines is available in a recent book [35].

29.5 Conclusions

Careful design of nanocarriers with a clear target product profile and clinical rationale is required for their successful development and commercialization into products. The experience and learning from the first nanomedicines, the modern R & D process, emerging science, and the developing infrastructure and support systems available from various sources should aid easier translation into successful medicines. The commercialization of nanomedicines needs to be interdisciplinary and will integrate biotechnology, academia, drug delivery companies, government laboratories, and traditional big pharma. It is an exciting time for nanopharmaceutical and drug delivery scientists as drug delivery is critical to the success of many new entities and will play a far more pivotal role in bringing new medicines from discovery through development to patients than ever before.

References

1 Cook, D., Brown, D., Alexander, R., March, R., Morgan, P., Satterthwaite, G., and Pangalos, M.N. (2014) Lessons learned from the fate of AstraZeneca's drug pipeline: a five-dimensional framework. *Nat. Rev. Drug Discov.*, **13**, 419–431.

2 Holohan, C., Van Schaeybroeck, S., Longley, D.B., and Johnston, P.G. (2013) Cancer drug resistance: an evolving paradigm. *Nat. Rev. Cancer*, **13**, 714–726.

3 Gao, J., Feng, S.S., and Guo, Y. (2012) Nanomedicine against multidrug resistance in cancer treatment. *Nanomedicine (Lond.)*, **7**, 465–468.

4 Iyer, A.K., Singh, A., Ganta, S., and Amiji, M.M. (2013) Role of integrated cancer nanomedicine in overcoming drug resistance. *Adv. Drug Deliv. Rev.*, **65**, 1784–1802.

5 Etheridge, M.L., Campbell, S.A., Erdman, A.G., Haynes, C.L., Wolf, S.M., and McCullough, J. (2013) The big picture on nanomedicine: the state of investigational and approved nanomedicine products. *Nanomedicine*, **9**, 1–14.

6 Hamill, R.J. (2013) Amphotericin B formulations: a comparative review of efficacy and toxicity. *Drugs*, **73**, 919–934.

7 Gabizon, A., Shmeeda, H., and Barenholz, Y. (2003) Pharmacokinetics of pegylated liposomal doxorubicin: review of animal and human studies. *Clin. Pharmacokinet.*, **42**, 419–436.

8 Barenholz, Y. (2012) Doxil(R)--the first FDA-approved nano-drug: lessons learned. *J. Control Release*, **160**, 117–134.

9 Miele, E., Spinelli, G.P., Miele, E., Tomao, F., and Tomao, S. (2009) Albumin-bound formulation of paclitaxel (Abraxane ABI-007) in the treatment of breast cancer. *Int. J. Nanomed.*, **4**, 99–105.

10 Jevsevar, S., Kunstelj, M., and Porekar, V.G. (2010) PEGylation of therapeutic proteins. *Biotechnol. J.*, **5**, 113–128.

11 Eaton, M.A., Levy, L., and Fontaine, O.M. (2015) Delivering nanomedicines to patients: a practical guide. *Nanomedicine*, **11**, 983–992.

12 Venditto, V.J. and Szoka, F.C., Jr. (2013) Cancer nanomedicines: so many papers and so few drugs!. *Adv. Drug Deliv. Rev.*, **65**, 80–88.

13 Dobrovolskaia, M.A. (2015) Pre-clinical immunotoxicity studies of nanotechnology-formulated drugs: challenges, considerations and strategy. *J. Control. Release*, **220**, 571–583.

14 Hare, J., Lammers, T., Ashford, M., Puri, S., Storm, G., and Barry, S. (2016) Challenges and strategies in anti-cancer nanomedicine development: an industry perspective, http://dx.doi.org/10.1016/j.addr.2016.04.025.

15 Moghimi, S.M. and Farhangrazi, Z.S. (2014) Just so stories: the random acts of

anti-cancer nanomedicine performance. *Nanomedicine*, **10**, 1661–1666.

16 Esch, M.B., Smith, A.S., Prot, J.M., Oleaga, C., Hickman, J.J., and Shuler, M.L. (2014) How multi-organ microdevices can help foster drug development. *Adv. Drug Deliv. Rev.*, **69–70**, 158–169.

17 Vladisavljevic, G.T., Khalid, N., Neves, M.A., Kuroiwa, T., Nakajima, M., Uemura, K., Ichikawa, S., and Kobayashi, I. (2013) Industrial lab-on-a-chip: design, applications and scale-up for drug discovery and delivery. *Adv. Drug Deliv. Rev.*, **65**, 1626–1663.

18 Karnik, R., Gu, F., Basto, P., Cannizzaro, C., Dean, L., Kyei-Manu, W., Langer, R., and Farokhzad, O.C. (2008) Microfluidic platform for controlled synthesis of polymeric nanoparticles. *Nano Lett.*, **8**, 2906–2912.

19 Rhee, M., Valencia, P.M., Rodriguez, M.I., Langer, R., Farokhzad, O.C., and Karnik, R. (2011) Synthesis of size-tunable polymeric nanoparticles enabled by 3D hydrodynamic flow focusing in single-layer microchannels. *Adv. Mater.*, **23**, H79–H83.

20 Liu, D., Cito, S., Zhang, Y., Wang, C.F., Sikanen, T.M., and Santos, H.A. (2015) A versatile and robust microfluidic platform toward high throughput synthesis of homogeneous nanoparticles with tunable properties. *Adv. Mater.*, **27**, 2298–2304.

21 Shi, J., Xiao, Z., Kamaly, N., and Farokhzad, O.C. (2011) Self-assembled targeted nanoparticles: evolution of technologies and bench to bedside translation. *Acc. Chem. Res.*, **44**, 1123–1134.

22 Bjornmalm, M., Roozmand, A., Noi, K.F., Guo, J., Cui, J., Richardson, J.J., and Caruso, F. (2015) Flow-based assembly of layer-by-layer capsules through tangential flow filtration. *Langmuir*, **31**, 9054–9060.

23 Rolland, J.P., Maynor, B.W., Euliss, L.E., Exner, A.E., Denison, G.M., and DeSimone, J.M. (2005) Direct fabrication and harvesting of monodisperse, shape-specific nanobiomaterials. *J. Am. Chem. Soc.*, **127**, 10096–10100.

24 D'Souza, S. (2014) A review of *in vitro* drug release test methods for nano-sized dosage forms. *Adv. Pharm.*, **2014**. doi: doi.org/10.1155/2014/304757

25 Skoczen, S., McNeil, S.E., and Stern, S.T. (2015) Stable isotope method to measure drug release from nanomedicines. *J. Control. Release*, **220**, 169–174.

26 Crist, R.M., Grossman, J.H., Patri, A.K., Stern, S.T., Dobrovolskaia, M.A., Adiseshaiah, P.P., Clogston, J.D., and McNeil, S.E. (2013) Common pitfalls in nanotechnology: lessons learned from NCI's Nanotechnology Characterization Laboratory. *Integr. Biol.*, **5**, 66–73.

27 Ehmann, F., Sakai-Kato, K., Duncan, R., Hernan Perez de la Ossa, D., Pita, R., Vidal, J.M., Kohli, A., Tothfalusi, L., Sanh, A., Tinton, S. *et al.* (2013) Next-generation nanomedicines and nanosimilars: EU regulators' initiatives relating to the development and evaluation of nanomedicines. *Nanomedicine (Lond.)*, **8**, 849–856.

28 Sainz, V., Conniot, J., Matos, A.I., Peres, C., Zupan, I.E., Moura, L., Silva, L.C., Florindo, H.F., and Gaspar, R.S. (2015) Regulatory aspects on nanomedicines. *Biochem. Biophys. Res. Commun.*, **468**, 504–510.

29 Meekings, K.N., Williams, C.S., and Arrowsmith, J.E. (2012) Orphan drug development: an economically viable strategy for biopharma R&D. *Drug Discov. Today*, **17**, 660–664.

30 Murday, J.S., Siegel, R.W., Stein, J., and Wright, J.F. (2009) Translational nanomedicine: status assessment and opportunities. *Nanomedicine*, **5**, 251–273.

31 Applications des nanotechnologies à la médecine, http://www.etp-nanomedicine.eu/public/press-documents/publications/public-documents/bionest-partners-2014-nanomedicine-study-leem/Rapport%20final%20version%20definitive.pdf/view, 2013.

32 www.transparencymarketresearch.com. Nanomedicine market (neurology, cardiovascular, anti-inflammatory, anti-infective, and oncology applications): global industry analysis, size, share, growth, trends and forecast, 2013–2019 (2013).

33 Finch, G., Havel, H., Analoui, M., Barton, R.W., Diwan, A.R., Hennessy, M., Reddy, V., Sadrieh, N., Tamarkin, L., Wolfgang,

M. *et al.* (2014) Nanomedicine drug development: a scientific symposium entitled "Charting a Roadmap to Commercialization". *AAPS J.*, **16**, 698–704.

34 Oberdorster, G. (2010) Safety assessment for nanotechnology and nanomedicine: concepts of nanotoxicology. *J. Intern. Med.*, **267**, 89–105.

35 Escoffier, L., Ganau, M., and Wong, J. (2015) *Commercialzing Nanomedicines: Industrial Applications, Patents, Ethics*, Pan Stanford, UK.

30
Future Outlook of Nanopharmacy: Challenges and Opportunities

Dan Peer,[1,2,3] *Jean Cornier,*[4] *and Marcel Van de Voorde*[5]

[1]*George S. Wise Faculty of Life Sciences, Tel Aviv University, Laboratory of NanoMedicine, Department of Cell Research and Immunology, Ramat Aviv, Tel Aviv 69978, Israel*
[2]*The Iby and Aladar Fleischman Faculty of Engineering, Tel Aviv University, Department of Materials Science and Engineering, P.O. Box 39040, Tel Aviv 6997801, Israel*
[3]*Tel Aviv University, Center for Nanoscience and Nanotechnology, Levanon st., Tel Aviv 69978, Israel*
[4]*VDL Consult, Seumestr. 7, 81379 Munich, Germany*
[5]*Rue du Rhodania, 5, BRISTOL A, Appartement 31, 3963 Crans-Montana, Switzerland*

The use of nanocarriers (NCs) for the delivery of drugs, termed here as Nanopharmacy, has emerged as a novel field in medicine integrating nanoscale technologies with materials sciences, chemistry, pharmacy, and biology.

Nanopharmacy has the potential to revolutionize diagnosis and therapy, and bring this new field from concept to reality while impacting on the lives of millions around the world.

NCs may have a huge impact on patient's outcomes by increasing the drug efficacy and reducing systemic toxicity. Yet, it seems that current NCs are far from fulfilling their therapeutic potential, not least given the enormous gap between the number of NCs, which are currently under preclinical and clinical evaluation compared with the number of FDA-approved NCs as anticancer drugs. Many bottlenecks exist from the Lab to the clinic and hence commercial translation becomes difficult and risky. The development of a faster, easier, cheaper, and more efficient route is needed.

Since 1995, when the first nanoscale liposomal anthracycline drugs were approved by the FDA (Doxil™ in 1995, DaunoXome™ in 1996), until today, 13 liposomal-based anticancer formulations have been approved by the regulatory agencies but none for polymeric nanoscale delivery systems.

Here, we discuss several potential explanations for why NCs as anticancer drugs do not fulfill their full potential:

Pharmaceutical Nanotechnology: Innovation and Production, First Edition. Edited by Jean Cornier, Arno Kwade, Andrew Owen, and Marcel Van de Voorde.

30.1 Matching the NC's Delivery Mode of Action (MoA) to the Tumor Type

Intracellular delivery of drugs via NCs remains challenging. It is essential to understand the particular tumor biology and match the best NCs available. Tumor heterogeneity with different cell milieu will add complexity to the already complex design of NCs.

Systemic administration of NCs could affect the encapsulated or nanostructured tagged drug and its effectiveness (e.g., a premature efflux of the therapeutic payload from the NCs – means that the NCs will most likely reach the tumor site as a drug-free carrier). In addition, several considerations must be taken into account when NCs are administrated systemically, among them the vast dilution of NCs into the bloodstream [1]. Beyond this, the sequestration and disaggregation on NP-enabled drugs remains a continuous challenge; the body truly regards such entities as host environment infringing materials, unlike soluble drug agents, and elimination of them is multitissue, multifunction, and multicapacity.

NC's pharmacokinetics and biodistribution will be determined based on several factors: the absorption, distribution, metabolism, and their excretion (ADME); the materials by which they are made of; their surface charge and their curvature that can be easily tagged by proteins in order to alert the immune system [2–9]. Moreover, how these carriers penetrate tumors, and by which MoA they release their payload is an additional factor that can determine the effectiveness of the treatment and relates to the tumor biology [5,10,11].

NC's MoA can be divided into passive tissue targeting or active cellular targeting strategies [3,12]. The passive tissue targeting MoA relays on the "leaky" nature of blood vessels next to the tumor and the ineffective lymphatic drainage known as enhanced permeability and retention (EPR) effect, which permits selective penetration of NCs into the tumor vicinity. It is crucial to choose the appropriate delivery strategy and match it to the specific tumor, since passive tissue delivery may be ineffective in cases of poor vascularization and may result in treatment failure. For example, prostate and pancreatic tumors as well as metastatic liver cancer are poorly vascularized and thus tumor penetration via EPR effect is likely to be ineffective [13,14]. However, even in highly vascularized tumors, the type of the tumor and its origin is not enough to rely solely on the EPR effect; since, in many cases the released drug will not reach the inner tumor layers where the cancer stem cells (CSCs) or tumor initiating cells are often located (necrotic inner core or deeper embedded CSC niches) [15], thus the NCs treatment modality should fit to the tumor vascular phenotype. Developing new methods in order to enhance tumor vascular permeability will attribute to efficient penetration of the NCs into the tumor microenvironment (TME) and will enhance treatment effectiveness. Currently, some efforts are being made to develop strategies to assess the EPR in an individual patient via imaging modalities such as MRI or PET/CT. These strategies are based on preinjecting patients with iron oxide NPs (in the case of MRI) or by injecting size-defined nanoliposomes with ^{64}Cu (in the case of PET/CT) in order to quantify the EPR dimensions and better fit patients with the appropriate NC modality.

NCs with active targeting capabilities, which present targeting molecules, such as natural ligands, peptides, antibodies, and nucleic acids on their surface, allow high affinity interactions with abundant tumor cell surface receptors, hence increasing binding and cellular uptake into the tumor cells and reducing off target effects or affecting bystander cells [3,7,8,16–19].

30.2 Nonpredictive Animal Models

Animal studies are essential preclinical models in the field of anticancer drugs development in order to measure the performance of the NCs and the encapsulated drug under whole animal conditions. However, developing animal models, which provide reliable prediction for human cancer, are hampered by the lack of understanding of the complexity of cancer. Most preclinical cancer research is performed in immune deficient animals, such as with use of xenograft models, which are mainly based on Nude/SCID/Rag mice that tend to give low correlation with the human clinical outcome, and so without an intact immune system it is hard to predict potential adverse effect such as immune suppression or activation [20,21] or removal and destruction. Patient-derived xenografts (PDXs) are potentially more reliable when implanted in mice. However, the real effects (both toxic and therapeutic) are more likely to be seen in larger animals and ultimately in humans.

30.3 The Lack of Reliable Techniques that can Efficiently Characterize NCs and Measure their Stability in the Human Body

Interactions with the biological environment such as body fluids, immune cells, complement fragments, proteins, and blood vessels can variously influence NC structure clearance rate, carrier structure, drug dissociation profile, and may lead to destabilization of the NCs; the functional consequence being noncontrollable release rates of the encapsulated drug, which decrease tissue specificity and overall efficiency. An attempt to prolong circulation half-life by increasing the NCs' plasma stability is illustrated by the wide-scale use of polyethylene glycol (PEG), which is mainly characterized by increased circulation time and improved evasion of the immune systems. Some FDA approved examples of clinically PEG composed lipid-based nanoparticles are Lipoplatin™, Mitoxantrone (Novantrone®), and Doxil®.

However, various examples are documented for drugs-based NCs, which were expected to be stable in body fluids according to *in vitro* stability studies such as critical micelle concentrations (CMC), colloidal stability, and drug release profile but exhibit poor drug retention in circulation, when the drug was quickly released (<1 h in blood). For example, Abraxene [22], PLGA particles coated with PEG entrapping doxorubicin [23], and others. This premature drug release into the circulation and not in the tumor vicinity or inside tumor cells causes limited therapeutic effect.

It is more than necessary to develop reliable techniques that allow an accurate determination of NC stability in biological fluids along with an "*in vivo* like blood medium," in order to bridge the gap between estimated stability performance *in vitro*/saline and body fluids.

Among the most important parameters are size distribution, surface charge, quantitative analysis of lipids composition, drug loading rate, and formulation stability [24]. Determination of drug delivery nanoscale systems characterization is being performed using satisfactory analytical methods such as size distribution, zeta potential based on dynamic light scattering measurement, electronic microscopy (ESEM, TEM), SAXS and WAXS (n the case of lipid based systems), gel exclusion chromatography, and determination of therapeutic payloads amounts and release by analytical HPLC and/or LC/MS. False positive results along with a significant difference between the loading efficiency evaluation data with the different determination methods must be taken under consideration. However, NP formulation stability measurement under different conditions and body fluids is still a hurdle.

30.4 The Challenge of Scaling Up NCs

Moving from drug entrapped in NCs at a lab scale to scale up production for clinical testing is a multilevel complex problem, which requires optimization steps or various parameters. The main issues concern the presence of organic solvent residues, formulation stability, endotoxins levels, sterility, and batch-to-batch reproducibility. In order to move from small-scale preparation of milligrams to a large-scale quantity of grams and beyond for drug carrier production, the science of chemistry, manufacturing and controls (CMC) should be employed. For example, problematic batch process mixing: In stirred vessel versus static mixer in lines; control solvent remove rate; control extraction step, and so on. Each step needs to be carefully monitored and controlled.

All of these variations in NCs and its formulations through scale up process production may change the original formulation and affect the effectiveness of the treatment.

In order to accomplish a successful scaling-up formulation production, researchers should adapt several important steps during the small-scale formulation preparation such as: monitoring the entire NCs preparation process (e.g., pH and temperature, ionic strength with detectors inside the preparation vessels), collect and analyze the data, define critical key parameters during the process, keep consistency of NCs constituents, and select a scalable equipment designated for NCs production measuring the active drug loading rate. For example, microfluidic mixers are an emerged technology for high-quality synthesis of clean-up drug loaded NPs since it enables a rapid screening of different formulations with a high encapsulation rate [7,8,25].

In addition, nanomedicine expert labs should consider to combine automated detectors equipment capable of simultaneously and continuously monitoring wide range of NCs constituents and associated analytes in order to reduce "human error" element and have a homogenous well defined product ready to use for preclinical and clinical testing.

For NCs mass production, an inevitable step is a state-of-the-art designated nano medicine manufacturing facility, which is essential but sometimes problematic. NCs production must be held in a manufacturing environment that meets good manufacturing practice (GMP) in order to produce hundreds to thousands of grams of high-quality formulated NCs for late stages of clinical trials. It needs a large financial investment in building and qualifying GMP facility, which means a considerable risk for a company before the nanomedicine has been assessed for efficacy in human clinical trials to support the regulatory agencies (FDA, MEA) approval. An alternative approach is to apply to a contract research organization (CRO) able to manufacturing drugs NCs in order to scale up processes and have the desired NCs amounts necessary for animal and/or clinical testing. Even here, with the concern of society and any possible risk of side effects being greater acts as a barrier to innovation. The development of new drugs is costly, but the development on NCs may not adequately reduce the cost barriers to the developer or to the health care system. It also does not help that regulation and standards are still under development and may impact downstream in an unexpected way to the protracted process on NC development.

The development of such facilities by governmental funding will accelerate the transition of these novel therapies to proof-of-concept human testing in clinical development.

In summary, the translation of NCs drugs from research into clinical modality, still have serious hurdles such as formulation stability and batch-to-batch variations when trying to produce large amounts of high-quality targeted NCs. These parameters need to be addressed before coming to approve new NCs entrapping drugs through regulatory process.

Other diseases such as inflammatory diseases and neurodegenerative diseases could benefit from using different NCs. These should be developed in the appropriate way with the relevant predictive animal models and with substantial understanding of the disease targeted.

In addition to the several specific reasons listed above the limited number of NCs commercialized as anticancer drugs, can also be related to more general deficits like the lack of established characterization and testing methods and protocols, which at the end prevents regulatory authorities to open the way for more clinical testing, the questionable reproducibility of preclinical studies performed in academia, the imperfect cooperation between academic and industrial drug

R&D, the limited knowledge in academia about the patent process, the lack of robust appropriate regulations, and other bottlenecks limiting access to funding. Therefore, the "bench to bedside" transition remains difficult and impedes commercialization. However, these limitations have been well identified and solutions are being worked out in Europe as well as in the USA. The collaborative structures between the many stakeholders involved are being improved with the set up of nanocharacterization labs, pilot lines for GMP manufacturing of nanomedicines as well as the mobilization and better coordination of the different sources of public and private investments.

To summarize, improving clinical success of NCs-loaded drugs with a better, less toxic, and long-term therapeutic effect is a complex and not a trivial task. Changing today's fashionable way of cancer treatment, for example, by moving from a short term "tumor shrinking effect" to a long term destruction of more aggressive tumor cell populations and future maintenance therapy, when they are from drug resistance cells will be based on developing smarter and more sophisticated drug NCs platforms. It requires massive changes, modifications, and multidiscipline attitudes in order to deal successfully with the range of complex diseases that theoretically might benefit the use of NCs.

In addition, the field of Nanopharmacy should devise specific tools to better understand safety and toxicology aspects and improve predictive models prior to clinical testing.

Finally, nanopharmacy opens new avenues and new potential markets for old and new drugs and could ultimately become novel therapeutic modality to many types of diseases.

References

1 Peer, D., Karp, J.M., Hong, S., Farokhzad, O.C., Margalit, R., and Langer, R. (2007) Nanocarriers as an emerging platform for cancer therapy. *Nat. Nanotechnol.*, **2**, 751–760.

2 Peer, D. and Lieberman, J. (2011) Special delivery: targeted therapy with small RNAs. *Gene Ther.*, **18**, 1127–1133.

3 Cohen, K., Emmanuel, R., Kisin-Finfer, E., Shabat, D., and Peer, D. (2014) Modulation of drug resistance in ovarian adenocarcinoma using chemotherapy entrapped in hyaluronan-grafted nanoparticle clusters. *ACS Nano*, **8**, 2183–2195.

4 Vorup-Jensen, T. and Peer, D. (2012) Nanotoxicity and the importance of being earnest. *Adv. Drug Deliv. Rev.*, **64**, 1661–1662.

5 Bogart, L.K., Pourroy, G., Murphy, C.J., Puntes, V., Pellegrino, T., Rosenblum, D., Peer, D., and Levy, R. (2014) Nanoparticles for imaging, sensing, and therapeutic intervention. *ACS Nano*, **8**, 3107–3122.

6 Peer, D. (2013) A daunting task: manipulating leukocyte function with RNAi. *Immunol. Rev.*, **253**, 185–197.

7 Ramishetti, S., Kedmi, R., Goldsmith, M., Leonard, F., Sprague, A.G., Godin, B., Gozin, M., Cullis, P.R., Dykxhoorn, D.M., and Peer, D. (2015) Systemic gene silencing in primary T lymphocytes using targeted lipid nanoparticles. *ACS Nano*, **9**, 6706–6716.

8 Cohen, Z.R., Ramishetti, S., Peshes-Yaloz, N., Goldsmith, M., Wohl, A., Zibly, Z., and Peer, D. (2015) Localized RNAi therapeutics of chemoresistant grade IV glioma using hyaluronan-grafted

lipid-based nanoparticles. *ACS Nano*, **9**, 1581–1591.
9 Moghimi, S.M., Hunter, A.C., and Peer, D. (2016) Platelet mimicry: the emperor's new clothes? *Nanomedicine*, **12** (1), 245–248.
10 Jain, R.K. and Stylianopoulos, T. (2010) Delivering nanomedicine to solid tumors. *Nat. Rev. Clin. Oncol.*, **7**, 653–664.
11 Jain, K.K. (2012) Role of biological therapies in the development of personalized medicine. *Expert Opin. Biol. Ther.*, **12**, 1–5.
12 Jacoby, G., Cohen, K., Barkan, K., Talmon, Y., Peer, D., and Beck, R. (2015) Metastability in lipid based particles exhibits temporally deterministic and controllable behavior. *Sci. Rep.*, **5**, 9481.
13 Matsumura, Y. and Maeda, H. (1986) A new concept for macromolecular therapeutics in cancer chemotherapy: mechanism of tumoritropic accumulation of proteins and the antitumor agent smancs. *Cancer Res.*, **46**, 6387–6392.
14 Maeda, H., Sawa, T., and Konno, T. (2001) Mechanism of tumor-targeted delivery of macromolecular drugs, including the EPR effect in solid tumor and clinical overview of the prototype polymeric drug SMANCS. *J. Control. Release*, **74**, 47–61.
15 Zhao, Y., Alakhova, D.Y., and Kabanov, A.V. (2013) Can nanomedicines kill cancer stem cells? *Adv. Drug Deliv. Rev.*, **65**, 1763–1783.
16 Hrkach, J., Von Hoff, D., Mukkaram Ali, M., Andrianova, E., Auer, J., Campbell, T., De Witt, D., Figa, M., Figueiredo, M., Horhota, A., Low, S., McDonnell, K., Peeke, E., Retnarajan, B., Sabnis, A., Schnipper, E., Song, J.J., Song, Y.H., Summa, J., Tompsett, D., Troiano, G., Van Geen Hoven, T., Wright, J., LoRusso, P., Kantoff, P.W., Bander, N.H., Sweeney, C., Farokhzad, O.C., Langer, R., and Zale, S. (2012) Preclinical development and clinical translation of a PSMA-targeted docetaxel nanoparticle with a differentiated pharmacological profile. *Sci. Transl. Med.*, **4**, 128ra39.
17 Farokhzad, O.C., Cheng, J., Teply, B.A., Sherifi, I., Jon, S., Kantoff, P.W., Richie, J.P., and Langer, R. (2006) Targeted nanoparticle-aptamer bioconjugates for cancer chemotherapy *in vivo*. *Proc. Natl. Acad. Sci. U. S. A.*, **103**, 6315–6320.
18 Mizrahy, S., Goldsmith, M., Leviatan-Ben-Arye, S., Kisin-Finfer, E., Redy, O., Srinivasan, S., Shabat, D., Godin, B., and Peer, D. (2014) Tumor targeting profiling of hyaluronan-coated lipid based-nanoparticles. *Nanoscale*, **6**, 3742–3752.
19 Davis, M.E. (2009) The first targeted delivery of siRNA in humans via a self-assembling, cyclodextrin polymer-based nanoparticle: from concept to clinic. *Mol. Pharm.*, **6**, 659–668.
20 Landesman-Milo, D. and Peer, D. (2014) Toxicity profiling of several common RNAi-based nanomedicines: a comparative study. *Drug Deliv. Transl. Res.*, **4**, 96–103.
21 Peer, D. (2012) Immunotoxicity derived from manipulating leukocytes with lipid-based nanoparticles. *Adv. Drug Deliv. Rev.*, **64**, 1738–1748.
22 Desai, N.P., Trieu, V., Hwang, L.Y., Wu, R., Soon-Shiong, P., and Gradishar, W.J. (2008) Improved effectiveness of nanoparticle albumin-bound (nab) paclitaxel versus polysorbate-based docetaxel in multiple xenografts as a function of HER2 and SPARC status. *Anticancer Drugs*, **19**, 899–909.
23 Gullotti, E. and Yeo, Y. (2012) Beyond the imaging: limitations of cellular uptake study in the evaluation of nanoparticles. *J. Control. Release*, **164**, 170–176.
24 Torchilin, V.P. (2014) Multifunctional, stimuli-sensitive nanoparticulate systems for drug delivery. *Nat. Rev. Drug Discov.*, **13**, 813–827.
25 Jayaraman, M., Ansell, S.M., Mui, B.L., Tam, Y.K., Chen, J., Du, X., Butler, D., Eltepu, L., Matsuda, S., Narayanannair, J.K., Rajeev, K.G., Hafez, I.M., Akinc, A., Maier, M.A., Tracy, M.A., Cullis, P.R., Madden, T.D., Manoharan, M., and Hope, M.J. (2012) Maximizing the potency of siRNA lipid nanoparticles for hepatic gene silencing in vivo. *Angew. Chem., Int. Ed. Engl.*, **51** 8529–8533.

Index

Pharmaceutical Nanotechnology: Innovation and Production, First Edition. Edited by Jean Cornier, Arno Kwade, Andrew Owen, and Marcel Van de Voorde.

b